Role of Essential Oils in the Management of COVID-19

Role of Essential Oils in the Management of COVID-19

Ahmed Al-Harrasi and Saurabh Bhatia

CRC Press
Taylor & Francis Group
Boca Raton London New York

CRC Press is an imprint of the
Taylor & Francis Group, an **informa** business

First edition published 2022
by CRC Press
6000 Broken Sound Parkway NW, Suite 300, Boca Raton, FL 33487-2742

and by CRC Press
2 Park Square, Milton Park, Abingdon, Oxon, OX14 4RN

CRC Press is an imprint of Taylor & Francis Group, LLC

Library of Congress Cataloging-in-Publication Data
Names: Al-Harrasi, Ahmed, author. | Bhatia, Saurabh, author. Title: Role of essential oils in the management of COVID-19 / Ahmed Al-Harrasi and Saurabh Bhatia. Description: First edition. | Boca Raton : CRC Press, 2022. | Includes bibliographical references. Identifiers: LCCN 2021027446 (print) | LCCN 2021027447 (ebook) | ISBN 9781032008172 (hardback) | ISBN 9781032008189 (paperback) | ISBN 9781003175933 (ebook)
Subjects: LCSH: COVID-19 (Disease)—Alternative treatment. | Essences and essential oils. Classification: LCC RA644.C67 A443 2022 (print) | LCC RA644.C67 (ebook) | DDC 614.5/92414—dc23
LC record available at https://lccn.loc.gov/2021027446
LC ebook record available at https://lccn.loc.gov/2021027447

ISBN: 978-1-032-00817-2 (hbk)
ISBN: 978-1-032-00818-9 (pbk)
ISBN: 978-1-003-17593-3 (ebk)

DOI: 10.1201/9781003175933

Typeset in Times
by codeMantra

Contents

Foreword

This ongoing pandemic state caused physical and psychological illness to public. Based on the extensive literature available it is widely known that essential oils have high therapeutic potentials. Aromatherapy is one of the alternative therapies which use natural essential oils to treat various conditions. This book is timely due to unprecedented interest in understanding the molecular basis of the therapeutic properties of essential oils derived from aromatic plants. I warmly welcome this book authored by Prof. Ahmed Al Harrasi, Dr. Saurabh Bhatia et al., for multiple reasons, primarily to explore the therapeutic significance of the components of essential oils against COVID-associated complications and to systematically report the molecular pathways followed by volatile/nonvolatile components to treat complications associated with different human organ systems. Prof. Harrasi and his teammates through this book succeed in debunking molecular roles, safety profile and clinical usage of essential oils and its possible role in COVID-19. Part I of this book offer enough understanding related with evolution, pathogenesis, pathophysiology and treatment of COVID-19, whereas Part II aims to provide fundamental knowledge about essential oils such as extraction procedures, chemistry, therapeutic effects on complications associated with different organ systems as well as a more practical approach of olfactory aromatherapy in the management of COVID-19. Also, the book presents other interesting topics such as stability, safety, pharmacokinetic as well as pharmacodynamic profile, relationship between interactions of essential oil components with main course medication and blends of oils with therapeutic profile. This book also explores possible strategies to effectively manage mental and physical health by using essential oils in the COVID-19 pandemic.

Despite the explosion of online COVID-19-related information with the single click of mouse, this is a handy and easy-to-read book that has been carefully conceived and crafted by Prof. Harrasi and his teammates, it will become an indispensable contribution to COVID-19 science. Finally, I congratulate Prof. Harrasi, Dr. Bhatia and other authors for bringing out this reference book and I am sure the book will find respectable space in the bookshelves of academicians, busy healthcare practitioners, herbalists, aromatherapists and to the libraries of pharmaceutical as well as cosmetic industries.

Dr. K. Hüsnü Can Başer
Near East University Faculty of Pharmacy
Department of Pharmacognosy
Nicosia (Lefkoşa), N. Cyprus

Preface

Coronavirus disease 2019, abbreviated as COVID-19, is a respiratory infection caused by SARS-CoV-2 (formerly called "2019 novel coronavirus" or "2019-nCoV") resulting in severe acute respiratory syndrome, with a high possibility of transmission and infection to humans as well as considerable death and morbidity worldwide. Initial clinical care is primarily supportive, with newer antiviral drugs/vaccines under clinical investigation. Lesser realistic development has been seen in the treatment of COVID-19, as so far there is no specific medication suggested for COVID-19, and certain vaccine candidates show undesirable effects. Thus, more understanding of the pathogenesis of COVID-19 is required to provide key insight for its management. However, on the other hand, much progress has been seen in the development of advanced diagnostics, supportive care systems, and personal protective equipment for COVID-19. Other measures such as social restriction by isolation and quarantine of suspected cases are recommended. When the entire human race worldwide is suffering from the COVID-19 outbreak and seeking a definite safe and effective vaccine or other reliable treatment and when most of the therapeutics are under investigation, it's essential to explore the role of complementary and alternative medicine in the prevention and treatment of COVID-19. Recently, a lot of research articles have been published on the possible role of essential oils (EOs) in viral respiratory tract infections. The 26,645 search results obtained from NCBI by using keywords "essential oils" and "viral infection" on September 23, 2020 clearly show the significant role EOs in play in the treatment of viral infections. For the keywords "essential oil" vs "respiratory infection," the 14,099 search results that appeared demonstrated the active role EOs play in the treatment of respiratory tract infections. Recently, various EOs have been tested against pathogenic viruses such as influenza and other respiratory viral infections. EOs are used by inhalation, which mainly uses the olfactory system, termed as olfactory aromatherapy. Olfactory aromatherapy is an approach to directly load safe and effective volatile compounds in infected lungs to achieve maximum therapeutic action. These volatile compounds present in EOs are therapeutically active and can also be utilized in synergy with main course medications. Based on this information, this book is divided into two parts: Part I "Evolution, Pathogenesis, Pathophysiology, and Treatment of COVID-19" (Chapters 1–7) and Part II "Introduction to Essential Oils and Its Role in the Management of COVID-19" (Chapters 8–25).

Part I of this book includes seven detailed chapters that offer a complete outline of the recent SARS-CoV-2 infection, its biology, and associated challenges for its treatment and prevention. This book begins with Chapter 1, on the role of olfactory aromatherapy for COVID-19, followed by detailed information (Chapters 2–7) on viral respiratory tract infections, the discovery, evolution, and morphology of SARS-CoV-2, and the global epidemiology of COVID-19, subsequent chapters (Chapters 2–7) continue with coverage of pathogenesis, pathophysiology, genome manipulation, study of virus–host interactions, prevention, transmission, diagnosis, treatment, and management of coronavirus infections. Part I of this book, especially Chapters 3 and 6, covers some other aspects of COVID-19 infection, including genome organization and immunopathogenesis, and highlights host immune response along with pathogen immune invasion approaches toward developing an immune intervention or preventive vaccine for COVID-19.

In addition to therapeutics, Chapter 4 discusses essential life support systems, personal protective equipment, and sanitization facilities available and under development for COVID-19. Besides treatment strategies, there is a need for rapid and accurate diagnostics to better monitor and prevent the spread of COVID-19. Thus, this chapter will also discuss diagnostic tools available and under development along with a clear justification on the diagnostic performance of the available tests and analysis of the major challenges faced by them based on current research. Chapter 5 summarizes the most current pharmacotherapeutics prescribed in the treatment of severe cases of COVID-19 patients. These include antiviral therapy, antibiotics, systemic corticosteroid and anti-inflammatory drugs (including antiarthritis drugs), neuraminidase inhibitors, RNA synthesis inhibitors, convalescent plasma, monoclonal antibodies, and traditional herbal medicines. Interestingly, the treatment section of COVID-19 includes a list of more than 600 phytochemicals and extracts that have been tested so far against different coronaviruses. This list is tabulated in a way that allows readers to understand the source, IC_{50}/EC_{50}, the mechanisms of action, and the assay used in each study based on phytochemical composition.

Although COVID-19 presents primarily as a lower respiratory tract infection transmitted via air droplets, increasing reports suggest multiorgan involvement in patients that are infected. Chapter 7 in Part I deals with organ-specific manifestations of COVID-19 infection including extra-pulmonary involvement of vital organs such as the brain, liver, heart, kidney, and gastrointestinal tract (GIT). In addition, systemic effects of COVID-19 such as implications of autoantibodies, thrombocytopenia, cytokine storm, hyperferritinemia, and blood group and its association with COVID-19 are discussed. This information is followed by description of the implications of organ crosstalk (referred to as mutual effects) that can lead to progression of multiorgan dysfunction syndrome in severe cases of COVID-19. Overall, Part I includes the knowledge needed to design strategies to protect the human race from further losses and harm due to COVID-19. Thus, Part I will serve as a valuable section to researchers working to identify and control viruses with increased potential to cross the species barrier and to develop the diagnostics, vaccines, and antiviral therapeutics that are required to manage future outbreaks in both humans and animals.

Part II (Chapters 8–25) primarily focuses on volatile oils and their use as olfactory aromatherapy to treat various viral respiratory infections. Volatile compounds present in EOs have biological potential to treat respiratory tract infections. In vitro and clinical studies have revealed extraordinary anti-inflammatory, antibacterial, and antiviral effects.

Part II offers an introduction to the volatile compounds present in EOs with their relevance in terms of treatment and management of COVID-19. EOs are volatile liquid substances usually extracted from aromatic plants by conventional extraction methods such as steam distillation or mechanical expression or by advanced supercritical fluid extraction. Therapeutically, these oils are used in the form of olfactory aromatherapy for the improvement of physical, emotional, and spiritual well-being. As clinical development and approval of novel therapeutics is taking more time, this is the time when effective alternative treatments against COVID-19 can be developed. Olfactory aromatherapy is used with other complementary treatments as well as with standard treatments for symptom management as well as to treat several diseases. Olfactory aromatherapy can also be utilized by ICU patients as supportive care for general well-being. Currently, the use of olfactory aromatherapy with mainstream medicine has gained momentum. Inhalation of oils via olfactory aromatherapy is considered as the main method that allows entry of volatile compounds to decongest the respiratory system, reduce inflammation, relieve sinuses, and exhibit antimicrobial effects at the site of infection. Once these volatile oils enter the system, they remodulate themselves and work at the affected area. This type of therapy utilizes various permutations and combinations to get relief from numerous ailments. With this in mind, various blends of volatile oils are being prepared, dispensed, and marketed in the form of inhalers to provide maximum therapeutic effects.

The objective of Part II (Chapters 8–25) is to provide a general overview of the therapeutic potential of EOs in the treatment of viral respiratory tract infections and to highlight some promising future directions. Part II integrates chemistry, pharmacology, and medicine while discussing bioactive EOs in experimental models and clinical studies of respiratory infections. The next objective of Part II is to explore the potential of olfactory aromatherapy in treating various respiratory illnesses, more specifically coronavirus-induced respiratory illness. Part II includes a comprehensive report of ~500 EOs as well as their chemical components that have been evidenced for their promising effects in respiratory tract infections. Tabulated information based on the antimicrobial properties of 400 EOs and their chemical compounds, the effect of inhalation of 250 EOs on the central nervous system, cardiovascular system, renal system, and lungs, and understanding related to biological interactions between EOs and mainstream drugs provides deep insight into the possible role of EOs in the treatment of COVID-19.

Part II (Chapters 8–13) begins with fundamental information related to sources, chemical composition, extraction, detection, and pharmacokinetics of EOs followed by their mechanism of action, pharmacological potential, stability (at solid/liquid/gas interfaces), blend (based on synergism and antagonism), safety profile, analytical methods (such as gas chromatography coupled to mass spectrometry), and their dispensing in the form of compatible inhalers (conventional and advanced inhalers). A large section (Chapter 14) is devoted to the possible role of EOs and olfactory aromatherapy in the treatment of COVID-19 along with the possible mechanism of action of olfactory aromatherapy and its potential targets in the pathogenesis of COVID-19. In addition, how inhalation of volatile oils or their blends could be helpful during the hyperinflammatory stage, resulting in multiple organ failure, is also explained. Thus, the effect of olfactory aromatherapy on different organ systems such as the liver, kidney, brain, and heart as well as their systemic and immunomodulatory, antimicrobial, antioxidant, and anti-inflammatory potential of EO inhalation are well discussed. The role of olfactory aromatherapy in psychological interventions for people affected by COVID-19 as well as implications of olfactory aromatherapy over neurochemistry, neurotoxicology, neurometabolism, psychophysiological activity, and electroencephalography are covered in depth in Chapter 5.

Both parts include 27 simplified illustrations that are imperative for visual learning and 24 tables for systematic learning.

Part I of this book covers all scientific aspects of COVID-19, mainly evolution, management, treatment, and diagnosis, which may be interesting to virologists/researchers/lab workers/medical staff working in the development of therapeutics, diagnostics, supportive systems, and personal protective equipment for COVID-19.

Part II will be of great interest to scientists, physicians, practitioners, academicians, and researchers working in the area of development of natural-product-based therapeutics against COVID-19 or any other viral respiratory infection. This part provides a clear and reliable introduction to aromatherapy as practiced in modern healthcare settings. It provides valuable information to healthcare professional wishing to develop their understanding of the subject, providing the in-depth knowledge needed to use EOs in practice to treat respiratory infections. Also, it is a valuable resource for everyone engaged in the study of natural products and dedicated to the discovery of useful agents for the therapy or prevention of COVID-19.

It is important for the readers to understand that all the information was compiled by the authors from June to July, 2020, which clearly signifies that authors have included information as well as the development of COVID-19 up to that period. Thus this book includes information related to progress made in terms of the development of therapeutics as well as safety and preventive measures against COVID-19 till the period of June to July, 2020. Also through this book, authors made efforts to explore the potential of essential oils against COVID-19; however, none of the statements claims that essential oils could be an effective treatment or remedy or preventive therapy. At the same time in some of the sections, authors specify that how essential oils can be used to reduce the severity of respiratory viral infections without their direct relation with viral pathogens. Thus considering the sanctity of information related to COVID-19, readers are requested not to correlate it with the current scenario. Also, we request readers to look these essential oil based therapies as other possible natural treatments proposed so far, however still clinical significance of such therapies require more clinical validation.

Acknowledgments

This is the moment of gratification and pleasure to look back with a sense of contentment at the long-traveled path, to be able to recapture some of the fine moments, and to be able to thank the infinite number of people who contributed to or support this book. Some were with us from the beginning and some who joined us later, whose love and blessing have made this day possible for us. Through this platform we would like to pay special tribute to frontline coronavirus disease 2019 warriors in Sultanate of Oman, especially those who have sacrificed their own lives in the line of duty. Also, the authors are highly thankful to researchers who are working day in and night out against all odds, hoping to find safe and effective treatment against this infection. During this odd time we would like to acknowledge University of Nizwa's offer of endless support to all the staff members. Natural and Medical Sciences Research Center housed at University of Nizwa offers a central resource of advanced analytical instrument for research and for promoting interdisciplinary research. Researchers at this center worked endlessly to find a way to deal with this pandemic. The authors are thankful to the Natural and Medical Sciences Research Center for providing excellent facilities required for the completion of our book project. Also we are thankful to the whole team of CRC Press for their active work and support.

Prof. Ahmed Al-Harrasi
Professor
Natural and Medical Sciences Research Center
University of Nizwa, Oman

Dr. Saurabh Bhatia
Associate Professor
Natural and Medical Sciences Research Center
University of Nizwa, Oman

Main Authors

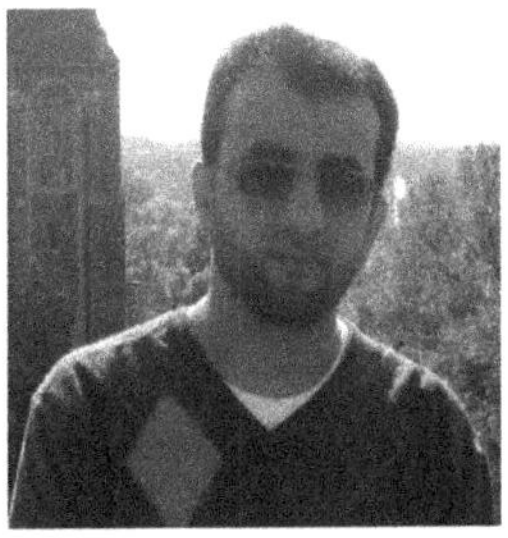

Prof. Ahmed Al-Harrasi received his BSc in Chemistry from Sultan Qaboos University (Oman) in 1997. He then moved to the University of Berlin from where he received his MSc. degree in Chemistry (2002) followed by PhD in Organic Chemistry (2005) as a DAAD fellow under the supervision of Prof. Hans-Ulrich Reissig. His PhD work was on New Transformations of Enantiopure 1,2-Oxazines. He received the Fulbright Award (2008) for postdoctoral research in chemistry for which he joined Prof. Tadhg Begely group at Cornell University to work on the synthesis of isotopically labeled thiamine pyrophosphate. After postdoctoral research from Cornell University (2009), he started his independent research at the University of Nizwa, Oman, where he founded the Natural and Medical Sciences Research Center merging chemistry and biology research that has now become a center of excellence in natural and medical sciences. He is currently Professor of Organic Chemistry and Vice Chancellor for Graduate Studies, Research and External Relations at the University of Nizwa. The budget of his interdisciplinary funded projects exceeds US$10 million. He was a chair and invited speaker in many international conferences. He is a referee for more than 15 international chemistry and biotechnology journals. He served as a guest editor in chemistry journals. While enduring his research aptitude, he has authored and co-authored over 400 scientific papers, 2 books, and 12 book chapters of high repute. He taught chemistry courses at both undergraduate and postgraduate levels.

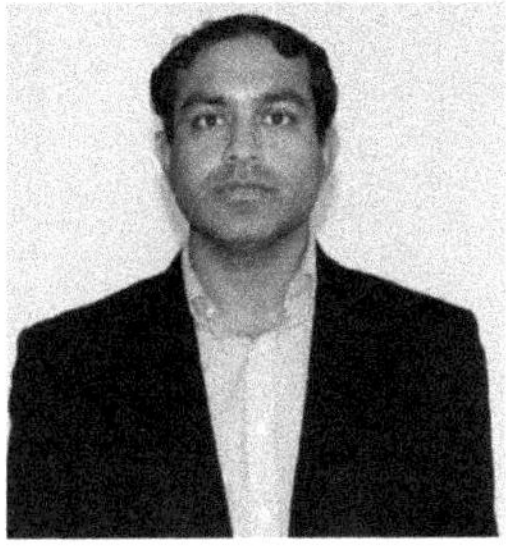

Dr. Saurabh Bhatia graduated from Kurukshetra University, India, in 2007, followed by postgraduation in 2009 from Bharati Vidyapeeth University, India. He successfully completed a PhD program in Pharmaceutical Technology at Jadavpur University, Kolkata, India (2015). Currently, he works as an Associate Professor at Natural and Medical Sciences Research Center, University of Nizwa, Nizwa, Sultanate of Oman, and Adjunct Associate Professor at School of Health Science, University of Petroleum and Energy Studies, India. He has 12 years of academic experience. His areas of interest include nanotechnology (drug delivery), biomaterials, natural products science, biotechnology (plant and animal), microbiology, modified drug delivery systems, analytical chemistry, parasitology (leishmaniasis), and marine science. He has promoted several marine algae and their derived polymers throughout India and has published more than 9 books and 75 articles in many areas of pharmaceutical science and filed 11 patents. He has participated in more than 30 national and international conferences.

Co-Authors

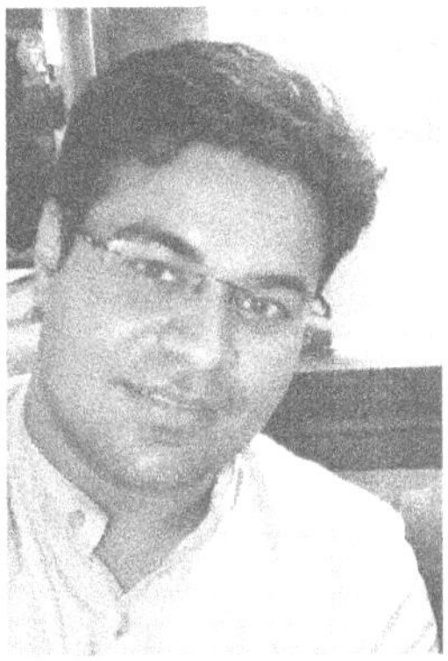

Tapan Behl
Chitkara College of Pharmacy
Chitkara University
Punjab, India

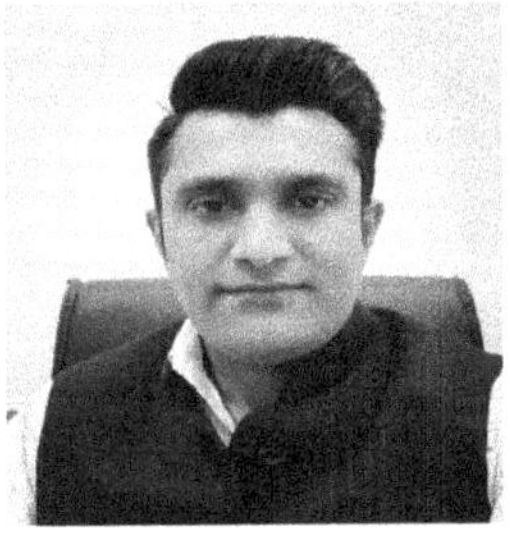

Deepak Kaushik
Dept. of Pharmaceutical Sciences
M.D. University
Haryana, India

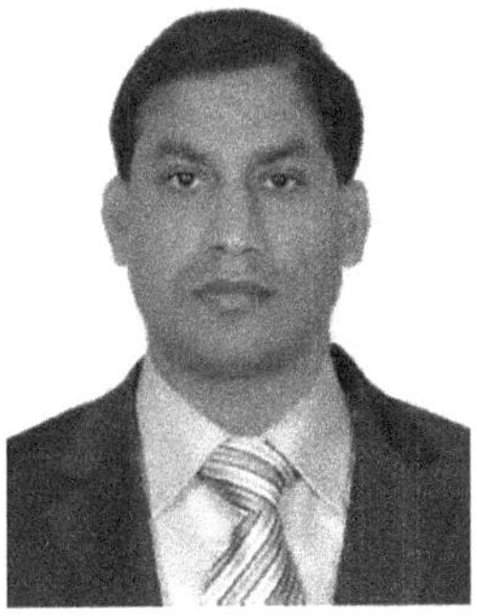

Md. Khalid Anwer
College of Pharmacy
Prince Sattam Bin Abdul Aziz
University
Al-Kharj, Kingdom of Saudi
Arabia

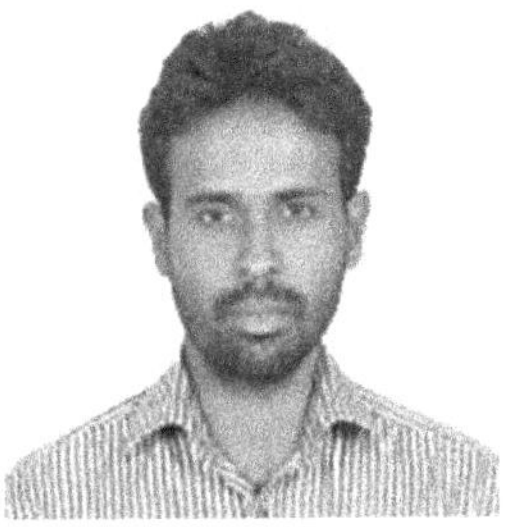

Mohammed Muqtader Ahmed
College of Pharmacy
Prince Sattam Bin Abdul Aziz
University
Al-Kharj, Kingdom of Saudi
Arabia

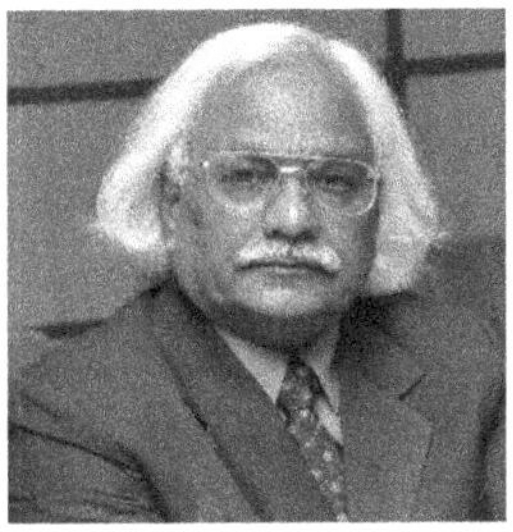

P.B. Sharma
Amity University Haryana
Haryana, India

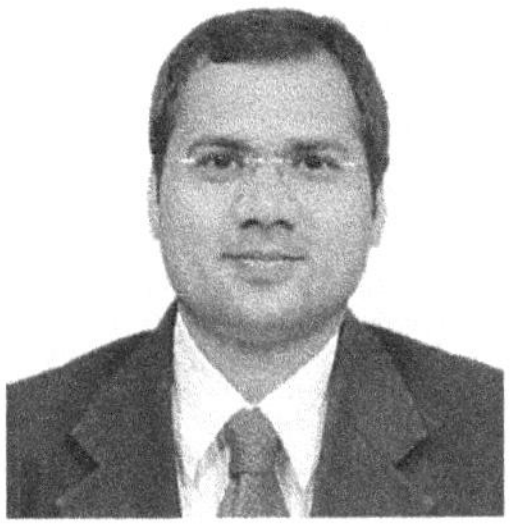

Ajay Sharma
Department of Pharmacognosy
and Phytochemistry
Delhi Pharmaceutical Sciences
and Research University
Delhi, India

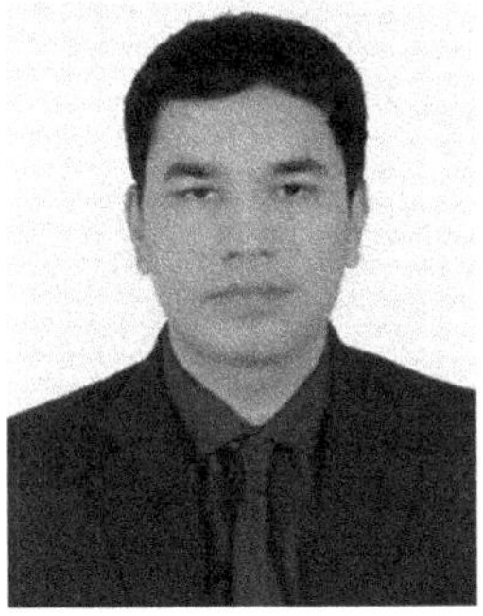

Md. Tanvir Kabir
Department of Pharmacy
BRAC University
Dhaka, Bangladesh

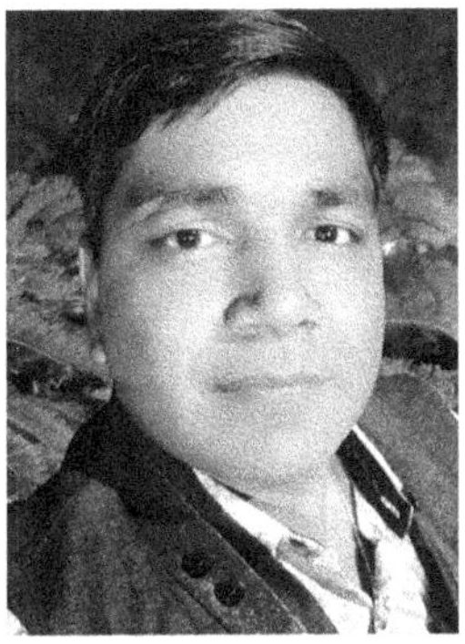

Vineet Mittal
Dept. of Pharmaceutical Sciences
M.D. University
Haryana, India

PART I

Evolution, Pathogenesis, Pathophysiology, and Treatment of COVID-19

1

Olfactory Aromatherapy vs COVID-19: A Systematic Review

Ahmed Al-Harrasi
Natural and Medical Sciences Research Center, University of Nizwa

Saurabh Bhatia
Natural and Medical Sciences Research Center, University of Nizwa
University of Petroleum and Energy Studies

CONTENTS

1.1 Introduction

Essential oils (EOs) are unorganized plant-based excretory products that contain complex mixtures of volatile chemicals responsible for different aromas and pharmacological activities. These odorous products are a complex combination of low-molecular-weight components that together create their distinctive fragrance and health benefits. The complex composition of EOs constitutes major classes of terpene hydrocarbons and oxygenated compounds. Volatile molecules responsible for aromatic characteristics are abundantly present in EOs. These volatile molecules contain monoterpenoids as well as sesquiterpenoids that are synthesized by the mevalonate pathway. Additionally, the presence of phenolic compounds in EOs further increases the therapeutic potential of the whole mixture. These phenolic compounds are synthesized via the shikimate pathway. EOs are extracted from plants using various procedures including distillation by using steam as well as water, maceration, solvent-mediated extraction, CO_2-based extraction, enfleurage, and cold-press extraction. These extraction methods affect the kinetics, chemical composition, and biological activities of EOs [1,2]. Moreover, the composition of EOs also varies due to the diversity of plants, geographical locations, harvesting seasons, and drying methods.

Recently, EOs have gained considerable importance in aromatherapy. Aromatherapy is a traditional curative procedure that uses EOs as the main therapeutic agents to support health and well-being. Aromatherapy is usually employed via inhalation or topical use or ingestion, which allows entry of EOs into the lungs, skin, and gastrointestinal tract from where they interact, cross physiological membranes and are carried to affected sites to show their potential effect. Based on the application, aromatherapy is classified as cosmetic, massage, medical, olfactory, and psycho-aromatherapy. Search results using the keywords "inhalation of essential oils" in the NCBI database on May 18, 2020, at 11:35 PM in India showed 7,764 results and 2,106 database NIH grants. These search results undoubtedly signify the importance of inhalation aromatherapy or olfactory aromatherapy (OA) in enhancing physical, emotional, and mental well-being. Inhalation of EOs stimulates olfaction, which is a sensory modality to carry volatile molecules present in EOs and transformed into the cerebral hemisphere of the central nervous system (CNS) to transduce certain chemosignals with high sensitivity in acuity or speed. OA is a non-invasive therapy used to not only reduce disease symptoms but also to rejuvenate the whole body by regulating the physiological, spiritual, and psychological processes of the body. In OA, blending of EOs is usually based on folk principles or the traditional formula, which have been used in traditional formulation like ayurvedic, unani, etc.; however, understanding of solubility, safety, aromatic behavior, chemical composition, the nature of metabolites, and therapeutic potential is required to prepare an effective and safe blend.

After evaporation, EOs are delivered by steam or various mechanical devices available in the form of portable inhaler or nasal sticks, diffuser, spray, etc. These inexpensive devices for vapor inhalation are available with different designs and applications. One report suggests that the loading of either essential oil or its components by using polymers decreases the volatility, improves the stability of the compounds and the stability of products, and extends the biological impact. Inhalation of vapors formed during the evaporation of EOs stimulates the olfactory system. The olfactory system is a part of the brain linked to smell, which includes the active physiological participation of the nose and the brain. After stimulation of the olfactory system, these volatile molecules interact with the limbic system to further trigger emotions, heart rate, hormone balance, blood pressure, stress, breathing, and memory. OA is of relevance in psycho-aromatherapy where EOs are being inhaled to evoke emotional well-being, tranquility, relaxation, pleasant memory, or regeneration of the human body. EOs in vapor phase comprise volatile components with a molecular

DOI: 10.1201/9781003175933-2

mass <300 Da, which can be recognized by the olfactory system containing 300 dynamic olfactory genes to distinguish thousands of different aromas. This olfaction plays a vital function in the determination of psychophysiological activities of people such as humor, tension, and working ability. Various reports also showed the role of fragrances in impulsive brain events as well as mental functions. Findings showed a substantial role for olfaction in the change of perception, feeling, and social conduct. In OA, inhalation of EOs reduces stress and depression and improves sleep quality (Figure 1.1). Inhalation of these volatile chemicals allows them to act at the site of injury where they can exert antioxidant, antibacterial, antiviral, and anti-inflammatory properties by stimulating the immune system. Inhalation of EOs results in the interaction of chemical compounds present in the EOs with receptors in the olfactory bulb. This interaction allows stimulation of the emotion center of the brain (i.e., amygdala) to stimulate biological responses of the cytokines, hormones, neurotransmitters, endocrine, as well as autonomic nerves (Figure 1.1).

Considerable levels of aromatic components have also been found in the blood following inhalation. This suggests the participation of inhaled aromatic compounds in direct therapeutic interaction in spite of involving in an indirect CNS relay. Various scientific studies and reports have shown the therapeutic efficacy of EOs in neurological disorders by their anxiolytic, antinociceptive, sedative, hypnotic, mood-stabilizing, sedative, analgesic, and anticonvulsive and neuroprotective actions. Anxiety as well as depression reducing properties of lavender ascribed to its volatile molecules might be because of antagonism on the N-methyl-D-aspartate (NMDA) protein and inhibition of serotonin transporter receptors [3].

An electroencephalography report obtained after the inhalation of rosemary oil demonstrated its stimulatory effect and provides proof that rosemary EO inhalation impact autonomic nervous system activity, brain wave activity, and mood states [4].

SuHeXiang Wan (Storax pill) EO is a recommendation commonly utilized in the treatment of epilepsy via inhalation. Inhalation of SuHeXiang Wan EO triggered suppressive effects on the CNS via modulating GABAergic (gamma-aminobutyric acid) pathway. EO extended the sleeping duration induced by pentobarbital as long as duration of inhalation of EO has been extended, and it prevented lipid peroxidation in the brain [5].

A similar effect of EOs obtained from *Acorus gramineus* on the CNS was reported. This finding suggests that preinhalation of EOs derived from *Acorus gramineus* delayed the appearance of convulsion and suppressed degrading enzyme for GABAtransaminase. This resulted in an increase in GABA level and a decrease in glutamate content, which supports the anticonvulsive effect of this AGR oil [6].

Apart from these psychological benefits, OA has also been used in the management of respiratory-related complications,

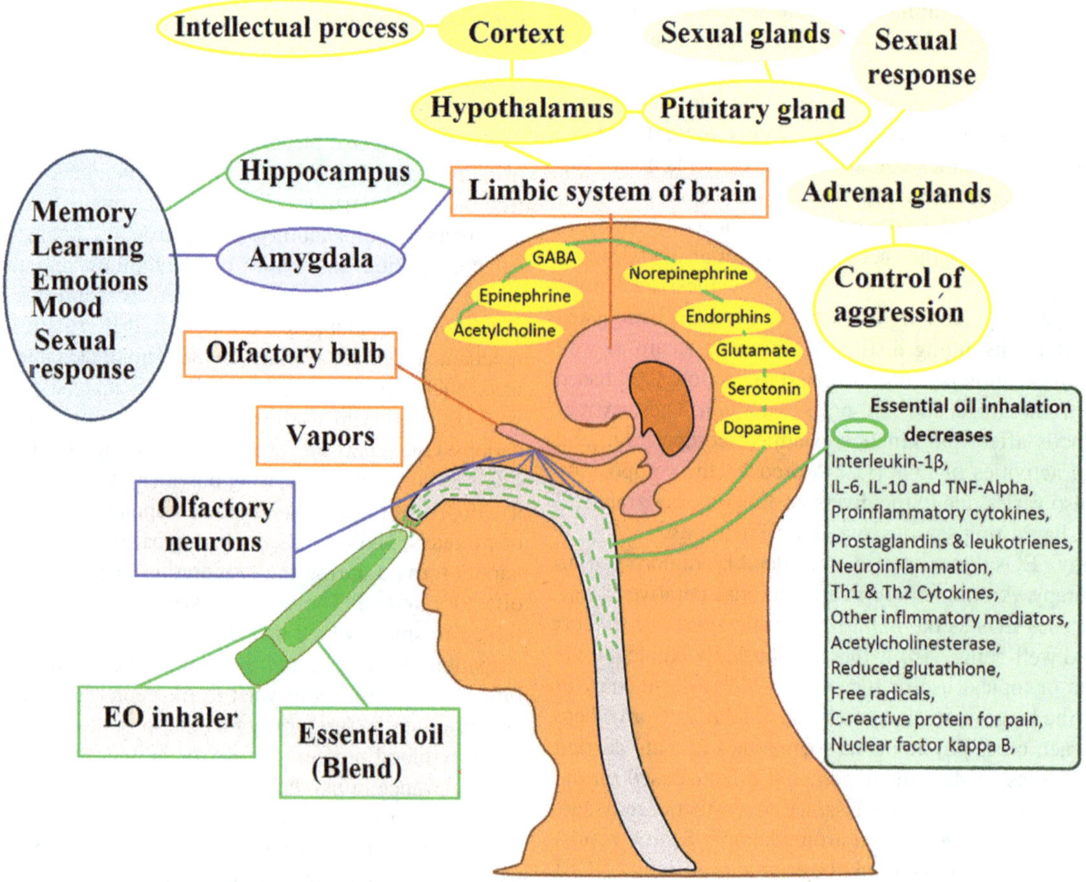

FIGURE 1.1 Effects of EOs and their components on the central nervous system (CNS).

mainly whooping cough, tuberculosis, bronchitis, and asthma. Unlike other natural products, one of the advantages of EOs is that they can be inhaled to reduce acute exacerbation in patients, mainly those associated with respiratory tract diseases (RTDs). RTDs related to viral and bacterial infections, pollutants, inflammation, and other intrinsic or extrinsic factors affect a large number of people from all age-group globally. Earlier studies suggested the importance of OA in the management of upper respiratory infections (acute and chronic) such as common cold, sinusitis, pharyngitis, and chronic obstructive pulmonary disease (COPD). These conditions can lead to the inflammation of bronchioles, which can be suppressed by EO inhalation. It was also observed that OA can be used to reduce the inflammation of lung tissue via decreasing interleukin (1β) as well as Th1 helper cells mediated immune effects in air pollutant-induced acute lung inflammation in rodent. OA also resulted in the inhibition of inflammation (caused by allergen) and hyperplasia of cells underlying mucosa with T-helper-2 cell inhibition as well as the expression of Muc5b in asthmatic rodent. The above reports and studies suggest the significant importance of OA in the treatment of various respiratory disorders and mental disorders.

Coronaviruses have been reported on due to their significant impact on health, economy, and society by causing different forms of infections including severe acute respiratory syndrome (SARS), Middle East respiratory syndrome (MERS), avian infectious bronchitis virus (IBV), and coronavirus disease 2019 (COVID-19). Severe acute respiratory syndrome coronavirus 2 (SARS-CoV-2) causes COVID-19, which was initially detected in late 2019, and may lead to mild-to-severe respiratory and systemic illness. This viral infection may progress to severe hypoxemia requiring some form of ventilator support in many suspected and confirmed cases. This highly infectious respiratory disease can lead to respiratory, physical, and psychological dysfunction in patients. At present (early 2020) no approved therapeutics or preventative therapeutic approaches are available. Various clinical studies are in progress to discover safe, effective, and inexpensive therapeutic agents against COVID-19. Chemical components derived from nature offer various biological effects such as anti-viral activity, anti-inflammatory activity, as well as immune-boosting effects, and therefore may be used as therapeutic agents against coronavirus infections. It has been known for a long time that EO inhalation or OA can be effectively used for the treatment of various respiratory infections. This antique wide range of natural EOs with multiple health benefits can be used against respiratory infections including viral infections such as COVID-19, bronchitis, asthma, or COPD. In contrast to other therapeutic agents EOs offer considerable benefits such as inhalation (of EOs) is more convenient for patients, and via inhalation the drug can be directly targeted at the infected site in the lungs with more retention or concentration in lungs than in blood. Thus, inhalation of EOs is usually linked to higher pulmonary effectiveness and minimum toxicity at a systemic level. Additionally, there are various studies available that report the immunological and psychological benefits of OA. Inhalation of suitable EOs disinfects lungs, boosts immunity, prevents and treats viral infections, and offers various psychological benefits. These biological properties make OA an ideal treatment strategy to combat against COVID-19 [7–28]. So far the anti-coronaviral potential of only a few EOs has been explored. Thus, the purpose of this chapter as well as other chapters is to describe the possible role of EOs in the treatment and management of COVID-19.

REFERENCES

1. Benmoussa H, Elfalleh W, Farhat A, Bachoual R, Nasfi Z, Romdhane M. Effect of extraction methods on kinetic, chemical composition and antibacterial activities of Tunisian Thymus vulgaris. L. essential oil. *Sep Sci Technol.* 2016;51(13):2145–2152.
2. Tongnuanchan, P, Benjakul, S. Essential oils: Extraction, bioactivities, and their uses for food preservation. *J Food Sci.* 2014;79:R1231–R1249. doi:10.1111/1750-3841.12492.
3. López V, Nielsen B, Solas M, Ramírez MJ, Jäger AK. Exploring pharmacological mechanisms of lavender (*Lavandula angustifolia*) essential oil on central nervous system targets. *Front Pharmacol.* 2017;8:280. doi:10.3389/fphar.2017.00280.
4. Sayorwan W, Ruangrungsi N, Piriyapunyporn T, Hongratanaworakit T, Kotchabhakdi N, Siripornpanich V. Effects of inhaled rosemary oil on subjective feelings and activities of the nervous system. *Sci Pharm.* 2013;81(2):531–542. doi:10.3797/scipharm.1209-05.
5. Koo BS, Lee SI, Ha JH, Lee DU. Inhibitory effects of the essential oil from SuHeXiang Wan on the central nervous system after inhalation. *Biol Pharm Bull.* 2004;27(4):515–519. doi:10.1248/bpb.27.515.
6. Koo BS, Park KS, Ha JH, Park JH, Lim JC, Lee DU. Inhibitory effects of the fragrance inhalation of essential oil from *Acorus gramineus* on central nervous system. *Biol Pharm Bull.* 2003;26(7):978–982. doi:10.1248/bpb.26.978.
7. Bhatia S, Namdeo AG, Nanda S. Factors effecting the gelling and emulsifying properties of a natural polymer. *SRP.* 2010;1(1):86–92.
8. Bhatia S, Sharma K, Bera T. Structural characterization and pharmaceutical properties of porphyran. *Asian J Pharm.* 2015;993–101.
9. Bhatia S, Sharma A, Sharma K, Kavale M, Chaugule BB, Dhalwal K, Namdeo AG, Mahadik KR. Novel algal polysaccharides from marine source: Porphyran. *Pharmacogn Rev.* 2008;4:271–276.
10. Bhatia S, Sharma K, Nagpal K, Bera T. Investigation of the factors influencing the molecular weight of porphyran and its associated antifungal activity. *Bioact Carb Diet Fiber* 2015;5:153–168.
11. Bhatia S, Kumar V, Sharma K, Nagpal K, Bera T. Significance of algal polymer in designing amphotericin B nanoparticles. *Sci World J.* 2014;2014:564573.
12. Bhatia S, Rathee P, Sharma K, Chaugule BB, Kar N, Bera T. Immuno-modulation effect of sulphated polysaccharide (Porphyran) from Porphyra vietnamensis. *Int J Biol Macromol.* 2013;57:50–56.
13. Bhatia S. *Natural Polymer Drug Delivery Systems: Marine Polysaccharides Based Nano-Materials and Its Applications.* Springer International Publishing, Switzerland; 2016:185–225.

14. Bhatia S. *Natural Polymer Drug Delivery Systems: Plant Derived Polymers, Properties, and Modification & Applications.* Springer International Publishing, Switzerland; 2016:119–184.
15. Bhatia S. *Natural Polymer Drug Delivery Systems: Nanotechnology and Its Drug Delivery Applications.* Springer International Publishing, Switzerland; 2016: 1–32.
16. Bhatia S. *Natural Polymer Drug Delivery Systems: Nanoparticles Types, Classification, Characterization, Fabrication Methods and Drug Delivery Applications.* Springer International Publishing; Switzerland; 2016:33–93.
17. Bhatia S. *Natural Polymer Drug Delivery Systems: Natural Polymers vs Synthetic Polymer.* Springer International Publishing, Switzerland; 2016:95–118.
18. Bhatia S. *Systems for Drug Delivery: Mammalian Polysaccharides and Its Nanomaterials.* Springer International Publishing, Switzerland; 2016:1–27.
19. Bhatia S. *Systems for Drug Delivery: Microbial Polysaccharides as Advance Nanomaterials.* Springer International Publishing, Switzerland; 2016:29–54.
20. Bhatia S. *Systems for Drug Delivery: Chitosan Based Nanomaterials and Its Applications.* Springer International Publishing, Switzerland; 2016:55–117.
21. Bhatia S. *Systems for Drug Delivery: Advance Polymers and Its Applications.* Springer International Publishing, Switzerland; 2016:119–146.
22. Bhatia S. *Systems for Drug Delivery: Advanced Application of Natural Polysaccharides.* Springer International Publishing, Switzerland; 2016:147–170.
23. Bhatia S. *Systems for Drug Delivery: Modern Polysaccharides and Its Current Advancements.* Springer International Publishing, Switzerland; 2016:171–188.
24. Bhatia S. *Systems for Drug Delivery: Toxicity of Nanodrug Delivery Systems.* Springer International Publishing, Switzerland; 2016:189–197.
25. Bhatia S. *Nanotechnology in Drug Delivery Fundamentals, Design, and Applications: Part 1: Protein and Peptide-Based Drug Delivery Systems.* Apple Academic Press, Palm Bay, FL; 2016:50–204.
26. Bhatia S. *Nanotechnology in Drug Delivery Fundamentals, Design, and Applications: Part 2: Peptide-Mediated Nanoparticle Drug Delivery System.* Apple Academic Press, Palm Bay, FL; 2016:205–280.
27. Bhatia S. *Nanotechnology in Drug Delivery Fundamentals, Design, and Applications: Part 3: CPP and CTP in Drug Delivery and Cell Targeting.* Apple Academic Press, Palm Bay, FL; 2016:309–312.
28. Bhatia S, Al-Harrasi A, Behl T, Anwer MK, Ahmed MM, Mittal V, Kaushik D, Chigurupati S, Kabir MT, Sharma PB, Chaugule B, Vargas-de-la-Cruz C. Unravelling the photoprotective effects of freshwater alga Nostoc commune Vaucher ex Bornet et Flahault against ultraviolet radiations. *Environ Sci Pollut Res Int.* 2021.

2

Epidemiology Respiratory Infections: Types, Transmission, and Risks Associated with Co-infections

Ahmed Al-Harrasi
Natural and Medical Sciences Research Center, University of Nizwa

Saurabh Bhatia
Natural and Medical Sciences Research Center, University of Nizwa
University of Petroleum and Energy Studies

CONTENTS

2.1 Introduction

Respiratory viruses have been reported for their capability in causing respiratory infections with considerable level of death as well as morbidity, more frequently than other classes of pathogens. Various respiratory viruses that have been reported among human beings usually cause infections among all age-groups. These viruses can have the capability to transmit in between or among different species with varying levels of virulence. Upper respiratory tract infections (URTIs) caused by a variety of viruses and bacteria are more common in infants and young children. The frequency of URTIs may vary from three to eight episodes per year; however, the number of episodes may increase for those who attend childcare centers [1]. URTIs can result in inflammation in the middle ear, swelling as well as inflammation of airways, and lower respiratory tract infections (LRTIs). LRTIs such as pneumonia, inflammation of airways, and inflammation of the bronchioles result in considerable mortality and morbidity across the globe. Thus, such complications increase healthcare costs causing more financial burden over the infected ones. Virus-based respiratory infections are usually restricted to mild upper and middle respiratory tract infections; however, in children they can reach the bronchioles and cause bronchiolitis. Among adults, bacteria are the main cause of pneumococcal pneumonia, which is caused by the *Streptococcus pneumoniae* germ that normally survives in the upper respiratory tract [2]. Respiratory viruses include influenza (A &B) (Orthomyxoviridae); parainfluenza virus (PIV) (type 1 to 3); adenovirus (ADV); rhinoviruses and enteroviruses (Picornaviridae); human metapneumovirus (hMPV) and respiratory syncytial viruses (RSVs) A and B (Paramyxoviridae); and Cov types (OC43 & 229E) (Coronaviridae) [3,4]. The rare respiratory viral pathogens consist of PIV-4, influenza virus C, as well as certain forms of enteroviruses. The implications of newly revealed viral pathogens including HKU1, human bocavirus (hBoV), and coronavirus NL63 in context with pathogenesis, molecular targets, and its associated pathways at cellular as well as genetic level hasn't been revealed more [7,8]. With the exception of ADVs, all of these viruses have the RNA genome. *Streptococcus pneumoniae*, *Haemophilus influenzae*, and *Moraxella catarrhalis* are the most common bacterial pathogens in URTIs and LRTIs [5]. The most common infectious agents that cause lower respiratory illness are bacteria such as *Streptococcus pneumoniae*, *Haemophilus influenzae*, and viruses such as RSV and influenza virus [5]. Pulmonary infection caused by viruses always results in the activation of cellular and humoral immunity [6]. Additionally, the vagal afferent neural pathway plays a dominant role in contributing to distant inflammatory effects. New viruses that have evolved recently are more pathogenic as most

DOI: 10.1201/9781003175933-3

people have not acquired immunity against them. Due to the shorter generation times and their quicker evolutionary rates, the prevalence of RNA virus-based infections to new host species is higher. The fast development of countless RNA viruses is because of the repeated error-prone replication cycles [7]. The rate of mutation of RNA viruses is also high, increasing the chances of development of new strains of the same family of virus [7]. Human coronaviruses (HCoVs), members of the family Coronaviridae (corona- or crown-like surface projections of proteins, also known as surface spike proteins, present over the lipid bilayer to envelop or protect single-stranded non-segmented RNA), cause the common cold as well as more severe respiratory diseases, specifically severe acute respiratory syndrome (SARS) and Middle East respiratory syndrome (MERS), which are both zoonoses [8]. Coronavirus disease (COVID-19) is considered an infectious disease caused by severe acute respiratory syndrome coronavirus 2 (SARS-CoV-2), which was first identified in 2019 in Wuhan [8].

The respiratory tract is the most common site for a number of viruses that can cause a variety of URTIs and LRTIs such as the common cold, influenza, ear infection, inflammation of the larynx, inflammation of the tissue lining the sinuses, pneumonia, inflammation of the bronchiol, and aggravations of chronic obstructive pulmonary disease as well as asthma [9]. Diagnostic virology has now become a part of social therapy and clinical medicine where the diagnosis of all kinds of respiratory illness is predominantly treated clinically and is further reinforced by lab-based procedures including identification of antigen, serological tests, identification of nucleic acid, and *in vitro* cultures. Viral antigens, nucleic acids, and antibodies (serology) have now become mainstream methods for the laboratory diagnosis of viral infections [9]. These immunologic and nucleic acid diagnostic techniques are now replacing viral culture. Treatment strategies include over-the-counter, non-specific medicines and a small number of specific antiviral medications. Other than treatment and diagnosis modalities, preventive strategies play an important role in the prevention of risk factors including vaccination when recommended [9].

Viruses are well adapted for their transmission from person to person; however, these pathogens acquire different patterns of transmission in human beings. Thus, it's very critical to understand how environmental factors affect person-to-person transmission. As per the Centers for Disease Control and Prevention (CDC), viral transmission is comprised of contact transmission that includes direct as well as indirect spread of infection, whereas transmission of infection by air encompasses via aerosol as well as by droplet mist [10]. Airborne transmission involves the direct transfer of viral pathogens from the air interface into the individual with no involvement of any medium. Virus transmission is generally mediated by large-droplet aerosol, airborne particles, or direct contact, through which viruses get a chance to enter into host cells. Aerosols are solid or liquid particles that are suspended in the air (e.g., fog, dust, and gas commonly used in medical procedures). These aerosols or droplets are the main carriers for respiratory viruses. Virus entry into the host cell is facilitated by specific viral surface proteins, which primarily results in the initiation of host intracellular pathogenic mechanisms [10]. This may cause tissue injury and ultimately result in clinical disease. In immune-compromised patients, virus-mediated complications are more severe as they can cause significant morbidity and mortality among such patients. Recently, it was noticed that the pattern of transmission of SARS-CoV-2 in its speed and effects is unique. Thus, more understanding is required to interrupt transmission to further prevent widespread community transmission. Based on the transmission rate, respiratory viruses can be limited to endemic or epidemic but can also result in pandemic. The rate of transmission is mainly determined by the rate of reproduction of a virus. The higher the reproduction rate, the higher the risk of transmission of virus. R0, a numerical term, which is referred to as the reproduction number, represents how communicable a contagious disease is, and hence, it is an important marker to study the progression of a disease [11]. As an infection is transmitted to new people, it reproduces itself; thus, it's represented as R0 [11]. It also represents the average number of individuals who can acquire a contagious disease from one person with that disease. Using the R0 value, the transmission rate of a disease or its decline can be calculated. It's exclusively relevant to a population that was previously free of infection and hasn't been vaccinated. Thus, the R0 value is only applied when each person in a homogeneous population is fully exposed to the infection, which means that no one has been vaccinated, no one has had the disease before, and there's no way to control the spread of the disease. If the typical R0 among the people is >1, transmission of infection will be augmented. If R0 is <1, the transmission of infection will be at slow rate, and it will ultimately disappear [12]. The greater the R0 value, the more rapidly an epidemic will continue. This also depends on the size of the population (i.e., the denser the population [population per unit area], the more people are vulnerable, and the more the chances of viral infection) [11,12]. In this case, the R0 value would be large for a particular viral pathogen. If the percentage of the decline in the number of infected is fast by showing more recovery or a higher death rate, the R0 would be small. Thus, the intensity of an infectious disease outbreak is determined by R0 since it approximately estimates pandemics or large publicized outbreaks [11,12]. Various factors such as biological, sociobehavioral, and environmental factors affect the transmission of a pathogen and ultimately affect R0. For this reason, R0 is represented by different complex mathematical equations, which can cause it to be distorted, misapprehended, and misapplied [11,12].

Virus mutations create genetic diversity that can lead to immune escape or drug-resistant viral mutants [13]. The type of antigenic proteins in the virus, the affinity of viral proteins toward the binding site (receptor), the expression of receptors/binding site, and many other factors determine the pathogenicity of a virus [14].

Respiratory viruses include diverse viral agents from different families. Among them, the most common respiratory viruses responsible for causing acute respiratory disease include rhinoviruses, RSVs, ADVs, bocaviruses, hMPVs, respiratory coronaviruses, PIVs, and influenza viruses [15]. Due to the lack of information concerning virus biology, host–parasite relationship, genomic sequence, and virus transmission under the influence of various environmental factors, effective treatments such as vaccines as well as antiviral agents are not still available. Virus-mediated respiratory infection can result in mild-to-severe illness depending on the healthy state of an infected individual as well as the type and pathogenicity of the virus. Acute respiratory infections (ARIs) represent one of the main causes of morbidity and mortality across the world. Respiratory viral agents are the most common etiological agents of respiratory disease in human beings. More than 60% of acute lower respiratory infections (ALRIs) are caused by viruses [16,17]. Among all etiological agents, enveloped viruses (syncytial viruses and PIVs) that are members of the paramyxovirus family are considered as an important cause of LRTIs, especially in infants and children [17]. Supportive care and antiviral therapy are the foundation of the treatment of viral infections in intensive care units [18]. Nebulization of beta-agonists, aminophylline, and steroids is considered one of the most common treatments used against viral respiratory infections [19]. Antiviral drugs such as ribavirin are approved by the Food and Drug Administration (FDA) against RSV infection. Acute viral respiratory infections require immediate medical assistance as well as examination because if not treated at the right time they may result in the development of secondary infections such as bacterial pneumonia, particularly staphylococcal pneumonia [20]. At the same time, it's also important to understand various stages of respiratory illness to know possible targets and the pathogenicity of a causative organism. During the onset of respiratory illness, infection is generally restricted to the upper respiratory tract and is self-limiting. However, in certain cases, infectious agents can travel to the lower respiratory tract and cause infections such as bronchiolitis and pneumonia. Various immune responses determine the severity or progression of infection from URTI to LRTI. Moreover, the rate of infiltration of immune cells at the site of infection, the rate of production of inflammatory mediators, the pathogenicity of infectious agent, the age of the host, and comorbidity factors also determine the severity of respiratory illnesses. Thus, variation in the severity of these illnesses, from mild or asymptomatic upper airway infections to severe wheezing, bronchiolitis, or pneumonia, is determined by many factors. Older adults and children are at increased risk of severe respiratory illness caused by viral pathogens [21]. Boncristiani et al. [15] have demonstrated several respiratory viruses, treatments, detection methods, and classification and principal syndromes as seen in Table 2.1 [15].

2.2 Epidemiology of Respiratory Infections

In 2016, it was reported that LRTIs caused ~6.52 million fatalities in children's <5 years, one million fatalities among adults (>70 years), and nearly 2.38 deaths among individuals of each age range worldwide [22]. This death rate makes LRTIs the sixth most important leading cause of death for all age groups and the most important cause of mortality in kids <5 years. The main causative agent responsible for respiratory illness that led to a large number deaths and other complications globally was found to be *Streptococcus pneumoniae.* Pneumonia or bronchiolitis is considered as the most important cause of death and other complications globally. However, until 2010, 5.8 million casualties due to ALRIs were reported worldwide [23]. Respiratory infections are very common among kids at certain age groups younger than age 5. RSV triggers the most acute LRTIs among children <1 year of age, with maximum occurrence at an average age of 3 months [24]. Similarly, hMPV causes URTI (such as a cold), clinical or subclinical infection in children by 2 years of age [25]. Likewise, human PIVs (HPIVs) are currently divided into five serotypes belonging to the Paramyxoviridae family, out of which HPIV (1-3) are the most common etiological agents for LRTI among newborns, young kids, the immunodeficient, individuals with considerable morbidity, and the elderly [26]. HPIV-1 causes LRTI mainly in infants aged 7–36 months, with highest incidence in the second or third year [27]. Seasonal HPIV-3 infection,

TABLE 2.1

Respiratory Viruses, Treatments, Detection Methods, Classifications, and Principal Syndromes [15]

Virus	Treatment	Virus Detection Methods	Classification[a]	Principal Syndromes
SARS-CoV	Ivermectin	Culture, RT-PCR	Type 1	SARS
HRV	Ribavirin, pleconaril	Culture, RT-PCR	Species A, B, and C with 100 serotypes	URTI; asthma and COPD exacerbation
HRSV	Ribavirin	Culture, Ag detection, RT-PCR	Groups A and B	URTI, bronchiolitis, croup, bronchitis, pneumonia
HPIV	Acetaminophen or ibuprofen	Culture, Ag detection, RT-PCR	Types 1, 2, 3, and 4	URTI, croup, bronchiolitis, bronchitis, pneumonia
hMPV	Ribavirin	Culture, RT-PCR	Groups A and B	URTI, bronchitis, pneumonia
HCoV	Dexamethasone	Culture, RT-PCR	Types OC43, 229E, NL(NH), and HKU1	URTI, bronchitis, pneumonia
HBoV	Bronchodilators	PCR	Two lineages	URTI, bronchiolitis, asthma exacerbation, bronchitis, pneumonia
ADV	Cidofovir and ribavirin	Culture, Ag detection, PCR	51 serotypes	URTI, PCF, bronchitis, pneumonia

Source: Boncristiani HF, Criado MF, Arruda E, Encycl Microbiol, 2009, 500–518, doi: 10.1016/B978-012373944-5. With permission.

ADV, adenovirus; Ag, antigen; COPD, Chronic obstructive pulmonary disease; HBoV, human bocavirus; HCoV, human coronavirus; hMPV, human metapneumovirus; HPIV, human parainfluenza virus; HRSV, human respiratory syncytial virus; HRV, human rhinovirus; PCF, pharyngoconjunctival fever; SARS, severe acute respiratory syndrome; SARS-CoV, coronavirus associated with SARS; URTI, upper respiratory tract infections; RT-PCR, reverse transcription polymerase chain reaction, which includes both conventional and real-time methods.

[a] This classification signify eight human respiratory viruses causing infection usually among all age groups.

which is mostly associated with pneumonia and bronchiolitis, infects patients aged 0–26 months, whereas HPIV-2 results in nearly 60% of infections among kids >5 years. The highest frequency is among children 1 and 2 years of age [27]. HPIV-2 peak incidence is usually age 2; however, peak incidence of HPIV-3 in children who experience the infection is age 1 [27,27]. Similarly, another respiratory virus, influenza, causes communicable viral diseases that affect both the upper and lower respiratory tracts. There are four types of influenza viruses: A, B, C, and D; however, only A and B cause human infections [28]. Influenza viruses (A and B) cause infections in all age-groups, but playschool (nursery, preschool, and kindergarten) kids and schoolchildren have the highest risk. Immunocompromised patients due to age, comorbid state, and weak immune system have impaired immunity [28]. Natural products (such as algal polysaccharides) and biotechnological products can be utilized with nanotechnological approaches to improve the immune response. Recently, several algal polysaccharides have been used to modulate the immune response of host cells [29–43].

Such patients are at higher risk of developing acute viral respiratory infections. Rhinoviruses and coronaviruses are another class of viruses that are considered as the main etiological agents for common cold syndrome and also participate in causing more serious respiratory infections that can result in increased morbidity and mortality. These viruses usually trigger URTI and affect people at several occasions during their live period. Rhinoviruses have been reported to cause LRTI among kids, but their exact pathophysiology hasn't been explored yet [44]. Except immunocompromised patients due to the comorbid state, these viruses are rarely associated with severe illnesses resulting in hospitalizations. This may be due to the limited virulence of these pathogens, the pathogenesis of their infections, the lack of detection or diagnostic tools, or challenges in the identification of these pathogens. SARS-CoV-2 is considered as one of the novel viruses that mainly target the human respiratory system and cause a respiratory illness that may result in severe pneumonia and acute respiratory distress syndrome (ARDS). This infectious agent was first identified in early January 2020 after it caused an outbreak of viral pneumonia in Wuhan, China. In December 2019, Wuhan, China, was the place where the first cases had their symptom of onset. SARS-CoV, MERS-CoV, and SARS-CoV-2 belong to the same genus, Betacoronavirus [45]. These viruses are characterized as great public health threats. One of the main distinguishing features among these viruses in terms of transmission is that SARS and MERS are linked mainly with nosocomial transmission, while SARS-CoV-2 is widely spread in the community with much higher transmission rate [45]. However, there is much more to understand about COVID-19, mainly its epidemiological features such as mortality and ability to spread on a pandemic level.

2.3 Types of Respiratory Infections

The upper and lower respiratory tracts are considered as the most common sites for viral infections. Thus, based on the site of infection or onset of infection, respiratory infections can be classified as URTIs and LRTIs. However, respiratory infections can also be classified on the basis of causative agents such as virus (e.g., influenza). Classification based on respiratory infections caused by virus (e.g., influenza) or classification based on clinical syndrome (e.g., the common cold) is common [46,47].

Influenza is caused by influenza viruses, RNA viruses of the *Orthomyxovirus* genus. Influenza viruses are classified into four types, A, B, C, and D, and can cause a wide range of complications such as the common cold, bronchiolitis, croup, and pneumonia. However, some specific pathogens cause characteristic clinical manifestations; for example, rhinovirus typically causes the common cold, whereas RSV typically causes bronchiolitis [46,47]. Each of these viruses can cause many of the viral respiratory syndromes and they have an important characteristic clinical manifestation that makes them distinct from each other [46,47]. Classification can also be based on the type of genetic material, morphology, binding site (receptor of host), nature of viral proteins, and cellular targets of the virus. The classification of respiratory tract infection is based on the symptomatology (symptoms of an illness exhibited by a patient) and anatomic involvement (the site where the pathogen is well adapted and causes pathogenicity). As viruses usually affect the upper or lower respiratory tracts, respiratory infections are classified based on the site of infection as URTI and LRTI as discussed below [46,47].

2.3.1 Upper Respiratory Tract Infections (URTIs)

URTIs are a major cause of mild morbidity both in children and in adults; "URTI" is perhaps a misnomer as it wrongly involves an absence of lower respiratory tract symptoms (Figure 2.1). Upper respiratory tract infection (URTI) or "the common cold" is a symptom complex usually caused by several families of virus which is more common during summer, fall, and winter. URTI are caused by invasion of a variety of viruses and bacteria directly into the upper airway mucosa of the host by inhalation of infected droplets where they can cause clinical syndromes such as the common cold, pharyngitis, epiglottitis, and laryngotracheitis [46]. Except for epiglottitis and laryngotracheitis, which can be serious in children and young infants, other infections are usually benign, temporary, and self-limited [46]. It's important to determine the incubation period of an infectious agent that can cause respiratory infections because the incubation period provides important information including when the infected individuals will be symptomatic and most likely to spread the disease. The incubation period, the time between exposure to the infectious agent and symptom onset, also provides important information about the growth, rate of multiplication, and toxin production and clues about the cause and source of an infection. Viruses, bacteria, mycoplasma, and fungi are the etiological agents associated with URTI; however, viruses and bacteria are the most common etiological agents that cause URTI [46]. The main etiological agents that are responsible for URTI are rhinovirus, coronavirus, PIV, RSV, ADV, hMPV, and influenza virus. Some of the URTI complications such as pharyngitis are also caused by bacteria such as *Streptococcus pyogenes*. A newly identified pathogen, that is, hBoV (belonging to human

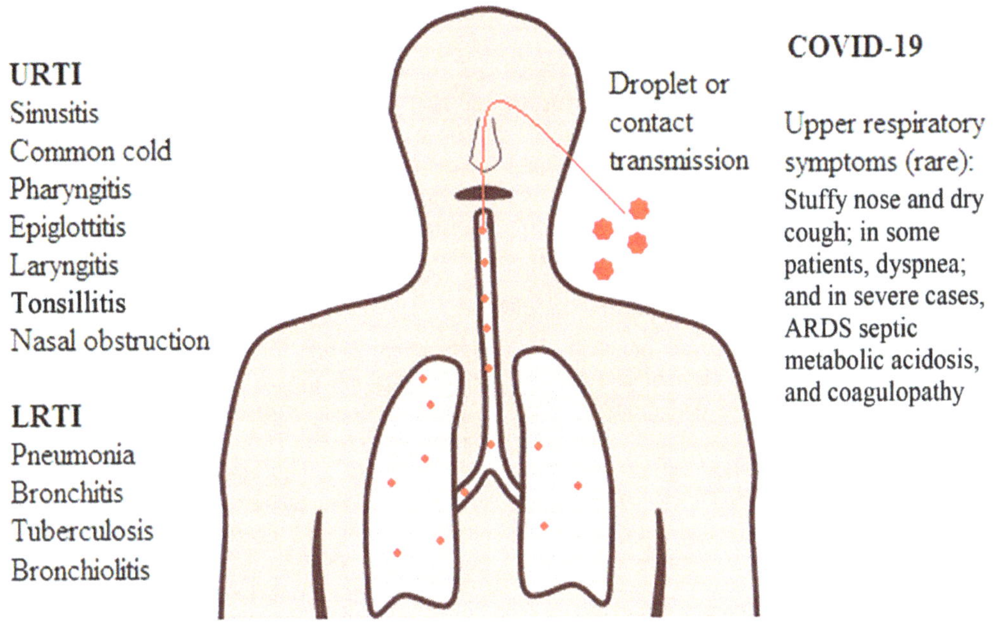

FIGURE 2.1 Upper and lower respiratory tract infections and respiratory symptoms of coronavirus infection.

parvovirus), can cause URTI and LRTI usually in children. Virus- and bacteria-based URTI include acute bronchitis, the common cold, influenza, and respiratory distress syndromes [46]. Due to the overlapping or close similarity between complications or symptoms and asymptomatic host response, it's often quite challenging to categorize patients. The diagnosis of URTI is usually based on a review of symptoms, physical examination, and occasionally, laboratory tests. During physical examination, inflammation and pain inside the wall of the nasal cavity and throat, enlargement of the tonsils and lymph nodes, nasal secretion as well as tonsillar exudate, ocular inflammation and sinusitis, halitosis, hoarseness of voice, cough, and fever are initially assessed [46]. Laboratory testing is usually not suggested in the diagnosis of URTI as the majority of URTI are caused by viruses. Thus, specific testing is not required as there is no specific treatment available for URTI. However, there are some critical situations in which infection can spread to the lower respiratory tract and can cause significant damage to lungs [47]. In such cases, numerous samples could be utilized for the identification of respiratory viral pathogens, such as nasopharyngeal (NP) washes/swabs/aspirates, lung aspirates, bronchoalveolar lavage, throat swab lung aspirates, and NP swabs. X-rays as well as CT scans are also recommended in these cases. The majority of URTIs involve self-limited irritation and inflammation of upper airways (nose, sinuses, pharynx, larynx) with persistent cough, which are usually caused by viruses and bacteria. As far as fungal infection is concerned, *Aspergillus* strains are considered as the most widespread fungal pathogen affecting upper as well as lower respiratory systems as their spores are everywhere and can cause chronic rhinosinusitis, cystic fibrosis, and allergic rhinitis [48].

HCoVs are associated with URTI that occasionally travel to the lower respiratory tract. COVID-19 affects different people in different ways. Most infected people will develop mild-to-moderate illness and recover without hospitalization. It can affect the upper respiratory tract, and in most serious cases, the most common symptoms include fever, dry cough, and tiredness. Droplet and contact transmission and high-concentration aerosols are considered as the main modes of transmission of COVID-19. SARS-CoV-2 in live form can be easily isolated by throat swabs, which suggests the active viral replication in upper respiratory tissues [49–51].

2.3.2 Lower Respiratory Tract Infections (LRTIs)

The most common LRTIs include bronchitis, bronchiolitis, and pneumonia (Figure 2.1) [22]. The development of these respiratory illnesses, mainly bacterial infection (pneumonia), can be extremely serious and even life-threatening. Severity can be explained by presenting the mortality rate. Based on a report published in 2016, LRTI caused 652,572 fatalities among kids <5 years, 1,080,958 among adults >70 years, and 2,377,697 fatalities among individuals of all ages globally [22]. One of the most common LRTIs caused by *Streptococcus pneumoniae* (i.e., pneumonia) can be serious and life-threatening with a high mortality rate of around 25% [51]. The most common etiological agents of LRTI are viruses or bacteria. In addition to these agents, mycoplasma, rickettsiae, and fungi can also cause LRTI [46]. Viruses are the most common cause of bronchitis and bronchiolitis. Acute bronchitis and pneumonia are the most common complications of LRTI; bronchitis is an inflammation of the airways characterized by cough, with or without sputum production, which can last up to 1–3 weeks, while pneumonia is an inflammation of the air sacs in the lungs and the surrounding tissue, which can last up to one month or sometimes even several months. Acute bronchitis is typically a viral infection. LRTIs, mainly pneumonia, bronchiolitis, and SARS, continue to be a major cause of morbidity and mortality worldwide disproportionately affecting adults ≥ 70 years old and children < 5 years old. Severe LRTIs develop only in immunocompromised patients [52].

SARS-CoV disease affects LRTI, with cytokine hyperproduction among individuals with poor outcomes. Mutated viruses that are well adapted to humans trigger more serious LRTI. Poor outcomes of individuals with SARS and MERS are usually linked with elevated amounts of proinflammatory mediators in the LRT as well as other organs. Among all etiological agents of LRTI, viruses cause an enormous disease burden in children, elderly individuals, patients with multiple comorbidities, and immunocompromised patients with serious LRTI. Infants and preschool children are more vulnerable and experience more viral respiratory illness than other age-groups. Electron microscopy, cell culture (tube culture and shell vial culture), antigen detection assays (rapid immunoassays such as latex fixation method, lateral flow tests detection by using optical immunosensors, and direct fluorescent antibody tests), serological tests (fluorescent antibody assay, and reverse transcription polymerase chain reaction (RT-PCR), IgM testing) are non-molecular procedures for the detection of respiratory viruses as well as other pathogens [53]. Molecular approaches to the assessment of respiratory pathogens include nucleic acid amplification examinations (i.e., real-time RT-PCR, multiplex microarray, competitive DNA hybridization, microarray hybridization, nested multiplex RT-PCR, isothermal RT-helicase-dependent amplification, loop-mediated isothermal DNA amplification, isothermal nucleic acid amplification) [53]. Nucleic acid amplification tests include high-complexity multiplex panel assays, moderate-complexity multiplex integrated systems, low-plex integrated test systems, and waived molecular point-of-care tests [53]. These tests are often used for the diagnosis of various viral respiratory infections. For these respiratory examinations for the detection of respiratory viruses, different types of specimens can be used as discussed above while the suitable sample form varies by patient [53]. Serological tests can be used to identify pathogen-specific antibodies. These antibodies usually appear within 14 days after the onset of infection. The detection of antibodies by different sera-based examinations can effectively detect antibodies against most active respiratory viruses including PIV (1–3), ADV, RSV, and influenza (A & B), and are able to identify mixed infections from ARI children (hospitalized) [53].

2.4 Transmission of Human Respiratory Viruses

As per the published information in 2012, there were almost 219 virus species identified as being able to cause human infection. Approximately 60% of human infections worldwide are caused by viruses [54]. Among all viruses, enteric and respiratory viruses are considered as the most common cause for human illness [20]. Transmission of respiratory viruses is dependent on their journey within the host and outside the host system. These viruses reproduce initially in the host respiratory system and then later are transmitted to other individuals via respiratory secretions. The duration of viral shedding varies significantly, and this may depend on severity, which is mainly determined by the pathogenicity of the virus and host immune response [47]. The duration of viral shedding is often increased in immunocompromised patients [55]. Thus, viral shedding is a contagious stage that determines the rate of removal and release of virus progeny from host cells to the environment. During this process, the virus replicates inside the host and forms more number in an exponential fashion. Transmission of the virus depends on many factors such as viral load or the amount of virus released from an infected individual, host–virus interaction, stability in the environment, transmission rate in a closed environment, and the rate of viral shedding via different body secretions (such as plasma, urine vomit, saliva, feces, and other respiratory excretions). The rate of transmission of respiratory tract infections is found to be high among young children, elderly people, and immunocompromised people [56].

Novel emerging viruses are the most important threats to community health. Transmission of such viruses from animals to human beings causes infectious diseases with a high transmission rate as found in SARS, Ebola fever, and influenza in humans [56]. There are several ways the virus transfers from the infected host to a new host. Transfer of viral infection among one or different species to an uninfected individual can occur via both direct or indirect means. Indirect routes such as the involvement of contaminated surfaces can play an important role in the transmission of viral infections. Based on transmission, the disease can be zoonotic, where it is transmitted between species from animals to humans (or from humans to animals), or epizootic, where the outbreak of disease affects many animals of one kind at the same time. Switching of virus from animals to humans may result in efficient and high transmissibility among humans but maintaining high-level pathogenicity. Viral transmission is based on the type of contact between two hosts of the same or different species [56]. Viruses can be transmitted from an infected host to a susceptible host by direct or indirect contact. Direct-contact transmission takes place when there is physical contact between an infected and a susceptible host, whereas indirect-contact transmission occurs when there is no direct human-to-human contact. Contact transmission occurs when a susceptible host comes in contact with an infected host or surfaces or objects. Transmission through surface or intermediate objects or via fomites, called fomite-based transmission, is common in a number of setups (e.g., schools, daycare centers, childcare centers, long-term care facilities) [56]. Droplet- or aerosol-mediated transmission of virus via air is also common. Based on the particle size, especially aerodynamic diameter, respiratory particles can be distinguished as droplets or aerosols. Respiratory droplets refer to droplets >5 μm in diameter; however, this varies significantly among reports varying up to 12 μm. Previous reports demonstrated that sneezing can generate 40,000 droplets of average size between 0.5–12 μm which could be ejected at rates up to 100 m/s, while coughing could generate equal to 3000 droplets [57,58]. Large-size droplets produced while coughing/sneezing/talking do not suspend for longer duration in an atmosphere and thus move <1 m prior to falling on the mucosa of nearby acquaintances or intermediate surfaces. On the contrary, aerosol droplets have a sluggish dropping rate; therefore, they stay in the atmosphere for an extended time and may move further. Respiratory viruses use fomites and large-particle-size aerosols in the form of respiratory droplets for their transmission from one person to another

[59]. These droplets are produced during expiratory events; for example, during normal exhalation, coughing or sneezing plays an important role in the transmission of viral respiratory infections [59]. The indirect mode of transmission (i.e., fomite transmission) takes place when virus-carrying droplets contaminate hands or non-living objects and surfaces. Except for measles virus or varicella zoster virus, the majority of respiratory viruses do not transmit by means of aerosols inside rooms. In most healthcare services, contact isolation and droplet precautions are sufficient to prevent the transmission of pathogens spread in surroundings. Droplet- and aerosol-based airborne transmission allows some infectious viruses to transmit easily in the community, causing community spread in the form of epidemics that are hard to manage [59]. Kutter et al. [60] demonstrated normally recognized respiratory modes of spread as mentioned in Table 2.2.

Different environmental factors such as temperature and humidity play a major role in the transmission of viral infections; however, other factors such as social distancing or crowding of people, hygiene level, and the availability of binding sites of virus inside the respiratory tract of the host equally affect the transmission of viruses. These variables factors affect the common route of respiratory virus transmission in a different way. Understanding of the transmission of infections within the host system and inter-host transmission may possibly be used to improve intervention approaches [60]. Kutter et al. [60] demonstrated transmission routes of respiratory viruses as seen in Table 2.3.

2.5 Respiratory Tract-Based Co-infections

Respiratory tract-based co-infections that involve both viral and bacterial pathogens are usually observed during severe acute infections and in the course of chronic respiratory diseases. One of the most common acute conditions, community-acquired pneumonia, often leads to the development of mixed infections; however, the immunopathology of co-infections hasn't been studied well so far. Other conditions such as exacerbation of chronic obstructive pulmonary disease often result in the development of mixed infections where both pathogenic bacteria and viruses have been found simultaneously.

TABLE 2.2

Commonly Accepted Respiratory Routes of Transmission [60]

Transmission Route	Particles Involved and Particle Characteristics	Characteristics/Definition of Transmission
Contact		Self-inoculation of mucous membranes by contaminated hands
Direct	Deposited on persons	Virus transfer from one infected person to another
Indirect	Deposited on objects	Virus transfer through contaminated intermediate objects (fomites)
Airborne		
Droplet	Droplets (>5 μm)	Short-range transmission
	Remain only shortly in air (<17 min)	Direct inoculation of the naïve person through coughing/sneezing/breathing of the infected person
	Dispersed over short distances (<1 m)	Deposition mainly on mucous membranes and the upper respiratory tract
Aerosol	Aerosols, droplet nuclei (<5 μm)	Long-range transmission
	Remain in air for an almost infinite amount of time	Inhalation of aerosols in respirable size range
	Dispersed over long distances (>1 m)	Deposition along the respiratory tract, including the lower airways

Source: Kutter JS, Spronken MI, Fraaij PL, Fouchier RA, Herfst S, Curr Opin Virol, 2018, 28, 142–151. With permission.

TABLE 2.3

Overview of the Evidence on Transmission Routes of Respiratory Viruses Based on Experimental Data and the Transmission Route According to Infection Prevention Guidelines [60]

		Transmission Route	
Virus	**Virus Family**	**Experimental and Observational Data**	**Guidelines**
Measles virus	*Paramyxoviridae*	Aerosol	Contact, aerosol
Parainfluenza virus	*Paramyxoviridae*	Limited data, contact (by fomite)	Contact, droplet, aerosol
hMPV	*Pneumoviridae*	Limited data, contact (by fomite)	Contact, droplet
RSV	*Pneumoviridae*	Contact, droplet, aerosol	Contact, droplet, aerosol
HCoV	*Coronaviridae*	Limited data, contact (by fomite)	Contact, droplet
MERS-CoV	*Coronaviridae*	Contact, droplet, aerosol	Contact, droplet
SARS-CoV	*Coronaviridae*	Contact, droplet, aerosol	Contact, droplet, aerosol
Rhinovirus	*Picornaviridae*	Contact, aerosol	Contact, droplet, aerosol
Adenovirus	*Adenoviridae*	Contact, droplet, aerosol	Contact, droplet, aerosol
Influenza virus	*Orthomyxoviridae*	Droplet/aerosol	Contact, droplet, aerosol

Several environmental factors such as temperature, humidity, and light can influence air quality, especially suspension of pollutants and microorganisms in the air. The risk of co-infections usually increases in winter. Procedures such as cell culture of isolates from respiratory secretions of the infected host can be utilized for their identification. It's interesting to note that co-infections can be insignificant, harmful, or even beneficial. Considering respiratory infections, co-infections could be both viral to bacterial or viral to viral infections as discussed below [61]. Such infections can also alter the distribution of infections caused by virus [62]. For instance, rhinovirus is a fast reproducing viral pathogen and can affect reproduction of other viruses, but rate of replication of PIV is low and its reproduction could be disrupted by the existence of other viral pathogens [62].

2.5.1 Simultaneous Virus Infections or Viral Interference

Single infections and infections with multiple respiratory viruses or simultaneous virus infections cause mortality worldwide. Respiratory viruses such as human enterovirus, RSV, influenza A and B, PIV, human rhinovirus (HRV), coronavirus, hMPV, ADV, and hBoV were reported to be capable of causing simultaneous infections [63]. The involvement of more than one virus in viral respiratory infections is known as viral interference, particularly when one virus inhibits the growth or action of the other virus. Simultaneous virus infections are most common among different age-groups of children. A report by Goka et al. [64] on people of age-groups from 0 to 105 years showed that kids <5 years were more susceptible to viral co-infections than others. Another report showed that children between 6 and 24 months old showed the rate of viral co-infection when compared with newborn babies (0–6 months old). One more study among 164 children under the age of 3 years showed that the rate of co-infection was significantly higher among the 13–24 month age-group than among the 8 to 12 month or 25 to 36 month age-groups [65]. However, the relationship between the acute infections caused by viral co-infections and the clinical effect is still unclear. Numerous reports claim that viral co-infections are not severe when compared to single-virus infections. It was also found that the severity of viral co-infections in terms of clinical impact was less when compared to single-virus infections. However, a number of studies also suggest that severity is more common among patients infected with simultaneous viral infections. Aberle et al., during his work on non-RSV respiratory viruses, suggested that the severity of simultaneous infection with non-RSV respiratory viral pathogen is equivalent to that of single infections [66]. They also suggested that the root cause of dual infection associated with RSV is the reduced immune response resulting from severe LRTI. On the contrary, it was also discovered that co-infections are more acute in comparison to infection caused by single RSV [67]. A study related to influenza showed that patients infected with both influenza A and B viruses had higher mortality rate and admission to intensive care units. Based on studies on animals, it was concluded that co-infections with reovirus and SARS coronavirus in guinea pigs resulted in rapid death of the animals. An *in vitro* study showed that co-infections caused by RSV, swine influenza, and porcine reproductive virus suggested that viral interference was dominant; however, the outcome of viral interference was based on the virus that caused the primary infection. Another report on viral interference suggested that influenza A virus potentially blocked the development of RSV if it is expected to cause infection to the host cells simultaneously. During this work, it was also observed that RSV infection caused a high viral load in a single infection in comparison with its simultaneous infection to influenza virus when both commenced at the same time [68]. Thus, from this work it was concluded that influenza growth and multiplication can be inhibited by RSV conditionally primary infection should be influenza, followed by RSV infection. It was also found that the inhibitory response of a virus over another started during the protein synthesis. On the contrary, a study based on immunofluorescence and scanning electron microscopy revealed selective release of specific surface antigens by viruses during co-infection, and showed no viral interference was involved during the inhibitory action.

2.5.2 Simultaneous Viral–Bacterial Infections

Acute respiratory co-infection based on simultaneous onset of viral–bacterial infections or co-existence of both infections at the same time or viral infection followed by bacterial infections or vice versa is an important cause of morbidity among different age-groups of children. The co-existence or co-detection of both virus- and bacteria-based respiratory infections is common among children with a significant clinical impact. However, due to the lack of understanding of the kind of interaction between virus/bacteria and the host, this mixed etiology or this co-infectious state remains a controversial topic. Early reports suggested that co-infectious stage caused severe bacterial pneumonia followed by the influenza infection [69,70]. This type of viral–bacterial infection is very common in young children, such as the co-infection caused by RSV. However, understanding the role of bacteria in influencing the severity of the infection is quite challenging unless information related to the role of viral/bacterial co-infection state and pathogenicity caused by the same virus and bacteria independently is not clear. Several reports have also revealed the association of higher severity of inflammatory disease with mixed infections, particularly in secondary pneumococcal infections followed by infection with influenza virus. Thus, it can be concluded that the type of pathogens involved during mixed infections or co-infections determines the severity of infection as the pathogenicity of all pathogens or a single pathogen can be decreased or increased under the influence of each other [69,70].

In a pandemic of viral infection, the focus is primarily on the treatment of the primary infection; however, it's also equally important to identify the risk of co-infections (instantaneous infection with another pathogenic agent) such as bacterial infections (primary followed by secondary infection). Moreover, co-infections can also occur and lead to patient sufferance from problems caused by more than one pathogen, which are completely different from each other [70,71]. Viral infections, mainly caused pulmonary viruses, often result in the multiplication of bacteria in virus-affected organs or tissues, resulting in high morbidity and death rates. This type of viral infection initially weakened the immune response and facilitated the entry of bacterial pathogen(s) inside the host [72]. As reported earlier, secondary bacterial infections or superinfections are mainly the result of immune system weakness triggered by primary viral infection. This can lead to co-infection where multiple pathogens take the opportunity to enter into the host resulting in many-infection state (viral-bacterial-yeast). Co-infections, secondary infections, or "superinfections" are widespread in a viral outbreak. Spanish flu outbreak (1918) data suggested that the deaths of millions of people were due to bacterial co-infections; similarly H1N1 influenza outbreak (2009) resulted in millions of deaths due to bacterial co-infections [73].

2.6 Symptomatic vs. Asymptomatic Infections

As per reports, significant morbidity and mortality across different human populations has been seen due to severe respiratory infections; however, the severity of illness is determined by different variants. The diagnosis of viral infection is often challenging because in some cases infection can be mild or severe or without symptoms and sometimes it presents clinical symptoms that are not serious but still require hospital care. Based on the severity of illness, pathogenicity of pathogen, symptomatology, anatomic involvement of infections, and host health condition, an illness can be symptomatic and asymptomatic. Infection without any considerable signs or symptoms of respective disease is known as asymptomatic infection, whereas infection with considerable signs or symptoms of illness is known as symptomatic infection. The meaning of symptomatic infection is not described evenly as most of the investigations described asymptomatic individuals as those free from symptoms during their active participation or enrollment in the study. This difference between asymptomatic and symptomatic terms underlines the requirement for more studies to better understand the patterns of symptoms across different respiratory infections. Viral infections can be treated on the basis of symptoms (symptomatic treatment). Symptomatic treatment of streptococcal pharyngitis and epiglottitis caused by *Haemophilus influenzae* is one of the common examples where antibacterials are considered as the first choice of drugs. Similarly, the treatment of the uncomplicated common cold and sinus is generally symptomatic. Symptomatic treatment is recommended for viral pharyngitis. However, almost 50% of infections with normal seasonal flu may be asymptomatic. This may be due to pre-existing partial immunity of the individual against a similar pathogen. The rate of transmission and its severity vary significantly among symptomatic and asymptomatic patients. The transmission rate of viral respiratory infections among symptomatic and asymptomatic patients varies as asymptomatic patients form an undetectable reservoir for the virus that can transmit the disease with a high rate of infection. As per the reports, the viral load detected in NP swabs of symptomatic and asymptomatic carriers remains unaffected or the same with a great possibility for transmission. Thus, advancements in molecular testing, mainly PCR assays, are required to detect viruses in the biological samples of asymptomatic individuals. Recent reports showed asymptomatic infections during the summer months caused by respiratory viruses such as coronavirus, ADV, HRV, hMPV, RSV, influenza virus, and PIV [74]. Based on the type of host and virus, asymptomatic infection rates may vary. An earlier study suggested that almost 52% of kids without symptoms from Anchorage, Alaska, were found to be transmitting viral infections caused by HRV and ADV. Another previous study demonstrated asymptomatic as well as symptomatic infants in Perth, Australia. During this study, 70% of the specimens collected from symptomatic infants were found to be infected with respiratory viruses, whereas 24.6% of the samples from asymptomatic infants were also found to be infected with the viruses. It was also discovered that 24.6%–64% of HRV-infected individuals were found to be asymptomatic. The pattern of asymptomatic infection and respective shedding or transmission rates varies among different age-groups of children. A previous report revealed that the shedding rate of HRVs was 12.3% among healthy children [74]. Van Benten et al. reported that 20% of asymptomatic infants (2 years old) were found to be positive for HRVs [75]. Another similar report demonstrated HRV or coronavirus infection among 20% of kids with no previous or new respiratory infection [76]. Some reports suggested viral respiratory infections among 40% and 42% of asymptomatic kids.

REFERENCES

1. Cotton M, Innes S, Jaspan H, Madide A, Rabie H. Management of upper respiratory tract infections in children. *S Afr Fam Pract.* 2008;50(2):6–12.
2. Weiser JN, Ferreira DM, Paton JC. Streptococcus pneumoniae: Transmission, colonization and invasion. *Nat Rev Microbiol.* 2018;16(6):355–367.
3. Crowe JE Jr. Human respiratory viruses. *Ref Module Biomed Sci.* 2014. doi:10.1016/B978-0-12-801238-3.02600-3.
4. Nichols WG, Peck Campbell AJ, Boeckh M. Respiratory viruses other than influenza virus: Impact and therapeutic advances. *Clin Microbiol Rev.* 2008;21(2):274–290.
5. Cappelletty D. Microbiology of bacterial respiratory infections. *Pediatr Infect Dis J.* 1998;17(8 Suppl):S55–S61.
6. Newton AH, Cardani A, Braciale TJ. The host immune response in respiratory virus infection: Balancing virus clearance and immunopathology. *Semin Immunopathol.* 2016;38(4):471–482.
7. Carrasco-Hernandez R, Jácome R, López Vidal Y, Ponce de León S. Are RNA viruses candidate agents for the next global pandemic? A review. *ILAR J.* 2017;58(3):343–358.
8. Pal M, Berhanu G, Desalegn C, Kandi V. Severe acute respiratory syndrome coronavirus-2 (SARS-CoV-2): An update. *Cureus.* 2020;12(3):e7423.
9. Thomas M, Bomar PA. *Upper Respiratory Tract Infection.* StatPearls Publishing, Treasure Island, FL; 2020. Available from: https://www.ncbi.nlm.nih.gov/books/NBK532961/.
10. Jayaweera M, Perera H, Gunawardana B, Manatunge J. Transmission of COVID-19 virus by droplets and aerosols: A critical review on the unresolved dichotomy. *Environ Res.* 2020;188:109819. doi: 10.1016/j.envres.2020.109819.

11. Delamater PL, Street EJ, Leslie TF, Yang YT, Jacobsen KH. Complexity of the basic reproduction number (R0). *Emerg Infect Dis.* 2019;25(1):1–4.
12. Ridenhour B, Kowalik JM, Shay DK. Unraveling R0: Considerations for public health applications. *Am J Public Health.* 2014;104(2):e32–e41.
13. Sanjuán R, Domingo-Calap P. Mechanisms of viral mutation. *Cell Mol Life Sci.* 2016;73(23):4433–4448.
14. Maginnis MS. Virus-receptor interactions: The key to cellular invasion. *J Mol Biol.* 2018;430(17):2590–2611.
15. Boncristiani HF, Criado MF, Arruda E. Respiratory viruses. *Encycl Microbiol.* 2009:500–518. doi: 10.1016/B978-012373944-5.00314-X. Epub 2009 Feb 17. https://www.ncbi.nlm.nih.gov/pmc/articles/PMC7149556/
16. Elliott SP, Ray CG. Viral infections of the lower respiratory tract. *Pediatr Respir Med.* 2008:481–489. https://www.ncbi.nlm.nih.gov/pmc/articles/PMC7152490/
17. Wright M, Piedimonte G. Respiratory syncytial virus prevention and therapy: Past, present, and future. *Pediatr Pulmonol.* 2011;46(4):324–347.
18. Kelesidis T, Mastoris I, Metsini A, Tsiodras S. How to approach and treat viral infections in ICU patients. *BMC Infect Dis.* 2014;14:321.
19. Walker TA, Khurana S, Tilden SJ. Viral respiratory infections. *Pediatr Clin North Am.* 1994;41(6):1365–1381. doi: 10.1016/s0031-3955(16)38876-9. Erratum in: *Pediatr Clin North Am.* 1995;42(4):xi.
20. Abed Y, Boivin G. Treatment of respiratory virus infections. *Antiviral Res.* 2006;70(2):1–16.
21. Rouse BT, Sehrawat S. Immunity and immunopathology to viruses: What decides the outcome? *Nat Rev Immunol.* 2010;10(7):514–526.
22. GBD. Lower respiratory infections collaborators. Estimates of the global, regional, and national morbidity, mortality, and aetiologies of lower respiratory infections in 195 countries, 1990–2016: A systematic analysis for the Global Burden of Disease Study 2016. *Lancet Infect Dis.* 2018;18(11):1191–1210.
23. Seidu AA, Dickson KS, Ahinkorah BO, Amu H, Darteh EKM, Kumi-Kyereme A. Prevalence and determinants of acute lower respiratory infections among children under-five years in sub-Saharan Africa: Evidence from demographic and health surveys. *SSM Popul Health.* 2019;8:100443. Erratum in: *SSM Popul Health.* 2020.
24. Piedimonte G, Perez MK. Respiratory syncytial virus infection and bronchiolitis. *Pediatr Rev.* 2014;35(12):519–530. doi: 10.1542/pir.35-12-519. Erratum in: *Pediatr Rev.* 2015;36(2):85.
25. Nokso-Koivisto J, Hovi T, Pitkäranta A. Viral upper respiratory tract infections in young children with emphasis on acute otitis media. *Int J Pediatr Otorhinolaryngol.* 2006;70(8):1333–1342.
26. Branche AR, Falsey AR. Parainfluenza virus infection. *Semin Respir Crit Care Med.* 2016;37(4):538–554.
27. Henrickson KJ. Parainfluenza viruses. *Clin Microbiol Rev.* 2003;16(2):242–264.
28. Boktor SW, Hafner JW. Influenza. StatPearls Publishing, Treasure Island, FL; 2020. Available from: https://www.ncbi.nlm.nih.gov/books/NBK459363/.
29. Bhatia S, Sardana S, Sharma A, Vargas De La Cruz CB, Chaugule B, Khodaie L. Development of broad spectrum mycosporine loaded sunscreen formulation from Ulva fasciata delile. *Biomedicine (Taipei).* 2019;9(3):17.
30. Bhatia S, Sardana S, Senwar KR, Dhillon A, Sharma A, Naved T. In vitro antioxidant and antinociceptive properties of Porphyra vietnamensis. *Biomedicine (Taipei).* 2019;9(1):3.
31. Bhatia S, Sharma K, Nagpal K, Bera T. Investigation of the factors influencing the molecular weight of porphyran and its associated antifungal activity. *Bioact Carb Diet Fiber* 2015;5:153–168.
32. Bhatia S, Sharma K, Sharma A, Nagpal K, Bera T. Anti-inflammatory, analgesic and antiulcer properties of Porphyra vietnamensis. *Avicenna J Phytomed.* 2015;5(1):69–77.
33. Bhatia S, Kumar V, Sharma K, Nagpal K, Bera T. Significance of algal polymer in designing amphotericin B nanoparticles. *Sci World J.* 2014;2014:564573.
34. Bhatia S, Rathee P, Sharma K, Chaugule BB, Kar N, Bera T. Immuno-modulation effect of sulphated polysaccharide (porphyran) from Porphyra vietnamensis. *Int J Biol Macromol.* 2013;57:50–56.
35. Bhatia S, Garg A, Sharma K, Kumar S, Sharma A, Purohit AP. Mycosporine and mycosporine-like amino acids: A paramount tool against ultra violet irradiation. *Pharmacogn Rev.* 2011;5(10):138–146.
36. Bhatia S, Sharma K, Namdeo AG, Chaugule BB, Kavale M, Nanda S. Broad-spectrum sun-protective action of Porphyra-334 derived from Porphyra vietnamensis. *Pharmacognosy Res.* 2010;2(1):45–49.
37. Bhatia S, Sharma K, Dahiya R, Bera T. *Modern Applications of Plant Biotechnology in Pharmaceutical Sciences.* Academic Press, Elsevier; 2015:164–174.
38. Bhatia S. *Nanotechnology in Drug Delivery: Fundamentals, Design, and Applications.* CRC Press, Boca Raton, FL; 2016:121–127.
39. Bhatia S, Goli D. *Leishmaniasis: Biology, Control and New Approaches for Its Treatment.* CRC Press, Boca Raton, FL; 2016:164–173.
40. Bhatia S. *Natural Polymer Drug Delivery Systems: Nanoparticles, Plants, and Algae.* Springer Nature, London; 2016:117–127.
41. Bhatia S. *Introduction to Pharmaceutical Biotechnology, Volume 2: Enzymes, Proteins and Bioinformatics.* IOP Publishing Ltd, Bristol, UK; 2018:1.
42. Bhatia S. *Introduction to Pharmaceutical Biotechnology, Volume 1: Basic Techniques and Concepts.* IOP Publishing Ltd, Bristol, UK; 2018:2.
43. Bhatia S. *Introduction to Pharmaceutical Biotechnology, Volume 3: Animal Tissue Culture Technology.* IOP Publishing Ltd, Bristol, UK; 2019:3.
44. Pattemore PK, Jennings LC. Epidemiology of respiratory infections. *Pediatr Respir Med.* 2008:435–452. doi: 10.1016/B978-032304048-8.50035-9.
45. Zheng J. SARS-CoV-2: An emerging coronavirus that causes a global threat. *Int J Biol Sci.* 2020;16(10):1678–1685.
46. Dasaraju PV, Liu C. Infections of the respiratory system, Chapter 93. In: Baron S, editor. *Medical Microbiology*, 4th edition. University of Texas Medical Branch, Galveston, TX; 1996.
47. Couch RB. Orthomyxoviruses, Chapter 58. In: Baron S, editor. *Medical Microbiology*, 4th edition. University of Texas Medical Branch, Galveston, TX; 1996. Available from: https://www.ncbi.nlm.nih.gov/books/NBK8611/.
48. Delfino E, Del Puente F, Briano F, Sepulcri C, Giacobbe DR. Respiratory fungal diseases in adult patients with cystic fibrosis. *Clin Med Insights Circ Respir Pulm Med.* 2019;13:1179548419849939.

49. Jayaweera M, Perera H, Gunawardana B, Manatunge J. Transmission of COVID-19 virus by droplets and aerosols: A critical review on the unresolved dichotomy. *Environ Res*. 2020;188:109819.
50. Nowicki J, Murray MT. Bronchitis and pneumonia. *Textbook Nat Med*. 2020:1196–1201.e1.
51. Mani CS, Murray DL. Acute pneumonia and its complications. *Principles Pract Pediatr Infect Dis*. 2008:245–257.
52. Selvaraj K, Chinnakali P, Majumdar A, Krishnan IS. Acute respiratory infections among under-5 children in India: A situational analysis. *J Nat Sci Biol Med*. 2014;5(1):15–20.
53. Das S, Dunbar S, Tang YW. Laboratory diagnosis of respiratory tract infections in children: The State of the art. *Front Microbiol*. 2018;9:2478.
54. Barker J, Stevens D, Bloomfield SF. Spread and prevention of some common viral infections in community facilities and domestic homes. *J Appl Microbiol*. 2001;91(1):7–21.
55. Widders A, Broom A, Broom J. SARS-CoV-2: The viral shedding vs infectivity dilemma. *Infect Dis Health*. 2020;25(3): 210–215.
56. Louten J. Virus transmission and epidemiology. *Essent Hum Virol*. 2016:71–92. doi:10.1016/B978-0-12-800947-5.00005-3.
57. Cole EC, Cook CE. Characterization of infectious aerosols in health care facilities: An aid to effective engineering controls and preventive strategies. *Am J Infect Control*. 1998;26(4):453–464.
58. Tang JW, Li Y, Eames I, Chan PK, Ridgway GL. Factors involved in the aerosol transmission of infection and control of ventilation in healthcare premises. *J Hosp Infect*. 2006;64(2):100–114.
59. Atkinson J, Chartier Y, Pessoa-Silva CL, et al., editors. *Natural Ventilation for Infection Control in Health-Care Settings*. World Health Organization, Geneva; 2009. Annex C, Respiratory droplets. Available from: https://www.ncbi.nlm.nih.gov/books/NBK143281/.
60. Kutter JS, Spronken MI, Fraaij PL, Fouchier RA, Herfst S. Transmission routes of respiratory viruses among humans. *Curr Opin Virol*. 2018;28:142–151.
61. Meskill SD, O'Bryant SC. Respiratory virus co-infection in acute respiratory infections in children. *Curr Infect Dis Rep*. 2020;22(1):3.
62. Kumar N, Sharma S, Barua S, Tripathi BN, Rouse BT. Virological and immunological outcomes of coinfections. *Clin Microbiol Rev*. 2018;31(4):e00111-17.
63. Pinky L, Dobrovolny HM. Coinfections of the respiratory tract: Viral competition for resources. *PLoS One*. 2016;11(5):e0155589.
64. Goka EA, Vallely PJ, Mutton KJ, Klapper PE. Single, dual and multiple respiratory virus infections and risk of hospitalization and mortality. *Epidemiol Infect*. 2015;143(1):37–47.
65. Zhang G, Hu Y, Wang H, Zhang L, Bao Y, Zhou X. High incidence of multiple viral infections identified in upper respiratory tract infected children under three years of age in Shanghai, China. *PLoS One*. 2012;7(9):e44568.
66. Aberle JH, Aberle SW, Pracher E, Hutter HP, Kundi M, Popow-Kraupp T. Single versus dual respiratory virus infections in hospitalized infants: impact on clinical course of disease and interferon-gamma response. *Pediatr Infect Dis J*. 2005;24(7):605–610.
67. Brand HK, de Groot R, Galama JM, Brouwer ML, Teuwen K, Hermans PW, Melchers WJ, Warris A. Infection with multiple viruses is not associated with increased disease severity in children with bronchiolitis. *Pediatr Pulmonol*. 2012;47(4):393–400.
68. Shinjoh M, Omoe K, Saito N, Matsuo N, Nerome K. In vitro growth profiles of respiratory syncytial virus in the presence of influenza virus. *Acta Virol*. 2000;44(2):91–97.
69. Bradley BT, Bryan A. Emerging respiratory infections: The infectious disease pathology of SARS, MERS, pandemic influenza, and legionella. *Semin Diagn Pathol*. 2019;36:152–159.
70. Morris DE, Cleary DW, Clarke SC. Secondary bacterial infections associated with influenza pandemics. *Front Microbiol*. 2017;8:1041.
71. Wang H, Anthony D, Selemidis S, Vlahos R, Bozinovski S. Resolving viral-induced secondary bacterial infection in COPD: A concise review. *Front Immunol*. 2018;9:2345.
72. Mallia P, Footitt J, Sotero R, et al. Rhinovirus infection induces degradation of antimicrobial peptides and secondary bacterial infection in chronic obstructive pulmonary disease. *Am J Respir Crit Care Med*. 2012;186:1117–1124.
73. Chertow DS, Memoli MJ. Bacterial coinfection in influenza: A grand rounds review. *JAMA*. 2013;309:275–282.
74. Calvo C, Casas I, García-García ML, Pozo F, Reyes N, Cruz N, García-Cuenllas L, Pérez-Breña P. Role of rhinovirus C respiratory infections in sick and healthy children in Spain. *Pediatr Infect Dis J*. 2010;29(8):717–720.
75. van Benten I, Koopman L, Niesters B, Hop W, van Middelkoop B, de Waal L, van Drunen K, Osterhaus A, Neijens H, Fokkens W. Predominance of rhinovirus in the nose of symptomatic and asymptomatic infants. *Pediatr Allergy Immunol*. 2003;14(5):363–370.
76. Nokso-Koivisto J, Kinnari TJ, Lindahl P, Hovi T, Pitkäranta A. Human picornavirus and coronavirus RNA in nasopharynx of children without concurrent respiratory symptoms. *J Med Virol*. 2002;66(3):417–420.

3

Origin, Morphology, Genome Organization, Growth, Replication, and Pathogenesis of SARS-CoV-2

Ahmed Al-Harrasi
Natural and Medical Sciences Research Center, University of Nizwa

Saurabh Bhatia
Natural and Medical Sciences Research Center, University of Nizwa
University of Petroleum and Energy Studies

CONTENTS

3.1 Introduction

Coronavirus disease is an infectious disease caused by virus of zoonotic origin, characteristically with a genomic material of positive-sense single-stranded ribonucleic acid (RNA) resulting into acute respiratory syndrome [1]. The disease, abbreviated as "COVID-19," is caused by a newly discovered coronavirus, namely severe acute respiratory syndrome coronavirus 2 (SARS-CoV-2). Clinical findings have shown that the majority of people infected with the COVID-19 virus experience mild-to-moderate respiratory illness and recover without requiring special treatment. The rate of COVID-19 infection and the number of infected patients were exponentially increased at a high rate since its emergence (until December 2020). COVID-19 has become one of the major communal health challenges in the world. Due to the lack of suitable treatment, clinical management of this infectious and communicable disease has been restricted to infection prevention and control methods related to supportive care including supplemental oxygen and mechanical ventilation [2]. As per the data published by the CDC on January 15, 2021, COVID-19 vaccine has been authorized and then recommended for use in the United States. Currently, two vaccines are authorized and recommended to prevent COVID-19: Pfizer-BioNTech COVID-19 vaccine and Moderna's COVID-19 vaccine. Additionally, there are a few vaccines in Phase 3 clinical trials (December 28, 2020) in the United States: AstraZeneca's COVID-19 vaccine, Janssen's COVID-19 vaccine, and Novavax's COVID-19 vaccine (https://www.cdc.gov/coronavirus/2019-ncov/vaccines/different-vaccines.html). As of August 11, 2020, 28 of these companies have advanced into clinical trials with Moderna, CanSino, with the University of Oxford, BioNTech, Sinovac, Sinopharm, Anhui Zhifei Longcom, Inovio, Novavax, Vaxine, Zydus Cadila, Institute of Medical Biology, and the Gamaleya Research Institute having moved beyond their initial safety and immunogenicity studies [3]. Different approaches for vaccine development are accessible specifically: virus-vectored vaccines, protein subunit vaccines, genetic vaccines, and monoclonal antibodies for passive immunization are under evaluations for SARS-CoV-2 [4]. This deadly novel virus emerged in December 2019, endured as a debatable topic of strong assumptions in context with its origin. As far as the origin of SARS-CoV-2 is concerned, coronaviruses are a large family of various viruses. Out of these, certain viruses cause the common cold in human beings and some animals, such as bats, camels, and cattle. Genetically, coronaviruses contain positive-sense RNA (large genome) and morphologically contain club-like spikes covering their surface with a distinct mechanism for replication [5]. There are four types (α, β, γ, and Δ), out of which only α-and β-types cross animal–human

DOI: 10.1201/9781003175933-4

barriers and arise as main human pathogens [6]. Previously, seven human coronaviruses (HCoVs) were identified: the β type of CoVs, specifically SARS-CoV, MERS-CoV, SARS-CoV HCoV-OC43, and HCoV-HKU1, and α-type of CoVs, which are HCoV-229E and HCoV-NL63 [7].

Coronavirus-2 has some common characteristics with SARS-CoV and MERS-CoV. Some of the viruses belonging to Coronaviridae show great resemblance to the receptor-binding domain (RBD) of SARS-CoV-2. Despite bat RaTG13 as well as coronavirus-2reveal the main homology in context with complete genetic sequence, coronavirus-2 displays the great sequence resemblance (97.4%) to pangolin CoVs in terms of RBD. Nevertheless, considering RBD sequence, resemblance among bat RaTG13 and SARS-CoV-2 is comparatively low (89.2%). Coronavirus-2 has around 79.5% of genetic homology with coronavirus-1, whereas it has a mere 50% resemblance with MERS-CoV, demonstrating that coronavirus-2 has more resemblance to coronavirus-1 [8]. SARS-CoV uses angiotensin-converting enzyme 2 (ACE2) as a receptor to mainly infect ciliated bronchial epithelial cells and type II pneumocytes [9,10], while MERS-CoV uses dipeptidyl peptidase 4 (DPP4; also known as CD26) as a receptor to infect unciliated bronchial epithelial cells and type II pneumocytes [11,12]. From a transmission (via aerosol) perspective, MERS-CoV shows greater potential in persisting out of the host and thus stays in the active phase until an hour after aerosol formation. As per WHO reports, SARS-CoV-2 infection can spread via contaminated surfaces or by droplets (in 1-meter distance) or aerosol transmission can occur in small and closed environments (indoor settings) [13–16]. The maximum distance of virus transmission could be 4 m in indoor settings such as hospitals. Nevertheless, in a number of reports, the maximum distance traveled has also been observed to be 8 m [13–16]. Recent reports showed aerosolization as well as surface stability of coronavirus-2 in comparison to coronavirus-1 [13–16]. This study demonstrated that coronavirus-2 can remain active in atmosphere for 3 h, with a comparable decrease in activity like coronavirus-1 [13–16]. Additionally, different characteristics of coronavirus-2 are comparable to coronavirus-1 with regard to its potential to remain stable in aerosol form and the stability of air particles. Nevertheless, the binding potential of coronavirus-2 to receptors in human beings is almost 10-fold greater than that of coronavirus-1 [13–16]. As far as morphology of this virus is concerned, coronavirus-2 show similarity with coronavirus-1 with the size varying from 70 to 90 nm. Genomic characterization of SARS-CoV-2 demonstrated the presence of four key essential proteins: spike (S), membrane (M), envelope (E), and the nucleocapsid (N) [17,18]. These four proteins are encoded in the 3′ end of the genome. Spike (S) protein allows the virus to bind to the cell membrane surface proteins of the host leading to viral invasion. M protein, which is also called membrane protein, is more predominant in the virus membrane and is vital for virus assembly and accounts for maintenance of the virion shape and architecture [17,18]. The E protein, or envelope protein, is the smallest protein of size 8–12 kDa, and is involved in a wide spectrum of functions and participates in viral assembly and budding. The N protein is the only one that binds to the RNA genome. The primary function of N protein is to bind to viral RNA genome and pack them into a long helical nucleocapsid structure or ribonucleoprotein (RNP) complex [17,18]. Genomic organization studies have revealed that the genomic size of coronavirus-2 lies between 26 and 32 kb and contains 6–11 open reading frames (ORFs) (which lack hemagglutinin-esterase gene) with 5′ and 3′ flanking untranslated areas (UTRs). No substantial variation is found in ORFs and non-structural proteins (nsps) of coronavirus-2 or coronavirus-1. The structural features of coronavirus-2 such as arrangements of the spike proteins are similar to that of the spike protein of coronavirus-1 with a root-mean-square deviation (RMSD) of 3.8 Å. Other comparable aspects of SARS-CoV and SARS-CoV-2 are that they both use ACE2 host receptor for internalization and transmembrane serine proteinase 2 (TMPRSS2) serine proteases for S protein priming [19]. This chapter considers the structural as well as genomic arrangements, pathogenesis, and replication of coronavirus-2 to better understand this infection.

3.2 Origin and Evolution of SARS-CoV-2

The World Health Organization declared the outbreak of novel coronavirus (SARS-CoV-2) as a pandemic [20]. SARS-CoV-2, which contains single-stranded positive-sense RNA with genome size of about 26–32 kb including a variable number of ORFs (6–11 ORFs encoded with 9,680 amino acid polyproteins), belongs to genus Coronavirus and family Coronaviridae [19]. In comparison with other RNA-based viruses, COVID viruses have a strangely large positive-sense RNA genome with a size ranging from 26 to 34 kb [19]. The genera of coronaviruses (subfamily Coronavirinae) is classified on the basis of the phylogenetic relationship and genomic organization, which includes alphacoronavirus (αCoV); betacoronavirus (βCoV); gammacoronavirus (γCoV); and deltacoronavirus (δCoV) [19]. Coronaviruses are of zoonotic origin (i.e., some have the capability to transmit from animals to humans, whereas some are limited to animals only as they have not yet infected humans) [21]. This tendency of coronaviruses to cross the species barricade has led to the development of more pathogenic novel coronaviruses. Moreover, the evolutionary roadmap of coronaviruses shows that both βCoV and αCoV originated from bats and rodents, whereas δCoV and γCoV originated from avian species [21]. To achieve the successful replication of their genomes, positive-stranded RNA viruses trigger the development of cytoplasmic membrane structures in their host cells. These cytoplasmic complex structures possibly allow the more systematic arrangement, coordination, and management of the replication process as well as the placement of the machinery essentials for RNA synthesis. These cytoplasmic structures also protect RNA intermediates from detection by the host cell's defense mechanisms. Structural integrity of these membranes can be obtained from different cellular compartments. A lot of viruses are genetically identical to known human viruses within the βCoV genus, which is further divided into four lineages: A–D. SARS-CoV and SARS-CoV-2 are part of lineage B, which has about 200 reported virus sequences, while lineage C that contains MERS-related coronavirus has more than 500 viral sequences [22,23]. The most common human coronaviruses including HKU1, NL63,

OC43, and 229E CoVs usually cause mild-to-moderate upper respiratory illness, while SARS-CoV as well as MERS-CoV have been identified as pathogens that trigger severe respiratory illness [24]. SARS-CoV virus which was emerged in 2002 from China and caused more than 8000 cases and 800 deaths (fatality rate of 9.6%) [25]. Both pathogens crossed the animal-to-human barrier and caused disease outbreaks with significant morbidity and mortality.

Genomic sequences of SARS-CoV-2 have shown their origin to be zoonotic (i.e., they have very close genetic similarity to the genomic sequence of bat coronaviruses [bat CoVs], which suggests that they emerged from a bat-borne virus) [21]. Investigation of a small number of patients (sample size=9) revealed that the genomic characteristics of coronavirus-2 were similar to SARS-like bat CoVs (i.e., bat-SL-CoVZC45 and bat-SL-CoVZXC21 from Zhoushan in eastern China) [8]. It was also found that genomic arrangements and characteristics are more similar to SARS-like bat CoVs than SARS-CoV and the MERS-CoV [8]. Whole genomic characterization revealed that the SARS-CoV-2 genomic sequences are 87.23% similar to bat-SL-CoVZXC2, but not very similar gnomically to SARS-CoV (almost 79%) and MERS-CoV (around 50%) [8]. Moreover, a number of investigations have indicated that the source of coronavirus-2 is linked with pangolins [26]. Considering the similarity of SARS-CoV-2 to bat SARS-CoV-like coronaviruses, genomic sequences of SARS-CoV-2 were found to be 87.99% similar to bat-SL-CoVZC45 and 87.23% similar to bat-SL-CoVZXC2 [27]. However, SARS-CoV-2 is genetically similar to the SARS-CoV that is almost 79%, whereas almost 50% similarity is reported with MERS-CoV [8]. In addition to similarity at the genetic level, its similarity at the protein level has also been reported in terms of similarity between protein size encoded by the 2019-nCoV, bat-SL-CoVZC45, and bat-SL-CoVZXC21 [27]. Thus, SARS-CoV-2 at the protein and genomic level is nearly identical to the bat-SL-CoVZC45 as well as -SL-CoVZXC21; however, the receptor-binding site of the 2019-nCoV is in lineage B, which is similar to CoV-1. Both SARS-CoV and SARS-CoV-2 have a common receptor domain (i.e., both bind to ACE2 receptor for their entry into the cell), whereas binding to TMPRSS2 serine protease for S protein priming is required for viral RNA synthesis [27]. Apart from the similarity between genetic sequences and length of encoded proteins, the morphology of SARS-CoV-2 closely resembles CoV-1 with virus particle size varying in between 70 and 90 nm [19]. Morphological characteristics of SARS-CoV-2 such as size, shape, and arrangement of spike, membrane (lipid bilayer), envelope surface viral proteins, and helical nucleocapsid containing viral RNA are almost identical to SARS-CoV [19]. The genomic sequence contains ORFs (6–11) with 5′ and 3′ extended untranslated deoxyribonucleic acid (DNA) sequences on either side of gene. Based on the difference in sequence among 2019-nCoV and CoV-1 in ORFs and nsps, it was observed that there is no considerable difference between SARS-CoV-2 and SARS-CoV. Nsps participate in various processes associated with viruses and human cells. Mutations in nsps and the ORF during virus transmission can affect virus intracellular survival and its pathogenicity, which may result in virus-induced cellular autophagy. As mentioned before, morphological characteristics such as arrangement of surface spike glycoprotein of SARS-CoV-2 closely resemble CoV-1 membrane surface protein (S protein) with an RMSD of 3.8 Å [19].

Emerging viral infections often result from host shift (via intermediate host), when viral infection transfers from its original host into other species. This event can result in dead-end (spillover infection) or mild or severe infections with sustained transmission in the new host. All human coronaviruses have animal origins (Figure 3.1). HCoV-OC43 and HKU1 probably originated from rodents, whereas SARS-CoV, MERS-CoV, HCoV-NL63, and HCoV-229E originated from bats. As mentioned earlier, numerous SARS-associated CoV (SARSr-CoV) have been found in bats. So, it has been extensively understood that bats are the natural pools of SARSr-CoV. 2019-nCoV is closely associated to various bat SARSr-CoVs (bat CoV, bat CoV RaTG13) with high nucleotide similarity of 96.2% [28–30]. While SARS and MERS are considered as highly infectious CoVs that developed among individuals but might also have bat sources, both have been transmitted to humans via intermediary hosts [28–30]. It has also been reported that 2019-nCoV transmitted to humans via intermediary host(s). Nevertheless, 2019-nCoV-associated viral pathogens have also been rarely found among mammals except humans as well as bats. Numerous investigations have evidenced the presence of SARS-CoV-2-related viruses in pangolins that were trafficked into southern China [28–30]. Notably, the Guangdong pangolin CoVs showed higher genomic similarity (97.4%) with 2019-nCoV than bat CoV RaTG13 (89.2%) considering RBD [28–30].

The rest of the genome of SARS-CoV-2 showed high similarity with bat CoV RaTG13 in comparison with Guangdong pangolin CoVs. Thus, close association in structural as well as sequential features represents convergent advancement between the 2019-nCoV and CoV-1 RBDs for enhanced attachment to ACE2. Thus, from these findings, it has been suggested that intermediate host of SARS-CoV-2 (i.e., Guangdong pangolin [28–30]) can be considered as a probable source of SARS-CoV-2. Based on the genomic studies except RBD, it has been assumed pangolin CoVs are not the immediate source of 2019-nCoV. On the basis of RBD analysis, it cannot be suggested that pangolins are the intermediate source of 2019-nCoV. Perhaps interspecies transmission of CoVs between pangolin and bats could be the reason behind this [28–30].

3.3 *In vitro* and *in vivo* Models for SARS-CoV-2

As per the previous report, more complex interactions occur between 2019-nCoV and human cells, resulting in the exploration of lead targets [32,33]. Because of the complexity associated with these interactions, choosing a suitable model is challenging so as to get significant results and to guarantee the rational use of animals. However, considering physiological, pathological, and therapeutic viewpoints, numerous animal models might respond like humans; thus, selection should be done carefully seeing association among the experimental models and the viral infection. In view of the present viral outbreak, it is important to select a suitable cell- or animal-based model that mimics the disease conditions more closely that

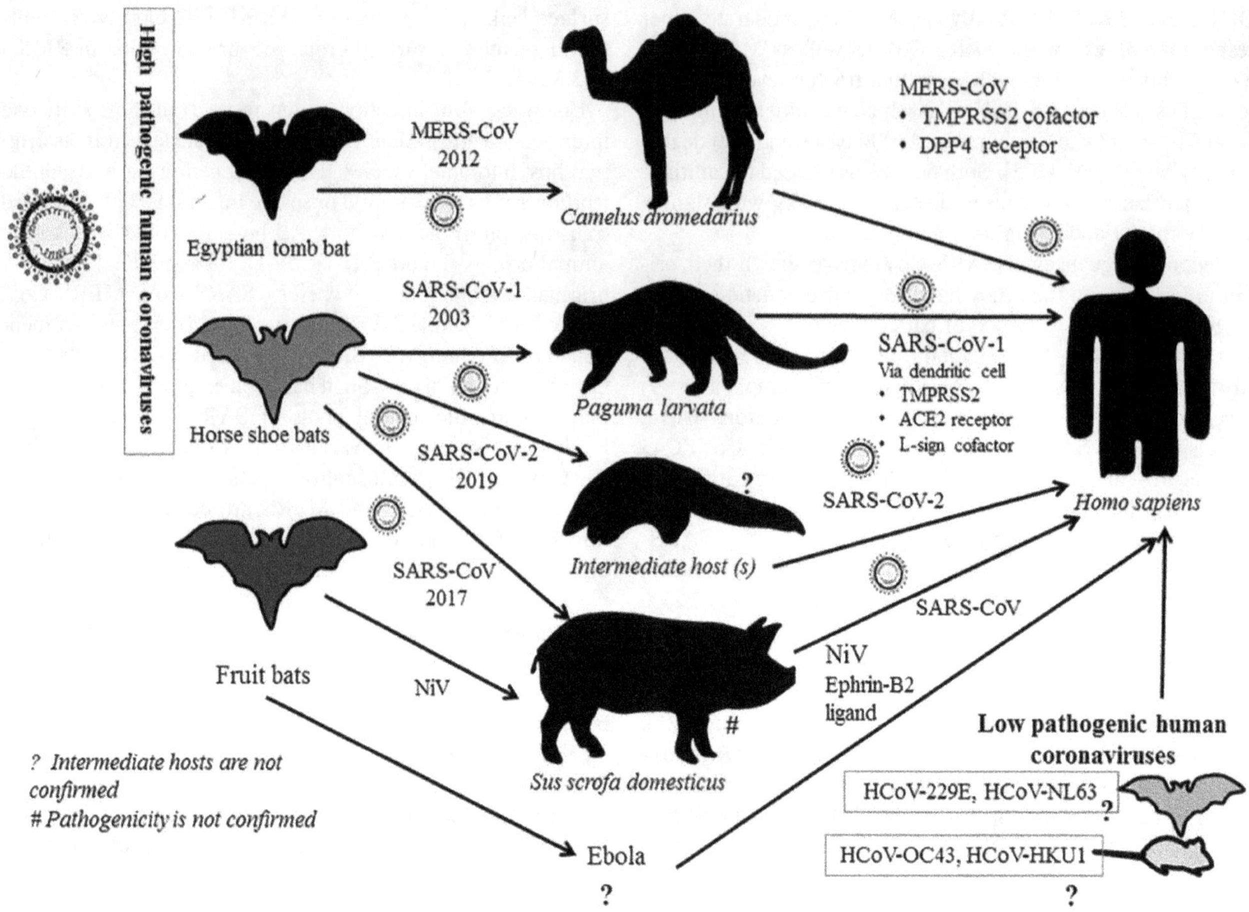

FIGURE 3.1 Evolutionary pathways of high and low pathogenic virus of bat and rodent origin MERS: Middle East respiratory syndrome, HCoV: Human coronavirus, SARS: Severe acute respiratory syndrome, SADS: Swine acute diarrhea syndrome coronavirus; SARS-CoV-2: Severe acute respiratory syndrome coronavirus 2 [28–31].

are common among COVID-19 patients with SARS-CoV-2. Viruses have complex and particular nutritional requirements in vitro culture process in form of particular cell line to mimic the in vitro environment. Isolation of the virus is essential for developing and evaluating diagnostic tools and therapeutics assays (Figure 3.2). This fastidious property of HCoVs on conventional cell lines was described during the mid-1960s and led to ex vivo culturing of human embryo respiratory tract explants [32,33]. Recently, replication and tissue tropism of two different SARS-CoV-2 isolates in the respiratory tract of cattle, sheep, and pigs using respiratory ex vivo organ cultures were investigated. Findings showed that a SARS-CoV-2 (D614G) replicated at higher magnitude in ex vivo tissues of both ruminant species [34].

Another investigation demonstrated that D614G variant (spike aspartic acid–614 to glycine) displays more efficient infection, replication, and competitive fitness in primary human airway epithelial cells but maintains similar morphology and in vitro neutralization properties as the ancestral wild-type virus [35]. SARS-CoV was initially identified in Vero E6 and FRhK cells administered with clinical samples as part of early efforts to identify the etiologic agent of SARS [36]. The first isolation of SARS-CoV-2 was done on human airway epithelial cells in China [37]. Then, like SARS-CoV and MERS-CoV, SARS-CoV-2 was isolated on Vero cells, which are kidney epithelial cells extracted from African green monkeys [38,39].

Recent investigation showed that cell line-based studies, kidney cells (Vero E6, HEK293 along with their clones), liver Huh7 cells, respiratory Calu-3 cells, and intestinal Caco-2 are the most extensively used in vitro models for SARS-CoV-2 [40]. Another report showed that cell lines such as Vero E6, Vero E6/TMPRSS2, HEK 293T, BHK-21, Huh7, LLC-MK2, Caco-2, and Calu-3 cell lines can be used as in vitro models to perform in vitro research mainly for diagnosis and isolation and to explore infection mechanisms of SARS-CoV-2 among these cell lines. CHO-K1, K-562, and PER.C6 have been used by various groups to develop cell-based vaccines against SARS-CoV-2. Numerous cell lines with suitable promoters vulnerable to transfection can also be utilized *in vitro* studies; for example, hACE2-HB-01 with mACE2 promoter, HFH4-hACE2 with forkhead transcription factor (HFH4/FOXJ1), K18-hACE2 with cytokeratin 18 (K18), AdV-hACE2 with HFH4, and humanized ACE2 with native mACE2 promoter have been used as animal and translational models of SARS-CoV-2 infection and COVID-19 [41].

In previous investigations, mouse and hamster strains were used as animal-based models for in vivo studies on CoV-1 and MERS-CoV [42]. As far as in vivo research on SARS-CoV-2 is concerned, mouse-adapted strains of SARS-CoV-2 that

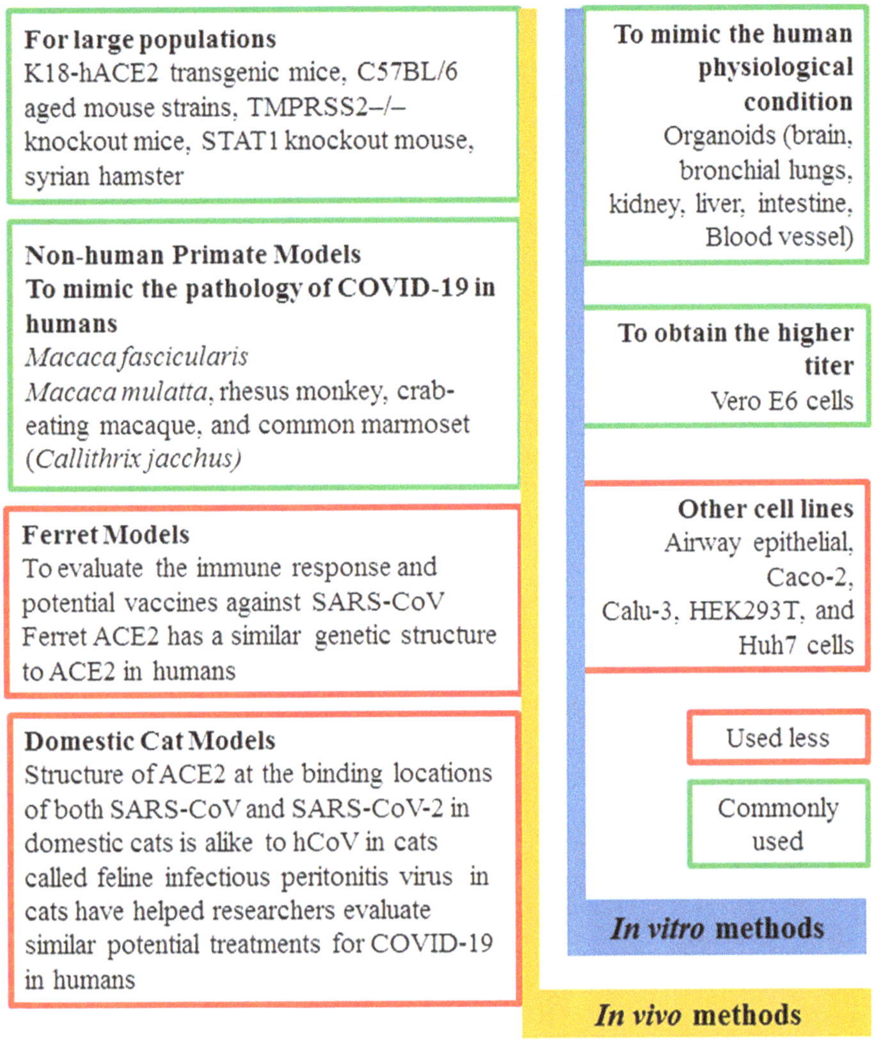
For large populations
K18-hACE2 transgenic mice, C57BL/6 aged mouse strains, TMPRSS2–/– knockout mice, STAT1 knockout mouse, syrian hamster
Non-human Primate Models
To mimic the pathology of COVID-19 in humans
Macaca fascicularis
Macaca mulatta, rhesus monkey, crab-eating macaque, and common marmoset (Callithrix jacchus)
Ferret Models
To evaluate the immune response and potential vaccines against SARS-CoV
Ferret ACE2 has a similar genetic structure to ACE2 in humans
Domestic Cat Models
Structure of ACE2 at the binding locations of both SARS-CoV and SARS-CoV-2 in domestic cats is alike to hCoV in cats called feline infectious peritonitis virus in cats have helped researchers evaluate similar potential treatments for COVID-19 in humans
To mimic the human physiological condition
Organoids (brain, bronchial lungs, kidney, liver, intestine, Blood vessel)
To obtain the higher titer
Vero E6 cells
Other cell lines
Airway epithelial, Caco-2, Calu-3, HEK293T, and Huh7 cells
Used less
Commonly used
In vitro methods
In vivo methods

FIGURE 3.2 Experimental (*in vitro* and *in vivo*) models for SARS-CoV-2.

showed the expression of the hACE2 protein with the main target of copying the pathways, implicated in human infection have been used [42]. K18-hACE2 transgenic mice have been used in order to show the expression of hACE2, which is regulated via gene promoter (K18) model that could be valuable for knowing facts related to disease, multiplication (intra or extracellularly), and pathogenicity of SARS-CoV-2 and for assessment of therapeutics. In a recent investigation, Sun et al. [43] utilized the CRISPR/Cas9 approach to design a murine-based hACE2 system among aged as well as young animals. A TMPRSS2–/– knockout-based rodent method has been created by directional vector to change exons (10–13), which collate the TMPRSS2 gene (serine protease domain) [43]. Likewise, the STAT1 knockout rodent approach (129S6/SvEv-STAT1tmRDS) containing a STAT1 mutation (homozygous) as well as fully needs functional STAT1 proteins (Pgm1c and Gpi1b alleles of 129S6) have been used to investigate the immune response, mainly coronavirus-2 induced inflammatory pathways [44,45].

Mouse-adapted approaches (BALB/c as well as C57BL/6 mice with adapted SARS-CoV-2 MA and SARS-CoV-2 MASCp6 strains) have been used to cause infection without any changes in the mice, since the developed viral strains can capably show binding with ACE2 protein among both young and aged mice, resulting in an infection similar to human COVID-19 [46]. BALB/c mice were also utilized for investigating the stimulation of neutralizing antibodies [47]. Moreover, Syrian hamster models have been used to reproduce the respiratory and enteric symptoms identified in COVID-19 patients [48]. Ferrets (Mustela putorius furo) have been used to inoculate the virus via intranasal route to further investigate their vulnerability against infection caused by two different SARS-CoV-2 strains [49]. SARS and MERS were also investigated among non-human primates [50]. Currently, the same models have been suggested for the coronavirus-2 [51], particularly with a focus on therapeutics development [52]. The following non-human primate models to inoculate the SARS-CoV-2 virus have been reported [42]:

- Intratracheal and intranasal inoculation of young and aged adult cynomolgus macaques (*Macaca fascicularis*);
- Young as well as aged rhesus monkeys inoculated intratracheally;

- Combined (intranasal, intratracheal, conjunctival, and oral) inoculation of rhesus monkeys;
- Inoculation of rhesus monkeys via conjunctival route;
- *Callithrix jacchus*, rhesus monkey, and crab-consuming macaque inoculation via intratracheal, intranasal, and conjunctival routes.

It was found that monkey (rhesus) is the more vulnerable against infection caused by virus and thus considered as a suitable experimental method for the investigation of SARS-Cov-2 infection as well as for the assessment and discovery of new therapeutics [53]. Additionally, in context with experimental approaches to study the effect of SARS-Cov-2 infection in CNS, CNS cell lines such as progenitor cells of the CNS, neurons, astrocytes, oligodendrocytes, and neuroglia (glial cell) from human-induced pluripotent stem cells were utilized to study the effect of SARS-CoV-2 infection (*in vitro*). These studies showed the extent of pathogenicity caused by the virus in CNS (central nervous system) cells [54]. Additionally, various organoids (of human origin) derived from vasculature, hepatic system, renal system, GIT, and cardiac system [55,56] have been used to study impact of coronavirus-2 infection more deeply.

Nasopharyngeal and oropharyngeal isolates of SARS-CoV-2 were inoculated on the Vero cells to prevent possible mutations during viral culture and isolation [57]. Viral culture is often based on cell tropism (i.e., the capability of the virus to infect single and specific host cells that support their growth) [58]. A number of viruses have a broad cell tropism as they have the ability to infect many types of cells. Based on this, it was found that SARS-CoV and SARS-CoV-2 can be easily cultured on Vero cells, the HAE culture system that facilitates complete characterization [58].

Recently, researchers identified several cell lines for the efficient replication of SARS-CoV and SARS-CoV-2; however, cytopathogenic effect (structural changes by virus in host cells after its invasion) was only observed in the Vero E6 and FRhK4 [58]. Inoculation of these SARS-CoV and SARS-CoV-2 with these non-human primate kidney cell lines offers a better understanding of cellular degeneration, mitotic cell rounding, and separation. Vero E6 is considered the ideal platform for cell culture-based viral infection where the virus can easily replicate to form multiple SARS-CoV-2. One important observation was made when both SARS-CoV and SARS-CoV-2 were separately cultured on Vero E6 cells followed by the subculturing of Vero E6 cells; only SARS-CoV-2 underwent tough selection pressure to acquire adaptive mutations in its spike protein gene [59]. This is also considered as the major difference between SARS-CoV and SARS-CoV-2. It was observed that cytopathogenic results obtained from Vero E6 cell line remain constant due to the sensitivity of Vero E6 cells against Cov-1 and CoV-2 infection [59]. Additionally, during the incubation period, inoculated Vero E6 cell lines release viral progeny in the medium containing gel [58]. Gel restricts transmission of virus from the infected cells to the surrounding cells. Thus, these gel-suspended viral particles create a circular zone of infected cells known as plaque. Use of Vero E6 cell line for culture of CoV and CoV-2 is suitable as it provides lower saturation density (optimal for plaque formation) and deficiency of immune interferon (α and β) production [58]. Other than Vero E6, FRhK4 cell line has also been investigated; however, limited information is available on SARS-CoV- and SARS-CoV-2-infected FRhK4 cell line as more information is required to demonstrate the cytopathic effects in relation to intact innate immune response [58]. Researchers also investigated the scope of these viruses among more epithelial renal cell lines (animal based) such as CRFK (from feline kidney), RK-13 (renal cells of a 5 week old rabbit), LLC-MK2 (renal tissue of adult rhesus monkeys), and PK-15 (porcine kidney) cell lines and found considerable rise in viral load (2–120 hpi) [58]. A number of bat cell lines such as Rhinolophus sinicus kidney (RSK) as well as Rhinolophus sinicus lung (RSL) cells were also investigated by researchers, and it was found that only SARS-CoV represents considerable increase in growth in RSK cell lines; however, relatively level of growth was less than other cell lines, and no growth was observed in RSL cell lines [58]. Furthermore, coronaviruses are usually identified by oral and anal swabs of bats; thus, bats' GIT epithelial cell lines must be examined further. Researchers also investigated the growth of SARS-CoV-2 in human lung cancer Calu3 and human epithelial Caco2 cell lines [58]. This study showed the ability of the invasion of the virus in pulmonary and intestinal cell lines as the integration of viral RNA has been seen in these cell lines. Growth of SARS-CoV-2 was also assessed in lung adenocarcinoma Calu3 and A549 cells [58]. It has been observed that coronavirus-2 showed considerable growth with more titer value than SARS-CoV in Calu3 cells; however, no sign of growth was reported in A549 cells. In spite of the considerable growth with higher titer range, SARS-CoV-2 avoids interferon release and causes decreased production of proinflammatory cytokines in comparison with SARS-CoV [58]. This suggests better evasion of SARS-CoV-2 in immune cells of the host where it can utilize different ways to avoid and antagonize the immune response of the host [58].

3.4 Morphology of Coronavirus

To determine the morphological characteristics of coronavirus, it is essential to understand the process of the identification of nCoV19. For identification of nCoV19, a desirable amount of specimen ranging from 200 to 1000 μL should be collected [58]. Initially, the specimen must be examined by real-time polymerase chain reaction for the confirmation of the presence of SARS-CoV-2 (positive test) [60]. This step can be further followed by centrifugation to remove debris. Afterward, the specimen can be fixed conventionally with 2% paraformaldehyde and 2.5% glutaraldehyde. Negative staining can be done with sodium phosphotungstic acid as reported earlier [61]. Later, transmission electron microscopy can be performed to determine morphology and ultrastructure of this virus [61]. Morphological features of a coronavirus based on TEM examination revealed its size ranging from 70 to 90 nm (Figure 3.3) [61]. This examination also confirmed the presence of SARS-CoV-2 under various intracellular organelles, mainly vesicles [61]. The structural pattern of nCoV19 was supposed to be the same like CoV-1. This is because of its high sequence similarity with SARS-CoV. Other structural features such as spike surface protein, membrane, and envelope of SARS-CoV-2 were compared with SARS-CoV in earlier reports (Figure 3.3) [19]. The majority of coronaviruses have common characteristics of containing several important proteins such as spike protein, a hemagglutinin-esterase dimer, a membrane glycoprotein, an envelope protein, and a nucleocapsid protein, to ease infection (Figure 3.3) [19]. The viral proteins (M as well as E) are important for viral development, envelopment by a membrane, and packaging of the virus genome and budding to form bud via ER-Golgi-cell membrane pathway and exit the host cell (Figure 3.3) [62]. Fusion S glycoprotein is a 1255-residue glycoprotein that contains two subunits (S1 and S2) [63]. As has been reported, S glycoprotein cleavage by either trypsin (R667 and S668) or endosomal cathepsin (T678 and M679) resulted in the development of S1 and S2 subunits (Figures 3.3 and 3.4). S1 subunit of S glycoprotein shares almost 70% uniqueness of amino acid sequence with Bt-SLCoVs and SARS-CoV [63]. This subunit consists of RBD, N-terminal domain, and signal peptide (Figures 3.3 and 3.4). Based on recent reports, the ectodomain of the majority of coronaviruses spike proteins has a similar association with the two domains [63] (Figures 3.3 and 3.4). The S1 (N-terminal) domain is responsible for receptor binding, whereas S2 (C-terminal domain) is responsible for fusion. S2 participates late in the fusion process. It includes amino acid sequences essential for ongoing infiltration. For fusion, the S protein needs to be chopped by proteases, which is generally mediated by furin responsible for the cleavage of precursor proteins, and allows their conversion to a biologically active state [63].

The ectodomain of type I transmembrane spike protein which contains more than 1,200 residues of amino acids have been replicated, allowed to express, and crystallized in order to crack structural features of the spike glycoprotein of SARS-CoV-2 [63]. The glycoprotein (spike) structural characteristics of n2019-CoV resemble the protein (spike) of CoV-1 (with a RMSD of 3.8 Å) [19]. This work suggested that the receptor-binding region shows the maximum structural variance [19]. The external subdomain in the RBD of SARS-CoV-2 that has been identified recently shares almost 40% amino acid identity with other SARS-CoV. CoV-1 RBD, found in the C-terminal domain of subunit C-terminal domain of subunit-1, with a length of 220 amino acids, is comprised of two subdomains: a core and an external (Figures 3.3 and 3.4) [64]. The center core contains central β-sheet comprised of strands (antiparallel) covered via polypeptide loop, whereas the external domain is comprised primarily of two β-strands and a big inter-strand loop [65]. CoV surprisingly showed the possibility of dimerization of protein that might cross-link S trimers, and thus it

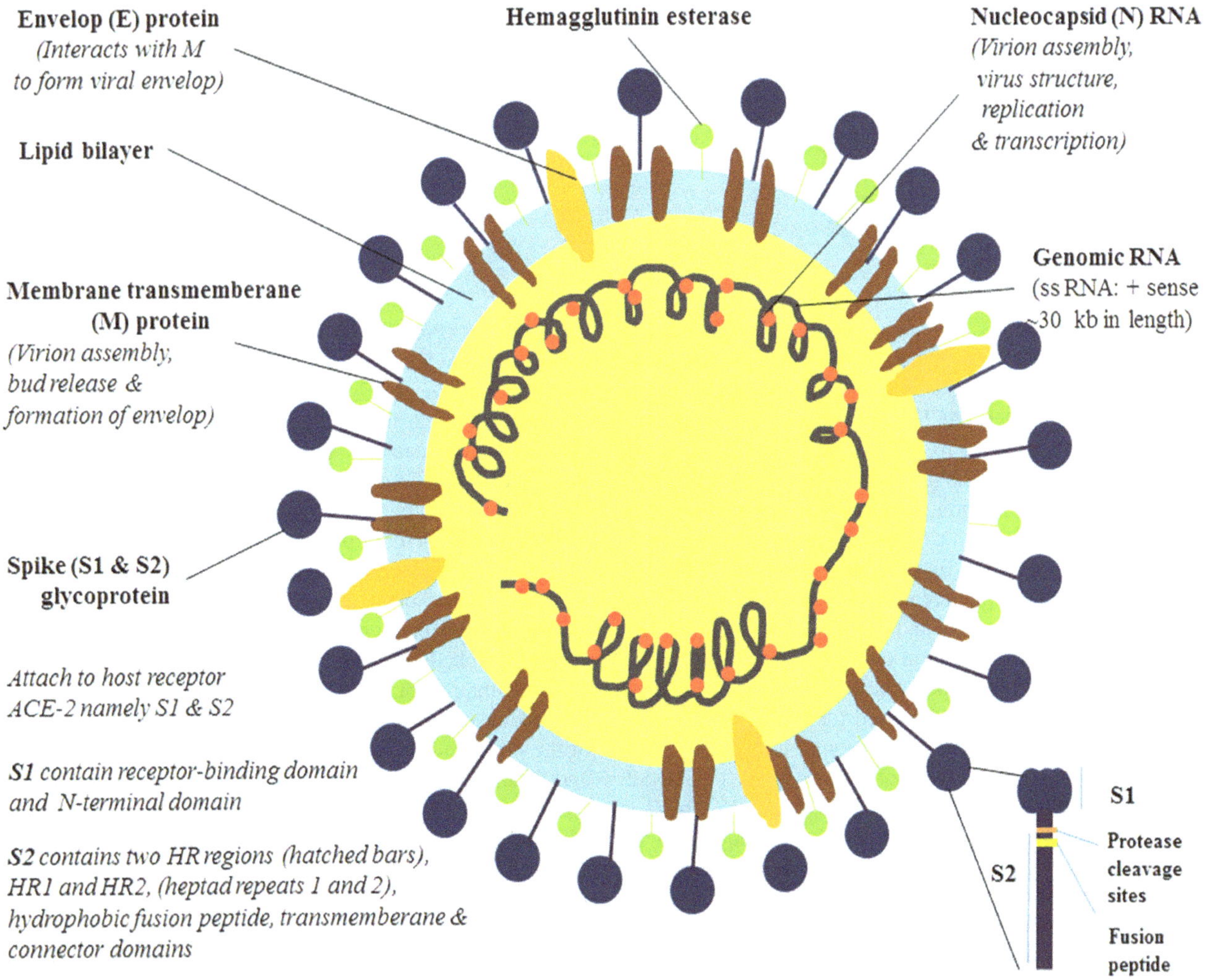

FIGURE 3.3 Morphology of SARS-CoV-2.

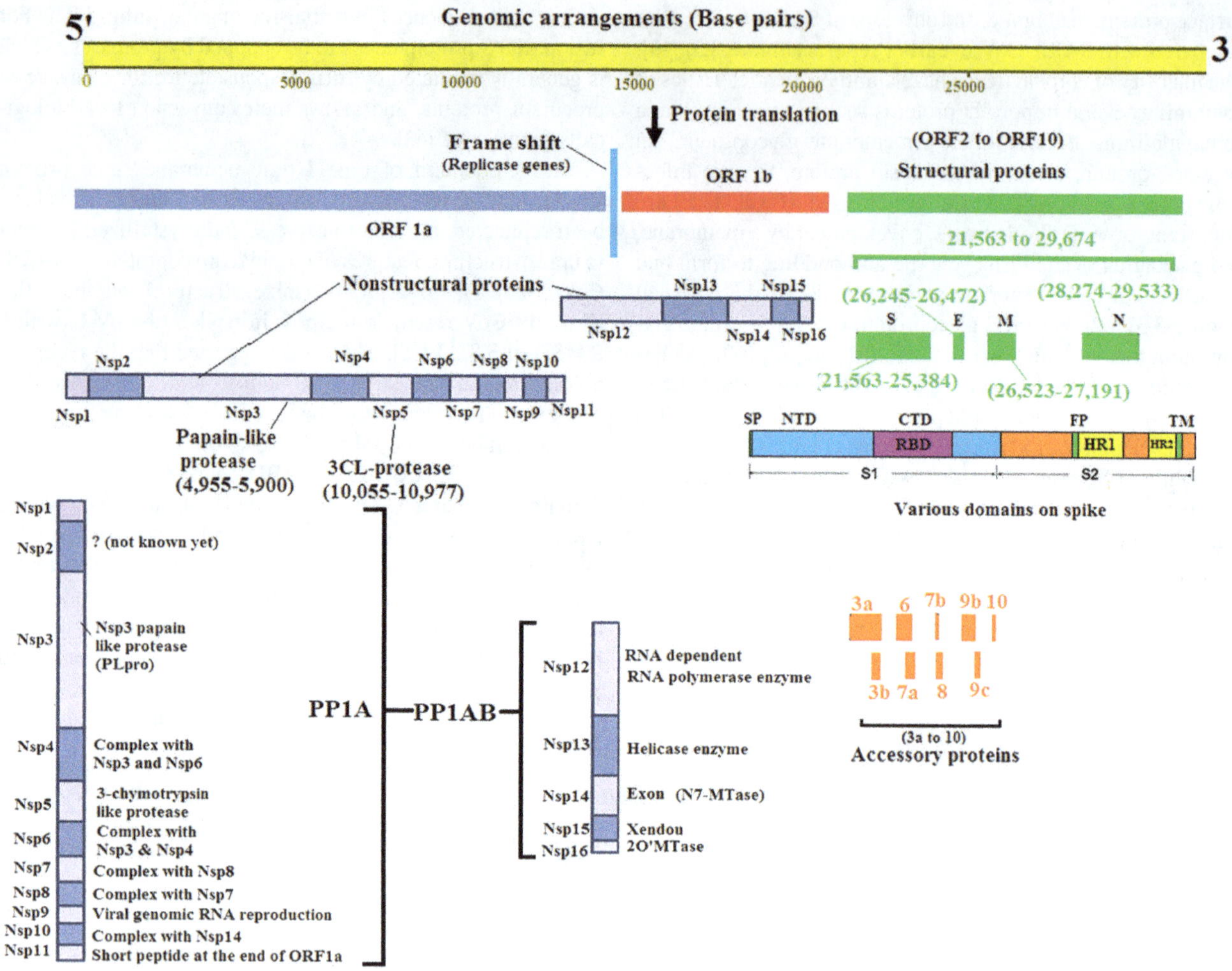

FIGURE 3.4 Genetic sequences of SARS-CoV-2 [72–75].

can affect virus stability and infectivity [66]. The subdomain (external) is mainly responsible for the spike binding with the ACE2. For host entry, SARS-CoV initially binds to the cell-surface glycoprotein (ACE2) that contains the N-terminal ectodomain. After binding to ACE2 via the viral RBD, fusion among the envelope of CoV-1 and the host cell membrane takes place [66]. This fusion process is carried out by the S2 subunit. SARS-CoV contains numerous fusion-related components in S2 including the fusion core made up of HR1 and HR2 and membranotropic areas (n=3) that are designated as the fusion-, internal fusion-, and pretransmembrane-peptides [66]. These fusion elements can create a hydrophobic region and are likely involved in the viral invasion event. A diverse array of proteases has been reported for priming proteolytic process of SARS-CoV such as endosomal cathepsin L, factor Xa, plasmin, trypsin, thermolysin, elastase, TMPRSS2, TMPRSS11a, and HAT. The S2 subunit of SARS-CoV-2 is highly conserved and reveals 99% identity of sequence with bat CoVs and CoV-1 [67]. S2 region contains two heptad HR-N and HR-C repeat regions. These regions help in the development of the twisted constructs enclosed by the ectodomain protein [68]. The spike glycoprotein of the newly emerged SARS-CoV-2 contains a potential cleavage site called the furin cleavage site (PRRARS'V) at the line sandwiched between subunits S1 and S2 that is handled through the biogenesis [69]. An envelope protein allows self-assembly as well as virus release within the host cell. Self-assembly of SARS-CoV-2 allows genetic reactions involving protein–protein associations and interactions between the viral genome and capsid proteins [19]. Membrane glycoprotein offers structure to the virus and binds to the N protein. This association between two proteins facilitates RNA binding with viral genome to form replicase–transcriptase complex. Based on immunoelectron microscopy techniques, it has been suggested that n2019-CoV-2 is embedded in the lipid membrane of the host [19]. This membrane encapsulates the protein coat of a virus and the genome in the form of viral RNA. The structural landscape of the protease and spike was determined by Yan et al. [70], and Zhang et al. [71] reported an approach to developing a possible drug for COVID-19 treatment [69,71]. Genomic size of positive-stranded RNA virus is in the scale of 26- 32 kb and contains 6–11 ORFs (Figure 3.4). Due to this positive-stranded RNA, SARS-CoV-2 shows high mutation rate. This is because of the lack of proofreading activity of polymerases. Primary ORFs contain about 67% of the genome. This 67% of genomic sequence encodes for 16 nsps, which roughly forms two-thirds of the genome (Figure 3.4). Other ORFs encode for accessory and structural proteins. Protease (viral 3C and papain) cleave nsps to form viral RNA-dependent RNA polymerase and helicase. These polymerase and helicase will further direct viral genome replication, transcription, and translation [19]. Thus, the 5′ end of the genomic material translates the nsps needed for replication as well as transcription and the 3′ end translates for four major proteins (structural), including spike, envelope, membrane, and nucleocapsid proteins as well as accessory proteins. Other than nsps of virus, four main structural proteins (envelope, membrane, spike surface glycoprotein, and nucleocapsid protein and) as well as other proteins (accessory) are encrypted by open reading fragments [19].

The SARS-CoV-2 has four structural proteins (top): E (stands for envelope protein that interacts with M to form envelope) and M (stands for membrane protein that determines the shape of viral envelope and central organizer of COVID virus assembly) proteins form the viral envelope, whereas S (spike) protein binds to human receptors to facilitate its entry into the host cell and N (nucleocapsid) protein binds to RNA to form nucleocapsid. The COVID virus genome is a single-stranded positive-sense RNA (+ssRNA) molecule containing genomic sequences of 29,000 bases that encode for 29 proteins. Whole genomic organization of SARS-CoV-2 is comprised of no less than six ORFs. ORF1ab positioned at the 5′ side of the genetic material and covers almost two-thirds of the entire genome size. ORF1a/b encodes for a polyprotein1a, b. In between ORF1a and ORF1b, there is a −1 change in the reading frame by bases resulting in the production of pp1a and pp1ab polypeptides. The virus processes these polypeptides by using virally encoded chymotrypsin-like protease (3CLpro) or main protease (Mpro) and one or two papain-like proteases into 16 nsps. These 16 nsps (nsp1-16), excluding Gamma-CoV that does not have nsp1, are important for viral replication. The rest of the ORFs are present at the 3′ end and encode four structural proteins (S, M, E, and N). In addition to the four main structural proteins, there are at least six or seven accessory proteins that are species-specific, such as HE protein, 3a/b protein, and 4a/b protein. After entry into the host cell the virus releases a +ssRNA virus. Later, it is translated into two pp1a and pp1b polypeptides. These polyproteins after translation into two extended polypeptides are further chopped by viral protease. The genome determines ORF1a and ORF1b genes that translate Nsp1–Nsp16, whereas other ORF2–ORF10 encode for four structural proteins (S, M, E, and N). These Nsp1–Nsp16 create a replication–transcription complex (RTC) that is engaged in transcription as well as replication of the genome. As a result, an array of subgenomic RNAs (sgRNAs) is produced by replication–transcription complex via discontinuous transcription.

The 2019-nCoV is a shrouded, non-segmented, +ssRNA virus genome (size: 29.9 kb) (Figure 3.3). 2019-nCoV has key surface proteins, such as spikeglycoprotein trimmer (S), which allows its binding with ACE2. S protein mediates viral attachment to the cell membrane receptor hACE2, membrane fusion, and eventually viral invasion into the host cell (Figure 3.3). Membrane (M) as well as envelope proteins (E) of CoV-2 are buried inside phospholipid bilayers encapsulating the helical nucleocapsid comprising viral genomic RNA (gRNA) and phosphorylated nucleocapsid (N) protein. M proteins in association with E proteins are responsible for the coronavirus membrane structure (Figure 3.3). Membrane fusion depends on S protein cleavage by host cell proteases at the S1/S2 and the S2′ site. The S protein is shaped like a bolt with a head (three spike proteins fused to form a trimer) and stalk (Figures 3.3 and 3.4). The stalk is introduced into the viral membrane and holds the head outward away from the virus. The head region and small part of the stalk are called the S1 region, whereas the left part of the stalk is called the S2 region (Figure 3.3). Numerous human proteases can cleave the S protein, such as TMPRSS2, furin, elastase, and trypsin (Figure 3.3). The proteolytic cleavage of the spike at S1/S2 and S2′ is essential for viral entry into target cells. This allows the activation of SARS-CoV-2 to generate the subunits S1 and S2 that remain non-covalently linked (Figures 3.3 and 3.4). A considerable difference between the spike protein of SARS-CoV-2 and SARS-CoV is that SARS-CoV-2 contains a multibasic cleavage site at the S1-S2 boundary. Several reports suggest that the protease responsible for the cleaving S protein in the case of SARS-CoV-2 virus is furin.

Different coronaviruses encode for different structural and accessory proteins. The genome of SARS-CoV-2 lacks the hemagglutinin-esterase gene that is characteristically found in human coronavirus HKU1, lineage A βCoVs) [76]. Nevertheless, the genome of coronavirus contains two flanking UTRs (5′ &3′ end of nucleotides) and long ORFs [76]. There are no considerable differences found in the ORFs and nsps of 2019-nCoV and CoV-1. However, both are reasonably distinct from each other when genetic sequences of orf3b, spike (spike S1), and orf8 are compared with each other (Figure 3.4). Spike S1 and orf8 were previously considered recombination sites. The SARS-CoV-2 genome is comprised of 29,811 nucleotides (Figure 3.4) [77]. These nucleotides encode for 29 proteins, while one may perhaps not get expressed. Out of these 29 proteins, four proteins form the virus actual structure, including the S protein, and of the remaining 25 proteins, one set of proteins regulates virus assembly and plays an important role in its replication process (Figure 3.4) [78]. These proteins also help the virus evade the host immune system. These sets of proteins are also known as nsps. They are always expressed as two huge polyproteins (pp1a and pp1ab) that are later chopped into 16 smaller proteins (Figure 3.4). Viral protease has been identified as promising drug target and is responsible for conversion of polypeptides into 11 smaller proteins [78]. To explore the possibility of a potential antiviral medication candidate against 2019-nCoV, important target sites must be identified such as 3C-like protease, coronavirus proteases, and papain-like protease (PLpro) as they are essential for coronaviral replication (Figure 3.4). The structure of this protein has recently been explored and identified as a main target to inhibit the growth of the virus. These proteases are responsible for processing the viral polyprotein into its functional units and competent in cleaving ubiquitin and ISG15 conjugates [78] (Figure 3.4). These functionalities due to the presence of unique protease allow SARS-CoV to evade the human immune system. Thus, more focus must be given to the development as well as optimization of an effective agent against the PLpro that triggers SARS-CoV infection [79]. As SARS-CoV replicates in a very complex manner, this replication process essentially requires a set of procedures for the coronaviral life cycle. Thus, it is very important to identify targets for the inhibition of viral replication. Viral nsps are components of the replication complex and are required for viral RNA replication, cell-to-cell movement as well as virion production. These nsps are formed by the cleavage of a multi-domain viral polyprotein that brings together into complexes to carry out viral RNA synthesis [79]. These viral polyproteins contain two cysteine proteases (PLpro and 3C-like protease) to activate their own release and initiate virus-mediated RNA replication [80]. Viral cysteine protease performs an important role in non-structural polyprotein processing and constitutes nsps that create the replication complex, thus becoming a potential drug target. In spite of many biochemical, structural, and inhibitor development investigations on 3C-like protease, an effective drug candidate that targets 3CLpro directly is still being investigated [73]. On the other hand, structural and functional investigations on PLpro are limited. However, reported studies have explored the role of PLpro (with the exception of viral peptide cleavage) including deubiquitination (process for the elimination and regulation of Ub), deISGylation (deconjugation from target proteins), and escape mechanism of the virus from immune cells of the host [81]. Modern investigations have also revealed that an enzyme similar to PLpro from the human coronavirus is vital for replication of the virus [81].

3.5 Mutations in SARS-CoV-2 Spike

DNA is more stable than RNA as the genetic material of DNA viruses allows proofreading check as a part of their reproductive process. DNA viruses infect the host by replicating its DNA. If the virus makes an error in copying the DNA, the host cell can often correct the error. Thus, DNA viruses do not alter or mutate in the same way as RNA viruses. Nevertheless, RNA is an unstable molecule and RNA virus lacks an inbuilt proofreading mechanism in their replication. Errors during replicating RNA occur frequently and the host cell does not correct these errors. Therefore, RNA virus mutations are very common and can have significant consequences for their hosts. Mutations in the structural proteins of SARS-CoV-2 are considered as the main obstacle for prevention and control of COVID-19. Due to inherent high mutations in its genome SARS-CoV-2 has formed numerous descendants from the original Wuhan strain and these descendants due to their new forms (genetic diversity) easily escape from the host immune responses. The complete protein reporting or genomic organization of the virus is very important for the development of a suitable drug or vaccine. Various researchers have successfully explored the complete or partial genome sequences of SARS-CoV-2 isolates that are accessible via the databases of the scientific community [72]. It has been reported that the genome size of SARS-CoV-2 varies from 29.8 to 29.9 kb. Specific genetic sites or characteristics in its genome have also been found [82]. The genome consists of four structural proteins out of which one is a spike protein (S) of size of around 180 kDa with two subunits S1 and S2. The S1 unit contains RBD (residues 319–541) that is responsible for interaction with ACE2 and offers strong attachment to the ACE2-peptidase domain [83].

Thus, RBD is an important site that plays a crucial role in virus–receptor interaction, tropism, and infectivity. However, the RBD site is one of the most variable regions in the sequence and has shown mutations among SARS-CoV-2 pandemic isolates [84,85]. Thus, understanding mutations in SARS-CoV-2 helps in correlating mutated strains found in pandemic samples with higher death rates and transmission forms [86]. It was found that the rate of mutation in RNA viruses is more than double-strand DNA viruses. Thus, this mutation can further alter virulence [84]. Certain mutagens cause amino acid alteration in the protein (surface) of the virus, which may considerably change viral properties and their capability to bind with neutralizing antibodies. Thus, genetic interpretation of mutations in the virus is valuable for evaluating the suitability of therapeutics (resistance offered by drugs), escape from immune response, and manner of disease caused by the virus. SARS-CoV-2 contains immunogenic spike proteins that have receptor-binding sites. These sites can be considered as a possible focus for development of the neutralizing antibodies and vaccines. It was found that single base pair changes in the amino acid sequences (conserved) in the RBD area fully stop the capability of S protein (full-length) to induce neutralizing antibodies [87]. Another study compared the mutation pattern of SARS-CoV-2 with HIV and found that SARS-CoV-2 changes much more slowly as its transmission. However, a single mutation in the gene encrypting the spike protein (which aids viral particles to enter host cells) was found more commonly among samples from COVID-19 patients. This single mutation was found at the 614th amino-acid position [the amino acid aspartate (D, in biochemical shorthand)] of the spike protein [88–91]. This missense mutation in the S-protein encoding gene leads to the replacement of amino acid from an aspartate to a glycine residue at the 614th amino acid position of the spike protein (D614G) [88–90]. This mutation results in a copying fault and causes an alteration of a single nucleotide in the virus 29,903-letter RNA code, and is called the D614G mutation [88–91]. In mid-2020, 329 variants in S protein were identified. During this period, a mere 13 amino acid sites with a percentage >0.1% were found. Several reports suggest that the enhanced mortality rate could be linked with the predominant variant (D614G). As discussed above, this type of alteration might have caused conformational changes of the S protein, causing increased infectivity. Nevertheless, it is still not clear whether these evidenced variants can directly affect infectivity of the virus, level of transmission, or its affinity against neutralizing antibodies. On the contrary, it is also evidenced that genetic changes influence viral proteins glycosylation that can severely influence viral development and its binding with host cell. Thus, some glycosylation site removal can prevent the viral protein interaction with the host cell receptor, which can ultimately stop the host cell infection [92]. Additionally, mutation of glycosylation sites has also been identified in reducing the resistance of virus against neutralization effect caused by the antibodies [93], while in certain virus proteins, deletion of glycosylation sites influences cleavage of hemagglutinin, replication, stability, and antigenicity [94]. S protein of coronavirus-2 is vastly glycosylated with 22 possible 1 N-glycosylation positions [95]. Thus, it is important to understand in what way these glycosylation patterns and glycosylation sites can influence infectivity and antibody-mediated neutralization of virus. Recent investigations have shown that deletion of both N331 and N343 glycosylation considerably decreased infectivity, indicating the significance of glycosylation for viral infectivity. Additionally, it was also found that N234Q was considerably resistant to neutralizing antibodies, while N165Q became more sensitive. This type of investigation could be important in the development of vaccine or any therapeutics against COVID-19 [19,74,96–102].

3.6 Cellular Invasion and Proliferation of SARS-CoV-2

Cellular invasion by 2019-nCoV is mediated by attachment of spike (S) protein to the host cell receptors, namely ACE2 and CD147. The spike protein of CoV-19 virus and SARS-CoV represents structural similarity and conserved ectodomains. Thus, advance approaches are required to avert binding of SARS-CoV and SARS-CoV-2 with cell host receptor (ACE2) [19,74,96–102]. SARS-CoV-2 spike protein present in the form of a trimer that contains several monomers of size ~1,300 amino acids. Out of these all amino acids, 300 amino acids form the RBD. These spike proteins of SARS-CoV-2 produce high immune response against the host immune system [19,74,96–102]. During the binding of SARS-CoV-2, the spike protein on the surface of SARS-CoV-2 mediates receptor recognition and membrane fusion (Figure 3.5). During this process, the structure of trimeric viral S protein is broken down into S1 and S2 subunits. During the conversion to the postfusion conformation, S1 subunits become free and released [19,74,96–102] (Figure 3.5). ACE2 protein contains N-terminal peptidase M2 domain and a C-terminal collectrin renal amino acid transporter domain. During the binding process, the RBD of S1 units directly binds to the N-terminal peptidase M2 domain of ACE2 (Figure 3.5). The other subunit S2 is responsible for membrane fusion. Binding of S1 to the ACE2 allows one more cleavage on S2 that is cleaved by host proteases. The spike protein present on the surface of SARS-CoV-2 takes over ACE2 for host infection where it inhibits the expression of ACE2 (Figure 3.5). This step is very important for viral infection as interaction between RBD and N-terminal peptidase domain is very strong, which makes this virus more infectious and pathogenic than SARS-CoV. This interaction also suggests a pharmacological target for a potential antiviral drug to limit 2019-nCoV invasion inside the host cell [19,74,96–102] (Figure 3.5).

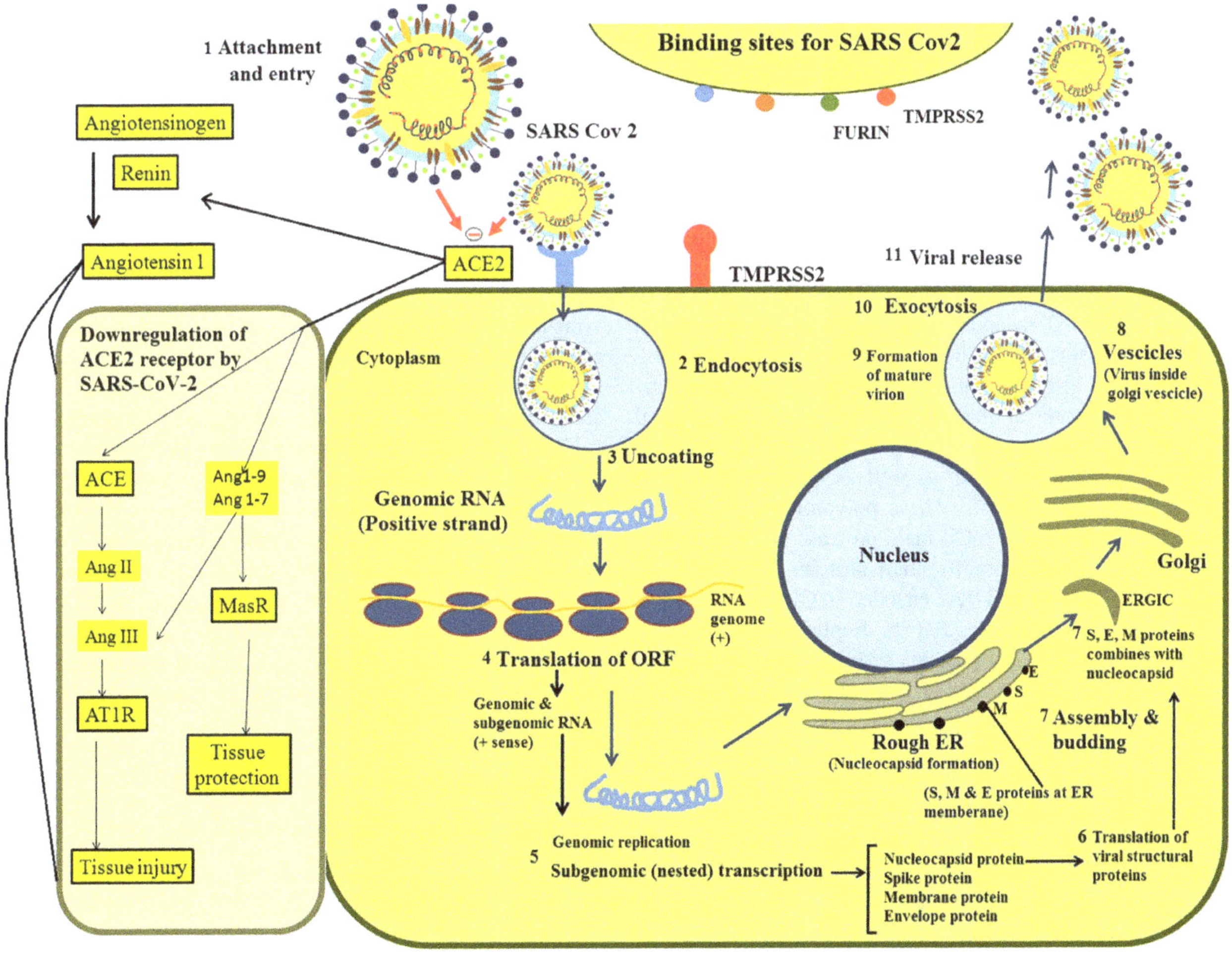

FIGURE 3.5 Entry and replication of SARS-CoV-2 in host cells [19,74,96–102].

In an animal experiment, it was observed that murine polyclonal antibodies against S protein of SARS-Co-V can possibly restrict SARS-CoV-2 spike protein-mediated cell entry. This shows that cross-reactivity and cross-neutralization potential of antibodies can be utilized to target conserved S epitopes that can be obtained upon vaccination. Like other SARS and MERS viruses, 2019-nCoV mainly infects pulmonary alveolar epithelium cells resulting in severe double pneumonia [19,74,96–102] (Figure 3.5). This can be diagnosed in CT scan image as ground-glass opacity. SARS-CoV-2 imitates invasion steps as followed by CoV-1. 2019-nCoV initially utilizes the ACE2 for invasion as well as uses the cellular serine protease TMPRSS2 for priming of S protein to initiate RNA synthesis (Figure 3.5). Colocalization of ACE2 and TMPRSS2 on host cell surfaces improves the entry of SARS-CoV-2 in host cell. ACE2, an exopeptidase, showing its expression on epithelial cells of the respiratory tract is recognized as a target for SARS-CoV-2 invasion into host cell. The spike protein of SARS-CoV-2 contains a RBD that particularly identifies ACE2 as its receptor [19,74,96–120] (Figure 3.5). Recently, residues in the SARS-CoV-2 RBD have been identified that are essential for ACE2 binding. Moreover, it has also been reported that the RBD present in the S protein of SARS-CoV-2 has 10–20 times higher affinity to ACE2 and in comparison with SARS RBD. As a result of its high affinity toward ACE2, SARS-CoV-2 is very infectious (Figure 3.5). Thus, SARS-CoV-2 S protein binding results in hijacking of ACE2, which causes a decrease in the expression of ACE2 with a restriction in maturation of angiotensin. ACE2 is usually expressed in lungs, heart, kidneys, and intestine. Thus, cardiovascular and other organ complications may occur in infected patients due to decreased expression of ACE2. Further respiratory spread of novel coronavirus to different organs or tissues is similar to SARS-CoV. This is due to the diverse expression of the ACE2 receptor among different tissues. Conformational changes of the spike protein occur when the spike protein binds to the ACE2 receptor. This results in the attachment of viral E proteins with cellular membrane of the host cell. This step of viral fusion with host membrane is followed by the endosomal pathway that later allows the release of viral RNA into the host cytoplasm (Figure 3.5). Afterward viral RNA experiences translation as well as produces pp1a and pp1b replicase polyproteins. These polyproteins are further sliced by viral proteases (3CL main protease and papain-like accessory proteinase) into 16 small proteins [19,74,96–102] (Figure 3.5). Nsp1 to nsp11 are encoded in ORF1a, and nsp12 to nsp16 are encoded in ORF1b. Replicase–transcriptase proteins along with viral proteins assemble into membrane-bound replication–transcription complexes [19,74,96–102] (Figure 3.5). These membrane-bound replication–transcription complexes collect at perinuclear regions and are coupled with double-membrane vesicles. Hydrophobic transmembrane domains are present in nsp3, nsp4, and nsp6 and likely serve to anchor the nascent pp1a/pp1ab polyproteins to membranes during the first step of RTC formation. SARS-CoV-2 replication entails programmed ribosomal frameshifting to regulate the expression of multiple genes during the translation process. Ribosomal frameshifting allows the single guide RNA production [19,74,96–102] (Figure 3.5). This is achieved by the irregular transcription that encodes for important viral proteins. Coronaviruses assemble after the interaction between viral RNA VS host protein present over endoplasmic reticulum (ER) and Golgi apparatus. Afterward, coronaviruses are released extracellularly by extracellular vesicle formation.

The SARS-CoV-2 host cell entry is primarily facilitated by the binding potential of spike protein to the ACE2 for cellular invasion. Infection of ciliated bronchial epithelial cells and type II pneumocytes by SARS-CoV-2 initiates binding of spike glycoprotein to the surface receptor, ACE2. After the S protein binding to the ACE2, cleavage of trimeric form of S protein is activated via cellular receptors, namely cathepsin and transmembrane protease serine2 (TMPRSS2). The spike protein contains two S1 and S2 domains. The S1 domain decides host cell tropism as well as enables binding of the virus to the targeted cells. The S2 domain allows viral and cellular membrane fusion, to ensure viral invasion via endocyte formation. Internalization via endosomal pathway (i.e., endocytosis formation) facilitates the release of viral RNA into cytoplasm. Viral invasion to the host cell is followed via the unveiling of the viral RNA in the cytoplasm. This viral genome (+ss RNA) containing ORF (1a as well as1ab) undergoes translation to yield two polyproteins (pp1a and pp1ab). These polyproteins are chopped via proteases of the RTC. The replication of 2019-nCov entails translational frameshifting, where RTC controls the production of RNA full-length (–) copies and is used as templates for full-length (+) RNA genomes. This process involves the translational recoding phenomenon and produces both genomic and various sgRNA copies via intermittent transcription necessary for appropriate structural proteins of the virus. A nested set of sgRNAs are produced via discontinuous (fragmented) transcription. These sets of sgRNAs might have a number of ORFs; however, only the closest ORF (to the 5′ end) will be translated. Intracellular assembling of nucleocapsids is required for the SARS-CoV-2 structural protein development. Assembly of virion occurs after the interaction between viral RNA as well as ER and Golgi apparatus protein. This results in the bud formation in the ER–Golgi lumen intermediate partition. Afterwards by using exocytosis pathway virions are released from the host cell (infected). Several binding sites (ACE2, TMPRSS2, CD147, and FURIN) have been identified by different researchers for the binding of viral spike proteins with these host cell receptors. Thus, it has been concluded that the number of binding affinity of spike protein SARS-CoV-2 to ACE2 receptor determines its host cell entry, transmissibility, and pathogenesis. SARS-CoV-2 downregulates ACE2 protein but not ACE via attachment between the spike glycoprotein and ACE2. However, it has been observed that blocking the renin–angiotensin pathway and ACE2 expression attenuates cellular injury [19,74,96–102].

3.7 Pathogenesis of SARS-CoV-2

Pathogenesis of viral respiratory disorders is usually determined by the virulence of causative agent, viral load, host immune response (healthy and unhealthy), asymptomatic state, upper airway and conducting airway response and hypoxia, ground-glass infiltrates, and progression to ARDS

[103–105]. Clinical results of SARS-CoV-2-infected patients are very close to SARS-CoV- and MERS-CoV-infected patients. In context with the molecular mechanism of SARS-CoV-2, it enters into the cell after binding to ACE2 primarily via the Toll-like receptor-7 (TLR-7) that is present in endosomes [103–105]. Activation of TLR-7 results in the generation of tumor necrosis factor-α (TNF-α), IL-12, and IL-6, which allows the production of specific cytotoxic CD8+ T cells. Cytokines play an important role in pathogenesis of COVID-19 and are considered as important mediators of the inflammatory response [103–105]. A number of cytokines, such as IL-6, IL-8, TNF-α, IL-1, gamma interferon (IFN-γ), and tumor growth factor beta (TGF-β), increase inflammation by causing cell injury, whereas other cytokines including IL-4 and IL-10 reduce the inflammatory process. It has been reported that circulating T lymphocyte counts including CD4 and CD8 were decreased in patients with SARS at the early stage [103–105]. A drop in CD4 and CD8 count was also linked with disease severity, which establishes the relationship between severity of disease vs. immune response of infected host cell. COVID-19 results in the production or suppression of certain inflammatory mediators that regulate the inflammatory process. During severe infection, COVID-19 gets worse by the high production of proinflammatory cytokines, such as IL-1, IL-6, IL-12, IFN-γ, and TNF-α, in lung tissue [103–105]. COVID-19-infected people usually have normal or decreased white cell levels along with lymphocytopenia. In acute cases, there may be a high concentration of urea, dimer-D, and neutrophils, in blood, with a continuous fall in lymph cell count. Increase in the production of chemokines (e.g., IL-6, IL-10, and TNF-α) as well as cytokines resulted in the development of a cytokine storm that can be injurious to host cells. Inflation in certain cytokine and chemokine (e.g., IL-6, IL-10, and TNF-α) counts among SARS-CoV-2-infected patients has been observed; however, elevated serum levels of IL-7, IL-10, IL-2 granulocyte-macrophage colony-stimulating factor, macrophage colony-stimulating factor, granulocyte colony-stimulating factor, 10kD interferon-gamma-induced protein, monocyte chemo-attractant protein-1, macrophage inflammatory protein 1-α, and TNF-α have been observed among critically ill SARS-CoV-2-infected intensive care unit patients [103–105]. Considerable drop in total T cells, CD4+, as well as CD8+ T lymphocytes, count with elevated level of the exhausted marker PD-1 was also reported among COVID-19 patients, especially in critically ill and mild cases [103–105].

Pathogenesis of COVID-19 is also determined by the manner in which COVID-19 pneumonia develops as it can be mild, moderate, or severe [103–105]. Rapid progression of COVID-19 pneumonia from mild-to-moderate state and then to severe acute severe pneumonia can lead to respiratory failure. Postmortem investigations on SARS-infected lungs revealed non-specific severe pulmonary injury features such as gross appearance of lungs with diffuse alveolar damage, secondary bacterial pneumonia, and multinucleated giant cell and macrophage infiltration of alveoli space and lung interstitium [103–105]. The presence of subpleural fibrosis and fibroplasia in small airways and air spaces was found to be common among critically ill COVID-19 patients [106]. Radiological examination of lungs plays a vital role in the diagnosis and management of SARS-CoV-2, especially in the case of pneumonia. Computed tomography (CT) examinations of SARS-CoV-2-infected lungs have revealed important features such as bilateral distribution of ground-glass opacities with or without consolidation in posterior and peripheral areas of lungs. These findings are one of the main hallmarks for the diagnosis of SARS-CoV-2-infected patients. On the contrary, routine chest X-ray examination to detect pneumonia in chest radiograph is again a commonly accessible radiological procedure [107].

Histopathological examination of SARS-CoV-2 patients (lung and extrapulmonary tissues) has revealed congestion in capillary, degeneration and necrosis of pneumocytes, hyaline membrane (collapsed and damaged cells of alveoli collected in the airways), interstitial edema, pneumocyte hyperplasia (hamartomatous proliferation of type II pneumocytes), and reactive atypia [108]. Intravascular coagulopathy observed in patients with severe COVID-19 resulted in platelet aggregation and fibrin formation via thrombin generation in small arterial vessels. In alveolar lumens infiltration of macrophages and infiltration of lymphocytes was also observed [109]. COVID-19 pathogenesis in terms of lung damage is evidenced in terms of diffuse alveolar disease with severe capillary congestion like SARS and MERS [110].

Detailed features of lung biopsy of COVID-19 patients have revealed development of soft tissue tumor with diffusion in both sides resulting in alveolar damage. Right lung biopsy examination showed elevated levels of macrophage infiltration in pneumocytes with the development of hyaline membrane [110–112]. This represents the hallmark of acute respiratory distress syndrome, while the left lung represents excess fluid accumulation with development of hyaline membrane. Moreover, infiltration of inflammatory mediators (mainly lymphocytes in both lungs) resulted in the development of patchy infiltrates accompanied by inflammation [110–112]. Also, the acute phase of illness represents ground-glass or interstitial filling with inflammation of alveoli following by the accumulation of fluid and edema. The space inside the alveoli was characterized by the accumulation of multinucleated syncytial cells formed by the fusion of alveolar epithelial cells with unusual inflamed pneumocytes that represent virus-induced cytopathic effect microvesicular steatosis (accumulation of small intracytoplasmic fat vacuoles in the liver cell) and signs of chronic hepatitis due to mild portal and lobular activity [110–112]. These biopsy findings suggest hepatic injury due to either virus or drug. Infiltration of mononuclear cells resulted in the development of inflammatory injuries in heart tissue, where mainly lymphocytes accumulate at the site of injury [110–112]. Human coronaviruses such as 229E, NL63, OC43, and HKU1 normally cause upper respiratory tract infection with somewhat minor symptoms [110–112]. Nevertheless, there are three other coronaviruses (SARS-CoV, MERS-CoV, and 2019 nCov) that can multiply in the lower respiratory tract and subsequently cause pneumonia, which can be one of the major reasons for respiratory failure [110–112]. Droplet transmission of SARS-CoV-2 is more common as it can primarily cause upper respiratory tract infection with an average incubation period of 4–5 days before COVID-19 symptoms. The majority of symptomatic patients showed symptoms within 11.5 days [110–112]. After incubation, symptomatic patients always suffer from influenza-like illness symptoms such as tiredness, dry cough, and fever. Other associated symptoms that are less common are difficulty breathing, pain in joints and muscles, head pain/feeling unsteady, diarrhea, nausea, and blood in cough [113]. Usually, after symptom onset, peak load of SARS-CoV-2 is reached within 5–6 days, whereas CoV-1 viral peak reached before ten days [114]. During the progression of COVID-19, severity can progress with acute respiratory distress syndrome around 8–9 days after symptom onset [114]. During this infection, the virus induces production of high level of inflammatory mediators (mainly cytokines), which can result in acute respiratory distress syndrome COVID-19. A virus-induced inflammatory storm is considered to be one of the main causes of ARDS and multiple organ failure and plays a significant role in the process of disease exacerbation [115]. These destructive virus-induced inflammatory reactions are powerfully associated with consequential injury to the airways. Thus, severity of the infection is not only due to the injury caused by the virus but also due to inflammatory host response [115]. Additionally, age and comorbid factors can also aggravate severity of the respiratory illness. COVID-19-related ARDS can be characterized by persistent dry cough, shortness of breath, and low blood oxygen level [115]. This may also result in bacterial and fungal co-infection in coronavirus-infected individuals, which may increase the mortality among these patients. Moreover, severity of COVID-19 can also be determined by the extent of production of inflammatory mediators such as cytokines [115]. Excess production of cytokines into blood spontaneously due to severe immune reaction (called a cytokine storm or hypercytokinemia) causes hyperinflammation of the lung tissue. A cytokine storm in the lung alveolar environment and systemic circulation is one of the main features of ARDS [115]. This continuous inflammatory response due to the release of proinflammatory cytokines and chemokines by immune cells results in infiltration of leucocytes, tissue destruction, and necrosis. Among COVID-19 patients, IL1-β, IL1RA, IL7, IL8, IL9, IL10, basic FGF2, GCSF, GMCSF, IFNγ, IP10, MCP-1, MIP1α, MIP1β, PDGFB, TNFα, and VEGFA are detected in high proportion [116]. The resulting aggressive cytokine storm due to the hyperactivation inflammatory immune response contributes to ARDS and can further cause multiple organ failure and death in severe cases of SARS-CoV-2 infection [116]. Multiple organ exhaustion due to the damage mainly caused by proinflammatory cytokines during viral infection and/or secondary infections can lead to states like sepsis (cardiac, hepatic, and renal systems failure), which is the cause of death among almost 28% of fatal COVID-19 cases [116].

In 2020, before COVID-19 vaccine availability, different nanomaterials were proposed by using various drug delivery systems to improve patient immune response, to target the antigenic viral proteins, and to improve the therapeutic efficacy as well as safety profile of drugs [123–150]. Various nano-based approaches were applied for the diagnosis, prevention as well as treatment of SARS-Cov-2 infection, including nano-based drug delivery systems, nanomaterial-based surface sterlants and face masks, adjuvants, nanotechnology-enabled vaccine, and point-of-care tests [123–150]. This safe and effective approach can be used via engineered nanocarriers to block the initial interactions of viral spike glycoprotein with host cell-surface receptors and disrupt virion construction. There are various approaches that can be utilized to design risk-free and effective immunization strategies for SARS-CoV-2 vaccine candidates such as protein constructs and nucleic acids [123–150]. Various biopolymers, especially algal polymers, can also be used; especially those having antiviral effects can also be explored. Algal polymers are natural polymers that are non-toxic, cheap, biodegradable, and biocompatible [117–122]. They have been tested for their antiviral efficacy against many viruses including human immunodeficiency virus (HIV) and dengue virus (DENV). Thus, they have acquired importance in biomedical and pharmaceutical industries and can be further explored to develop drug molecules targeting SARS-CoV-2 [123–150].

3.8 COVID-19 (SARS Coronavirus 2) Pathophysiology (ARDS)

As discussed above, the severity of COVID-19 varies significantly among different infected individuals. This variation of progression of COVID-19 among different individuals has not been studied properly so far. Factors like comorbid state, viral load, timely diagnosis impacts, multiplication rate of virus and its virulence inside host cell, immune response, and negative impact of immune response such as overproduction of cytokines determine the development of disease and its severity [115]. ARDS and pneumonia are considered as the two major illnesses caused by SARS-CoV-2 that can lead to hypoxemic respiratory failure of infected individuals. Thus, more research is required to understand the root causes of hypoxemia in COVID-19 [115]. However, research is often complicated because of low availability of hemodynamic and autopsy data. Hypoxemic respiratory failure in ARDS usually results from large intrapulmonary ventilation-perfusion mismatch or shunt and generally requires mechanical ventilation. Intrapulmonary ventilation-perfusion is defined as the phase when ventilation fails to attain the perfused region due to the accumulation of fluid in alveoli [151]. These complications result in malfunction of the body's homeostatic oxygen-sensing system [152] (Figures 3.6 and 3.7). This means that oxygen uptake capability and its systemic delivery regulated by homeostatic O2-sensing system (HOSS) are considerably influenced in COVID-19-induced acute respiratory distress syndrome (ARDS). Failure of HOSS can result in homeostatic reaction against airway hypoxia in the form of hypoxic pulmonary vasoconstriction. Human airway epithelial cell (HPV) causes pulmonary artery constriction and represents lung tissue deprived of sufficient oxygen supply. This can lead to diversion of blood supply to better ventilated alveoli [152]. The carotid arteries (supply blood to the brain) recognize hypoxemia and increase intensity of the output of the respiratory centers to further improve breathing effort [152]. A mitochondria-based oxygen-sensing system in the form of redox sensors (proteins) is available in the carotid to control oxygen-sensitive potassium and voltage-gated calcium channels that keep mitochondria from oxygen starvation [152] (Figures 3.6 and 3.7). As has been reported, SARS-CoV-2 infection can cause considerable

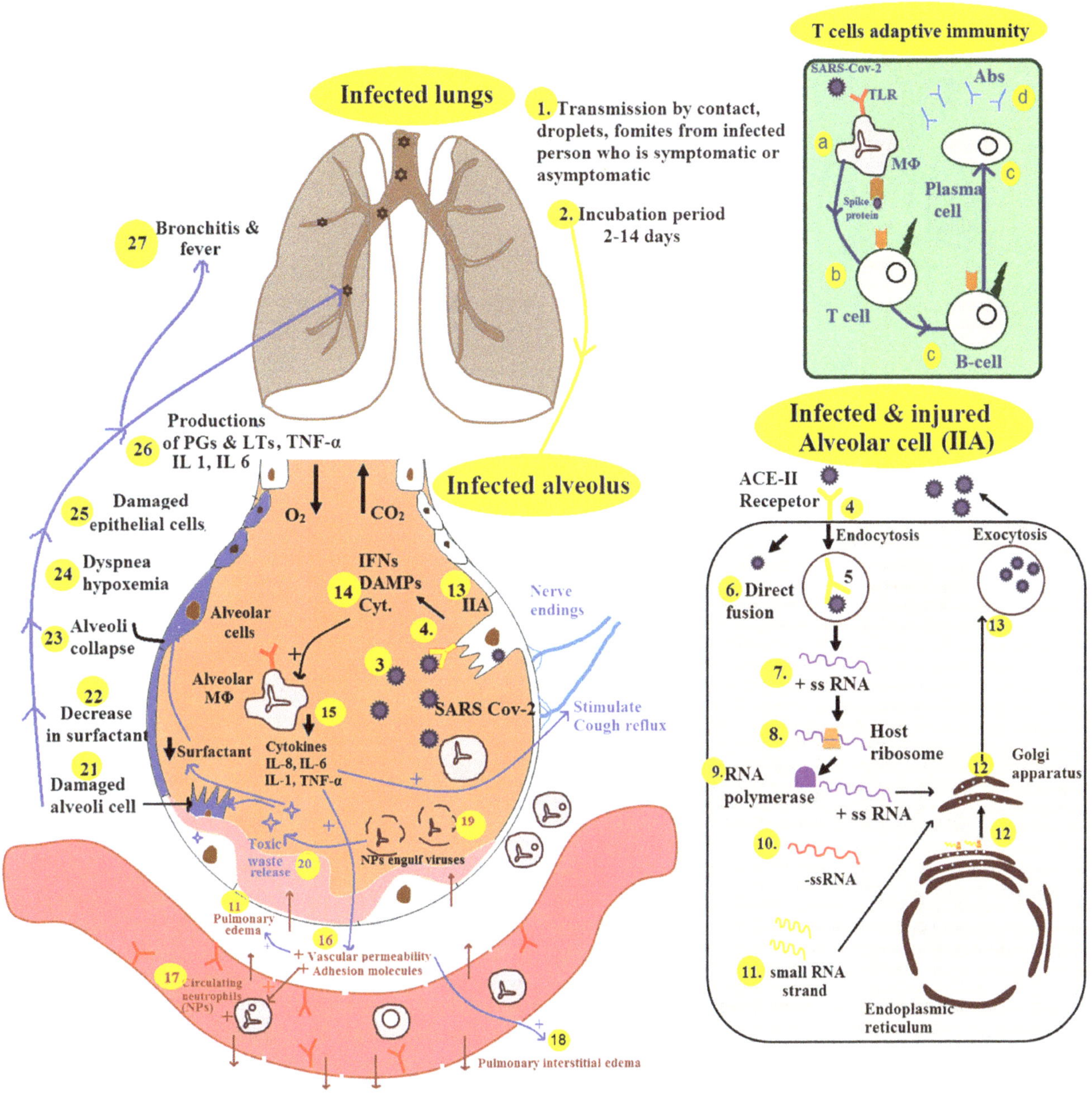

FIGURE 3.6 Pathophysiology of COVID-19 and SARS-CoV-2 infection. Mφ: Macrophages, Abs: Antibodies, TLRs: Toll-like receptors, IL: Interleukin, TNF: tumor necrosis factor, IFNs: cytokines, DAMPs: Damage-associated molecular patterns, ACE2: angiotensin-converting enzyme 2, ss RNA: single-stranded ribonucleic acid, NPs: neutrophils [1–26,164].

change in the expression of various proteins including mitochondrial proteins that are involved in apoptosis and mechanism of oxygen-sensing. However, no direct evidence has been reported so far that supports the involvement of SARS-CoV-2 in the suppression of proteins responsible for mitochondrial oxygen-sensing [152] (Figures 3.6 and 3.7). This possibility was recently hypothesized by Archer et al. [152]. Thus, to explore more possibilities for treatment, better understanding related to the pathophysiology of COVID-19 is required. COVID-19 is an infectious viral disease that can progress into ARDS and pneumonia. These viral infections can prove to be fatal among infected individuals with impaired immune system or any comorbid state. Persistent dry cough, difficulty in breathing, and increased heart rate are the major signs of acute respiratory distress syndrome; however, these symptoms can be mild among healthy individuals. In severe cases, this viral infection can develop into severe ARDS, which can eventually lead to pneumonia. After its transmission via droplets or fomites, SARS-CoV-2 displays an incubation period (time from infection to appearance of symptoms) of about 2–14 days, which can be symptomatic or even asymptomatic [153]. Through the incubation phase, the virus slowly stimulates a response within the respiratory tract as mentioned in Figure 3.6. Surfactant (surface-active lipoprotein complex) produces by alveoli sacs (specifically by type II alveolar cells) of the lungs, forms the inner lining of the alveoli to allow

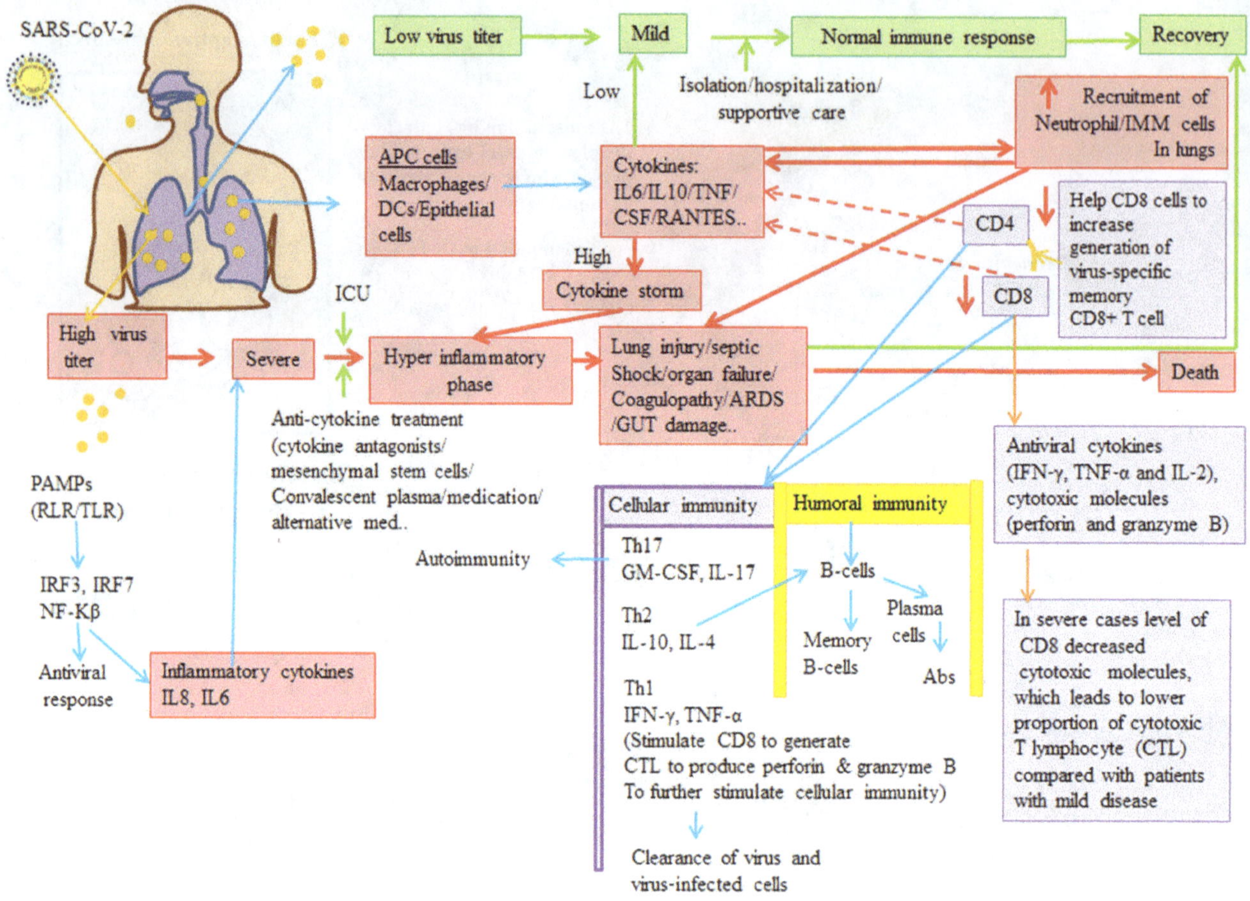

FIGURE 3.7 Phases of COVID-19 pathogenesis in context with CoV-2-induced immune responses (pathogenic inflammatory cytokine response) [167].

gaseous exchange [154]. Invasion of SARS-CoV-2 into alveolar epithelial cells results in the development of respiratory symptoms. To gain entry inside the host cell, initially the virus targets and binds onto ACE receptor present over alveolar cell membrane (type 2) via their surface proteins called spikes. This process of spike-ACE2 protein binding is exposed to enzyme-based changes via transmembrane serine protease, which further allows the conformational changes of S protein to facilitate its fusion with the plasma membrane and to initiate endocytosis. Endocytic pathway used by SARS-CoV-2 allows direct fusion of the viral envelope with the host membrane [102]. This is followed by the release and uncoating of viral nucleocapsid to the cytoplasm. During attachment as well as the release of viral RNA genome (+single-stranded gRNA) in host cell, the virion experience several changes (Figures 3.6 and 3.7). These modifications are done by cysteine proteases (lysosomal), cathepsin (L and B), present in the endolysosomal system [155]. This critical phase is more dependent on pH. The acidic environment of endolysosomes is required for the fusion and finally uncoating of the envelope. +ssRNA contain ORF1a and ORF1b genes (21,291 nt in length) initially synthesize two large polyproteins, pp1a and pp1ab [156]. Pp1a and pp1ab syntheses involve programmed ribosomal frameshifting, which is a strongly controlled phenomenon used by a SARS-CoV-2 to synthesize various proteins during the translation of ORF1a and ORF1b from the input genome RNA [156] (Figures 3.6 and 3.7). During this process, host ribosomes translate the viral ssRNA (particularly ORF1a and ORF1b genes) into pp1a (nsp1–11) as well as pp1ab (nsp1–16) polyproteins, which translate non-structural and accessory proteins as well as form replication–transcription complex (RTC) [156]. Thus, through this process, gRNAs produce their own proteins and new genomes in the cytoplasm by attaching to the host ribosomes. These proteins (nsp1–16) perform different tasks. RNA-dependent RNA polymerase (RdRp) is a vital enzyme for the life cycle of RNA viruses and mainly responsible for the replication of RNA from an RNA template [157,158]. Consequently, RNA polymerase converts the positive strand of RNA of the virus to make a negative RNA strand. The negative strand will be used by the RNA polymerase again to make a positive RNA strand as well as other small positive RNA strands [157,158] (Figures 3.6 and 3.7). These small RNA strands (sgRNAs) will be translated via the ribosomes of the host again in the ER to help get the viral structural elements. These cuddled collections of sgRNAs are continuously produced via polymerase and in the end change into related proteins of the virus [157–159]. The ER transport these accessory and structural proteins into the Golgi apparatus where they are adequately packed with the positive RNA strands to create new vesicles in the form of virus progeny [157–159] (Figures 3.6 and 3.7). Packing of positive RNA strands and structural proteins is followed by the release of newly assembled viruses from the host cell via exocytic pathway by forming secretary vesicles. However, before its release from alveolar cells, it causes enormous damage to the cell, which initiates uncontrolled production of proinflammatory mediators such as interferon's cytokines as well as its intracellular components. Through cell signaling or cell–cell communication, interferons exert many impacts over the neighboring cells and prepare these cells to prevent against infection caused by the virus. Simultaneously macrophages (alveolar) recognize cellular damage caused by the virus via damage-associated molecular patterns (DAMPs) from the alveolar cells [157–159] (Figures 3.6 and 3.7). Pathogen-associated molecular patterns are present on the surface of pathogens that are recognized by pattern recognition receptors in antigen-presenting cells (APCs) such as macrophages and dendritic cells. APCs have pattern recognition receptors (PRR) including RIG-I-like receptors (RLRs), TLRs, and NOD-like receptors (NLRs) that are present in several sites of the host cells [160] (Figures 3.6 and 3.7). Each one of the PRRs might create a distinct response against consequent activation of protein. Immune reaction against SARS-CoV-2 by alveolar macrophages is mediated by the detection of the virus by using its special receptors called TLRs in order to engulf the virus particles via a phagocytosis process and later present it on their surface. As has been reported, the spike protein of the virus could be presented to specific T cells to stimulate adaptive immune response containing B cells or the plasma cells to further initiate the production of antibodies (IgG and IgM) against the viral spike proteins. SARS-CoV-2 infections also cause lymphopenia (i.e., decrease in NK cells and T- lymphocytes) [161]. Recent reports have shown that nearly 85% of acute COVID-19 individuals presented lymphopenia [162,163]. It has also been reported that RNA containing SARS-CoV can be identified by RNA sensors in cytosol such as RIG-I/MDA5 and TLR-3 and TLR-7 [165].

These pathogen-associated molecular patterns help the immune cells such as macrophages and dendritic cells to differentiate host cells from infected host cells or any other pathogens in order to protect healthy host cells from its own immune system [165]. This step is important to protect surrounding infected cells from viral infection. SARS-CoV-2 RNA and S protein may be evolved as foremost pathogen-associated molecular patterns as they can participate in intracellular signaling cascades during innate immune response of the host cell. CoV antigens once presented by APCs to the CD4 helper T lymphocytes by MHC class I resulted in the production of IL-12 [19,97,161,166] (Figures 3.6 and 3.7). Simultaneously, CD4 T cell-mediated humoral immune responses can also increase the production of antigen-specific IgM and IgG antibodies by the activation of T-dependent B cells. IgM can only last up to 12 weeks, whereas IgG can relatively last longer. IL-12 stimulates Th1 responses to produce IFNγ production by T and NK cell activation. Simultaneously, it increases the MHC class I expression and mediators production via NF-κB route [19,97,161,166] (Figures 3.6 and 3.7). On the contrary, IL-17 and GM-CSF production via activation of T-helper cell 17 (Th17) further causes tissue inflammation and tissue destruction by recruitment of more monocytes as well as neutrophils to the infected site and further trigger numerous more proinflammatory mediators including IL (–1, –6, –8, –21), TNF-β, and MCP-1 [19,97,161,167–171] (Figures 3.6 and 3.7). Alveolar macrophages (APC cells) also act in response to the cytokines produced by injured alveolus cells. This causes the alveolar macrophages themselves to secrete cytokines such as TNF-α, interleukin 1, interleukin 6, and interleukin 8 as well as other chemokines [167–171] (Figures 3.6 and 3.7).

2019-nCov affects the cellular expression surface receptors ACE2 and TMPRSS2 via binding to cellular receptors ACE2. After its entry into cells, the SARS-CoV-2 actively replicates and releases out of the host cell. These events encourage pyroptotic cell death as well as release damage-associated molecular patterns, such as adenosine triphosphates (ATPs), nucleic acids, and apoptosis-associated speck-like protein containing a CARD (ASC) oligomers. Simultaneously, the innate immune response instigates the recognition of pathogen-associated molecular patterns by the RLR and TLR and stimulates IRF3, IRF7, and NF-κB, which can further result in antiviral response and the generation of inflammatory cytokines. On the contrary, APC along with T cells possesses various immune responses by different immune effectors. This event finally results in the recruitment of IMM and neutrophil in the lung tissue to secrete high amounts of cytokines that can lead to the hyperinflammatory state. This inflammatory state due to secretion of multiple cytokines, also termed cytokine release syndrome, causes enormous damage not only to lungs but also to other organs. As illustrated above, apart from factors like immune condition of an individual exposed to the virus and many other factors, titer value as well as viral load also determines severity of the disease. COVID-19 can be asymptomatic, mild, or severe depending on immune condition, titer value as well as many other factors that can trigger uncontrolled production of different cytokines to cause lungs damage, multiple organ damage, and many other complications. T cells, CD4+, and CD8+ decreased in severe patients, whereas infiltration of neutrophils along with IMM cells increased. Figure 3.7 also outlined different roles of CD4+ and CD8+ in stimulating cellular and humoral immunity [167].

The inflammatory process that takes place inside the lung parenchyma stimulates vagal afferent nerves which are abundantly present in various regions of lungs, to initiate the cough reflex, and as a result infected people may present with a dry cough early. Production of proinflammatory cytokines such as TNFα and Interleukin 1β increases vascular permeability and expression of adhesion molecules [167–171] (Figures 3.6 and 3.7). These cytokines further recruit other immune cells such as monocytes as well as neutrophils as these cells will interact with these adhesion proteins and enter the site of injury. In addition to IL17, IL8 is responsible for the recruitment of more neutrophils as well as more inflammatory mediators triggered by monocytes resulting in the increase in vascular permeability (Figures 3.6 and 3.7). This increase in vascular permeability allows the leakage of the fluids into the interstitial edema and later into the alveoli resulting in pulmonary edema. Development of pulmonary edema leads to shortness of breath and impaired oxygenation resulting in low oxygen levels in the blood. Simultaneously, continuous recruitment of more macrophages and neutrophils at the site of injury can be detrimental, since after a while they can produce more proinflammatory cytokines, which can damage the surrounding tissue, especially alveolar type II cells [167–171] (Figures 3.6 and 3.7).

As a result, damaged alveolar type II cells result in less surfactant (surface-active agent) being available. Pulmonary surfactant is secreted by alveolar epithelial cells (type II) and encompasses the epithelium (alveolar). Pulmonary surfactant is responsible for stabilizing alveolar dimensions and thus is required for typical alveolar and lung performance (Figures 3.6 and 3.7). However, depletion of surfactant causes disintegration of alveolar sacs by a surface-area-mediated decrease of surface tension in alveolar sacs. This can further result in the impaired oxygenation state or hypoxemia. In addition to the production of proinflammatory cytokines (IL-6, IL-1 β, TNF-α), reports are also available on the stimulation of arachidonic acid (AA) pathway resulting in the production of eicosanoids (prostaglandins and leukotrienes), which are released by white blood cells and damaged endothelial cells [167–171] (Figure 3.6). Leukotriene production causes bronchoconstriction with impaired ventilation leading to hypoxemia, whereas prostaglandins, interleukin 1, interleukin 6, and TNFα are responsible for causing fever, which is one of the main characteristics of COVID-19 [167–171]. Hypoxemia state stimulates chemoreceptors in the aortic arch. Carotid bodies are the chemoreceptors in the aortic arch that detect any variation in arterial blood oxygen levels, and the ensuing chemoreflex is an effective regulator of blood pressure. Abnormal low pO2 stimulates these chemoreceptors to send afferent impulses to cardiopulmonary centers in the brain stem to convey to the lungs to breathe more mainly to recover normal pO2 [167–171] (Figures 3.6 and 3.7). This leads to the increase in respiratory rate and tidal volume, increases in blood flow toward the kidneys and the brain, and increases in cardiac output in order to maintain blood flow to the body's tissues. To achieve more cardiac output the heart pumps faster to deliver oxygen to the body and thus COVID-19 patients who have hypoxemia are usually tachycardic. However, due to differences among host immune response against this virus and other factors, COVID-19 can be asymptomatic when patients only develop minor symptoms such as coughing, low fever, and temporary dyspnea. In coronaviruses, just like in the case of other viral agents, the adaptive immune system plays an important part in the infection. NK cells, cytotoxic T lymphocytes, stimulated circulating helper T cells, stimulated CD8 T adaptive immune response, and antibodies play an important role during viral infection; however, cytokine over production via the stimulation of extremely inflammatory macrophages can inhibit adaptive immune response against COVID-19 infection [167–171] (Figures 3.6 and 3.7). Elderly patients with compromised immune systems with decreased antimicrobial potential of neutrophils and macrophages, decreased antigen presentation by dendritic cells, decreased natural killer cell cytotoxicity, and compromised adaptive lymphocyte responses have higher mortality rates [167–171]. A recent report by Du and Yuan [172] postulated by using a mathematical model that severity and mortality in COVID-19 patients are somehow more dependent on the interaction between host innate and adaptive immune response. Moreover, it has been also postulated that disease progression of COVID-19 is in one way or another related to a mismatch in the timing between the active involvement of innate and adaptive immune response. As per postulates, adaptive immune response among coronavirus-infected patients can appear earlier than the peak viral load. This early involvement of adaptive immune response can result in the late depletion of susceptible epithelial cells of the lungs in COVID-19 patients. Thus, mismatch in timing as well as the resulting intervention with innate immunity can result in the incomplete clearance of the infected cells and thus act as an epicenter for the transmission of infection to surrounding cells. These events can lead to overactive immune responses and other complications with high mortality.

3.9 COVID-19 Transmission with Variation in Climatic Conditions

Earlier reports have suggested the role and significance of climatic variables in the transmission of viral infection such as SARS [173]. Previous reports have suggested that sudden variation in ambient temperature was linked with an increased risk of SARS [174]. Similarly, a decrease in temperature or dry air can increase the risk of viral infection such as influenza [175]. The virus activity of influenza virus was enhanced in northern Europe during low temperature and low ultraviolet indexes in the period of 2010–2018 [176]. Thus, it was initially assumed that coronavirus transmission may reduce or even vanish when the temperature as well as the UV radiation increases during the summer [177]. The stability of SARS-CoV-2 in different environmental conditions has also been reported on recently, and it has been suggested that SARS-CoV-2 is highly stable at 4°C, however sensitive it is to heat [178]. Data for several nations except China suggested that humidity (relative) as well as temperature have been not directly associated with new cases and death rates of COVID-19 [179]. Sanchez-Lorenzo et al. [180] reported that lower temperatures (8°C to 11°C) with humidity (<6 g/Kg) in Spain and Italy have been associated with more cases of infection as well as rate of mortality. Sajadi et al. [181] based on worldwide meteorological data suggested that regions with constant spread of infection had variable humidity (44% to 84%), however constantly low specific (3to6 g/kg) and absolute humidity (4to7 g/cubic mt). Qi et al. [182] reported in China (during the winter season) that 1°C increase in the daily average temperature with humidity in the range of 67% to 86% resulted in a decrease in COVID-19 patients. Luo et al. [183], based on its study in Asian countries, postulated a positive association among humidity (absolute) and rise in cases and a low negative association between weather temperature and case increase. Juni (2020) based on a report on 144 global areas (excluding China) suggested that COVID-19 transmission is correlated with higher public health interventions; however, it is poorly correlated with relative or absolute humidity and with latitude and temperature [184]. Islam (2020) based on climatic conditions worldwide in association with transmission of COVID-19 suggested that calm, cold, dry, and overcast climatic circumstances have been supportive to COVID-19 transmission [185]. Recent findings demonstrated that climatic conditions on the COVID-19 outbreak play different roles in different countries, suggesting dissimilar climatic zones. Accordingly, COVID-19 can be intensified by increases of the upward long-wave radiation flux and temperature in an arid region, whereas it can be alleviated by increases of these factors in a temperate area [186]. A recent study also showed that temperature and relative humidity are negatively correlated with COVID-19 transmission across the globe [187]. This study also demonstrated that climate conditions are not the significant factors in COVID-19 transmission, but government intervention as well as public awareness to mitigate COVID-19 transmission in winter must be considered [187]. Another report studied the effect of population density, temperature, and absolute humidity on spread and decay durations of COVID-19 in China, England, Germany, and Japan. Parameters like spread duration and decay duration of COVID-19 can be determined in a specific model with its correlation with certain factors such as population density, absolute humidity, and maximum temperature. Population and meteorological factors correlated with spread duration and decay duration of COVID-19 will be helpful in finding the mortality rate. The results showed a significant correlation of the transmission and decay durations with population density in the four analyzed countries. Specifically, spread duration showed a high correlation with population density and absolute humidity, whereas decay duration demonstrated the highest correlation with population density, absolute humidity, and maximum temperature [188]. On the contrary, the influence of population density was nearly absent in China due to the strict implementation of lockdown. Thus, higher population density can prolong spread and decay durations, though fewer correlations were established with the population and meteorological factors [188]. Thus, these and many other reports support as well as contradict the association of transmission rate of COVID-19 with different meteorological parameters including precipitation, temperature, speed of the wind, and humidity (relative). Due to the lack of concrete experimental evidence, existence of an association between transmission rate of COVID-19 and different meteorological conditions is still a myth.

REFERENCES

1. Weiss SR. Forty years with coronaviruses. *J Exp Med.* 2020;217:e20200537.
2. Dos Santos WG. Natural history of COVID-19 and current knowledge on treatment therapeutic options. *Biomed Pharmacother.* 2020;129:110493.
3. Chung YH, Beiss V, Fiering SN, Steinmetz NF. COVID-19 vaccine frontrunners and their nanotechnology design. *ACS Nano.* 2020;14(10):12522–12537.
4. Kaur SP, Gupta V. COVID-19 vaccine: A comprehensive status report. *Virus Res.* 2020;288:198114.
5. Sofi MS, Hamid A, Bhat SU. SARS-CoV-2: A critical review of its history, pathogenesis, transmission, diagnosis and treatment. *Biosaf Health.* 2020;2(4):217–225.
6. Coleman CM, Frieman MB. Coronaviruses: Important emerging human pathogens. *J Virol.* 2014;88(10):5209–5212.
7. Coronaviridae Study Group of the International Committee on Taxonomy of Viruses. The species severe acute respiratory syndrome-related coronavirus: Classifying 2019-nCoV and naming it SARS-CoV-2. *Nat Microbiol.* 2020;5:536–544.
8. Lu R, Zhao X, Li J, Niu P, Yang B, Wu H, Wang W, Song H, Huang B, Zhu N, Bi Y, Ma X, Zhan F, Wang L, Hu T, Zhou H, Hu Z, Zhou W, Zhao L, Chen J, Meng Y, Wang J, Lin Y, Yuan J, Xie Z, Ma J, Liu WJ, Wang D, Xu W, Holmes EC, Gao GF, Wu G, Chen W, Shi W, Tan W. Genomic characterisation and epidemiology of 2019 novel coronavirus: implications for virus origins and receptor binding. *Lancet.* 2020;395(10224):565–574.
9. Li W, Moore MJ, Vasilieva N, Sui J, Wong SK, Berne MA, Somasundaran M, Sullivan JL, Luzuriaga K, Greenough TC, Choe H, Farzan M. Angiotensin-converting enzyme 2 is a functional receptor for the SARS coronavirus. *Nature.* 2003;426(6965):450–454.
10. Qian Z, Travanty EA, Oko L, Edeen K, Berglund A, Wang J, Ito Y, Holmes KV, Mason RJ. Innate immune response of human alveolar type II cells infected with severe acute respiratory syndrome-coronavirus. *Am J Respir Cell Mol Biol.* 2013;48(6):742–748.
11. Lu G, Hu Y, Wang Q, Qi J, Gao F, Li Y, Zhang Y, Zhang W, Yuan Y, Bao J, Zhang B, Shi Y, Yan J, Gao GF. Molecular basis of binding between novel human coronavirus MERS-CoV and its receptor CD26. *Nature.* 2013;500(7461):227–231.
12. Raj VS, Mou H, Smits SL, Dekkers DH, Müller MA, Dijkman R, Muth D, Demmers JA, Zaki A, Fouchier RA, Thiel V, Drosten C, Rottier PJ, Osterhaus AD, Bosch BJ, Haagmans BL. Dipeptidyl peptidase 4 is a functional receptor for the emerging human coronavirus-EMC. *Nature.* 2013;495(7440):251–254.
13. van Doremalen N, Bushmaker T, Morris DH, Holbrook MG, Gamble A, Williamson BN, Tamin A, Harcourt JL, Thornburg NJ, Gerber SI, Lloyd-Smith JO, de Wit E, Munster VJ. Aerosol and surface stability of SARS-CoV-2 as compared with SARS-CoV-1. *N Engl J Med.* 2020;382(16):1564–1567.
14. Guo ZD, Wang ZY, Zhang SF, Li X, Li L, Li C, Cui Y, Fu RB, Dong YZ, Chi XY, Zhang MY, Liu K, Cao C, Liu B, Zhang K, Gao YW, Lu B, Chen W. Aerosol and surface distribution of severe acute respiratory syndrome coronavirus 2 in hospital wards, Wuhan, China, 2020. *Emerg Infect Dis.* 2020;26(7):1583–1591.
15. Bourouiba L. Turbulent gas clouds and respiratory pathogen emissions: Potential implications for reducing transmission of COVID-19. *JAMA.* 2020;323(18):1837–1838.
16. Bourouiba L. Images in clinical medicine. *A Sneeze N Engl J Med.* 2016;375(8):e15.
17. Malik YA. Properties of coronavirus and SARS-CoV-2. *Malays J Pathol.* 2020;42(1): 3–11.
18. Kang S, Yang M, Hong Z, Zhang L, Huang Z, Chen X, He S, Zhou Z, Zhou Z, Chen Q, Yan Y, Zhang C, Shan H, Chen S. Crystal structure of SARS-CoV-2 nucleocapsid protein RNA binding domain reveals potential unique drug targeting sites. *Acta Pharm Sin B.* 2020;10(7):1228–1238.
19. Kumar S, Nyodu R, Maurya VK, Saxena SK. Morphology, genome organization, replication, and pathogenesis of severe acute respiratory syndrome coronavirus 2 (SARS-CoV-2). Coronavirus Disease 2019 (COVID-19). 2020:23–31.
20. Cucinotta D, Vanelli M. WHO declares COVID-19 a pandemic. *Acta Biomed.* 2020;91(1):157–160.
21. Ye ZW, Yuan S, Yuen KS, Fung SY, Chan CP, Jin DY. Zoonotic origins of human coronaviruses. *Int J Biol Sci.* 2020;16(10):1686–1697.

22. Pal M, Berhanu G, Desalegn C, Kandi V. Severe acute respiratory syndrome coronavirus-2 (SARS-CoV-2): An update. *Cureus*. 2020;12(3):e7423.
23. Letko M, Marzi A, Munster V. Functional assessment of cell entry and receptor usage for SARS-CoV-2 and other lineage B betacoronaviruses. *Nat Microbiol*. 2020;5(4):562–569.
24. Liu DX, Liang JQ, Fung TS. Human coronavirus-229E, -OC43, -NL63, and -HKU1. In: Roitberg BD, editor. *Reference Module in Life Sciences*. Elsevier, Amsterdam, Netherlands; 2020: 180 p.
25. Cascella M, Rajnik M, Cuomo A, Dulebohn SC, Di Napoli R. Features, *Evaluation, and Treatment of Coronavirus*. StatPearls Publishing, Treasure Island, FL; 2020.
26. Lam TT, Jia N, Zhang YW, Shum MH, Jiang JF, Zhu HC, Tong YG, Shi YX, Ni XB, Liao YS, Li WJ, Jiang BG, Wei W, Yuan TT, Zheng K, Cui XM, Li J, Pei GQ, Qiang X, Cheung WY, Li LF, Sun FF, Qin S, Huang JC, Leung GM, Holmes EC, Hu YL, Guan Y, Cao WC. Identifying SARS-CoV-2-related coronaviruses in Malayan pangolins. *Nature*. 2020;583(7815):282–285.
27. Wang H, Li X, Li T, Zhang S, Wang L, Wu X, Liu J. The genetic sequence, origin, and diagnosis of SARS-CoV-2. *Eur J Clin Microbiol Infect Dis*. 2020;39(9):1629–1635.
28. Han GZ. Pangolins harbor SARS-CoV-2-related coronaviruses. *Trends Microbiol*. 2020;28(7):515–517.
29. Tang X, Wu C, Li X, Song Y, Yao X, Wu X, Duan Y, Zhang H, Wang Y, Qian Z, Cui J, Lu J. On the origin and continuing evolution of SARS-CoV-2. *Natl Sci Rev*. 2020:nwaa036.
30. Cyranoski D. Did pangolins spread the China coronavirus to people? *Nature*. 2020. https://www.nature.com/articles/d41586-020-00364-2
31. Cui J, Li F, Shi ZL. Origin and evolution of pathogenic coronaviruses. *Nat Rev Microbiol*. 2019;17(3):181–192.
32. Hamre D, Procknow JJ. A new virus isolated from the human respiratory tract. *Proc Soc Exp Biol Med*. 1966;121: 190–193.
33. Tyrrell DAJ, Bynoe ML. Cultivation of novel type of common-cold virus in organ cultures. *Br Med J*. 1965;1:1467–1470.
34. Di Teodoro G, Valleriani F, Puglia I, Monaco F, Di Pancrazio C, Luciani M, Krasteva I, Petrini A, Marcacci M, D'Alterio N, Curini V, Iorio M, Migliorati G, Di Domenico M, Morelli D, Calistri P, Savini G, Decaro N, Holmes EC, Lorusso A. SARS-CoV-2 replicates in respiratory ex vivo organ cultures of domestic ruminant species. *Vet Microbiol*. 2021;252:108933.
35. Hou YJ, Chiba S, Halfmann P, Ehre C, Kuroda M, Dinnon KH 3rd, Leist SR, Schäfer A, Nakajima N, Takahashi K, Lee RE, Mascenik TM, Graham R, Edwards CE, Tse LV, Okuda K, Markmann AJ, Bartelt L, de Silva A, Margolis DM, Boucher RC, Randell SH, Suzuki T, Gralinski LE, Kawaoka Y, Baric RS. SARS-CoV-2 D614G variant exhibits efficient replication ex vivo and transmission in vivo. *Science*. 2020;370(6523):1464–1468.
36. Ksiazek TG, Erdman D, Goldsmith CS, Zaki SR, Peret T, Emery S, Tong S, Urbani C, Comer JA, Lim W, Rollin PE, Dowell SF, Ling AE, Humphrey CD, Shieh WJ, Guarner J, Paddock CD, Rota P, Fields B, DeRisi J, Yang JY, Cox N, Hughes JM, LeDuc JW, Bellini WJ, Anderson LJ; SARS Working Group. A novel coronavirus associated with severe acute respiratory syndrome. *N Engl J Med*. 2003;348(20):1953–1966.
37. Zhu N, Zhang D, Wang W, Li X, Yang B, Song J, Zhao X, Huang B, Shi W, Lu R, Niu P, Zhan F, Ma X, Wang D, Xu W, Wu G, Gao GF, Tan W; China Novel Coronavirus Investigating and Research Team. A novel coronavirus from patients with pneumonia in China, 2019. *N Engl J Med*. 2020;382(8):727–733.
38. Matsuyama S, Nao N, Shirato K, Kawase M, Saito S, Takayama I, Nagata N, Sekizuka T, Katoh H, Kato F, Sakata M, Tahara M, Kutsuna S, Ohmagari N, Kuroda M, Suzuki T, Kageyama T, Takeda M. Enhanced isolation of SARS-CoV-2 by TMPRSS2-expressing cells. *Proc Natl Acad Sci U S A*. 2020;117(13):7001–7003.
39. Park WB, Kwon NJ, Choi SJ, Kang CK, Choe PG, Kim JY, Yun J, Lee GW, Seong MW, Kim NJ, Seo JS, Oh MD. Virus isolation from the first patient with SARS-CoV-2 in Korea. *J Korean Med Sci*. 2020;35(7):e84.
40. Kumar S, Sarma P, Kaur H, Prajapat M, Bhattacharyya A, Avti P, Sehkhar N, Kaur H, Bansal S, Mahendiratta S, Mahalmani VM, Singh H, Prakash A, Kuhad A, Medhi B. Clinically relevant cell culture models and their significance in isolation, pathogenesis, vaccine development, repurposing and screening of new drugs for SARS-CoV-2: A systematic review. *Tissue Cell*. 2021;70: 101497.
41. Johansen MD, Irving A, Montagutelli X, Tate MD, Rudloff I, Nold MF, Hansbro NG, Kim RY, Donovan C, Liu G, Faiz A, Short KR, Lyons JG, McCaughan GW, Gorrell MD, Cole A, Moreno C, Couteur D, Hesselson D, Triccas J, Neely GG, Gamble JR, Simpson SJ, Saunders BM, Oliver BG, Britton WJ, Wark PA, Nold-Petry CA, Hansbro PM. Animal and translational models of SARS-CoV-2 infection and COVID-19. *Mucosal Immunol*. 2020;13(6):877–891.
42. Sanclemente-Alaman I, Moreno-Jiménez L, Benito-Martín MS, Canales-Aguirre A, Matías-Guiu JA, Matías-Guiu J, Gómez-Pinedo U. Experimental models for the study of central nervous system infection by SARS-CoV-2. *Front Immunol*. 2020;11:2163.
43. Sun SH, Chen Q, Gu HJ, et al. A mouse model of SARS-CoV-2infection and pathogenesis. *Cell Host Microbe*. 2020;28:1–10.
44. Sugawara I, Yamada H, Mizuno S. STAT1 knockout mice are highly susceptible to pulmonary mycobacterial infection. *Tohoku J Exp Med*. 2004;202(1):41–50.
45. Meraz MA, White JM, Sheehan KC, et al. Targeted disruption of the STAT1 gene in mice reveals unexpected physiologic specificity in the JAK-STAT signaling pathway. *Cell*. 1996;84:431–442.
46. Dinnon KH, Leist SR, Schäfer A, Edwards CE, Martinez DR, Montgomery SA, West A, Yount BL, Hou YJ, Adams LE, Gully KL, Brown AJ, Huang E, Bryant MD, Choong IC, Glenn JS, Gralinski LE, Sheahan TP, Baric RS. A mouse-adapted SARS-CoV-2 model for the evaluation of COVID-19 medical countermeasures. bioRxiv. 2020, Preprint.
47. Gao Q, Bao L, Mao H, et al. Rapid development of an inactivated vaccine for SARS-CoV-2. bioRxiv. 2020, Preprint.
48. Roberts A, Vogel L, Guarner J, Hayes N, Murphy B, Zaki S, Subbarao K. Severe acute respiratory syndrome coronavirus infection of golden Syrian hamsters. *J Virol*. 2005;79(1):503–511.

49. Zhang Q, Shi J, Deng G, Guo J, Zeng X, He X, Kong H, Gu C, Li X, Liu J, Wang G, Chen Y, Liu L, Liang L, Li Y, Fan J, Wang J, Li W, Guan L, Li Q, Yang H, Chen P, Jiang L, Guan Y, Xin X, Jiang Y, Tian G, Wang X, Qiao C, Li C, Bu Z, Chen H. H7N9 influenza viruses are transmissible in ferrets by respiratory droplet. *Science*. 2013;341(6144):410–414.
50. Gretebeck LM, Subbarao K. Animal models for SARS and MERS coronaviruses. *Curr Opin Virol*. 2015;13:123–129.
51. Rockx B, Kuiken T, Herfst S, Bestebroer T, Lamers MM, Oude Munnink BB, de Meulder D, van Amerongen G, van den Brand J, Okba NMA, Schipper D, van Run P, Leijten L, Sikkema R, Verschoor E, Verstrepen B, Bogers W, Langermans J, Drosten C, Fentener van Vlissingen M, Fouchier R, de Swart R, Koopmans M, Haagmans BL. Comparative pathogenesis of COVID-19, MERS, and SARS in a nonhuman primate model. *Science*. 2020;368(6494):1012–1015.
52. Munster VJ, Feldmann F, Williamson BN, van Doremalen N, Pérez-Pérez L, Schulz J, Meade-White K, Okumura A, Callison J, Brumbaugh B, Avanzato VA, Rosenke R, Hanley PW, Saturday G, Scott D, Fischer ER, de Wit E. Respiratory disease in rhesus macaques inoculated with SARS-CoV-2. *Nature*. 2020;585(7824): 268–272.
53. Le Bras A. SARS-CoV-2 causes COVID-19-like disease in cynomolgus macaques. *Lab Anim (NY)*. 2020;49(6):174.
54. Yang L, Han Y, Nilsson-Payant BE, Gupta V, Wang P, Duan X, Tang X, Zhu J, Zhao Z, Jaffré F, Zhang T, Kim TW, Harschnitz O, Redmond D, Houghton S, Liu C, Naji A, Ciceri G, Guttikonda S, Bram Y, Nguyen DT, Cioffi M, Chandar V, Hoagland DA, Huang Y, Xiang J, Wang H, Lyden D, Borczuk A, Chen HJ, Studer L, Pan FC, Ho DD, tenOever BR, Evans T, Schwartz RE, Chen S. A human pluripotent stem cell-based platform to study SARS-CoV-2 tropism and model virus infection in human cells and organoids. *Cell Stem Cell*. 2020;27(1):125–136.e7.
55. Han Y, Yang L, Duan X, Duan F, Nilsson-Payant BE, Yaron TM, Wang P, Tang X, Zhang T, Zhao Z, Bram Y, Redmond D, Houghton S, Nguyen D, Xu D, Wang X, Uhl S, Huang Y, Johnson JL, Xiang J, Wang H, Pan FC, Cantley LC, tenOever BR, Ho DD, Evans T, Schwartz RE, Chen HJ, Chen S. Identification of candidate COVID-19 therapeutics using hPSC-derived lung organoids. bioRxiv. 2020, Preprint.
56. Zhao B, Ni C, Gao R, Wang Y, Yang L, Wei J, Lv T, Liang J, Zhang Q, Xu W, Xie Y, Wang X, Yuan Z, Liang J, Zhang R, Lin X. Recapitulation of SARS-CoV-2 infection and cholangiocyte damage with human liver ductal organoids. *Protein Cell*. 2020;11(10):771–775.
57. Kim JM, Chung YS, Jo HJ, Lee NJ, Kim MS, Woo SH, Park S, Kim JW, Kim HM, Han MG. Identification of coronavirus isolated from a patient in Korea with COVID-19. *Osong Public Health Res Perspect*. 2020;11(1):3–7.
58. Cagno V. SARS-CoV-2 cellular tropism. *Lancet Microbe*. 2020;1(1):e2–e3.
59. Ogando NS, Dalebout TJ, Zevenhoven-Dobbe JC, Limpens RWAL, van der Meer Y, Caly L, Druce J, de Vries JJC, Kikkert M, Bárcena M, Sidorov I, Snijder EJ. SARS-coronavirus-2 replication in Vero E6 cells: Replication kinetics, rapid adaptation and cytopathology. *J Gen Virol*. 2020;101(9):925–940.
60. Wang W, Xu Y, Gao R, Lu R, Han K, Wu G, Tan W. Detection of SARS-CoV-2 in different types of clinical specimens. *JAMA*. 2020;323(18):1843–1844.
61. Prasad S, Potdar V, Cherian S, Abraham P, Basu A; ICMR-NIV NIC Team. Transmission electron microscopy imaging of SARS-CoV-2. *Indian J Med Res*. 2020;151(2 & 3):241–243.
62. Ruch TR, Machamer CE. The coronavirus E protein: Assembly and beyond. *Viruses*. 2012;4(3):363–382.
63. Du L, He Y, Zhou Y, Liu S, Zheng BJ, Jiang S. The spike protein of SARS-CoV--a target for vaccine and therapeutic development. *Nat Rev Microbiol*. 2009;7(3):226–236.
64. Jaimes JA, André NM, Chappie JS, Millet JK, Whittaker GR. Phylogenetic analysis and structural modeling of SARS-CoV-2 spike protein reveals an evolutionary distinct and proteolytically sensitive activation loop. *J Mol Biol*. 2020;432(10):3309–3325.
65. Li F. Structure, function, and evolution of coronavirus spike proteins. *Annu Rev Virol*. 2016;3(1):237–261.
66. Ou X, Liu Y, Lei X, Li P, Mi D, Ren L, Guo L, Guo R, Chen T, Hu J, Xiang Z, Mu Z, Chen X, Chen J, Hu K, Jin Q, Wang J, Qian Z. Characterization of spike glycoprotein of SARS-CoV-2 on virus entry and its immune cross-reactivity with SARS-CoV. *Nat Commun*. 2020;11(1):1620.
67. Shulla A, Heald-Sargent T, Subramanya G, Zhao J, Perlman S, Gallagher T. A transmembrane serine protease is linked to the severe acute respiratory syndrome coronavirus receptor and activates virus entry. *J Virol*. 2011;85(2):873–882.
68. Bosch BJ, Martina BE, Van Der Zee R, Lepault J, Haijema BJ, Versluis C, Heck AJ, De Groot R, Osterhaus AD, Rottier PJ. Severe acute respiratory syndrome coronavirus (SARS-CoV) infection inhibition using spike protein heptad repeat-derived peptides. *Proc Natl Acad Sci U S A*. 2004;101(22):8455–8460.
69. Coutard B, Valle C, de Lamballerie X, Canard B, Seidah NG, Decroly E. The spike glycoprotein of the new coronavirus 2019-nCoV contains a furin-like cleavage site absent in CoV of the same clade. *Antiviral Res*. 2020;176:104742.
70. Yan R, Zhang Y, Li Y, Xia L, Guo Y, Zhou Q. Structural basis for the recognition of SARS-CoV-2 by full-length human ACE2. *Science*. 2020;367(6485):1444–1448.
71. Zhang L, Lin D, Sun X, Curth U, Drosten C, Sauerhering L, Becker S, Rox K, Hilgenfeld R. Crystal structure of SARS-CoV-2 main protease provides a basis for design of improved α-ketoamide inhibitors. *Science*. 2020;368(6489): 409–412.
72. Khailany RA, Safdar M, Ozaslan M. Genomic characterization of a novel SARS-CoV-2. *Gene Rep*. 2020;19:100682.
73. Prajapat M, Sarma P, Shekhar N, Avti P, Sinha S, Kaur H, Kumar S, Bhattacharyya A, Kumar H, Bansal S, Medhi B. Drug targets for corona virus: A systematic review. *Indian J Pharmacol*. 2020;52(1):56–65.
74. V'kovski P, Kratzel A, Steiner S, Stalder H, Thiel V. Coronavirus biology and replication: Implications for SARS-CoV-2. *Nat Rev Microbiol*. 2020:1–16.
75. Alanagreh L, Alzoughool F, Atoum M. The human coronavirus disease COVID-19: Its origin, characteristics, and insights into potential drugs and its mechanisms. *Pathogens*. 2020;9(5):331.
76. Chan JF, Kok KH, Zhu Z, Chu H, To KK, Yuan S, Yuen KY. Genomic characterization of the 2019 novel human-pathogenic coronavirus isolated from a patient with atypical pneumonia after visiting Wuhan. *Emerg Microbes Infect*. 2020;9(1):221–236.

77. Satarker S, Nampoothiri M. Structural proteins in severe acute respiratory syndrome coronavirus-2. *Arch Med Res.* 2020;51(6):482–491.
78. Shamsi A, Mohammad T, Anwar S, Amani S, Khan MS, Husain FM, Rehman MT, Islam A, Hassan MI. Potential drug targets of SARS-CoV-2: From genomics to therapeutics. *Int J Biol Macromol.* 2021;177:1–9.
79. Ratia K, Pegan S, Takayama J, Sleeman K, Coughlin M, Baliji S, Chaudhuri R, Fu W, Prabhakar BS, Johnson ME, Baker SC, Ghosh AK, Mesecar AD. A noncovalent class of papain-like protease/deubiquitinase inhibitors blocks SARS virus replication. *Proc Natl Acad Sci U S A.* 2008;105(42):16119–16124.
80. Báez-Santos YM, St John SE, Mesecar AD. The SARS-coronavirus papain-like protease: Structure, function and inhibition by designed antiviral compounds. *Antiviral Res.* 2015;115:21–38.
81. Zong Z, Zhang Z, Wu L, Zhang L, Zhou F. The functional deubiquitinating enzymes in control of innate antiviral immunity. *Adv Sci (Weinh).* 2020;8(2):2002484.
82. Schoeman D, Fielding BC. Coronavirus envelope protein: Current knowledge. *Virol J.* 2019;16(1):69.
83. Shang J, Wan Y, Liu C, Yount B, Gully K, Yang Y, Auerbach A, Peng G, Baric R, Li F. Structure of mouse coronavirus spike protein complexed with receptor reveals mechanism for viral entry. *PLoS Pathog.* 2020;16(3):e1008392.
84. Pachetti M, Marini B, Benedetti F, Giudici F, Mauro E, Storici P, Masciovecchio C, Angeletti S, Ciccozzi M, Gallo RC, Zella D, Ippodrino R. Emerging SARS-CoV-2 mutation hot spots include a novel RNA-dependent-RNA polymerase variant. *J Transl Med.* 2020;18(1):179.
85. Starr TN, Greaney AJ, Hilton SK, Crawford KHD, Navarro MJ, Bowen JE, Tortorici MA, Walls AC, Veesler D, Bloom JD. Deep mutational scanning of SARS-CoV-2 receptor binding domain reveals constraints on folding and ACE2 binding. bioRxiv. 2020, Preprint.
86. Baud D, Qi X, Nielsen-Saines K, Musso D, Pomar L, Favre G. Real estimates of mortality following COVID-19 infection. *Lancet Infect Dis.* 2020;20(7):773.
87. Yi CE, Ba L, Zhang L, Ho DD, Chen Z. Single amino acid substitutions in the severe acute respiratory syndrome coronavirus spike glycoprotein determine viral entry and immunogenicity of a major neutralizing domain. *J Virol.* 2005;79(18):11638–11646.
88. Zhang L, Jackson CB, Mou H, Ojha A, Rangarajan ES, Izard T, Farzan M, Choe H. The D614G mutation in the SARS-CoV-2 spike protein reduces S1 shedding and increases infectivity. bioRxiv. 2020, Preprint.
89. Rahman MS, Hoque MN, Islam MR, Islam I, Mishu ID, Rahaman MM, Sultana M, Hossain MA. Mutational insights into the envelope protein of SARS-CoV-2. *Gene Rep.* 2021;22:100997.
90. Onder G, Rezza G, Brusaferro S. Case-fatality rate and characteristics of patients dying in relation to COVID-19 in Italy. *JAMA.* 2020;323(18):1775–1776.
91. Guruprasad L. Human SARS CoV-2 spike protein mutations. *Proteins.* 2021;89(5):569–576.
92. François KO, Balzarini J. The highly conserved glycan at asparagine 260 of HIV-1 gp120 is indispensable for viral entry. *J Biol Chem.* 2011;286(50):42900–42910.
93. Wang W, Zirkle B, Nie J, Ma J, Gao K, Chen XS, Huang W, Kong W, Wang Y. N463 glycosylation site on V5 loop of a mutant gp120 regulates the sensitivity of HIV-1 to neutralizing monoclonal antibodies VRC01/03. *J Acquir Immune Defic Syndr.* 2015;69(3):270–277.
94. Zhang X, Chen S, Yang D, Wang X, Zhu J, Peng D, Liu X. Role of stem glycans attached to haemagglutinin in the biological characteristics of H5N1 avian influenza virus. *J Gen Virol.* 2015;96(Pt 6):1248–1257.
95. Kumar S, Maurya VK, Prasad AK, Bhatt MLB, Saxena SK. Structural, glycosylation and antigenic variation between 2019 novel coronavirus (2019-nCoV) and SARS coronavirus (SARS-CoV). *Virusdisease.* 2020;31(1):13–21.
96. Hoffmann M, Kleine-Weber H, Schroeder S, Krüger N, Herrler T, Erichsen S, Schiergens TS, Herrler G, Wu NH, Nitsche A, Müller MA, Drosten C, Pöhlmann S. SARS-CoV-2 cell entry depends on ACE2 and TMPRSS2 and is blocked by a clinically proven protease inhibitor. *Cell.* 2020;181(2):271–280.e8.
97. Astuti I, Ysrafil. Severe Acute Respiratory Syndrome Coronavirus 2 (SARS-CoV-2): An overview of viral structure and host response. *Diabetes Metab Syndr.* 2020;14(4):407–412.
98. Mahmoud IS, Jarrar YB, Alshaer W, Ismail S. SARS-CoV-2 entry in host cells-multiple targets for treatment and prevention. *Biochimie.* 2020;175:93–98.
99. Shang J, Wan Y, Luo C, Ye G, Geng Q, Auerbach A, Li F. Cell entry mechanisms of SARS-CoV-2. *Proc Natl Acad Sci U S A.* 2020;117(21):11727–11734.
100. Harrison AG, Lin T, Wang P. Mechanisms of SARS-CoV-2 transmission and pathogenesis. *Trends Immunol.* 2020;41(12):1100–1115.
101. Li H, Liu SM, Yu XH, Tang SL, Tang CK. Coronavirus disease 2019 (COVID-19): Current status and future perspectives. *Int J Antimicrob Agents.* 2020;55(5):105951.
102. Tang T, Bidon M, Jaimes JA, Whittaker GR, Daniel S. Coronavirus membrane fusion mechanism offers a potential target for antiviral development. *Antiviral Res.* 2020;178:104792.
103. Greenland JR, Michelow MD, Wang L, London MJ. COVID-19 infection: Implications for perioperative and critical care physicians. *Anesthesiology.* 2020;132(6):1346–1361.
104. Cevik M, Kuppalli K, Kindrachuk J, Peiris M. Virology, transmission, and pathogenesis of SARS-CoV-2. *BMJ.* 2020;371:m3862.
105. Rothan HA, Byrareddy SN. The epidemiology and pathogenesis of coronavirus disease (COVID-19) outbreak. *J Autoimmun.* 2020;109:102433.
106. Ojo AS, Balogun SA, Williams OT, Ojo OS. Pulmonary fibrosis in COVID-19 survivors: Predictive factors and risk reduction strategies. *Pulm Med.* 2020;2020:6175964.
107. Ippolito D, Maino C, Pecorelli A, Allegranza P, Cangiotti C, Capodaglio C, Mariani I, Giandola T, Gandola D, Bianco I, Ragusi M, Franzesi CT, Corso R, Sironi S. Chest X-ray features of SARS-CoV-2 in the emergency department: A multicenter experience from northern Italian hospitals. *Respir Med.* 2020;170:106036.
108. Tabary M, Khanmohammadi S, Araghi F, Dadkhahfar S, Tavangar SM. Pathologic features of COVID-19: A concise review. *Pathol Res Pract.* 2020;216(9):153097.

109. Connors JM, Levy JH. COVID-19 and its implications for thrombosis and anticoagulation. *Blood.* 2020;135(23): 2033–2040.
110. Becker RC. COVID-19 update: COVID-19-associated coagulopathy. *J Thromb Thrombolysis.* 2020;50(1):54–67.
111. Xu Z, Shi L, Wang Y, Zhang J, Huang L, Zhang C, Liu S, Zhao P, Liu H, Zhu L, Tai Y, Bai C, Gao T, Song J, Xia P, Dong J, Zhao J, Wang FS. Pathological findings of COVID-19 associated with acute respiratory distress syndrome. *Lancet Respir Med.* 2020;8(4):420–422.
112. Matthay MA, Zemans RL. The acute respiratory distress syndrome: Pathogenesis and treatment. *Annu Rev Pathol.* 2011;6:147–163.
113. Struyf T, Deeks JJ, Dinnes J, Takwoingi Y, Davenport C, Leeflang MM, Spijker R, Hooft L, Emperador D, Dittrich S, Domen J, Horn SRA, Van den Bruel A; Cochrane COVID-19 Diagnostic Test Accuracy Group. Signs and symptoms to determine if a patient presenting in primary care or hospital outpatient settings has COVID-19 disease. *Cochrane Database Syst Rev.* 2020;7(7):CD013665.
114. Walsh KA, Jordan K, Clyne B, Rohde D, Drummond L, Byrne P, Ahern S, Carty PG, O'Brien KK, O'Murchu E, O'Neill M, Smith SM, Ryan M, Harrington P. SARS-CoV-2 detection, viral load and infectivity over the course of an infection. *J Infect.* 2020;81(3):357–371.
115. Ye Q, Wang B, Mao J. The pathogenesis and treatment of the 'Cytokine Storm' in COVID-19. *J Infect.* 2020;80(6): 607–613.
116. Nile SH, Nile A, Qiu J, Li L, Jia X, Kai G. COVID-19: Pathogenesis, cytokine storm and therapeutic potential of interferons. *Cytokine Growth Factor Rev.* 2020;53:66–70.
117. Sami N, Ahmad R, Fatma T. Exploring algae and cyanobacteria as a promising natural source of antiviral drug against SARS-CoV-2. *Biomed J.* 2020;44(1):54–62.
118. Bhatia S, Sardana S, Sharma A, Vargas De La Cruz CB, Chaugule B, Khodaie L. Development of broad spectrum mycosporine loaded sunscreen formulation from Ulva fasciata delile. *Biomedicine (Taipei).* 2019;9(3):17.
119. Bhatia S, Sardana S, Senwar KR, Dhillon A, Sharma A, Naved T. In vitro antioxidant and antinociceptive properties of Porphyra vietnamensis. *Biomedicine (Taipei).* 2019;9(1):3.
120. Bhatia S, Sharma K, Nagpal K, Bera T. Investigation of the factors influencing the molecular weight of porphyran and its associated antifungal activity bioact. *Carb Diet Fiber* 2015;5:153–168.
121. Bhatia S, Sharma K, Sharma A, Nagpal K, Bera T. Anti-inflammatory, analgesic and antiulcer properties of Porphyra vietnamensis. *Avicenna J Phytomed.* 2015;5(1):69–77.
122. Bhatia S, Kumar V, Sharma K, Nagpal K, Bera T. Significance of algal polymer in designing amphotericin B nanoparticles. *Sci World J.* 2014;2014:564573.
123. Bhatia S, Rathee P, Sharma K, Chaugule BB, Kar N, Bera T. Immuno-modulation effect of sulphated polysaccharide (porphyran) from Porphyra vietnamensis. *Int J Biol Macromol.* 2013;57:50–56.
124. Bhatia S, Garg A, Sharma K, Kumar S, Sharma A, Purohit AP. Mycosporine and mycosporine-like amino acids: A paramount tool against ultra violet irradiation. *Pharmacogn Rev.* 2011;5(10):138–146.
125. Bhatia S, Sharma K, Namdeo AG, Chaugule BB, Kavale M, Nanda S. Broad-spectrum sun-protective action of Porphyra-334 derived from Porphyra vietnamensis. *Pharmacognosy Res.* 2010;2(1):45–49.
126. Bhatia S, Sharma K, Dahiya R, Bera T. *Modern Applications of Plant Biotechnology in Pharmaceutical Sciences.* Academic Press, Elsevier, Cambridge, MA; 2015:164–174.
127. Bhatia S. *Nanotechnology in Drug Delivery: Fundamentals, Design, and Applications.* CRC Press, Boca Raton, FL; 2016:121–127.
128. Bhatia S, Goli D. *Leishmaniasis: Biology, Control and New Approaches for Its Treatment.* CRC Press, Boca Raton, FL; 2016:164–173.
129. Bhatia S. *Natural Polymer Drug Delivery Systems: Nanoparticles, Plants, and Algae.* Springer Nature, Basingstoke, UK; 2016:117–127.
130. Bhatia S. *Introduction to Pharmaceutical Biotechnology, Volume 2: Enzymes, Proteins and Bioinformatics.* IOP Publishing Ltd, Bristol, UK; 2018:1.
131. Bhatia S. *Introduction to Pharmaceutical Biotechnology, Volume 1: Basic Techniques and Concepts.* IOP Publishing Ltd, Bristol, UK; 2018:2.
132. Bhatia S. *Introduction to Pharmaceutical Biotechnology, Volume 3: Animal Tissue Culture Technology.* IOP Publishing Ltd, Bristol, UK; 2019:3.
133. Bhatia S. *Natural Polymer Drug Delivery Systems: Nanotechnology and Its Drug Delivery Applications.* Springer International Publishing, Switzerland; 2016: 1–32.
134. Bhatia S. *Natural Polymer Drug Delivery Systems: Nanoparticles Types, Classification, Characterization, Fabrication Methods and Drug Delivery Applications.* Springer International Publishing, Switzerland; 2016: 33–93.
135. Bhatia S. *Natural Polymer Drug Delivery Systems: Natural Polymers vs Synthetic Polymer.* Springer International Publishing, Switzerland; 2016:95–118.
136. Bhatia S. *Natural Polymer Drug Delivery Systems: Plant Derived Polymers, Properties, and Modification & Applications.* Springer International Publishing, Switzerland; 2016:119–184.
137. Bhatia S. *Natural Polymer Drug Delivery Systems: Marine Polysaccharides Based Nano-Materials and Its Applications.* Springer International Publishing, Switzerland; 2016:185–225.
138. Bhatia S. *Systems for Drug Delivery: Mammalian Polysaccharides and Its Nanomaterials.* Springer International Publishing, Switzerland; 2016:1–27.
139. Bhatia S. *Systems for Drug Delivery: Microbial Polysaccharides as Advance Nanomaterials.* Springer International Publishing, Switzerland; 2016:29–54.
140. Bhatia S. *Systems for Drug Delivery: Chitosan Based Nanomaterials and Its Applications.* Springer International Publishing, Switzerland; 2016:55–117.
141. Bhatia S. *Systems for Drug Delivery: Advance Polymers and Its Applications.* Springer International Publishing, Switzerland; 2016:119–146.
142. Bhatia S. *Systems for Drug Delivery: Advanced Application of Natural Polysaccharides.* Springer International Publishing, Switzerland; 2016:147–170.

143. Bhatia S. *Systems for Drug Delivery: Modern Polysaccharides and Its Current Advancements.* Springer International Publishing, Switzerland; 2016:171–188.
144. Bhatia S. *Systems for Drug Delivery: Toxicity of Nanodrug Delivery Systems.* Springer International Publishing, Switzerland; 2016:189–197.
145. Bhatia S, Sharma K, Bera T. Structural characterization and pharmaceutical properties of porphyran. *Asian J Pharm* 2015;9:93–101.
146. Bhatia S, Sharma A, Sharma K, Kavale M, Chaugule BB, Dhalwal K, Namdeo AG, Mahadik KR. Novel algal polysaccharides from marine source: Porphyran. *Pharmacogn Rev.* 2008;4:271–276.
147. Bhatia S. *Nanotechnology in Drug Delivery Fundamentals, Design, and Applications: Part 1: Protein and Peptide-Based Drug Delivery Systems.* Apple Academic Press, Palm Bay, FL; 2016:50–204.
148. Bhatia S. *Nanotechnology in Drug Delivery Fundamentals, Design, and Applications: Part 2: Peptide-Mediated Nanoparticle Drug Delivery System.* Apple Academic Press, Palm Bay, FL; 2016:205–280.
149. Bhatia S. *Nanotechnology in Drug Delivery Fundamentals, Design, and Applications: Part 3: CPP and CTP in Drug Delivery and Cell Targeting.* Apple Academic Press, Palm Bay, FL; 2016:309–312.
150. Bhatia S. *Systems for Drug Delivery: Safety, Animal, and Microbial Polysaccharides.* Springer Nature, Basingstoke, UK; 2016:122–127.
151. Diamond M, Peniston Feliciano HL, Sanghavi D, et al. *Acute Respiratory Distress Syndrome.* StatPearls Publishing, Treasure Island, FL; 2020. Available from: https://www.ncbi.nlm.nih.gov/books/NBK436002/.
152. Archer SL, Sharp WW, Weir EK. Differentiating COVID-19 pneumonia from acute respiratory distress syndrome and high altitude pulmonary edema: Therapeutic implications. *Circulation.* 2020;142(2):101–104.
153. Tan J, Liu S, Zhuang L, Chen L, Dong M, Zhang J, Xin Y. Transmission and clinical characteristics of asymptomatic patients with SARS-CoV-2 infection. *Future Virol.* 2020. doi: 10.2217/fvl-2020-0087.
154. Knudsen L, Ochs M. The micromechanics of lung alveoli: Structure and function of surfactant and tissue components. *Histochem Cell Biol.* 2018;150(6):661–676.
155. Yang N, Shen HM. Targeting the endocytic pathway and autophagy process as a novel therapeutic strategy in COVID-19. *Int J Biol Sci.* 2020;16(10):1724–1731.
156. Mousavizadeh L, Ghasemi S. Genotype and phenotype of COVID-19: Their roles in pathogenesis. *J Microbiol Immunol Infect.* 2020;54(2):159–163.
157. Romano M, Ruggiero A, Squeglia F, Maga G, Berisio R. A structural view of SARS-CoV-2 RNA replication machinery: RNA synthesis, proofreading and final capping. *Cells.* 2020;9(5):1267.
158. Wang Y, Anirudhan V, Du R, Cui Q, Rong L. RNA-dependent RNA polymerase of SARS-CoV-2 as a therapeutic target. *J Med Virol.* 2021;93(1):300–310.
159. Wiersinga WJ, Rhodes A, Cheng AC, Peacock SJ, Prescott HC. Pathophysiology, transmission, diagnosis, and treatment of coronavirus disease 2019 (COVID-19): A review. *JAMA.* 2020;324(8):782–793.
160. Li G, Fan Y, Lai Y, Han T, Li Z, Zhou P, Pan P, Wang W, Hu D, Liu X, Zhang Q, Wu J. Coronavirus infections and immune responses. *J Med Virol.* 2020;92(4):424–432.
161. Shah VK, Firmal P, Alam A, Ganguly D, Chattopadhyay S. Overview of immune response during SARS-CoV-2 infection: Lessons from the past. *Front Immunol.* 2020;11:1949.
162. Huang C, Wang Y, Li X, Ren L, Zhao J, Hu Y, Zhang L, Fan G, Xu J, Gu X, Cheng Z, Yu T, Xia J, Wei Y, Wu W, Xie X, Yin W, Li H, Liu M, Xiao Y, Gao H, Guo L, Xie J, Wang G, Jiang R, Gao Z, Jin Q, Wang J, Cao B. Clinical features of patients infected with 2019 novel coronavirus in Wuhan, China. *Lancet.* 2020;395(10223):497–506.
163. Huang C, Wang Y, Li X, Ren L, Zhao J, Hu Y, Zhang L, Fan G, Xu J, Gu X, Cheng Z, Yu T, Xia J, Wei Y, Yang X, Yu Y, Xu J, Shu H, Xia J, Liu H, Wu Y, Zhang L, Yu Z, Fang M, Yu T, Wang Y, Pan S, Zou X, Yuan S, Shang Y. Clinical course and outcomes of critically ill patients with SARS-CoV-2 pneumonia in Wuhan, China: A single-centered, retrospective, observational study. *Lancet Respir Med.* 2020;8(5):475–481.
164. Hu D, Zhu C, Ai L, He T, Wang Y, Ye F, Yang L, Ding C, Zhu X, Lv R, Zhu J, Hassan B, Feng Y, Tan W, Wang C. Genomic characterization and infectivity of a novel SARS-like coronavirus in Chinese bats. *Emerg Microbes Infect.* 2018;7(1):154. doi: 10.1038/s41426-018-0155-5. Erratum in: *Emerg Microbes Infect.* 2020;9(1):2727.
165. Carty M, Guy C, Bowie AG. Detection of viral infections by innate immunity. *Biochem Pharmacol.* 2021;183:114316.
166. Kumar S, Nyodu R, Maurya VK, Saxena SK. Host immune response and immunobiology of human SARS-CoV-2 infection. Coronavirus Disease 2019 (COVID-19). 2020:43–53.
167. Wang J, Jiang M, Chen X, Montaner LJ. Cytokine storm and leukocyte changes in mild versus severe SARS-CoV-2 infection: Review of 3939 COVID-19 patients in China and emerging pathogenesis and therapy concepts. *J Leukoc Biol.* 2020;108(1):17–41.
168. Costela-Ruiz VJ, Illescas-Montes R, Puerta-Puerta JM, Ruiz C, Melguizo-Rodríguez L. SARS-CoV-2 infection: The role of cytokines in COVID-19 disease. *Cytokine Growth Factor Rev.* 2020;54:62–75.
169. Tufan A, Avanoğlu Güler A, Matucci-Cerinic M. COVID-19, immune system response, hyperinflammation and repurposing antirheumatic drugs. *Turk J Med Sci.* 2020;50(SI-1):620–632.
170. Del Valle DM, Kim-Schulze S, Huang HH, Beckmann ND, Nirenberg S, Wang B, Lavin Y, Swartz TH, Madduri D, Stock A, Marron TU, Xie H, Patel M, Tuballes K, Van Oekelen O, Rahman A, Kovatch P, Aberg JA, Schadt E, Jagannath S, Mazumdar M, Charney AW, Firpo-Betancourt A, Mendu DR, Jhang J, Reich D, Sigel K, Cordon-Cardo C, Feldmann M, Parekh S, Merad M, Gnjatic S. An inflammatory cytokine signature predicts COVID-19 severity and survival. *Nat Med.* 2020;26(10):1636–1643.
171. Merad M, Martin JC. Author correction: Pathological inflammation in patients with COVID-19: A key role for monocytes and macrophages. *Nat Rev Immunol.* 2020;20(7):448. doi: 10.1038/s41577-020-0353-y. Erratum for: *Nat Rev Immunol.* 2020;20(6):355–362.
172. Du SQ, Yuan W. Mathematical modeling of interaction between innate and adaptive immune responses in COVID-19 and implications for viral pathogenesis. *J Med Virol.* 2020;92(9):1615–1628.

173. Sobral MFF, Duarte GB, da Penha Sobral AIG, Marinho MLM, de Souza Melo A. Association between climate variables and global transmission of SARS-CoV-2. *Sci Total Environ.* 2020;729:138997.
174. Tan J, Mu L, Huang J, Yu S, Chen B, Yin J. An initial investigation of the association between the SARS outbreak and weather: With the view of the environmental temperature and its variation. *J Epidemiol Community Health.* 2005;59(3):186–192.
175. Davis RE, Dougherty E, McArthur C, Huang QS, Baker MG. Cold, dry air is associated with influenza and pneumonia mortality in Auckland, New Zealand. *Influenza Other Respir Viruses.* 2016;10(4):310–313.
176. Ianevski A, Zusinaite E, Shtaida N, Kallio-Kokko H, Valkonen M, Kantele A, Telling K, Lutsar I, Letjuka P, Metelitsa N, Oksenych V, Dumpis U, Vitkauskiene A, Stašaitis K, Öhrmalm C, Bondeson K, Bergqvist A, Cox RJ, Tenson T, Merits A, Kainov DE. Low temperature and low UV indexes correlated with peaks of influenza virus activity in Northern Europe during 2010–2018. *Viruses.* 2019;11(3):207.
177. Yao Y, Pan J, Liu Z, Meng X, Wang W, Kan H, Wang W. No association of COVID-19 transmission with temperature or UV radiation in Chinese cities. *Eur Respir J.* 2020;55(5):2000517.
178. Chin AWH, Chu JTS, Perera MRA, Hui KPY, Yen HL, Chan MCW, Peiris M, Poon LLM. Stability of SARS-CoV-2 in different environmental conditions. *Lancet Microbe.* 2020;1(1):e10.
179. Wu Y, Jing W, Liu J, Ma Q, Yuan J, Wang Y, Du M, Liu M. Effects of temperature and humidity on the daily new cases and new deaths of COVID-19 in 166 countries. *Sci Total Environ.* 2020;729:139051.
180. Sanchez-Lorenzo A, Vaquero-Martínez J, Calbó J, Wild M, Santurtún A, Lopez-Bustins JA, Vaquero JM, Folini D, Antón M. Did anomalous atmospheric circulation favor the spread of COVID-19 in Europe? *Environ Res.* 2020;194:110626.
181. Sajadi MM, Habibzadeh P, Vintzileos A, Shokouhi S, Miralles-Wilhelm F, Amoroso A. Temperature, humidity, and latitude analysis to estimate potential spread and seasonality of coronavirus disease 2019 (COVID-19). *JAMA Netw Open.* 2020;3(6):e2011834.
182. Qi H, Xiao S, Shi R, Ward MP, Chen Y, Tu W, Su Q, Wang W, Wang X, Zhang Z. COVID-19 transmission in Mainland China is associated with temperature and humidity: A time-series analysis. *Sci Total Environ.* 2020;728:138778.
183. Luo W, Maimuna S. Majumder, Diambo Liu, Canelle Poirier, Kenneth D Mandl, Marc Lipsitch, Mauricio Santillana. The role of absolute humidity on transmission rates of the COVID-19 outbreak. medRxiv. 2020.
184. Jüni P, Rothenbühler M, Bobos P, Thorpe KE, da Costa BR, Fisman DN, Slutsky AS, Gesink D. Impact of climate and public health interventions on the COVID-19 pandemic: A prospective cohort study. *CMAJ.* 2020;192(21): E566–E573.
185. Islam N, Shabnam S, Erzurumluoglu AM. Temperature, humidity, and wind speed are associated with lower COVID-19 incidence. medRxiv. 2020.
186. Mansouri Daneshvar MR, Ebrahimi M, Sadeghi A, Mahmoudzadeh A. Climate effects on the COVID-19 outbreak: A comparative analysis between the UAE and Switzerland. *Model Earth Syst Environ.* 2021:1–14. https://pubmed.ncbi.nlm.nih.gov/33521243/
187. Zhang C, Liao H, Strobl E, Li H, Li R, Jensen SS, Zhang Y. The role of weather conditions in COVID-19 transmission: A study of a global panel of 1236 regions. *J Clean Prod.* 2021;292:125987.
188. Diao Y, Kodera S, Anzai D, Gomez-Tames J, Rashed EA, Hirata A. Influence of population density, temperature, and absolute humidity on spread and decay durations of COVID-19: A comparative study of scenarios in China, England, Germany, and Japan. *One Health.* 2020; 12:100203.

4

Epidemiology, Clinical Manifestations, Diagnostic Approaches, and Preventive Measures for COVID-19

Ahmed Al-Harrasi
Natural and Medical Sciences Research Center, University of Nizwa

Saurabh Bhatia
Natural and Medical Sciences Research Center, University of Nizwa
University of Petroleum and Energy Studies

Md. Tanvir Kabir
BRAC University

Tapan Behl
Chitkara University

Deepak Kaushik
M.D. University

CONTENTS

4.1 Introduction

The emergence of coronavirus disease 2019 (COVID-19) was initially reported in the Wuhan South China Seafood Wholesale Market, where almost 49%–66% of patients were infected due to their contact history of the Wuhan Seafood Wholesale Market [1]. This emergence of SARS-CoV-2 from Wuhan, China, and its clinical expression in the form of COVID-19 has now spread across the world, and resulted in fear of global outbreak, a pandemic, or death [1]. Based on the previous reports, the COVID-19 was originally correlated with bats, as they are host to more than 30 coronaviruses [1]. RNA-dependent RNA polymerase (RdRp) of RaTG13, which is a SARS-related coronavirus found in bats, is close to that of the

DOI: 10.1201/9781003175933-5

SARS-CoV-2 virus with 96.2% to 98.7% similarity in genomic sequences [2]. bat-SL-CoVZXC21 and bat-SL-CoVZC45 are other bat-originated SARS-like viruses that are closer to coronavirus 2 than coronavirus 1 and MERS-CoV, with almost 88% similarity in genome sequences [2]. Recent studies also revealed Pangolin-CoV is 91.02% and 90.55% similar to coronavirus 2 and BatCoV RaTG13 [3]. Apart from the similarity of the SARS-CoV-2 genome with RaTG13, Pangolin-CoV is the most closely related to SARS-CoV-2 [3]. Moreover, it was found that the surface spike protein (S1 protein) of Pangolin-CoV is more similar to SARS-CoV-2 than to RaTG13 [3]. Five key amino acid residues participating in the interaction with human ACE2 are consistent with Pangolin-CoV and SARS-CoV-2; however, four amino acid mutations have been found in RaTG13 [4]. Thus, based on current reports, it is accepted that bats are considered as the original host for SARS-CoV-2; nevertheless, the Wuhan Huanan Seafood Marketplace is not the single reason SARS-CoV-2 is increasing worldwide. The transmission of SARS-CoV-2 in an indoor as well as outdoor environment is a critical component of an epidemic as transmission rate determines the extent of outbreak of any disease. In nature, survival of a virus depends on its transmission from one host to another, whether of the same or another species. Its transmission among human beings is mediated by droplet and/or infected surface or fomite, fecal–oral, and blood-borne [5]. However, it is still uncertain whether transmission between human beings can be effected via the aforementioned modes. The World Health Organization (WHO) revealed that SARS-CoV-2 might also spread through aerosols in the absence of aerosol-generating procedures, mainly in indoor settings with poor ventilation [5]. The R0 value, already discussed in the previous chapter, is 2.1; and it could be as high as 5.7 [6]. The R0 (reproduction number/rate) is a valuable parameter of transmission that is used to determine the contagiousness and transmissibility of infectious pathogens [6,7]. The R0 value is usually estimated to detect the average number of cases caused by person (infected) in a fully susceptible community [6,7]. If $R0 > 1$, then human-to-human transmission may occur. It was noticed that asymptomatic patients are considered as super communicator as they infect more than 100 individuals at times. The virus mortality rate varies among different ages and counties [8]. According to the WHO, globally, as of 2:19 pm CEST, August 2, 2020, there have been 17,660,523 confirmed cases of COVID-19, including 680,894 deaths (WHO [9]). Data that were available until March 3, 2020, also suggested that out of the 90,870 confirmed cases with 3.4% mortality, the average age of individuals ranged from 41 to 57 years, whereas based on gender, male confirmed cases were more (50%–75%). It was also found that almost 25.2%–50.5% SARS-CoV-2-affected individuals have one or more health complications. The mean incubation period of COVID-19 patients from the time of its introduction to illness inception was 3.0 days among 1,099 cases and 4.0 days among 62 cases, whereas the longest incubation period reported so far was 24 days [10]. This chapter discusses the distribution, clinical presentation, diagnosis, treatment, medical conditions of COVID-19, preventive measures, life support systems, vaccine development, biotechnological interventions, and imaging findings of COVID-19.

4.2 Epidemiology of COVID-19

The WHO announced the outbreak caused by coronavirus-2 as coronavirus infection 2019 (COVID-19). This infectious disease has been transmitted extensively worldwide, impacting more than 70 nations. Various phases, clinical manifestations, diagnostic tools, and imaging findings of COVID-19 progression are illustrated in Figure 4.1 [11–18].

Figure 4.1 demonstrates four important advanced phases of the viral infection, based on stage of disease, clinical manifestations and symptoms, host response against infection, diagnostic as well as imaging outcomes. This illustration is divided into five different sections representing different phases of COVID-19 in context with its severity (clinical manifestations) and development of imaging as well as diagnostic tools. Depending upon the severity of the disease, the progression of COVID-19 is represented in different phases. The initial incubation phase for this viral infection is the first stage, which is the time interval between exposure of an individual to SARS-CoV-2 (becoming infected) and symptom onset. This interval varies between 5 and 10 days but can extend up to 14 days. During this phase, some individuals present symptoms and some do not; however, both types of individuals remain contagious and can transfer infection to others. In phase I (4–10 days), virus replication and shedding quickly accelerate (phase I) along with structural changes in the host cells resulting from viral infection. Cytopathic effect caused by the virus triggers various immunological reactions in phase II. Stimulation of immune reaction results in the progression of an infection from mild to moderate to eventually severe multisystem inflammatory syndrome (MIS). Phase II includes shortness of breath with or without hypoxia with clinical signs of pneumonia. This viral pneumonia due to hyperinflammation can turn into severe pneumonia or acute respiratory distress syndrome (ARDS). Cytokine storm further promotes the inflammatory phase resulting in hyperinflammation. This stage can progress into phase III resulting in the production of non-neutralizing antibodies, which can further lead to antibody-dependent increase of inflammation with local thrombosis and sepsis resulting in the following:

- multiple organ dysfunction syndrome (MODS)
- ARDS
- acute kidney injury (AKI)
- deep vein thrombosis (DVT)
- pulmonary embolism (PE)

Various molecular markers such as white blood count (WBC), procalcitonin (PCT), non–vitamin K antagonist oral anticoagulant (NOAC), natrium (Na), natural killer (NK), low-molecular-weight heparin (LMWH), lactate dehydrogenase (LDH), interleukin (IL), immunoglobulin G (IgG), immunoglobulin (Ig), high-sensitivity cardiac troponin I (hs-cTnI), erythrocyte sedimentation rate (ESR), creatinine (C), creatine kinase (CK), C-reactive protein (CRP), B-type natriuretic peptide (BNP), blood urea nitrogen (BUN), aspartate aminotransferase (AST), and alanine aminotransferase (ALT) as well as their respective expression varies among different individuals; however, some

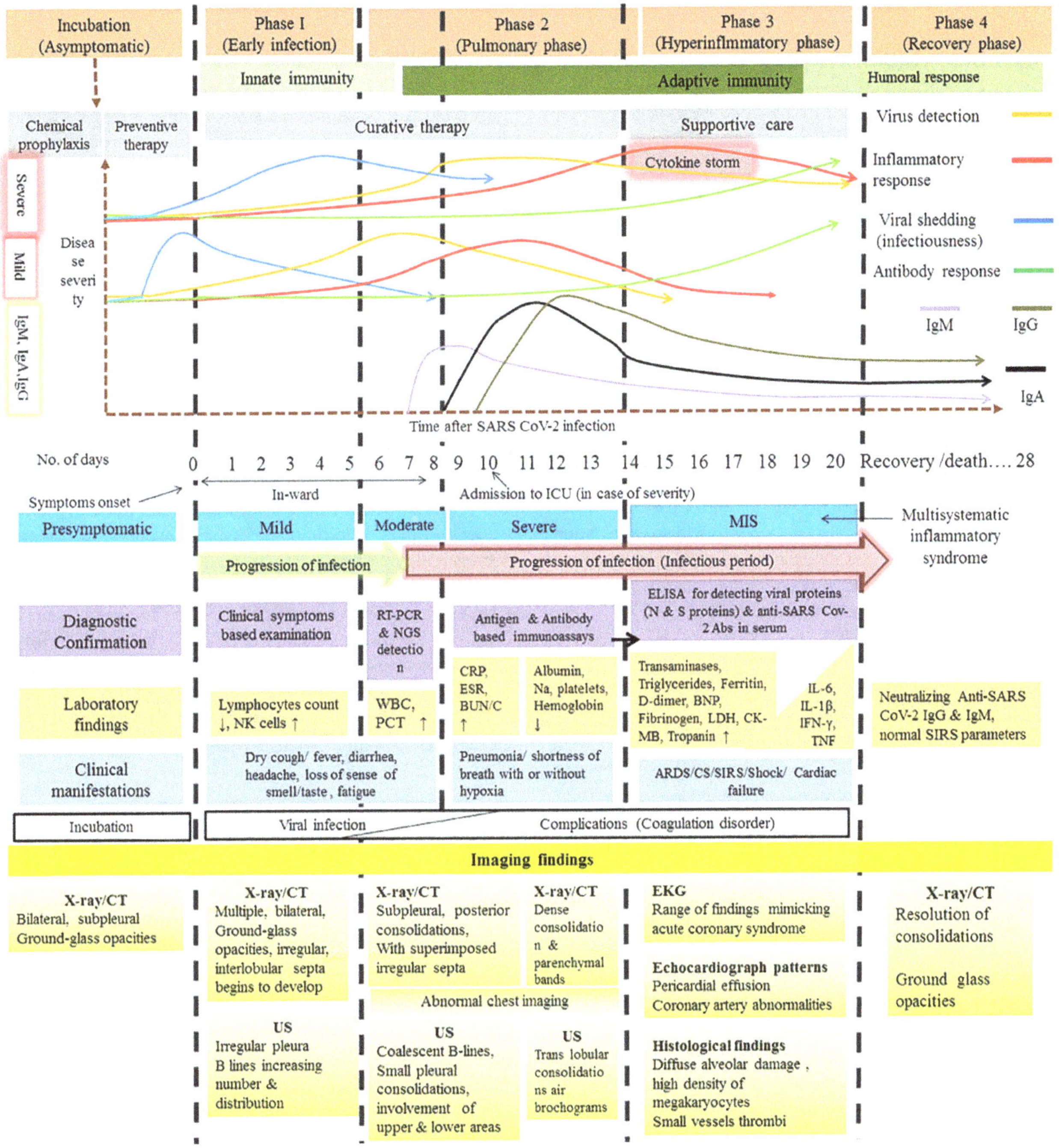

FIGURE 4.1 Different phases, clinical manifestations, diagnostic tools, and imaging findings of COVID-19 progression [11–18].

of the common findings are illustrated above. These are widely used biomarkers to assess the risk of COVID infection and its progression to systemic inflammatory response syndrome (SIRS), for example.

Most importantly, specific antibodies' response (IgM, IgA, IgG) to SARS-CoV-2 starts after the 7th day of infection. The onset of IgM-mediated specific response starts and peaks within 7 days of infection, and production persists as far as the acute infection continues. The onset of IgA and IgG antibody production usually takes place numerous days after IgM. Presently, the detection of coronavirus-2 RNAs is considered as a usual method for COVID-19 diagnosis. Nevertheless, there is a serious requirement for consistent and quick serological diagnostic methods to screen SARS-CoV-2-infected individuals including asymptomatic. Most test kits contain indicator lines for both IgM and IgG antibodies, which are important for the determination of immunity titers months and years after COVID-19 infection or vaccination. The majority of investigations have demonstrated serological examination based on the detection of SARS-CoV-2-specific IgM and IgG. However, the examination of SARS-CoV-2-specific IgA in the serum of COVID-19 patients has been done only in a few studies. Thus, serological (blood) detection of IgM, IgA, and IgG is essential in determining recovery of the patients as well as progression or severity of infection. It was found that among mild as well as acute COVID-19 patients, serum IgM and IgG were considerably higher in comparison with mild cases; however, no major difference has been seen between severe and moderate patients. It has been discovered that the levels of IgA in acute cases are considerably higher in comparison with mild cases. Another study showed that coronavirus-2-specific antibodies reactions include IgG, IgM, and IgA, IgA is responsible for the neutralization of SARS-CoV-2 to a greater extent than IgG. It has also been found that specific IgA serum levels reduced considerably one month after the onset of symptoms; however, neutralizing IgA remained detectable in saliva for a longer period [11–13].

Figure 4.1 also shows the importance of imaging and diagnostic procedures such as X-rays, ultrasound (US), reverse transcription polymerase chain reaction (RT-PCR), CRP, level of triglycerides (TG), and computer-based tomography (CT) in determining the progression of infection [14–18].

Presently, there are various studies which have been reported by different researchers in an attempt to explore effective diagnostic and treatment strategies against COVID-19. However, this chapter focuses on transmission, clinical manifestations, diagnosis, treatment, and medical conditions associated with COVID-19. Additionally, various biotechnological interventions against COVID-19 are also discussed.

4.3 Clinical Manifestations

The reported clinical symptoms and radiological abnormalities may vary among SARS-CoV-2 infected indviduals as the severity of this infection vary from moderate infection to acute pneumonia with multiple organ failure and can also asymptomatic.

Lirong Zou et al. [19] suggested that symptomatic and asymptomatic patients showed similar viral load and viral RNA in the respiratory secretions of asymptomatic patients. Therefore, asymptomatic or symptomatic patients both have transmission potential. The most common clinical symptoms reported so far are cough (59.4%–81.8%), dyspnea (3.2%–55.0%), fatigue (38.1%–69.6%), fever (77.4%–98.6%), muscle pain (11.1%–34.8%), production of sputum (28.25–56.5%), and head pain (6.55–33.9%) [20–22]. However, some of the symptoms evidenced are diarrhea, vomiting, nausea, chest pain, hemoptysis, conjunctival congestion, rhinorrhea, and sore throat. One report showed that out of 140 confirmed COVID-19 cases 39.6% showed gastrointestinal (GI) symptoms [36] and in Wang's study [22] 10.1% of patients had GI discomfort. In some confirmed COVID-19 cases, did not have a fever initially but did so after hospitalization and a number of severe patients did not have fever at all [23]. Similar clinical symptoms such as fever, cough, myalgia, and dyspnea were found among SARS-CoV-2, SARS-CoV, and MERS-CoV patients. Nevertheless, GI complications among SARS and MERS patients are more common than among SARS-CoV-2 patients. It was found that out of 95 patients, 61% of patients presented GI symptoms and 49.5% developed the GI symptoms during hospitalization. Diarrhea was one of the most common clinical symptoms presented by 24.2% of cases, whereas other patients also presented anorexia (17.9%) and nausea (17.9%). Moreover, episodes of diarrhea substantially increased after using various drugs including antibiotics. Stool examination of 65 hospitalized patients revealed that 42 showed GI symptoms out of which 22 were COVID positive [24]. Endoscopy data obtained from the same study revealed that few patients showed esophageal bleeding with erosions and ulcers. Based on the examination of esophagus, stomach, duodenum, and rectum specimens in two severe patients, it was revealed that SARS-CoV-2 RNA was detected in all specimens. As far as the effects on the renal system are concerned, the frequency of renal failure among MERS patients is high, as it has become one of the main clinical features of MERS, which is not often presented by coronavirus patients [25,26].

Based on several reports, it has been concluded that individuals of all age groups are vulnerable to COVID-19 infection; nevertheless, elderly age groups with comorbidities are more vulnerable and subsequently develop severe symptoms of acute pneumonia, pulmonary edema, ARDS, multiple organ failure, and death. It was also found that in comparison with non-pregnant women, pregnant women are more severely affected by SARS viruses. White blood cell counts increased and levels of CRP in the serum were found to be higher than the levels found in common pregnancy, whereas a considerable decrease in lymphocyte counts was also observed.

COVID-19 immunopathology is the response of the immune system against coronavirus 2. SARS-CoV-2 invades the host via triggering the immune system resulting in uncontrolled inflammatory responses, lymphocytopenia, high cytokine levels, and increased antibodies. The most prominent immuno-invasion processes observed in patients and their associated clinical outcomes and associated manifestations are illustrated in Figure 4.2.

4.4 Laboratory and Radiologic Characteristics

Laboratory investigations have revealed that during the initial stage of the infection patient blood samples present normal or decreased WBC with a considerable drop in lymphocyte count. Out of positive cases, a higher number of the patients presented with lymphopenia (35.3%–82.1%); however, 5.0%–36.2% suffered from thrombocytopenia and 9.1%–33.7% had leucopenia [20,27,34–36]. Chen's research showed that some of the COVID-19 patients also showed a high range of serum ferritin, CRP, interleukin-6, and ESR[21]. A lot of COVID-19 patients also presented high levels of ALT, AST, CK, LDH, D-dimer, and prolonged prothrombin time [37]. Nevertheless, patients also showed rare laboratory findings such as high creatinine, procalcitonin, and troponin I levels [38]. Radiological examination based on CT of lungs showed typical characteristics for novel SARS-CoV-2 pneumonia such as ground-glass like opacity (hazy opacity of lungs parenchyma through which underlying airway and pulmonary blood vessels remain visible), bilateral patchy shadows (air sacs of the lungs that often appear patchy or opaque), and subsegmental areas of consolidation (compressible lung tissue that has filled with liquid instead of air) occasionally with a rounded structure as well as a peripheral distribution [39,40]. A CT scan examination reported on 21 novel coronavirus pneumonia cases revealed that the complications in lungs were serious for almost 10 days following the onset of early symptoms. Radiological-based examination of lungs revealed the information in the form of image

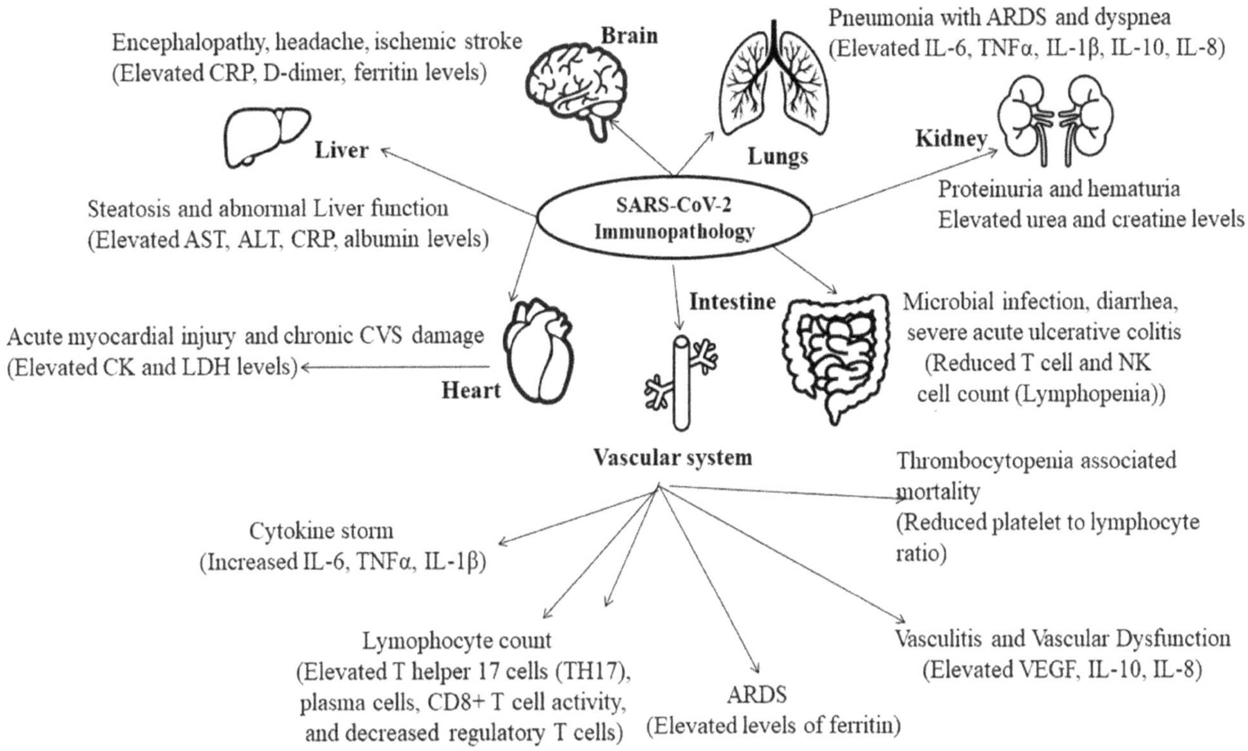

FIGURE 4.2 Immunopathology of SARS-CoV-2 in humans [20,27–34].

or radiograph done by a more suitable technique, chest CT (particularly high resolution CT) then X-ray plays an important role in screening and diagnosis of COVID-19 patients. Radiographic changes help in diagnosis and to check the development of disease, mainly its severity in terms of implications of the inflammatory storm caused by the viral replication over lung tissue exudation, proliferation, and metamorphism. Some of the important implications are as follows [41]:

- Ground-glass opacity is due to the leakage of the alveolar cavity caused by the invasion of the virus, which may lead to inflammation in the alveoli.
- Consolidation and air bronchi sign is an inflammatory progression due to patient response against hyperinflammatory reaction, which can lead to significant exudation in the alveolar sacs of lungs, presented by "white lung" performance.
- Halo appearance is a lesion in the center represented by cloud-like ground-glass shadow may be due to virus replication in epithelial cells and its implications.
- Paving stone sign can be detected by high-resolution CT that involves pathological findings such as lobular intervals and interlobular interstitial thickening and suggesting interstitial changes.
- Fibrous lesions form during lung tissue repair and heal during chronic inflammation or enlargement of lung tissue when normal cellular components are slowly replaced by fibrous components to form scars.
- Vascular thickening can be observed at the periphery or in the center of the lesion during the progression of disease.

CT examination for COVID-19 patients is required to reveal the occurrence of lesions in the lungs and the progression of the illness, and it is a reliable method to diagnose when virus nucleic acid test fails to detect viral RNA [42]. Assesment of image can be compared from nucleic acid detection (with high specificity and a low sensitivity of 30%–50%) which is considered as one of the main diagnostic tools for diagnosis of COVID-19 [43]. Because of the low sensitivity of the nucleic acid test, other clinical and imaging-based findings are supportive in the screening of COVID-19 patients so that suspected patients should not be housed with positive cases of COVID-19 to avoid the transmission of this disease. As a nucleic acid test can be negative in positive COVID-19 patients, overdependence on nucleic acid tests can result in misdiagnosis of patients who are actually COVID-19 positive. Moreover, this can also be utilized to study the effects of various therapeutics over the lungs of infected patients [43].

4.5 Pathological Studies

A lung biopsy investigation of a COVID-19 patient revealed the release of fluid from low-grade sarcoma with fibrous and myxoid areas, represented as cellular fibromyxoid exudates along with diffuse alveolar damage caused by acute interstitial pneumonia [44,45]. The formation of hyaline membrane along the walls of the alveoli (restricting the exchange of gasses), pulmonary edema, acute diffuse alveolar damage, fibrin deposition, desquamation of pneumocytes, and proteinaceous exudates are the severe or acute pulmonary stage signs of COVID-19 [46]. Flow cytometric findings of blood samples revealed the low value of peripheral CD4 as well as CD8 T cells but a hyperactivated level [47]. It was also reported that the extent of lymphocytopenia as well as hyperproduction of cytokines is higher among patients suffering from acute COVID-19 in comparison to those with mild disease and is associated with the severity of the disease. Neutrophil: CD8+ T lymphocytes as well as neutrophil: lymphocyte ratio can be considered as an important factor for the early detection of acute COVID-19 individuals [48]. Moreover, a considerable drop in the number of T lymphocytes, particularly CD8+ T lymphocytes, with a rise in neutrophil counts and high levels of interleukins (–6, –10, –2, –γ) in blood samples has also been found [49]. Systemic anatomy investigation based on autopsy from the other patient showed gray, white patchy injuries in lungs, scarring across the lungs, white viscous fluid spread out in the lung tissue, and appearance of fiber bands [49]. This indicates damage caused by SARS-CoV-2-induced inflammatory responses to deep airways and alveolar space of infected lungs. Pathological findings were found to be similar among SARS-CoV and MERS-CoV patients, but it was later found that pulmonary scarring across the lungs as well as consolidation were not more acute than found with SARS, but leakage of fluid was more visible [49].

4.6 Diagnostic Tools

The COVID-19 pandemic has had a major effect on clinical microbiology-based diagnostic centers as they have faced major difficulties in the lab-based diagnosis of infectious COVID-19. International health organizations are updating and issuing new regulations for all the laboratories in order to develop and implement COVID-19 reliable diagnostic tests. Based on the progression of the disease, the diagnosis of COVID-19 is categorized as preanalytical, analytical, and postanalytical [50,51]. During the preanalytical stage, timely and safe collection of a suitable sample from the respiratory tract is important for a quick and exact diagnosis of COVID-19. Collection of nasopharyngeal specimens requires special sampling room facility, stringent sterilization procedures, proper guidance of paramedical staff, development of personal precautionary measures, standardization of procedures for collection of sample (or swab), and submission of samples in a timely manner with all safety precautions [50,51]. Apart from swabs from nasal and throat routes, swabs collected from nasopharyngeal is a key procedure of nucleic acid-based assessment of SARS Cov-2 infection. This approach of sampling requires proper training of those are in close contact with the patient [50,51]. The report [52] recommends that the best approach for detecting or screening of COVID-19 is real-time fluorescence-based PCR of samples from the upper respiratory tract (such as nasal, throat and nasopharyngeal swabs), samples from the lower respiratory tract (such as bronchoalveolar lavage), as well as blood or samples from urine, stool, etc. Presently, the nucleic acid-based analysis of COVID-19 primarily entails nasopharyngeal swabs. Sample collection from susceptible individual is done via nasopharyngeal swab in an open setting, which can cause production or droplets or aerosol. During this procedure, close contact between COVID-19 patients and medical staff can increase the risk of transmission. Most healthcare settings use special rooms for collection of samples. Procedures for the collection of different respiratory tract samples (lower as well as upper) and from other routes are also mentioned [52]. Thus, suitable measures must be used to keep lab and medical staff safe as well as to produce reliable test results.

During the analytical stage, most sensitive and specific method for the amplification and detection of viral RNA, i.e., modification of PCR technique, termed as reverse transcription (RT)-PCR, is used [50,51]. This procedure involves using RNA-dependent DNA polymerase (reverse transcriptase) to copy RNA into DNA (cDNA) and Taq polymerase to amplify the cDNA. RT-PCR is a molecular test to qualitatively detect the nucleic acid from SARS-CoV-2 in both upper and lower respiratory specimens [50,51]. Accessed specimens can be from nasopharyngeal or oropharyngeal swabs, sputum, tracheal secretions, and bronchoalveolar washing [50,51]. In addition, serological examinations such as antibody-based techniques can be used in supplementation with RT-PCR. The analytical stage is followed by the postanalytical stage where the interpretation of the results is based on RT-PCR and serological results. A number of procedures as well as the portable devices are currently available and some are in development for rapid as well as correct detection of COVID-19 infections [53]. Finally, random-access integrated, point-of-care molecular devices for quick and accurate diagnosis of SARS-CoV-2 infections are available for this stage. Laboratory procedures for SARS-CoV-2 diagnosis, especially recommendations on the interpretation of laboratory results and laboratory test result criteria for confirming or rejecting the diagnosis of SARS, are available on the WHO website [54] so that COVID-19 infected individuals across the world can be detected on the basis of these criteria. Confirmed cases or positive cases with SARS-CoV-2 infection were defined on the basis of positive report diagnosed from either high-throughput sequencing or real-time RT-PCR test of samples from susceptible COVID-19 cases. Considering the radiological examinations, CT scan or radiograph is considered as a diagnostic tool for COVID-19 with a high sensitivity, is being given more important value for diagnosis [55]. In one study based on the examination of 1,014 susceptible patients, 601 (59%) had positive RT-PCR reports and 888 (88%) had positive chest CT scans, suggesting that for the diagnosis of COVID-19, chest CT has greater sensitivity and can be considered as a key technique for the diagnosis of COVID-19 [56]. Another study conducted on 106 susceptible patients showed that estimating the volume of disease by CT technique along with the help of clinical data predicts SARS-CoV-2 burden, which allows precise forecast of short-term clinical outcome [57].

4.7 Therapeutics, Sanitization, Personal Protective Equipment (PPE), and Life Support Systems for the Prevention and Treatment of COVID-19

Presently due to the lack of availability of potential antiviral therapy and vaccine, actual pathogenesis and proliferation pathways followed by SARS-CoV-2 are still a mystery. Due to this, more emphasis is given on prevention via PPE as well as sanitization. Life support systems, mainly oxygen-based treatment via ventilator, are required to support the respiratory system of severely ill hypoxemic patients [58]. However, patients with whom COVID-19 caused acute respiratory (hypoxemic) collapse, conventional oxygen therapy may not be adequate to fulfill oxygen demands [59]. Thus, other approaches such as high-flow nasal cannula (HFNC), non-invasive positive pressure ventilation (NIPPV), or intubation and invasive mechanical ventilation (IMV) can be used to provide immediate support system [59]. Just like oxygen therapy and artificial ventilation are the primary tools used during respiratory failure, hemodynamic and renal support systems are also important for septic shock management [60]. Ventilation is considered as a life-supporting therapy that involves mainly non-invasive ventilation (NIV) and invasive mechanical ventilation (IMV) support for the treatment of ARDS. As per reports NIV offer less unfavorable outcomes for patients in contrast to IMV [61]. Nevertheless, NIV increases the chances of transmission of infection to healthcare workers dealing with infected patients due to the chances of SARS-CoV-2 transmission by aerosols [62,63]. However, the scale of this risk of transmission of COVID-19 via NIV is not yet well evidenced. On the contrary, IMV reduces the risk of transmission via aerosols as it usually uses a closed system [62,63]. However, nations with higher numbers of COVID-19 cases experience shortage of ventilators (mechanical ventilation) and thus rely more on NIV. As has been reported, HFNC oxygen and NIPPV are preferable to conventional oxygen therapy as these procedures reduce the need for intubation (insertion of a tube via mouth for the placement of a patient on a ventilator) and therapeutic escalation in patients [64]. According to unblinded clinical trial reports (conducted before the COVID-19 pandemic) available on patients with acute hypoxemic respiratory failure, HFNC is preferred over NIPPV [65]. Early intubation among ARDS patients is suitable when patients have chronic comorbidities or acute organ dysfunction or if HFNC and NIPPV are not available [66]. It was also reported that the failure rate of NIPPV among non-COVID-19 viral pneumonia and ARDS patients is high. This is due to the production of aerosols, which can spread from an infected patient to others, and thus increases the risk of transmission of COVID-19; however, transmission from patients who underwent HFNC is still not clear. To improve oxygenation and decrease the risk for intubation and mortality among COVID-19 patients with severe hypoxic respiratory failure, an adjunct therapy, namely prone positioning (lying facing chest down), which has been used since the 1970s to treat severe hypoxemia patients, was explored [67]. Proning, or prone positioning, enhances the level of oxygen at a systemic level and improves patient outcomes among ARDS patients as it increases ventilation-perfusion fitting and involves damaged alveoli in the lungs (dorsal site) [67]. However, prone positioning is not suitable for individuals in respiratory distress (acute) mainly ARDS and those who need instant endotracheal intubation. Moreover, this therapy is also not recommended for patients with hemodynamically instability, patients with complications related to the spine, or those who have just had stomach surgery [67]. Thus, for proning, patients who can change positions on their own and those who can tolerate lying face down position are considered good candidates for this therapy. For pregnant patients, awake prone positioning is acceptable and possible as it can be carried out in the left lateral decubitus position when the surface of the body is closest to the flat surface or else the completely prone anatomical position [68]. To avoid the risk of transmission to healthcare workers while administering oxygen via nasal cannula/HFNC/CPAP/NIV/nebulization of drugs with jet nebulizer and ventilatory support, exhaled air dispersion distance from human patient simulator can be determined by means of a laser smoke visualization procedure in a negative pressure room [69]. This estimates the minimum distance required to maintain distance from an infected patient. However, transmission is also dependent on other factors such as the duration of exposure, the level of hygiene and sanitization, the availability of PPE, air condition, and spacing of rooms where infected patients are placed. Thus, as per the recommendations of the WHO and other scientific bodies, three categories have been made to minimize the risk of spread of infection [69]:

- Standard oxygen therapy or HFNC oxygen therapy, positive airway pressure (CPAP) therapy, and invasive artificial airway therapy (NIV).
- Precautions to reduce transmission of infection via contact/droplets.
- Safety measures to reduce the risk of transmission from aerosol-generating procedures (such as endotracheal intubation, suctioning, and nasopharyngeal aspiration/swabbing) among COVID-19 patients.

Maximum exhaled air dispersion distance must be carefully measured especially when using oxygen and ventilatory support given to infected patients by health care workers those are caring or in close contact with them [69]. This can be studied in a negative-pressure room or isolation rooms (where lower air pressure guarantees that air from rooms with infected patients is not recirculated into other areas of the hospital) on a human patient simulator that represents a 70 kg (adult male) in a semi-sitting position on a hospital bed inclined at the 45° angle [69]. Exhaled air dispersion space from the human patient simulator is assessed by means of laser smoke visualization procedure [70]. It is always recommended to place infected patients in a quarantine facility with negative pressure (no less than 12 air shifts per hour); however, if this facility is not available, then a quarantine facility with normal ventilation (minimum airflow 160 L/s per patient) should be considered [69]. The transmission rate of nosocomial infection is dependent on the exhaled aerosol size, which is further dependent on environmental conditions such as air flow, air pressure, temperature humidity of the rook and attributes of the fluid, as well as the force applied by the patient during coughing or emission [69]. Various precautionary steps in or outside hospital settings must be taken to minimize transmission of COVID-19 via aerosol.

PPE such as gloves, disposable shirts, goggles, masks, and respirators are considered as an effective means to prevent infection [71,72]. Medical or surgical masks could be used whereas masks made with cotton or gauze fabric are not recommended as they do not guarantee protection from the virus [71,72]. To seal the wearer's face and to protect from dust or fibers suspended in the air, tight masks in the form of respirators are recommended. Ventilators are classified on the basis of pressure, volume, or flow controller, whereas masks are classified on the basis of their filtration efficiency [73,74]. The American system categorizes ventilators mainly based on the proportion of particles with a size (dia. >0.3 μm) that can be passed via material of the masks, whereas the European system classified on the basis of filtration efficiency in the form of filtering face piece mask (FFP1/2/3 based on European standard 2009) [75]. The American and European classifications for face masks depending upon their respirator filtration efficiency are illustrated in Figure 4.3 [76]. Until now, no potential vaccine and antiviral treatment are available against SARS-CoV-2, and the prevention of further transmission is a practical approach to controlling the ongoing and future outbreaks. Another measure to eliminate or minimize SARS-CoV-2 transmission from vehicles, skin, mucosa (oral or nasal), atmosphere, and surfaces is sanitization. Other than transmission of infection from infected COVID-19 patients, SARS-CoV-2-contaminated dry surfaces can also serve as a source for transmission of coronaviruses. Thus, the inactivation of coronaviruses over animate or inanimate objects by disinfectants or biocides agents approved by the EPA is a good approach to decreasing virus spread. US EPA-certified disinfecting and sanitizing products, nasal sprays, and mouthwashes can be utilized to minimize human-to-human spread [77]. As per reports, povidone-iodine, ethanol at high proportion (>70%), hypochlorite, as well as quaternary ammonium compounds mixed with alcohol are effective against coronavirus 2 for disinfection of surfaces, whereas ozone, chlorine dioxide, hydrogen peroxide vapor, and ultraviolet radiations can be used to minimize viral load in air with suitable safety measures to avoid contact of susceptible individual against these agents [78]. Social distancing, hand washing, and sanitization are commonly implemented practices to prevent transmission of the COVID-19 infection from asymptomatic people with high load of virus in their nasal cavity. Nevertheless, therapeutic treatment which should be safe and effective is immediately required at this stage for the treatment of COVID-19. The various therapeutics available, such as standard medications, monoclonal antibodies,

Clinical development of the therapeutics for COVID-19

THERAPEUTICS UNDER DEVELOPMENT

Antiparasitic (chloroquine or hydroxychloroquine)
Antiviral (Remdesivir, Favipiravir, Ribavirin, Galidesivir, Interferon α/β, Nitazoxanide, Umifenovir, Clevudine, Arbidol, Ivermectin, Nitazoxanide, Darunavir, Lopinavir, ritonavir, BLD-2660, SARS-CoV-2 main protease inhibitor 11a and 11b)
Renin-angiotensin-aldosterone system inhibitors
Recombinant human angiotensin-converting enzyme 2
ACE/ACE receptor inhibitors (Losartan, Telmisartan)
Angiotensin II receptor-blocker (Camostat mesylate)
Janus kinases inhibitor (Baricitinib, Ruxolitinib, upadacitinib and filgotinib)
Anti-influenza (Umifenovir/Arbidol)
Interleukin-6 inhibitors (IL-6 monoclonal antibodies, Tocilizumab)
Interleukin-1 inhibitors (IL-1 monoclonal antibodies)
Interleukin-17 inhibitors (IL-17 monoclonal antibodies)
Interleukin (IL)-1β blocker (Canakinumab)
Steroids (Tacrolimus, Prednisolone, Dexamethasone, Methylprednisolone)
Vaccine (ChAdOx1 nCoV-19 Vaccine, Artificial Antigen Presenting Cell Vaccine, BCG vaccine, Bifidobacteria monovalent SARS-CoV-2 DNA oral vaccine, INO-4800, vaccine mRNA-1273, trimerized SARS-CoV-2 S protein, RBD-based SARS-CoV vaccine, live influenza vaccine, adenovirus-vectored vaccine using AdVac®/PER.C6® vaccine, Ad5-nCoV, two lentivirus vector-based vaccine candidates, COVID-19/aAPC and LV-SMENP-DC, COVID-19/aAPC, LV-SMENP DC vaccine, adjuvants including MF59, AS03 and CpG 1018, Huaier Granule)
Bruton's tyrosine kinase inhibitor (Acalabrutinib)
Convalescent plasma or hyperimmune immunoglobulin therapy (Plasma containing Abs, cytokines, protein C&S, albumin, clotting or anti clotting factors)
Stem cell therapy (Human Mesenchymal Stem Cells, Allogeneic Mesenchymal Stromal Cells, FT516 - induced pluripotent stem cell)
Antipsychotics (Chlorpromazine)
Antiangiogenic (Lenalidomide)
Anti-inflammatory (Piclidenoson)
Phosphodiesterase inhibitor (Sildenafil citrate)
Cholesterol lowering drugs (Atorvastatin)
Alpha-blockers and Antihypertensive drug (Prazosin)
Anticancer (Bortezomib)

Personal protective, sanitization and life supportive facilities

LIFE SUPPORTIVE & PPE facilities

Noninvasive ventilation via full-face mask (via helmets)
O_2 therapy via nasal cannula [via oronasal mask; via Venturi mask via non-rebreathing mask}; High-flow nasal cannula therapy; Continuous Positive Airway Pressure (via oronasal mask, via nasal cannula); Bilevel positive airway pressure

Invasive mechanical ventilation (lower tidal volumes, lower inspiratory pressure, prone position, conservative fluid management strategy, extracorporeal membrane oxygenation)
Restrictive fluid resuscitation

PPE (personal protective equipment) masks and respirators:
American classification system [N95 (≥95), N99 (≥99)}
European classification system [FFP1 (≥80), FFP2 (≥94), FFP3 (≥99)]
Components of personal protective equipment (PPE)
- Respiratory protection (FFP2 or FFP3 respirator)
- Eye protection (Goggles or face shield)
- Body protection (Long-sleeved water-resistant gown)
- Hand protection (Gloves)
- Others: gown, boots or closed work shoes, double non-sterile gloves, disposable gown, medical mask

SANITIZATION

Disinfectants, foams, sprays, gel, soap, sanitizer, radiations
Chemical based: Ethanol concentrations of 60% to 95% (v/v) with or without Propylene glycol, glycerol, carboxypolymethylene, Hydroxyethyl cellulose, Hydroxypropyl cellulose, Hydroxypropyl methylcellulose, Sodium carboxymethyl cellulose
Ethanol (78–95%)30 s; 2-Propanol (70–100%)30s; 2-Propanol and 1-propano (45%)30s; Glutardialdehyde (0.5–2.5%)2–5min; Formaldehyde (0.7–1.0%)2min; Povidone iodine (0.23–7.5%) 15–60s; Sodium hypochlorite (0.21%)30s; Hydrogen peroxide (0.5%)1s; Benzalkonium chloride (0.05%)10 min
Radiations based: UVC-based disinfection trolley, honeycomb air heater and a fogging chamber using UVC germicidal lamps, dry heat sterilization and HOCl-based chemical disinfectant

FIGURE 4.3 Availability and clinical development of therapeutics, sanitization, personal protective equipment (PPE), and life support systems (especially for critically ill patients) for COVID-19.

small-molecule medication, vaccines, oligonucleotide-based formulations, peptides-based preparations, and interferon-based therapy are tested for the treatment of COVID-19 [79]. Nevertheless, possibly it takes long period to discover new drug/vaccine-candidates and it take more time to assess its safety and efficacy profile . Considering the severity of COVID-19, drug repurposing procedures can be experimented with to test the potential of currently available therapeutics against COVID-19. This may require persistent efforts in repositioning, repurposing, or redirecting to redevelop possible safe and effective compound/drug for the different disease than its main use. This approach of classifying accepted, suspended, shelved, and experimental drugs for novel utilization that are approved for the cure of other ailments such as COVID-19 could be a wonderful strategy in terms of safety assessment, preclinical testing, and formulation development which takes less time, thus decreasing the overall duration for the drug development.

4.8 COVID-19 Vaccines

COVID-19 vaccines have been developed with an aim to develop a key immune response via presenting modified or attenuated antigens (or parts thereof) that commonly trigger pathogenicity, so as to improve immune response without causing any harm to the host [80]. Apart from their safety profiles, these vaccine candidates must be able to produce antigen-specific antibodies and trigger B- and T-cell responses. Thus, the level of antibodies in biological samples as well as affinity, specificity, and/or neutralizing capacity of the antibodies determines the efficacy of a vaccine. Development of antigen-specific antibodies in biological samples up to safe limits/or the maintenance and reactivation of human memory B cells after successive introduction are essential for long periods of protection [80]. Latest reports showed that vaccine candidates do not cause disease-specific effects and have promising non-specific effects against unrelated pathogens [81]. So far, 233 vaccine candidates have been developed for COVID-19 out of which 170 have been assessed in the preclinical studies and 63 are under clinical examination (Figure 4.4) [82]. The majority of vaccine candidates are in the initial stages of clinical studies (phase I or I/II), whereas 15 vaccine agents are under phase III. Some vaccines are in the last stages of clinical studies (phase III) (Table 4.1). During the initial assessment of a vaccine under phase III trial, young healthy volunteers are involved. Based on the safety profile obtained from these studies, elder volunteers and patients with comorbidities are further examined. A number of vaccine candidates who are in advanced stages have been tested on people around the whole world. The effectiveness as well as dose of these vaccines over racial and ethnic diversity is important as COVID-19 disproportionally toll on people with different racial as well as ethnic background. For example, in the United States, COVID-19-associated disease and death rates are higher among certain people with the same ethnic background [83–85]. Thus, it is essential to include in studies individuals from different ethnic or racial background so as to understand safety and efficacy of developed therapeutics. As per US FDA guidelines, volunteers involved have not been essentially symbolic of groups from all racial/ethnic background [86]. As illustrated in Figure 4.4, COVID-19 vaccines are now being assessed at preclinical and clinical levels by using 12 different platforms. Various vaccine candidates have been assessed including protein subunits, nucleic acid, virus, and viral vector as shown in Figure 4.4 [87].

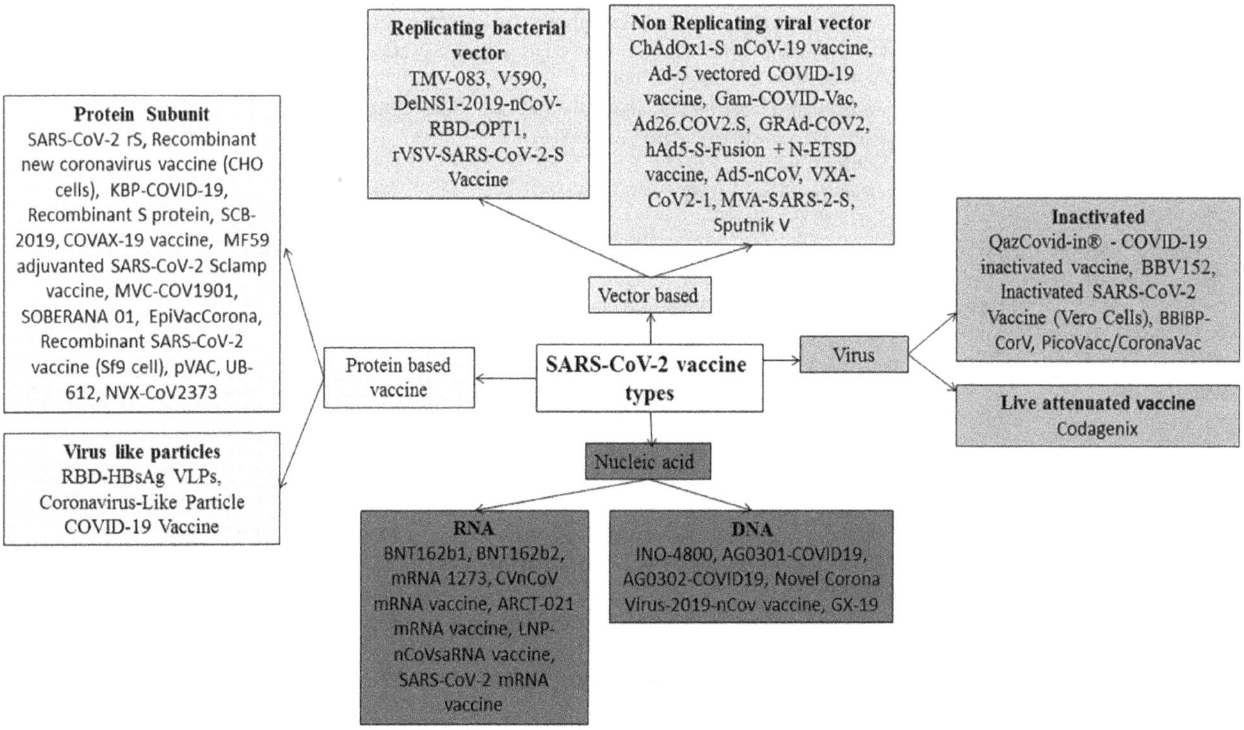

FIGURE 4.4 COVID-19 vaccines under preclinical and clinical trials [90].

TABLE 4.1
Candidate Vaccines in Phase III of Clinical Evaluation [89–95]

Platform	Candidate	Vaccine Characteristics	Clinical Stage
Inactivated	PicoVacc/CoronaVac	Inactivated SARS-CoV-2 alum adjuvant	Phase I/II (NCT04551547), phase III (NCT04456595)
	Inactivated SARS-CoV-2 vaccine	-	Phase I/II (ChiCTR2000032459), phase III (NCT04560881)
	Inactivated SARS-CoV-2 vaccine	-	Phase I/II (ChiCTR2000031809), phase III (ChiCTR2000034780)
	BBV152	Inactivated whole virion	Phase I/II (CTRI/2020/07/026300, CTRI/2020/09/027674, NCT04471519), phase III (CTRI/2020/11/028976 NCT04641481)
	BBIBP-CorV	Inactivated SARS-CoV-2 virus	Phase III (ChiCTR2000034780 NCT04560881)
Non-replicating viral vector	ChAdOx1 nCoV-19/ AZD1222/Covishield	Chimpanzee adenovirus containing the genetic sequence of the SARS-CoV-2 surface spike protein	Phase I (PACTR202005681895696), phase I/II (PACTR202006922165132), phase II/III (NCT04400838), phase III (ISRCTN89951424)
	Ad5-nCoV	Ad5 vector	Phase I (ChiCTR2000030906), phase II (ChiCTR2000031781), phase III (NCT04526990)
	Sputnik V	Recombinant adenovirus type 26 (rAd26) and type 5 (rAd5) vectors carrying the gene for SARS-CoV-2 spike glycoprotein (rAd26-S and rAd5-S)	Phase I/II (NCT04436471), phase III (NCT04530396)
	Ad26.COV2.S	Ad26 vector	Phase I (NCT04509947), phase I/II (NCT04436276), phase II (EUCTR2020-002584-63-DE), phase III (NCT04505722)
	Gam-COVID-Vac	Adeno-based vectored combined (rAd26-S + rAd5-S) vector expressing the SARS-CoV-2 S spike protein	Phase III (NCT04530396 NCT04564716)
	GRAd-CoV2	Replication defective Gorilla Adenovirus that encodes for SARS-COV-2 spike protein	Phase I (NCT04528641)
	hAd5-S-Fusion + N-ETSD vaccine	Virus serotype 5 (hAd5) vector with E1/E2b/E3 deletions expressing viral S fusion protein and nucleocapsid with an enhanced T-cell stimulation domain (ETSD)	Phase I (NCT04591717)
	Ad5-nCoV	Recombinant Novel Coronavirus Vaccine (Adenovirus Type 5 Vector)	Phase I (NCT04552366)
	VXA-CoV2-1	Ad5-vector-based vaccine expressing a SARS-CoV-2 antigen and dsRNA adjuvant given as oral tablets	Phase I (NCT04563702)
	MVA-SARS-2-S	Modified vaccinia virus Ankara (MVA) vector expressing the SARS-CoV-2 spike protein (S)	Phase I (NCT04569383)
Replicating viral vector	TMV-083	Live-attenuated recombinant measles vaccine virus vector expressing a modified surface glycoprotein of SARS-CoV-2	Phase I (NCT04497298)
	V590	Replication-competent VSV delivering the SARS-CoV-2 spike	Phase I (NCT04569786)
	DelNS1-2019-nCoV-RBD-OPT1	Intranasal flu-based RBD	Phase I (ChiCTR2000037782)
	rVSV-SARS-CoV-2-S vaccine	Replication-competent SARS-CoV-2 spike protein	Phase I (NCT04608305)
Protein subunit	NVX-CoV2373	Full-length recombinant SARS-CoV-2 glycoprotein nanoparticle vaccine adjuvanted with Matrix-M	Phase I/II (NCT04368988), phase II (NCT04533399), phase III (2020-004123-16, NCT04611802)
		Recombinant SARS-CoV-2 vaccine (CHO cell)	Phase I (NCT04445194), phase I/II (NCT04550351), phase II (NCT04466085), phase III (ChiCTR2000040153)
	SARS-CoV-2 rS	Full-length recombinant SARS-CoV-2 glycoprotein nanoparticle vaccine adjuvanted with Matrix-M	Phase III (2020-004123-16)
	KBP-COVID-19	RBD-based	Phase I/II (NCT04473690)
	Recombinant S protein	Recombinant S protein (baculovirus production) with different adjuvants	Phase I/II (NCT04537208)
	COVAX-19 vaccine	Recombinant spike protein with Advax™ adjuvant	Phase I (NCT04453852)

(*Continued*)

TABLE 4.1 (*Continued*)

Candidate Vaccines in Phase III of Clinical Evaluation [89–95]

Platform	Candidate	Vaccine Characteristics	Clinical Stage
	MF59 adjuvanted SARS-CoV-2 Sclamp vaccine	Molecular clamp stabilized Spike protein with MF59 adjuvant	Phase I (ACTRN12620000674932p ISRCTN51232965)
	MVC-COV1901	Spike protein with CpG 1018 and aluminum content as adjuvant	Phase I (NCT04487210)
	SOBERANA 01	RBD+adjuvant	Phase I (IFV/COR/04)
	EpiVacCorona	Peptide antigens of SARS-CoV-2 proteins, conjugated to a carrier protein and adsorbed on an aluminum-containing adjuvant (aluminum hydroxide)	Phase I (NCT04527575)
	Recombinant SARS-CoV-2 vaccine (Sf9 cell)	RBD (baculovirus production expressed in Sf9 cells)	Phase I (ChiCTR2000037518)
	pVAC	SARS-CoV-2 HLA-DR peptides	Phase I (NCT04546841)
	UB-612	High-precision designer S1-RBD-protein-based vaccine containing a Th/CTL epitope peptide pool that could bind to human MHC-I and MHC-II to activate T cells	Phase I (NCT04545749)
RNA	mRNA-1273	LNP-encapsulated mRNA encoding the surface spike protein	Phase I (NCT04283461), phase II (NCT04405076), phase II/III (NCT04649151), phase III (NCT04470427)
	BNT162b2	LNP nucleoside-modified mRNA encoding an optimized SARS-CoV-2 RBD antigen	Phase I/II (2020-001038-36, ChiCTR2000034825, NCT04537949), phase III (NCT04368728)
	BNT162b1	RBD trimer, LNP-mRNA	Phase I/II
DNA	INO-4800	DNA plasmid encoding S protein with electroporation delivery mechanism	Phase I: Inovio Pharmaceuticals (NCT04336410)
	Plasmid DNA oral vaccine (bacTRL-IL-Spike-1)	-	Phase I: Symvivo (NCT04334980), participants: 19 = 55 years; $n = 84$
	AG0301-COVID19 AG0302-COVID19	DNA plasmid vaccine administered with adjuvant	Phase I/II (NCT04463472, NCT04527081)
	Novel Coronavirus-2019	DNA plasmid vaccine expressing S protein	Phase I/II (CTRI/2020/07/026352)
	GX-19	DNA vaccine expressing SARS-CoV-2 S-protein antigen	Phase I/II (NCT04445389)
Virus-like particle	RBD-HBsAg VLPs	RBD antigen is conjugated to the hepatitis B surface antigen that stimulates immune system to produce anti-RBD antibodies	Phase I/II (ACTRN12620000817943)
	Coronavirus-like particle COVID-19 vaccine	Plant-derived VLP unadjuvanted or adjuvanted with either CpG 1018 or AS03	Phase I (NCT04450004)

Source: Mellet J, Pepper MS, *MDPI Vaccines*, 2021, 9(1), 39; Rawat K, Kumari P, Saha L, *European Journal of Pharmacology*, 2021, 892, 173751. With permission.

CHO, Chinese hamster ovary; LNP, lipid nanoparticle; mRNA, messenger RNA; NIAID, National Institute of Allergy and Infectious Diseases; RBD, receptor-binding domain; RNA, ribonucleic acid; S, spike.

These therapeutic agents against coronavirus-2 are assessed at clinical as well as preclinical levels by using various approaches such as nucleic acid-, viral vector-, virus-, and protein subunit-based vaccines (Figure 4.4). Almost 70 vaccine candidates are based on protein subunit, 30 are based on non-replicating vector, and 29 are based on RNA (Figure 4.4). Overall, ten different vaccine types are being assessed during clinical trials, mainly protein subunits, non-replicating vector-based, killed vaccine, and viral DNA (Figure 4.4) [88,89]. Different vaccine candidates under phase III trial of clinical assessment [89–95], their properties, and stages of development are listed in Table 4.1.

4.9 Biotechnological Interventions against COVID-19

4.9.1 DNA Science

Modern biotechnology, especially DNA science, can be used to create potential vaccines against COVID-19. In an effort to better understand COVID-19, genetic engineering can also be utilized to create a virus that is non-replicating. This type of virus could not multiply by its own inside a host cell, as it uses host cell machinery for its own development [96,97].

4.9.2 Stem Cell Therapy

Several reports have shown that stem cell therapy can be used to treat COVID-19. Various studies have reported on the active role of stem cells in treating ARDS during the cytokine storm. This is mainly due to the immune-modulatory role of mesenchymal stromal cells [98,99]. A report from China also showed that UC-MSCs can also be utilized to treat elderly COVID-19 patients on ventilation. Currently, researchers are focusing on developing a way to stimulate host-specific resident stem cells in order to resolve site-specific ARDS [98,99].

4.9.3 Nucleic Acid-Based Therapy

Additionally, nucleic acid-based therapy can also be utilized to regulate the level of gene expression inside target cells to restore genetic stability via overexpression of protective genes and silencing of damaged genes. So far, various nucleic acid-based therapies have been proposed out of which some showed satisfactory results against pulmonary diseases [100]. RNA-based therapies such as small interfering RNAs (siRNAs), RNA interference (RNAi) and RNA aptamers, ribozymes, and antisense oligonucleotides (ASOs) have shown promising results in neutralizing antigenic proteins present in the virus such as virus-like specific mRNA molecules; viral proteins such as E (envelope), M (membrane), or N (nucleocapsid); or SARS helicase. Earlier reports showed that these RNA-based therapies were effective in treating previous epidemic due to SARS-CoV [100].

4.9.4 Transgenic Animals

Various researchers are also seeking an animal model that closely resembles the clinical manifestation of SARS-CoV-2. A transgenic approach to developing and creating a genetically engineered animal model could be the most reliable approach considered so far. One of the most reliable transgenic animal models used for COVID-19 studies is the K18-hACE2 transgenic mouse model [101–103].

4.9.5 Role of Enzymes Such as Proteolytic Enzymes

Additionally, the role of enzymes such as proteolytic enzymes in the COVID-19 infection has been also reported. Various proteolytic enzymes of either host or virus regulate viral replication and assembly, which could be considered as promising targets for the development of antiviral strategies for SARS-CoV-2 [104–107].

4.9.6 Bioinformatics

The complex genetic profile of coronavirus 2 has imposed various challenges in discovering potential drug/vaccine candidates. However, the knowledge of bioinformatics in viral research can be used to interpret viral genomics architecture [108–112]. A number of major in silico investigations such as computer-aided drug design, genome-wide association studies, and next-generation sequencing have been successfully used in SARS-CoV-2-based research methods and revealed new report on SARS-CoV-2 in different forms. The application of computational simulation-based investigations in the study of SARS-CoV-2 has not only explored the sequence of SARS-CoV-2 genetic makeup but also precisely analyzed the genetic variations, sequencing faults, putative drug candidates, and evolutionary relationship of coronavirus-2 genes and other components. This understanding would be helpful in knowing several aspects related to COVID-19 outbreak and also important for the vaccine development against coronavirus-2 SARS-CoV-2 [108–112].

4.9.7 Cell-based Models

Cell-based models are also important for understanding SARS-CoV-2-based pathogenesis, developmental cycle, tropism, rate of transmission, genetic profile, as well as growth kinetics. As human lung cells are the primary target of SARS-CoV-2, cell-based models such as Vero E6, Calu-3, and A549 cells can be used for isolation, growth, as well as screening therapeutics against SARS-CoV-2 [113–120]. However, Vero E6 cells express ACE2, a host cell protein that allows SARS-CoV-2 entry, and these proteins are also present in immortalized monkey kidney cell line but do not show the same response as human primary airway cells. These models can provide better understanding of SARS-CoV-2 pathogenesis. Moreover, several mucosal tissue-based cell culture (such as the mouth, nasal epithelium, upper as well as lower airway epithelium), primary cells, or organoids can be used to examine coronavirus-2 pathogenesis.

4.9.8 Organoids

Organoids systems can also be an interesting model for assessing coronavirus-2 infection, tropism, as well as for assessing novel therapeutics against coronavirus-2. ACE2 has high expression in human kidney and thus SARS-CoV-2 can easily infect human kidney. Therefore, human kidney organoids have been used as a model to screen SARS-CoV-2 inhibitors. More recently, 3D-based organoids derived from lung tissue and presenting SCGB1A1+ club cells have been considered as new coronavirus-2 infection targets. Organoid-based models offer various advantages over immortalized cell lines as they closely mimic the in vivo environment of related vulnerable cell types. Additionally, an organoid-based platform can also be utilized in identifying SARS-CoV-2-permissive cell types [117,121].

REFERENCES

1. Jiang F, Deng L, Zhang L, Cai Y, Cheung CW, Xia Z. Review of the clinical characteristics of coronavirus disease 2019 (COVID-19). *J Gen Intern Med.* 2020;35(5):1545–1549.
2. Lau SKP, Luk HKH, Wong ACP, Li KSM, Zhu L, He Z, Fung J, Chan TTY, Fung KSC, Woo PCY. Possible bat origin of severe acute respiratory syndrome coronavirus 2. *Emerg Infect Dis.* 2020;26(7):1542–1547.
3. Zhang T, Wu Q, Zhang Z. Probable pangolin origin of SARS-CoV-2 associated with the COVID-19 outbreak. *Curr Biol.* 2020;30(7):1346–1351.e2. doi: 10.1016/j.cub.2020.03.022. Epub 2020 March 19. Erratum in: *Curr Biol.* 2020;30(8):1578.

4. Zhai X, Sun J, Yan Z, Zhang J, Zhao J, Zhao Z, Gao Q, He WT, Veit M, Su S. Comparison of severe acute respiratory syndrome coronavirus 2 spike protein binding to ACE2 receptors from human, pets, farm animals, and putative intermediate hosts. *J Virol.* 2020;94(15):e00831–20.
5. Arslan M, Xu B, Gamal El-Din M. Transmission of SARS-CoV-2 via fecal-oral and aerosols-borne routes: Environmental dynamics and implications for wastewater management in underprivileged societies. *Sci Total Environ.* 2020;743:140709.
6. Bulut C, Kato Y. Epidemiology of COVID-19. *Turk J Med Sci.* 2020;50(SI-1):563–570.
7. Delamater PL, Street EJ, Leslie TF, Yang YT, Jacobsen KH. Complexity of the basic reproduction number (R0). *Emerg Infect Dis.* 2019;25(1):1–4.
8. Liu J, Xie W, Wang Y, Xiong Y, Chen S, Han J, Wu Q. A comparative overview of COVID-19, MERS and SARS: Review article. *Int J Surg.* 2020;81:1–8.
9. WHO. 2009. www.who.int/20200502-covid-19-sitrep-103.
10. Ge H, Wang X, Yuan X, Xiao G, Wang C, Deng T, Yuan Q, Xiao X. The epidemiology and clinical information about COVID-19. *Eur J Clin Microbiol Infect Dis.* 2020;39(6):1011–1019.
11. Sterlin D, Mathian A, Miyara M, Mohr A, Anna F, Claër L, Quentric P, Fadlallah J, Devilliers H, Ghillani P, Gunn C, Hockett R, Mudumba S, Guihot A, Luyt CE, Mayaux J, Beurton A, Fourati S, Bruel T, Schwartz O, Lacorte JM, Yssel H, Parizot C, Dorgham K, Charneau P, Amoura Z, Gorochov G. IgA dominates the early neutralizing antibody response to SARS-CoV-2. *Sci Transl Med.* 2021;13(577):eabd2223. doi: 10.1126/scitranslmed.abd2223. Epub 2020 December 7.
12. Ma H, Zeng W, He H, Zhao D, Jiang D, Zhou P, Cheng L, Li Y, Ma X, Jin T. Serum IgA, IgM, and IgG responses in COVID-19. *Cell Mol Immunol.* 2020;17(7):773–775.
13. Jacofsky D, Jacofsky EM, Jacofsky M. Understanding antibody testing for COVID-19. *J Arthroplasty.* 2020;35(7S):S74–S81. doi: 10.1016/j.arth.2020.04.055. Epub 2020 April 27.
14. Cevik M, Kuppalli K, Kindrachuk J, Peiris M. Virology, transmission, and pathogenesis of SARS-CoV-2. *BMJ.* 2020;371:m3862.
15. Azkur AK, Akdis M, Azkur D, Sokolowska M, van de Veen W, Brüggen MC, O'Mahony L, Gao Y, Nadeau K, Akdis CA. Immune response to SARS-CoV-2 and mechanisms of immunopathological changes in COVID-19. *Allergy.* 2020;75(7):1564–1581.
16. Kowalik MM, Trzonkowski P, Łasińska-Kowara M, Mital A, Smiatacz T, Jaguszewski M. COVID-19 -toward a comprehensive understanding of the disease. *Cardiol J.* 2020;27(2):99–114.
17. Simon Junior H, Sakano TMS, Rodrigues RM, Eisencraft AP, Carvalho VEL, Schvartsman C, Reis AGADC. Multisystem inflammatory syndrome associated with COVID-19 from the pediatric emergency physician's point of view. *J Pediatr (Rio J).* 2020;S0021–7557(20):30203–3025.
18. Siordia JA Jr. Epidemiology and clinical features of COVID-19: A review of current literature. *J Clin Virol.* 2020;127:104357.
19. Zou L, Ruan F, Huang M, Liang L, Huang H, Hong Z, Yu J, Kang M, Song Y, Xia J, Guo Q, Song T, He J, Yen HL, Peiris M, Wu J. SARS-CoV-2 viral load in upper respiratory specimens of infected patients. *N Engl J Med.* 2020;382(12):1177–1179.
20. Huang C, Wang Y, Li X, Ren L, Zhao J, Hu Y, Zhang L, Fan G, Xu J, Gu X, Cheng Z, Yu T, Xia J, Wei Y, Wu W, Xie X, Yin W, Li H, Liu M, Xiao Y, Gao H, Guo L, Xie J, Wang G, Jiang R, Gao Z, Jin Q, Wang J, Cao B. Clinical features of patients infected with 2019 novel coronavirus in Wuhan, China. *Lancet.* 2020;395(10223):497–506.
21. Chen N, Zhou M, Dong X, Qu J, Gong F, Han Y, Qiu Y, Wang J, Liu Y, Wei Y, Xia J, Yu T, Zhang X, Zhang L. Epidemiological and clinical characteristics of 99 cases of 2019 novel coronavirus pneumonia in Wuhan, China: A descriptive study. *Lancet.* 2020;395(10223):507–513.
22. Wang D, Hu B, Hu C, Zhu F, Liu X, Zhang J, Wang B, Xiang H, Cheng Z, Xiong Y, Zhao Y, Li Y, Wang X, Peng Z. Clinical characteristics of 138 hospitalized patients with 2019 novel coronavirus-infected pneumonia in Wuhan, China. *JAMA.* 2020;323(11):1061–1069. doi: 10.1001/jama.2020.1585. Erratum in: *JAMA.* 2021;325(11):1113.
23. Wang XW, Li JS, Guo TK, Zhen B, Long QX, Yi B, et al. Concentration and detection of SARS coronavirus in sewage from Xiao Tang Shan Hospital and the 309th Hospital. *J Virol Methods.* 2005;128:156–161.
24. Lin L, Jiang X, Zhang Z, Huang S, Zhang Z, Fang Z, Gu Z, Gao L, Shi H, Mai L, Liu Y, Lin X, Lai R, Yan Z, Li X, Shan H. Gastrointestinal symptoms of 95 cases with SARS-CoV-2 infection. *Gut.* 2020 Jun;69(6):997–1001. doi: 10.1136/gutjnl-2020-321013. Epub 2020 Apr 2. PMID: 32241899; PMCID: PMC7316116.
25. Al-Omari A, Rabaan AA, Salih S, Al-Tawfiq JA, Memish ZA. MERS coronavirus outbreak: Implications for emerging viral infections. *Diagn Microbiol Infect Dis.* 2019;93(3):265–285.
26. Yeung ML, Yao Y, Jia L, Chan JF, Chan KH, Cheung KF, Chen H, Poon VK, Tsang AK, To KK, Yiu MK, Teng JL, Chu H, Zhou J, Zhang Q, Deng W, Lau SK, Lau JY, Woo PC, Chan TM, Yung S, Zheng BJ, Jin DY, Mathieson PW, Qin C, Yuen KY. MERS coronavirus induces apoptosis in kidney and lung by upregulating Smad7 and FGF2. *Nat Microbiol.* 2016;1(3):16004.
27. Zhou F. Clinical course and risk factors for mortality of adult inpatients with COVID-19 in Wuhan, China: A retrospective cohort study. *Lancet.* 2020;395:1054–1062.
28. Qin C, Zhou L, Hu Z. et al. Dysregulation of immune response in patients with COVID-19 in Wuhan, China. *Clin Infect Dis.* 2020;71:762–768.
29. Lippi G, Plebani M, Henry BM. Thrombocytopenia is associated with severe coronavirus disease 2019 (COVID-19) infections: A meta-analysis. *Clin Chim Acta.* 2020;506:145–148.
30. Beyrouti R. Characteristics of ischaemic stroke associated with COVID-19. *J Neurol Neurosurg Psychiatry.* 2020;91:889–891.
31. D'Amico F, Baumgart DC, Danese S, Peyrin-Biroulet L. Diarrhea during COVID-19 infection: Pathogenesis, epidemiology, prevention and management. *Clin Gastroenterol Hepatol.* 2020;18:1663–1672.
32. Ling W. C-reactive protein levels in the early stage of COVID-19. *Med Maladies Infect.* 2020;50:332–334.
33. Xu Z. Pathological findings of COVID-19 associated with acute respiratory distress syndrome. *Lancet Respir Med.* 2020;8:420–422.
34. Wu A. Genome composition and divergence of the novel Coronavirus (2019-nCoV) originating in China. *Cell Host Microbe.* 2020;27:325–328.

35. Xu XW, Wu XX, Jiang XG, Xu KJ, Ying LJ, Ma CL, Li SB, Wang HY, Zhang S, Gao HN, Sheng JF, Cai HL, Qiu YQ, Li LJ. Clinical findings in a group of patients infected with the 2019 novel coronavirus (SARS-Cov-2) outside of Wuhan, China: Retrospective case series. *BMJ.* 2020;368:m606. doi: 10.1136/bmj.m606. Erratum in: *BMJ.* 2020;368:m792.
36. Zhang JJ, Dong X, Cao YY, Yuan YD, Yang YB, Yan YQ, Akdis CA, Gao YD. Clinical characteristics of 140 patients infected with SARS-CoV-2 in Wuhan, China. *Allergy.* 2020;75(7):1730–1741.
37. Mardani R, Ahmadi Vasmehjani A, Zali F, Gholami A, Mousavi Nasab SD, Kaghazian H, Kaviani M, Ahmadi N. Laboratory parameters in detection of COVID-19 patients with positive RT-PCR; a diagnostic accuracy study. *Arch Acad Emerg Med.* 2020;8(1):e43.
38. Ponti G, Maccaferri M, Ruini C, Tomasi A, Ozben T. Biomarkers associated with COVID-19 disease progression. *Crit Rev Clin Lab Sci.* 2020;57(6):389–399.
39. Cui N, Zou X, Xu L. Preliminary CT findings of coronavirus disease 2019 (COVID-19). *Clin Imaging.* 2020;65: 124–132.
40. Ye Z, Zhang Y, Wang Y, Huang Z, Song B. Chest CT manifestations of new coronavirus disease 2019 (COVID-19): A pictorial review. *Eur Radiol.* 2020;30(8):4381–4389.
41. Chen H, Ai L, Lu H, Li H. Clinical and imaging features of COVID-19. *Radiol Infect Dis.* 2020;7(2):43–50.
42. Li X, Zeng W, Li X, Chen H, Shi L, Li X, Xiang H, Cao Y, Chen H, Liu C, Wang J. CT imaging changes of corona virus disease 2019(COVID-19): A multi-center study in Southwest China. *J Transl Med.* 20206;18(1):154.
43. Afzal A. Molecular diagnostic technologies for COVID-19: Limitations and challenges. *J Adv Res.* 2020;26:149–159.
44. Xu Z, Shi L, Wang Y, Zhang J, Huang L, Zhang C, Liu S, Zhao P, Liu H, Zhu L, Tai Y, Bai C, Gao T, Song J, Xia P, Dong J, Zhao J, Wang FS. Pathological findings of COVID-19 associated with acute respiratory distress syndrome. *Lancet Respir Med.* 2020;8(4):420–422. doi: 10.1016/S2213-2600(20)30076-X. Epub 2020 February 18. Erratum in: *Lancet Respir Med.* 2020.
45. Tian S, Xiong Y, Liu H, Niu L, Guo J, Liao M, Xiao SY. Pathological study of the 2019 novel coronavirus disease (COVID-19) through postmortem core biopsies. *Mod Pathol.* 2020;33(6):1007–1014.
46. Batah SS, Fabro AT. Pulmonary pathology of ARDS in COVID-19: A pathological review for clinicians. *Respir Med.* 2021;176:106239.
47. Chen Z, John Wherry E. T cell responses in patients with COVID-19. *Nat Rev Immunol.* 2020;20(9):529–536.
48. Kong M, Zhang H, Cao X, Mao X, Lu Z. Higher level of neutrophil-to-lymphocyte is associated with severe COVID-19. *Epidemiol Infect.* 2020;148:e139.
49. Zhang C, Wu Z, Li JW, Zhao H, Wang GQ. Cytokine release syndrome in severe COVID-19: Interleukin-6 receptor antagonist tocilizumab may be the key to reduce mortality. *Int J Antimicrob Agents.* 2020;55(5):105954.
50. Tang YW, Schmitz JE, Persing DH, Stratton CW. Laboratory diagnosis of COVID-19: Current issues and challenges. *J Clin Microbiol.* 2020;58(6):e00512–20.
51. Pizzol JLD, Hora VPD, Reis AJ, Vianna J, Ramis I, Groll AV, Silva PAD. Laboratory diagnosis for COVID-19: A mini-review. *Rev Soc Bras Med Trop.* 2020;53:e20200451.
52. National Administration of Traditional Chinese Medicine Internet. The national health commission of the People's Republic of China: corona virus disease 2019 diagnosis and treatment plan (5th trial edition revised version) 2020–02–08. http://www.gov.cn/zhengce/zhengceku/2020-02/09/5476407/files/765d1e65b7d1443081053c29ad37fb07.pdf.
53. Loeffelholz MJ, Tang YW. Laboratory diagnosis of emerging human coronavirus infections: The state of the art. *Emerg Microbes Infect.* 2020;9(1):747–756.
54. https://www.who.int/csr/sars/diagnostictests/en/.
55. Kovács A, Palásti P, Veréb D, Bozsik B, Palkó A, Kincses ZT. The sensitivity and specificity of chest CT in the diagnosis of COVID-19. *Eur Radiol.* 2021:31(5):2819–2824.
56. Ai T, Yang Z, Hou H, Zhan C, Chen C, Lv W, Tao Q, Sun Z, Xia L. Correlation of chest CT and RT-PCR testing for coronavirus disease 2019 (COVID-19) in China: A report of 1014 cases. *Radiology.* 2020;296(2):E32–E40.
57. Matos J, Paparo F, Mussetto I, Bacigalupo L, Veneziano A, Perugin Bernardi S, Biscaldi E, Melani E, Antonucci G, Cremonesi P, Lattuada M, Pilotto A, Pontali E, Rollandi GA. Evaluation of novel coronavirus disease (COVID-19) using quantitative lung CT and clinical data: Prediction of short-term outcome. *Eur Radiol Exp.* 2020;4(1):39.
58. Scala R, Ciarleglio G, Maccari U, Granese V, Salerno L, Madioni C. Ventilator support and oxygen therapy in palliative and end-of-life care in the elderly. *Turk Thorac J.* 2020;21(1):54–60.
59. Price S, Singh S, Ledot S, Bianchi P, Hind M, Tavazzi G, Vranckx P. Respiratory management in severe acute respiratory syndrome coronavirus 2 infection. *Eur Heart J Acute Cardiovasc Care.* 2020;9(3):229–238.
60. Shang Y, Pan C, Yang X, Zhong M, Shang X, Wu Z, Yu Z, Zhang W, Zhong Q, Zheng X, Sang L, Jiang L, Zhang J, Xiong W, Liu J, Chen D. Management of critically ill patients with COVID-19 in ICU: Statement from front-line intensive care experts in Wuhan, China. *Ann Intensive Care.* 2020;10(1):73.
61. Dobler CC, Murad MH, Wilson ME. Noninvasive positive pressure ventilation in patients with COVID-19. *Mayo Clin Proc.* 2020;95(12):2594–2601.
62. Harding H, Broom A, Broom J. Aerosol-generating procedures and infective risk to healthcare workers from SARS-CoV-2: The limits of the evidence. *J Hosp Infect.* 2020;105(4):717–725.
63. Mas A, Masip J. Noninvasive ventilation in acute respiratory failure. *Int J Chron Obstruct Pulmon Dis.* 2014;9:837–852.
64. Frat JP, Coudroy R, Marjanovic N, Thille AW. High-flow nasal oxygen therapy and noninvasive ventilation in the management of acute hypoxemic respiratory failure. *Ann Transl Med.* 2017;5(14):297.
65. Agarwal A, Basmaji J, Muttalib F, Granton D, Chaudhuri D, Chetan D, Hu M, Fernando SM, Honarmand K, Bakaa L, Brar S, Rochwerg B, Adhikari NK, Lamontagne F, Murthy S, Hui DSC, Gomersall C, Mubareka S, Diaz JV, Burns KEA, Couban R, Ibrahim Q, Guyatt GH, Vandvik PO. High-flow nasal cannula for acute hypoxemic respiratory failure in patients with COVID-19: Systematic reviews of effectiveness and its risks of aerosolization, dispersion, and infection transmission. *Can J Anaesth.* 2020;67(9):1217–1248.
66. Scala R, Pisani L. Noninvasive ventilation in acute respiratory failure: Which recipe for success? *Eur Respir Rev.* 2018;27(149):180029.

67. Ghelichkhani P, Esmaeili M. Prone position in management of COVID-19 patients; a commentary. *Arch Acad Emerg Med.* 2020;8(1):e48.
68. Khan S, Choudry E, Mahmood SU, Mulla AY, Mehwish S. Awake proning: A necessary evil during the COVID-19 pandemic. *Cureus.* 2020;12(7):e8989.
69. Ferioli M, Cisternino C, Leo V, Pisani L, Palange P, Nava S. Protecting healthcare workers from SARS-CoV-2 infection: Practical indications. *Eur Respir Rev.* 2020;29(155):200068.
70. Hui DS, Chow BK, Chu L, Ng SS, Lee N, Gin T, Chan MT. Exhaled air dispersion during coughing with and without wearing a surgical or N95 mask. *PLoS One.* 2012;7(12):e50845.
71. Escombe AR, Oeser CC, Gilman RH, Navincopa M, Ticona E, Pan W, Martínez C, Chacaltana J, Rodríguez R, Moore DA, Friedland JS, Evans CA. Natural ventilation for the prevention of airborne contagion. *PLoS Med.* 2007;4(2):e68.
72. Park SH. Personal protective equipment for healthcare workers during the COVID-19 pandemic. *Infect Chemother.* 2020;52(2):165–182.
73. Carter C, Osborn M, Agagah G, Aedy H, Notter J. COVID-19 disease: Invasive ventilation. *Clin Integr Care.* 2020;1:100004.
74. Chua MH, Cheng W, Goh SS, Kong J, Li B, Lim JYC, Mao L, Wang S, Xue K, Yang L, Ye E, Zhang K, Cheong WCD, Tan BH, Li Z, Tan BH, Loh XJ. Face masks in the new COVID-19 normal: Materials, testing, and perspectives. *Research (Wash D C).* 2020;2020:7286735.
75. Lee SA, Hwang DC, Li HY, Tsai CF, Chen CW, Chen JK. Particle size-selective assessment of protection of European standard FFP respirators and surgical masks against particles-tested with human subjects. *J Healthc Eng.* 2016;2016:8572493.
76. Forouzandeh P, O'Dowd K, Pillai SC. Face masks and respirators in the fight against the COVID-19 pandemic: An overview of the standards and testing methods. *Saf Sci.* 2021;133:104995.
77. Dev Kumar G, Mishra A, Dunn L, Townsend A, Oguadinma IC, Bright KR, Gerba CP. Biocides and novel antimicrobial agents for the mitigation of coronaviruses. *Front Microbiol.* 2020;11:1351.
78. McDonnell G, Russell AD. Antiseptics and disinfectants: Activity, action, and resistance. *Clin Microbiol Rev.* 1999;12(1):147–179. Erratum in: *Clin Microbiol Rev* 2001;14(1):227.
79. Ahamad S, Branch S, Harrelson S, Hussain MK, Saquib M, Khan S. Primed for global coronavirus pandemic: Emerging research and clinical outcome. *Eur J Med Chem.* 2021;209:112862. doi: 10.1016/j.ejmech.2020.112862. Epub 2020 September 19.
80. Siegrist CA. Vaccine immunology. In: Plotkin SA, Orenstein WA, Offit PA, Edwards KM, editors. *Plotkin's Vaccines.* Elsevier Inc., Philadelphia, PA; 2018:16–34.e7.
81. Benn CS, Netea MG, Selin LK, Aaby P. A small jab: A big effect: Nonspecific immunomodulation by vaccines. *Trends Immunol.* 2013;34:431–439.
82. World Health Organization. Draft landscape of COVID-19 candidate vaccines. 5 January 2021. Available online: https://www.who.int/who-documents-detail/draft-landscape-of-covid-19-candidate-vaccines (accessed on 7 January 2021).
83. Yancy CW. COVID-19 and African Americans. *JAMA.* 2020;323:1891.
84. Centre for Disease Control and Prevention. COVID-19 hospitalization and death by race/ethnicity. Available online: https://www.cdc.gov/coronavirus/2019-ncov/covid-data/investigations-discovery/hospitalization-death-by-race-ethnicity.html (accessed on 21 December 2020).
85. Bassett MT, Chen JT, Krieger N. Variation in racial/ethnic disparities in COVID-19 mortality by age in the United States: A cross-sectional study. *PLoS Med.* 2020;17:e1003402.
86. US Food and Drug Association. Drug Trials Snapshot: Summary Report. 2019. Available online: https://www.fda.gov/media/135337/download (accessed on 5 November 2020).
87. Walsh EE, Frenck RW Jr, Falsey AR, Kitchin N, Absalon J, Gurtman A, Lockhart S, Neuzil K, Mulligan MJ, Bailey R, Swanson KA, Li P, Koury K, Kalina W, Cooper D, Fontes-Garfias C, Shi PY, Türeci Ö, Tompkins KR, Lyke KE, Raabe V, Dormitzer PR, Jansen KU, Şahin U, Gruber WC. Safety and immunogenicity of two RNA-based COVID-19 vaccine candidates. *N Engl J Med.* 2020;383(25):2439–2450.
88. Zhao J, Zhao S, Ou J, Zhang J, Lan W, Guan W, Wu X, Yan Y, Zhao W, Wu J, Chodosh J, Zhang Q. COVID-19: Coronavirus vaccine development updates. *Front Immunol.* 2020;11:602256.
89. Kaur SP, Gupta V. COVID-19 vaccine: A comprehensive status report. *Virus Res.* 2020;288:198114.
90. Sharma O, Sultan AA, Ding H, Triggle CR. A review of the progress and challenges of developing a vaccine for COVID-19. *Front Immunol.* 2020;11:585354.
91. National Library of Medicine. 2020. https://clinicaltrials.gov/ct2/results?cond=COVID-19&term=vaccines&cntry=&state=&city=&dist=&Search=Search WWW Document (accessed on 28 October 2020).
92. World Health Organization. Draft landscape of COVID-19 candidate vaccines. 2020. https://www.who.int/who-documents-detail/draft-landscape-of-covid-19-candidate-vaccines WWW Document (accessed on 30 October 2020).
93. Cochrane. Cochrane COVID-19 study register. 2020. https://covid-19.cochrane.org/WWWDocument (accessed on 29 October 2020).
94. Rawat K, Kumari P, Saha L. COVID-19 vaccine: A recent update in pipeline vaccines, their design and development strategies. *Eur J Pharmacol.* 2021;892:173751.
95. Chen WH, Strych U, Hotez PJ, Bottazzi ME. The SARS-CoV-2 vaccine pipeline: An overview. *Curr Trop Med Rep.* 2020:1–4. doi:10.1007/s40475-020-00201-6.
96. Bhatia S. Modern DNA science and its applications. In: *Introduction to Pharmaceutical Biotechnology, Volume 1 Basic Techniques and Concepts.* IOP Publishing Ltd, Bristol, UK; 2018;1(3):1–70.
97. Bhatia S. Introduction to genetic engineering. In: *Introduction to Pharmaceutical Biotechnology, Volume 1 Basic Techniques and Concepts.* IOP Publishing Ltd, Bristol, UK; 2018;1(3):1–63.
98. Shetty R, Murugeswari P, Chakrabarty K, et al. Stem cell therapy in coronavirus disease 2019: Current evidence and future potential. *Cytotherapy.* 2021;23(6):471–482.
99. Bhatia S. Applications of stem cells in disease and gene therapy. In: *Introduction to Pharmaceutical Biotechnology, Volume 1 Basic Techniques and Concepts.* IOP Publishing Ltd, Bristol, UK; 2018;1:1–40.

100. Chen J, Tang Y, Liu Y, Dou Y. Nucleic acid-based therapeutics for pulmonary diseases. *AAPS PharmSciTech.* 2018;19(8):3670–3680.
101. Bhatia S. Transgenic animals in biotechnology. In: *Introduction to Pharmaceutical Biotechnology, Volume 1 Basic Techniques and Concepts.* IOP Publishing Ltd, Bristol, UK; 2018;1:1–67.
102. Takayama K. In vitro and animal models for SARS-CoV-2 research. *Trends Pharmacol Sci.* 2020;41(8):513–517.
103. Johansen MD, Irving A, Montagutelli X, Tate MD, Rudloff I, Nold MF, Hansbro NG, Kim RY, Donovan C, Liu G, Faiz A, Short KR, Lyons JG, McCaughan GW, Gorrell MD, Cole A, Moreno C, Couteur D, Hesselson D, Triccas J, Neely GG, Gamble JR, Simpson SJ, Saunders BM, Oliver BG, Britton WJ, Wark PA, Nold-Petry CA, Hansbro PM. Animal and translational models of SARS-CoV-2 infection and COVID-19. *Mucosal Immunol.* 2020;13(6):877–891.
104. Gioia M, Ciaccio C, Calligari P, et al. Role of proteolytic enzymes in the COVID-19 infection and promising therapeutic approaches. *Biochem Pharmacol.* 2020;182: 114225.
105. Bhatia S. Industrial enzymes and their applications. In: *Introduction to Pharmaceutical Biotechnology, Enzymes, Proteins and Bioinformatics.* IOP Publishing Ltd, Bristol, UK; 2018;2:21.
106. Bhatia S. Introduction to enzymes and their applications. In: *Introduction to Pharmaceutical Biotechnology, Enzymes, Proteins and Bioinformatics.* IOP Publishing Ltd, Bristol, UK; 2018;2:1–29.
107. Bhatia S. Biotransformation and enzymes. In: *Introduction to Pharmaceutical Biotechnology, Enzymes, Proteins and Bioinformatics.* IOP Publishing Ltd, Bristol, UK; 2018;3:1–13.
108. Ray M, Sable MN, Sarkar S, Hallur V. Essential interpretations of bioinformatics in COVID-19 pandemic. *Meta Gene.* 2021;27:100844.
109. Rana R, Rathi V, Ganguly NK. A comprehensive overview of proteomics approach for COVID 19: New perspectives in target therapy strategies. *J Proteins Proteom.* 2020;11:223–232.
110. Bhatia S. Bioinformatics. In: *Introduction to Pharmaceutical Biotechnology, Enzymes, Proteins and Bioinformatics.* IOP Publishing Ltd, Bristol, UK; 2018;3:1–16.
111. Bhatia S. Protein and enzyme engineering. In: *Introduction to Pharmaceutical Biotechnology, Enzymes, Proteins and Bioinformatics.* IOP Publishing Ltd, Bristol, UK; 2018;2:1–15.
112. Bhatia S. Introduction to genomics. In: *Introduction to Pharmaceutical Biotechnology, Enzymes, Proteins and Bioinformatics.* IOP Publishing Ltd, Bristol, UK; 2018;,2:1–39.
113. Monteil V, Kwon H, Prado P, Hagelkrüys A, Wimmer RA, Stahl M, Leopoldi A, Garreta E, Hurtado Del Pozo C, Prosper F, Romero JP, Wirnsberger G, Zhang H, Slutsky AS, Conder R, Montserrat N, Mirazimi A, Penninger JM. Inhibition of SARS-CoV-2 infections in engineered human tissues using clinical-grade soluble human ACE2. *Cell.* 2020;181(4):905–913.e7.
114. Bhatia S. Characterization of cultured cells. In: *Introduction to Pharmaceutical Biotechnology, Volume 3: Animal Tissue Culture and Biopharmaceuticals.* IOP Publishing Ltd, Bristol, UK; 2019:3;1–47.
115. Bradley BT, Maioli H, Johnston R, Chaudhry I, Fink SL, Xu H, Najafian B, Deutsch G, Lacy JM, Williams T, Yarid N, Marshall DA. Histopathology and ultrastructural findings of fatal COVID-19 infections in Washington State: A case series. *Lancet.* 2020;396(10247):320–332. doi: 10.1016/S0140-6736(20)31305-2. Epub 2020 July 16. Erratum in: *Lancet.* 2020;396(10247):312.
116. Bhatia S. Animal tissue culture facilities. In: *Introduction to Pharmaceutical Biotechnology, Volume 3: Animal Tissue Culture and Biopharmaceuticals.* IOP Publishing Ltd, Bristol, UK; 2019;3:1–32.
117. Salahudeen AA, Choi SS, Rustagi A, et al. Progenitor identification and SARS-CoV-2 infection in long-term human distal lung organoid cultures. bioRxiv 2020.
118. Bhatia S. Culture media for animal cells. In; *Introduction to Pharmaceutical Biotechnology, Volume 3: Animal Tissue Culture and Biopharmaceuticals.* IOP Publishing Ltd, Bristol, UK; 2019:3;1–33.
119. Leist SR, Schäfer A, Martinez DR. Cell and animal models of SARS-CoV-2 pathogenesis and immunity. *Dis Model Mech.* 2020;13(9):dmm046581.
120. Bhatia S. Stem cell culture. In: *Introduction to Pharmaceutical Biotechnology, Volume 3: Animal Tissue Culture and Biopharmaceuticals.* IOP Publishing Ltd, Bristol, UK; 2019;3:1–24.
121. Bhatia S. Organ culture. In: *Introduction to Pharmaceutical Biotechnology, Volume 3: Introduction to Animal Tissue Culture Science.* IOP Publishing Ltd, Bristol, UK; 2019;3:1–28.

5

Role of Drug Repurposing and Natural Products

Ahmed Al-Harrasi
Natural and Medical Sciences Research Center, University of Nizwa

Saurabh Bhatia
Natural and Medical Sciences Research Center, University of Nizwa
University of Petroleum and Energy

Md. Tanvir Kabir
BRAC University

Tapan Behl
Chitkara University

Deepak Kaushik
M.D. University

CONTENTS

5.1 Introduction

Drug repositioning is an important and general approach employed in the development of novel therapeutics due to various advantages such as cost-effectiveness, the possibility to bypass some clinical trials, shorter timeframes mainly in relation to phases I and II, established supply chains for its formulation and distribution, lowers chances of toxicity due to available safety profiles, and the fact that it can be potentially used in combination with other therapeutics rather than as a single therapeutic [1,2]. Using this approach, new uses for available drugs can be explored to treat conditions that are different from their original therapeutic purpose. However, repurposing has some considerable disadvantages such as more access to data from other industry-sponsored clinical trials, challenges associated with regulatory pathways, lack of funding, patent-associated limitations, and the heterogeneity of populations for new clinical studies [1,3]. However, this approach is still considered as a way to find completely new classes of drugs when other treatments are not available [1]. This approach of using already accepted or investigational medications has been found as more promising way for

DOI: 10.1201/9781003175933-6

screening and development of effective drug [4]. This chapter focuses on the effectiveness of repurposing already approved medications including tocilizumab, interferons remdesivir, ribavirin, ritonavir, lopinavir, favipiravir, hydroxychloroquine, darunavir, chloroquine and arbidol in the treatment of SARS Cov-2 infection [5]. Various reports based on computational approaches, *in vitro, in vivo,* clinical investigations among human subjects, as well as case studies have shown that several drugs have shown effectiveness against the coronavirus [5]. These therapeutics can target viral pathogenic proteins via different molecular pathways to neutralize pathogenesis caused by the virus, especially by targeting its genome (ribonucleic acid), polypeptide packing, and virus entry routes or act on host-related pathways especially those targets (proteins) which faciltates invasion as well as development of virus and progression of disease such as angiotensin-converting enzyme-2 (ACE2) protein as well its associated inflammatory markers [5]. Further using information based on viral pathogenesis, bioinformatics tools as well as pharmacodynamics of various drugs are presently in line to be retasked [5]. However, in the context of COVID-19, additional drawbacks of using of repurposed drug molecules include dosage regimen and challenges such as localized delivery in respiratory tract [6]. Natural products such as medicinal herbs like *Hypericum perforatum*, *Zingiber officinale*, *Nigella sativa*, *Scutellaria baicalensis*, *Camellia sinensis*, *Echinacea spp.*, *Allium sativum*, and *Glycyrrhiza glabra* can boost and strengthen immune system and are being studied as a way to treat COVID-19 [7,8]. Natural products like terpenoids have shown effectiveness in inhibiting viral replication, whereas alkaloids like homoharringtonine, lycorine, and emetine have shown significant anticoronavirus effects. Some phytochemicals have been reported for their effects against certain molecular targets of virus such as iguesterin against viral enzymes such as 3CLpro, cryptotanshinone act against papain-like protease (PLpro), silvestrol against helicase, sotetsuflavone against RdRp [7,8]. Thus, these natural products can be used as therapeutic agents against coronavirus [7,8].

As has also been reported, phytochemicals can also be used as preventive and therapeutic agents in the combating against COVID infection. Furthermore, certain therapeutics, such as antiviral (remdesivir), glucocorticoid (dexamethasone), antimalarial (chloroquine/hydroxychloroquine), and IL-6 receptor blocking monoclonal antibodies (tocilizumab), have been utilized in different permutations to treat coronavirus infection [7,8]. An important class of natural products (i.e., essential oils (EOs)) have been used for decades to reduce inflammation, trigger immune reactions, cause bronchiodilation, and trigger viral inhibition and are now seen as possible effective agents against coronavirus. Due to their hydrophobic property, EOs can easily infiltrate viral membranes resulting in disruption of the membrane [9]. Additionally, EOs have diverse chemical components that can act collectively in various phases of viral replication and have beneficial properties on the human respiratory system due their bronchodilation and mucolytic effects [9]. This chapter discusses the role of drug repurposing, natural products, and EOs in the prevention and treatment of COVID-19 [9].

5.2 Therapeutics under Investigation

Researchers are striving to discover reliable, safe, and effective drugs/compounds to treat COVID-19. However, till date no approved therapeutics to fight against COVID-19 is available. It is still necessary to develop safe, effective, and reliable treatments to cure and prevent the disease at this stage. Various therapeutic approaches have been adopted so far to treat the various complications associated with COVID-19 such as follows:

- Antiviral drugs to inhibit viral replication [10].
- Ang II receptor blockers or ACE inhibitors; however, this strategy might have possible side effects such as systemic hypotension [10].
- Soluble forms of recombinant ACE2 receptor protein (e.g., human recombinant-soluble ACE2 (hrsACE2) attaches to viral particles and prevents its entry into host cell) [11].
- Serum therapy based on passive immunotherapy via convalescent serum, convalescent plasma, inactivated convalescent plasma, immunoglobulin of cured patients, and immunoglobulins obtained with double-filtration plasmapheresis (DFPP). Passive antibody administration (passive immunotherapy) through transfusion of convalescent plasma by using serum of immunized individuals [12].
- Monoclonal antibodies such as B38, H4, and 47D11 to neutralize the coronavirus and to reduce cytokines such as IL-6 accountable for inflammation [13].
- Natural killer cells secrete cytokines, including IFN-γ, which have key antiviral properties. This type of natural killer cell-based adoptive immunotherapy can be used to flatten the COVID-19 curve [14].
- Mesenchymal stromal cells to balance the inflammatory response, thus playing an essential role in immunomodulation of severe immune response [15].
- Drug-based nanoparticles to encourage specific drug targeting and controlled drug-release rate. Nanoencapsulation of antimicrobial drugs can be utilized to bind onto the viral envelope or its protein to prevent its interaction with the host cell [16].
- 3C-like protease inhibitors against the serine protease TMPRSS2 to prevent spike protein cleavage, which is necessary for viral fusion into the host cell. 3C-like protease is necessary for SARS-CoV-2 replication. This protein is considered as a key target for infection caused by SARS-CoV-2 [17].
- Natural products such as carolacton (from myxobacterium Sorangium cellulosum), Homoharringtonine (from Cephalotaxus harringtonii), and Emetine (from Psychotria ipecacuanha) [18]. EOs with antibacterial and antiviral qualities can also be utilized as possible therapies against COVID-19 [10].

Various clinical trials registered for COVID-19 and development stages of different therapeutics are illustrated in Figure 5.1.

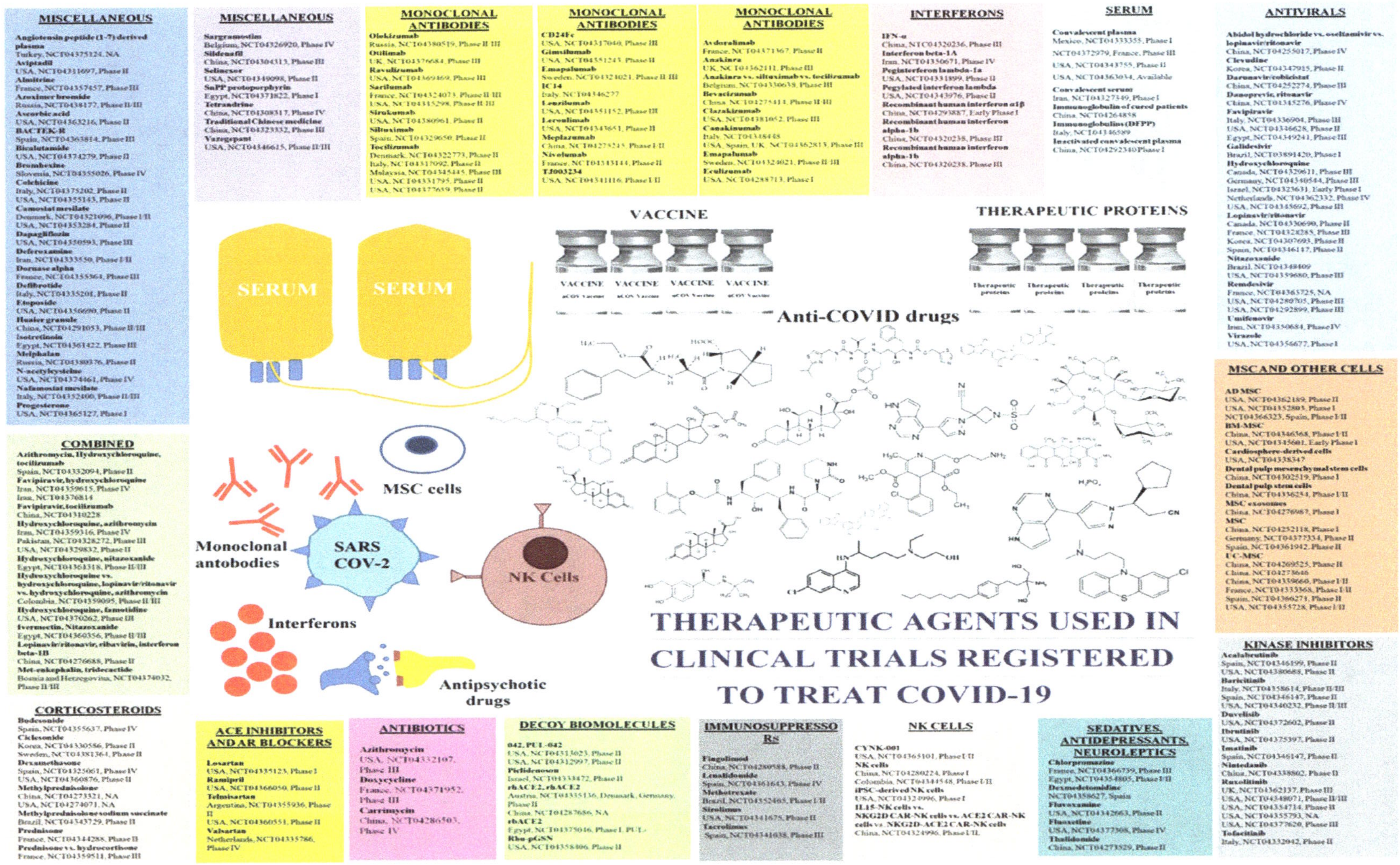

FIGURE 5.1 Registered clinical trials for COVID-19 and development stages of different therapeutics in the pipeline. WJ-MSC: Wharton jelly–derived MSC, UC-MSC: umbilical cord–derived MSC, Rhu-pGSN: recombinant human plasma gelsolin, rhACE2: recombinant human angiotensin-converting enzyme-2, rbACE2: recombinant bacterial angiotensin-converting enzyme-2, NK cells: natural killer cells, MSC: mesenchymal stem (stromal) cells; DFPP: double-filtration plasmapheresis, BM-MSC: bone marrow–derived MSC, AR: angiotensin receptor, AD MSC: adipose-derived MSC, ACE: angiotensin-converting enzyme.

5.3 Drug Repositioning for COVID-19 Treatment

Due to unavailability of safe and effective antiviral treatment at this stage, none of vaccine candidate passed all the phases of clinical trials. This is mainly due to the several pathogenesis, and proliferation pathways of COVID-19 are still unknown [1–5]. Current treatment of critically ill patients is based on the symptoms and oxygen therapy. Due to its various advantages, drug repositioning could be a reliable strategy to to treat COVID-19 [1–5]. Due to considerable advantages such as less time consumed during safety evaluation as well as preclinical assessment of medication during their development cycle, drug repositioning is always preferred for the treatment of new infection [1–5]. Additionally, less criteria for the preliminary screening of drug/compound on the basis of drug efficacy and safety and also availability of drug candidates that have shown adequate safety in preclinical and human trials make drug repositioning desirable [1–5].

5.3.1 Antimalarial Drugs

Chloroquine, a 4-aminoquinoline, is an inexpensive and potent alkaloid therapeutic (from the bark of Remija and Cinchona species) that is primarily used as approved antimalarial as well as immuno-modulator medication and has been recently studied for its effectiveness as a potential antiviral drug. This drug has been used for the last 70 years [19]. Chloroquine prevents viral infection by elevating pH in endosomes that are essential for virus/cell fusion, as well as interferes with the terminal glycosylation of ACE2 receptor of the host cell [20]. Chloroquine, also known for its anti-inflammatory response, can decrease the progression of COVID-19 due to hyperinflammatory response [21]. Both chloroquine and hydroxychloroquine have immunomodulatory effects and can suppress immune response as they inhibit the toll-like receptor pathway involved in pro-inflammatory cytokine signaling [22]. A recent study of Vero E6 cells showed that chloroquine demonstrates inhibitory activity against SARS-CoV-2 ($EC50 = 1.13\,\mu M$). In contrast, in other investigations chloroquine showed no significant results and also caused cardiac complications [23]. Thus, utilization of this drug can be unsafe for COVID-19 patients, especially when there is dose error [23]. Several clinical trials were registered and performed in China to determine the safety and efficacy of chloroquine for the treatment of COVID-19-associated pneumonia [24]. Chloroquine was found to be effective against SARS-CoV-2; however, other reports claimed some undesirable effects. Because of unexpected outcomes in some trials, the WHO delayed further clinical trials on hydroxychloroquine; nevertheless, this repurposed drug has been considered for re-evaluation of certain parameters such as active dose, time of administration, and unfavorable effects as well as its preventive effect over COVID-19 [25]. Guangdong region suggested chloroquine (500 mg, twice a day) for 10 days for any COVID-19 patient without contraindications to chloroquine [26]. High dose or overdose of chloroquine (>5 g) has been linked with mortality because of ventricular dysrhythmias and hypokalemia. Overdose can also lead to cardiovascular and neurological complications [26]. Recently, an Arizona man died and his wife was hospitalized after consumption of chloroquine phosphate [27]. Other cases of chloroquine poisoning have been reported in Nigeria [28].

Hydroxychloroquine, a chloroquine analog, can be explored as a safe and effective therapy for SARS-CoV-2 infection, as it represents potential in vitro antiviral activity against SARS-CoV with a better clinical profile [29]. In addition to its in vitro potential, hydroxychloroquine showed better viral inhibitory effects against SARS-CoV-2 in comparison with chloroquine [29]. Various clinical trials have been registered and performed to determine the safety and efficacy of hydroxychloroquine. The optimal amount of hydroxychloroquine (400 mg/d, 200 mg bid) was evaluated in a previous clinical study (ChiCTR2000029559) for COVID-19 [30]. Sixty-two COVID-19 patients (31 treated with hydroxychloroquine and another 31 considered as the control group) were treated [31]. After 5 days, it was found that the clinical improvement period of the hydroxychloroquine-treated group was signfiicantly reduced with considerable relief from fever, cough, and pneumonia when compared to control group. Clinical trial ($n = 36$ COVID-19 patients) based on the combination of hydroxychloroquine with azithromycin was also performed, which showed better effects than hydroxychloroquine alone [31,32]. Just like chloroquine, hydroxychloroquine showed a similar mechanism of action whereby it interacts with glycosylation of ACE2 and reduces the interaction among ACE2 and surface protein of SARS-CoV-2 [33]. Also, hydroxychloroquine increases endosomal pH to avert SARS-CoV-2 fusion with host cells and subsequent replication [34]. Moreover, hydroxychloroquine also restricts antigen presentation mediated by major histocompatibility complex (MHC)-II to CD4 T cells that suppresses stimulation of T cells and other inflammatory mediators, mainly CD154 expression [35]. Hydroxychloroquine can possibly the nucleic acid sensors cGAS and TLR9 via alteration of the structural configuration of the DNA substrate [36]. Thus, both chloroquine and hydroxychloroquine can prevent the progression of inflammatory responses among COVID-19 patients by inhibiting replication and invasion as well as decreasing the possibility of cytokine storm by suppressing T-cell stimulation. Utilization of chloroquine and hydroxychloroquine in combination with azithromycin or oseltamivir can increase mortality and adverse cardiac events. Hydroxychloroquine has a better clinical safety profile than chloroquine that allows a high daily dose [35]. However, more information related to the safety and efficacy of chloroquine and hydroxychloroquine is required before its utilization in the treatment of COVID-19 [35].

5.3.2 Antiviral Drugs

Until now, no antiviral drug has been recommended for COVID-19 patients with a suspected or confirmed infection. However, preclinical data suggest the antiviral potential of many antiviral drugs. Antiviral drugs, lopinavir as well as ritonavir, have been utilized to treat human immunodeficiency virus and have been tested against COVID-19 infection. It was found that amount of SARS-CoV-2 in an infected blood sample was considerably reduced post-treatment [37]. Preclinical data also suggest that lopinavir inhibits the protease activity of SARS-CoV-2 under *in vitro* and *in vivo* conditions [37]. It was also found during a matched-cohort study that involved 1,052 SARS patients that initial treatment with lopinavir/ritonavir decreased mortality rate (2.3% vs. 11.0%) [38]. These protease inhibitors were hypothesized to inhibit the 3-chymotrypsin-like and PL proteases of SARS-CoV-2 [38]. This led to controversy because HIV protease is from the aspartic protease family, while the 3-chymotrypsin-like and PLpros are from the family of cysteine protease [39]. Furthermore, HIV protease inhibitors target HIV protease, which is a C2-symmetrical dimeric enzyme and considered as a site of action for potent inhibitors; nevertheless, this C2-symmetric pocket is not present in coronavirus proteases [40]. To hinder coronavirus infection, if these HIV protease inhibitors are modifying host pathways, then their effectiveness remains a concern [41]. On July 4, 2020, the WHO considered the suggestion from the solidarity trial's international steering committee (a multinational phase III-IV clinical trial organized by the WHO) to stop the trial's hydroxychloroquine and lopinavir/ritonavir arms [42].

The potent broad-spectrum antiviral agent remdesivir (nucleoside analog) that acts against several RNA viruses and was initially used for the Ebola disease has been claimed to be an alternative to treat SARS-CoV-2 infection [43]. Remdesivir efficiently reduces the amount of virus in the tissue of lungs and improves lungs performance in animal model infected with Middle East respiratory syndrome (MERS-CoV) [44]. Recently, remdesivir with emetine presented 64.9% inhibition of SARS-CoV-2 under in vitro conditions [45]. As far as its clinical usage is concerned, Grein et al. described excellent recovery in patients suffering from severe COVID-19 treated with remdesivir [46]. Similar findings were also observed in the United States for treatment of COVID-19 patients [47]. Remdesivir and IFN-b also showed an excellent antiviral potential in comparison with lopinavir and ritonavir in vitro [5]. Based on cell-based assay findings, remdesivir induced RNA chain that demonstrates its high potency against RNA [48]. Also, in the United States, remdesivir-treated COVID-19 patients and showed improvement in clinical condition [49]. Nevertheless, remdesivir did not show significant clinical benefits during a randomized, double-blind, placebo-controlled, multicenter trial, as reported by Wang et al., due to which its effectiveness in COVID-19 is still doubted [44]. Phase II and III clinical trial of remdesivir carried out by the University of Nebraska Medical Center, Omaha, Nebraska, USA, and China-Japan Friendship Hospital showed improvement in mortality and recovery rate. Preliminary data also showed that remdesivir has more potential than lopinavir/ritonavir–IFN-b [50].

Favipiravir, a nucleoside and pyrazine carboxamide derivative, is a RNA-dependent RNA polymerase inhibitor that is accepted for the management of novel or re-emerging pandemic influenza among different nations [51]. Intracellularly favipiravir is metabolized into its active form (i.e., phosphoribosylated form (favipiravir-RTP)) and considered as a substrate by viral RNA polymerase and as a result suppresses RNA polymerase activity [51]. Preliminary findings on 35 COVID-19 patients revealed that favipiravir takes less time to reduce viral load (4 days vs. 11 days) and also shows higher improvement rates of chest image than lopinavir and ritonavir and with fewer adverse reactions when compared to control group [52]. A study (ChiCTR2000030254) on 240 COVID-19 patients performed by Zhongnan Hospital of Wuhan University showed that favipiravir showed considerably better results than control group. Favipiravir is an agent that causes physical or functional defects in the human fetus and thus was banned for its use in pregnancy as well lactation [52]. Ribavirin, an antiviral guanosine derivative, alone as well in combination was utilized effectively in the treatment SARS and MERS [53]. Earlier findings proved its effectiveness in rhesus macaques infected with MERS-CoV [54]. It was also utilized to treat several virus infections, such as hepatitis C virus, respiratory syncytial virus, and some viral hemorrhagic fevers [55]. Moreover, targeting RNA-dependent RNA polymerase of COVID-19 virus by ribavirin on the basis of sequence analysis, modeling, and docking to build a suitable model was done [56]. This showed increased antiviral potential against COVID-19 virus [56]. Moreover, ribavirin also showed direct in vitro antiviral activity against SARS-CoV-2; in particular, it has beneficial effects in the treatment of COVID-19-induced pneumonia and before sepsis or organ system failure [53]. The effect of ribavirin in combination with interferon-α was tested over SARS-CoV-2-infected Vero and LLC-MK2 cells. Findings from this study showed that ribavirin inhibits the replication of SARS-CoV-2 at very low concentration (both ribavirin and interferon-α) [57].

Arbidol or Umifenovir is a broad-spectrum antiviral medication currently approved in both China as well as Russia against respiratory illness (upper) triggered via influenza viruses (A and B) [58]. The antiviral activity of this drug is based on the inhibition of hemagglutinin present as surface protein in influenza virus. Hemagglutinin shows its high binding affinity against human cells' sialic acid receptors that facilitate its entry inside human cells via endocytosis. Inhibition of hemagglutinin by Arbidol prevents its entry and subsequent infections caused by influenza virus to human cells [58]. This drug has shown its antiviral effects against several more viruses such as Ebola virus, Zika virus, herpes simplex Lassa virus, and flavivirus [59]. Additionally, it has shown activity against COVID-19 virus. Due to its direct virucidal activity and action on single or multiple phases of the life cycle of the virus, Arbidol offers broad-spectrum action. Apart from its ability to show its interaction with amino acid residues, it also inhibits viral lipid envelope, trafficking pathways inside cell, and clathrin-facilitated endocytosis [60]. Direct involvement of Arbidol with virus aromatic residues of the glycoprotein, which are accountable for cellular identification and fusion, is the major cause of antiviral activity. Thus, Arbidol alone or in a combination treatment approach for COVID-19 patients can be considered as a potential therapy. Various clinical trials have been registered and performed to evaluate the safety and efficacy of Arbidol. An *in vitro* study performed in China showed that Arbidol efficiently suppresses coronavirus infection at small dose (10–30 μM). On the basis of its efficacy in COVID-19 infection, the National Health Commission, People's Republic of China, introduced Arbidol in recent procedures for the inhibition, identification, as well treatment of novel coronavirus-induced pneumonia as a provisional therapy of COVID-19. As far as bioavailability is concerned Arbidol is quickly absorbed when administered orally and has shown maximum plasma concentration (415–467 ng/mL) that needs time of 0.65–1.8 h [61]. Arbidol plasma half-life (which is 17–21 h) is dependent on how quickly it is eliminated from the plasma via feces. For the treatment of COVD-19 infection, 200 mg of Arbidol is administered thrice daily for up to 10 days [62]. Darunavir is an antiretroviral second-generation protease inhibitor for the effective management of HIV-1 infection. On February 4th, 2020, scientists in China claimed that darunavir inhibited *in vitro* COVID-19 illness. It was also reported that darunavir prevents replication of the virus at 300 μM concentration under in vitro conditions, with an inhibition efficacy of 280 times in comparison with control group [63]. Among COVID-19-induced pneumonia patients, darunavir is used in combination with cobicistat (NCT04252274) [64]. This combination of darunavir (protease inhibitor) and cobicistat is an approved treatment for AIDS. Cobicistat is added to improve darunavir pharmacokinetics as well as pharmacodynamics profile via suppressing cyt.P450 [65,66]. Thus, effectiveness as well as safety profile of this combination therapy is limited to HIV settings. So far, no report is available over the use of darunavir in combination with other drugs in SARS-CoV-2.

Oseltamivir is an antiviral neuraminidase inhibitor and suitable for the treatment of acute and uncomplicated influenza A or B by selective inhibition of the influenza virus neuraminidase. Oseltamivir acts by inhibiting the release of viral particles from host cells and its replication thereby reduces its subsequent transmission in the respiratory tract. In China, oseltamivir was tested with or without antibiotics and corticosteroids for the treatment of COVID-19 [67]. Moreover, it was also used in combination with favipiravir as well as chloroquine during clinical studies [68].

5.3.3 Antibiotics

Azithromycin is a broad-spectrum antibiotic that has demonstrated potential action against COVID-19 virus by interacting with its surface (S) protein as well as ACE2 protein. This prevents viral invasion into cells. Various reports suggest that chloroquine with azithromycin is effective effective in decreasing the viral load during the SARS Cov-2 infection treatment. For COVID-19 treatment, azithromycin (1–2 g) in with chloroquine/hydroxychloroquine is usually used. So far more than 80 clinical trials have been recorded for investigating the potential of azithromycin with various medications in the treatment of COVID-19. Gautret et al. performed clinical studies on COVID-19 patients to determine the effectiveness of combination therapy (azithromycin and hydroxychloroquine) [69] and found that hydroxychloroquine (500 mg/day) as well as azithromycin (250 mg/day for 5 days) effectively decreased the load of virus.

Tetracyclines are therapeutics having bacteriostatic action. Many investigations have suggested that in addition to bacterial inhibitory effects, tetracyclines also have antiviral properties against viruses such as COVID-19 [70]. As has been reported, tetracycline possibly shows antiviral activity by three mechanisms against COVID-19 virus. Tetracyclines (e.g., tetracycline, doxycycline, and minocycline) act by chelating with the zinc compound present over matrix metalloproteinases. Coronaviruses are dependent on host matrix metalloproteinases for their survival, replication, and invasion. Also, tetracyclines have been reported to inhibit the expression of pro-inflammatory mediators via decreasing expression of proteins involved NFKB pathways and also to cause direct inhibition of the replication in the pulmonary tissue, which is primarily due to its lipophilic nature as well as tissue-penetrating capability [71].

Teicoplanin is a therapeutic approved for the treatment of bacterial infections (mainly Gram-positive) such as infections caused by staphylococcus strains and has shown antiviral effects against various viruses [72].

Effectiveness of molecular targets of teicoplanin against coronavirus is determined based on the prevention of release of the viral genome and prevention of its replication [72]. This is due to the inhibition of viral spike protein cleavage at low pH via endopeptidase enzyme called as cathepsin L [73]. One investigation also revealed that teicoplanin effectively prevents the invasion of the SARS-CoV-2 spike pseudovirus into the cytoplasm [74].

5.3.4 Interferons

Antiviral interferons, also known as clusters of cytokines, play an important role in the innate immune system in human beings [75]. During viral infection, these cytokines are primarily produced by host cells; however, among SARS-CoV as well as MERS-CoV patients, interferon generation is inhibited. Interferon fixation over interferon receptors present on most of the cells is responsible for the activation of interferon stimulating genes that can further initiate immunomodulatory and inflammatory reactions by downregulating the secretion or metabolism of cytokines via inhibiting with replication of virus [76]. Interferon-stimulating genes also avoid fusion of the membrane via diminishing the fluidity of the membrane and provoke the host cells against pathogenic microbes [77]. Monotherapy based on the interferons or its combination with ribavirin, which was tested under in vitro conditions and animal models, did not show good results, which may be due to delay in administration via subcutaneous route or due to the multiple organ injury. Interferon administration via inhalation was recommended at the beginning of the pandemic to ensure increased amounts of the drug in lung tissue and to bypass delay caused via subcutaneous administration. However, in view of the risk of transmission of infectious aerosols, lack of availability of clinical data, contraindication with some patients and doubtful pharmacokinetics profile, it is challenging to recommend IFN inhalation for the treatment of COVID-19 patients. The pharmacokinetic profile of interferon has not been determined yet; however, pegylated IFN has the half-life of 4.6–22 h. Clinical studies were performed to study the efficacy of pegylated IFN-α for the SARS-Cov-2 infection treatment. Clinical studies (open-label, controlled, randomized phase II) with pegylated IFN λ (NCT04343976) and IFN λ (pegylated form) - (NCT04388709) among COVID-19 patients were also initiated [78,79].

5.3.5 Corticosteroids

Corticosteroids are recognized for their immunosuppressant potential, which is needed to suppress lung inflammation and cytokine storms to prevent the development of pneumonia and also for acute respiratory syndrome treatment. Other than its immunosuppressant effect, corticosteroids also exhibit anti-inflammatory effect by reducing systemic inflammation and accumulation of fluid in the lung, and prevent alveolar injury to prevent subsequent hypoxemia. The role of corticosteroids was also investigated among COVID-19 patients being treated with steroids for longer duration, and it was observed that there was no increased frequency of development of severe pneumonia. However, the role of corticosteroids in COVID-19 is still controversial as their administration can increase risks of secondary infection and delay virus clearance among SARS and influenza pneumonia patients [80]. Earlier reports that showed low-dose corticosteroid administration among COVID-19 patients showed potential benefits in spite of any improvement in survival rate [81,82]. However, reports also showed that the treatment of severe COVID-19 patients with corticosteroids can improve mortality [81,82]. Corticosteroids can be utilized to suppress a host's immune response caused by the pathogen to prevent sepsis shock. The incidence of sepsis shock is extremely low among COVID-19 patients (<5% of cases) and treatment of such critically ill patients with corticosteroids showed variable results [81,82]. Thus, because of its negative effect on the immune system, their use in COVID-19 treatment is still debated. The Centers for Disease Control and Prevention and the WHO also recommend against corticosteroids use among COVID-19 patients for immune modulation.

5.4 Immunotherapy (Passive)

Following approaches have been used for development of therapeutics such as vaccines and antibodies against SARS-CoV-2:

5.4.1 Convalescent Plasma Transfusion

Convalescent plasma treatment involves giving sick patients blood transfusions with pooled plasma or immunoglobulins donated by infected patients who have been recovered from a disease. This therapy does not always show significant results as was seen among Ebola patients, where the convalescent plasma transfusions also did not show significant results [83]. However, in the case of COVID-19 patients, it was found that the transfusion of convalescent plasma reduced hypoxia (improved oxygenation) and immediately decreased viral load among a small group of patients (intubated and non-intubated) with acute lung injury [84]. However, there are some considerable adverse effects caused by plasma transfusion such as allergic/anaphylactic reactions, transfusion reaction due to volume excess (led to the development of pulmonary edema), and transfusion-associated acute lung injury [85]. Moreover, chances of transmission of infections, RBC (red blood cell) alloimmunization, and transfusion reaction due to fever but not directly with hemolysis and transfusion reactions due to hemolysis were less common. Several reports suggested that convalescent plasma transfusion showed no major adverse effects except reactions such as chills and fevers due to minor infusion reactions [86]. Anti-Ebola virus antibodies such as MAb114 and REGN-EB3 developed for Ebola treatment considerably decreased death rate from Ebola virus disease. As monoclonal antibodies have monovalent affinity, which means they can only recognize a single antigen epitope, this feature restricted MAb114 and REGN-EB3 use for the treatment of COVID-19 [87].

Antibody administration among infected and vulnerable individuals offers instant immunity or boosts the immune system in order to prevent or treat the infection [88–90]. Thus, identification of recovered individuals with high titer of neutralizing antibodies in sera and its extraction from these individuals to further transfuse neutralizing antibodies to infected patients can neutralize antigens of the virus [91]. Nevertheless, more research is required to understand the neutralization potential of these antibodies. It was found that these neutralizing antibodies must be extracted from recently recovered patients because these antibodies do not last long [91]. Also, titer volume of neutralizing antibodies among elderly patients was found to be higher than recovered individuals. It was also assumed that transfusion of convalescent serum may lead to phagocytosis and antibody-mediated cellular cytotoxicity [92]. Convalescent serum therapy has considerable disadvantages as this treatment can increase chances for antibody-dependent enhancement [93]. As per earlier assumptions, neutralizing antibodies can increase chances for other viral infections. Also, donor availability is always a concern as most of the recovered patients are not easily convinced to donate plasma [88].

5.4.2 Monoclonal Antibodies

Monoclonal antibody-based therapy possibly is an active technique for COVID-19 treatment [94]. Various methods are available to develop monoclonal antibodies including single isolation of B lymphocytes, hybridoma, transgenic mice, and phage display library [94]. Monoclonal antibodies, such as LCA60, 80R, m396, and S3.1, were developed for the treatment of MERS and SARS infections [94]. Monoclonal antibody-based therapy inhibited replication of virus as well as allowed rapid recovery of lungs in an experimental animal model [95]. As found in earlier investigations, S protein (type I transmembrane protein contains two subunits, S1 and S2; S1 contains a RBD) is considered as the most immunogenic protein in coronaviruses [96].

Receptor-binding domain of S protein encourages viral invasions into host cells by first binding to a host receptor. A number of SARS-CoV-specific human monoclonal antibodies such as S230, 80R, F26G18, F26G19, CR3014, CR3022, M396, and S230.15 can bind to RBD in the virus spike glycoproteins and prevent virus entry into the cells [97]. However, it was suggested that out of these human monoclonal antibodies, CR3022 might represent the highest binding affinity with SARS-CoV-2 S-protein RBD [98]. CR3022 can be considered as a potential therapeutic human monoclonal antibody (independently or with other neutralizing antibodies) for the treatment and prevention of COVID-19 infection [99]. Moreover, it was also suggested that monoclonal antibodies against SARS-CoV-1 could cross-react with SARS-CoV-2 [100]. It was found that monoclonal antibodies 1A9 that can target the S protein of SARS-CoV-1 might also target the S protein in SARS-CoV-2 [101]. Therefore, CR3022 antibody can potentially bind with the SARS-CoV-2 RBD; however, other antibodies such as 230, m396, and 80R (those are effective against SARS-CoV RBD) cannot bind to the SARS-CoV-2 RBD [101].

Tocilizumab is a humanized monoclonal antibody also known as antihuman IL-6 receptor antibody due to its capability to act against the IL-6 receptor cytokine, which is responsible for immune responses and inflammatory reactions [102]. Tocilizumab inhibits IL-6 from binding to both membrane-bound and soluble receptor and can be administered via intravenous and subcutaneous routes. Except for the risk of complications like malignancy, gastrointestinal perforation, and dose-dependent neutropenia, tocilizumab showed a good safety profile. Tocilizumab can possibly be an effective treatment for COVID-19 as when COVID-19 becomes severe (ARDS), it led to the production of a high amount of interleukin-6 and interleukin-8 [103]. A study on a small number of COVID-19 patients ($n=21$) showed that tocilizumab therapy could be an effective treatment [104]. A recent report also showed that tocilizumab treatment caused a rise in body temperature, whereas C-reactive protein resumed to the normal range with improvement in lung function [103]. Many trials have been conducted on the safety and effectiveness of tocilizumab against COVID-19.

Vascular endothelial growth factor covalently linked homodimeric angiogenic protein responsible for acute lung injury and acute respiratory distress syndrome. Plasma levels of vascular endothelial growth factor were found to be considerably higher among intensive care unit patients, non-intensive care unit patients, and COVID-19 patients than in normal individuals. Promising humanized monoclonal antibodies like bevacizumab for critical COVID-19 patients can target and bind vascular endothelial growth factor. Clinical trials have also reported the safety and effectiveness of this antivascular endothelial growth factor against COVID-19 (NCT04275414). As COVID-19 infection also leads to a decrease in T lymphocytes and natural killer cells, regain cell numbers, monoclonal antibodies can be utilized to prevent the TIM3 as well as PD-1/PD-L1 associated pathways [105].

5.5 Vaccines

Various drug candidates have been clinically tested via clinical trials to decrease the progression of infection as well as mortality; however, none of them proved to be 100% effective. One of the most successful approaches to controlling COVID-19 is to develop a vaccine.A lot of scientific institutes are competing to develop vaccines; however, all are experiencing several challenges. Positive-side structure of SARS-CoV-2 S protein is now well known which will accelerate the development of safe and effective vaccine candidates. Till now (July 2, 2020), more than 158 vaccine candidates have entered into clinical pipeline; however, majority of them are at initial or preclinical trials. Currently, pathogen-specific aAPC (Shinzen Genoimmune Medical Institute), Ad5-nCoV (CanSino Biologics), LV-SMENP-DC, mRNA-1273 (Moderna), INO-4800 (Inovio, Inc.), and ChAdOx1 (University of Oxford) are under phase I/II clinical trials [106,107]. Vaccines that are under clinical pipeline are based on the DNA/RNA, nanoparticles, protein subunit, inactivated or live attenuated viruses, viral vectors (replicating and non-replicating), virus-like particles, etc. [108]. Currently, numerous adjuvant technologies are available such as CpG 1018 (Dynavax), MF-59 (Novartis), and AS03 (GSK) for effective immunization, which can further accelerate the vaccine development [109]. Other strategies such as immuno-informatics involve the application of computational methods for multi-epitope vaccine designing against SARS-CoV-2 [110]. This method is utilized in detection of epitope for the SARS-CoV-2 vaccines and also utilized to identify important cytotoxic T as well as B lymphocytes epitopes in the viral spike protein. One hundred and thirty-six vaccine candidates based on the mRNA, DNA, adenoviral/lentiviral/bacterial vector-based vaccines, and inactivated SARS-CoV-2 has entered into clinical trial (June 19, 2020) [107]. DNA- and mRNA-based vaccines always carry an advantage in terms of ease in manufacturing and manipulation of antigen; however, no approved DNA/mRNA-based vaccines are available for use in humans [111]. mRNA offers more advantages than DNA-based vaccine as these candidates can trigger a much wider variety of innate as well as adaptive immune reactions that are required against SARS-CoV-2. Moderna, an American biotechnology company, developed mRNA vaccine (SARS-CoV-2 mRNA-1273) that is now under phase II clinical trials and sooner enters into phase III trials [112]. Adenoviral vector vaccines via targeting dendritic cells could be another approach against COVID-19. Recently, a Chinese vaccine company (CanSino Biologics) and Chinese military medical research institute have developed a non-replicating vector based on the human adenovirus serotype-5 containing spike gene and clinical trials are in process in Wuhan, China [113,114]. Similarly, ChAdOx1 weakened and non-replicating versions of common cold virus have been engineered to carry SARS-CoV-2 spike gene and experimented to show immune response against SARS-CoV-2, now under phase III clinical trials. These vaccines are made by adding genetic material of SARS-CoV-2 spike and considered as safe even people have weak immunity. Another approach for immunization is the modification of dendritic cells/antigen-presenting cells via lentiviral vector (LV-SMENP-DC vaccine) [109]. The subcutaneous administration of the vaccine activates the cytotoxic T cells and triggers the immune response via the presentation of the antigens on antigen-presenting cells. Some of the vaccines that are entered into clinical trials and considered as promising candidates: ZyCoV-D in Phase I/II: CTRI/2020/07/026352 (CTRI/2020/07/026352, 2020) [115] by Zydus Cadila; BNT162 [116] in Phase III: NCT04368728 by BioNTech, Fosun Pharma, Pfizer; adenovirus type5 vector/non-replicating viral vaccine in Phase II: ChiCTR2000031781 [117] by CanSino Biological Inc./Beijing Institute of Biotechnology; BBV152 (A-C) in Phase I/II: NCT04471519 [115] by Bharat Biotech/ICMR/NIV; PiCoVacc [118] in Phase III: NCT04456595 by Sinovac; mRNA-1273 in Phase III: NCT04470427 [119] by Moderna/NIAID; and ChAdOx1, Phase III: ISRCTN89951424 [120] by the University of Oxford/AstraZeneca.

- As far as the development of safe and effective SARS-CoV-2 vaccine is concerned, USFDA and WHO already laid down standards for their development, as they have to pass through minimum three placebo-controlled clinical trials, this may take more than years to successfully complete. Preliminary investigation is based on the laboratory animal models as these animals respond in a same manner as like human beings. Nevertheless, as a result of the dissimilarity between humans and mice ACE2 receptors, mice of an inbred strain are not susceptible to the SARS-CoV-2 infection (Anon [121]). This encourages the development and involvement of transgenic mice such as K18-hACE2 transgenic mouse for the expression of hACE2 protein in order to perform coronavirus research. hACE2 transgenic mice model and rhesus macaques model have been developed before for the SARS-CoV; however, to fulfill global demands, steady breeding is required. It was also found that transmissibility as well as pathogenicity of SARS-CoV-2 in golden (Syrian) hamsters mimick pattern of COVID-19 among human. Thus, the Syrian hamster can also be considered as a suitable model to understand the pathogenesis of coronavirus, and assessment of vaccines, antiviral medications, and immune-based treatment. However, evaluation of the vaccine based on immune stimulation cannot be merely estimated on the basis of animal models and thus requires a valid investigation of stage III human trials. Another approach, namely immune enhancement or antibody-dependent enhancement, can be utilized as an another approach of causing infection among range of host cells. In this approach, preexisting antibodies developed from primary infection do not neutralize secondary viral infection, but enhance it, possibly by triggering Fcγ receptor-mediated virus uptake. The virus-antibody complex may bind to the Fcprotein, trigger the complement system, or cause structural changes in viral envelope glycoprotein [122]. Several clinical studies based on SARS-CoV vaccine presented the excaberation of the infection because of the progression of ADE. Another challenge during the development of the vaccine is viral genome that is always at the risk of genomic alterations and may experience the antigenic shift and the antigenic drift. Findings from large size of samples (n=7,500) of theinfected patients showed 198 mutations that represent the development of the virus in the host. Mutation resulted in the generation of different subtypes that can allow the virus to escape from the host immune response even after treatment with a suitable vaccine [123].

5.6 Natural Products

Keywords such as extract, plant, natural products, SARS-CoV, COVID-19, and coronavirus were used to locate articles in the PubMed database (www.ncbi.nlm.nih.gov/pubmed/). Reports mainly aimed at the antiviral activity of either phytochemicals or plant-based extracts were considered. All articles up to August 27, 2020 were studied, comprising a total of 1,226 results. After screening, out of these 1,266 articles, many articles were excluded on the basis of relevance producing a total of 67 main articles including both human as well as animal coronaviruses vs. natural products included in this review. Relevant information received from these articles is tabulated in Table 5.1, which summarizes the suitable investigations based on the suppression of different human coronavirus strains using phytochemicals isolated from plant sources. Table 5.1 includes phytochemicals or extracts with their respective biological source and IC50 or EC50 and type of assay used in the study along with the possible mechanism of action. The information in Table 5.1 is arranged in such a manner so that the antiviral activity of extract or compound can be compared among different phytochemicals or extracts vs. different viral strains. Phytochemicals isolated from the plant materials have been resported for viral inhibitory effects via following specific pathways as presented in Table 5.1. EC50 (effective concentration) and IC50 (inhibitory concentration) of various phytochemicals or plant extracts derived from different cell-based assays and enzyme- or biochemical-based assays are also presented.

5.6.1 Role of Essential Oils in Treatment of COVID-19

Essential oils (EOs) are the complex mixture of various active volatile (mono- and sesquiterpenoids, and phenylpropanoids) as well as nonvolatile components. The majority of the oxygenated terpenoids present in EOs such as ketones, peroxides, alcohols, aldehydes, esters, and phenols exhibit strong antimicrobial activity. These active chemical constituents such as eugenol, geranic, citronellol, geraniol, linalool, citronellyl formate, citral, myrtenol, terpineol, methone, and sabinene are responsible for various biological activities. EOs are isolated from the plant material by various conventional and advanced distillation techniques or by supercritical fluid extraction methods. The chemical profiles of EOs are usually determined by gas chromatography–mass spectrometry. Yield and chemical composition of EOs can vary and is dependent on several factors such as isolation procedure used, environmental conditions of plant, nature of soil, part of plant, chemotype, and genotype of plant species. Chemical composition and amount of chemical constituents determine the biological activity of EOs. Due to the development of various multidrug-resistant strains and increasing antibiotic resistance, various researchers are now focused on antimicrobial phytochemicals/extracts with the hope of finding novel antimicrobials. Recently, a numbers of report based on in vitro antimicrobial effects of EOs have been published. Based on the data reported by the WHO, lower respiratory infections are cause for about 5% of deaths across the globe. Various treatments such as antibiotics and vaccine candidates have been developed; however, existing treatments are not effective against novel pathogenic strains. Aromatherapy is a natural therapy that has been practiced for centuries to prevent and treat various respiratory disorders. This EO-based treatment can be considered as an effective alternative approach to the treatment of respiratory tract infections (Figure 5.1). EO-based treatment of respiratory viral infections via inhalation can be considered as the most effective method. Due to their volatile properties, EOs and their components can reach the desirable site in the respiratory tract where they can exhibit their biological actions. The safety and efficacy of EOs can be assessed by various in vitro (such as broth dilution, disk diffusion, and agar diffusion) and

TABLE 5.1
Anti-SARS-CoV-1 Natural Metabolites Tested *in vitro*

Natural Source	Compound/Extract Type	IC_{50}/EC_{50}	Mechanism of Action	Method to Assess Activity	Test System	References
(−)-Catechin gallate and (−)-gallocatechin gallate	Pure compounds were used	0.05 μg/mL	Nanoparticle-based RNA oligonucleotide inhibition	Fluorescent assay in a confocal laser-scanning microscope	SARS-CoV	[124]
Cladistris-lectins isolated from diaminopropane extracts, Man/Glc-specific	*Cladrastis lutea*	7.4±0.2 μg/mL	Inhibition of viral binding and another target at the end of the replication cycle	CPE assay	SARS-CoV	[125]
EHA-Man-specific agglutinins	*Epipactis helleborine*	1.8±0.3 μg/mL	Inhibition of viral binding and another target at the end of the replication cycle	CPE assay	SARS-CoV	[126]
Glechoma-GalNAc-specific agglutinins	*Glechoma hederacea*	>100 μg/mL	Inhibition of viral binding and another target at the end of the replication cycle	CPE assay	SARS-CoV	[127]
Hevein-(GlcNAc)n-specific agglutinins	*Hevea brasiliensis*	>100 μg/mL	Inhibition of viral binding and another target at the end of the replication cycle	CPE assay	SARS-CoV	[126]
IRA B-Lectins isolated from diaminopropane extracts, GalNAcα(1.3)Gal>Gal NAc>Gal-specific agglutinins	*Iris* hybrid	4.4±3.1 μg/mL	Inhibition of viral binding and another target at the end of the replication cycle	CPE assay	SARS-CoV	[125]
IRA r-Lectins isolated from diaminopropane extracts, GalNAcα(1.3)Gal>Gal NAc>Gal-specific agglutinins	*Iris* hybrid	3.4±2.0 μg/mL	Inhibition of viral binding and another target at the end of the replication cycle	CPE assay	SARS-CoV	[125]
IRA-Lectins isolated from diaminopropane extracts, GalNAcα(1.3)Gal>Gal NAc>Gal-specific agglutinins	*Iris* hybrid	2.2±0.9 μg/mL	Inhibition of viral binding and another target at the end of the replication cycle	CPE assay	SARS-CoV	[125]
Jacalin-Gal-specific agglutinins	*Artocarpus integrifolia*	>100 μg/mL	Inhibition of viral binding and another target at the end of the replication cycle	CPE assay	SARS-CoV	[126]
ML II Gal/GalNAc-specific agglutinins	*Viscum album*	0.015±0.003 μg/mL	Inhibition of viral binding and another target at the end of the replication cycle	CPE assay	SARS-CoV	[126]
ML III GalNAc (>Gal)-specific agglutinins	*Viscum album*	28±11 μg/mL	Inhibition of viral binding and another target at the end of the replication cycle	CPE assay	SARS-CoV	[126]
3′-(3-methylbut-2-enyl)-3′,4′,7-trihydroxyflavane5	*Broussonetia papyrifera*	30.2±6.8μM, 35.8±6.7 μM	Non-competitive inhibition of protease	SARS-CoV 3CLpro and PLpro inhibition assays	3-Chymotrypsin-like and papain-like coronavirus cysteine proteases	[128]

(Continued)

TABLE 5.1 (*Continued*)

Anti-SARS-CoV-1 Natural Metabolites Tested *in vitro*

Natural Source	Compound/Extract Type	IC_{50}/EC_{50}	Mechanism of Action	Method to Assess Activity	Test System	References
3′-(3-methylbut-2-enyl)-3′,4′,7-trihydroxyflavane5	*Broussonetia papyrifera*	34.7±2.0μM, 48.8±6.6μM	Inhibition of protease	MERS-CoV 3CLpro and PLpro inhibition assays	3-Chymotrypsin-like and papain-like coronavirus cysteine proteases	[128]
3′-O-Methyldiplacol	*Paulownia tomentosa*	9.5±0.10μM	Reversible, mixed-type (allosteric) inhibitors of PLpro	SARS-CoV PLpro inhibition assay	SARS-CoV PLpro	[129]
3′-O-Methyldiplacone	*Paulownia tomentosa*	13.2±0.14μM	Reversible, mixed-type (allosteric) inhibitors of PLpro	SARS-CoV PLpro inhibition assay	SARS-CoV PLpro	[129]
3-Isotheaflavin-3-gallate	Black tea	7μm	Inhibition of 3CLpro	3CLpro inhibition assay	SARS 3CLpro	[129]
3β,12-Diacetoxyabieta-6,8,11,13-tetraene (PCWU)	Labdane derivatives	1.57μM	Inhibits 50% of Vero E6 cell proliferation and viral replication	CPE on Vero E6 cells via SARS-CoV infection, SARS-CoV 3CL protease inhibition assay	SARS-CoV	[130]
3β-Acetoxy friedelane	*Euphorbia neriifolia*	80.9[h] (Cell survival (%))	ND	Anti-HCoV assay (MRC-5 system)	HCoV-229E	[131]
3β-friedelanol	*Euphorbia neriifolia*	132.4[h] (Cell survival (%))	ND	Anti-HCoV assay (MRC-5 system)	HCoV-229E	[131]
4,4′-O-Benzoylisolariciresinol (PCWU)	Neolignans	N.T.	Inhibits 50% of Vero E6 cell proliferation and viral replication	CPE on Vero E6 cells via SARS-CoV infection, SARS-CoV 3CL protease inhibition assay	SARS-CoV	[130]
4′-O-Methylbavachalcone	*Psoralea corylifolia*	10.1±1.2μM	Mixed inhibitor of SARS-CoV PLpro	Fluorogenic PLpro inhibition assay	SARS-CoV PLpro	[132]
4′-O-Methyldiplacol	*Paulownia tomentosa*	9.2±0.13μM	Reversible, mixed-type (allosteric) inhibitors of PLpro	SARS-CoV PLpro inhibition assay	SARS-CoV PLpro	[129]
4′-O-Methyldiplacone	*Paulownia tomentosa*	12.7±0.19μM	Reversible, mixed-type (allosteric) inhibitors of PLpro	SARS-CoV PLpro inhibition assay	SARS-CoV PLpro	[129]
4-Hydroxyisolonchocarpin3	*Broussonetia papyrifera*	202.7±3.9μM, 35.4±11.3μM	Non-competitive inhibition of protease	SARS-CoV 3CLpro and PLpro inhibition assays	3-Chymotrypsin-like and papain-like coronavirus cysteine proteases	[128]
4-Hydroxyisolonchocarpin3	*Broussonetia papyrifera*	193.7±15.6μM, 171.6±10.2μM	Inhibition of protease	MERS-CoV 3CLpro and PLpro inhibition assays	3-Chymotrypsin-like and papain-like coronavirus cysteine proteases	[128]
6,7-Dehydro royleanone (PCWU)	Abietane derivatives	5.55μM	Inhibits 50% of Vero E6 cell proliferation and viral replication	CPE on Vero E6 cells via SARS-CoV infection, SARS-CoV 3CL protease inhibition assay	SARS-CoV	[130]
6,7-Dihydroxyflavone	*Scutellaria baicalensis*	59.1±1.9 (% inhibition at 50μM)	Inhibits SARS-CoV-2 3CLpro activity	SARS-CoV 3CLpro assay	SARS-CoV-2 3CLpro activity	[133]
6-Geranyl-4′,5,7-trihydroxy-3′,5′-dimethoxyflavanone	*Paulownia tomentosa*	13.9±0.18μM	Reversible, mixed-type (allosteric) inhibitors of PLpro	SARS-CoV PLpro inhibition assay	SARS-CoV PLpro	[129]

(*Continued*)

TABLE 5.1 (*Continued*)
Anti-SARS-CoV-1 Natural Metabolites Tested *in vitro*

Natural Source	Compound/Extract Type	IC_{50}/EC_{50}	Mechanism of Action	Method to Assess Activity	Test System	References
7-Methoxycryptopleurine	*Tylophora indica*	20±1 nM	Inhibition of viral replication	CoV-infected swine testicular cells	SARS-CoV	[134]
7-Methoxycryptopleurine	*Tylophora indica*	<0.005 μM	Inhibition of protease	CoV-infected swine testicular cells	SARS-CoV	[134]
7-Phloroeckol	*Ecklonia cava*	18.6±2.3 μM (Simultaneous-treatment)	Prevents the viral binding of virus to cells	Simultaneous treatment assay	Porcine epidemic diarrhea CoV	[135]
7β-Hydroxy Deoxycryptojaponol (PCWU)	Abietane derivatives	1.15 μM	Inhibits 50% of Vero E6 cell proliferation and viral replication	CPE on Vero E6 cells via SARS-CoV infection, SARS-CoV 3CL protease inhibition assay	SARS-CoV	[130]
8β-Hydroxyabieta-9(11),13-dien-12-one) (PCWU)	Pure compound was used	1.47 μM	Inhibits 50% of Vero E6 cell proliferation and viral replication	CPE on Vero E6 cells via SARS-CoV infection, SARS-CoV 3CL protease inhibition assay	SARS-CoV	[130]
95% EtOH (contain lycorine)	*Lycoris radiata*	2.1–2.4 (all μg/mL)	ND	CPE/MTS assay	SARS-CoV (BJ001 and BJ006	[136]
Aescin, reserpine, valinomycin	*Aesculus hippocastanum and Rauvolfia serpentina*	3.4, 6.0, 0.85 μM	Inhibition of viral replication	SARS-CoV 3CL protease inhibition assay	SARS-CoV 3CL protease	[137]
Aloe emodin	*Isatis indigotica*	8.3 μM	Inhibition of 3CL protease	Protease inhibition test	SARS-CoV	[138]
Aloe-emodin	*Isatis indigotica*	132 μM	3CLpro inhibition	3CLpro cleavage assay	SARS-CoV 3CLpro	[138]
Amentoflavone	*Torreya nucifera*	8.3±1.2 μM	Non-competitive inhibition of CoV CLpro	CLpro inhibition assay	SARS-CoV CLpro	[139]
Amentoflavone	*Torreya nucifera*	8.3 μM	Inhibition of 3CL protease	3CLpro inhibition test	SARS-CoV	[139]
Apigenin	*Torreya nucifera*	280.8 μM	Inhibition of 3CL protease	3CLpro inhibition test	SARS-CoV	[139]
Baicalein	*Scutellaria baicalensis*	0.39±0.12 μM	Inhibits SARS-CoV-2 3CLpro activity	SARS-CoV 3CLpro assay	SARS-CoV-2 3CLpro activity	[133]
Baicalin	*Scutellaria baicalensis*	41.5±0.6 (% inhibition at 50 μM)	Inhibits SARS-CoV-2 3CLpro activity	SARS-CoV 3CLpro assay	SARS-CoV-2 3CLpro activity	[133]
Bavachinin	*Psoralea corylifolia*	38.4±2.4 μM	Mixed inhibitor of SARS-CoV PLpro	Fluorogenic PLpro inhibition assay	SARS-CoV PLpro	[132]
BDA-GalNAc-specific agglutinins	*Bryonia dioica*	>100 μg/mL	Inhibition of viral binding and another target at the end of the replication cycle	CPE assay	SARS-CoV	[126]
Berbamine	Purified compound	1.48 μM (HCoV-OC43 EC50); 9.46 μM (HCoV-NL63)	Antihypertensive, skeletal muscle relaxant	Indirect immunofluorescence assay	HCoV-OC43, HCoV-NL63	[140]
Berbamine		*1.48 μM*	ND		*HCoV-NL63*	[140]
Beta-sitosterol	*Isatis indigotica*	1.210 μM	Inhibition of 3CL protease	Protease inhibition test	SARS-CoV	[138]
Betulinic acid	*Isatis indigotica*	10 μM	3CL protease inhibition	Protease inhibition test	SARS-CoV	[130]
Betulinic acid (PCWU)	Triterpenes usually obtained from birch tree	>10 μM	Competitive inhibitors of SARS-CoV 3CL protease	CPE on Vero E6 cells via SARS-CoV infection, SARS-CoV 3CL protease inhibition assay	SARS-CoV	[130]

(Continued)

TABLE 5.1 (*Continued*)
Anti-SARS-CoV-1 Natural Metabolites Tested *in vitro*

Natural Source	Compound/Extract Type	IC_{50}/EC_{50}	Mechanism of Action	Method to Assess Activity	Test System	References
Betulonic acid	*Isatis indigotica*	0.63 µM	Inhibition of viral replication	Protease inhibition test	SARS-CoV	[130]
Betulonic acid	*Isatis indigotica*	>100 µM	3CL protease inhibition	Protease inhibition test	SARS-CoV	[130]
Betulonic acid (PCWU)	Pentacyclic triterpenoid	0.63 µM	Inhibits 50% of Vero E6 cell proliferation and viral replication	CPE on Vero E6 cells via SARS-CoV infection, SARS-CoV 3CL protease inhibition assay	SARS-CoV	[130]
Bilobetin	*Torreya nucifera*	72.3±4.5 µM	Non-competitive inhibition of CoV CLpro	CLpro inhibition assay	SARS-CoV CLpro	[139]
Black tea extract	Extract	70 µM	ND	3CLpro inhibition assay	SARS 3CLpro	[141]
Blancoxanthone	*Calophyllum blancoi*	3 µg/mL	Not determined	XTT assay-MRC-5 cells	HCoV-229E	[142]
Broussochalcone A2	*Broussonetia papyrifera*	88.1±13.0 µM to 9.2±1.5 µM	Non-competitive inhibition of protease	SARS-CoV 3CLpro and PLpro inhibition assays	3-Chymotrypsin-like and papain-like coronavirus cysteine proteases	[128]
Broussochalcone A2	*Broussonetia papyrifera*	36.2±0.4 µM, 42.1±5.0 µM	Inhibition of protease	MERS-CoV 3CLpro and PLpro inhibition assays	3-Chymotrypsin-like and papain-like coronavirus cysteine proteases	[128]
Broussochalcone B1	*Broussonetia papyrifera*	57.8±0.5 µM and 11.6±0.7 µM	Non-competitive inhibition of protease	SARS-CoV 3CLpro and PLpro inhibition assays	3-Chymotrypsin-like and papain-like coronavirus cysteine proteases	[128]
Broussochalcone B1	*Broussonetia papyrifera*	27.9±1.2 µM, 112.9±10.1 µM	Inhibition of protease	MERS-CoV 3CLpro and PLpro inhibition assays	3-Chymotrypsin-like and papain-like coronavirus cysteine proteases	[128]
Broussoflavan A8	*Broussonetia papyrifera*	125.7±17.4 µM, 49.1±7.5 µM	Non-competitive inhibition of CoV PLpro	MERS-CoV 3CLpro and PLpro inhibition assays	MERS-COV PLpro	[128]
Broussoflavan A8	*Broussonetia papyrifera*	92.4±2.1 µM to 30.4±5.5 µM	Non-competitive inhibition of protease	SARS-CoV 3CLpro and PLpro inhibition assays	3-Chymotrypsin-like and papain-like coronavirus cysteine proteases	[128]
Caffeic acid	*Sambucus formosana*	3.54±0.77	Inhibits cell docking	Virus yield reduction assay	HCoV-NL63	[143]
Cedrane-3β,12-diol (PCWU)	Sesquiterpenes	>10 µM	Inhibits 50% of Vero E6 cell proliferation and viral replication	CPE on Vero E6 cells via SARS-CoV infection, SARS-CoV 3CL protease inhibition assay	SARS-CoV	[130]
Celastrol	*Tripterygium regelii*	10.3±0.2 µM	Competitive inhibition of CoV protease	CLpro inhibition assay	SARS-CoV CLpro	[144]
Cepharanthine	*Stephania tetrandra*	729.7 nM	ND	MRC-5 system	SARS-CoV-1	[145]
Cepharanthine	*Stephania tetrandra* and related species (present in)	0.83±0.07 µM	Inhibition of viral replication and expression of viral S and N protein	MTS assay and *q*RT-PCR, MRC-5 system	HCoV-OC43	[145]

(*Continued*)

TABLE 5.1 (*Continued*)
Anti-SARS-CoV-1 Natural Metabolites Tested *in vitro*

Natural Source	Compound/Extract Type	IC_{50}/EC_{50}	Mechanism of Action	Method to Assess Activity	Test System	References
Cepharanthine	Present in Stephania (*Stephania tetrandra*)	9.5 µg/mL	Inhibition of protease	Protease inhibition test	SARS-CoV	[146]
Chloroform extract	*Pyrrosia lingua*	BJ001: 43.2 (±14.1) ; BJ006: 40.5 (±3.7)	ND	MTS assays	SARS-CoV-1	[136]
Chlorogenic acid	*Sambucus formosana*	43.5±6.0	Not determined	Virus yield reduction assay	HCoV-NL63	[143]
Chrysin (5,7-dihydroxyflavone)	Pure compound	400 µM	Inhibited interaction of SARS-CoV (S) protein and ACE2 (400 µM) Stimulated the binding of S protein to ACE2 (50 µM)	Immunofluorescence assay	SARS-CoV	[147]
Cinanserin (1 dpi)	*Houttuynia cordata*	31.25 µg/mL	Broad-spectrum antiviral activity by inhibiting eIF4A-dependent viral mRNA translation	CPE assay	Murine coronavirus (mouse hepatitis virus)	[148]
Cinanserin (2 dpi)	*Houttuynia cordata*	62.50 µg/mL	Broad-spectrum antiviral activity by inhibiting eIF4A-dependent viral mRNA translation	CPE assay	Murine coronavirus (mouse hepatitis virus)	[148]
Cinnamtannin B1	*Cinnamomi cortex*	32.9±3.9 Mm	Pseudovirus infection inhibition Inhibition of viral entry via clathrin-dependent endocytosis pathway	Plaque reduction assay	SARS-CoV	[149]
Conessine	Purified compound	2.34 µM (HCoV-OC43 EC50); 10.75 µM (HCoV-NL63)	Antiviral, antimalarial, antihistamine	Indirect immunofluorescence assay	HCoV-OC43, HCoV-NL63	[140]
Corylifol A	*Psoralea corylifolia*	32.3±3.2 µM (rest in µM)	Mixed inhibitor of SARS-CoV PLpro	Fluorogenic PLpro inhibition assay	SARS-CoV PLpro	[132]
Cryptojaponol (PCWU)	Abietane derivatives	>10 µM	Inhibits 50% of Vero E6 cell proliferation and viral replication	CPE on Vero E6 cells via SARS-CoV infection, SARS-CoV 3CL protease inhibition assay	SARS-CoV	[130]
Cryptotanshinone	*Salvia miltiorrhiza*	226.7±6.2 µM	Non-competitive enzyme isomerization inhibitor of protease	CLpro inhibition assay	SARS-CoV CLpro	[150]
Cryptotanshinone	*Salvia miltiorrhiza*	0.8±0.2 µM	Non-competitive enzyme isomerization inhibitor of protease	PLpro inhibition assay	SARS-CoV PLpro	[150]
Curcumin (PCWU)	Usually obtained from *Curcuma longa*	>10 µM	Inhibits 50% of Vero E6 cell proliferation and viral replication	CPE on Vero E6 cells via SARS-CoV infection, SARS-CoV 3CL protease inhibition assay	SARS-CoV	[130]
Dehydroabieta-7-one (PCWU)	Abietane derivatives	4 µM	Inhibits 50% of Vero E6 cell proliferation and viral replication	CPE on Vero E6 cells via SARS-CoV infection, SARS-CoV 3CL protease inhibition assay	SARS-CoV	[130]
Dieckol	*Ecklonia cava*	14.6±1.3 µM (posttreatment)	Inhibition of viral replication	Posttreatment assay	Porcine epidemic diarrhea CoV	[135]

(*Continued*)

TABLE 5.1 (*Continued*)
Anti-SARS-CoV-1 Natural Metabolites Tested *in vitro*

Natural Source	Compound/Extract Type	IC_{50}/EC_{50}	Mechanism of Action	Method to Assess Activity	Test System	References
Dihydromyricetin	*Scutellaria baicalensis*	1.20±0.09 µM	Inhibits SARS-CoV-2 3CLpro activity	SARS-CoV 3CLpro assay	SARS-CoV-2 3CLpro activity	[133]
Dihydrotanshinone I	*Salvia miltiorrhiza*	14.4±0.7 µM	Non-competitive enzyme isomerization inhibitor of protease	CLpro inhibition assay	SARS-CoV CLpro	[150]
Dihydrotanshinone I	*Salvia miltiorrhiza*	4.9±1.2 µM	Non-competitive enzyme isomerization inhibitor of protease	PLpro inhibition assay	SARS-CoV PLpro	[150]
Diplacone	*Paulownia tomentosa*	10.4±0.16 µM	Reversible, mixed-type (allosteric) inhibitors of PLpro	SARS-CoV PLpro inhibition assay	SARS-CoV PLpro	[129]
Eckol	*Ecklonia cava*	22.5±2.2 µM (simultaneous treatment)	Inhibits viral entry and/or viral replication	Simultaneous treatment assay	Porcine epidemic diarrhea CoV	[135]
Emetine	Purified compound	0.30 µM (HCoV-OC43 EC50); 1.43 µM (HCoV-NL63)	Inhibits RNA, DNA, and protein synthesis Broad-spectrum antiviral activity against HCoV	Indirect immunofluorescence assay	HCoV-OC43, HCoV-NL63	[140]
Emodin (1,3,8-trihydroxy-6-methylanthraquinone)	Pure compound	200 µM	Inhibit interaction between SARS-CoV (S) protein and ACE2 was inhibited	Immunofluorescence assay (IFA)	SARS-CoV	[147]
Epigallocatechin gallate, epicatechin gallate and gallocatechin-3-gallate	*Green tea*	ND	Interaction with catalytic residues of major protease (Mpro)	in silico docking and molecular dynamics simulation study	SARS-CoV-2	[151]
Epitaraxerol	*Euphorbia neriifolia*	111.0 [b](Cell survival (%))	ND	Anti-HCoV assay (MRC-5 system)	HCoV-229E	[131]
EPs® 7630 (formulation), approved drug for the treatment of acute bronchitis, Germany	*Pelargonium sidoides extract*	44.50±15.84 µg/mL	Possibly interference of virus surface resulting in viral inactivation	CPE assay	HCov-229E	[152]
Ethanol extract of seeds	*Psoralea corylifolia*	15 µg/mL	Mixed inhibitor of SARS-CoV PLpro	Fluorogenic PLpro inhibition assay	SARS-CoV PLpro	[132]
Ethanol extract of stem	*Sambucus formosana*	1.17±0.75 (µg/mL)	Not determined	Virus yield reduction assay	HCoV-NL63	[143]
Ethanol extract(95% EtOH)	*Lindera aggregate Ethanol*	BJ001: 88.2 (±7.7) µg mL−1BJ006: 80.6 (±5.2) µg m/L	ND	CPE/MTS assay	SARS-CoV-1	[136]
Ethanolic extract	*Artemisia annua*	BJ001: 34.5 (±2.6) µg/mL; BJ006: 39.2 (±4.1)µg/mL	ND	CPE/MTS assay	SARS-CoV-1	[136]
EtOH extract	*Ecklonia cava*	12.4±2.2 lg/mL	Inhibits viral entry and/or viral replication	Simultaneous treatment assay	Porcine epidemic diarrhea CoV	[135]
EtOH extract	*Ecklonia cava*	19.5±3.8 lg/mL	Inhibits viral entry and/or viral replication	Posttreatment assay	Porcine epidemic diarrhea CoV	[135]

(*Continued*)

TABLE 5.1 (*Continued*)
Anti-SARS-CoV-1 Natural Metabolites Tested *in vitro*

Natural Source	Compound/Extract Type	IC_{50}/EC_{50}	Mechanism of Action	Method to Assess Activity	Test System	References
Extract	*Radix et Rhizoma Rhei, Radix Polygoni multiflori, and Caulis Polygoni multiflori*	1–10 µg/mL	Prevents interaction between S protein and ACE2	Immunofluorescence assay (IFA)	SARS-CoV S protein	[147]
Extract	*Cibotium barometz*	8.42 µg/mL to >10 µg/mL (of two fractions)	Inhibition of SARS-CoV 3CL protease activity	CPE assay	SARS-CoV (Hong Kong strain)	[147]
Extract	*Taxillus chinensis*	5.39 µg/mL	May inhibit fatty acid synthase and viral entry	CPE assay	SARS-CoV (Hong Kong strain)	[153]
Extract	*Cassia tora*	8.43 µg/mL	ND	CPE assay	SARS-CoV (Hong Kong strain)	[153]
Extract	*Gentiana scabra*	8.7	ND	CPE assay	SARS-CoV (Hong Kong strain)	[153]
Extract	*Anthemis hyalina*, *Nigella sativa*, and *Citrus sinensis* extracts	Decreased viral load at 6-8hpi by *Anthemis hyalina*	Increased IL-8 level Considerably changed the expression of TRPA1, TRPC4, TRPM6, TRPM7, TRPM8, and TRPV4 genes	Coronavirus-infected HeLa-epithelial carcinoembryonic antigen-related cell adhesion molecule 1a cells inoculated with MHV-A59 (mouse hepatitis virus–A59)	ELISA for quantitative analysis of IL-8	[154]
Extract part of traditional Chinese medicines	*Ganoderma lucidum*	41.9 µg/mL	Inhibition against SARS-CoV RNA polymerase enzyme and viral replication	SARS-CoV RNA polymerase enzyme inhibition assay	SARS-CoV RNA polymerase enzyme	[155]
Extract part of traditional Chinese medicines	*Coriolus versicolor*	IC50:108.4 µg/mL	Inhibition against SARS-CoV RNA polymerase enzyme and viral replication	SARS-CoV RNA polymerase enzyme inhibition assay	SARS-CoV RNA polymerase enzyme	[155]
Extract part of traditional Chinese medicines	*Sinomenium acutum*	(IC50:198.6 µg/mL)	Inhibition against SARS-CoV RNA polymerase enzyme and viral replication	SARS-CoV RNA polymerase enzyme inhibition assay	SARS-CoV RNA polymerase enzyme	[155]
Fangchinoline	*Stephania tetrandra* and related species (present in)	1.01 ± 0.07 µM	Inhibition of viral replication and expression of viral S and N protein	MTS assay and *q*RT-PCR, MRC-5 system	HCoV-OC43	[145]
Ferruginol (PCWU)	Abietane derivatives	1.39 µM	Inhibits 50% of Vero E6 cell proliferation and viral replication	CPE on Vero E6 cells via SARS-CoV infection, SARS-CoV 3CL protease inhibition assay	SARS-CoV	[130]
Ferulic acid	*Tribulus terrestris fruits*	200 < µM	ND	PLpro inhibition assay	SARS-CoV CLpro	[156]
Forskolin (PCWU)	Labdane derivatives	7.5 µM	Inhibits 50% of Vero E6 cell proliferation and viral replication	CPE on Vero E6 cells via SARS-CoV infection, SARS-CoV 3CL protease inhibition assay	SARS-CoV	[130]
Friedelin	*Euphorbia neriifolia*	109.0^{h}(Cell survival (%))	ND	Anti-HCoV assay (MRC-5 system)	HCoV-229E	[131]
Gallic acid	*Sambucus formosana*	71.5 ± 18.4	Not determined	Virus yield reduction assay	HCoV-NL63	[143]
Ginkgetin	*Torreya nucifera*	32.0 ± 1.7 µM	Non-competitive inhibition of CoV CLpro	CLpro inhibition assay	SARS-CoV CLpro	[139]
Glycyrrhetinic acid	*Glycyrrhiza radix*	>20	ND	Immunocytochemical staining and visual CPE assay	SARS-CoV FFM1	[157]

(Continued)

TABLE 5.1 (*Continued*)
Anti-SARS-CoV-1 Natural Metabolites Tested *in vitro*

Natural Source	Compound/Extract Type	IC_{50}/EC_{50}	Mechanism of Action	Method to Assess Activity	Test System	References
Glycyrrhizic acid	*Glycyrrhiza radix*	365±12	ND	Immunocytochemical staining and visual CPE assay	SARS-CoV FFM1	[157]
Glycyrrhizin	Liquorice (present in)	EC50 300 mg/L	Inhibition of SARS-CoV in Vero cells	SARS-CoV inhibition assay	SARS-CoV	[158]
Glycyrrhizin	Liquorice (present in)	>607.6 µM	ND	Wild-type SARS-CoV infection inhibition assay (BJ01 strain)	SARS-CoV-1	[159]
Griffithsin	*Griffithsia* sp. (found in)	0.44, 2.5 µg/mL	Direct binding to spike protein	CPE assay and neutral red assay	MHV (JHM) in mouse embryonic liver cells (BNL)	[160]
Griffithsin	*Griffithsia* sp. (Found in)	68, >100 µg/mL	Direct binding to spike protein	CPE assay and neutral red assay	IBV (Connecticut A5968) in chicken embryonic fibroblast cells (UMNSAH/DF-1)	[160]
Griffithsin	*Griffithsia* sp. (found in)	32, >100 µg/mL	Direct binding to spike protein	CPE assay and neutral red assay	BCoV in human ileocecal colorectal human adenocarcinoma cells (HRT-18G)	[160]
Griffithsin	*Griffithsia* sp. (found in)	57, 46 µg/mL	Direct binding to spike protein	CPE assay and neutral red assay	PCoV (Miller) in pig testis fibroblast cells (ST)	[160]
Griffithsin	*Griffithsia* sp. (found in)	>100 µg/mL	Direct binding to spike protein	CPE assay	*Urbani* strain SARS-CoV	[160]
Griffithsin	*Griffithsia* sp. (found in)	>100 µg/mL	Direct binding to spike protein	CPE assay	*Tor-II* strain SARS-CoV	[160]
Griffithsin	*Griffithsia* sp. (found in)	>100 µg/mL	Direct binding to spike protein	CPE assay	*CuHK* strain SARS-CoV	[160]
Griffithsin	*Griffithsia* sp. (found in)	>100 µg/mL	Direct binding to spike protein	CPE assay	*Frank* strain SARS-CoV	[160]
Griffithsin	*Griffithsia* sp. (present in)	52, >100 µg/mL	Direct binding to surface envelope glycoprotein spike	CPE assay and neutral red assay	HCoV (OC43) in human ileocecal colorectal human adenocarcinoma cells (HCT-8)	[160]
Griffithsin	*Griffithsia* sp. (present in)	>10, >10 µg/mL	Direct binding to surface envelope glycoprotein spike	CPE assay and neutral red assay	HCoV (229E) in human diploid fibroblast cells (MRC-5)	[160]
Griffithsin	*Griffithsia* sp. (present in)	10, >10 µg/mL	Direct binding to surface envelope glycoprotein spike	CPE assay and neutral red assay	HCoV-NL63 in rhesus monkey kidney cells (LLC-MK2)	[160]

(*Continued*)

TABLE 5.1 (*Continued*)

Anti-SARS-CoV-1 Natural Metabolites Tested *in vitro*

Natural Source	Compound/Extract Type	IC_{50}/EC_{50}	Mechanism of Action	Method to Assess Activity	Test System	References
Harmine	Purified compound	1.90 μM (HCoV-OC43 EC50); 13.46 μM (HCoV-NL63)	Antiparkinsonian, CNS stimulant, antiviral	Indirect immunofluorescence assay	HCoV-OC43, HCoV-NL63	[140]
Herbacetin	*Scutellaria baicalensis*	56.7±2.0 (% Inhibition at 50 μM)	Inhibits SARS-CoV-2 3CLpro activity	SARS-CoV 3CLpro assay	SARS-CoV-2 3CLpro activity	[133]
Herbal extracts	*Cibotium barometz*	39, 44 μg/mL (two extracts of *Cibotium barometz*)	Inhibition of 3CL protease	Protease inhibition test	SARS-CoV	[153]
Hesperetin	*Isatis indigotica*	60 μM	3CLpro inhibition	3CLpro cleavage assay	SARS-CoV 3CLpro	[138]
Hesperetin	*Isatis indigotica*	365 μM	3CL protease inhibition	Protease inhibition test	SARS-CoV	[138]
Hexachlorophene	*Isatis indigotica*	1.2 μM	ND	Protease inhibition test	Murine CoV (MHV-2aFLS)	[161]
Hinokinin	*Isatis indigotica*	>100 μM	3CL protease inhibition	Protease inhibition test	SARS-CoV	[130]
Hinokinin (PCWU)	Dibenzylbutyrolactone lignin	>10 μM	Inhibits 50% of Vero E6 cell proliferation and viral replication	CPE on Vero E6 cells via SARS-CoV infection, SARS-CoV 3CL protease inhibition assay	SARS-CoV	[130]
Hirsutanonol	Diarylheptanoid from Alnus japonica	105.6±6.5; 24.1±2.0 μM	ND	SARS-CoV 3CLpro inhibition assay Deubiquitination activity	SARS-CoV 3CLpro	[162]
Hirsutenone	Diarylheptanoid from Alnus japonica	36.2±2.0; 3.0±1.1 μM	ND	SARS-CoV 3CLpro inhibition assay, Deubiquitination activity	SARS-CoV 3CLpro	[162]
Homoharringtonine	*Isatis indigotica*	12 nM	ND	3CLpro cleavage assay	Murine CoV (MHV-2aFLS)	[161]
Honokiol (PCWU)	Usually obtained from Magnolia sp. (neolignans)	6.50 μM	Inhibits 50% of Vero E6 cell proliferation and viral replication	CPE on Vero E6 cells via SARS-CoV infection, SARS-CoV 3CL protease inhibition assay	SARS-CoV	[130]
Hygromycin B	*Streptomyces hygroscopicus*	MHV antigen Expression reduced at 12.5 μM	Virus replication was reduced and reduced necrotic liver foci	Immunofluorescence assay	Mouse hepatitis virus (MHV-A59)	[163]
Iguesterin	*Tripterygium regelii*	2.6±0.3 μM	Competitive inhibition of CoV protease	CLpro inhibition assay	SARS-CoV CLpro	[144]
Iguesterin	*Celastrus orbiculatus*	2.6 mM	ND	3CLpro assay	SARS-CoV-3CLpro	[164]
Indigo	*Isatis indigotica*	300 μM	3CLpro inhibition	3CLpro cleavage assay	SARS-CoV 3CLpro	[138]
Indigo	*Isatis indigotica*	752 μM	Inhibition of 3CL protease	3CLpro cleavage assay	SARS-CoV	[138]
Indigodole B	*Strobilanthes cusia* leaf	2.09 μM	Blocking viral RNA genome synthesis and papain-like protease 2 activity	Plaque virucidal assay	HCoV-NL63	[165]
Isobavachalcone	*Psoralea corylifolia*	7.3±0.8 μM	Mixed inhibitor of SARS-CoV PLpro (also reversible)	Fluorogenic PLpro inhibition assay	SARS-CoV PLpro	[132]
Isolated lycorine	Pure compound	48.8±3.6 nM	ND	CPE/MTS assay	SARS-CoV (BJ001 and BJ006	[136]

(Continued)

TABLE 5.1 (*Continued*)
Anti-SARS-CoV-1 Natural Metabolites Tested *in vitro*

Natural Source	Compound/Extract Type	IC_{50}/EC_{50}	Mechanism of Action	Method to Assess Activity	Test System	References
Isolinoleic acid	*Mucuna pruriens*	50 µM		n.i	SARS-CoV-1	[164]
Isopsoralen (pure compound was considered)	*Psoralea corylifolia*	>150	Mixed inhibitor of SARS-CoV PLpro	Fluorogenic PLpro inhibition assay	SARS-CoV PLpro	[132]
Isotheaflavin-3-gallate	Black tea	7 µm	ND	3CLpro inhibition assay	SARS 3CLpro	[141]
Jubanine G	Alkaloid	13.41 ± 1.1 µM 3	Showed potent inhibitory effects on PEDV replication	CPE assay	PEDV	[166]
Jubanine H	Alkaloid	4.49 ± 0.67 µM	Showed potent inhibitory effects on PEDV replication	CPE assay	PEDV	[166]
Juglanin	Pure compound	2.3 µM	Inhibition of the 3a channel	Voltage–clamp experiments	3a Channel protein of coronavirus	[167]
Kazinol A6	*Broussonetia papyrifera*	84.8 ± 10.4 to 66.2 ± 6.8 µM	Non-competitive inhibition of protease	SARS-CoV 3CLpro and PLpro inhibition assays	3-Chymotrypsin-like and papain-like coronavirus cysteine proteases	[128]
Kazinol A6	*Broussonetia papyrifera*	88.5 ± 3.9 µM	Non-competitive inhibition of CoV 3CLpro	MERS-CoV 3CLpro and PLpro inhibition assays	MERS-COV 3CLpro	[128]
Kazinol B7	*Broussonetia papyrifera*	94.9 ± 13.1 µM	Non-competitive inhibition of CoV PLpro	MERS-CoV 3CLpro and PLpro inhibition assays	MERS-COV PLpro	[128]
Kazinol B7	*Broussonetia papyrifera*	233.3 ± 6.7 to 31.4 ± 2.9 µM	Non-competitive inhibition of protease	SARS-CoV 3CLpro and PLpro inhibition assays	3-Chymotrypsin-like and papain-like coronavirus cysteine proteases	[128]
Kazinol F9	*Broussonetia papyrifera*	135.0 ± 5.1, 39.5 ± 5.1 µM	Non-competitive inhibition of CoV PLpro	MERS-CoV 3CLpro and PLpro inhibition assays	SARS-CoV PLpro	[128]
Kazinol F9	*Broussonetia papyrifera*	43.3 ± 10.4 to 27.8 ± 2.5 µM	Non-competitive inhibition of protease	SARS-CoV 3CLpro and PLpro inhibition assays	3-Chymotrypsin-like and papain-like coronavirus cysteine proteases	[128]
Kazinol J10	*Broussonetia papyrifera*	109.2 ± 3.7, 55.0 ± 1.3		MERS-CoV 3CLpro and PLpro inhibition assays	MERS-CoV 3CLpro, MERS-CoV PLpro	[128]
Kazinol J10	*Broussonetia papyrifera*	64.2 ± 1.7 to 15.2 ± 1.6 µM	Non-competitive inhibition of protease	SARS-CoV 3CLpro and PLpro inhibition assays	3-Chymotrypsin-like and papain-like coronavirus cysteine proteases	[128]
Lectins isolated from diaminopropane extracts (Man/GalNAc-specific agglutinins)	*Tulipa* hybrid	38 µg/mL	Inhibition of viral binding and another target at the end of the replication cycle	CPE assay, Vero E6 cells	SARS-CoV	[126]

(*Continued*)

TABLE 5.1 (*Continued*)

Anti-SARS-CoV-1 Natural Metabolites Tested *in vitro*

Natural Source	Compound/Extract Type	IC_{50}/EC_{50}	Mechanism of Action	Method to Assess Activity	Test System	References
Lectins isolated from diaminopropane extracts GalNAc(>Gal)-specific	*Multiflorum*	18±13 μg/mL	Inhibition of viral binding and another target at the end of the replication cycle	CPE assay	SARS-CoV	[125]
Lectins isolated from diaminopropane extracts-Man-specific agglutinins	*Listera ovata*	2.2±1.3 μg/mL	Inhibition of viral binding and another target at the end of the replication cycle	CPE assay	SARS-CoV	[126]
Lectins isolated from diaminopropane extracts, Agglutinins: mannose-specific	*Hippeastrum* hybrid	3.2±2.8 μg/mL	Inhibition of viral binding and another target at the end of the replication cycle	CPE assay	SARS-CoV	[125]
Lectins isolated from diaminopropane extracts-Man-specific agglutinins	*Morus nigra*	1.6±0.5	Inhibition of viral binding and another target at the end of the replication cycle	CPE assay	SARS-CoV	[168]
Luteolin	Present in *Rhodiola kirilowii*	10.6 μM	Prevents the viral entry	SARS-CoV (wild-type) inhibition assay and SARS pseudotyped virus entry inhibition assays	SARS-CoV	[159]
Luteolin	*Torreya nucifera*	20.2 μM	Inhibition of 3CL protease	3CLpro inhibition test	SARS-CoV	[139]
Lycorine	Purified compound	0.15 μM (HCoV-OC43 EC50); 0.47 μM (HCoV-NL63)	Broad-spectrum antiviral activity against HCoV	Indirect immunofluorescence assay	HCoV-OC43, HCoV-NL63	[140]
Lycorine (ethanol extract)	*Lycoris radiate*	BJOO1: 2.4 (±0.2) μg/mL; BJ006: 2.1 (±0.2) μg/mL	ND	CPE/MTS assay	SARS-CoV-1	[136]
Magnolol (PCWU)	Usually obtained *Houpu magnolia (Magnolia officinalis)* or in *M. grandiflora(neolignans)*	3.80 μM	Inhibits 50% of Vero E6 cell proliferation and viral replication	CPE on Vero E6 cells via SARS-CoV infection, SARS-CoV 3CL protease inhibition assay	SARS-CoV	[130]
Mannose-specific agglutinins	*Allium porrum*	0.45±0.0 μg/mL	Inhibition of viral binding and another target at the end of the replication cycle	CPE assay	SARS-CoV	[125]
Mannose-specific agglutinins	*Allium ursinum*	18±4 μg/mL	Inhibition of viral binding and another target at the end of the replication cycle	CPE assay	SARS-CoV	[125]
Mannose-specific agglutinins	*Allium sativum*	>100 μg/mL	Inhibition of viral binding and another target at the end of the replication cycle	CPE assay	SARS-CoV	
Mannose-specific agglutinins	*Narcissus pseudonarcissus*	5.7±4.4 μg/mL	Inhibition of viral binding and another target at the end of the replication cycle	CPE assay	SARS-CoV	[125]

(*Continued*)

TABLE 5.1 (*Continued*)
Anti-SARS-CoV-1 Natural Metabolites Tested *in vitro*

Natural Source	Compound/Extract Type	IC_{50}/EC_{50}	Mechanism of Action	Method to Assess Activity	Test System	References
Mannose-specific agglutinins–lectins	*Cymbidium* hybrid	4.9±0.8 µg/mL	Inhibition of viral binding and another target at the end of the replication cycle	CPE assay	SARS-CoV	[125]
Man-specific agglutinins	*Lycoris radiate*	48 µg/mL	Inhibition of viral binding and another target at the end of the replication cycle	CPE assay	SARS-CoV	[125]
Man-specific agglutinins–lectins	*Galanthus nivalis*	6.2±0.6 µg/mL	Inhibition of viral binding and another target at the end of the replication cycle	CPE assay	SARS-CoV	[125]
Methanol extract	*Strobilanthes cusia* leaf	0.64 µg/mL	Blocking viral RNA genome synthesis and papain-like protease 2 activity	Plaque virucidal assay	HCoV-NL63	[165]
Methyl tanshinonate	*Salvia miltiorrhiza*	21.1±0.8 µM	Non-competitive enzyme isomerization inhibitor of protease	CLpro inhibition assay	SARS-CoV CLpro	[150]
Methyl tanshinonate	*Salvia miltiorrhiza*	9.2±2.8 µM	Non-competitive enzyme isomerization inhibitor of protease	PLpro inhibition assay	SARS-CoV PLpro	[150]
Mimulone	*Paulownia tomentosa*	14.4±0.27 µM	Reversible, mixed-type (allosteric) inhibitors of PLpro	SARS-CoV PLpro inhibition assay	SARS-CoV PLpro	[129]
Monensin sodium	Purified compound	3.81 µM (HCoV-OC43 EC50); 1.54 µM (HCoV-NL63)	Broad-spectrum antiviral activity against HCoV	Indirect immunofluorescence assay	HCoV-OC43, HCoV-NL63	[140]
Morniga G II-lectins isolated from diaminopropane extracts, Gal-specific agglutinins	*Morus nigra*	50±13 µg/mL	Inhibition of viral binding and another target at the end of the replication cycle	CPE assay	SARS-CoV	[168]
Mycalamide A	*Mycale* sp. (sponge)	0.2 µg k/g		n.i	SARS-CoV-1	[169]
Mycophenolate mofetil	Purified compound	1.58 µM (HCoV-OC43 EC50); 0.3 µM (HCoV-NL63)	Broad-spectrum antiviral activity against HCoV	Indirect immunofluorescence assay	HCoV-OC43, HCoV-NL63	[140]
Mycophenolic acid	Purified compound	1.95 µM (HCoV-OC43 EC50); 0.18 µM (HCoV-NL63)	Broad-spectrum antiviral activity against HCoV	Indirect immunofluorescence assay	HCoV-OC43, HCoV-NL63	[140]
Myricetin	*Scutellaria baicalensis*	2.74±0.31 µM	Inhibits SARS-CoV-2 3CLpro activity	SARS-CoV 3CLpro assay	SARS-CoV-2 3CLpro activity	[133]
Myricetin	*Purified compound*	2.71±0.19 µM	Inhibits the SARS-CoV helicase protein in vitro by affecting the ATPase activity	Fluorescence resonance energy transfer (FRET)-based double-stranded (ds) DNA unwinding assay	SARS-CoV helicase	[170]

(*Continued*)

TABLE 5.1 (*Continued*)
Anti-SARS-CoV-1 Natural Metabolites Tested *in vitro*

Natural Source	Compound/Extract Type	IC_{50}/EC_{50}	Mechanism of Action	Method to Assess Activity	Test System	References
Essential oil	*Thuja orientalis*	270±1.5 µg/mL	Inhibits viral replication	CPE assay	SARS-CoV FFM1	[171]
Essential oil	*Cupressus sempervirens*	700±2.3 µg/mL	Inhibits viral replication	CPE assay	SARS-CoV FFM1	[171]
Essential oil	*Pistacia palaestina*	>1,000 µg/mL	Inhibits viral replication	CPE assay	SARS-CoV FFM1	[171]
Essential oil	*Salvia officinalis*	8 70±1.5 µg/mL	Inhibits viral replication	CPE assay	SARS-CoV FFM1	[171]
Essential oil	*Satureja thymbra*	641±1.5 µg/mL	Inhibits viral replication	CPE assay	SARS-CoV FFM1	[171]
Neobavaisoflavone	*Psoralea corylifolia*	18.3 ± 1.1 µM	Mixed inhibitor of SARS-CoV PLpro	Fluorogenic PLpro inhibition assay	SARS-CoV PLpro	[132]
Niclosamide	Pure compound was used	<0.1 µM	Inhibits 50% of Vero E6 cell proliferation and viral replication	CPE on Vero E6 cells via SARS-CoV infection, SARS-CoV 3CL protease inhibition assay	SARS-CoV	[130]
Nictaba-lectins isolated from diaminopropane extracts, GlcNAc-specific agglutinins	*Nicotiana tabacum*	1.7±0.3 µg/mL	Inhibition of viral binding and another target at the end of the replication cycle	CPE assay	SARS-CoV	[172]
N-trans-coumaroyltyramine	*Tribulus terrestris Fruits*	70.1±0.7 µM	ND	PLpro inhibition assay	SARS-CoV CLpro	[156]
N-trans-feruloyloctopamine	*Tribulus terrestris Fruits*	26.6±0.5 µM	ND	PLpro inhibition assay	SARS-CoV CLpro	[156]
Nummularine	Alkaloid	6.17±0.50 µM	Showed potent inhibitory effects on PEDV replication	CPE assay	PEDV	[166]
Oregonin	Diarylheptanoid from *Alnus japonica*	129.5±3.1; 44.5±5.3 µM	ND	SARS-CoV 3CLpro inhibition assay Deubiquitination activity	SARS-CoV 3CLpro	[162]
Ouabain	*Acokanthera schimperi* and *Strophanthus gratus* (can be present in these plants)	143±13 nM	Reduced both viral load and viral yields Reduction of the number of viral RNA copies	Cell lines (Swine testicular), viruses, immunofluorescence assay	Transmissible gastroenteritis CoV	[173]
Papaverine	Purified compound	1.61 µM (HCoV-OC43 EC50); 7.32 µM (HCoV-NL63)	Muscle relaxant, cerebral vasodilator	Indirect immunofluorescence assay	HCoV-OC43, HCoV-NL63	[140]
Papyriflavonol A4	*Broussonetia papyrifera*	103.6±17.4 to 3.7±1.6 µM	Non-competitive inhibition of protease	SARS-CoV 3CLpro and PLpro inhibition assays	3-chymotrypsin-like and papain-like coronavirus cysteine proteases	[128]
Papyriflavonol A4	*Broussonetia papyrifera*	64.5±4.9, 112.5±7.3 µM	Inhibition of protease	MERS-CoV 3CLpro and PLpro inhibition assays	3-chymotrypsin-like and papain-like coronavirus cysteine proteases	[128]
Phenazopyridine	NI	1.90, 2.02, 1.93, and 0.77 µM	Potent broad-spectrum inhibitors of coronaviruses	High-throughput screening	HCoV-OC43, HCoV-NL63, MERS-CoV, and MHV-A59	[140]
Phloroglucinol	*Ecklonia cava*	12.2±2.8 µM (posttreatment)	Inhibits viral entry and/or viral replication	Posttreatment assay	Porcine epidemic diarrhea CoV	[135]

(*Continued*)

TABLE 5.1 (*Continued*)

Anti-SARS-CoV-1 Natural Metabolites Tested *in vitro*

Natural Source	Compound/Extract Type	IC_{50}/EC_{50}	Mechanism of Action	Method to Assess Activity	Test System	References
Pinusolidic acid (PCWU)	Labdane derivatives	4.71 µM	Inhibits 50% of Vero E6 cell proliferation and viral replication	CPE on Vero E6 cells via SARS-CoV infection, SARS-CoV 3CL protease inhibition assay	SARS-CoV	[130]
Platyphyllenone	Diarylheptanoid from Alnus japonica	>200, >200 µM	ND	SARS-CoV 3CLpro inhibition assay Deubiquitination activity	SARS-CoV 3CLpro	[162]
Platyphylline	Diarylheptanoid from Alnus japonica	>200, >202 µM	ND	SARS-CoV 3CLpro inhibition assay Deubiquitination activity	SARS-CoV 3CLpro	[162]
Platyphyllonol-5-xylopyranosid	Diarylheptanoid from Alnus japonica	>200, >201 µM	ND	SARS-CoV 3CLpro inhibition assay Deubiquitination activity	SARS-CoV 3CLpro	[162]
PMRIP m-Lectins isolated from diaminopropane extracts, Gal/GalNAc-specific agglutinins	*Polygonatum multiflorum monomer*	18±13 µg/mL	Inhibition of viral binding and another target at the end of the replication cycle	CPE assay	SARS-CoV	[126]
Polysaccharides	*Dioscorea batatas*	8.06 µg/mL	Inhibition of SARS-CoV 3CL protease activity	CPE assay	SARS-CoV (Hong Kong strain)	[153]
Possibly anthraquinones	*Rheum palmatum*	13.76±0.03 µg/mL	3CLpro inhibition	3CLpro inhibition test	SARS-CoV 3CLpro	[174])
Pristimerin	*Tripterygium regelii*	5.5±0.7 µM	Competitive inhibition of CoV protease	CLpro inhibition assay	SARS-CoV CLpro	[144]
Pristimerin	*Celastrus orbiculatus*	5.5 Mm	ND	3CLpro assay	SARS-CoV-3CLpro	[164]
Procyanidin A2	*Cinnamomi cortex*	29.9±3.3 µM	Pseudovirus infection inhibition , inhibition of viral entry via clathrin-dependent endocytosis pathway	Plaque reduction assay	SARS-CoV	[149]
Procyanidin B1	*Cinnamomi cortex*	41.3±3.4 µM	Pseudovirus infection inhibition, inhibition of viral entry via clathrin-dependent endocytosis pathway	Plaque reduction assay	SARS-CoV	[149]
Psoralen (pure compound was considered)	Present in *Psoralea corylifolia*	>150	Mixed inhibitor of SARS-CoV PLpro	Fluorogenic PLpro inhibition assay	SARS-CoV PLpro	[132]
Psoralidin	*Psoralea corylifolia*	4.2±1.0 µM	Mixed inhibitor of SARS-CoV PLpro (also reversible)	Fluorogenic PLpro inhibition assay	SARS-CoV PLpro	[132]
Pu-erh tea extract	*Extract*	25 µM	ND	3CLpro inhibition assay	SARS 3CLpro	
Pyranojacareubin	*Calophyllum blancoi*	15 µg/ML	Not determined	XTT assay-MRC-5 cells	HCoV-229E	[142]
Quercetagetin	*Scutellaria baicalensis*	1.27±0.15 µM	Inhibits SARS-CoV-2 3CLpro activity	SARS-CoV 3CLpro assay	SARS-CoV-2 3CLpro activity	[133]
Quercetin	*Houttuynia cordata*	125.00 µg/mL	Broad-spectrum antiviral activity by inhibiting eIF4A-dependent viral mRNA translation	CPE assay	Murine coronavirus (mouse hepatitis virus)	[148]
Quercetin	*Torreya nucifera*	23.8 µM	Inhibition of 3CL protease	3CLpro inhibition test	SARS-CoV	[139]
Quercetrin	*Houttuynia cordata*	-	Broad-spectrum antiviral activity by inhibiting eIF4A-dependent viral mRNA translation	CPE assay	Murine coronavirus (mouse hepatitis virus)	[148]
Rosmariquinone	*Salvia miltiorrhiza*	21.1±0.8 µM	Exhibits simple reversible slow-binding inhibition	CLpro inhibition assay	SARS-CoV CLpro	[150]

(*Continued*)

TABLE 5.1 (*Continued*)

Anti-SARS-CoV-1 Natural Metabolites Tested *in vitro*

Natural Source	Compound/Extract Type	IC_{50}/EC_{50}	Mechanism of Action	Method to Assess Activity	Test System	References
Rosmariquinone	*Salvia miltiorrhiza*	30.0±5.5 µM	Showed simple reversible slow-binding inhibition	PLpro inhibition assay	SARS-CoV PLpro	[150]
Rubranol	Diarylheptanoid from Alnus japonica	144.6±4.8; 35.2±1.7 µM	ND	SARS-CoV 3CLpro inhibition assay Deubiquitination activity	SARS-CoV 3CLpro	[162]
Rubranoside	*Diarylheptanoid*	IC50=7.2±2.2 µM			SARS-CoV	[162]
Rubranoside A	Diarylheptanoid from Alnus japonica	102.1±2.5 µM; 14.4±3.0 µM	ND	SARS-CoV 3CLpro inhibition assay Deubiquitination activity	SARS-CoV 3CLpro	[162]
Rubranoside B	Diarylheptanoid from Alnus japonica	105.3±1.7 µM; 7.2±2.2 µM	ND	SARS-CoV 3CLpro inhibition assay Deubiquitination activity	SARS-CoV 3CLpro	[162]
Saikosaponin A	*Bupleurum* spp., *Heteromorpha* spp., *Scrophularia scorodonia* (present in)	8.6±0.3 µmol/L	Likely interference in the early stage of viral replication, e.g., absorption and penetration	XTT assay	HCoV-229E	[175]
Saikosaponin B_2	*Bupleurum* spp., *Heteromorpha* spp., *Scrophularia scorodonia* (present in)	1.7±0.1 µmol/L	Possible interference in the early stage of viral replication, e.g., absorption and penetration	XTT assay	HCoV-229E	[175]
Saikosaponin C	*Bupleurum* spp., *Heteromorpha* spp., *Scrophularia scorodonia* (present in)	19.9±0.1 µmol/L	Possible interference in the early stage of viral replication, e.g., absorption and penetration	XTT assay	HCoV-229E	[175]
Saikosaponin D	*Bupleurum* spp., *Heteromorpha* spp., *Scrophularia scorodonia* (present in)	13.2±0.3 µmol/L	Possible interference in the early stage of viral replication, e.g., absorption and penetration	XTT assay	HCoV-229E	[175]
Savinin		25 µM	Inhibition of 3C-like protease	3CLpro inhibition test	SARS-CoV	[130]
Savinin (PCWU)	Lignan derivatives usually obtained from *Pterocarpus santalinus*	1.13 µM	Competitive inhibitors of SARS-CoV 3CL protease	CPE on Vero E6 cells via SARS-CoV infection, SARS-CoV 3CL protease inhibition assay	SARS-CoV	[130]
Schimperinone	Triterpene	0.28±0.09 µM	Significantly reduce the RNA levels; potent inhibitory effects on PEDV replication by inhibiting PEDV genes encoding GP6 nucleocapsid, GP2 spike, and GP5 membrane protein	CPE assay	SARS-CoV, 3CLpro, PLpro	[176]
Sciadopitysin	*Torreya nucifera*	38.4±0.2 µM	Non-competitive inhibition of CoV CLpro	CLpro inhibition assay	SARS-CoV CLpro	[139]
Scutellarein	*Scutellaria baicalensis*	5.80 ±0.22 µM	Inhibits SARS-CoV-2 3CLpro activity	SARS-CoV 3CLpro assay	SARS-CoV-2 3CLpro activity	[133]
Scutellarein	Purified compound (present in Scutellaria baicalensis)	0.86±0.48 µM	Inhibits the SARS-CoV helicase protein in vitro by affecting the ATPase activity	FRET-based dsDNA unwinding assay	SARS-CoV helicase nsP13	[170]
Silvestrol	*Aglaia* sp. (found in)	1.3 nM	Specific inhibitor of RNA helicase eIF4A	Cellular dual-luciferase reporter assay	MERS-CoV EMC/2012	[177]

(*Continued*)

TABLE 5.1 (*Continued*)
Anti-SARS-CoV-1 Natural Metabolites Tested *in vitro*

Natural Source	Compound/Extract Type	IC_{50}/EC_{50}	Mechanism of Action	Method to Assess Activity	Test System	References
Silvestrol	*Aglaia foveolata*	3 nM	Broad-spectrum antiviral activity by inhibiting eIF4A-dependent viral mRNA translation	MRC-5 system	HCoV-229E	[177]
Silvestrol	*Aglaia foveolata*	2.8 nM	Broad-spectrum antiviral activity by inhibiting eIF4A-dependent viral mRNA translation	PBMC system	HCoV-229E	[177]
Silvestrol	Pure compound (purity >98%)	40 nM	Inhibition of cap-dependent viral mRNA translation; Broad-spectrum antiviral activity by inhibiting eIF4A-dependent viral mRNA translation	Dual-luciferase assay via plaque assays (Huh-7 system)	HCoV-229E	[177]
Sinigrin	*Isatis indigotica*	121 µM	3CLpro inhibition	3CLpro cleavage assay	SARS-CoV 3CLpro	[138]
Sinigrin	*Isatis indigotica*	217 µM	Inhibition of 3C-like protease	3CLpro inhibition test	SARS-CoV	[138]
SNA I-Neu5Acα(2.6)Gal/GalNAc-specific agglutinins	*Sambucus nigra*	>100 µg/mL	Inhibition of viral binding and another target at the end of the replication cycle	CPE assay	SARS-CoV	[136]
Tannic acid	Black tea	3 µM	3CL protease inhibition	3CLpro inhibition assay	SARS-CoV	[141]
Tanshinone I	*Salvia miltiorrhiza*	38.7±8.2 µM	Non-competitive enzyme isomerization inhibitor of protease	CLpro inhibition assay	SARS-CoV CLpro	[150]
Tanshinone I	*Salvia miltiorrhiza*	8.8±0.4 µM	Non-competitive enzyme isomerization inhibitor of protease	PLpro inhibition assay	SARS-CoV PLpro	[150]
Tanshinone I	*Salvia miltiorrhiza*	0.7 µM	Non-competitive inhibition	SARS-CoV = deubiquitination activity	SARS-CoV	[150]
Tanshinone IIA	*Salvia miltiorrhiza*	89.1±5.2 µM	Non-competitive enzyme isomerization inhibitor of protease	CLpro inhibition assay	SARS-CoV CLpro	[150]
Tanshinone IIA	*Salvia miltiorrhiza*	1.6±0.5 µM	Non-competitive enzyme isomerization inhibitor of protease	PLpro inhibition assay	SARS-CoV PLpro	[150]
Tanshinone IIB	*Salvia miltiorrhiza*	24.8±0.8 µM	Non-competitive enzyme isomerization inhibitor of protease	CLpro inhibition assay	SARS-CoV CLpro	[150]
Tanshinone IIB	*Salvia miltiorrhiza*	10.7±1.7 µM	Non-competitive enzyme isomerization inhibitor of protease	PLpro inhibition assay	SARS-CoV PLpro	[150]
Terrestriamide	*Tribulus terrestris Fruits*	21.5±0.5 µM	ND	PLpro inhibition assay	SARS-CoV CLpro	[156]
Terrestrimine	*Tribulus terrestris Fruits*	15.8±0.6 µM	ND	PLpro inhibition assay	SARS-CoV CLpro	[156]
Tetrandrine	Purified compound	0.29 µM (HCoV-OC43 EC50); 2.05 µM (HCoV-NL63)	Analgesic, antineoplastic, antihypertensive	Indirect immunofluorescence assay	HCoV-OC43, HCoV-NL63	[140]
Tetrandrine	*Stephania tetrandra* and related species (present in)	0.33±0.03 µM	Inhibition of viral replication and expression of viral S and N protein, suppressed the replication of HCoV-OC43	MTS assay and *q*RT-PCR, MRC-5 system	HCoV-OC43-infected MRC-5 human lung cells	[145]

(*Continued*)

TABLE 5.1 (*Continued*)

Anti-SARS-CoV-1 Natural Metabolites Tested *in vitro*

Natural Source	Compound/Extract Type	IC_{50}/EC_{50}	Mechanism of Action	Method to Assess Activity	Test System	References
Tetra-O-galloyl-beta-D-glucose	Can be present in *P. emblica, Galla chinensis*	4.5 µM	Prevents the viral entry	HIV-luc/SARS pseudotyped virus entry inhibition assays	SARS-CoV	[149]
Tetra-O-galloyl-beta-D-glucose	Can be present in *P. emblica*	2.86 µM	Prevents the viral invasion	HIV-luc/SARS pseudotyped virus entry inhibition assays	HIV-luc/SARS pseudo type virus	[159]
Theaflavin (TF1)	Black tea	56 µm	ND	3CLpro inhibition assay	SARS-CoV CLpro	[141]
Theaflavin-3,3′ -digallate	Black tea	9.5 µm	3CL protease inhibition	3CLpro inhibition assay	SARS 3CLpro	[141]
Tingenone	*Tripterygium regelii*	9.9±0.1 µM	Competitive inhibition of CoV protease	CLpro inhibition assay	SARS-CoV CLpro	[164]
TL M I-Man-specific agglutinins	*Tulipa* hybrid	22±6 µg/mL	Inhibition of viral binding and another target at the end of the replication cycle	CPE assay, Vero E6 cells	SARS-CoV	[126]
Tomentin A	*Paulownia tomentosa*	6.2±0.04µM	Reversible, mixed-type (allosteric) inhibitors of PLpro	SARS-CoV PLpro inhibition assay	SARS-CoV *Urbani* strain PLpro	[129]
Tomentin B	*Paulownia tomentosa*	6.1±0.02µM	Reversible, mixed-type (allosteric) inhibitors of PLpro	SARS-CoV PLpro inhibition assay	SARS-CoV *Urbani* strain PLpro	[129]
Tomentin C	*Paulownia tomentosa*	11.6±0.13 µM	Reversible, mixed-type (allosteric) inhibitors of PLpro	SARS-CoV PLpro inhibition assay	SARS-CoV *Urbani* strain PLpro	[129]
Tomentin D	*Paulownia tomentosa*	12.5±0.22 µM	Reversible, mixed-type (allosteric) inhibitors of PLpro	SARS-CoV PLpro inhibition assay	SARS-CoV *Urbani* strain PLpro	[129]
Tomentin E	*Paulownia tomentosa*	5.0±0.06µM	Reversible, mixed-type (allosteric) inhibitors of PLpro	SARS-CoV PLpro inhibition assay	SARS-CoV *Urbani* strain PLpro	[129]
Tryptanthrin	*Strobilanthes cusia*	1.52 µM	Inhibits HCoV-NL63 replication	Cytopathic effect reduction and virus yield inhibition assays	SARS-CoV-1	[165]
Tryptanthrin	*Strobilanthes cusia* leaf	0.06 µM	Blocking viral RNA genome synthesis and papain-like protease 2 activity	Plaque virucidal assay	HCoV-NL63	[165]
Tylophorine	Found in *Tylophora indica*	NI	Targeting viral RNA replication and cellular JAK2-mediated dominant NF-κB activation	Anti-TGEV activity and the end point dilution assay	CoV	[178]
Tylophorine	*Tylophora indica*	0.018 µM	Inhibition of protease and viral replication	CoV-infected swine testicular cells	SARS-CoV	[134]
UDA-Lectins isolated from diaminopropane extracts, $(GlcNAc)_n$-specific agglutinins	*Urtica dioica*	1.3±0.1 µg/mL	Inhibition of viral binding and another target at the end of the replication cycle	CPE assay	SARS-CoV	[126]

(*Continued*)

TABLE 5.1 (*Continued*)

Anti-SARS-CoV-1 Natural Metabolites Tested *in vitro*

Natural Source	Compound/Extract Type	IC_{50}/EC_{50}	Mechanism of Action	Method to Assess Activity	Test System	References
Urtica dioica agglutinin	*Urtica dioica* (found in)	0.6±0.6 μg/mL	Inhibition of viral replication and binds to spike protein and N-acetylglucosamine-like residues on the glycosylated envelope	Neutral red uptake assay	Mouse-adapted virus, SARS-CoV replication in Vero 76 cells	[179]
Urtica dioica agglutinin	*Urtica dioica* (found in)	2.0±1.1 μg/mL	Inhibition of viral replication and binds to spike protein and N-acetylglucosamine-like residues on the glycosylated envelope	Neutral red uptake assay	Frankfurt v1940, SARS-CoV replication in Vero 76 cells	[179]
Urtica dioica agglutinin	*Urtica dioica* (found in)	1.7±0.2 μg/mL	Inhibition of viral replication and binds to spike protein and N-acetylglucosamine-like residues on the glycosylated envelope	Neutral red uptake assay	Hong Kong v2157, SARS-CoV replication in Vero 76 cells	[179]
Urtica dioica agglutinin	*Urtica dioica* (found in)	0.9±1.2 μg/mL	Inhibition of viral replication and binds to spike protein and N-acetylglucosamine-like residues on the glycosylated envelope	Neutral red uptake assay	Toronto-2 v2147, SARS-CoV replication in Vero 76 cells	[179]
Urtica dioica agglutinin	*Urtica dioica* (found in)	2.6±3.7 μg/mL	Inhibition of viral replication and binds to spike protein and N-acetylglucosamine-like residues on the glycosylated envelope	Neutral red uptake assay SARS-CoV-infected BALB/c mouse model	SARS-CoV *Urbani* strain (200,300,592)	[179]
Valinomycin	Usually obtained from Streptomyces species	1.63 μM	Inhibits 50% of Vero E6 cell proliferation and viral replication	CPE on Vero E6 cells via SARS-CoV infection, SARS-CoV 3CL protease inhibition assay	SARS-CoV	[130]
Xanthoangelol	Chalcone isolated from Angelica keiskei	11.4±1.4; 13.0±0.9 μM		SARS-CoV 3CLpro and PLpro inhibition assays	SARS-CoV 3CLpro, SARS-CoV PLpro.	[162]
α-Pinene and β-myrcene	*Juniperus oxycedrus*	270 μg/mL	Inhibits viral replication	CPE assay	SARS-CoV FFM1	[171]
α-Pinene, δ-3-carene, α-cedrol	*Thuja orientalis*	130±0.4 μg/mL	Inhibits viral replication	CPE assay	SARS-CoV FFM1	[171]
β-Cadinol (PCWU)	Sesquiterpenes	4.44 μM	Inhibits 50% of Vero E6 cell proliferation and viral replication	CPE on Vero E6 cells via SARS-CoV infection, SARS-CoV 3CL protease inhibition assay	SARS-CoV	[130]
β-Ocimene, 1,8-cineole, α-pinene, β-pinene	*Laurus nobilis*	120±1.2 μg/mL	Inhibits viral replication	CPE assay	SARS-CoV FFM1	[171]
β-Sitosterol	*Isatis indigotica*	115 μM	3CLpro inhibition	3CLpro cleavage assay	SARS-CoV 3CLpro	[138]

Source: Mani JS, Johnson JB, Steel JC, Broszczak DA, Neilsen PM, Walsh KB, Naiker M, *Virus Res*, 2020, 284, 197989. With permission.

CLpro, chymotrypsin-like protease; CPE assay, cytopathogenic effect assay; n/a, not applicable to this study; ND, no data; PLpro, papain-like protease; PCWS: Pure compound was used in the study; Effective concentration (EC50) for the inhibition of viral replication to 50% of the untreated (control) cell cultures; N.T., not tested; h, Exposure to the tested compound improved cell viability resulting in the multiplication and survival of a larger number of cells with inhibited virus in vivo assays. Due to their non-polar and volatile characteristics, common in vitro screening assays such as disk diffusion or agar absorption are not suitable for their antimicrobial assessment. Since only polar constituents can dispert into agar medium, various researchers have determined that this method is not suitable for screening of EOs. An assay based on liquid medium such as broth dilution method is suitable; however, tween concentration (added to increase the solubility of EOs) should be optimized as tween can encourage bacterial growth or alter cell permeability. Tween can also interact with EO components to show antagonistic or synergistic effects, which can lead to either a decrease or increase in pharmacological activity. Thus, it is important to develop suitable methods such as vapor phase test (VPT) to screen for effective EOs. Modified methods such as modification of disk volatilization method by using four-section Petri dish, large filter paper disk consistently saturated with EO and medium containing lid have been used to determine the composition of EOs in vapour phase.

Both solid and vapor diffusion tests can be used with solid-phase microextraction combined with gas chromatography–ion trap mass spectrometry to analyze the atmosphere generated from EOs.

Certain factors determine the effectiveness of olfactory aromatherapy (OA) as demonstrated in Figure 5.2. Dilution, stability in vapor and solid phases, EO–EO interaction, EO–antibiotic interaction, nature of pathogen (Gram-positive or Gram-negative, resistant, or normal strain), chemical composition, percentage of active substance, and other parameters determine the significance of biological activity of an EO and its components. Due to their volatile nature, EOs can easily reach both the upper and lower parts of the respiratory tract via inhalation. This alternative approach to avoid antibiotic use or abuse is an effective and safe treatment. The stability of EOs should be monitored in different phases. For example, lemon grass oil showed more antifungal activity and greater potency in the vapor phase and has been used as air purifier in hospitals.

5.6.2 Marine-Based Natural Products

Synthetic medication-based side effects and toxicity have attracted scientific attention to natural product-based drugs. Marine organisms offer a wide range of natural products with significant biological activities. These natural products contain a diverse range of chemical compounds with broad-spectrum antiviral properties. The chemodiversity of marine as well freshwater organisms represents a unique approach and can be considered as an important source for the development of a future natural "antiviral drug." Alga-based natural products are one of the richest sources of bioactive compounds and possess potential antiviral properties. Alga-based metabolites have been reported for their potential in inhibiting proteins like 3CLpro, transmembrane serine protease 2 (TMPRSS2), and ACE2 involved in the replication of COVID-19. Consequently,

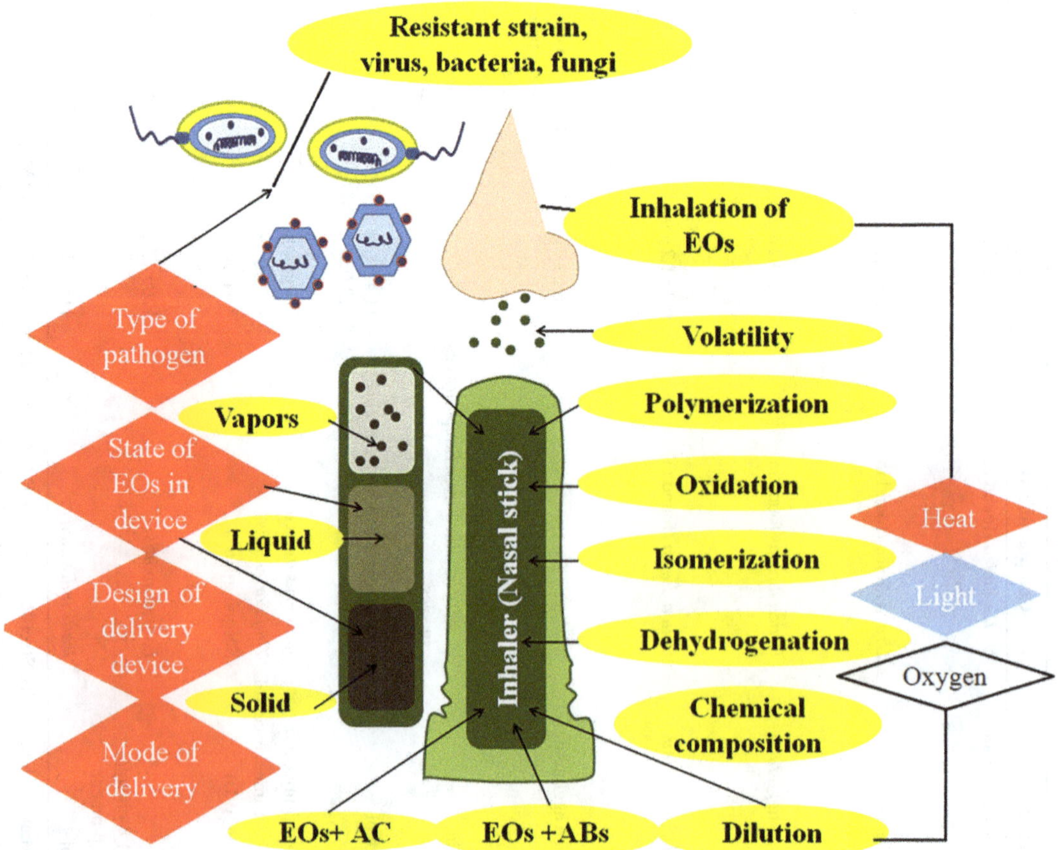

FIGURE 5.2 Factors that determine the effectiveness of OA.

the antiviral compounds present in algae and cyanobacteria need to be explored as a therapy for SARS-CoV-2. These potential marine-based antiviral natural products can be used against SARS-CoV-2 as a possible candidate to suppress SARS-CoV-2 antigenic proteins. In our previous research, we explored various natural products from marine as well as freshwater algae [180–193]. Therefore, the development of a broad-spectrum class of natural antiviral products that bind to these specific targets to reduce pathogenesis caused by this virus should be pursued.

5.7 Polymeric Nanoparticles

Nanotechnology has a wide range of advantages by using core medication in nanoform such as polymeric and lipid nanoparticles (NPs), metallic NPs, liposomes, and micelles for drug encapsulation as well as for improving its biological properties [194–207]. Nanomedicines can easily cross biological membranes without affecting host functions such as the immune system. Polymeric NPs have been reported for their quick mucous penetration, acting with little toxicity in the lungs and effective in treating respiratory diseases [194–207]. Viral diseases such as respiratory syncytial were treated with NPs carrying RSV fusion proteins to activate immune cells including natural killer cells, IFN-γ, and TNF-α. So far various nanosystems such as polymeric NPs (200–300 nm), self-assembling proteins, and peptide-based NPs (15 nm) and inorganic NPs (100 nm) have been studied against respiratory viruses. Polymer-based nanoformulations, which are fabricated by using natural (marine, plant, and mammalian sources) as well as synthetic polymers decrease the non-specific interaction in the serum; thus, the pharmacokinetic parameters of the drug improve and side effects reduce via overcoming early drug degradation [194–207]. These types of nanoformulations have been effectively used against HIV, HSV, and hepatitis B. For efavirenz, darunavir, indinavir, acyclovir, and lamivudine, polymeric micelles have been effectively used [194–207]. Polymeric NPs have considerable advantages; for example, they can be used to target monocytes and macrophages in the brain and lymphatic system and tackle viral diseases like HIV. Subunit vaccines via polymeric nanoparticulate systems have been developed to improve vaccine potency by modifying their physicochemical properties to integrate various immunological cues to mimic pathogenic microbes and viruses [194–207]. Recent advancement in polymeric nanostructure-based delivery systems allows effective development of particulate vaccines to produce desirable immune response. These particulate vaccines are prepared by considering various parameters such as effect of microbe mimicry on modulation of the nanoparticle delivery, trafficking, and targeting antigen-presenting cells to elicit potent, humoral, and cellular immune responses [194–207]. These polymeric nanostructures loaded with antigens and immunostimulatory molecules are available in diverse forms such as particles, micelles, nanogels, and polymersomes to the advanced core–shell structures where polymeric particles are coated with lipids, cell membranes, or proteins [194–207].

REFERENCES

1. Pushpakom S, Iorio F, Eyers PA, Escott KJ, Hopper S, Wells A, Doig A, Guilliams T, Latimer J, McNamee C, Norris A, Sanseau P, Cavalla D, Pirmohamed M. Drug repurposing: Progress, challenges and recommendations. *Nat Rev Drug Discov.* 2019;18(1):41–58.
2. Mercorelli B, Palù G, Loregian A. Drug repurposing for viral infectious diseases: How far are we? *Trends Microbiol.* 2018;26(10):865–876.
3. Breckenridge A, Jacob R. Overcoming the legal and regulatory barriers to drug repurposing. *Nat Rev Drug Discov.* 2019;18(1):1–2.
4. Ashburn TT, Thor KB. Drug repositioning: Identifying and developing new uses for existing drugs. *Nat Rev Drug Discov.* 2004;3(8):673–683.
5. Singh TU, Parida S, Lingaraju MC, Kesavan M, Kumar D, Singh RK. Drug repurposing approach to fight COVID-19. *Pharmacol Rep.* 2020;72(6):1479–1508.
6. Parvathaneni V, Gupta V. Utilizing drug repurposing against COVID-19-efficacy, limitations, and challenges. *Life Sci.* 2020;259:118275.
7. Boozari M, Hosseinzadeh H. Natural products for COVID-19 prevention and treatment regarding to previous coronavirus infections and novel studies. *Phytother Res.* 2021;35(2):864–876.
8. Pamuru RR, Ponneri N, Damu AG, Vadde R. Targeting natural products for the treatment of COVID-19- an updated review. *Curr Pharm Des.* 2020;26(41):5278–5285.
9. Asif M, Saleem M, Saadullah M, Yaseen HS, Al Zarzour R. COVID-19 and therapy with essential oils having antiviral, anti-inflammatory, and immunomodulatory properties. *Inflammopharmacology.* 2020;28(5):1153–1161. doi: 10.1007/s10787-020-00744-0. Epub 2020. Erratum in: Inflammopharmacology.
10. Goyal A, Cusick AS, Thielemier B. *ACE Inhibitors.* StatPearls Publishing, Treasure Island, FL, 2021. Available from: https://www.ncbi.nlm.nih.gov/books/NBK430896/.
11. Abd El-Aziz TM, Al-Sabi A, Stockand JD. Human recombinant soluble ACE2 (hrsACE2) shows promise for treating severe COVID-19. *Signal Transduct Target Ther.* 2020;5(1):258.
12. Focosi D, Anderson AO, Tang JW, Tuccori M. Convalescent plasma therapy for COVID-19: State of the art. *Clin Microbiol Rev.* 2020;33(4):e00072–20.
13. Jahanshahlu L, Rezaei N. Monoclonal antibody as a potential anti-COVID-19. *Biomed Pharmacother.* 2020;129:110337. doi: 10.1016/j.biopha.2020.110337. Epub 2020 June 4.
14. Wang X, Gui J. Cell-mediated immunity to SARS-CoV-2. *Pediatr Investig.* 2020;4(4):281–291.
15. Ellison-Hughes GM, Colley L, O'Brien KA, Roberts KA, Agbaedeng TA, Ross MD. The role of MSC therapy in attenuating the damaging effects of the cytokine storm induced by COVID-19 on the heart and cardiovascular system. *Front Cardiovasc Med.* 2020;7:602183.
16. Mainardes RM, Diedrich C. The potential role of nanomedicine on COVID-19 therapeutics. *Ther Deliv.* 2020;11(7):411–414.
17. Bestle D, Heindl MR, Limburg H, Van Lam van T, Pilgram O, Moulton H, Stein DA, Hardes K, Eickmann M, Dolnik O, Rohde C, Klenk HD, Garten W, Steinmetzer T,

Böttcher-Friebertshäuser E. TMPRSS2 and furin are both essential for proteolytic activation of SARS-CoV-2 in human airway cells. *Life Sci Alliance.* 2020;3(9):e202000786.
18. Wang Z, Yang L. Turning the tide: Natural products and natural-product-inspired chemicals as potential counters to SARS-CoV-2 infection. *Front Pharmacol.* 2020;11:1013.
19. Achan J, Talisuna AO, Erhart A, Yeka A, Tibenderana JK, Baliraine FN, Rosenthal PJ, D'Alessandro U. Quinine, an old anti-malarial drug in a modern world: Role in the treatment of malaria. *Malar J.* 2011;10:144.
20. Al-Bari MAA. Targeting endosomal acidification by chloroquine analogs as a promising strategy for the treatment of emerging viral diseases. *Pharmacol Res Perspect.* 2017;5(1):e00293.
21. Zhang W, Zhao Y, Zhang F, Wang Q, Li T, Liu Z, Wang J, Qin Y, Zhang X, Yan X, Zeng X, Zhang S. The use of anti-inflammatory drugs in the treatment of people with severe coronavirus disease 2019 (COVID-19): The perspectives of clinical immunologists from China. *Clin Immunol.* 2020;214:108393.
22. Pal A, Pawar A, Goswami K, Sharma P, Prasad R. Hydroxychloroquine and COVID-19: A cellular and molecular biology based update. *Indian J Clin Biochem.* 2020;35(3):274–284.
23. Wang M, Cao R, Zhang L, Yang X, Liu J, Xu M, Shi Z, Hu Z, Zhong W, Xiao G. Remdesivir and chloroquine effectively inhibit the recently emerged novel coronavirus (2019-nCoV) in vitro. *Cell Res.* 2020;30(3):269–271.
24. Khuroo MS. Chloroquine and hydroxychloroquine in coronavirus disease 2019 (COVID-19). Facts, fiction and the hype: A critical appraisal. *Int J Antimicrob Agents.* 2020;56(3):106101.
25. Acharya Y, Sayed A. Chloroquine and hydroxychloroquine as a repurposed agent against COVID-19: A narrative review. *Ther Adv Infect Dis.* 2020;7:2049936120947517.
26. Qiu T, Liang S, Dabbous M, Wang Y, Han R, Toumi M. Chinese guidelines related to novel coronavirus pneumonia. *J Mark Access Health Policy.* 2020;8(1):1818446.
27. Waldrop T, Alsup D, McLaughlin EC. Fearing coronavirus, Arizona man dies after taking a form of chloroquine used in aquariums. CNN Internet. 2020 March 23. https://www.cnn.com/2020/03/23/health/arizona-coronavirus-chloroquine-death/index.html (accessed on 24 March 2020).
28. Busari S, Bukola A. Nigeria records chloroquine poisoning after Trump endorses it for coronavirus treatment. CNN Internet. 2020 March 23. https://www.cnn.com/2020/03/23/africa/chloroquine-trump-nigeria-intl/index.html (accessed on 24 March 2020).
29. Zou L, Dai L, Zhang X, Zhang Z, Zhang Z. Hydroxychloroquine and chloroquine: A potential and controversial treatment for COVID-19. *Arch Pharm Res.* 2020;43(8):765–772.
30. Yao X, Ye F, Zhang M, Cui C, Huang B, Niu P, Liu X, Zhao L, Dong E, Song C, Zhan S, Lu R, Li H, Tan W, Liu D. In vitro antiviral activity and projection of optimized dosing design of hydroxychloroquine for the treatment of severe acute respiratory syndrome coronavirus 2 (SARS-CoV-2). *Clin Infect Dis.* 2020;71(15):732–739.
31. Kumar R, Sharma A, Srivastava JK, Siddiqui MH, Uddin MS, Aleya L. Hydroxychloroquine in COVID-19: Therapeutic promises, current status, and environmental implications. *Environ Sci Pollut Res Int.* 2021:1–14. https://pubmed.ncbi.nlm.nih.gov/33447984/
32. Chen Z, Hu J, Zhang Z, et al. Efficacy of hydroxychloroquine in patients with COVID-19: Results of a randomized clinical trial. *J Zhejiang Univ (Med Sci)* 2020;49(2):215–219.
33. Kalra RS, Tomar D, Meena AS, Kandimalla R. SARS-CoV-2, ACE2, and hydroxychloroquine: Cardiovascular complications, therapeutics, and clinical readouts in the current settings. *Pathogens.* 2020;9(7):546.
34. Oscanoa TJ, Romero-Ortuno R, Carvajal A, Savarino A. A pharmacological perspective of chloroquine in SARS-CoV-2 infection: An old drug for the fight against a new coronavirus? *Int J Antimicrob Agents.* 2020;56(3):106078.
35. Zhou D, Dai SM, Tong Q. COVID-19: A recommendation to examine the effect of hydroxychloroquine in preventing infection and progression. *J Antimicrob Chemother.* 2020;75(7):1667–1670.
36. Gies V, Bekaddour N, Dieudonné Y, Guffroy A, Frenger Q, Gros F, Rodero MP, Herbeuval JP, Korganow AS. Beyond anti-viral effects of chloroquine/hydroxychloroquine. *Front Immunol.* 2020;11:1409.
37. Cao B, Wang Y, Wen D, Liu W, Wang J, Fan G, Ruan L, Song B, Cai Y, Wei M, Li X, Xia J, Chen N, Xiang J, Yu T, Bai T, Xie X, Zhang L, Li C, Yuan Y, Chen H, Li H, Huang H, Tu S, Gong F, Liu Y, Wei Y, Dong C, Zhou F, Gu X, Xu J, Liu Z, Zhang Y, Li H, Shang L, Wang K, Li K, Zhou X, Dong X, Qu Z, Lu S, Hu X, Ruan S, Luo S, Wu J, Peng L, Cheng F, Pan L, Zou J, Jia C, Wang J, Liu X, Wang S, Wu X, Ge Q, He J, Zhan H, Qiu F, Guo L, Huang C, Jaki T, Hayden FG, Horby PW, Zhang D, Wang C. A trial of lopinavir-ritonavir in adults hospitalized with severe COVID-19. *N Engl J Med.* 2020;382(19):1787–1799.
38. Yao TT, Qian JD, Zhu WY, Wang Y, Wang GQ. A systematic review of lopinavir therapy for SARS coronavirus and MERS coronavirus-A possible reference for coronavirus disease-19 treatment option. *J Med Virol.* 2020;92(6):556–563.
39. Magro P, Zanella I, Pescarolo M, Castelli F, Quiros-Roldan E. Lopinavir/ritonavir: Repurposing an old drug for HIV infection in COVID-19 treatment. *Biomed J.* 2021;44(1):43–53.
40. Ghosh AK, Osswald HL, Prato G. Recent progress in the development of HIV-1 protease inhibitors for the treatment of HIV/AIDS. *J Med Chem.* 2016;59(11):5172–5208.
41. Kumar S, Zhi K, Mukherji A, Gerth K. Repurposing antiviral protease inhibitors using extracellular vesicles for potential therapy of COVID-19. *Viruses.* 2020;12(5):486.
42. https://www.who.int/news/item/04-07-2020-who-discontinues-hydroxychloroquine-and-lopinavir-ritonavir-treatment-arms-for-covid-19.
43. Cao YC, Deng QX, Dai SX. Remdesivir for severe acute respiratory syndrome coronavirus 2 causing COVID-19: An evaluation of the evidence. *Travel Med Infect Dis.* 2020;35:101647.
44. Wang Y, Zhang D, Du G, Du R, Zhao J, Jin Y, Fu S, Gao L, Cheng Z, Lu Q, Hu Y, Luo G, Wang K, Lu Y, Li H, Wang S, Ruan S, Yang C, Mei C, Wang Y, Ding D, Wu F, Tang X, Ye X, Ye Y, Liu B, Yang J, Yin W, Wang A, Fan G, Zhou F, Liu Z, Gu X, Xu J, Shang L, Zhang Y, Cao L, Guo T, Wan Y, Qin H, Jiang Y, Jaki T, Hayden FG, Horby PW, Cao B, Wang C. Remdesivir in adults with severe COVID-19: A randomised, double-blind, placebo-controlled, multicentre trial. *Lancet.* 2020;395(10236):1569–1578. doi: 10.1016/S0140–6736(20)31022-9. Epub 2020 April 29. Erratum in: *Lancet.* 2020;395(10238):1694.

45. Choy KT, Wong AY, Kaewpreedee P, Sia SF, Chen D, Hui KPY, Chu DKW, Chan MCW, Cheung PP, Huang X, Peiris M, Yen HL. Remdesivir, lopinavir, emetine, and homoharringtonine inhibit SARS-CoV-2 replication in vitro. *Antiviral Res.* 2020;178:104786.
46. Grein J, Ohmagari N, Shin D, Diaz G, Asperges E, Castagna A, Feldt T, Green G, Green ML, Lescure FX, Nicastri E, Oda R, Yo K, Quiros-Roldan E, Studemeister A, Redinski J, Ahmed S, Bernett J, Chelliah D, Chen D, Chihara S, Cohen SH, Cunningham J, D'Arminio Monforte A, Ismail S, Kato H, Lapadula G, L'Her E, Maeno T, Majumder S, Massari M, Mora-Rillo M, Mutoh Y, Nguyen D, Verweij E, Zoufaly A, Osinusi AO, DeZure A, Zhao Y, Zhong L, Chokkalingam A, Elboudwarej E, Telep L, Timbs L, Henne I, Sellers S, Cao H, Tan SK, Winterbourne L, Desai P, Mera R, Gaggar A, Myers RP, Brainard DM, Childs R, Flanigan T. Compassionate use of remdesivir for patients with severe COVID-19. *N Engl J Med.* 2020;382(24):2327–2336.
47. Sheahan TP, Sims AC, Leist SR, Schäfer A, Won J, Brown AJ, Montgomery SA, Hogg A, Babusis D, Clarke MO, Spahn JE, Bauer L, Sellers S, Porter D, Feng JY, Cihlar T, Jordan R, Denison MR, Baric RS. Comparative therapeutic efficacy of remdesivir and combination lopinavir, ritonavir, and interferon beta against MERS-CoV. *Nat Commun.* 2020;11(1):222.
48. Malin JJ, Suárez I, Priesner V, Fätkenheuer G, Rybniker J. Remdesivir against COVID-19 and other viral diseases. *Clin Microbiol Rev.* 2020;34(1):e00162–20.
49. Lin HXJ, Cho S, Meyyur Aravamudan V, Sanda HY, Palraj R, Molton JS, Venkatachalam I. Remdesivir in coronavirus disease 2019 (COVID-19) treatment: A review of evidence. *Infection.* 2021;49(3):401–410.
50. Beigel JH, Tomashek KM, Dodd LE, Mehta AK, Zingman BS, Kalil AC, Hohmann E, Chu HY, Luetkemeyer A, Kline S, Lopez de Castilla D, Finberg RW, Dierberg K, Tapson V, Hsieh L, Patterson TF, Paredes R, Sweeney DA, Short WR, Touloumi G, Lye DC, Ohmagari N, Oh MD, Ruiz-Palacios GM, Benfield T, Fätkenheuer G, Kortepeter MG, Atmar RL, Creech CB, Lundgren J, Babiker AG, Pett S, Neaton JD, Burgess TH, Bonnett T, Green M, Makowski M, Osinusi A, Nayak S, Lane HC; ACTT-1 Study Group Members. Remdesivir for the treatment of COVID-19-final report. *N Engl J Med.* 2020;383(19):1813–1826.
51. Furuta Y, Komeno T, Nakamura T. Favipiravir (T-705), a broad spectrum inhibitor of viral RNA polymerase. *Proc Jpn Acad Ser B Phys Biol Sci.* 2017;93(7):449–463.
52. Cai Q, Yang M, Liu D, Chen J, Shu D, Xia J, Liao X, Gu Y, Cai Q, Yang Y, Shen C, Li X, Peng L, Huang D, Zhang J, Zhang S, Wang F, Liu J, Chen L, Chen S, Wang Z, Zhang Z, Cao R, Zhong W, Liu Y, Liu L. Experimental treatment with favipiravir for COVID-19: An open-label control study. *Engineering (Beijing).* 2020;6(10):1192–1198.
53. Khalili JS, Zhu H, Mak NSA, Yan Y, Zhu Y. Novel coronavirus treatment with ribavirin: Groundwork for an evaluation concerning COVID-19. *J Med Virol.* 2020;92(7):740–746.
54. Falzarano D, de Wit E, Rasmussen AL, Feldmann F, Okumura A, Scott DP, Brining D, Bushmaker T, Martellaro C, Baseler L, Benecke AG, Katze MG, Munster VJ, Feldmann H. Treatment with interferon-α2b and ribavirin improves outcome in MERS-CoV-infected rhesus macaques. *Nat Med.* 2013;19(10):1313–1317.
55. Beaucourt S, Vignuzzi M. Ribavirin: A drug active against many viruses with multiple effects on virus replication and propagation. Molecular basis of ribavirin resistance. *Curr Opin Virol.* 2014;8:10–15.
56. Elfiky AA. Anti-HCV, nucleotide inhibitors, repurposing against COVID-19. *Life Sci.* 2020;248:117477.
57. Falzarano D, de Wit E, Martellaro C, Callison J, Munster VJ, Feldmann H. Inhibition of novel β coronavirus replication by a combination of interferon-α2b and ribavirin. *Sci Rep.* 2013;3:1686.
58. Blaising J, Polyak SJ, Pécheur EI. Arbidol as a broad-spectrum antiviral: An update. *Antiviral Res.* 2014;107:84–94.
59. Hulseberg CE, Fénéant L, Szymańska-de Wijs KM, Kessler NP, Nelson EA, Shoemaker CJ, Schmaljohn CS, Polyak SJ, White JM. Arbidol and other low-molecular-weight drugs that inhibit Lassa and Ebola viruses. *J Virol.* 2019;93(8):e02185–18.
60. Teissier E, Zandomeneghi G, Loquet A, Lavillette D, Lavergne JP, Montserret R, Cosset FL, Böckmann A, Meier BH, Penin F, Pécheur EI. Mechanism of inhibition of enveloped virus membrane fusion by the antiviral drug arbidol. *PLoS One.* 2011;6(1):e15874.
61. Liu MY, Wang S, Yao WF, Wu HZ, Meng SN, Wei MJ. Pharmacokinetic properties and bioequivalence of two formulations of arbidol: An open-label, single-dose, randomized-sequence, two-period crossover study in healthy Chinese male volunteers. *Clin Ther.* 2009;31(4):784–792.
62. Jin YH, Cai L, Cheng ZS, Cheng H, Deng T, Fan YP, Fang C, Huang D, Huang LQ, Huang Q, Han Y, Hu B, Hu F, Li BH, Li YR, Liang K, Lin LK, Luo LS, Ma J, Ma LL, Peng ZY, Pan YB, Pan ZY, Ren XQ, Sun HM, Wang Y, Wang YY, Weng H, Wei CJ, Wu DF, Xia J, Xiong Y, Xu HB, Yao XM, Yuan YF, Ye TS, Zhang XC, Zhang YW, Zhang YG, Zhang HM, Zhao Y, Zhao MJ, Zi H, Zeng XT, Wang YY, Wang XH; for the Zhongnan Hospital of Wuhan University Novel Coronavirus Management and Research Team, Evidence-Based Medicine Chapter of China International Exchange and Promotive Association for Medical and Health Care (CPAM). A rapid advice guideline for the diagnosis and treatment of 2019 novel coronavirus (2019-nCoV) infected pneumonia (standard version). *Mil Med Res.* 2020;7(1):4.
63. Researchers find two new drugs that can effectively inhibit coronavirus,(n.d.).https://news.cgtn.com/news/2020-02-04/Researchers-find-two-drugs-that-can-effectively-inhibit-coronavirus-NOFpci7NJK/index.html (accessed on May 17 2020).
64. Lu H. Efficacy and safety of darunavir and cobicistat for treatment of COVID-19, clinicaltrials.gov. 2020. https://clinicaltrials.gov/ct2/show/NCT04252274.
65. Santos JR, Curran A, Navarro-Mercade J, Ampuero MF, Pelaez P, Pérez-Alvarez N, Clotet B, Paredes R, Moltó J. Simplification of antiretroviral treatment from darunavir/ritonavir monotherapy to darunavir/cobicistat monotherapy: Effectiveness and safety in routine clinical practice. *AIDS Res Hum Retroviruses.* 2019;35(6):513–518.
66. Mathias AA, German P, Murray BP, Wei L, Jain A, West S, Warren D, Hui J, Kearney BP. Pharmacokinetics and pharmacodynamics of GS-9350: A novel pharmacokinetic enhancer without anti-HIV activity. *Clin Pharmacol Ther.* 2010;87(3):322–329.

67. Wang D, Hu B, Hu C, Zhu F, Liu X, Zhang J, Wang B, Xiang H, Cheng Z, Xiong Y, Zhao Y, Li Y, Wang X, Peng Z. Clinical characteristics of 138 hospitalized patients with 2019 novel coronavirus-infected pneumonia in Wuhan, China. *JAMA*. 2020;323(11):1061–1069. doi: 10.1001/jama.2020.1585. Erratum in: *JAMA*. 2021 Mar 16;325(11):1113.
68. Kongsaengdao DS. A 6week prospective, open label, randomized, in Multicenter Study of, Oseltamivir Plus Hydroxychloroquine Versus Lopinavir/Ritonavir Plus Oseltamivir Versus Darunavir/Ritonavir Plus Oseltamivir Plus Hydroxychloroquine in Mild COVID-19 AND Lopipinavir/Ritonavir Plus Oseltamivir Versus Favipiravir Plus Lopipinavir/Ritonavir Versus Darunavir/Ritonavir Plus Oseltamivir Plus Hydroxychloroquine Versus Favipiravir Plus Darunavir and Ritonavir Plus Hydroxychloroquine in Moderate to Critically Ill COVID-19, clinicaltrials.gov. 2020.
69. Gautret P, Lagier JC, Parola P, Hoang VT, Meddeb L, Mailhe M, Doudier B, Courjon J, Giordanengo V, Vieira VE, Tissot Dupont H, Honoré S, Colson P, Chabrière E, La Scola B, Rolain JM, Brouqui P, Raoult D. Hydroxychloroquine and azithromycin as a treatment of COVID-19: results of an open-label non-randomized clinical trial. *Int J Antimicrob Agents*. 2020;56(1):105949.
70. Griffin MO, Fricovsky E, Ceballos G, Villarreal F. Tetracyclines: A pleitropic family of compounds with promising therapeutic properties. Review of the literature. *Am J Physiol Cell Physiol*. 2010;299(3):C539–48.
71. Henehan M, Montuno M, De Benedetto A. Doxycycline as an anti-inflammatory agent: Updates in dermatology. *J Eur Acad Dermatol Venereol*. 2017;31(11):1800–1808.
72. Parenti F, Beretta G, Berti M, Arioli V. Teichomycins, new antibiotics from Actinoplanes teichomyceticus Nov. Sp. I. Description of the producer strain, fermentation studies and biological properties. *J Antibiot (Tokyo)*. 1978;31(4):276–283.
73. Zhou N, Pan T, Zhang J, Li Q, Zhang X, Bai C, Huang F, Peng T, Zhang J, Liu C, Tao L, Zhang H. Glycopeptide antibiotics potently inhibit cathepsin L in the late endosome/lysosome and block the entry of ebola virus, middle east respiratory syndrome coronavirus (MERS-CoV), and severe acute respiratory syndrome coronavirus (SARS-CoV). *J Biol Chem*. 2016;291(17):9218–9232.
74. Zhang J, Ma X, Yu F, Liu J, Zou F, Pan T, Zhang H. Teicoplanin potently blocks the cell entry of 2019-nCoV. *Microbiology*. 2020;55(4):105944.
75. Liu YJ. IPC: Professional type 1 interferon-producing cells and plasmacytoid dendritic cell precursors. *Annu Rev Immunol*. 2005;23:275–306.
76. Totura AL, Baric RS. SARS coronavirus pathogenesis: Host innate immune responses and viral antagonism of interferon. *Curr Opin Virol*. 2012;2(3):264–275.
77. Schneider WM, Chevillotte MD, Rice CM. Interferon-stimulated genes: A complex web of host defenses. *Annu Rev Immunol*. 2014;32:513–545.
78. U.S. National Institutes of Health. Pegylated interferon lambda treatment for COVID-19- full text view, ClinicalTrials.gov, (n.d.). https://clinicaltrials.gov/ct2/show/NCT04343976 (accessed on May 23 2020).
79. U.S. National Institutes of Health. Interferon lambda therapy for COVID-19- full text view, ClinicalTrials.gov, (n.d.). https://clinicaltrials.gov/ct2/show/NCT04388709 (accessed on May 23, 2020).
80. Singh AK, Majumdar S, Singh R, Misra A. Role of corticosteroid in the management of COVID-19: A systemic review and a Clinician's perspective. *Diabetes Metab Syndr*. 2020;14(5):971–978.
81. WHO Rapid Evidence Appraisal for COVID-19 Therapies (REACT) Working Group, Sterne JAC, Murthy S, Diaz JV, Slutsky AS, Villar J, Angus DC, Annane D, Azevedo LCP, Berwanger O, Cavalcanti AB, Dequin PF, Du B, Emberson J, Fisher D, Giraudeau B, Gordon AC, Granholm A, Green C, Haynes R, Heming N, Higgins JPT, Horby P, Jüni P, Landray MJ, Le Gouge A, Leclerc M, Lim WS, Machado FR, McArthur C, Meziani F, Møller MH, Perner A, Petersen MW, Savovic J, Tomazini B, Veiga VC, Webb S, Marshall JC. Association between administration of systemic corticosteroids and mortality among critically Ill patients with COVID-19: A meta-analysis. *JAMA*. 2020;324(13):1330–1341.
82. Wu C, Hou D, Du C, Cai Y, Zheng J, Xu J, Chen X, Chen C, Hu X, Zhang Y, Song J, Wang L, Chao YC, Feng Y, Xiong W, Chen D, Zhong M, Hu J, Jiang J, Bai C, Zhou X, Xu J, Song Y, Gong F. Corticosteroid therapy for coronavirus disease 2019-related acute respiratory distress syndrome: A cohort study with propensity score analysis. *Crit Care*. 2020;24(1):643.
83. van Griensven J, Edwards T, de Lamballerie X, Semple MG, Gallian P, Baize S, Horby PW, Raoul H, Magassouba N, Antierens A, Lomas C, Faye O, Sall AA, Fransen K, Buyze J, Ravinetto R, Tiberghien P, Claeys Y, De Crop M, Lynen L, Bah EI, Smith PG, Delamou A, De Weggheleire A, Haba N; Ebola-Tx consortium. Evaluation of convalescent plasma for ebola virus disease in Guinea. *N Engl J Med*. 2016;374(1):33–42.
84. Tobian AAR, Shaz BH. Earlier the better: Convalescent plasma. *Blood*. 2020;136(6):652–654. doi: 10.1182/blood.2020007638.
85. Pandey S, Vyas GN. Adverse effects of plasma transfusion. *Transfusion*. 2012;52(Suppl 1):65S–79S.
86. Nguyen FT, van den Akker T, Lally K, Lam H, Lenskaya V, Liu STH, Bouvier NM, Aberg JA, Rodriguez D, Krammer F, Strauss D, Shaz BH, Rudon L, Galdon P, Jhang JS, Arinsburg SA, Baine I; Mount Sinai Health System Convalescent Plasma Team. Transfusion reactions associated with COVID-19 convalescent plasma therapy for SARS-CoV-2. *Transfusion*. 2021;61(1):78–93.
87. Abraham J. Passive antibody therapy in COVID-19. *Nat Rev Immunol*. 2020;20(7):401–403.
88. Casadevall A, Pirofski LA. The convalescent sera option for containing COVID-19. *J Clin Invest*. 2020;130(4):1545–1548.
89. Wu XX, Gao HN, Wu HB, Peng XM, Ou HL, Li LJ. Successful treatment of avian-origin influenza A (H7N9) infection using convalescent plasma. *Int J Infect Dis*. 2015;41:3–5.
90. Beigel JH, Voell J, Kumar P, Raviprakash K, Wu H, Jiao JA, Sullivan E, Luke T, Davey RT Jr. Safety and tolerability of a novel, polyclonal human anti-MERS coronavirus antibody produced from transchromosomic cattle: A phase 1 randomised, double-blind, single-dose-escalation study. *Lancet Infect Dis*. 2018;18(4):410–418.

91. Duan K, Liu B, Li C, Zhang H, Yu T, Qu J, Zhou M, Chen L, Meng S, Hu Y, Peng C, Yuan M, Huang J, Wang Z, Yu J, Gao X, Wang D, Yu X, Li L, Zhang J, Wu X, Li B, Xu Y, Chen W, Peng Y, Hu Y, Lin L, Liu X, Huang S, Zhou Z, Zhang L, Wang Y, Zhang Z, Deng K, Xia Z, Gong Q, Zhang W, Zheng X, Liu Y, Yang H, Zhou D, Yu D, Hou J, Shi Z, Chen S, Chen Z, Zhang X, Yang X. Effectiveness of convalescent plasma therapy in severe COVID-19 patients. *Proc Natl Acad Sci U S A*. 2020;117(17):9490–9496.
92. Tiberghien P, de Lamballerie X, Morel P, Gallian P, Lacombe K, Yazdanpanah Y. Collecting and evaluating convalescent plasma for COVID-19 treatment: Why and how? *Vox Sang*. 2020;115(6):488–494.
93. Wang SF, Tseng SP, Yen CH, Yang JY, Tsao CH, Shen CW, Chen KH, Liu FT, Liu WT, Chen YM, Huang JC. Antibody-dependent SARS coronavirus infection is mediated by antibodies against spike proteins. *Biochem Biophys Res Commun*. 2014;451(2):208–214.
94. Jin Y, Lei C, Hu D, Dimitrov DS, Ying T. Human monoclonal antibodies as candidate therapeutics against emerging viruses. *Front Med*. 2017;11(4):462–470.
95. Corti D, Zhao J, Pedotti M, Simonelli L, Agnihothram S, Fett C, Fernandez-Rodriguez B, Foglierini M, Agatic G, Vanzetta F, Gopal R, Langrish CJ, Barrett NA, Sallusto F, Baric RS, Varani L, Zambon M, Perlman S, Lanzavecchia A. Prophylactic and postexposure efficacy of a potent human monoclonal antibody against MERS coronavirus. *Proc Natl Acad Sci U S A*. 2015;112(33):10473–10478.
96. Yu F, Du L, Ojcius DM, Pan C, Jiang S. Measures for diagnosing and treating infections by a novel coronavirus responsible for a pneumonia outbreak originating in Wuhan, China. *Microbes Infect*. 2020;22(2):74–79. doi: 10.1016/j.micinf.2020.01.003. Epub 2020 February 1.
97. Hussain A, Hasan A, Nejadi Babadaei MM, Bloukh SH, Chowdhury MEH, Sharifi M, Haghighat S, Falahati M. Targeting SARS-CoV2 spike protein receptor binding domain by therapeutic antibodies. *Biomed Pharmacother*. 2020;130:110559.
98. Tian X, Li C, Huang A, Xia S, Lu S, Shi Z, Lu L, Jiang S, Yang Z, Wu Y, Ying T. Potent binding of 2019 novel coronavirus spike protein by a SARS coronavirus-specific human monoclonal antibody. *Emerg Microbes Infect*. 2020;9(1):382–385.
99. Wang C, Li W, Drabek D, Okba NMA, van Haperen R, Osterhaus ADME, van Kuppeveld FJM, Haagmans BL, Grosveld F, Bosch BJ. A human monoclonal antibody blocking SARS-CoV-2 infection. *Nat Commun*. 2020;11(1):2251.
100. Tai W, Zhang X, He Y, Jiang S, Du L. Identification of SARS-CoV RBD-targeting monoclonal antibodies with cross-reactive or neutralizing activity against SARS-CoV-2. *Antiviral Res*. 2020;179:104820.
101. Zheng Z, Monteil VM, Maurer-Stroh S, Yew CW, Leong C, Mohd-Ismail NK, Cheyyatraivendran Arularasu S, Chow VTK, Lin RTP, Mirazimi A, Hong W, Tan YJ. Monoclonal antibodies for the S2 subunit of spike of SARS-CoV-1 cross-react with the newly-emerged SARS-CoV-2. *Euro Surveill*. 2020;25(28):2000291.
102. Zumla A, Hui DS, Azhar EI, Memish ZA, Maeurer M. Reducing mortality from 2019-nCoV: Host-directed therapies should be an option. *Lancet*. 2020;395(10224):e35–e36.
103. Xu X, Han M, Li T, Sun W, Wang D, Fu B, Zhou Y, Zheng X, Yang Y, Li X, Zhang X, Pan A, Wei H. Effective treatment of severe COVID-19 patients with tocilizumab. *Proc Natl Acad Sci U S A*. 2020;117(20): 10970–10975.
104. Colaneri M, Bogliolo L, Valsecchi P, Sacchi P, Zuccaro V, Brandolino F, Montecucco C, Mojoli F, Giusti EM, Bruno R, The COVID IRCCS San Matteo Pavia Task Force. Tocilizumab for treatment of severe COVID-19 patients: Preliminary results from SMAtteo COVID19 REgistry (SMACORE). *Microorganisms*. 2020;8(5):695.
105. Chiappelli F, Khakshooy A, Greenberg G. COVID-19 immunopathology and immunotherapy. *Bioinformation*. 2020;16(3):219–222.
106. Kaur SP, Gupta V. COVID-19 vaccine: A comprehensive status report. *Virus Res*. 2020;288:198114.
107. Wang N, Shang J, Jiang S, Du L. Subunit vaccines against emerging pathogenic human coronaviruses. *Front Microbiol*. 2020;11:298.
108. Thanh Le T, Andreadakis Z, Kumar A, Gómez Román R, Tollefsen S, Saville M, Mayhew S. The COVID-19 vaccine development landscape. *Nat Rev Drug Discov*. 2020;19(5):305–306.
109. Baruah V, Bose S. Immunoinformatics-aided identification of T cell and B cell epitopes in the surface glycoprotein of 2019-nCoV. *J Med Virol*. 2020;92(5):495–500.
110. World Health Organization (WHO). Draft landscape of COVID-19 candidate vaccines (accessed on 17th June 2020).
111. Liu MA. A comparison of plasmid DNA and mRNA as vaccine technologies. *Vaccines (Basel)*. 2019;7(2):37.
112. Baden LR, El Sahly HM, Essink B, Kotloff K, Frey S, Novak R, Diemert D, Spector SA, Rouphael N, Creech CB, McGettigan J, Khetan S, Segall N, Solis J, Brosz A, Fierro C, Schwartz H, Neuzil K, Corey L, Gilbert P, Janes H, Follmann D, Marovich M, Mascola J, Polakowski L, Ledgerwood J, Graham BS, Bennett H, Pajon R, Knightly C, Leav B, Deng W, Zhou H, Han S, Ivarsson M, Miller J, Zaks T; COVE Study Group. Efficacy and safety of the mRNA-1273 SARS-CoV-2 vaccine. *N Engl J Med*. 2021;384(5):403–416.
113. Poland GA, Ovsyannikova IG, Kennedy RB. SARS-CoV-2 immunity: Review and applications to phase 3 vaccine candidates. *Lancet*. 2020;396(10262):1595–1606.
114. Bakhiet M, Taurin S. SARS-CoV-2: Targeted managements and vaccine development. *Cytokine Growth Factor Rev*. 2021;58:16–29.
115. Myupchar. 2020. Race for COVID-19 vaccine: Covaxin and ZyCoV-D begin human trials in India, Moderna publishes preliminary data from phase 1. https://www.firstpost.com/health/race-for-covid-19-vaccine-covaxin-and-zycov-d-begin-human-trials-in-india-moderna-publishes-preliminary-data-from-phase-1-8600211.html/amp, https://www.firstpost.com/.
116. Anon. 2020. UW–Madison, FluGen, Bharat Biotech to develop CoroFlu, a coronavirus vaccine. https://www.businesswire.com/news/home/20200402005666/en/UW%E2%80%93Madison-FluGen-Bharat-Biotech-develop-CoroFlu-coronavirus https://www.businesswire.com.

117. Zhu FC, Guan XH, Li YH, Huang JY, Jiang T, Hou LH, Li JX, Yang BF, Wang L, Wang WJ, Wu SP, Wang Z, Wu XH, Xu JJ, Zhang Z, Jia SY, Wang BS, Hu Y, Liu JJ, Zhang J, Qian XA, Li Q, Pan HX, Jiang HD, Deng P, Gou JB, Wang XW, Wang XH, Chen W. Immunogenicity and safety of a recombinant adenovirus type-5-vectored COVID-19 vaccine in healthy adults aged 18 years or older: A randomised, double-blind, placebo-controlled, phase 2 trial. *Lancet.* 2020;396(10249):479–488.
118. Anon 2020. Coronavirus resource center, Johns Hopkins University, August 05, 2020. https://coronavirus.jhu.edu/ [Online].
119. Jackson LA, Anderson EJ, Rouphael NG, Roberts PC, Makhene M, Coler RN, McCullough MP, Chappell JD, Denison MR, Stevens LJ, Pruijssers AJ, McDermott A, Flach B, Doria-Rose NA, Corbett KS, Morabito KM, O'Dell S, Schmidt SD, Swanson PA 2nd, Padilla M, Mascola JR, Neuzil KM, Bennett H, Sun W, Peters E, Makowski M, Albert J, Cross K, Buchanan W, Pikaart-Tautges R, Ledgerwood JE, Graham BS, Beigel JH; mRNA-1273 Study Group. An mRNA vaccine against SARS-CoV-2-preliminary report. *N Engl J Med.* 2020;383(20):1920–1931.
120. Folegatti PM, Ewer KJ, Aley PK, Angus B, Becker S, Belij-Rammerstorfer S, Bellamy D, Bibi S, Bittaye M, Clutterbuck EA, Dold C, Faust SN, Finn A, Flaxman AL, Hallis B, Heath P, Jenkin D, Lazarus R, Makinson R, Minassian AM, Pollock KM, Ramasamy M, Robinson H, Snape M, Tarrant R, Voysey M, Green C, Douglas AD, Hill AVS, Lambe T, Gilbert SC, Pollard AJ; Oxford COVID Vaccine Trial Group. Safety and immunogenicity of the ChAdOx1 nCoV-19 vaccine against SARS-CoV-2: A preliminary report of a phase 1/2, single-blind, randomised controlled trial. *Lancet.* 2020;396(10249):467–478. doi: 10.1016/S0140–6736(20)31604-4. Epub 2020 July 2020. Erratum in: Lancet. 2020 August 15;396(10249):466.
121. Anon. 2020. COVID-19/SARS-CoV-2. http://www.animalresearch.info/en/medical-advances/diseases-research/sars-cov-2/, http://www.animalresearch.info/.
122. Yip MS, Leung HL, Li PH, Cheung CY, Dutry I, Li D, Daëron M, Bruzzone R, Peiris JS, Jaume M. Antibody-dependent enhancement of SARS coronavirus infection and its role in the pathogenesis of SARS. *Hong Kong Med J.* 2016;22(3 Suppl 4):25–31.
123. van Dorp L, Acman M, Richard D, Shaw LP, Ford CE, Ormond L, Owen CJ, Pang J, Tan CCS, Boshier FAT, Ortiz AT, Balloux F. Emergence of genomic diversity and recurrent mutations in SARS-CoV-2. *Infect Genet Evol.* 2020;83:104351.
124. Roh C. A facile inhibitor screening of SARS coronavirus N protein using nanoparticle-based RNA oligonucleotide. *Int J Nanomed.* 2012;7:2173–2179.
125. Keyaerts E, Vijgen L, Pannecouque C, Van Damme E, Peumans W, Egberink H, Balzarini J, Van Ranst M. Plant lectins are potent inhibitors of coronaviruses by interfering with two targets in the viral replication cycle. *Antiviral Res.* 2007;75(3):179–187.
126. Van Damme E, Peumans W, Pusztai A, Bardocz S. *Handbook of Plant Lectins: Properties and Biomedical Applications.* John Wiley & Sons, Chichester, West Sussex, England; 1998.
127. Wang W, Peumans WJ, Rougé P, Rossi C, Proost P, Chen J, Van Damme EJ. Leaves of the Lamiaceae species Glechoma hederacea (ground ivy) contain a lectin that is structurally and evolutionary related to the legume lectins. *Plant J.* 2003;33(2):293–304.
128. Park JY, Yuk HJ, Ryu HW, Lim SH, Kim KS, Park KH, Ryu YB, Lee WS. Evaluation of polyphenols from Broussonetia papyrifera as coronavirus protease inhibitors. *J Enzyme Inhib Med Chem.* 2017;32(1):504–515.
129. Cho JK, Curtis-Long MJ, Lee KH, Kim DW, Ryu HW, Yuk HJ, Park KH. Geranylated flavonoids displaying SARS-CoV papain-like protease inhibition from the fruits of Paulownia tomentosa. *Bioorg Med Chem.* 2013;21(11):3051–3057. doi: 10.1016/j.bmc.2013.03.027. Epub 2013 March 29. Erratum in: *Bioorg Med Chem.* 2013;21(22):7229.
130. Wen CC, Kuo YH, Jan JT, Liang PH, Wang SY, Liu HG, Lee CK, Chang ST, Kuo CJ, Lee SS, Hou CC, Hsiao PW, Chien SC, Shyur LF, Yang NS. Specific plant terpenoids and lignoids possess potent antiviral activities against severe acute respiratory syndrome coronavirus. *J Med Chem.* 2007;50(17):4087–4095.
131. Chang FR, Yen CT, Ei-Shazly M, et al. Anti-human coronavirus (anti-HCoV) triterpenoids from the leaves of Euphorbia neriifolia. *Nat Prod Commun.* 2012;7(11):1415–1417.
132. Kim DW, Seo KH, Curtis-Long MJ, Oh KY, Oh JW, Cho JK, Lee KH, Park KH. Phenolic phytochemical displaying SARS-CoV papain-like protease inhibition from the seeds of Psoralea corylifolia. *J Enzyme Inhib Med Chem.* 2014;29(1):59–63.
133. Liu H, Ye F, Sun Q, Liang H, Li C, Li S, Lu R, Huang B, Tan W, Lai L. Scutellaria baicalensis extract and baicalein inhibit replication of SARS-CoV-2 and its 3C-like protease in vitro. *J Enzyme Inhib Med Chem.* 2021;36(1):497–503.
134. Yang CW, Lee YZ, Kang IJ, Barnard DL, Jan JT, Lin D, Huang CW, Yeh TK, Chao YS, Lee SJ. Identification of phenanthroindolizines and phenanthroquinolizidines as novel potent anti-coronaviral agents for porcine enteropathogenic coronavirus transmissible gastroenteritis virus and human severe acute respiratory syndrome coronavirus. *Antiviral Res.* 2010;88(2):160–168.
135. Kwon HJ, Ryu YB, Kim YM, Song N, Kim CY, Rho MC, Jeong JH, Cho KO, Lee WS, Park SJ. In vitro antiviral activity of phlorotannins isolated from Ecklonia cava against porcine epidemic diarrhea coronavirus infection and hemagglutination. *Bioorg Med Chem.* 2013;21(15):4706–4713.
136. Li SY, Chen C, Zhang HQ, Guo HY, Wang H, Wang L, Zhang X, Hua SN, Yu J, Xiao PG, Li RS, Tan X. Identification of natural compounds with antiviral activities against SARS-associated coronavirus. *Antiviral Res.* 2005;67(1):18–23.
137. Wu CY, Jan JT, Ma SH, Kuo CJ, Juan HF, Cheng YS, Hsu HH, Huang HC, Wu D, Brik A, Liang FS, Liu RS, Fang JM, Chen ST, Liang PH, Wong CH. Small molecules targeting severe acute respiratory syndrome human coronavirus. *Proc Natl Acad Sci U S A.* 2004;101(27):10012–10017.
138. Lin CW, Tsai FJ, Tsai CH, Lai CC, Wan L, Ho TY, Hsieh CC, Chao PD. Anti-SARS coronavirus 3C-like protease effects of Isatis indigotica root and plant-derived phenolic compounds. *Antiviral Res.* 2005;68(1):36–42.

139. Ryu YB, Jeong HJ, Kim JH, Kim YM, Park JY, Kim D, Nguyen TT, Park SJ, Chang JS, Park KH, Rho MC, Lee WS. Biflavonoids from Torreya nucifera displaying SARS-CoV 3CL(pro) inhibition. *Bioorg Med Chem.* 2010;18(22):7940–7947.
140. Shen L, Niu J, Wang C, Huang B, Wang W, Zhu N, Deng Y, Wang H, Ye F, Cen S, Tan W. High-throughput screening and identification of potent broad-spectrum inhibitors of coronaviruses. *J Virol.* 2019;93(12):e00023–19.
141. Chen CN, Lin CP, Huang KK, Chen WC, Hsieh HP, Liang PH, Hsu JT. Inhibition of SARS-CoV 3C-like protease activity by theaflavin-3,3′-digallate (TF3). *Evid Based Complement Alternat Med.* 2005;2(2):209–215.
142. Shen YC, Wang LT, Khalil AT, Chiang LC, Cheng PW. Bioactive pyranoxanthones from the roots of Calophyllum blancoi. *Chem Pharm Bull (Tokyo).* 2005;53(2):244–247.
143. Weng JR, Lin CS, Lai HC, Lin YP, Wang CY, Tsai YC, Wu KC, Huang SH, Lin CW. Antiviral activity of Sambucus FormosanaNakai ethanol extract and related phenolic acid constituents against human coronavirus NL63. *Virus Res.* 2019;273:197767.
144. Ryu YB, Park SJ, Kim YM, Lee JY, Seo WD, Chang JS, Park KH, Rho MC, Lee WS. SNM SARS-CoV 3CLpro inhibitory effects of quinone-methide triterpenes from Tripterygium regelii. *Bioorg Med Chem Lett.* 2010;20(6):1873–1876.
145. Kim DE, Min JS, Jang MS, Lee JY, Shin YS, Song JH, Kim HR, Kim S, Jin YH, Kwon S. Natural bis-benzylisoquinoline alkaloids-tetrandrine, fangchinoline, and cepharanthine, inhibit human coronavirus OC43 infection of MRC-5 human lung cells. *Biomolecules.* 2019;9(11):696.
146. Zhang CH, Wang YF, Liu XJ, Lu JH, Qian CW, Wan ZY, Yan XG, Zheng HY, Zhang MY, Xiong S, Li JX, Qi SY. Antiviral activity of cepharanthine against severe acute respiratory syndrome coronavirus in vitro. *Chin Med J (Engl).* 2005;118(6):493–496.
147. Ho TY, Wu SL, Chen JC, Li CC, Hsiang CY. Emodin blocks the SARS coronavirus spike protein and angiotensin-converting enzyme 2 interaction. *Antiviral Res.* 2007;74(2):92–101.
148. Chiow KH, Phoon MC, Putti T, Tan BK, Chow VT. Evaluation of antiviral activities of Houttuynia cordata Thunb extract, quercetin, quercetrin and cinanserin on murine coronavirus and dengue virus infection. *Asian Pac J Trop Med.* 2016;9(1):1–7.
149. Zhuang M, Jiang H, Suzuki Y, Li X, Xiao P, Tanaka T, Ling H, Yang B, Saitoh H, Zhang L, Qin C, Sugamura K, Hattori T. Procyanidins and butanol extract of Cinnamomi Cortex inhibit SARS-CoV infection. *Antiviral Res.* 2009;82(1):73–81.
150. Park JY, Kim JH, Kim YM, Jeong HJ, Kim DW, Park KH, Kwon HJ, Park SJ, Lee WS, Ryu YB. Tanshinones as selective and slow-binding inhibitors for SARS-CoV cysteine proteases. *Bioorg Med Chem.* 2012;20(19): 5928–5935.
151. Ghosh R, Chakraborty A, Biswas A, Chowdhuri S. Evaluation of green tea polyphenols as novel corona virus (SARS CoV-2) main protease (Mpro) inhibitors: An in silico docking and molecular dynamics simulation study. *J Biomol Struct Dyn.* 2020:1–13. https://pubmed.ncbi.nlm.nih.gov/32568613/
152. Michaelis M, Doerr HW, Cinatl J Jr. Investigation of the influence of EPs® 7630, a herbal drug preparation from Pelargonium sidoides, on replication of a broad panel of respiratory viruses. *Phytomedicine.* 2011;18(5): 384–386.
153. Wen CC, Shyur LF, Jan JT, Liang PH, Kuo CJ, Arulselvan P, Wu JB, Kuo SC, Yang NS. Traditional Chinese medicine herbal extracts of Cibotium barometz, Gentiana scabra, Dioscorea batatas, Cassia tora, and Taxillus chinensis inhibit SARS-CoV replication. *J Tradit Complement Med.* 2011;1(1):41–50.
154. Ulasli M, Gurses SA, Bayraktar R, Yumrutas O, Oztuzcu S, Igci M, Igci YZ, Cakmak EA, Arslan A. The effects of Nigella sativa (Ns), Anthemis hyalina (Ah) and Citrus sinensis (Cs) extracts on the replication of coronavirus and the expression of TRP genes family. *Mol Biol Rep.* 2014;41(3):1703–1711.
155. Fung KP, Leung PC, Tsui KW, Wan CC, Wong KB, Waye MY, Au WN, Wong CK, Lam WK, Lau BS. Immunomodulatory activities of the herbal formula Kwan Du Bu Fei Dang in healthy subjects: A randomised, double-blind, placebo-controlled study. *Hong Kong Med J.* 2011;17 Suppl 2:41–43.
156. Song YH, Kim DW, Curtis-Long MJ, Yuk HJ, Wang Y, Zhuang N, Lee KH, Jeon KS, Park KH. Papain-like protease (PLpro) inhibitory effects of cinnamic amides from Tribulus terrestris fruits. *Biol Pharm Bull.* 2014;37(6):1021–1028.
157. Hoever G, Baltina L, Michaelis M, Kondratenko R, Baltina L, Tolstikov GA, Doerr HW, Cinatl J Jr. Antiviral activity of glycyrrhizic acid derivatives against SARS-coronavirus. *J Med Chem.* 2005;48(4):1256–1259.
158. Cinatl J, Morgenstern B, Bauer G, Chandra P, Rabenau H, Doerr HW. Glycyrrhizin, an active component of liquorice roots, and replication of SARS-associated coronavirus. *Lancet.* 2003;361(9374):2045–2046.
159. Yi L, Li Z, Yuan K, Qu X, Chen J, Wang G, Zhang H, Luo H, Zhu L, Jiang P, Chen L, Shen Y, Luo M, Zuo G, Hu J, Duan D, Nie Y, Shi X, Wang W, Han Y, Li T, Liu Y, Ding M, Deng H, Xu X. Small molecules blocking the entry of severe acute respiratory syndrome coronavirus into host cells. *J Virol.* 2004;78(20):11334–11339.
160. O'Keefe BR, Giomarelli B, Barnard DL, Shenoy SR, Chan PK, McMahon JB, Palmer KE, Barnett BW, Meyerholz DK, Wohlford-Lenane CL, McCray PB Jr. Broad-spectrum in vitro activity and in vivo efficacy of the antiviral protein griffithsin against emerging viruses of the family Coronaviridae. *J Virol.* 2010;84(5):2511–2521.
161. Cao J, Forrest JC, Zhang X. A screen of the NIH clinical collection small molecule library identifies potential anti-coronavirus drugs. *Antiviral Res.* 2015;114:1–10.
162. Park JY, Jeong HJ, Kim JH, Kim YM, Park SJ, Kim D, Park KH, Lee WS, Ryu YB. Diarylheptanoids from Alnus japonica inhibit papain-like protease of severe acute respiratory syndrome coronavirus. *Biol Pharm Bull.* 2012;35(11):2036–2042.
163. Macintyre G, Curry B, Wong F, Anderson R. Hygromycin B therapy of a murine coronaviral hepatitis. *Antimicrob Agents Chemother.* 1991;35(10):2125–2127.
164. Kumar V, Jung YS, Liang PH. Anti-SARS coronavirus agents: A patent review (2008- present). *Expert Opin Ther Pat.* 2013;23(10):1337–1348.

165. Tsai YC, Lee CL, Yen HR, Chang YS, Lin YP, Huang SH, Lin CW. Antiviral action of tryptanthrin isolated from strobilanthes cusia leaf against human coronavirus NL63. *Biomolecules.* 2020;10(3):366.
166. Kang KB, Ming G, Kim GJ, Ha TK, Choi H, Oh WK, Sung SH. Jubanines F-J, Cyclopeptide alkaloids from the roots of Ziziphus jujuba. *Phytochemistry.* 2015;119:90–95.
167. Schwarz S, Sauter D, Wang K, Zhang R, Sun B, Karioti A, Bilia AR, Efferth T, Schwarz W. Kaempferol derivatives as antiviral drugs against the 3a channel protein of coronavirus. *Planta Med.* 2014;80(2–3):177–182.
168. Van Damme EJ, Hause B, Hu J, Barre A, Rougé P, Proost P, Peumans WJ. Two distinct jacalin-related lectins with a different specificity and subcellular location are major vegetative storage proteins in the bark of the black mulberry tree. *Plant Physiol.* 2002;130(2):757–769.
169. Donia M, Hamann MT. Marine natural products and their potential applications as anti-infective agents. *Lancet Infect Dis.* 2003;3(6):338–348.
170. Yu MS, Lee J, Lee JM, Kim Y, Chin YW, Jee JG, Keum YS, Jeong YJ. Identification of myricetin and scutellarein as novel chemical inhibitors of the SARS coronavirus helicase, nsP13. *Bioorg Med Chem Lett.* 2012;22(12):4049–4054.
171. Loizzo MR, Saab AM, Tundis R, Statti GA, Menichini F, Lampronti I, Gambari R, Cinatl J, Doerr HW. Phytochemical analysis and in vitro antiviral activities of the essential oils of seven Lebanon species. *Chem Biodivers.* 2008;5(3):461–470.
172. Chen Y, Peumans WJ, Hause B, Bras J, Kumar M, Proost P, Barre A, Rougé P, Van Damme EJ. Jasmonic acid methyl ester induces the synthesis of a cytoplasmic/nuclear chitooligosaccharide binding lectin in tobacco leaves. *FASEB J.* 2002;16(8):905–907.
173. Yang CW, Chang HY, Lee YZ, Hsu HY, Lee SJ. The cardenolide ouabain suppresses coronaviral replication via augmenting a Na+/K+-ATPase-dependent PI3K_PDK1 axis signaling. *Toxicol Appl Pharmacol.* 2018;356:90–97.
174. Luo W, Su X, Gong S, Qin Y, Liu W, Li J, Yu H, Xu Q. Anti-SARS coronavirus 3C-like protease effects of *Rheum palmatum L.* extracts. *Biosci Trends.* 2009;3(4):124–126.
175. Cheng PW, Ng LT, Chiang LC, Lin CC. Antiviral effects of saikosaponins on human coronavirus 229E in vitro. *Clin Exp Pharmacol Physiol.* 2006;33(7):612–616.
176. Yang JL, Ha TK, Dhodary B, Pyo E, Nguyen NH, Cho H, Kim E, Oh WK. Oleanane triterpenes from the flowers of Camellia japonica inhibit porcine epidemic diarrhea virus (PEDV) replication. *J Med Chem.* 2015;58(3): 1268–1280.
177. Müller C, Schulte FW, Lange-Grünweller K, Obermann W, Madhugiri R, Pleschka S, Ziebuhr J, Hartmann RK, Grünweller A. Broad-spectrum antiviral activity of the eIF4A inhibitor silvestrol against corona- and picornaviruses. *Antiviral Res.* 2018;150:123–129.
178. Yang CW, Lee YZ, Hsu HY, Shih C, Chao YS, Chang HY, Lee SJ. Targeting coronaviral replication and cellular JAK2 mediated dominant NF-κB activation for comprehensive and ultimate inhibition of coronaviral activity. *Sci Rep.* 2017;7(1):4105.
179. Kumaki Y, Wandersee MK, Smith AJ, Zhou Y, Simmons G, Nelson NM, Bailey KW, Vest ZG, Li JK, Chan PK, Smee DF, Barnard DL. Inhibition of severe acute respiratory syndrome coronavirus replication in a lethal SARS-CoV BALB/c mouse model by stinging nettle lectin, Urtica dioica agglutinin. *Antiviral Res.* 2011;90(1):22–32.
180. Bhatia S, Sharma A, Vargas De La Cruz CB, Chaugule B, Ahmed Al-Harrasi. Nutraceutical, antioxidant, antimicrobial properties of pyropia vietnamensis (Tanaka et Pham-Hong Ho) J.E. Sutherl. et Monotilla. *Curr Bioact Compd.* 2020;16:1.
181. Bhatia S, Sardana S, Senwar KR, Dhillon A, Sharma A, Naved T. In vitro antioxidant and antinociceptive properties of Porphyra vietnamensis. *Biomedicine (Taipei).* 2019;9(1):3.
182. Bhatia S, Sharma K, Namdeo AG, Chaugule BB, Kavale M, Nanda S. Broad-spectrum sun-protective action of Porphyra-334 derived from Porphyra vietnamensis. *Pharmacognosy Res.* 2010;2(1):45–49.
183. Bhatia S, Sharma K, Sharma A, Nagpal K, Bera T. Anti-inflammatory, analgesic and antiulcer properties of Porphyra vietnamensis. *Avicenna J Phytomed.* 2015;5(1):69–77.
184. Bhatia S, Sardana S, Sharma A, Vargas De La Cruz CB, Chaugule B, Khodaie L. Development of broad spectrum mycosporine loaded sunscreen formulation from Ulva fasciata delile. *Biomedicine (Taipei).* 2019;9(3):17.
185. Bhatia S, Garg A, Sharma K, Kumar S, Sharma A, Purohit AP. Mycosporine and mycosporine-like amino acids: A paramount tool against ultra violet irradiation. *Pharmacogn Rev.* 2011;5(10):138–146.
186. Bhatia S, Namdeo AG, Nanda S. Factors effecting the gelling and emulsifying properties of a natural polymer. *SRP.* 2010;1(1):86–92.
187. Bhatia S, Sharma K, Bera T. Structural characterization and pharmaceutical properties of porphyran. *Asian J Pharm* 2015;9:93–101.
188. Bhatia S, Sharma A, Sharma K, Kavale M, Chaugule BB, Dhalwal K, Namdeo AG, Mahadik KR. Novel algal polysaccharides from marine source: Porphyran. *Pharmacognosy Review* 2008;4;271–276.
189. Bhatia S, Sharma K, Nagpal K, Bera T. Investigation of the factors influencing the molecular weight of porphyran and its associated antifungal activity Bioact. *Carb Diet Fiber* 2015;5:153–168.
190. Bhatia S, Kumar V, Sharma K, Nagpal K, Bera T. Significance of algal polymer in designing amphotericin B nanoparticles. *Sci World J.* 2014;2014:564573.
191. Bhatia S, Rathee P, Sharma K, Chaugule BB, Kar N, Bera T. Immuno-modulation effect of sulphated polysaccharide (porphyran) from Porphyra vietnamensis. *Int J Biol Macromol.* 2013;57:50–56.
192. Bhatia S. *Natural Polymer Drug Delivery Systems: Marine Polysaccharides Based Nano-Materials and Its Applications.* Springer International Publishing, Switzerland; 2016:185–225.
193. Bhatia S. *Natural Polymer Drug Delivery Systems: Plant Derived Polymers, Properties, and Modification & Applications.* Springer International Publishing, Switzerland; 2016:119–184.
194. Bhatia S. *Natural Polymer Drug Delivery Systems: Nanotechnology and Its Drug Delivery Applications.* Springer International Publishing, Switzerland; 2016:1–32.
195. Bhatia S. *Natural Polymer Drug Delivery Systems: Nanoparticles Types, Classification, Characterization, Fabrication Methods and Drug Delivery Applications.* Springer International Publishing, Switzerland; 2016:33–93.

196. Bhatia S. *Natural Polymer Drug Delivery Systems: Natural Polymers vs Synthetic Polymer.* Springer International Publishing, Switzerland; 2016:95–118.
197. Bhatia S. *Systems for Drug Delivery: Mammalian Polysaccharides and Its Nanomaterials.* Springer International Publishing, Switzerland; 2016:1–27.
198. Bhatia S. *Systems for Drug Delivery: Microbial Polysaccharides as Advance Nanomaterials.* Springer International Publishing, Switzerland; 2016:29–54.
199. Bhatia S. *Systems for Drug Delivery: Chitosan Based Nanomaterials and Its Applications.*Springer International Publishing, Switzerland; 2016:55–117.
200. Bhatia S. *Systems for Drug Delivery: Advance Polymers and Its Applications.* Springer International Publishing, Switzerland; 2016:119–146.
201. Bhatia S. *Systems for Drug Delivery: Advanced Application of Natural Polysaccharides.* Springer International Publishing, Switzerland; 2016;147–170.
202. Bhatia S. *Systems for Drug Delivery: Modern Polysaccharides and Its Current Advancements.* Springer International Publishing, Switzerland; 2016:171–188.
203. Bhatia S. *Systems for Drug Delivery: Toxicity of Nanodrug Delivery Systems.* Springer International Publishing, Switzerland; 2016:189–197.
204. Bhatia S. *Nanotechnology in Drug Delivery Fundamentals, Design, and Applications: Part 1: Protein and Peptide-Based Drug Delivery Systems.* Apple Academic Press, Palm Bay, FL; 2016:50–204.
205. Bhatia S. *Nanotechnology in Drug Delivery Fundamentals, Design, and Applications: Part 2: Peptide-Mediated Nanoparticle Drug Delivery System.* Apple Academic Press, Palm Bay, FL; 2016:205–280.
206. Bhatia S. *Nanotechnology in Drug Delivery Fundamentals, Design, and Applications: Part 3: CPP and CTP in Drug Delivery and Cell Targeting.* Apple Academic Press, Palm Bay, FL; 2016:309–312.
207. Wibowo D, Jorritsma SHT, Gonzaga ZJ, Evert B, Chen S, Rehm BHA. Polymeric nanoparticle vaccines to combat emerging and pandemic threats. *Biomaterials.* 2021;268:120597.

6

Host Immune Response vs. COVID-19

Ahmed Al-Harrasi
Natural and Medical Sciences Research Center, University of Nizwa

Saurabh Bhatia
Natural and Medical Sciences Research Center, University of Nizwa
University of Petroleum and Energy Studies

Tapan Behl
Chitkara University

Deepak Kaushik
M.D. University

CONTENTS

6.1 Introduction

Severe acute respiratory syndrome coronavirus 2 (SARS-CoV-2) causes infection in the lung cells, specifically type 2 alveolar epithelial cells that are expressing angiotensin-converting enzyme 2 (ACE2). After invasion of SARS-CoV-2 these ACE2-expressing cells enroll dendritic cells, neutrophils, monocytes, and macrophages, resulting in the production of lymphocytes (CD4+ and CD8+ T cells) [1]. The activation of these cells results in the activation of the antiviral immune response. This lymphocyte-mediated activation of immune reaction causes the overall inhibition of viral replication or affects vial development in a restricted percentage of diseased patients. However, in some individuals inhibition of the virus is partial, due to which the proportion of circulating B and T lymphocytes are successively decreased via unidentified pathways [1]. Continued viral replication in some patients results in a severe condition known as a cytokine storm. Generally, therapeutics, mainly antiviral medication, must be used at the initial level of infection to avoid disease advancement; however, due to the unavailability of effective antiviral drugs to considerably inhibit viral replication in vivo and suppress the production of pro-inflammatory mediators, chances of disease advancement in severe cases are found to be high. Thus, it's important to understand the kinetics of the pathogenic virus and the immunopathology of coronavirus disease 2019 (COVID-19) [1].

6.2 Host Innate Non-Specific Response against Viral Infections

Host innate non-specific response against viral infections usually involves macrophages, neutrophils, and dendritic cells [2]. These cells always attempt to decrease further progression of the virus in terms of its replication and pathogenicity. This non-specific innate defense mechanism of the host is followed by an adaptive immune response where the host produces antibodies or immunoglobulins to neutralize specific antigen action present in the pathogen via antibody–antigen interaction. Another type of immune response against viruses can be achieved by cell-mediated immunity where the infected

DOI: 10.1201/9781003175933-7

site stimulates the production of T cells. Thus, these combined immune adaptive responses can eliminate the pathogen from the infected individual; however, when the immune response is weak, the virus can cause severe illness or re-infection.

6.3 Host Immune Response vs COVID-19 Infection

COVID-19 infection causes recruitment of more immune cells, mainly macrophages and monocytes, in response to the injury and infection caused by the SARS-CoV-2 in the lungs [2]. This immune response further leads to the production of pro-inflammatory mediators such as cytokines and also stimulates prime adaptive T- and B-cell immune responses [3]. In the majority of cases, the host immune response itself is capable enough to resolve the infection; however, any imbalance in immune response can lead to further progression of the disease in the form of acute respiratory distress syndrome (ARDS). Thus, from a treatment perspective, greater understanding of the structure of SARS-CoV-2 and its interaction with host cells is required to identify possible drug targets. SARS-CoV-2 is a type of cytopathic virus that causes structural modifications in host cells after its invasion [4]. These modifications in host cells can lead to cellular injury and death. In addition, infected tissues become a part of the virus replicative cycle. In COVID-19-positive patients, replication and expression of SARS-CoV-2 increase several fold, which can further increase virus-associated pyroptosis with considerable vascular leakage [5]. This type of response is also common among SARS-CoV patients.

6.4 COVID-19-Associated Hyper-inflammation

The hyper-inflammatory stage of programmed cell death (i.e., pyroptosis) further triggers inflammatory responses such as the production of high levels of IL-1β [6]. With the help of various pattern recognition receptors (i.e., proteins that are able to identify molecules often present in pathogenic organism), lung alveolar macrophages and epithelial cells identify distinct evolutionarily structures present over pathogens known as pathogen-associated molecular patterns (PAMPs) and cell-based molecules that can trigger immunity in response to cellular injury known as damage-associated molecular patterns (DAMPs) (Figure 3.7) [7]. Damaged tissues locally release inflammatory mediators such as pro-inflammatory cytokines and chemokines interleukin (IL)-6, interferon-gamma (IFN-γ), monocyte chemoattractant protein-1 (MCP-1), and 10kD interferon-gamma-induced protein (IP-10) in systemic circulation of COVID-19 patients [8]. High levels of pro-inflammatory cytokines and chemokines display polarized T-helper 1 (Th1) cell reaction, which is also found during SARS-CoV and Middle East respiratory syndrome (MERS)-CoV infections [9] (Figure 3.7). Secretion of high levels of cytokines and chemokines encourages the migration of monocytes and T lymphocytes from systemic circulation to the site of infection (infected lung tissue) [10]. This migration allows more enrolment of immune cells in the lungs from the systemic circulation and also lymphocytes infiltration at the site of infection, resulting in a high level of neutrophil–lymphocyte ratio, which is common among ~80% of COVID-19 patients. Among the majority of patients, this type of infiltration and migration of immune cells results in elimination of the infection. Immunity development against viral infection, especially SARS-CoV-2, involves various steps that usually take ~1–2 weeks. Nevertheless, in a number of COVID-19 patients, an imbalance or dysfunction in immune response can result in excess production of cytokines (called a cytokine storm), which can lead to the hyper-inflammatory stage of lungs. In most severe or critically ill COVID-19 patients, increased levels of interleukins such as IL-2, IL-7, and IL-10, granulocyte colony-stimulating factor (G-CSF), IP-10, macrophage inflammatory protein-1α (MIP-1α), and tumor necrosis factor (TNF) in blood plasma have been found [8] (Figure 3.7). Among all interleukins, IL-6 in COVID-19 patients in ICUs increases continuously and the IL-6 level in non-survivors is higher than that in survivors [11]. Some researchers have shown that the severity of COVID-19 is linked with a high level of inflammatory (FCN1+ and SPP1+) macrophages but a low level of FABP4+ alveolar macrophages in comparison with COVID-19 patients suffering from mild infection (Figure 3.7) [12]. Since these inflammatory macrophages (mainly FCN1+ macrophages) are responsible for the increase in the expression of interferon genes and multiple chemokines, they may be responsible for the hyper-inflammatory state seen in critically ill COVID-19 patients [12]. It was also reported that a low level of FABP4+ alveolar macrophages among controls and patients with mild COVID-19 could be responsible for the failure of lung function when disease progresses into the severe form [12]. Periodic examination of FCN1+ macrophages in severe patients is important, and is usually done by the bronchoalveolar lavage method [13] (Figure 3.7). This procedure is performed to examine the lower respiratory system by means of a bronchoscope that is passed via the mouth or nose into an appropriate airway to collect the fluid. It was also observed that severe patients in the ICU showed a considerable increase in the level of inflammatory CD14+ CD16+ blood monocytes. These inflammatory monocytes can further stimulate the production of inflammatory cytokines that are responsible for the violent cytokine storm (Figure 3.7). Based on reports, blood examination of severe COVID-19 patients showed high levels of IL-1β, IL-1RA, IL-7, IL-8, IL-9, IL-10, basic FGF2, G-CSF, granulocyte–macrophage colony-stimulating factor (GM-CSF), IFN-γ, IP-10, MCP-1, MIP-1α, MIP-1β, PDGFB, tumor necrosis factor-alpha (TNF-α), and VEGFA [14] (Figure 3.7). This type of hyper-inflammatory response can lead to ARDS and multiple organ failure and can also result in death in severe cases of SARS-CoV-2 infection. It's still not clear how SARS-CoV-2 undermines the host innate antiviral cytokine responses; however, various reports suggest that interferon responses are suppressed by structural as well as non-structural proteins of the virus. This suppression caused by proteins of SARS-CoV-2 involves various steps of the interferon signaling pathway. An imbalance in host immune response, mainly characterized by low production of type I interferons along with the exacerbated release of pro-inflammatory cytokines, can lead to the development of severe respiratory illness. SARS-CoV-2 proteins such as ORF6, ORF8, and N proteins suppress the expression of interferon, mainly IFN-β, by inhibiting RIG-I-like signaling pathways [15] (Figure 3.7). RIG-I-like receptors are pattern recognition receptors (PRRs), express in both immune and non-immune cells and regulate signaling pathways to promote expression of interferon (type I and type III) [16]. In addition, RIG-I-like receptors also promote NF-kappa B-dependent expression of pro-inflammatory cytokines. Inhibition of interferon expression takes place at different steps of its respective signaling pathways via averting pattern recognition receptors detection of viral genome [16]. Additionally, SARS-CoV-2 also adopts other strategies to inhibit interferon by averting the PRR signaling via TANK-binding kinase and I-kappa-B kinase epsilon [17] (Figure 3.7). This is performed by preventing the phosphorylation of interferon regulatory factor 3. Similarly, SARS-CoV-2 inhibits phosphorylation of STAT1 and promotes mRNA degradation and suppresses host protein translation [15]. Possibly SARS-CoV-2 proteins follow any of these pathways to inhibit interferon expression. SARS-CoV-2 protein-based suppression of interferon supports viral replication, which may lead to an increase in pyroptosis-based end products, which can ultimately trigger abnormal inflammatory responses [15]. Besides direct damage caused by viral infection, this uncontrolled infiltration of inflammatory cells can cause immense damage to the lung tissue via unnecessary release of proteases and reactive oxygen species (Figure 3.7). Collectively, these factors can cause alveolar injury by desquamation of alveolar epithelial cells, extensive pulmonary edema, fibrous tissue in alveolar spaces, and alveoli collapse, which may result in the increase of damaged cells in the alveolar sacs to form hyaline membrane [18]. Hyaline formation restricts gaseous exchange through the airways causing difficulty in breathing and subsequently decreasing blood oxygen levels. This pathological finding is defined as diffuse alveolar damage, which can be caused by both direct viral effects and immunopathogenetic factors [18]. This state results in the impairment of the phagocytic capacity of macrophages, which may render damaged lungs more vulnerable to secondary infections [19]. Moreover, the prevalence of the hyper-inflammatory state across the body due to cytokine storm increases cytokines including TNF, which may result in life-threatening organ dysfunction known as sepsis [20]. Due to this, many COVID-19 patients experience myocardial injury and peripheral circulatory collapse. Because of the dysfunctional immune response, elderly people and people with comorbidities are at higher risk. Aging has considerable implications over both lung function and architecture. Also, it has significant effects on the pulmonary surfactant, which can directly affect the lung microenvironment [21]. Alterations in the lung microenvironment can lead to a change in the maturation of dendritic cells and their relocation to the lymphoid organs, thus resulting in activation of malfunctioned T-cell. This occurs when dendritic cells, also called potent antigen-presenting cells (which are capable of activating T-cell responses), present viral antigens to native T cells [22] (Figure 3.7). To achieve this, dendritic cells have to migrate from the injured site to the neighboring lymph nodes by afferent lymphatic vessels that carry lymph to a lymph node. In contrast, based on recent reports, children do not develop severe disease in spite of having high viral titers, due to which >50% of kids faced slight symptoms or remain asymptomatic [23]. Thus, variable immune responses of different hosts against viral infection are not yet well understood. Even the relationship between virus persistence (viral titers), viral load, and disease outcome is not yet clear. Several reports suggested the peak of viral titers before the onset of symptoms; however, viral RNA was noticeable in non-survivors [24]. It was concluded that viral RNA possibly will remain even after active infection, which doesn't represent the infectivity of the virus. It was also speculated that the presence of a higher range of viral particles could be directly associated with a poor disease outcome [24]. Previous studies have also suggested SARS-CoV can also infect other organs besides lung cells, which can result in multiple-organ infection. As per earlier reports, virus particles of SARS and its respective genomic makeup have been identified in a substantial proportion among lymph cells as well as monocytes, and also found in lymphoid [25]. In addition, they were found in the mucosa of the intestine, the neurons of the brain, the epithelium of the renal distal tubules, epithelial cells of the respiratory tract, and macrophages in different organs. As per earlier reports, SARS virus can infect different cells, mainly immune cells, in quite a few organs, whereas pulmonary epithelium is considered as the main site of injury. Thus, immune cells, including monocyte-derived dendritic cells, macrophages, and lymphocytes, were found to be infected by the virus, whereas the continuous drop in lymphocytes (COVID-19-associated lymphopenia) could be linked with direct killing of lymph cells by SARS-CoV-2 [26]. Abnormal cytokine production in the form of acute reaction resulting from viral infection in immune cells causes enormous damage to the infected tissue. Moreover, the binding affinity and the mechanism adopted by SARS-CoV-2 to target different cells are still not clearly understood. Thus, immunomodulatory treatment can't be effective until the particular drivers of immune dysfunction are clearly known.

6.5 Immunomodulatory Therapy for COVID-19

Various immunosuppressants have recently been discovered to prevent immune-mediated injury caused by SARS-CoV-2 [27]. At present, clinical trials for determining the safety and efficacy of corticosteroids for the treatment of infection caused by SARS-CoV-2 are in progress. However, corticosteroids were not suggested during the outbreak caused by SARS-CoV-1 in 2003 [27]. Currently, clinical trials have been conducted determine the safety and efficacy of IL-6 antagonists (tocilizumab and sarilumab) [27]. In addition, clinical examinations are also underway to evaluate the potential of monoclonal antibodies targeting GM-CSF such as namilumab, lenzilumab, and gimsilumab [28]. Anti-cytokine treatment could be supportive to avert tissue injury. Anti-inflammatory drugs also have the potential to inhibit the organ injury; however, their use augments chances of concurrent infection. Moreover, the role of adjunctive treatments such as CytoSorb® (CytoSorbents Corporation, USA), which is a blood sorbent medical device for extracorporeal cytokine removal in COVID-19, was also studied [29]. This device acts by absorbing diverse cytokines (DAMPs and PAMPs) so as to diminish their levels and prevent cytokine-induced damage to tissue [29]. The anti-cancer drug thalidomide was also tested for its potential to decrease lung injury.

6.6 Anti-TNF Treatment and Other Approaches to Treat COVID-19

Anti-TNF treatment to treat patients suffering from COVID-19 could be a reliable strategy [30]. Recently, an argument related to the potential of TNF inhibitors in acute COVID-19 patients was published in an article authored by Markus F. Neurath [31]. In particular, TNF may worsen lymphopenia via modulating TNF/TNFR1 signaling among T-lymphocytes. TNFR1 as well as TNFR2 are two different membrane proteins that act as the binding sites on target cells [32]. TNFR1 is expressed on nearly every cell type, while TNFR2 is limited to immune cells and a number of tumor cells. As T-cell killing appears as the key target for immunomodulatory interventions, anti-TNF approaches could be a remarkable choice in acute COVID-19. This is supported by information collected from inflammatory bowel disease (IBD) patients who underwent anti-TNF treatment. As reported, in contrast to various anti-inflammatory drug candidates available, the safety data obtained from anti-TNF therapy seem to be more significant and effective. Recently, anti-TNF therapy based on infliximab, a monoclonal antibody, was tested among patients with severe COVID-19, and promising results were obtained initially [33]. Additionally, hydroxychloroquine with azithromycin was tested in a small open-label, non-randomized studies, and the results showed that this combination could be helpful in the treatment of severe COVID-19 patients [34]. The immunomodulatory, anti-inflammatory, and SARS-CoV-2 inhibition potential of hydroxychloroquine was already reported; however, its mechanism of action against COVID-19 has yet to be determined [34]. This section gives a detailed account of immune dysregulation or abnormalities and new cytokine networks contributing to the pathophysiology of COVID-19 patients.

6.7 SARS-CoV-2-Specific T-Cell Immunity

Blood examination of COVID-19 patients ~1 week after the onset of COVID-19 symptoms revealed active responses of B and T cells against SARS-CoV-2. CD8+ T cells, which are responsible for direct attacking and killing of virus-infected cells, showed a continuous drop in number, especially in severe cases. Moreover, SARS-CoV-2 infection was linked with a considerable drop in the activation of T-cell, mediated via CD expression [CD (25, 28,69)] over CD4+ and CD8+ T lymphocytes subsets [35]. Thus, it's important to understand the overall mechanism and factors that contribute to lymphopenia. This understanding might be helpful in developing a novel treatment against COVID-19. Based on the previous reports, various factors are speculated to contribute to the root causes of lymphopenia in COVID-19 patients:

- COVID-19 infection can cause immense damage to central lymphoid organs such as bone marrow (for B cells) and thymus (for T cells), resulting in abnormal function of these organs.
- Lymphocytes are trapped in infected tissues.
- Massive production of inflammatory cytokines can result in lymphocyte apoptosis.
- Direct infection caused by SARS-CoV-1 to lymphocytes leads to lymphocyte death [36].

However, more understanding is required to prove these hypotheses. In some SARS cases, loss of lymphocytes (CD8+ T as well memory CD4+ T cells) was temporary. This transient loss was regained in two to twelve months following illness; however, other CD4+ T-cell subsets remained lower in comparison with healthy controls [37]. Alternatively, a decrease in CD4+ T cells among SARS-infected individuals resulted in decreased neutralizing antibodies as well as Th1 cytokine production and caused low enrollment of monocytes in the lung tissue. CD4+ T lymphocytes are required to activate both CD8+ T as well as B lymphocytes. As discussed above, these lymphocytes are also responsible for production of cytokines to recruit immune cells at the site of infection. A post-mortem examination of COVID-19 patients suggested an increase in monocytes as well as T lymphocytes in the pulmonary tissue, along with a drop in hyperactive T lymphocytes in the peripheral systemic circulation [38]. Thus, a report based on lymphopenia and a drop in T-cell levels in systemic circulation among non-survivors suggested that T lymphocytes are migrated from the systemic circulation to the site of infection to control the viral infection [38]. Greater T-cell exhaustion among COVID-19 patients can be responsible for severity among COVID-19 patients. In spite of weak immune response, SARS-CoV infected individuals developed SARS-CoV-2s-specific memory T lymphocytes, which were present until 2 years after recovery [38]. It was also observed that coronavirus disease showed T helper type 1 cells effects primarily mediated by SARS-CoV-specific CD4+ T lymphocytes that further showed expression IFN-γ, TNF, and IL-2 (i.e., cell-based immunity was used to control the infection) [39]. It was also speculated that depletion of CD4+ T cells reduces the clearance of virus particles from SARS patients, which may further aggravate inflammation of lungs. Thus, a decrease in CD4+ T cells can indirectly aggravate immunopathogenesis [39].

It's well known that coronavirus causes a highly lethal emerging disease, namely SARS. For the effective treatment of this lethal disease, preclinical trials on animal models are essential to determining the safety and efficacy of new antiviral drug candidates. Thus, for the initial screening of antiviral drugs, novel lethal animal models for SARS are required. Recently, a new rodent-designed strain from SARS-CoV, Urbani, for assessing antiviral therapeutics was reported. In this study, a novel SARS-CoV strain (strain v2163) has been found to be more dangerous, as it showed nine mutants [40]. This novel strain (v2163) elevated IL (-1α,-6), IL-6, macrophage inflammatory protein-1 α, monocyte chemoattractant protein-1, and RANTES in rodents and increases IL-6 expression [40]. This developed model showed almost the same physiological response; nevertheless, it lacked alveolar hyaline membrane formation [40]. As per an earlier report, using this novel model, mice were immunized with SARS-CoV peptides containing dendritic cells, resulting in an increase in virus-specific CD4+ and CD8+ T cells [40]. This accumulation of virus stimulated T cells (CD4+ and CD8+) increased in the pulmonary tissue, which ultimately enhanced survival. Improved immunity against a rodent-designed strain (SARS-CoV) was reported when SARS-CoV-stimulated CD4+ and CD8+ T cells were transferred to immune-deficient rodent [40].

Apart from the reports available on the significance of T cells in the treatment of infection, several vaccine candidates against SARS-CoV were developed earlier in animal models that demonstrated signs of immunopathology linked with TH2 cell-mediated eosinophil infiltration. Particularly, immunization of aged mice appeared to exhibit augmented immunopathology rather than protection. Thus, it's important to understand the protective and detrimental effects of T-cells in order to determine the most favorable T-lymphocytes action approaches for vaccine development. Coronavirus-specific T-cells can be considered as an effective approach to clearing the virus to further control disease progression and must be considered in vaccine strategies.

6.8 B-Cell Immunity against COVID-19

B lymphocytes acts simultaneously with T follicular helper cells among COVID-19 patients. This response of B-cell initiates after onset of symptoms. B lymphocytes activity has been found to increase initially against the nucleocapsid protein of virus in the samples of SARS-CoV infected individuals. During the 4 to 8 days after inception of symptoms activity of antibody against S protein increased [41]. Usually, during the second or third week neutralizing action of antibody against surface protein developed [42]. It was also found that peak concentration of SARS-CoV-2 particles than SARS-CoV, at initial phase was more. Also, SARS-CoV-2 individuals have not developed lifelong antibodies against virus particles [43]. It has not been revealed whether these patients are vulnerable against reinfection or not [44]. Convalescent-based plasma treatments earlier used against SARS received considerable attention for their effectiveness against SARS-CoV-2 [45]. However, apart from their neutralizing effects deep understanding related to the mechanism of action of these antibodies has not been established.

The neutralization capability of these antibodies is seen by its high binding affinity against binding receptor-binding domain (RBD), which contain 193 amino acids from 318 to 510, over the surface protein of SARS-CoV. These surface proteins have been reported for their binding to human ACE2 protein. As was reported, only limited monoclonal antibodies have been identified against SARS-CoV. Out of these few antibodies have shown binding affinity against SARS-CoV-2 [46]. This is mainly because of the variation in the RBDs of both viruses. More specifically, the surface protein of SARS-CoV, which contains 33 amino acids (from 460 to 492), shows high affinity against ACE2 [47], out of which only some (15/33) are conserved in SARS-CoV-2. It has also been found that rodent anti-serum used to neutralize SARS-CoV protein can cross-neutralize the SARS-CoV-2 pseudovirus, suggesting corresponding neutralizing epitopes among these viral strains [48]. Convalescent plasma was used in China as potential therapeutics for the treatment of SARS-Cov-2 infection, and it was found that this treatment showed positive results in terms of respiratory viral load and mortality [49].

Various research studies using the following strategies are going on to discover safe and effective monoclonal antibodies against SARS-CoV-2: using approaches including [50]:

- phage-display immune libraries
- traditional mouse model for antibodies production immunization
- isolation of monoclonal hybridoma
- B lymphocyte sequence cloning

As is known from previous research, SARS-CoV perhaps lacks a potential mechanistic approach to avoiding or inhibiting the neutralizing effect of antibodies such as glycan shield of the RBD (proximal glycosylation sites). This was confirmed by the evidence that SARS-CoV-infected individuals usually have a tendency to produce neutralizing antibodies. In comparison to other S recombinant fragments, maximum immunogenicity has been shown by a fragment of recombinant surface protein of SARS-CoV comprising the RBD region. This indicates that immune cells can efficiently target the neutralizing epitopes [51]. It was also revealed that changes in surface protein can lead to the development of SARS-CoV-2-resistant strains against

monoclonal antibodies, which can ultimately affect its pattern of transmission and mutation. Its also known that, till yet the complete RBD remain conserved, except four identified unique non-synonymous variations in the surface protein: V483A, L455I, F456V, and G476S135. The V483A variation pattern has been found to be similar to MERS-CoV (I529T). Similarly, G476S as well as F456V variation patterns were found to be similar as the variation shown by SARS-CoV (L443R and D463G)[52]. To avoid undesirable side effects or toxicity, development as well as selection of these therapeutics must be done carefully since previous antibodies against other coronaviruses can worsen SARS-CoV infections via stimulating antibody-dependent inflammatory pathways [53]. Previous reports have shown that SARS-CoV-infected animals those who developed neutralizing antibodies against surface protein can possibly enhance acute pulmonary injury via worsening inflammatory reactions [53].

Additionally, a connection between IgG level and progression of ARDS has been reported among 80% of patients. As per this report infected individuals who developed neutralizing antibodies at the early phase of infection presented more mortality than those who presented a peak level of antibody at a later phase of infection [54]. Likewise, patients infected with MERS showed the same pattern (i.e., high antibody titer value patients at early phase of infection presented more severity than others) [55], while one report also claimed that a pause in the development of antibody response could be linked to the progression of infection [56]. Inflammatory responses triggered by these antibodies generally via binding to viral protein (to form complex) in order to stimulate Fc receptors present on macrophages (alveolar) can trigger the production of pro-inflammatory mediators [57]. These complexes can further stimulate the complementary system resulting in the stimulation of undesirable inflammatory responses. Thus it's important to develop safe antibodies with the capability to neutralize virulence factors of the virus instead of stimulating inflammatory pathways associated with the production of pro-inflammatory mediators. Certain approaches such as glycosylation or any other possible alteration of Fc site in order to prevent its interaction with Fc receptors can be adopted [58].

6.9 Biotechnological Approaches for Treatment of COVID-19

6.9.1 Role of Animal Biotechnology

Modern biotechnology, especially DNA science, can be used to create potential vaccines against COVID-19. In an effort to understand the COVID-19 virus more deeply, genetic engineering can also be utilized to create a virus that is non-replicating. This type of virus couldn't multiply by itself inside a human cell, as it requires essential components for replication that are not present in the human body [59–73].

Several reports have shown that stem cell therapy can also be utilized to treat COVID-19. Various scientists have reported the active role of stem cells in treating ARDS during the cytokine storm. This is mainly due to the immunomodulatory role of mesenchymal stromal cells [59–73]. A previous report from China also showed that Umbilical Cord Mesenchymal Stem Cells can also be utilized to treat elderly COVID-19 patients on ventilation. Currently, various researchers are focusing on developing a way to stimulate host-specific resident stem cells in order to resolve site-specific ARDS [59–73].

Additionally, nucleic acid-based therapy can also be utilized to modulate the extent of genetic expression in investigated cells mainly to restore genetic stability via upregulation of protective genes and downregulation or inactivation of defective or damaged genes. So far, various nucleic acid-mediated therapies have been proposed, out of which some showed satisfactory results against pulmonary diseases [59–73]. RNA-based therapies such as siRNA (small interfering RNA), RNAi (RNA interference), and RNA aptamers, ribozymes, and antisense oligonucleotides (ASOs) have shown more promising results in neutralizing antigenic proteins present in virus such as virus-like specific mRNA molecules, viral proteins such as E (envelope), M (membrane), or N (nucleocapsid), or SARS helicase. Earlier reports showed that these RNA-based therapies had promising results in the treatment of SARS-CoV [59–73].

Various researchers are also seeking an animal model that closely resembles the clinical manifestation of SARS-CoV-2. Transgenic approaches to developing or creating a genetically engineered animal model could be the most reliable approaches considered so far. One of the most reliable transgenic animal models used for COVID-19 studies is the K18-hACE2 transgenic mouse model [59–73].

Additionally, the role of enzymes such as proteolytic enzymes in COVID-19 infection has also been reported. Various proteolytic enzymes of either host or virus regulate viral replication and assembly, which could be considered as promising targets for the development of antiviral strategies for SARS-CoV-2 [59–73].

The complex genetic characteristics of SARS-CoV-2 have imposed various challenges in discovering potential drug/vaccine candidates. In the meantime, the knowledge of bioinformatics in viral research can be used to interpret viral genomics architecture [59–73]. A number of major in silico investigations such as computer-aided drug design, genome-wide association studies, and next-generation sequencing were successfully used in SARS-CoV-2 infection associated research Currently, the application of computational-based investigations over SARS-CoV-2 mediated infection has not only revealed the SARS-CoV-2 genomic sequence but also accurately examined the genetic variations, errors in sequencing, putative drug candidates, and the evolutionary relationship of the COVID-19 virus genome and other components in a very short time period. This can help understand specific aspects related to the COVID-19 outbreak and also help vaccine development for SARS-CoV-2 [59–73].

Further, cell-based models are considered as an important for gaining knowledge regarding the biology of SARS-CoV-2 infection, growth patterns, and virus tropism at cellular and tissue levels. As human lung cells are the primary target of SARS-CoV-2, cell-based models such as Vero E6, Calu-3, and A549 cells can be utilized for isolating, growing, and screening inhibitors against SARS-CoV-2 [59–73]. However, Vero E6 cells express ACE2, an entry receptor of SARS-CoV-2, and they are an immortalized monkey kidney cell line and might not behave as human primary airway cells. Nonetheless, these models can provide better understanding of SARS-CoV-2 pathogenesis. In addition, cell cultures based on mucosal tissues such as the mouth, nasal, and alveolar epithelium, as well as primary cells or organoids, can also be used to study coronavirus-associated pathogenesis.-Organoid systems can also be an interesting model for assessing coronavirus infection and tropism, and for screening coronavirus inhibitors. As the human renal system has shown considerable expression of ACE2 and thus is vulnerable to being infected by SARS-CoV-2, recently human kidney organoids have been used as a model to screen SARS-CoV-2 inhibitors. More recently, 3D lung organoids presenting SCGB1A1+ club cells were considered as a new model for SARS-CoV-2 infection. Organoid-based models offer various advantages over immortalized cell lines as they closely mimic the in vivo makeup of the related vulnerable cell types. Additionally, organoids can also be utilized to distinguish SARS-CoV-2-permissive cell types [59–73].

6.9.2 Role of Plant Biotechnology

To offer a wide range of therapeutics in the form of novel proteins, vaccines, and anti-viral agents against various pathogenic viral strains including SARS-CoV-2 and their transient expression in plants could be an outstanding approach [74–86]. Development of these proteins via transgenesis using plant systems is considered as a platform to produce a wide array of therapeutic proteins with antiviral properties that could be further used as modules of assays as well as kits [74–86]. Transient expression to produce proteins can allow clinical testing in less time, and large-scale production in a cost-effective manner can be done [74–86]. Plants such as tobacco, legumes, or cereal plants can be cultivated in numerous environmental conditions and thus therapeutics such as antigens, antibodies, or antivirals can be developed. Plant molecular-based farming includes a diversity of expression tools such as stable nuclear transformation (transgenic plants) or plastid transformation (transplastomic plants) to transient expression without stable transgene integration [74–86]. Considering the urgent requirement of therapeutic proteins for the development of safe and effective antiviral therapeutics for COVID-19 pandemic, transient expression of plant-based systems can offer the needed pace and scalability [74–86].

REFERENCES

1. Shimizu Y. Understanding the immunopathogenesis of COVID-19: Its implication for therapeutic strategy. *World J Clin Cases.* 2020;8(23):5835–5843.
2. Felsenstein S, Herbert JA, McNamara PS, Hedrich CM. COVID-19: Immunology and treatment options. *Clin Immunol.* 2020;215:108448.
3. Acharya D, Liu G, Gack MU. Dysregulation of type I interferon responses in COVID-19. *Nat Rev Immunol.* 2020;20(7):397–398.
4. Gorshkov K, Chen CZ, Bostwick R, Rasmussen L, Xu M, Pradhan M, Tran BN, Zhu W, Shamim K, Huang W, Hu X, Shen M, Klumpp-Thomas C, Itkin Z, Shinn P, Simeonov A, Michael S, Hall MD, Lo DC, Zheng W. The SARS-CoV-2 cytopathic effect is blocked with autophagy modulators. bioRxiv, 2020, Preprint.
5. Morris G, Bortolasci CC, Puri BK, Olive L, Marx W, O'Neil A, Athan E, Carvalho AF, Maes M, Walder K, Berk M. The pathophysiology of SARS-CoV-2: A suggested model and therapeutic approach. *Life Sci.* 2020;258:118166.
6. Li S, Zhang Y, Guan Z, Li H, Ye M, Chen X, Shen J, Zhou Y, Shi ZL, Zhou P, Peng K. SARS-CoV-2 triggers inflammatory responses and cell death through caspase-8 activation. *Signal Transduct Target Ther.* 2020;5(1):235.
7. Mogensen TH. Pathogen recognition and inflammatory signaling in innate immune defenses. *Clin Microbiol Rev.* 2009;22(2):240–273.
8. Costela-Ruiz VJ, Illescas-Montes R, Puerta-Puerta JM, Ruiz C, Melguizo-Rodríguez L. SARS-CoV-2 infection: The role of cytokines in COVID-19 disease. *Cytokine Growth Factor Rev.* 2020;54:62–75.
9. Coperchini F, Chiovato L, Croce L, Magri F, Rotondi M. The cytokine storm in COVID-19: An overview of the involvement of the chemokine/chemokine-receptor system. *Cytokine Growth Factor Rev.* 2020;53:25–32.
10. Sokol CL, Luster AD. The chemokine system in innate immunity. *Cold Spring Harb Perspect Biol.* 2015;7(5):a016303.
11. Gorham J, Moreau A, Corazza F, Peluso L, Ponthieux F, Talamonti M, Izzi A, Nagant C, Ndieugnou Djangang N, Garufi A, Creteur J, Taccone FS. Interleukine-6 in critically ill COVID-19 patients: A retrospective analysis. *PLoS One.* 2020;15(12):e0244628.
12. Hajivalili M, Hosseini M, Haji-Fatahaliha M. Gaining insights on immune responses to the novel coronavirus, COVID-19 and therapeutic challenges. *Life Sci.* 2020;257:118058.
13. Zhang F, Mears JR, Shakib L, Beynor JI, Shanaj S, Korsunsky I, Nathan A, Donlin LT, Raychaudhuri S. IFN-γ and TNF-α drive a CXCL10+CCL2+macrophage phenotype expanded in severe COVID-19 and other diseases with tissue inflammation. bioRxiv. 2020 August 5, Preprint.
14. Nile SH, Nile A, Qiu J, Li L, Jia X, Kai G. COVID-19: Pathogenesis, cytokine storm and therapeutic potential of interferons. *Cytokine Growth Factor Rev.* 2020;53:66–70.
15. Xia H, Shi PY. Antagonism of type i interferon by severe acute respiratory syndrome coronavirus 2. *J Interferon Cytokine Res.* 2020;40(12):543–548.
16. Li G, Fan Y, Lai Y, Han T, Li Z, Zhou P, Pan P, Wang W, Hu D, Liu X, Zhang Q, Wu J. Coronavirus infections and immune responses. *J Med Virol.* 2020;92(4):424–432.
17. Kindler E, Thiel V, Weber F. Interaction of SARS and MERS coronaviruses with the antiviral interferon response. *Adv Virus Res.* 2016;96:219–243.
18. Matthay MA, Zemans RL. The acute respiratory distress syndrome: Pathogenesis and treatment. *Annu Rev Pathol.* 2011;6:147–163.
19. Meidaninikjeh S, Sabouni N, Marzouni HZ, Bengar S, Khalili A, Jafari R. Monocytes and macrophages in COVID-19: Friends and foes. *Life Sci.* 2021;269:119010.
20. Chaudhry H, Zhou J, Zhong Y, Ali MM, McGuire F, Nagarkatti PS, Nagarkatti M. Role of cytokines as a double-edged sword in sepsis. *In Vivo.* 2013;27(6):669–684.
21. Fara A, Mitrev Z, Rosalia RA, Assas BM. Cytokine storm and COVID-19: A chronicle of pro-inflammatory cytokines. *Open Biol.* 2020;10(9):200160.
22. Desch AN, Henson PM, Jakubzick CV. Pulmonary dendritic cell development and antigen acquisition. *Immunol Res.* 2013;55(1–3):178–186. doi: 10.1007/s12026-012-8359-6.
23. Zimmermann P, Curtis N. Coronavirus infections in children including COVID-19: An overview of the epidemiology, clinical features, diagnosis, treatment and prevention options in children. *Pediatr Infect Dis J.* 2020;39(5):355–368.
24. Tay MZ, Poh CM, Rénia L, MacAry PA, Ng LFP. The trinity of COVID-19: Immunity, inflammation and intervention. *Nat Rev Immunol.* 2020;20(6):363–374.
25. Gu J, Gong E, Zhang B, Zheng J, Gao Z, Zhong Y, Zou W, Zhan J, Wang S, Xie Z, Zhuang H, Wu B, Zhong H, Shao H, Fang W, Gao D, Pei F, Li X, He Z, Xu D, Shi X, Anderson VM, Leong AS. Multiple organ infection and the pathogenesis of SARS. *J Exp Med.* 2005;202(3):415–424.
26. Fathi N, Rezaei N. Lymphopenia in COVID-19: Therapeutic opportunities. *Cell Biol Int.* 2020;44(9):1792–1797.
27. Florindo HF, Kleiner R, Vaskovich-Koubi D, Acúrcio RC, Carreira B, Yeini E, Tiram G, Liubomirski Y, Satchi-Fainaro R. Immune-mediated approaches against COVID-19. *Nat Nanotechnol.* 2020;15(8):630–645. doi: 10.1038/s41565-020-0732-3.
28. Berthelot JM, Lioté F, Maugars Y, Sibilia J. Lymphocyte changes in severe COVID-19: Delayed over-activation of STING? *Front Immunol.* 2020;11:607069.
29. Safari S, Salimi A, Zali A, Jahangirifard A, Bastanhagh E, Aminnejad R, Dabbagh A, Lotfi AH, Saeidi M. Extracorporeal hemoperfusion as a potential therapeutic option for severe COVID-19 patients; a narrative review. *Arch Acad Emerg Med.* 2020;8(1):e67.

30. Khalil A, Kamar A, Nemer G. Thalidomide-revisited: Are COVID-19 patients going to be the latest victims of yet another theoretical drug-repurposing? *Front Immunol.* 2020;11:1248.
31. Neurath MF. COVID-19 and immunomodulation in IBD. *Gut.* 2020;69(7):1335–1342.
32. Wajant H, Siegmund D. TNFR1 and TNFR2 in the control of the life and death balance of macrophages. *Front Cell Dev Biol.* 2019;7:91.
33. Robinson PC, Liew DFL, Liew JW, Monaco C, Richards D, Shivakumar S, Tanner HL, Feldmann M. The potential for repurposing anti-TNF as a therapy for the treatment of COVID-19. *Med (N Y).* 2020;1(1):90–102.
34. Gautret P, Lagier JC, Parola P, Hoang VT, Meddeb L, Mailhe M, Doudier B, Courjon J, Giordanengo V, Vieira VE, Tissot Dupont H, Honoré S, Colson P, Chabrière E, La Scola B, Rolain JM, Brouqui P, Raoult D. Hydroxychloroquine and azithromycin as a treatment of COVID-19: Results of an open-label non-randomized clinical trial. *Int J Antimicrob Agents.* 2020;56(1):105949.
35. Neidleman J, Luo X, Frouard J, Xie G, Gill G, Stein ES, McGregor M, Ma T, George AF, Kosters A, Greene WC, Vasquez J, Ghosn E, Lee S, Roan NR. SARS-CoV-2-specific T cells exhibit phenotypic features of helper function, lack of terminal differentiation, and high proliferation potential. *Cell Rep Med.* 2020;1(6):100081.
36. Wang, A. Muneer, L. Xie, F. Zhang, B. Wu, L. Mei, E.M. Lenarcic, E.H. Feng, J. Song, Y. Xiong, Novel gene-specific translation mechanism of dysregulated, chronic inflammation reveals promising, multifaceted COVID-19 therapeutics. bioRxiv, 2020.
37. Yip CYC, Yap ES, De Mel S, Teo WZY, Lee CT, Kan S, Lee MCC, Loh WNH, Lim EL, Lee SY. Temporal changes in immune blood cell parameters in COVID-19 infection and recovery from severe infection. *Br J Haematol.* 2020;190(1):33–36.
38. Carsana L, Sonzogni A, Nasr A, Rossi RS, Pellegrinelli A, Zerbi P, Rech R, Colombo R, Antinori S, Corbellino M, Galli M, Catena E, Tosoni A, Gianatti A, Nebuloni M. Pulmonary post-mortem findings in a series of COVID-19 cases from northern Italy: A two-centre descriptive study. *Lancet Infect Dis.* 2020;20(10):1135–1140.
39. Zhang YY, Li BR, Ning BT. The comparative immunological characteristics of SARS-CoV, MERS-CoV, and SARS-CoV-2 coronavirus infections. *Front Immunol.* 2020;11:2033.
40. Day CW, Baric R, Cai SX, Frieman M, Kumaki Y, Morrey JD, Smee DF, Barnard DL. A new mouse-adapted strain of SARS-CoV as a lethal model for evaluating antiviral agents in vitro and in vivo. *Virology.* 2009;395(2):210–222.
41. Tan YJ, Goh PY, Fielding BC, Shen S, Chou CF, Fu JL, Leong HN, Leo YS, Ooi EE, Ling AE, Lim SG, Hong W. Profiles of antibody responses against severe acute respiratory syndrome coronavirus recombinant proteins and their potential use as diagnostic markers. *Clin Diagn Lab Immunol.* 2004;11(2):362–371.
42. Nie Y, Wang G, Shi X, Zhang H, Qiu Y, He Z, Wang W, Lian G, Yin X, Du L, Ren L, Wang J, He X, Li T, Deng H, Ding M. Neutralizing antibodies in patients with severe acute respiratory syndrome-associated coronavirus infection. *J Infect Dis.* 2004;190(6):1119–1126.
43. CGTN. Expert: Recovered coronavirus patients are still prone to reinfection. 2020. YouTube https://www.youtube.com/watch?v=GZ99J7mlaIQ.
44. The Straits Times. Japanese woman reinfected with coronavirus weeks after initial recovery. *The Straits Times*, 2020. https://www.straitstimes.com/asia/east-asia/japanese-woman-reinfected-with-coronavirus-weeks-after-initial-recovery.
45. Xinhua. China puts 245 COVID-19 patients on convalescent plasma therapy. Xinhuanet, 2020. http://www.xinhuanet.com/english/2020-02/28/c_138828177.htm.
46. Wang C, Li W, Drabek D., et al. A human monoclonal antibody blocking SARS-CoV-2 infection. bioRxiv, 2020, Preprint. doi: 10.1101/2020.03.11.987958.
47. Li F, Li W, Farzan M, Harrison SC. Structure of SARS coronavirus spike receptor-binding domain complexed with receptor. *Science.* 2005;309(5742):1864–1868.
48. Tai W, He L, Zhang X, et al. Characterization of the receptor-binding domain (RBD) of 2019 novel coronavirus: Implication for development of RBD protein as a viral attachment inhibitor and vaccine. *Cell Mol Immunol.* 2020. doi: 10.1038/s41423-020-0400-4.
49. Li XY, Du B, Wang, YS, et al. The keypoints in treatment of the critical coronavirus disease 2019 patient. *Chin J Tuberculosis Respir Dis.* 2020;43:E026.
50. Johnson RF, Bagci U, Keith L, Tang X, Mollura DJ, Zeitlin L, Qin J, Huzella L, Bartos CJ, Bohorova N, Bohorov O, Goodman C, Kim DH, Paulty MH, Velasco J, Whaley KJ, Johnson JC, Pettitt J, Ork BL, Solomon J, Oberlander N, Zhu Q, Sun J, Holbrook MR, Olinger GG, Baric RS, Hensley LE, Jahrling PB, Marasco WA. 3B11-N, a monoclonal antibody against MERS-CoV, reduces lung pathology in rhesus monkeys following intratracheal inoculation of MERS-CoV Jordan-n3/2012. *Virology.* 2016;490:49–58.
51. Qiu M, Shi Y, Guo Z, Chen Z, He R, Chen R, Zhou D, Dai E, Wang X, Si B, Song Y, Li J, Yang L, Wang J, Wang H, Pang X, Zhai J, Du Z, Liu Y, Zhang Y, Li L, Wang J, Sun B, Yang R. Antibody responses to individual proteins of SARS coronavirus and their neutralization activities. *Microbes Infect.* 2005;7(5–6):882–889.
52. Rockx B, Donaldson E, Frieman M, Sheahan T, Corti D, Lanzavecchia A, Baric RS. Escape from human monoclonal antibody neutralization affects in vitro and in vivo fitness of severe acute respiratory syndrome coronavirus. *J Infect Dis.* 2010;201(6):946–955.
53. Tetro JA. Is COVID-19 receiving ADE from other coronaviruses? *Microbes Infect.* 2020;22(2):72–73.
54. Zhang L, Zhang F, Yu W, He T, Yu J, Yi CE, Ba L, Li W, Farzan M, Chen Z, Yuen KY, Ho D. Antibody responses against SARS coronavirus are correlated with disease outcome of infected individuals. *J Med Virol.* 2006;78(1):1–8.
55. Drosten C, Meyer B, Müller MA, Corman VM, Al-Masri M, Hossain R, Madani H, Sieberg A, Bosch BJ, Lattwein E, Alhakeem RF, Assiri AM, Hajomar W, Albarrak AM, Al-Tawfiq JA, Zumla AI, Memish ZA. Transmission of MERS-coronavirus in household contacts. *N Engl J Med.* 2014;371(9):828–835.
56. Park WB, Perera RA, Choe PG, Lau EH, Choi SJ, Chun JY, Oh HS, Song KH, Bang JH, Kim ES, Kim HB, Park SW, Kim NJ, Man Poon LL, Peiris M, Oh MD. Kinetics of serologic responses to MERS coronavirus infection in humans, South Korea. *Emerg Infect Dis.* 2015;21(12):2186–2189.

57. Nimmerjahn F, Ravetch JV. Fcgamma receptors as regulators of immune responses. *Nat Rev Immunol.* 2008;8(1):34–47.
58. Kaneko Y, Nimmerjahn F, Ravetch JV. Anti-inflammatory activity of immunoglobulin G resulting from Fc sialylation. *Science.* 2006;313(5787):670–673.
59. Bhatia S. Modern DNA science and its applications. In: *Introduction to Pharmaceutical Biotechnology, Volume 1 Basic Techniques and Concepts.* IOP Publishing Ltd, Bristol, UK; 2018;1:1–70.
60. Bhatia S. Introduction to genetic engineering. In: *Introduction to Pharmaceutical Biotechnology, Volume 1 Basic Techniques and Concepts.* IOP Publishing Ltd, Bristol, UK; 2018;3: 1–63.
61. Bhatia S. Applications of stem cells in disease and gene therapy. In: *Introduction to Pharmaceutical Biotechnology, Volume 1 Basic Techniques and Concepts.* IOP Publishing Ltd, Bristol, UK; 2018;1:1–40.
62. Bhatia S. Transgenic animals in biotechnology. In: *Introduction to Pharmaceutical Biotechnology, Volume 1 Basic Techniques and Concepts.* IOP Publishing Ltd, Bristol, UK; 2018;1:1–67.
63. Bhatia S. Industrial enzymes and their applications. In: *Introduction to Pharmaceutical Biotechnology, Enzymes, Proteins and Bioinformatics.* IOP Publishing Ltd, Bristol, UK; 2018;2:1–21.
64. Bhatia S. Introduction to enzymes and their applications. In: *Introduction to Pharmaceutical Biotechnology, Enzymes, Proteins and Bioinformatics.* IOP Publishing Ltd, Bristol, UK; 2018:2;1–29.
65. Bhatia S. Biotransformation and enzymes. In: *Introduction to Pharmaceutical Biotechnology, Enzymes, Proteins and Bioinformatics.* IOP Publishing Ltd, Bristol, UK; 2018;2:1–13.
66. Bhatia S. Bioinformatics. In: *Introduction to Pharmaceutical Biotechnology, Enzymes, Proteins and Bioinformatics.* IOP Publishing Ltd, Bristol, UK; 2018;2:1–16.
67. Bhatia S. Protein and enzyme engineering. In: *Introduction to Pharmaceutical Biotechnology, Enzymes, Proteins and Bioinformatics.* IOP Publishing Ltd, Bristol, UK; 2018;2:1–15.
68. Bhatia S. Introduction to genomics. In: *Introduction to Pharmaceutical Biotechnology, Enzymes, Proteins and Bioinformatics.* IOP Publishing Ltd, Bristol, UK; 2018;3:1–39.
69. Bhatia S. Characterization of cultured cells. In: *Introduction to Pharmaceutical Biotechnology: Animal Tissue Culture and Biopharmaceuticals.* IOP Publishing Ltd, Bristol, UK; 2019;3:1–47.
70. Bhatia S. Animal tissue culture facilities. In: *Introduction to Pharmaceutical Biotechnology: Animal Tissue Culture and Biopharmaceuticals.* IOP Publishing Ltd, Bristol, UK; 2019;3:1–32.
71. Bhatia S. Culture media for animal cells. In: *Introduction to Pharmaceutical Biotechnology: Animal Tissue Culture and Biopharmaceuticals.* IOP Publishing Ltd, Bristol, UK; 2019;3:1–33.
72. Bhatia S. Stem cell culture. In: *Introduction to Pharmaceutical Biotechnology: Animal Tissue Culture and Biopharmaceuticals.* IOP Publishing Ltd, Bristol, UK; 2019;3:1–24.
73. Bhatia S. Organ culture. In: *Introduction to Pharmaceutical Biotechnology: Introduction to Animal Tissue Culture Science.* IOP Publishing Ltd, Bristol, UK; 2019;3:1–28.
74. Sharma K, Bhatia S, Dahiya R, Bera T. Plant tissue culture. In: *Modern Applications of Plant Biotechnology in Pharmaceutical Sciences.* Academic Press, Cambridge, MA; 2015:31–107.
75. Sharma K, Bhatia S, Dahiya R, Bera T. Laboratory organization. In: *Modern Applications of Plant Biotechnology in Pharmaceutical Sciences.* Academic Press, Cambridge, MA; 2015:109–120.
76. Sharma K, Bhatia S, Dahiya R, Bera T. Concepts and techniques of plant tissue culture science. In: *Modern Applications of Plant Biotechnology in Pharmaceutical Sciences.* Elsevier, Amsterdam; 2015:121–156.
77. Sharma K, Bhatia S, Dahiya R, Bera T. Application of plant biotechnology. In: *Modern Applications of Plant Biotechnology in Pharmaceutical Sciences.* Academic Press, Cambridge, MA; 2015:157–207.
78. Sharma K, Bhatia S, Dahiya R, Bera T. Somatic embryogenesis and organogenesis. In: *Modern Applications of Plant Biotechnology in Pharmaceutical Sciences.* Academic Press, Cambridge, MA; 2015:209–230.
79. Sharma K, Bhatia S, Dahiya R, Bera T. Classical and non-classical techniques for secondary metabolite production in plant cell culture. In: *Modern Applications of Plant Biotechnology in Pharmaceutical Sciences.* Academic Press, Cambridge, MA; 2015:231–291.
80. Sharma K, Bhatia S, Dahiya R, Bera T. Plant-based biotechnological products with their production host, modes of delivery systems, and stability testing. In: *Modern Applications of Plant Biotechnology in Pharmaceutical Sciences.* Academic Press, Cambridge, MA; 2015:293–331.
81. Sharma K, Bhatia S, Dahiya R, Bera T. Edible vaccines. In: *Modern Applications of Plant Biotechnology in Pharmaceutical Sciences.* Academic Press, Cambridge, MA; 2015:333–343.
82. Sharma K, Bhatia S, Dahiya R, Bera T. Microenvironmentation in micropropagation. In: *Modern Applications of Plant Biotechnology in Pharmaceutical Sciences.* Academic Press, Cambridge, MA; 2015:345–360.
83. Sharma K, Bhatia S, Dahiya R, Bera T. Micropropagation. In: *Modern Applications of Plant Biotechnology in Pharmaceutical Sciences.* Academic Press, Cambridge, MA; 2015:361–368.
84. Sharma K, Bhatia S, Dahiya R, Bera T. Laws in plant biotechnology. In: *Modern Applications of Plant Biotechnology in Pharmaceutical Sciences.* Academic Press, Cambridge, MA; 2015:369–391.
85. Sharma K, Bhatia S, Dahiya R, Bera T. Technical glitches in micropropagation. In: *Modern Applications of Plant Biotechnology in Pharmaceutical Sciences.* Academic Press, Cambridge, MA; 2015:393–404.
86. Sharma K, Bhatia S, Dahiya R, Bera T. Plant tissue culture-based industries. In: *Modern Applications of Plant Biotechnology in Pharmaceutical Sciences.* Academic Press, Cambridge, MA; 2015:405–417.

7

Effect of COVID-19 on Different Organ Systems

Ahmed Al-Harrasi
Natural and Medical Sciences Research Center, University of Nizwa

Saurabh Bhatia
Natural and Medical Sciences Research Center, University of Nizwa
University of Petroleum and Energy Studies

Tapan Behl
Chitkara University

Deepak Kaushik
M.D. University

Mohammed Muqtader Ahmed and Md. Khalid Anwer
Prince Sattam Bin Abdul Aziz University

CONTENTS

DOI: 10.1201/9781003175933-8

7.1 Introduction

As we have learned from the COVID-19 outbreak this disease can be either restricted to the respiratory system or transmitted to other organs where it can lead to multiple-organ failure. Confirmed COVID-19 cases can be asymptomatic or presenting only a few symptoms (paucisymptomatic form) to severe respiratory involvement such as acute viral pneumonia with respiratory or multiorgan failure [1]. Thus, it is now clear that COVID-19 represents broad clinical manifestations that range from common cold or flu-like symptoms to more severe diseases such as bronchitis, pneumonia, acute respiratory distress syndrome (ARDS), multiorgan failure, and even death. Multiple-organ involvement in COVID-19 can be severe, which can not only lead to respiratory failure, but also can cause life-threatening multiorgan and systemic dysfunctions (due to systemic inflammatory response) or multiple-organ failure in terms of sepsis and septic shock and death. Thus, based on clinical findings, COVID-19 patients with comorbidities or underlying uncontrolled medical conditions (e.g., diabetes, hypertension, smokers, patients taking steroids chronically, transplant recipients, lung, liver, and kidney disease, and cancer patients on chemotherapy) are at high risk of COVID-19 infection. In addition, COVID-19 can be severe, resulting in hospitalization in the ICU and possibly death among older patients (>65 years old) with comorbidities [2]. Thus, patients with comorbidities must take all safety measures to avoid the chances of being affected with severe acute respiratory syndrome coronavirus 2 (SARS-CoV-2). Possible direct effects of severe acute respiratory syndrome (SARS) over multiple organs through angiotensin-converting enzyme 2 along with hyperinflammatory response of the host can be associated with complications of the disease.

7.2 Cardiovascular Complications Associated with COVID-19

Recent investigations have shown that people with cardiovascular complications are usually at high chances for mortality as well as morbidity associated with COVID-19 than the average population [2]. As reported, the most common comorbidity was hypertension (16.9%), followed by diabetes (8.2%) among 1,590 hospitalized patients from China between December 11, 2019, and January 31, 2020 [3,4]. The study based on a small number of COVID-19 patients ($n=21$) showed that congestive heart failure was considered as the second most prevalent comorbidity with 42.9%. Another report also showed that SARS-CoV-2 infection can also cause heart injury among people with or without underlying cardiovascular complications [5]. Nevertheless, clinical findings from COVID-19 patients showed that respiratory complications caused by SARS-CoV-2 are more dominant and cardiovascular complications can take place via a number of other mechanisms. It was suggested that about 8%–12% out of all COVID-19 patients had cardiovascular abnormality [6]. Comorbid patients with cardiovascular complications and cardiac abnormality caused by SARS-CoV-2 infection can increase the risk of mortality. A study on COVID-19 patients associated with cardiovascular abnormality showed that 4.1% had heart failure, 5.3% had cerebrovascular disease, and 10.6% patients had coronary heart disease. It was observed that out of all patients, 35% had primary cardiovascular complications such as coronary heart disease, cardiomyopathy, and hypertension, whereas 28% demonstrated proof of acute myocardial injury (high cardiac biomarkers with high-level of -sensitivity towards troponin I or troponin T) [7]. Additionally, death rate was considerably high among individuals with high troponin T levels in comparison with those with normal troponin T levels. These CVD complications among COVID-19 patients can cause the worst prognosis. Figure 7.1 demonstrates the cardiovascular complications caused by SARS-CoV-2.

7.2.1 Cardiac Implications for COVID-19 Patients and Its Pathogenic Considerations

The primary target for COVID-19 caused by SARS-CoV-2 (a novel non-segmented and enveloped positive-sense RNA betacoronavirus) is the respiratory tract; however, the cardiovascular system may possibly also be affected in a number of different ways [8]. Some prevalent pathway mechanisms responsible for cardiovascular abnormalities among COVID-19 patients are as follows:

- Direct myocardial damage: Coronavirus 2 invasion in human cells is based on the binding of spike protein to ACE2 receptor, which is highly expressed in heart (cardiomyocytes, coronary endothelial cells, cardiac fibroblasts, vascular mural cells, and epicardial adipose cells) and lungs (type II alveolar cells). However, ACE2 is also expressed in the vascular system (endothelial cells, migratory angiogenic cells, and vascular smooth muscle cells) and kidneys (endothelial cells of glomerular capillaries, epithelial cells of the Bowman capsule, and proximal tubule epithelial cells). The cardiovascular system is partially regulated by neural (autonomic) and humoral (circulating or hormonal) factors. ACE2, homologue of ACE, plays an important role in central negative regulation of the renin–angiotensin system and also plays an important role in neurohumoral regulation of the cardiovascular system. Coronavirus 2 binding to ACE2 can alter ACE2 expression or activity, which may further result in the alteration of signaling pathways, resulting in the progression of heart disease such as acute myocardial injury [9]. Additionally, ACE2 is an important mediator of hypertension; as a result, ACE2 is speculated to be a possible modulator of blood pressure. ACE2 is expressed in various heart cells where it counteracts angiotensin II activities and is also responsible for the activation of cellular signaling pathways of the Ang 1–7/MasR signaling [10]. ACE2 expression is greatly affected by COVID-19, which has demonstrated its responsibility in counter-regulating the progression of cardiac complications. Among human beings, genetic changes in the *ACE2* gene associate with propensity for cardiovascular

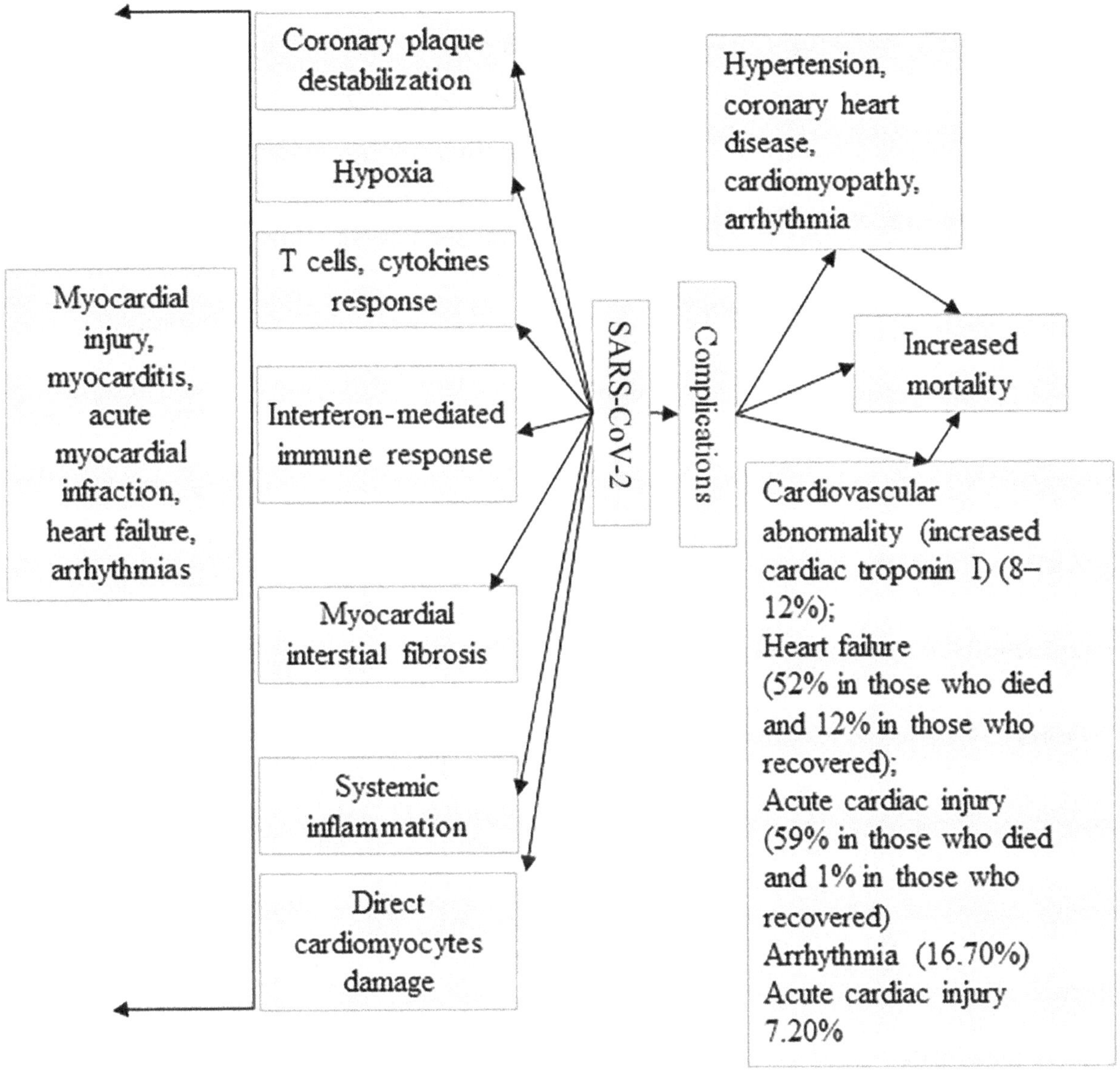

FIGURE 7.1 Cardiovascular complications in COVID-19.

complications. It was observed that single-nucleotide polymorphisms of *ACE2* are linked with changes in ventricular hypertrophy, septal wall thickness, and coronary artery disease [10–12].

- Systemic inflammatory response: Progression and severity of COVID-19 are usually associated with acute systemic inflammatory response mainly characterized by the overactivation of the systemic immune cells that result in cytokine storm due to sudden crease in circulatory levels of proinflammatory cytokines among critically ill COVID-19 patients. This hyperinflammatory response can damage multiple organs, resulting in multiple-organ failure. The circulatory system is also impacted badly, with various abnormalities such as dysrhythmias, myocarditis, acute myocardial infarction, heart failure, myocardial injury, and venous thromboembolic events [11–14].
- Impairment in myocardial oxygen supply/demand: Hypoxia and oxidative stress-induced decreased oxygen transport to the tissues among COVID-19 patients increases cardiometabolic demand. Prevailed hypoxic state due to acute system infection can further interfere with myocardial oxygen demand supply, which results in acute myocardial injury [11–14].
- Plaque disruption and multivessel coronary thrombosis: Plaque erosion among the most likely patients with cardiovascular complications can be increased by severe systemic inflammation and can be further aggravated by prothrombotic state. Higher local immune response due to SARS-CoV-2 infection is the leading cause of local inflammation in the plaques. This can further increase the collagenase production to degrade and weaken the fibrous cap, which can stimulate plaque rupture and thrombotic acute coronary syndrome, leading to acute

myocardial infarction. Systemic inflammation-induced prothrombotic milieu can further elevate the risk of cardiovascular complications [11–14].

- Adverse effects of various therapies: Several medications used for the treatment of COVID-19 such as antiviral drugs, corticosteroids, and other therapeutics can also have harmful effects on the cardiovascular system.
- Electrolyte imbalances: Previous investigations have shown various electrolyte imbalances in patients who progress to the severe form of COVID-19. As reported, COVID-19-associated progression is related to low levels of calcium, sodium, and potassium in serum. Electrolyte imbalances can occur in patients with underlying cardiac complications. One of the major concerns associated with cardiovascular complications, especially tachyarrhythmias induced by hypokalemia in COVID-19 because of the interaction of SARS-CoV-2 with RAS system, has also been evidenced. Hypernatremia (i.e., plasma sodium concentration ≥150 mmol/L) among critically severe COVID-19 patients is also evidenced. Unusual elevation in renal sodium reabsorption is perhaps due to the increased angiotensin II activity. COVID-19 patients with hyponatremia, hypochloride, or hypocalcemia with cardiovascular complications require stays in the ICU and mechanical ventilation and also have increased death rates [11–14].

The development of cardiovascular disorders among COVID-19 patients is still not clear; however, coexistence of cardiovascular complications (CVD comorbidity) and viral infection might be linked with a severe form of COVID-19 infection. A systematic review of 1,527 COVID-19 patients showed the prevalence of hypertension (17.1%) and cardiac complications (16.4%). This suggests that such individuals were more apt to need intensive care [12]. One more report on 44,672 COVID-19 patients suggested that patients with cardiovascular disorders showed mortality almost five times greater than patients without cardiovascular disorders (10.5% vs. 2.3%). Findings from previous reports also showed that COVID-19 patients with prior cardiovascular complications had higher chances of mortality. Further progression in COVID-19-associated complications among patients was found to be <20% [11–14]. These critically ill patients may show symptoms of acute pneumonia, ARDS, multiple-organ injury or dysfunction, and hemodynamic instability, with a number of cardiovascular complications. Acute heart failure and cardiogenic shock are the most severe cardiac complications and may occur among critically ill patients.

7.2.2 Cardiovascular Impact of COVID-19 Infection

7.2.2.1 Myocardial Damage and Inflammation of the Heart Muscle in COVID-19

Before the first evidence of myocardial damage linked with SARS-CoV-2, Middle East respiratory syndrome coronavirus (MERS-CoV) also showed its association with myocardial damage as well as inflammation of the heart muscle with increase in cardiac troponin T [16]. These cardiac complications associated with MERS-CoV were earlier thought to be due to elevated physiological cardiac stress, low level of oxygen in tissues, or immediate myocardial damage. The first report of myocardial damage linked with coronavirus 2 included 41 COVID-19 affected individuals in Wuhan, China, where 12% of patients showed more sensitivity against elevated level of troponin I (28 pg/mL). In a later investigation, it was found that myocardial damage with increased level of troponin presented among 7%–17% of COVID-19 hospitalized patients, out of which 22% to 31% were admitted to the ICU. A high viral load was found in patients suffering from myocarditis, whereas inflammatory lesions due to mononuclear infiltration were found after autopsy examination of a number of COVID-19 patients. A subsequent study recommended that up to 7% of COVID-19-associated mortality was because of myocarditis [14–16].

COVID-19 patients with acute myocarditis can present symptoms like dyspnea, acute left ventricular dysfunction, dysrhythmia, and chest pain. Among COVID-19 patients with myocardial damage and myocarditis, the level of serum troponin was found to be unusual. ECG reports have shown a variety of outcomes similar to acute coronary syndrome in a number of patients. Some of these reports showed abnormalities in the form of myocarditis as well as non-specific ST-T wave, defects, inversion of a T wave and ST segment as well as PR-segment variations [14–16]. Considering these ECG reports, it is difficult to differentiate myocarditis and acute coronary syndrome, but echocardiographic reports have revealed focal wall-motion defects with acute coronary syndrome. These echocardiographic reports did not show wall motion abnormalities among COVID-19-induced myocarditis patients. ECG and echocardiographic reports together can be essential markers to determine the progression of disease. Additionally, increases in serum troponin level among severe COVID-19 patients can be directly linked with higher probability of cardiovascular disorders with higher risk of mortality [14–16].

7.2.2.2 Acute Myocardial Infarction

As mentioned before, systemic hyperinflammatory state can increase the chances of atherosclerotic plaque erosion, which can result in acute myocardial infarction. A report published in 2018 revealed that viral infection caused by influenza and other viruses was linked with an elevated risk of acute myocardial infarction in the first week of disease diagnosis. Additionally, for influenza, prevalence ratio was 6.1 and 2.8 was reported for other viruses. Subsequent investigation revealed that individuals admitted to the hospital with pneumonia (community-acquired) presented more possibility of cardiovascular disorders that persisted for a number of years after hospitalization [14–16]. Because of this hyperinflammatory state and hypercoagulability, higher chances of acute myocardial infarction are possibly present with COVID.

7.2.2.3 Cardiac Involvement of COVID-19 Mainly Acute Heart Failure and Cardiomyopathy

SARS-CoV-2 infection can lead to or aggravate heart failure via an array of mechanisms such as myocarditis, pulmonary embolism, cardiomyopathy, increased oxygen demand, myocardial ischemia or infarction, stress, elevations in pulmonary pressures, and diffuse cytokine release. These clinical manifestations can concomitantly result in cardiac arrhythmia, cardiogenic shock, and acute heart failure [14–16]. COVID-19 patients are usually at high risk for thrombosis in the arterial and venous circulations. This is because of oxidative stress, platelet activation, inflammation, and endothelial dysfunction. Plaque erosion associated with acute coronary syndromes can result in type I myocardial infarction, whereas type II myocardial infarction can be caused by hypoxemic respiratory failure and increased myocardial oxygen demand. Both type I and type II myocardial infarction can activate the functional deterioration of already existing heart failure or development of *de novo* acute heart failure. SARS-CoV-2 infection linked with myocarditis was identified by the presence of SARS-CoV-2 particles on endomyocardial biopsy and the presence of diffuse myocardial edema on cardiac magnetic resonance. Treatment approaches may include systemic glucocorticoid treatment, lopinavir/ritonavir, hydroxychloroquine, and intravenous immunoglobulin. Various reports suggest that the prevalence of cardiomyopathy is high in COVID-19 patients. A recent US report revealed that 21 severe COVID-19 patients developed cardiomyopathy (33%), which was called decreased left ventricular systolic function [14–16].

Primary clinical findings of COVID-19 infection can be acute heart failure with cardiomyopathy. One report revealed that acute cardiac collapse was found among 23% of COVID-19 patients, whereas cardiomyopathy was present among 33% of patients. Another investigation showed that acute cardiac collapse found among 24% of patients increased the risk of death [14–16]. It was also noticed that patients admitted in these studies did not have any history of hypertension or cardiovascular complications. It is not clear yet whether cardiac failure is associated with new cardiomyopathy due to viral infection or if it is an aggravation of earlier undiagnosed cardiac complications. Thus, it is critical to know possible cardiac complications before providing fluid replacement therapy or intravenous fluid treatment. Among ARDS and acute lung injury patients, right heart failure was found to be common and can be an important clinical manifestation during the treatment of patients.

7.2.2.4 Arrhythmia in COVID-19

COVID-19 patients presenting dysrhythmias showed palpitations as one of the most common symptoms among almost 7% of patients [17]. However, a variety of dysrhythmias has been experienced by COVID-19 patients, out of which the most common was sinus tachycardia. A previous investigation revealed that 17% of patients after hospitalization and 44% of ICU COVID-19 infected individuals experienced dysrhythmias [17]. This may be due to inflammatory stress, abnormal metabolism, and hypoxia. Various pathological findings should be carefully monitored and diagnosed such as acute coronary syndrome, myocardial injury, and acute myocarditis in the case of dysrhythmias due to increase in serum troponin.

7.2.2.5 Venous Thromboembolic Events in COVID-19 Patients

Venous thromboembolic is a state in which a clot is formed in the deep veins and passed through circulation to further cause complication in the lungs. COVID-19 patients are at high risk of venous thromboembolic events as abnormal coagulation status, multiorgan dysfunction, and systemic inflammation make patients more vulnerable to them. Various reports suggest that considerable abnormal coagulation pathways are found among COVID-19 patients such as increased level of D-dimer. One investigation of 25 COVID-19 patients with acute pneumonia revealed that increased level of D-dimer was present among all individuals, out of which ten patients had pulmonary embolism. It was also noticed that D-dimer levels were >1 μg/mL, which was directly related to the possibility of death after hospitalization among COVID-19 patients [18]. Another study suggested that treatment with an anticoagulant such as heparin reduced death among severe COVID-19-infected individuals or among individuals presenting D-dimer more than six times the normal range [19].

7.2.2.6 Potential Drug–Drug Interactions in COVID-19 Patients

Some of the drugs investigated for the treatment of COVID-19 showed significant interaction with other cardiovascular drugs, which should be carefully considered, and suitable dose adjustments should be made to avoid any adverse effects of the medication. Recently, one of the most significant drug interactions, chloroquine/hydroxychloroquine, can potentially extend the QT interval on ECG [20]. This extension of QT interval can further escalate the chances for cardiac complications such as arrhythmias. Chloroquine/hydroxychloroquine and azathioprine have been recently suggested as potential treatment; however, based on earlier reports, both medications are known to extend QT interval [16,21–23]. Thus, necessary precaution should be taken before prescribing these drugs. Moreover, combination of these drugs must not be prescribed, and during administration of chloroquine/hydroxychloroquine alone, on a daily basis, ECG for examination of QT interval is essential, mainly among critically ill patients with liver and kidney complications and among those who are using another drug with the possibility to extend QT interval. There are several drugs that are under investigation for COVID-19 such as antimalarials (e.g., chloroquine, hydroxychloroquine), antivirals (e.g., favipiravir, ribavirin, remdesivir, and lopinavir/ritonavir), antibiotics (e.g., azithromycin), and corticosteroids [16, 21–23]. Out of these, some of them might trigger PR as well as QT extension such as lopinavir/ritonavir. Interactions of these drugs with other drugs such as anticoagulants and antiplatelets should be evaluated before administration. A prednisolone derivative glucocorticoid, namely methylprednisolone, can cause electrolyte imbalance, hypertension, and fluid retention; thus, such drugs and their associated drug interactions must be determined before use [16,21–23].

7.2.3 COVID-19 in the Heart and the Lungs (Notch)

7.2.3.1 COVID-19 and the Heart

It has been observed that certain COVID-19 patients experience cardiac-associated complications such as heart pounding or pain in chest rather than pulmonary complications [24]. During the flu epidemic in the United States (1990), flu-based secondary pneumonia caused myocardial infarction in some infected patients because severe inflammation caused destabilization of plaques present in coronary artery [25]. This complication of myocardial infarction can also be due to a variety of reasons such as release of inflammatory cytokines, tachycardia, increased wall stress, hypoxia, and thrombophilia. Thus, more investigation is required to identify the exact possible mechanism.

7.2.3.2 Cardiovascular Drugs and COVID-19

Angiotensin is a peptide hormone and important part of the renin–angiotensin system, responsible for vasoconstriction that leads to the elevation of blood pressure, which makes the heart pump harder. In addition to its expression over many tissues, ACE2 is also expressed highly over the cell surface of lungs and myocardium [24]. ACE2 is primarily expressed in the inner track of the respiratory system where the flu virus binds to these receptors to cause severe respiratory problems.

The main role of ACE2 is to efficiently cleave Ang II, resulting in the formation of cardioprotective peptides Ang (1–7), while the role of ACE1 is to catalyze the formation of angiotensin (Ang) II. Ang II is involved in the regulation of blood pressure and cardiorenal function as it is the main component of the renin–angiotensin system. Therefore, ACE2 antagonizes ACE1 activity. Angiotensin II receptor blockers (ARBs) are known to treat high blood pressure and congestive heart failure and also to enhance the level of Ang II [26] and, circuitously, can trigger ACE2. The main role of ARBs is to facilitate the relaxation of blood vessels to decrease blood pressure. It was suspected that patients using Ang II receptor blockers are more likely to have COVID-19 [27] infection. Thus, it was also projected that patients who are using Ang II receptor blockers for various cardiac ailments must change medication. However, this suggestion was not supported by any of the facts. The following points must be considered in case patient is using Ang II receptor blockers:

- In hypertension models, ACE2 expression is decreased.
- As such, there are no concrete proofs that Ang II receptor blockers can increase ACE2 expression in the lung.
- Also, ARBs-based treatment and hypertension did not influence earlier coronavirus infections.

Thus, based on the above findings, ACE2 is a potential target to prevent SARS-CoV-2 invasion inside the host cell. To achieve this, one of the researchers has developed a novel recombinant protein via appending the ACE2 extracellular domain to the fragment crystallizable region (tail region of an antibody that interacts with cell surface receptors) of the human immunoglobulin IgG1 to neutralize severe acute respiratory syndrome coronavirus (SARS-CoV) and SARS-CoV-2 spike pseudotyped virus in vitro [27]. One more strategy to avoid viral invasion might be to suppress ACE2 expression over cellular membranes. ACE2 contains N-glycosylated N-terminal ectodomain, which contains the active site (amino acids 1–740), a hydrophobic transmembrane region (amino acids 741–762), and a short C-terminal cytoplasmic tail (amino acids 763–805). ACE2 can experience an ADAM17 (a metalloproteinase)-mediated "shedding of surface proteins" from endothelial cells, ensuing in the release of the ectodomain. ADAM17 considerably showed its expression in the cardiac as well as pulmonary tissue and was also responsible for surface proteins shedding of such as ACE2 [28]. Thus, decrease in ADAM17 expression ultimately decreases ACE2 shedding, whereas increase in expression of ADAM17 considerably enhances its shedding [28]. Also, translocation of membrane protein (ADAM17) resulted in considerable decrease in ACE2 protein expression present at myocardial region but ADAM17 activation is linked with elevation in activity of plasma ACE2 [29]. This information supports the speculation that elevation in levels of ADAM17 will increase the surface protein (such as ACE2) shedding, whereas rise in soluble/plasma ACE2 levels might contribute to a mode to block SARS-CoV-2 invasion into cells. In this context, 5-fluorouracil treatment efficiently triggered ADAM17 in a colorectal cancer animal model [30]. In addition, estradiol increased the expression of ADAM17 in lung cancer cell lines [31].

In addition to ACE2, furin, a human protease, is also essential to support the invasion of the virus into the host cell [32]. Furin is expressed in various cells and organs such as the lungs. The spike glycoprotein of the SARS-CoV-2 contains a polybasic furin-like cleavage site between the S1/S2 subunits, which is absent in SARS-CoV. The binding of virus spike protein to ACE2 is mediated by furin, which allows the cleavage of S protein to enter into the cell [32]. Thus, for SARS-CoV-2 binding, the inhibition of furin can be a likely approach. In this regard, based on the cleavage of furin of the avian influenza A H5N1 virus, a novel peptide was designed to prevent the binding and further invasion of furin-dependent pathogens [33]. Based on an evolutionarily conserved system, it was also suggested that these two important targets (i.e., furin and ADAM17) are interconnected with each other by Notch. Thus, targeting Notch can be considered as an option to inhibit furin and upregulate ADAM17. In this context, a recent study hypothesized that an association between human proteins and SARS-CoV-2 involves 66 potential molecular proteins, which can be considered as potential targets to prevent viral entry. Considering this, it is not possible to distinguish those host proteins that are important for viral invasion, especially those that do not have direct association with viral proteins such as furin and ADAM17. Thus, these speculations require more experimental evidence to explore the understanding regarding possible targets involved during virus–cell interaction.

7.3 COVID-19 and Kidney Damage

In this section, we discuss possible molecular pathways as well as treatment approaches to COVID-19-associated acute kidney injury. Previous reports suggested that the incidence of acute renal damage among COVID-19 patients is low. For instance, a study on 1,099 COVID-19 patients from China showed that only 0.5% had acute kidney injury, whereas 93.6% were hospitalized, 91.1% had pneumonia, 5.3% were admitted to the ICU, and 3.4% had ARDS [34]. Possible mechanisms of kidney involvement among COVID-19 patients include:

- Cytokine associated renal injury
- Inflammatory pathways of organ cross talk during viral infection
- Role of systemic effect

These possible pathways are greatly interrelated and have significant implications for extracorporeal treatment such as hemofiltration, dialysis, and extracorporeal membrane oxygenation for the treatment of critically ill patients with sepsis. Possible pathways that are responsible for renal injuries with possible treatment approaches in COVID-19 are shown in Figure 7.2.

7.4 Liver vs COVID-19

Liver impairment in COVID-19 patients can be due to the following possible mechanisms [35,36]:

- Direct cytopathic effect caused by viral invasion
- Uncontrolled immune reaction leading to systemic hyperinflammatory response
- Sepsis (hemodynamic changes or via direct or indirect assault on the hepatocytes)
- Drug-induced liver injury

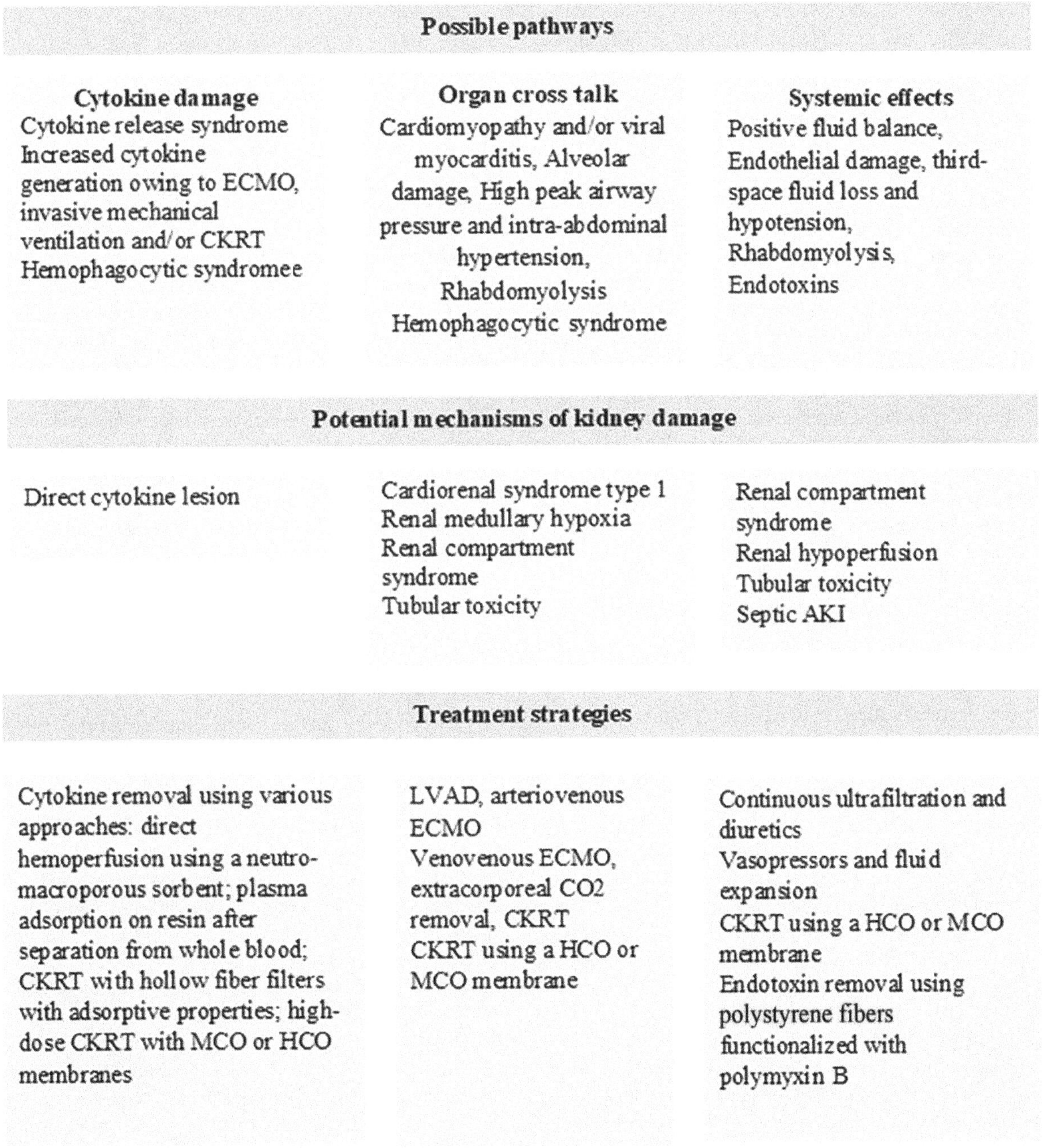
Possible pathways
Cytokine damage
Cytokine release syndrome
Increased cytokine generation owing to ECMO, invasive mechanical ventilation and/or CKRT
Hemophagocytic syndromee
Organ cross talk
Cardiomyopathy and/or viral myocarditis, Alveolar damage, High peak airway pressure and intra-abdominal hypertension, Rhabdomyolysis
Hemophagocytic syndrome
Systemic effects
Positive fluid balance, Endothelial damage, third-space fluid loss and hypotension, Rhabdomyolysis, Endotoxins
Potential mechanisms of kidney damage
Direct cytokine lesion
Cardiorenal syndrome type 1
Renal medullary hypoxia
Renal compartment syndrome
Tubular toxicity
Renal compartment syndrome
Renal hypoperfusion
Tubular toxicity
Septic AKI
Treatment strategies
Cytokine removal using various approaches: direct hemoperfusion using a neutro-macroporous sorbent; plasma adsorption on resin after separation from whole blood; CKRT with hollow fiber filters with adsorptive properties; high-dose CKRT with MCO or HCO membranes
LVAD, arteriovenous ECMO
Venovenous ECMO, extracorporeal CO2 removal, CKRT
CKRT using a HCO or MCO membrane
Continuous ultrafiltration and diuretics
Vasopressors and fluid expansion
CKRT using a HCO or MCO membrane
Endotoxin removal using polystyrene fibers functionalized with polymyxin B

FIGURE 7.2 Potential mechanisms of kidney damage and treatment strategies in COVID-19 [34]. MCO: Medium cutoff, LVAD: left ventricular assist device, HCO: high cutoff, ECMO: extracorporeal membrane oxygenation, CKRT: continuous kidney replacement therapy, AKI: acute kidney injury.

Earlier findings suggest that hepatic dysfunction is evidenced among almost 60% of SARS patients and is also evidenced in MERS-CoV-infected patients. ACE2 is considerably expressed in the majority of cholangiocytes (~59.7%); thus, liver can also be a possible target for SARS-CoV-2 to dysregulate liver function [35,36]. Considering the high expression ACE2 receptor-enriched cholangiocytes, COVID-19 infection can exacerbate cholestasis among patients with primary biliary cholangitis, or it can elevate alkaline phosphatase and gamma-glutamyl-transferase [35,36]. However, hepatic tissue-based pathological manifestations from a COVID-19 patient who died showed that viral inclusion was not observed in the hepatic tissue. In addition, COVID-19 can also aggravate underlying chronic liver disease, leading to decompensated cirrhosis and acute decompensation of chronic liver disease, with high death rate. Liver dysfunction was considerably higher in critically ill COVID-19 patients and was related to poor outcomes [35,36]. As per the previous report, 2%–11% of COVID-19 patients were shown to have underlying chronic liver disease (liver comorbidities), whereas 14%–53% of COVID-19 patients developed liver dysfunction, mainly those with severe COVID-19. This information suggests that 14%–53% of cases reported unusual levels of alanine aminotransferase and aspartate aminotransferase during disease progression. Thus, based on reports, it can be concluded that severe COVID-19 patients appear to have higher rates of liver complications. Increase in aspartate aminotransferase was found in 62% out of all ICU patients (n=13), compared with 25% of all (n=28) non-ICU patients in a report published by Lancet (Huang and colleagues) [35,36]. In a study that included large groups of individuals (1,099 patients from 552 hospitals), it was observed that critically ill patients with COVID-19 had unusual liver aminotransferase levels when compared to non-severe patients with COVID-19. Thus, liver dysfunction is more common in critical patients than in mild cases of COVID-19 [35,36].

Direct damage to liver can be caused by SARS-CoV-2 by causing direct infection to liver cells. Patients with COVID-19 (almost 2%–10%) present loose or watery stools with the presence of SARS-CoV-2 RNA in feces and blood samples [35,36]. This shows the possibility of direct infection caused by coronavirus to liver cells. Hepatic tissue-based pathological investigations of SARS patients revealed the presence of the virus in liver tissue. However, viral titer was comparatively lower as viral inclusion was not observed. Similarly, hepatic tissue-based pathological investigations in the case of Middle East respiratory syndrome (MERS) patients' viral titer were not measurable in examined liver tissue. Elevated gamma-glutamyl transferase that presents cholangiocyte injury was found among 54% of COVID-19 patients (n=56) during hospitalization. Additionally, increase in alkaline phosphatase levels was observed in 18% of COVID-19 patients (n=56) during hospitalization [35,36].

Hepatotoxicity can be due to drug-induced liver impairment or drug–drug interactions, which were observed in large groups of individuals. Moreover, liver injury or failure among critically ill COVID-19 patients can be due to the hyperinflammatory response caused by cytokine storm and hypoxia state (due to pneumonia-associated). Liver dysfunction is also observed among COVID-19 patients with mild forms of COVID-19; however, liver dysfunction is transient in mild form, and goes away without any treatment. Chronic hepatitis B patients or patients under long-term treatment with nucleos(t)ide analogues must be carefully monitored after COVID-19 infection as this can have the worst prognosis. COVID-19 patients with liver morbidities such as autoimmune hepatitis and their treatment with glucocorticoids must be investigated. In addition, patients with liver morbidities like liver cirrhosis or cancer may be more susceptible to COVID-19 infection due to their systemic immunocompromised status. Considering progression of COVID-19 infection and its severity, immune response, drug hepatotoxicity, and liver morbidity such as any advanced liver disease, hepatic encephalopathy should be carefully studied in large groups of individuals. Immunocompromised patients, especially older patients, with other comorbidities with COVID-19 infection require critical care to tailor safe as well as effective therapeutic approaches [35,36].

It was also noticed that COVID-19 infection caused mild to moderate hepatic injury, resulting in increase in prolongation of prothrombin time, aminotransferases, and hypoproteinemia. Moreover, ~60% of patients suffering from SARS had liver impairment, which clearly suggests the direct involvement of liver during COVID-19 infection. Percutaneous liver biopsy examination and detection of viral nucleic acids in hepatic tissue of SARS patients revealed the direct infection caused by coronavirus in liver. Pathological manifestation also revealed noticeable mitoses and apoptosis with unusual characteristics, including councilman hyaline bodies, hepatocytes death with increase in size, and lobular effects with no accumulation of fibrin. It was speculated that SARS-related liver impairment might be due to the viral hepatitis or toxicity caused by prescribed drug/s (antiviral medications, antibiotics, and steroids) usage at high dose along with hyperinflammatory response. Recently, single-cell RNA sequencing data from two separate groups of people showed considerable increase in expression of ACE2 in cholangiocytes (59.7% of cells) in comparison with hepatocytes (2.6% of cells). This proposes that COVID-19 infection can directly cause damage to the intrahepatic bile ducts [35,36].

7.5 COVID-19 Associated Gastrointestinal Tract Complications

A recent report showed that respiratory symptoms are the most common symptoms seen among COVID-19, MERS, and SARS patients [35–40]. Nevertheless, the risk of some common features associated with gastrointestinal tract (GIT) complications varies considerably among different patients as well populations. It was found that onset of GIT complications can be mild, which can be followed by respiratory complications. Several reports showed that GIT changes during SARS-CoV infection were confirmed by the detection of viral particles in the biopsy sample and stool samples obtained from recovered patients, which can suggest direct involvement of SARS-CoV in causing GIT complications [35–40]. A report obtained from the first COVID-19 patient in the United States revealed GIT complications such as nausea and vomiting during hospitalization, followed by loose bowel movements in the hospital for 2 days. Stool and respiratory sample reports of the same patient was later found to be positive, which suggests the existence of viral nucleic acids [35–40]. Moreover, COVID-19 sequence can also be found during the examination of saliva samples of nearly all infected patients. However, nasopharyngeal aspirate test for the same patients was found to be negative and it was also found that serial monitoring of saliva samples revealed a drop in viral load after hospitalization. This information is important to understand that extrapulmonary detection of viral nucleic acid does not mean the presence of virus or that the test for COVID-19 is positive. Further examination of viral culture obtained from saliva samples can also suggest the chances of infection in salivary gland along with its likely transmission [35–40]. Data obtained from two China-based laboratories revealed the presence of viral particles in the stool samples of infected patients (unpublished). This information is useful to take precautions, while clinical examination of stool or saliva samples should be obtained from COVID-19 patients, as the GIT system in addition to the respiratory system can be considered as another route of infection. Paramedical staff must take necessary precaution to quickly diagnose the patients with initial onset of gastrointestinal symptoms and also look at the time period of infection with late viral conversion. In addition, necessary precautions are required when uninfected individuals are in close contact with infected patients with mild GIT symptoms at an early stage [35–40]. This involvement of GIT should not be neglected or underestimated. Bioinformatics data based on single-cell transcriptomes (i.e., gene expression level of individual cells) from lung (normal) and GIT recently showed that expression of ACE2 is not limited to only alveolar type II pneumocyte; it was also expressed in upper esophagus and stratified epithelial cells and simple columnar intestinal absorptive cells from ileum and colon. Due to the increased permeability of GIT membrane against different pathogens once infected, the virus invades enterocytes and causes abnormality, resulting in GIT symptoms like diarrhea [35–40]. As reported, examination of SARS-CoV-2 RNA in a stool sample of a COVID-19 patient in the United States revealed the presence of SARS-CoV-2 RNA, which can suggest direct involvement of GIT during COVID-19 infection [41]. GIT association was found in COVID infections of animals as well as humans. Recently, it was also suggested that coexistence of GIT symptoms is not rare among COVID-19 patients. Earlier investigations of COVID-19 patients revealed that GIT symptoms such as vomiting or nausea, or both, along with diarrhea were observed among infected patients [42]. A cohort investigation of 204 COVID-19 patients revealed that 99 patients (48.5%) showed GIT symptoms, out of which seven patients did not have respiratory symptoms [43]. This report clearly suggests caution for hospital staff to spread awareness about the involvement of GIT in COVID-19 infection and its related clinical symptoms in spite of the general consensus that COVID can only cause respiratory complications. These reports can facilitate early diagnosis of COVID-19 infection to quarantine as well as provide suitable treatment to infected patients [44].

A report on a group of individuals (n=84) by Wei et al. showed that 31% of individuals had diarrhea associated with other symptoms like pain in the head, muscle aches and pain, production of sputum, cough, nausea, and vomiting more often in contrast to those without diarrhea [45]. One more report suggested that COVID-19 patients without digestive symptoms were possibly cured at a higher rate than patients with digestive symptoms. Perhaps this is because GIT involvement during this infection can be a sign of progression of disease severity, or respiratory symptoms will typically present after GIT symptoms among such patients. Several suggestions have been made regarding underlying cause of GIT involvement among COVID-19 infection. The first speculation is based on the interaction between SARS-CoV-2 and ACE2, which can be the leading cause of diarrhea as a bioinformatics study recently revealed that alveolar type II cells in lungs are enriched not only with ACE2 but also in the glandular cells of stomach as well as duodenum epithelium [46]. Likewise, Liang et al. suggested that ACE2 showed high expression in proximal as well as distal cells of the intestinal lining, which are in direct contact with food and pathogenic microorganisms [47]. Thus, ACE2-enriched enterocytes allow the invasion of COVID-19 virus, resulting in unstable fluid secretion in gut, malabsorption of enterocytes, and activated enteric nervous system, ultimately leading to diarrhea [46]. Second, enteric injury can be indirectly caused by hyperinflammatory response due to SARS-CoV-2 infection. Additionally, the likely cause of diarrhea among COVID-19 patients may be antibiotic-associated diarrhea. Various investigations have also suggested that antiviral therapy can affect microbiota of gut, its composition, and function. This can indirectly affect lungs via an immunomodulation process known as gut-lung axis by which the gut and lungs involve each compartment in a two-way manner, with both microbial and immune interactions ultimately regulating host health and disease. More autopsy examination should be done to understand the association of GIT during COVID-19 infection. An autopsy examination of an elderly COVID-19 patient (85-year-old man) suggested segmental (dilatation) and abnormal narrowing in the small intestine [48]. These outcomes and speculations might have a considerable effect in terms of spread of infection mainly during hospitalization of infected patients and necessary precaution required thereof. Detection of SARS-CoV and MERS-CoV in fecal samples of infected patients clearly presents the possibility of GIT involvement as another route of COVID-19 infection. Likewise, RT-PCR-based SARS-CoV-2 detection in stool samples of COVID-19 patients also supports GIT involvement [41]. During onset of a disease outbreak in Wuhan, the majority of the patients were evidenced for their connection to a Huanan Seafood Wholesale Market, which is believed to be the source of COVID-19. This connection raises an important concern in relation to transmission of SARS-CoV-2 via contaminated food at the small intestine [47]. One more concern of possible consideration is that the GIT might shed the virus for a longer duration in feces. Another investigation suggested that fecal samples of almost half of patients were found to be positive for SARS-CoV-2 RNA even after clearance of virus from the specimens obtained from respiratory tract [49]. In accordance with current guidelines, COVID-19 patients are usually discharged from the hospital on the basis of negative findings obtained from RT-PCR examination for SARS-CoV-2 [50]. As a result, based on the above reports, it is also advisable for regular fecal sample examination with RT-PCR before discharge from the hospital as transmission can continue if fecal samples are found to be positive [49].

Usually, COVID-19 shows poorer outcomes in patients with the presence of comorbidities. Thus, this can play a considerable role in the treatment of individuals with prior digestive complaints. It is now known that cancer patients are at higher risk of COVID-19 infection; nevertheless, whether patients suffering from GIT cancers are at higher risk to be infected with COVID-19 virus than normal individuals is still not known. A report from China revealed that 1% (n=18) out of 1,590 COVID-19 patients had a history of cancer. Out of this 1% of patients, three had colorectal cancer history. It was also suggested that COVID-19 patients with previous history of colorectal cancer had a higher risk of severe events [51]. Similarly, inflammatory bowel disease patients using medications such as immunosuppressive agents are more susceptible to severe infections and might be more vulnerable to COVID-19 infection. As per a report registered in Wuhan, out of 318 IBD individuals [ulcerative colitis patients (n = 204) and Crohn's disease patients (n = 114)], none of the samples from respective individuals were found positive for COVID-19 [52]. This information can be utilized while prescribing agents that can cause immunosuppression and biologic drugs, dietary intake, and deliberate delay of optional surgery and endoscopy. In this context, the risk of coexistence of *Clostridioides difficile* and SARS-CoV-2 infections suggests that stool samples must be screened properly as the chances of SARS-CoV-2 transmission can be higher during transplantation of this tissue [53].

7.6 Pulmonary Fibrosis in COVID-19 Patients

Based on the postmortem examination of cases, the main pathological feature among SARS patients is diffuse alveolar damage [54]. The underlying mechanism of diffuse alveolar damage is lung microvascular endothelial and alveolar epithelial cell injury, which is a hallmark of acute lung injury caused by direct injury by virus itself and other indirect factors [55]. The initial phase of SARS includes SARS development (7–10 days), presented by characteristics of diffuse alveolar damage. Diffuse alveolar damage is a non-specific reaction of the lung to a multitude of injurious agents, leading to endothelial and alveolar cell injury, which can progress into exudation of fluid and inflammatory mediators with extensive edema as well as formation of diffuse hyaline membrane that ultimately result in alveoli collapse and alveolar epithelium desquamated massively into the alveolus. Simultaneously, these pathological events can result in the deposition of fibrous tissue in alveolar spaces, which is designated as the severe progression of the disease. When the early stage progresses into the acute phase, this leads to the onset of the middle phase (10–14 days), which presents pulmonary fibrous organization such as interstitial and airspace fibrosis, intra-alveolar proliferation of fibroblast, and enlargement with continuous proliferation of type II pneumocyte. Fibrous organization is more common among the SARS patients and will increase further as long as the illnesses extend further. This is called the proliferative/organizing phase. Recently, it was revealed that SARS viral proteins essential for viral replication can further increase pulmonary fibrosis by the inhibition of the action of the enzyme responsible for connective tissue cleavage. The middle phase is followed by the late phase of SARS infection, the duration of which varies between 2 and 3 weeks, also called the fibrotic phase. The fibrotic phase is presented by dense septal and alveolar fibrosis in the lungs. Progression from the first stage to the third stage in diffuse alveolar damage varies as the progression of disease does not constantly develop during all three stages but can stop or improve at any stage [56]. It was concluded that the level of pulmonary fibrosis is definitely associated with the period of the SARS infection. Clinical investigation of SARS patients suggests that fibrous organization of lung tissue is more frequent among patients who are in the last stage than among patients in the early or middle stages.

On the contrary, diffuse alveolar damage is more common among patients who are going through the early or middle phases in contrast to patients who are in the late stage. As a result, pulmonary fibrosis can also present without diffuse alveolar damage [57]. Lung fibrosis usually evolves within a week; however, at first, it might not be apparent on chest radiographs. Nevertheless, noticeable architectural distortion and honeycomb lung are usually seen among patients with progressive fibrosis. It was also noticed that lung fibrosis was even found among recovered SARS patients. In addition, it was found that out of 200 recovered patients, 42 patients developed lung fibrosis after 9 months of discharge. The glucocorticoid and hormone-based conventional treatment for lung fibrosis has no influence on the SARS-induced lung fibrosis apart from the dose, mode of administration, or duration of medicine use. It was remarkable that patients suffering from lung fibrosis demonstrate spontaneous recovery [58].

Lung fibrosis usually resulted in the formation of scar in the lungs, which is due to the acute as well as chronic interstitial pulmonary disease. Pulmonary fibrosis is presented by failure in restoration of normal alveolar architecture and its function, which is mainly due to the unnecessary accumulation of collagen and other extracellular matrix components, failure in restoration of alveolar epithelial cells, proliferation of more fibroblast as well as damage to the normal lung architecture [59]. Further development of lung fibrosis can result in more severe complications such as expansion of interstitial matrix and destruction of normal pulmonary parenchyma, which can ultimately cause injury to the blood capillaries resulting in decrease in ventilation [60]. There are several causes of lung fibrosis; however, chronic inflammation is considered as the major cause of lung fibrosis, which can lead to epithelial damage as well as stimulation of fibroblast. Nevertheless, latest investigations revealed that damage to the alveolar epithelium and formation of myofibroblast foci (active) are the major causes for the majority of lung fibrotic processes [61]. This pulmonary tissue damage leads to the onset of inflammatory reaction by overexpression and release of growth factors and cytokines, such as tumor necrosis factor-α (TNF-α), monocyte chemoattractant protein-1 (MCP-1) and transforming growth factor-β1 (TGF-β1), interleukin-1β (IL-1β), and interleukin-6 (IL-6) by the cells. The main source of fibrogenic factors is type II alveolar epithelial cells. These factors are capable enough to initiate the following set of processes such as:

- Activation of fibroblasts into myofibroblasts
- Recruitment of fibroblasts to the fibrotic foci

- Stimulation of uncontrolled proliferation of alveolar epithelial (type II) cells
- Transdifferentiation of pulmonary fibroblasts into myofibroblasts

Due to the unnecessary deposition of extracellular matrix in the interstitial tissues (thin layer of interstitial space lying between the capillary endothelium and the alveolar epithelium) and basement membranes, there would be considerable changes in three-dimensional scaffold of the alveolar wall, leading to loss of their function, mainly exchange of gas between alveoli and capillaries. This unnecessary deposition of extracellular matrix is due to the overactivation of myofibroblasts. These cascades of events affect ventilation capacity of lungs, which may ultimately affect the overall performance of lungs [60]. Overdeposition of extracellular matrix can lead to higher production or low breakdown of ECM or both. Pulmonary fibrosis is a pulmonary pathological condition, and represents activation and proliferation of fibroblasts, leading to the instability of extracellular matrix protein accumulation. Extent of expression and deposition of collagen regulate ECM accumulation. Thus, overexpression of collagen usually results in lung fibrosis. Collagen types including type (I, III, and VI) are responsible for pulmonary fibrotic scars. Both fibronectins and plasminogen activators are involved in damage to extracellular matrix, out of which the plasminogen activator causes more deterioration of extracellular matrix. Plasminogen activity is mediated by plasminogen activator inhibitor 1, the expression of which is often increased among fibrotic lungs of patients. An investigation on mouse model of pulmonary fibrosis revealed that plasminogen activator inhibitor 1 gene deletion can decrease the vulnerability of rodent against pulmonary fibrosis, while overexpression of plasminogen activator inhibitor 1 protein increases the extent of lung fibrosis. This indicates that PAI-1 plays an important role in the development of lung fibrosis [62]. Other than this protein, additional proteases including matrix metalloproteinases, disintegrin, as well as metalloproteinase domain also cause the degradation of extracellular matrix. On the other hand, tissue inhibitors of metalloproteinases speed up extracellular matrix deposition by neutralizing matrix metalloproteinases activities [63]. Increase in the expression of tissue inhibitors of metalloproteinases and then matrix metalloproteinases in fibrotic lungs of patients suggested that during pulmonary fibrosis, the overall extracellular matrix breakdown is decreased [63].

7.6.1 Role of Transforming Growth Factor-beta in SARS-Stimulated Fibrosis of Lungs

7.6.1.1 Transforming Growth Factor-β (TGF-β) Signaling Pathway

Transforming growth factor-beta is a superfamily of multifunctional cytokines that elicit their effects on cells such as growth as well as differentiation of the cell migration and changes in extracellular matrix along with cellular death. Mutational inactivation or dysregulated expression of TGF-β signaling can lead to an array of human disorders including cardiovascular disorders, cancer, and tissue fibrosis. TGF-β signaling is commenced by the binding of TGF-β to TβRI and TβRII. TGF-β transduces signals through single-pass transmembrane receptors.

7.6.1.2 The Impact of TGF-β Activation on Lung Fibrosis

Various transgenic animal models suggest the role of TGF-β stimulation in pulmonary fibrosis. Adenovirus vectors-mediated complementary DNA (isolated from TGF-β) transfer to rodent lung revealed that temporary TGF-β1 overexpression leads to the acute pulmonary fibrosis [64]. Another animal model suggested the role of soluble TGF-β type II receptor with extracellular domain as a TGF-β antagonist to suppress lung fibrosis [65]. The detection of considerable levels of TGF-β mRNA and TGF-β protein in lung fibrotic tissue indicates TGF-β activation-mediated lung fibrosis [66]. Further, TGF-β is responsible for the accumulation of extracellular matrix proteins by eliciting the ECM protein production, increasing the secretion of protease inhibitor as well as decreasing the proteases secretion. Thus, the suppression of TGF-β expression or dysregulating TGF-β pathways events may perhaps prevent matrix production and inhibit pulmonary fibrosis in animal [66].

TGF-β1 can also elevate pulmonary fibrosis via spreading out of myofibroblast populations, which are considered as important effector cells in lung fibrogenesis responsible for increase in extracellular matrix production. TGF-β is directly involved in the differentiation of lung fibroblasts into myofibroblasts. TGF-β1-mediated differentiation of fibroblasts involves sequential events in which epithelial cells experience alterations to produce fibroblasts, which are further differentiated into myofibroblasts. This process is known as epithelial–mesenchymal transition. TGF-β1-mediated epithelial–mesenchymal transition of alveolar epithelial cells was reported in both in vitro and in animal models. Co-expression of epithelial and mesenchymal markers in a cell derived from biopsy sample of fibrotic lungs suggested the subsistence of the epithelial–mesenchymal transition state in fibrotic lungs [67]. Thus, this and many other reports revealed that the TGF-β activation plays an important role in lung fibrotic processes via multiple mechanisms.

7.6.1.3 Transforming Growth Factor-beta and SARS-Induced Pulmonary Fibrosis

Considering the impact of TGF-β in causing fibrosis, upregulation of TGF-β expression or TGF-β-modulated signaling due to viral infection has been reported in various tissues [68]. Increase in TGF-β1 level in the early phase of SARS was reported during SARS-CoV infection. As per the previous report, SARS-CoV-infected pulmonary cells such as alveolar and bronchial epithelial cells and monocytes/macrophages showed higher levels of TGF-β than uninfected pulmonary cells [69]. Virus infection also causes increase in TGF-β ligand number *in situ* and in serum, resulting in TGF-β overexpression of the signaling to elevate the pulmonary fibrosis. Nevertheless, the way through which coronavirus alters TGF-β level in tissue is still not clear.

Notably, SARS-CoV also directly modulates TGF-β expression via SARS-CoV nucleocapsid protein. During TGF-β signaling, contact to ligand increases nuclear localization of Smad proteins. These proteins further regulate targeted gene expression. The viral nucleocapsid protein, a protein that binds to RNA, can interact with Smad3, thereby preventing the complex formation between Smad3 and Smad4 [70]. In addition, SARS-CoV N proteins encourage the association among transcriptional co-activator p300 and Smad3 to trigger genes toward the 3′ end. Overexpression of nucleocapsid protein stimulates the TGF-β-mediated expression of collagen I as well as PAI-1, and this stimulation of TGF-β-mediated activation of collagen I as well as PAI-1 is independent of Smad4. Notably, nucleocapsid protein reduces Smad4-mediated cell programmed death, which corroborates with the fact that nucleocapsid protein not present in the cells underwent programmed cell death [70]. Therefore, SARS-CoV can encourage pulmonary fibrosis by its nucleocapsid protein.

7.6.2 Possible Role of ACE2/Angiotensin II in Lung Injury Caused by SARS

The renin–angiotensin II system, abbreviated as RAS, plays an important role in fluid homeostasis and regulation of blood pressure. Angiotensin-converting enzyme (ACE) is an ectoenzyme that plays a critical role in the production of angiotensin II (Ang II) by catalyzing the extracellular conversion from decapeptide Ang I, which has no therapeutic effects. ACE2 is a newly described novel angiotensin-converting enzyme homologue that reduced the level of Ang II via breakdown of Ang II. ACE2 works in an opposite manner in comparison with ACE in order to decrease the level of Ang II. In the pulmonary system, the ACE2 protein shows its expression in airway epithelial cells and tracheal epithelial cell [71]. It has been reported that ACE2 provides protection against lung fibrosis via restricting the local deposition of the profibrotic peptide Ang II. In addition, ACE2 also has a protective effect against a range of other lung diseases. In one report, lung biopsy sample derived from individuals with pulmonary fibrosis revealed a decrease in mRNA level of ACE2 and activity of the enzyme. ACE2 protects lungs from pulmonary fibrosis via negative regulation of the local Ang II level, which is reported for stimulating the synthesis as well as release of TGF-β cytokine in tissue and upregulating connective tissue growth factor [72]. Connective tissue growth factor can further encourage the accumulation of extracellular matrix as well as pulmonary fibrosis via the Ras-Raf-MEK-ERK pathway.

Several investigations have confirmed that ACE2 acts as key binding site for SARS-CoV. As mentioned earlier, alveolar epithelial cells in lungs are enriched with ACE2 proteins, which are considered as main targets of SARS-CoV. Therefore, ACE2 is not only responsible for providing protection to lungs against lung fibrosis but also acts as an important cellular receptor for viral invasion and infection. Notably, the expression of ACE2 protein is reduced during SARS-CoV infection (by the spike protein) and leads to the increase in Ang II level, which can subsequently cause lung fibrosis, and ultimately, the development of pulmonary fibrosis can result in the failure of lung. A previous study on an *in vivo* model of Ace2 knockout mice revealed that spike protein administration does not influence the progression of respiratory failure. In addition, spike protein administration in rodent model results in considerable increase in Ang II expression in the lung tissue. Thus, ARBs can prevent pathogenicity caused by spike protein [73]. In conclusion, SARS-CoV spike protein downregulates ACE2 expression on cells, thereby causing upregulation of Ang II and triggering TGF-β pathways and subsequently causing severe organ injury.

7.6.3 Possible Pathways of SARS-Mediated Pulmonary Fibrosis

In addition to TGF-β and ACE2 mediated pathways, there are other possible pathways that can be followed by SARS virus to cause lung fibrosis. One pathway that is based on MCP-1, pro-inflammatory chemokine, may play a significant role in promoting lung fibrosis. MCP-1 level was found to be increased among patients with pulmonary fibrosis [74]. Upregulation of the MCP-1 level has been reported among SARS-CoV-infected patients. Sudden increase in MCP-1 level takes place 2 weeks after disease inception. As far as the treatment is concerned, treatment with corticosteroid downregulates monocyte chemoattractant protein-1level.

The p38 MAPK signaling and its expression play an important role in the release of pro-inflammatory cytokines including IL-6. p38 MAPK expression is also associated with acute lung injury and myocardial dysfunction. As per previous reports, p38 MAPK is often activated during viral infection; however, in some of the reports, it was found that viral proteins sometimes downregulate p38 MAPK. Therefore, the stimulation or inactivation of p38 MAPK signaling or its expression determines the progression of viral infection. MAPK p38 activation in reponse to the viral infection regulates cell differentiation and ECM production. Sample analysis of lung fibrosis patients revealed that the hyperactivation of p38 and p38 phosphorylation was responsible for lung myofibroblast activation and α-SMA expression [75]. It was also suggested that p38 phosphorylation mediated by SARS-CoV in pulmonary epithelial resulted in restructuring of actin. Thus, these reports suggested the possible involvement of p38 in SARS-CoV-facilitated pulmonary fibrosis.

7.7 Organ Cross-talk

Organ cross-talk is can demonstrate the development of multi-organ dysfunction syndrome. Abnormalities or dysfunction or infection of an independent organ can impact the physiological condition of other organs leading to multiorgan dysfunction or failure. For instance, acute kidney injury can lead to multiple-organ failure leading to high mortality rate [76–79]. The primary cause of acute kidney injury is ischemia–reperfusion injury that provokes the release of proinflammatory mediators with serious systemic implications for remote organ injury [76–79].

Previous reports suggested close association between lungs (alveoli) and renal (tubular) impairment in ARDS patients.

A recent report based on 357 ARDS patients who did not have a previous history of chronic kidney disease before ARDS presentation revealed that acute pneumonia was the main reason for ARDS among 83% of patients; however, 68% of patients presented acute kidney injury [76–79]. It was also observed that developed acute kidney injury was found to be severe (Stage 3) among half of patients. Many factors are directly associated with acute kidney injury development such as comorbidity (e.g., cardiac complications, diabetes mellitus, and positive fluid balance), age, and severity of illness [76–79]. All these factors are associated with worse health outcomes and more complex clinical management. The severity of acute kidney injury is directly linked with older age, diabetes mellitus, previous cardiac complications, obesity, elevated peak inspiratory pressures, and elevated score of sequential organ failure assessment. No association of positive end-expiratory pressure (PEEP), nephrotoxic agents, and prone position with kidney impairment has been found [76–79]. Overproduction of proinflammatory cytokines and its direct association with bidirectional damage of lung and kidney have also been reported. As suggested earlier, renal damage, mainly tubular epithelium damage, upregulates the production of IL-6. Several reports also suggest that acute kidney injury elevates IL-6 level in serum, which can enhance alveolar-capillary permeability and subsequently increase the risk of pulmonary hemorrhage. ARDS also might cause renal medullary hypoxia, which is an additional insult to renal tubular cells. However, implications of IL-6 over acute kidney injury and lung epithelial cells and lung endothelial cells should be further explored. Another study from China including 201 COVID-19 patients with pneumonia revealed that 41.8% developed ARDS and 4.5% developed acute kidney injury. It was noted that older age, cardiac complications, hypertension, and diabetes were associated with ARDS development [76–79]. However, the high level of IL-6 in serum was not associated with ARDS; it was associated with high mortality among patients who developed ARDS. In one more investigation including 41 patients with confirmed COVID-19 pneumonia, 27% patients presented ARDS and 7% showed acute kidney injury. Thus, IL-6 level can be considered as a marker to relate acute kidney injury and ARDS. It was also observed that the level of IL-6 was almost comparable among ICU (39%) patients and those not admitted to ICU, while IL-10 level in plasma was high among ICU patients. The prevalence of acute kidney injury was found to be higher among patients with ARDS due to pneumonia with other causes (68%) than ARDS patients due to severe COVID pneumonia (4.5%) [76–79]. Cross-talk between heart and kidney can also lead to acute kidney injury among COVID-19 patients. Cardiac complications such as acute cardiorenal syndrome cardiomyopathy and acute viral myocarditis can lead to acute kidney injury due to low blood pressure, increased venous pressure (renal congestion), and renal hypoperfusion, resulting in decrease in glomerular performance. Lifesaving interventions for critically ill patients such as extracorporeal membrane oxygenation (extracorporeal life support system) can be used to provide cardiac as well as respiratory support and can be used in conjugation with continuous kidney replacement therapy [76–79].

7.8 CNS Complications Associated with SARS-CoV-2

Several reports are available that support that SARS-CoV-2 infection affects the central nervous system (CNS) in addition to other organs/systems. Recently, a number of secondary symptoms caused by viral infection in the nervous system have been identified such as fever, pain in any region of the head, nausea, vomiting, feeling faint, muscle aches as well as pain and fatigue. These symptoms are in addition to the primary symptoms of respiratory viral infection such as fever, coldness accompanied by shivering cough, production of phlegm, shortness of breath, irritation of the throat, vomiting, nausea, and congestion in the respiratory tract. However, some clinical symptoms are perhaps due to digestive system upset or disturbances in nervous system resulting in nausea and vomiting. These symptoms if in case are present with constant head pain or intracranial hypertension might be linked with infection of the CNS. Several studies have suggested that coronavirus 2 has the ability to cause infection in the nervous system. An observational research based on investigation of 214 hospitalized COVID-19 individuals in China revealed that 36.4% of individuals presented nervous system complications such as stroke or severe cerebrovascular infection, impaired perception, and injury of skeletal muscle as well as CNS-related symptoms, including nausea, hypogeusia, dizziness, hyposmia, and pain in head [80]. One patient also experienced maxillofacial musculoskeletal disease with constant hiccups after the onset of illness. Findings from cerebrospinal fluid analysis of the same patient revealed high pressure (330 mmH_2O), and later on, patient was diagnosed with inflammation of the brain. Massively parallel or deep sequencing of cerebrospinal fluid revealed the presence of COVID-19 infection in the CNS [81]. One more case of brain inflammation triggered by coronavirus 2 has been published [82]. Neurological manifestations such as stiffness in the neck, transient generalized seizures, unconsciousness on the 9th day after the inception of symptoms, and high pressure of cerebrospinal fluid (320 mmH_2O) suggest CNS involvement during COVID-19 infection. Surprisingly, specific SARS-CoV-2 RNA was not detected in the nasopharyngeal swab but was detected in a CSF [82]. This case of meningitis associated with SARS-CoV-2 suggested the direct involvement of the brain during the COVID-19 infection. Moreover, anti-herpes simplex virus 1 as well as varicella-zoster antibodies were not found in the samples of serum. Radiological examination based on MRI of the brain revealed possible signs of SARS-CoV-2 meningitis. This issue can be considered as caution for the patients who have CNS symptoms. Other reports suggested the development of neurological associated symptoms like dizziness, fatigue, and insanity with some common symptoms like headache, nausea, and vomiting [80]. Based on recent investigations, several neurological manifestations such as inflammation of the brain, inflammation of the meninges, ischemic as well as hemorrhagic stroke have been identified among SARS-CoV-2-infected patients [80].

Cerebrovascular disease has high incidence, disability rate, and fatality rate, and considering all neurological complications, acute cerebrovascular disease has been found to be more common among COVID-19 patients. COVID-19 patient outcomes may also be complicated with acute stroke.

Earlier reports based on SARS outbreak revealed that symptoms related to psychological disturbances such as stress, post-traumatic stress disorder, anxiety, and depression were found among SARS survivors [83]. Sudden execution of unprecedented firm quarantine measures, social distancing, and other strict precautionary protocols across the world have kept a number of people in isolation and influenced a lot of aspects of people's lives. At the same time, it has also caused several psychological complications including panic disorder, anxiety, and depression. COVID-19 outbreak has caused serious risks to the physical and mental health of people, even more than the SARS epidemic. COVID-19 has caused significant distress with negative psychological outcomes around the globe, which should be considered seriously [84]. Psychological complications, including anxiety, distress, sleep disorder, and depression, have been reported with some cases of mental derangement (9%). Recently, psychological investigation of 89 COVID-19 patients revealed that 52% had no psychological symptoms, 35% had only mild symptoms, whereas 13 had moderate to severe symptoms [85]. The psychological effect of COVID-19 over mental and health balance in terms of anxiety was examined in 230 medical staff, and it was found that the prevalence of anxiety was about 23%, whereas the occurrence of acute anxiety, moderate as well as mild anxiety was almost between 2% and 16%. It was also found that in comparison with anxiety, the incidence of stress conditions between hospital officials was higher (27%), wherein females had higher prevalence than men [86]. One more study reported psychological problems such as anticipation, irritability, unwillingness to sleep, and emotional distress among medical staff. During SARS upsurge, post-traumatic stress disorder and psychological distress were observed among hospitalized individuals and medical care workers. Thus, during the COVID-19 outbreak, psychological as well as neurological disorders have been major concerns among hospitalized individuals and medical staff, which can lead to inadequate prognosis, exacerbated medical state, and unexpected loss of life.

7.8.1 Possible Mechanisms of Neurological Complications Caused by SARS-CoV-2

Due to the 79.5% resemblance of genomic material (sequences of the RNA) among SARS-CoV as well as SARS-CoV-2 [87], the mechanisms of infection followed by SARS-CoV-2 might be related to SARS-CoV infection. As mentioned before, ACE2, a membrane protein, showed more expression over cells on the surface of many cell types [88] and is considered as a main focus for the treatment of SARS-CoV infection. ACE2 is expressed in several cell types and tissues such as the lungs, heart, blood vessels, kidneys, liver, and GIT. ACE2 is a hydrolytic enzyme that produces small proteins by the cleavage of the large protein angiotensinogen. After cleavage, these small proteins enter to regulate the functions in the cell. One investigation revealed that ACE2 is identified as an active protein for the invasion of SARS-CoV-2 and is used by the virus surface spike-like protein to bind and for the further invasion into infected cells. Thus, ACE2 is considered as a receptor in the form of cellular doorway for the entry of virus into cells that causes COVID-19. However, this process of virus binding to ACE-2 and its invasion involves multiple events, which are mediated by type II transmembrane serine proteases TMPRSS2 and histone acetyltransferase HAT enzymes. These proteases cleave and activate the spike protein (S) of the SARS-CoV for membrane fusion. Moreover, these proteases also cleave the ACE2, and it is suspected that ACE2 breakdown enhances viral infectivity. Just like influenza virus, binding with ACE2 and cleavage done by proteases allows the virus to cause infection and shed its RNA from the host to transmit; however, its mechanism of detachment is not like SARS-CoV [89]. After specific binding between the S protein of coronavirus and ACE2 receptor, the virus enters into infected cells via clathrin-mediated endocytosis. Different coronaviruses can use different cell receptors to complete the invasion. Due to the strong binding between SARS-CoV-2 and ACE2, pathogenicity and transmissibility of SARS-CoV-2 are more dominant than SARS-CoV and MERS-CoV [89].

Earlier reports suggested that under physiological conditions, ACE2 and its receptors are also present in the CNS neurons of glial cells [88]. It was also found that ACE2 is an enzyme that is expressed almost all over the brain and particularly in the areas of controlling central BP. However, in comparison with lungs, ACE2 expression is low in the brain. In a mouse model, it was clear that cell membrane protein ACE2 and protease TMPRSS2 are expressed in sustentacular cells of the olfactory epithelium; however, their expression is very low in most olfactory receptor neurons, which suggests direct involvement of sustentacular cells during SARS-CoV-2 infection, resulting in the impairment of the sense of smell in COVID-19 patients. Due to the presence of ACE2 in the CNS, there might always be a possibility of SARS-CoV-2 invasion via ACE2 leading to injury in brain and neurological manifestations. Since an important function of ACE2 in the brain is the central regulation of cardiovascular function, virus binding with ACE2 localized in the brain can lead to cardiovascular or cerebrovascular complications. Based on the previous studies, binding of surface protein to the neuronal ACE2 receptor and TMPRSS2-mediated activation of the spike protein facilitates virus invasion into the neuron. Moreover, it is also known that endothelial cells that lines the blood vessels are enriched with a high level of ACE2, which can facilitate SARS-CoV-2 invasion into endothelial cells and subsequently invade to the cerebral blood vessels via ACE2 receptor and disrupt the blood–brain barrier (BBB). These cascades of events lead to the increase in permeability of the BBB, cerebral edema or microhemorrhages, and intracranial hypertension. Brain or cerebrospinal fluid analysis recently suggested the presence of CoV, which can cause inflammation that resulted in intracranial hypertension. As per previous reports, downregulation of ACE2 causes neuroinflammation and BBB disruption, which can further enhance the expression of the TMPRSS2 and cathepsin L. Viral invasion also leads to the upregulation of proinflammatory genes, which can lead to excess production of cytokines/chemokines with the production of reactive oxygen species (ROS). These sequential events can lead to the progression of SARS-CoV-2-induced cerebral injury. Moreover, abnormal regulation of hormones and neurotransmitters can be considered as primary mechanism of the neuropathogenic condition of SARS-CoV-2 neuroinvasion. In addition, damage to BBB induced by SARS-CoV-2 can further support invasion into brain tissues and neurons. This pathway of coronavirus invasion into brain is followed by many coronaviruses [90]. Since ACE2 and TMPRSS2 are present in human hypothalamic neurons, tanycytes, and olfactory sensory neurons, a recent report based on the samples collected from cortical neurons as well as hypothalamus of patients with SARS suggested the detection of SARS-CoV, which can result in neuronal histopathological changes. Besides virus invasion via blood vessels, viruses can also invade into CNS through the terminals of the olfactory nerve. Notably, axoplasmic flow also promotes the fast spread from neuron to neuron [91]. Recent publication revealed that more or less no viral presence was identified in nonneuronal cells in infected brain areas [92]. Thus, brain injury can be due to neuroinflammation caused by the cytokines released by the infected neurons. This may occur mainly when there is invasion of virus in the nervous system of the infected patients (i.e., with low immunity). Pathogenies of SARS-CoV-2 is enlisted below:

- SARS-CoV-2 invasion inside the brain can be mediated via olfactory nerve endings, and thereby, SARS-CoV-2 directly binds to surface receptors (ACE2 protein) of neurons. This binding is regulated by serine protease enzyme TMPRSS2 for S protein priming. Axonal transport can encourage the fast transmission of SARS-CoV-2 from neurons to neurons. In addition, this viral invasion subsequently results in cytokine production, which ultimately causes damage to surroundings neurons and glial cells.
- SARS-CoV-2 shows high binding affinity toward ACE2, a protein that shows its expression among endothelial cells, disrupting endothelial cells and the BBB and resulting in an increase in intracranial pressure inside brain, which can further result in intracranial hypertension.
- Anti-SARS-CoV-2 IgG, IgM, and IgA antibodies produced by humoral immune response to SARS-CoV-2 infection, mainly against SARS-CoV-2 nucleoprotein and spike (S) protein antigens, play an important role in neutralizing and preventing further transmission of the infection. However, the underlying mechanism of the humeral response against SARS-CoV-2 is not completely understood; usually, IgM antibodies are produced at the early stages of infection, whereas IgG participates in immune reaction later to set up long-term immune memory. Previous investigations also revealed that IgA mainly exists in the mucosal tissue and may play an important role during the viral infection. These anti-SARS-CoV-2 IgG, IgM, and IgA antibodies unusually can act as autoantibodies and possibly attack endothelial cells that form the inner lining of blood vessels and also attack neurons, leading to autoimmune encephalitis.
- There is also the possibility of stress-induced behavioral changes mediated by the activation and release of corticotrophin-releasing factor, which stimulates the release of adrenocorticotropic hormone from the pituitary gland. Stimulation of hypothalamic–pituitary–adrenal axis led to the hyperstimulation of the glucocorticoid synthesis and its release from the zona fasciculate to regulate physiological changes and show different behaviors. Stress can be directly caused by SARS-CoV-2 infection or by anxiety due to the outbreak. This can also turn into oxidative stress phase due to the overproduction of ROS, which can further increase the severity of neuroinflammation caused by cytokines. Simultaneously, stress caused by several environmental factors due to COVID-19 outbreak leads to the epigenetic changes of stress-associated genes, which subsequently result in unusual gene expression. This atypical gene expression results in psychiatric disorders including anxiety, psychiatric symptoms, depression, or post-traumatic stress disorder.

Several reports are available that show how autoimmune encephalitis takes place when antibodies of host by mistake attack its own healthy neurons, leading to neuroinflammation with various neurologic and/or psychiatric manifestations [93]. Autoimmune reaction can be triggered by various factors such as genetic predisposition, viral disease, and traumatic conditions and hyperimmune response of the host itself or pathogen-mediated hyperimmune responses [94].

SARS-CoV-associated antibodies produced by the host against the CoV surface protein were found to react with human epithelial cells and endothelial cells [95]. This reaction results in the damage of epithelial cells and endothelial cells, which can lead to the progression of cytotoxic reaction [95]. As a result, likewise, patients suffering from COVID-19 infection can make antibodies to neutralize the pathogenicity caused by SARS-CoV-2; however, these antibodies can also attack antigenic proteins present among endothelial cells lining cerebral vessels or neurons by disrupting BBB. This may result in increased intracranial pressure, resulting in autoimmune encephalitis. However, these assumptions require more investigation to explore the underlying causes, mechanisms, and potential targets during SARS-CoV-2-mediated brain injury.

7.8.2 Psychosocial Impact of COVID-19

Due to the COVID-19 outbreak, communities across the world have been changed. Strict lockdowns have restricted people to their homes and badly affected their mental and physical health. Reports have suggested that anxiety, depression, and insomnia are the widespread psychological conditions resulting from the COVID-19 pandemic. These adverse psychological reactions with poor mental health outcomes will further progress as long as lockdowns continue. Thus, COVID-19 has the potential to cause permanent psychological disorders, and it is very important to identify how the virus affects mental health.

Early reports suggested that the psychological impact of quarantine includes panic of spreading infection, anxiety, depression, insomnia, annoyance, confusion, irritation, isolation, and even extremes such as suicide. Isolated people can also experience anxiety due to doubt related to health status and develop intrusive thoughts and compulsive behavior including frequent temperature monitoring and sanitization. Development of more severe complications such as post-traumatic stress disorder has been identified, manifestations of which have been linked with the period of quarantine. Psychological disorders after quarantine may include various socioeconomic factors, which can further aggravate psychological illness. The post-quarantine phase may also lead to public rejection and non-acceptance of recovered patients, which can further promote discrimination, suspicion, and avoidance in communities.

7.8.2.1 Psychiatric Manifestations of COVID-19

Psychological disorders during the COVID-19 pandemic can lead to the secretion of stressor-dependent corticotrophin-releasing hormone from hypothalamus in people. Stimulation of hypothalamic paraventricular nucleus in hypothalamus can subsequently stimulate the hypothalamic–pituitary–adrenal axis after interacting with the corticotrophin-releasing hormone proteins in the pituitary gland (anterior). This binding of corticotrophin-releasing hormone with their respective proteins in the pituitary gland (anterior lobe) further increases the secretion of adrenocorticotropic hormone in serum [96]. Rise in serum adrenocorticotropic hormone level further increases glucocorticoids level in the systemic circulation [97]. These systemic glucocorticoids ultimately bind to glucocorticoid receptors present in various organs such as the brain [98]. Hyperstimulation of hypothalamic–pituitary–adrenal axis can lead to the overproduction of effectors glucocorticoids, which can promote its binding with glucocorticoid receptors. This binding can lead to the overexpression or dysfunction of stress-related gene, which may be responsible for the development of different behaviors [98]. Dysfunction of stress-related gene elevates the vulnerability of several genes against environmental stress resulting in polymorphism of genes such as SERT, FKBP5, CRHR1, etc. Environmental stress-dependent epigenetic modifications of these genes use various possible ways such as methylation of DNA, changes in chromatinmaterial, and deacetylation of histone protein. These epigenetic modifications of several genes ultimately cause the transcriptional modifications of their genetic expression, leading to various stress-related disorders. In conclusion, harsh environmental stress such as mental stress can lead to the development of various psychiatric disorders via the stimulation of the hypothalamic–pituitary–adrenal axis to heritable in stress-related genes. In addition, mental stress can also enhance vulnerability to SARS-CoV-2 infection and elevate the severity of the disease process [99].

7.8.3 Neurological Manifestations of COVID-19 and Their Treatment

SARS-CoV can cause considerable neurological complications via targeting neurons. As is seen in several reports of neuro-invasion as well as neurodegeneration caused by SARS Cov-2, this virus causes considerable neurological complications. Recently, the neuroinvasive and neurodegeneration-like potential of COVID-19 is well reported. As reported, CoV can be present in the brain or cerebrospinal fluid. Pathophysiology of neuroinvasive viruses including coronaviruses is still not understood clearly, and as a result, it is essential to discover the exact mechanisms by which it causes pathogenesis in the brain. As far as the treatment is concerned, at the moment, the most reliable treatment during this pandemic is vaccines against COVID-19 [100]; nevertheless, the development of safe and effective vaccine candidate usually takes some time. Thus, it is essential to explore the other approaches such as drug repurposing, natural products-based treatment, and testing of earlier treatments, which were proved to be effective against SARS-CoV or other coronaviruses, combination therapy, antibodies-based treatment, exploration of important class of drugs such as antibiotics, antiviral, immunomodulatory, and antimalarial. Until now, none of the effective treatments has been developed. On the other hand, much progress has been seen in the development of diagnostics for coronaviruses. Neuroimaging (radiological techniques such advanced MRI, CT scan) and cerebrospinal fluid examination can be more reliable in the diagnosis of the extent of damage caused by virus in the brain. Previous reports suggested that medications used for CNS infection caused by virus demonstrated less penetration in the CNS and as a result showed less promising results (Figure 7.3). This much concentration was found to be less effective in inhibiting or preventing viral RNA replication. Drug analysis of these CNS-acting drugs demonstrated

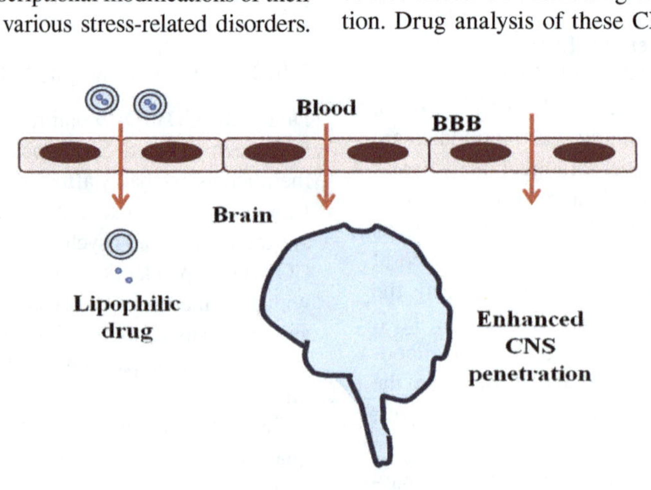

FIGURE 7.3 Therapeutic strategies to improve drug delivery across the BBB.

that these medications have lower log P values (partition coefficient), which is considered as an important parameter for CNS penetration and thus was not capable to cross the BBB. The low log P value may be because of the existence of additional water-soluble atoms such as O, N, S, P, and F in functional groups. Delay in antibiotic, antiviral, or other suitable drug treatment can lead to the worst disease outcomes mainly in the case of bacterial meningitis and herpes simplex virus encephalitis.

In 2005, SARS-CoV neuroinvasion and its associated pathogenesis including polyneuropathy, encephalitis, and aortic ischemic stroke [101] have been reported. Postmortem examination of SARS patients revealed pathological signs of cerebral edema and meningeal vasodilation. In addition, monocytes and lymphocytes infiltration within blood vessel wall, changes of neurons due to ischemia, damage to the myelin sheath surrounding nerve fiber, and presence of SARS-CoV virus particles and genome sequences in the nervous system have been reported [102].

Acute transverse myelitis (inflammation of the spinal cord), viral encephalitis and meningitis, infectious toxic encephalopathy (acute toxic encephalitis), acute hemorrhagic necrotizing encephalopathy (cerebral white matter, brain stem, and cerebellum are affected), and leukoencephalopathy (group of diseases that affect the white matter of the CNS) are some of the neurological manifestations experienced by coronavirus patients. After appearance and diagnosis of CNS manifestations in SARS-CoV-2 associated illness, immediately suitable antiviral medications with other life supportive care system must be provided to recover and alleviate the physiological conditions of the brain. More monitoring and attention must be given to reduce intracranial pressure caused by hypertension (within the cranium) by administering dehydrating agents including mannitol and furosemide. It has been also suggested that CNS infection caused by COVID-19 was in some measure responsible for acute respiratory failure in patients (Li et al. [92]). Thus, it is important to provide immediate treatment and supportive care to patients suffering from CNS infection to prevent respiratory complications and severe respiratory failure in addition to further improve the likely course of COVID-19. Moreover, the imbalance caused due to COVID-19 must be reduced to avoid aggravation of the disease [103]. Polytherapy including combination of medication and psychotherapy may improve healing efficiency and offer better outcomes [103]. A number of investigators have reported combination therapy. One study of 69 patients revealed an effectiveness rate of treatment of 82.3% [103].

7.9 COVID-19 and Its Systemic Effects

As has been reported, there is a possible association between blood type and a higher risk for COVID-19 infection and mortality. Zhao et al. found probable correlation between blood group A and significant possibility for SARS-CoV-2 infection and death rate, whereas blood type O was correlated with a minimum possibility of infection and death rate. Zietz and Tatonetti reported that blood group A was associated with higher odds of testing positive for disease [104]. Various reports suggested that SARS infection can cause hematological changes such as lymphopenia, thrombocytopenia, and leukopenia. These hematological changes might be due to:

- Direct infection of blood cells and bone marrow stromal cells mediated by CD13 or CD66a
- Destruction caused by auto-antibodies

Moreover, injury to lungs in SARS patients can also cause thrombocytopenia due to:

- Increase in the utilization of platelets
- Decreased production of platelets in the lungs

As lymphopenia and immunodeficiency are the most common hematological changes experienced by SARS patients, these patients can be possibly treated with hematopoietic growth factors to stimulate the immune system against these viruses.

Renin–angiotensin–aldosterone system activation can increase sodium uptake by the renal system, which may result in the decreased loss of water into the urine and ultimately lead to increase in blood volume. Patients with sepsis or shock often experience blood volume expansion, which can result in positive fluid balance. This expansion of blood volume can lead to the worst outcomes among ARDS patients, because it promotes alveolar-capillary leakage, whereas in acute kidney injury patients, the expansion of blood volume further aggravates renal vein congestion due to the elevation of renal vein pressure, resulting in renal compartment syndrome. One researcher suggested a correlation between rhabdomyolysis, metabolic acidosis, and hyperkalemia with COVID-19 due to hemodynamic instability.

7.9.1 Cytokine-Induced Damage

COVID-19 patients often experience inflammation of alveoli leading to interstitial pneumonia, which can subsequently lead to ARDS and SIRS (systemic inflammatory response syndrome). There are a number of factors that can aggravate ARDS as well as SIRS, out of which comorbidity is one of the common causes for the progression of acute COVID-19 associated systemic inflammatory response. Cardiac complications and diabetes (type 2) are considered as the most common comorbidities among COVID-19 patients who require hospitalization. In this context, enhanced expression of one more protein, known as human dipeptidyl peptidase 4, among type 2 diabetes patients has been reported. As this can enhance the expression of human dipeptidyl peptidase-4 which can lead to most undesirable effect as it can increase possibility of SARS-CoV-2 to cause infection at cellular level via binding to dipeptidyl peptidase-4 protein. The similar pathways it is already reported during MERS-CoV infection.

The cytokine storm is a condition in which there is hyperproduction of pro-inflammatory cytokines. It is considered as the main cause of death and also responsible for worsening disease outcomes. The cytokine storm is seen in various diseases triggered by pathogenic coronaviruses. During this event, inflammatory cytokines (IL-6, IL-10, and TNF-α) secreted by macrophages increase in patients, which can often augment the severity of COVID-19 infection, leading to injury to multiple organs but mainly the lungs. Recent reports showed that SARS-CoV-2 patients have presented some stages of inflammatory markers including serum amyloid A, erythrocyte sedimentation rate, C-reactive protein, and procalcitonin. Nevertheless, less focus has been given to ferritin and finding a correlation between ferritin level and COVID-19 pathogenesis. Ferritin is a pro-inflammatory mediator responsible for release of pro-inflammatory molecules; however, it works in an opposite manner as a pro-inflammatory and as an immunosuppressant. In vitro studies revealed that ferritin can be vigorously released by hepatic cells and macrophages via non-classical pathways.

One publication suggested an association between COVID-19-induced inflammatory reaction and hyperferritinemic syndromes. Both events are interlinked with each other in terms of the overproduction of IL-1βs in systemic circulation. There is an overproduction of cytokine (i.e., IL-1βs that are associated with hyperferritinemia), suggesting that COVID-19 is part of the hyperferritinemic syndrome spectrum. To discover this correlation, levels of serum ferritin among infected individuals with severe and non-severe COVID-19 infection, and other inflammatory markers can be evaluated. While going through some reports based on ferritin examinations in COVID-19 patients, it was found that the level of ferritin is usually in the normal range (ferritin concentration 30–400 μg/L) among individuals with non-severe infection, whereas the increased level of ferritin (ferritin concentration >400 μg/L) was found in patients with acute illness on hospitalization. This condition is called hyperferritinemia. Actually, the average level of ferritin was found to be >800 μg/L among patients with severe disease. Furthermore, during the admission of patients with severe disease, the concentration of ferritin was found to be 5.3 times greater than patients with less severe COVID-19 disease. The severity of COVID-19 can be correlated with high concentration of ferritin 1,400 μg/L in non-survivors, which is four times higher than that found in surviving COVID-19 patients. Simultaneously, these researchers also observed the high concentration of serum cytokines including IL-6, which are mainly high among the patients those who have developed severe disease. It was also found that in contrast to discharged patients, higher levels of ferritin and IL-6 were found among non-survivors. On the contrary, a considerable drop in the level of ferritin and IL-6 concentrations was found once patients started to recover. This evidence may establish a clear relationship between the co-emergence of inflammatory state during COVID-19 infection and hyperferritinemia; thus, both may directly be associated with each other. As a result, ferritin can be a considered as an important inflammatory marker to forecast disease progression along with the level of the cytokine storm.

In spite of its vigorous release during the cytokine storm, the main part of serum ferritin can be obtained during cellular death, mainly during hepatic cell death. After secretion, ferritin gives up central iron part, resulting in high proportion of free iron in serum. High free iron content in serum, especially during hyperinflammatory state, can lead to worsening of the inflammatory state, which may further lead to noticeable pro-coagulant state. This pro-coagulant state can result in a variety of arterial and venous thromboses by altering morphology of RBC. Also, free iron stimulates fibrin to increase the production of hydroxyl radical, resulting in oxidative stress on red blood cells. Simultaneously, continuous production of fibrin can promote dense clots production responsible for increase risks of stroke development. These fibrin clots are comparatively more resistant to lysis. Thus, medication like Desferal (Deferoxamine, NCT04333550, Iran) is an iron-chelating agent used in the treatment of a condition when excess iron is present in biological fluids, which may help reduce the inflammatory response and ROS production and may promote antiviral activity. Thus, this type of therapeutic approach among COVID-19 patients may be effective.

7.10 Role of Nanomedicine in COVID-19

Novel structure, strains, life cycle in host cells, and functional sites have attracted the attention of various pharma industries to study and discover novel therapeutic agents such as drugs, vaccines, and antibodies to effectively suppress the growth of SARS-CoV-2 [105–125]. One of the most reliable approaches to possibly treating SARS-CoV-2 is nanotechnology for site-specific delivery of a therapeutic agent and to eliminate SARS-CoV-2, and also improve the human immune response [105–125]. Using a nanoparticulate system, the efficacy of new drugs can be improved, toxicity can be reduced, and targeted sustained pulmonary release of drugs can be achieved [105–125]. The development of nano-based immunizations to improve humoral and cellular immune responses can also be done. Polymeric engineered nanoparticles can allow the safe and effective delivery of available therapeutics, which can inhibit early interactions of viral spike glycoprotein with host receptors and disrupt virion construction [105–125]. Recently, nanomedicine has been used to deal with various virus-based infectious diseases, such as SARS-CoV, MERS-CoV, influenza A virus subtype H1N1 (A/H1N1), and, more recently, SARS-CoV-2 [105–125]. Various polymeric nanostructures loaded with antigens and immunostimulatory molecules, ranging from particles, micelles, nanogels, and polymersomes to advanced core–shell structures coated with lipids, cell membranes, or proteins can be used against COVID-19 [105–125].

REFERENCES

1. Zaim S, Chong JH, Sankaranarayanan V, Harky A. COVID-19 and multiorgan response. *Curr Probl Cardiol.* 2020;45(8):100618.
2. Sanyaolu A, Okorie C, Marinkovic A, Patidar R, Younis K, Desai P, Hosein Z, Padda I, Mangat J, Altaf M. Comorbidity and its impact on patients with COVID-19. *SN Compr Clin Med.* 2020:1–8. https://www.ncbi.nlm.nih.gov/pmc/articles/PMC7314621/

3. Guan WJ, Liang WH, Zhao Y, et al. Comorbidity and its impact on 1590 patients with COVID-19 in China: A nationwide analysis. *Eur Respir J.* 2020;55(5):2000547.
4. Wu L, O'Kane AM, Peng H, Bi Y, Motriuk-Smith D, Ren J. SARS-CoV-2 and cardiovascular complications: From molecular mechanisms to pharmaceutical management. *Biochem Pharmacol.* 2020;178:114114.
5. Arentz M, Yim E, Klaff L, Lokhandwala S, Riedo FX, Chong M, Lee M. Characteristics and outcomes of 21 critically Ill patients With COVID-19 in Washington State. *JAMA.* 2020;323(16):1612–1614.
6. Lippi G, Plebani M. Laboratory abnormalities in patients with COVID-2019 infection. *Clin Chem Lab Med.* 2020;58(7):1131–1134.
7. Madjid M, Safavi-Naeini P, Solomon SD, Vardeny O. Potential effects of coronaviruses on the cardiovascular system: A review. *JAMA Cardiol.* 2020;5(7):831–840.
8. Driggin E, Madhavan MV, Bikdeli B, Chuich T, Laracy J, Biondi-Zoccai G, Brown TS, Der Nigoghossian C, Zidar DA, Haythe J, Brodie D, Beckman JA, Kirtane AJ, Stone GW, Krumholz HM, Parikh SA. Cardiovascular considerations for patients, health care workers, and health systems during the COVID-19 pandemic. *J Am Coll Cardiol.* 2020;75(18):2352–2371.
9. Babapoor-Farrokhran S, Gill D, Walker J, Rasekhi RT, Bozorgnia B, Amanullah A. Myocardial injury and COVID-19: Possible mechanisms. *Life Sci.* 2020;253:117723.
10. Gheblawi M, Wang K, Viveiros A, Nguyen Q, Zhong JC, Turner AJ, Raizada MK, Grant MB, Oudit GY. Angiotensin-converting enzyme 2: SARS-CoV-2 receptor and regulator of the renin-angiotensin system: Celebrating the 20th anniversary of the discovery of ACE2. *Circ Res.* 2020;126(10):1456–1474.
11. Guzik TJ, Mohiddin SA, Dimarco A, Patel V, Savvatis K, Marelli-Berg FM, Madhur MS, Tomaszewski M, Maffia P, D'Acquisto F, Nicklin SA, Marian AJ, Nosalski R, Murray EC, Guzik B, Berry C, Touyz RM, Kreutz R, Wang DW, Bhella D, Sagliocco O, Crea F, Thomson EC, McInnes IB. COVID-19 and the cardiovascular system: Implications for risk assessment, diagnosis, and treatment options. *Cardiovasc Res.* 2020;116(10):1666–1687.
12. Ortega-Paz L, Capodanno D, Montalescot G, Angiolillo DJ. Coronavirus disease 2019-associated thrombosis and coagulopathy: Review of the pathophysiological characteristics and implications for antithrombotic management. *J Am Heart Assoc.* 2021;10(3):e019650.
13. Xiong TY, Redwood S, Prendergast B, Chen M. Coronaviruses and the cardiovascular system: Acute and long-term implications. *Eur Heart J.* 2020;41(19):1798–1800.
14. Bansal M. Cardiovascular disease and COVID-19. *Diabetes Metab Syndr.* 2020;14(3):247–250.
15. Chang WT, Toh HS, Liao CT, Yu WL. Cardiac involvement of COVID-19: A comprehensive review. *Am J Med Sci.* 2021;361(1):14–22.
16. Long B, Brady WJ, Koyfman A, Gottlieb M. Cardiovascular complications in COVID-19. *Am J Emerg Med.* 2020;38(7):1504–1507.
17. Liu K, Fang YY, Deng Y, Liu W, Wang MF, Ma JP, Xiao W, Wang YN, Zhong MH, Li CH, Li GC, Liu HG. Clinical characteristics of novel coronavirus cases in tertiary hospitals in Hubei Province. *Chin Med J (Engl).* 2020;133(9):1025–1031.
18. Tang N, Bai H, Chen X, Gong J, Li D, Sun Z. Anticoagulant treatment is associated with decreased mortality in severe coronavirus disease 2019 patients with coagulopathy. *J Thromb Haemost.* 2020;18(5):1094–1099.
19. Zhou F, Yu T, Du R, Fan G, Liu Y, Liu Z, Xiang J, Wang Y, Song B, Gu X, Guan L, Wei Y, Li H, Wu X, Xu J, Tu S, Zhang Y, Chen H, Cao B. Clinical course and risk factors for mortality of adult inpatients with COVID-19 in Wuhan, China: A retrospective cohort study. *Lancet.* 2020;395(10229):1054–1062. Erratum in: *Lancet.* 2020 March 28;395(10229):1038.
20. Tönnesmann E, Kandolf R, Lewalter T. Chloroquine cardiomyopathy: A review of the literature. *Immunopharmacol Immunotoxicol.* 2013;35(3):434–442.
21. Krittanawong C, Kumar A, Hahn J, Wang Z, Zhang HJ, Sun T, Bozkurt B, Ballantyne CM, Virani SS, Halperin JL, Jneid H. Cardiovascular risk and complications associated with COVID-19. *Am J Cardiovasc Dis.* 2020;10(4):479–489.
22. Samidurai A, Das A. Cardiovascular complications associated with COVID-19 and potential therapeutic~strategies. *Int J Mol Sci.* 2020;21(18):6790.
23. Bandyopadhyay D, Akhtar T, Hajra A, Gupta M, Das A, Chakraborty S, Pal I, Patel N, Amgai B, Ghosh RK, Fonarow GC, Lavie CJ, Naidu SS. COVID-19 pandemic: Cardiovascular complications and future implications. *Am J Cardiovasc Drugs.* 2020;20(4):311–324.
24. Zheng YY, Ma YT, Zhang JY, Xie X. COVID-19 and the cardiovascular system. *Nat Rev Cardiol.* 2020;17(5):259–260.
25. Rizzo P, Vieceli Dalla Sega F, Fortini F, Marracino L, Rapezzi C, Ferrari R. COVID-19 in the heart and the lungs: Can we "Notch" the inflammatory storm? *Basic Res Cardiol.* 2020;115(3):31.
26. Schneider CS, Xu Q, Boylan NJ, Chisholm J, Tang BC, Schuster BS, Henning A, Ensign LM, Lee E, Adstamongkonkul P, Simons BW, Wang SS, Gong X, Yu T, Boyle MP, Suk JS, Hanes J. Nanoparticles that do not adhere to mucus provide uniform and long-lasting drug delivery to airways following inhalation. *Sci Adv.* 2017;3(4):e1601556.
27. Fang L, Karakiulakis G, Roth M. Are patients with hypertension and diabetes mellitus at increased risk for COVID-19 infection? *Lancet Respir Med.* 2020;8(4):e21. doi: 10.1016/S2213-2600(20)30116-8. Epub 2020 Mar 11. Erratum in: *Lancet Respir Med.* 2020;8(6):e54.
28. Lambert DW, Yarski M, Warner FJ, Thornhill P, Parkin ET, Smith AI, Hooper NM, Turner AJ. Tumor necrosis factor-alpha convertase (ADAM17) mediates regulated ectodomain shedding of the severe-acute respiratory syndrome-coronavirus (SARS-CoV) receptor, angiotensin-converting enzyme-2 (ACE2). *J Biol Chem.* 2005;280(34):30113–30119.
29. Patel VB, Clarke N, Wang Z, Fan D, Parajuli N, Basu R, Putko B, Kassiri Z, Turner AJ, Oudit GY. Angiotensin II induced proteolytic cleavage of myocardial ACE2 is mediated by TACE/ADAM-17: A positive feedback mechanism in the RAS. *J Mol Cell Cardiol.* 2014;66:167–176.

30. Kyula JN, Van Schaeybroeck S, Doherty J, Fenning CS, Longley DB, Johnston PG. Chemotherapy-induced activation of ADAM-17: A novel mechanism of drug resistance in colorectal cancer. *Clin Cancer Res.* 2010;16(13):3378–3389.
31. Ren J, Nie Y, Lv M, Shen S, Tang R, Xu Y, Hou Y, Zhao S, Wang T. Estrogen upregulates MICA/B expression in human non-small cell lung cancer through the regulation of ADAM17. *Cell Mol Immunol.* 2015;12(6):768–776.
32. Walls AC, Park YJ, Tortorici MA, Wall A, McGuire AT, Veesler D. Structure, function, and antigenicity of the SARS-CoV-2 spike glycoprotein. *Cell.* 2020;181(2):281–292.e6.
33. Shiryaev SA, Remacle AG, Ratnikov BI, Nelson NA, Savinov AY, Wei G, Bottini M, Rega MF, Parent A, Desjardins R, Fugere M, Day R, Sabet M, Pellecchia M, Liddington RC, Smith JW, Mustelin T, Guiney DG, Lebl M, Strongin AY. Targeting host cell furin proprotein convertases as a therapeutic strategy against bacterial toxins and viral pathogens. *J Biol Chem.* 2007;282(29):20847–20853.
34. Ronco C, Reis T. Kidney involvement in COVID-19 and rationale for extracorporeal therapies. *Nat Rev Nephrol.* 2020;16(6):308–310.
35. Wu J, Song S, Cao HC, Li LJ. Liver diseases in COVID-19: Etiology, treatment and prognosis. *World J Gastroenterol.* 2020;26(19):2286–2293.
36. Alqahtani SA, Schattenberg JM. Liver injury in COVID-19: The current evidence. *U Eur Gastroenterol J.* 2020;8(5):509–519.
37. Villapol S. Gastrointestinal symptoms associated with COVID-19: Impact on the gut microbiome. *Transl Res.* 2020;226:57–69.
38. Samanta J, Dhar J, Khaliq A, Kochhar R. Novel coronavirus infection: Gastrointestinal manifestations. *J Digestive Endosc.* 2020;11(1):13–18.
39. Cha MH, Regueiro M, Sandhu DS. Gastrointestinal and hepatic manifestations of COVID-19: A comprehensive review. *World J Gastroenterol.* 2020;26(19):2323–2332.
40. Galanopoulos M, Gkeros F, Doukatas A, Karianakis G, Pontas C, Tsoukalas N, Viazis N, Liatsos C, Mantzaris GJ. COVID-19 pandemic: Pathophysiology and manifestations from the gastrointestinal tract. *World J Gastroenterol.* 2020;26(31):4579–4588.
41. Holshue ML, DeBolt C, Lindquist S, Lofy KH, Wiesman J, Bruce H, Spitters C, Ericson K, Wilkerson S, Tural A, Diaz G, Cohn A, Fox L, Patel A, Gerber SI, Kim L, Tong S, Lu X, Lindstrom S, Pallansch MA, Weldon WC, Biggs HM, Uyeki TM, Pillai SK; Washington State 2019-nCoV case investigation team. First case of 2019 novel coronavirus in the United States. *N Engl J Med.* 2020;382(10):929–936.
42. Guan WJ, Ni ZY, Hu Y, et al. Clinical characteristics of coronavirus disease 2019 in China. *N Engl J Med.* 2020;382(18):1708–1720.
43. Leung WK, To KF, Chan PK, Chan HL, Wu AK, Lee N, Yuen KY, Sung JJ. Enteric involvement of severe acute respiratory syndrome-associated coronavirus infection. *Gastroenterology.* 2003;125(4):1011–1017.
44. Pan L, Mu M, Yang P, Sun Y, Wang R, Yan J, Li P, Hu B, Wang J, Hu C, Jin Y, Niu X, Ping R, Du Y, Li T, Xu G, Hu Q, Tu L. Clinical characteristics of COVID-19 patients with digestive symptoms in Hubei, China: A descriptive, cross-sectional, multicenter study. *Am J Gastroenterol.* 2020;115(5):766–773.
45. Wei XS, Wang X, Niu YR, et al. Clinical characteristics of SARS-CoV-2 infected pneumonia with diarrhea. *Lancet Respir Med-Manuscript Draft.* 2020. https://papers.ssrn.com/sol3/papers.cfm?abstract_id=3546120
46. Zhang H, Kang ZJ, Gong HY, et al. The digestive system is a potential route of 2019-nCov infection: A bioinformatics analysis based on single-cell transcriptomes. bioRxiv 927806. January 30, 2020. Preprint.
47. Liang W, Feng Z, Rao S, Xiao C, Xue X, Lin Z, Zhang Q, Qi W. Diarrhoea may be underestimated: A missing link in 2019 novel coronavirus. *Gut.* 2020;69(6):1141–1143.
48. Liu Q, Wang R, Qu G. Macroscopic autopsy findings in a patient with COVID-19. *J Forensic Med.* 2020;36:1–3 (in Chinese).
49. Wu Y, Guo C, Tang L, Hong Z, Zhou J, Dong X, Yin H, Xiao Q, Tang Y, Qu X, Kuang L, Fang X, Mishra N, Lu J, Shan H, Jiang G, Huang X. Prolonged presence of SARS-CoV-2 viral RNA in faecal samples. *Lancet Gastroenterol Hepatol.* 2020;5(5):434–435.
50. Xiao F, Tang M, Zheng X, Liu Y, Li X, Shan H. Evidence for gastrointestinal infection of SARS-CoV-2. *Gastroenterology.* 2020;158(6):1831–1833.e3.
51. Liang W, Guan W, Chen R, Wang W, Li J, Xu K, Li C, Ai Q, Lu W, Liang H, Li S, He J. Cancer patients in SARS-CoV-2 infection: A nationwide analysis in China. *Lancet Oncol.* 2020;21(3):335–337.
52. An P, Ji M, Ren H, et al. Protection of 318 inflammatory bowel disease patients from the outbreak and rapid spread of COVID-19 infection in Wuhan, China. Available at SSRN: https://ssrn.com/abstract=3543590.
53. Ianiro G, Mullish BH, Kelly CR, Sokol H, Kassam Z, Ng SC, Fischer M, Allegretti JR, Masucci L, Zhang F, Keller J, Sanguinetti M, Costello SP, Tilg H, Gasbarrini A, Cammarota G. Screening of faecal microbiota transplant donors during the COVID-19 outbreak: Suggestions for urgent updates from an international expert panel. *Lancet Gastroenterol Hepatol.* 2020;5(5):430–432. doi: 10.1016/S2468-1253(20)30082-0. Epub 2020 March 17. Erratum in: *Lancet Gastroenterol Hepatol.* 2020;5(6):e5.
54. Chan KS, Zheng JP, Mok YW, Li YM, Liu YN, Chu CM, Ip MS. SARS: Prognosis, outcome and sequelae. *Respirology.* 2003;8(Suppl 1):S36–S40.
55. Nicholls J, Dong XP, Jiang G, Peiris M. SARS: Clinical virology and pathogenesis. *Respirology.* 2003;8(Suppl 1):S6–S8.
56. Guo Y, Korteweg C, McNutt MA, Gu J. Pathogenetic mechanisms of severe acute respiratory syndrome. *Virus Res.* 2008;133(1):4–12.
57. Hwang DM, Chamberlain DW, Poutanen SM, Low DE, Asa SL, Butany J. Pulmonary pathology of severe acute respiratory syndrome in Toronto. *Mod Pathol.* 2005;18(1):1–10.
58. Xie L, Liu Y, Fan B, Xiao Y, Tian Q, Chen L, Zhao H, Chen W. Dynamic changes of serum SARS-coronavirus IgG, pulmonary function and radiography in patients recovering from SARS after hospital discharge. *Respir Res.* 2005;6(1):5.
59. Sime PJ, O'Reilly KM. Fibrosis of the lung and other tissues: New concepts in pathogenesis and treatment. *Clin Immunol.* 2001;99(3):308–319.
60. Razzaque MS, Taguchi T. Pulmonary fibrosis: Cellular and molecular events. *Pathol Int.* 2003;53(3):133–145.

61. Scotton CJ, Chambers RC. Molecular targets in pulmonary fibrosis: The myofibroblast in focus. *Chest.* 2007;132(4):1311–1321.
62. Izuhara Y, Takahashi S, Nangaku M, Takizawa S, Ishida H, Kurokawa K, van Ypersele de Strihou C, Hirayama N, Miyata T. Inhibition of plasminogen activator inhibitor-1: Its mechanism and effectiveness on coagulation and fibrosis. *Arterioscler Thromb Vasc Biol.* 2008;28(4):672–677.
63. Gill SE, Parks WC. Metalloproteinases and their inhibitors: Regulators of wound healing. *Int J Biochem Cell Biol.* 2008;40(6–7):1334–1347.
64. Sime PJ, Xing Z, Graham FL, Csaky KG, Gauldie J. Adenovector-mediated gene transfer of active transforming growth factor-beta1 induces prolonged severe fibrosis in rat lung. *J Clin Invest.* 1997;100(4):768–776.
65. Lee CG, Homer RJ, Zhu Z, Lanone S, Wang X, Koteliansky V, Shipley JM, Gotwals P, Noble P, Chen Q, Senior RM, Elias JA. Interleukin-13 induces tissue fibrosis by selectively stimulating and activating transforming growth factor beta(1). *J Exp Med.* 2001;194(6):809–821.
66. Rube CE, Uthe D, Schmid KW, Richter KD, Wessel J, Schuck A, Willich N, Rube C. Dose-dependent induction of transforming growth factor beta (TGF-beta) in the lung tissue of fibrosis-prone mice after thoracic irradiation. *Int J Radiat Oncol Biol Phys.* 2000;47(4):1033–1042.
67. Willis BC, Liebler JM, Luby-Phelps K, Nicholson AG, Crandall ED, du Bois RM, Borok Z. Induction of epithelial-mesenchymal transition in alveolar epithelial cells by transforming growth factor-beta1: Potential role in idiopathic pulmonary fibrosis. *Am J Pathol.* 2005;166(5):1321–1332.
68. Lin WY, Weinberg E, Kim KA, Peng LF, Kim SS, Brockman M, Lopez-Marra H, De Sa Borges CB, Hyppolite G, Shao RX, Chung RT. HIV and GP120 enhance HCV replication and upregulate TGF-beta 1. *Hepatology.* 2007;46:447a.
69. Baas T, Taubenberger JK, Chong PY, Chui P, Katze MG. SARS-CoV virus-host interactions and comparative etiologies of acute respiratory distress syndrome as determined by transcriptional and cytokine profiling of formalin-fixed paraffin-embedded tissues. *J Interferon Cytokine Res.* 2006;26(5):309–317.
70. Zhao X, Nicholls JM, Chen YG. Severe acute respiratory syndrome-associated coronavirus nucleocapsid protein interacts with Smad3 and modulates transforming growth factor-beta signaling. *J Biol Chem.* 2008;283(6):3272–3280.
71. Kuba K, Imai Y, Penninger JM. Angiotensin-converting enzyme 2 in lung diseases. *Curr Opin Pharmacol.* 2006;6(3):271–276.
72. Rodríguez-Vita J, Sánchez-López E, Esteban V, Rupérez M, Egido J, Ruiz-Ortega M. Angiotensin II activates the SMAD pathway in vascular smooth muscle cells by a transforming growth factor-beta-independent mechanism. *Circulation.* 2005;111(19):2509–2517.
73. Imai Y, Kuba K, Penninger JM. Angiotensin-converting enzyme 2 in acute respiratory distress syndrome. *Cell Mol Life Sci.* 2007;64(15):2006–2012.
74. Emad A, Emad V. Elevated levels of MCP-1, MIP-alpha and MIP-1 beta in the bronchoalveolar lavage (BAL) fluid of patients with mustard gas-induced pulmonary fibrosis. *Toxicology.* 2007;240(1–2):60–69.
75. Yoshida K, Kuwano K, Hagimoto N, Watanabe K, Matsuba T, Fujita M, Inoshima I, Hara N. MAP kinase activation and apoptosis in lung tissues from patients with idiopathic pulmonary fibrosis. *J Pathol.* 2002;198(3):388–396.
76. Zaim S, Chong JH, Sankaranarayanan V, Harky A. COVID-19 and multiorgan response. *Curr Probl Cardiol.* 2020;45(8):100618.
77. Jain U. Effect of COVID-19 on the organs. *Cureus.* 2020;12(8):e9540.
78. Mokhtari T, Hassani F, Ghaffari N, Ebrahimi B, Yarahmadi A, Hassanzadeh G. COVID-19 and multiorgan failure: A narrative review on potential mechanisms. *J Mol Histol.* 2020;51(6):613–628.
79. Ronco C, Reis T. Kidney involvement in COVID-19 and rationale for extracorporeal therapies. *Nat Rev Nephrol.* 2020;16(6):308–310.
80. Mao L, Jin H, Wang M, Hu Y, Chen S, He Q, Chang J, Hong C, Zhou Y, Wang D, Miao X, Li Y, Hu B. Neurologic manifestations of hospitalized patients with coronavirus disease 2019 in Wuhan, China. *JAMA Neurol.* 2020;77(6):683–690.
81. Xiang P et al. First case of 2019 novel coronavirus disease with encephalitis. ChinaXiv T202003000015. 2020.
82. Moriguchi T, Harii N, Goto J, Harada D, Sugawara H, Takamino J, Ueno M, Sakata H, Kondo K, Myose N, Nakao A, Takeda M, Haro H, Inoue O, Suzuki-Inoue K, Kubokawa K, Ogihara S, Sasaki T, Kinouchi H, Kojin H, Ito M, Onishi H, Shimizu T, Sasaki Y, Enomoto N, Ishihara H, Furuya S, Yamamoto T, Shimada S. A first case of meningitis/encephalitis associated with SARS-Coronavirus-2. *Int J Infect Dis.* 2020;94: 55–58.
83. Yang SL, Liu LJ, Dai L, Zhang C, Li JT, Chen C, Liu H. Analysis of anxiety in 78 SARS patients. *Nanfang J Nurs.* 2003;10:27–28.
84. Kang L, Li Y, Hu S, Chen M, Yang C, Yang BX, Wang Y, Hu J, Lai J, Ma X, Chen J, Guan L, Wang G, Ma H, Liu Z. The mental health of medical workers in Wuhan, China dealing with the 2019 novel coronavirus. *Lancet Psychiatry.* 2020;7(3):e14.
85. Xu K, Cai H, Shen Y, Ni Q, Chen Y, Hu S, Li J, Wang H, Yu L, Huang H, Qiu Y, Wei G, Fang Q, Zhou J, Sheng J, Liang T, Li L. Management of corona virus disease-19 (COVID-19): The Zhejiang experience. *Zhejiang Da Xue Xue Bao Yi Xue Ban (Journal of Zhejiang University).* 2020;49(1):147–157. In Chinese.
86. Huang JZ, Han MF, Luo TD, Ren AK, Zhou XP. Mental health survey of medical staff in a tertiary infectious disease hospital for COVID-19. *Zhonghua Lao Dong Wei Sheng Zhi Ye Bing Za Zhi.* 2020;38(3):192–195. In Chinese.
87. Zhou P, Yang XL, Wang XG, Hu B, Zhang L, Zhang W, Si HR, Zhu Y, Li B, Huang CL, Chen HD, Chen J, Luo Y, Guo H, Jiang RD, Liu MQ, Chen Y, Shen XR, Wang X, Zheng XS, Zhao K, Chen QJ, Deng F, Liu LL, Yan B, Zhan FX, Wang YY, Xiao GF, Shi ZL. A pneumonia outbreak associated with a new coronavirus of probable bat origin. *Nature.* 2020;579(7798):270–273.
88. Hamming I, Timens W, Bulthuis ML, Lely AT, Navis G, van Goor H. Tissue distribution of ACE2 protein, the functional receptor for SARS coronavirus. A first step in understanding SARS pathogenesis. *J Pathol.* 2004;203(2):631–637.

89. Zou L, Ruan F, Huang M, Liang L, Huang H, Hong Z, Yu J, Kang M, Song Y, Xia J, Guo Q, Song T, He J, Yen HL, Peiris M, Wu J. SARS-CoV-2 viral load in upper respiratory specimens of infected patients. *N Engl J Med.* 2020;382(12):1177–1179.
90. Bleau C, Filliol A, Samson M, Lamontagne L. Brain invasion by mouse hepatitis virus depends on impairment of tight junctions and beta interferon production in brain microvascular endothelial cells. *J Virol.* 2015;89(19):9896–9908.
91. Dubé M, Le Coupanec A, Wong AHM, Rini JM, Desforges M, Talbot PJ. Axonal transport enables neuron-to-neuron propagation of human coronavirus OC43. *J Virol.* 2018;92(17):e00404–18.
92. Li YC, Bai WZ, Hashikawa T. The neuroinvasive potential of SARS-CoV2 may play a role in the respiratory failure of COVID-19 patients. *J Med Virol.* 2020;92(6):552–555.
93. Dubey D, Pittock SJ, Kelly CR, McKeon A, Lopez-Chiriboga AS, Lennon VA, Gadoth A, Smith CY, Bryant SC, Klein CJ, Aksamit AJ, Toledano M, Boeve BF, Tillema JM, Flanagan EP. Autoimmune encephalitis epidemiology and a comparison to infectious encephalitis. *Ann Neurol.* 2018;83(1):166–177.
94. Karagianni P, Alexopoulos H, Sourdi A, Papadimitriou D, Dimitrakopoulos AN, Moutsopoulos HM. West Nile Virus infection triggering autoimmune encephalitis: Pathophysiological and therapeutic implications. *Clin Immunol.* 2019;207:97–99.
95. Lin YS, Lin CF, Fang YT, Kuo YM, Liao PC, Yeh TM, Hwa KY, Shieh CC, Yen JH, Wang HJ, Su IJ, Lei HY. Antibody to severe acute respiratory syndrome (SARS)-associated coronavirus spike protein domain 2 cross-reacts with lung epithelial cells and causes cytotoxicity. *Clin Exp Immunol.* 2005;141(3):500–508.
96. Soria V, González-Rodríguez A, Huerta-Ramos E, Usall J, Cobo J, Bioque M, Barbero JD, García-Rizo C, Tost M, Monreal JA; PNECAT Group, Labad J. Targeting hypothalamic-pituitary-adrenal axis hormones and sex steroids for improving cognition in major mood disorders and schizophrenia: A systematic review and narrative synthesis. *Psychoneuroendocrinology.* 2018;93:8–19.
97. Curtin NM, Boyle NT, Mills KH, Connor TJ. Psychological stress suppresses innate IFN-gamma production via glucocorticoid receptor activation: Reversal by the anxiolytic chlordiazepoxide. *Brain Behav Immun.* 2009;23(4):535–547.
98. Herman JP, McKlveen JM, Ghosal S, Kopp B, Wulsin A, Makinson R, Scheimann J, Myers B. Regulation of the hypothalamic-pituitary-adrenocortical stress response. *Compr Physiol.* 2016;6(2):603–621.
99. Glaser R, Kiecolt-Glaser JK. Stress-induced immune dysfunction: Implications for health. *Nat Rev Immunol.* 2005;5(3):243–251.
100. Patel A, Jernigan DB; 2019-nCoV CDC Response Team. Initial public health response and interim clinical guidance for the 2019 novel coronavirus outbreak - United States, December 31, 2019-February 4, 2020. MMWR Morb Mortal Wkly Rep. 2020;69(5):140–146.
101. Tsai LK, Hsieh ST, Chang YC. Neurological manifestations in severe acute respiratory syndrome. *Acta Neurol Taiwan.* 2005;14(3):113–119.
102. Gu J, Gong E, Zhang B, Zheng J, Gao Z, Zhong Y, Zou W, Zhan J, Wang S, Xie Z, Zhuang H, Wu B, Zhong H, Shao H, Fang W, Gao D, Pei F, Li X, He Z, Xu D, Shi X, Anderson VM, Leong AS. Multiple organ infection and the pathogenesis of SARS. *J Exp Med.* 2005;202(3):415–424.
103. Duan L, Zhu G. Psychological interventions for people affected by the COVID-19 epidemic. *Lancet Psychiatry.* 2020;7(4):300–302.
104. Zietz M, Tatonetti NP. Testing the association between blood type and COVID-19 infection, intubation, and death. medRxiv. 2020. doi: 10.1101/2020.04.08.20058073.
105. Bhatia S, Namdeo AG, Nanda S. Factors effecting the gelling and emulsifying properties of a natural polymer. *SRP.* 2010;1(1):86–92.
106. Bhatia S, Sharma K, Bera T. Structural characterization and pharmaceutical properties of porphyran. *Asian J Pharm* 2015;993–101.
107. Bhatia S, Sharma A, Sharma K, Kavale M, Chaugule BB, Dhalwal K, Namdeo AG, Mahadik KR. Novel algal polysaccharides from marine source: Porphyran. *Pharmacogn Rev* 2008;4:271–276.
108. Bhatia S, Sharma K, Nagpal K, Bera T. Investigation of the factors influencing the molecular weight of porphyran and its associated antifungal activity Bioact. *Carb Diet Fiber* 2015;5:153–168.
109. Bhatia S, Kumar V, Sharma K, Nagpal K, Bera T. Significance of algal polymer in designing amphotericin B nanoparticles. *Sci World J.* 2014;2014:564573.
110. Bhatia S, Rathee P, Sharma K, Chaugule BB, Kar N, Bera T. Immuno-modulation effect of sulphated polysaccharide (Porphyran) from Porphyra vietnamensis. *Int J Biol Macromol.* 2013;57:50–56.
111. Bhatia S. *Natural Polymer Drug Delivery Systems: Marine Polysaccharides Based Nano-Materials and Its Applications.* Springer International Publishing, Switzerland; 2016:185–225.
112. Bhatia S. *Natural Polymer Drug Delivery Systems: Plant Derived Polymers, Properties, and Modification & Applications.* Springer International Publishing, Switzerland; 2016:119–184.
113. Bhatia S. *Natural Polymer Drug Delivery Systems: Nanotechnology and Its Drug Delivery Applications.* Springer International Publishing, Switzerland; 2016:1–32.
114. Bhatia S. *Natural Polymer Drug Delivery Systems: Nanoparticles Types, Classification, Characterization, Fabrication Methods and Drug Delivery Applications.* Springer International Publishing; Switzerland; 2016:33–93.
115. Bhatia S. *Natural Polymer Drug Delivery Systems: Natural Polymers vs Synthetic Polymer.* Springer International Publishing, Switzerland; 2016;95–118.
116. Bhatia S. *Systems for Drug Delivery: Mammalian Polysaccharides and Its Nanomaterials.* Springer International Publishing, Switzerland; 2016;1–27.
117. Bhatia S. *Systems for Drug Delivery: Microbial Polysaccharides as Advance Nanomaterials.* Springer International Publishing, Switzerland; 2016:29–54.
118. Bhatia S. *Systems for Drug Delivery: Chitosan Based Nanomaterials and Its Applications.* Springer International Publishing, Switzerland; 2016:55–117.

119. Bhatia S. *Systems for Drug Delivery: Advance Polymers and Its Applications*. Springer International Publishing, Switzerland; 2016:119–146.
120. Bhatia S. *Systems for Drug Delivery: Advanced Application of Natural Polysaccharides*. Springer International Publishing, Switzerland; 2016:147–170.
121. Bhatia S. *Systems for Drug Delivery: Modern Polysaccharides and Its Current Advancements*. Springer International Publishing, Switzerland; 2016:171–188.
122. Bhatia S. *Systems for Drug Delivery: Toxicity of Nanodrug Delivery Systems*. Springer International Publishing, Switzerland; 2016:189–197.
123. Bhatia S. *Nanotechnology in Drug Delivery Fundamentals, Design, and Applications: Part 1: Protein and Peptide-Based Drug Delivery Systems*. Apple Academic Press, Palm Bay, FL; 2016:50–204.
124. Bhatia S. *Nanotechnology in Drug Delivery Fundamentals, Design, and Applications: Part 2: Peptide-Mediated Nanoparticle Drug Delivery System*. Apple Academic Press, Palm Bay, FL; 2016:205–280.
125. Bhatia S. *Nanotechnology in Drug Delivery Fundamentals, Design, and Applications: Part 3: CPP and CTP in Drug Delivery and Cell Targeting*. Apple Academic Press, Palm Bay, FL; 2016:309–312.

PART II

Introduction to Essential Oils and Its Role in the Management of COVID-19

8

Essential Oil Chemistry vs. Aromatherapy

Ahmed Al-Harrasi
Natural and Medical Sciences Research Center, University of Nizwa

Saurabh Bhatia
Natural and Medical Sciences Research Center, University of Nizwa
University of Petroleum and Energy Studies

Md. Tanvir Kabir
BRAC University

Tapan Behl
Chitkara University

Deepak Kaushik
M.D. University

Mohammed Muqtader Ahmed and Md. Khalid Anwer
Prince Sattam Bin Abdul Aziz University

CONTENTS

8.1 Introduction

Essential oil-based treatment has been utilized in traditional medicine as a non-invasive approach with few side effects and low toxicity . These natural oils have been extensively utilized in the management of various ailments related to mind and body [1]. Apart from their considerable psychological and physiological effects, recent reports have shown that these essential oils (EOs) can be directly utilized to treat various problems associated with the respiratory, circulatory, and nervous systems [2,3]. To exert their therapeutic effects, EOs are generally administered via skin (massage therapy) or inhalation. Systemic availability of these components of EOs, those are responsible for therapeutic effects varies as per their route of administration. After their systemic availability, it can reach other organs to exert physiological effects. Various reports have suggested inter-connection between the limbic system (brain) and olfaction, which may be the key mechanism of action of aromatherapy [4,5]. Molecular proteins, so-called receptors, present in the nasal chamber are responsible for transmitting chemical information via olfactory neurons to the limbic system to further control physiological as well as psychological activities such as blood pressure, breathing rate, and emotional balance [6]. Though, earlier beliefs over the mechanism of action of EOs are often debated. Previous reports suggested that upregulation of gamma-aminobutyric acid (GABA) might be considered as the underlying mechanism of action of lavender oil in improving tremors in rodent model [7]. However, few studies based on exploring the molecular targets of phytochemicals present in EOs are available. Also, due to their complex chemical composition and high volatility it is sometimes difficult to establish the exact mechanism of action of EOs, especially the compound responsible for therapeutic effects and their respective molecular targets. This complex constitution is comprised of monoterpenoids and also sesquiterpenoidal compounds. Furthermore, additional components including phenolic compounds are also present in the oils, often to improve the biological effects.

DOI: 10.1201/9781003175933-10

8.2 Olfactory Aromatherapy (OA)

EOs are unorganized plant-based excretory products constituting complex mixtures of volatile as well as aromatic organic compounds that are responsible for various therapeutic properties. They are made up of various low-molecular-weight organic compounds that are classified as secondary metabolites. EOs are synthesized by plants via various pathways such as:

- Terpenes (five-carbon isoprene unit): Mono- and diterpenes are synthesized via methyl-erythritol pathway; sesquiterpenes are synthesized via the mevalonate pathway.
- Phenylpropenes (six-carbon ring) are synthesized via the shikimic acid pathway [7].

However, not all EOs are synthesized via these pathways. Some new EOs that have been discovered recently might not follow these pathways. Chemically, EOs contain a diverse range of organic compounds, mainly terpene hydrocarbons and oxygenated compounds, predominantly alcohols, aldehydes, esters, ketones, oxides, and phenols [8–10]. The complex composition of EOs offers a wide range of biological activities, which are often mediated by active chemical compounds alone or the synergy between different components. Chemical interaction or synergy between these chemical compounds may have agonist or antagonist effects over the overall biological activity or when alternatively used with main course medication. Volatile compounds are abundantly present in EOs and provide the distinguished or unique aromas to plants. These volatile compounds are categorized as monoterpenes (acyclic, bicyclic, monocyclic), sesquiterpenes (acyclic, bicyclic, monocyclic, tricyclic), and aromatic compounds. Moreover, the phenolic components of EOs that are synthesized via the shikimate pathway contribute to additional therapeutic potential of the whole mixture. So far, several extraction procedures have been employed to extract EOs from various aromatic plants. These extraction procedures are broadly categorized as conventional (hydrodistillation, simple-, fractional-, steam-, or vacuum-distillation, hydrodiffusion, solvent extraction, enfleurage, and cold-press extraction) and modern (supercritical fluid extraction, subcritical extraction liquid, and solvent-free microwave extraction) [11]. Several environmental factors (biotic as well as abiotic) can influence the biosynthetic pathways responsible for the synthesis of compounds present in EOs. Apart from these, extraction procedures can also influence the kinetic effect, chemical composition, and pharmacological properties of EOs [12,13].

One of the most interesting therapeutic applications of EOs is aromatherapy, which has become popular in recent years. Aromatherapy is used to treat various ailments and promote a feeling of well-being. These procedures (such as cosmetic, massage, medical, olfactory, and psycho-based aromatherapies) may involve inhalation or topical application or oral administration. After the administration of EOs via any route, their respective chemical compounds cross biological membranes and exhibit various biological properties via different mechanisms of action.

Search results based on "inhalation of essential oils" in the NCBI database on December 23, 2020, at 11:35 PM in India included 8,760 filter results and 2,234 database NIH grants in PubMed central. PubMed search results during the same time period included 464 results from 1963 to 2020, book shelf search results: 279; NLM catalog: 04; BioProject: 01; clinical trials: 36; dbGaP studies: 07; and gene: 07. These findings undoubtedly suggest the significance of inhalation aromatherapy or OA in augmenting physical, emotional, and mental well-being. OA is mediated by a complex olfaction process that initiates when volatile compounds present in EOs bind to specific receptors called olfactory proteins. The olfactory limbic system that includes the olfactory cortex (important for the processing and perception of odor) is a part of the temporal lobe of the brain linked to smell, which requires the active physiological involvement of the nose and the brain. Inhalation of EOs containing volatile components with low molecular weight <300 Da can be identified as well as distinguished by the olfactory system containing 300 active olfactory receptor genes to differentiate thousands of dissimilar odors.

OA mediated by inhalation of EOs triggers a complex olfaction process, which is a stimulus-based modality to transmit information carried by volatile molecules (their synergy) from the EO to the cerebral hemisphere of the CNS where these chemical stimuli of significance are transduced. OA is a non-invasive treatment used to treat disease symptoms and to revitalize the whole system by influencing the physiological, spiritual, and psychological processes of the body. OA involves blending of EOs based on traditional concepts or formulas; however, recently, more interest has been raised in predetermining their chemical nature, chemical interaction, safety, solubility, or other physical properties such as aromatic characteristics as well as biological potential to prepare effective and safe blends. EO administration can be done via various means such as inhalation by using steam, via using advanced mechanical devices available in form of portable inhalers or nasal sticks, diffusers, sprays, etc. These economical, safe, and easy-to-use devices for EO inhalation are present in different designs with many potential applications [14].

Recent investigations have shown that nanoparticles functionalized with EOs or nanoencapsulation have considerable advantages such as increase in chemical stability as well as solubility, reduced fast evaporation, reduced toxicity as well as rapid degradation of EO components as well as allow controlled and sustained release to enhance their absorption and effectiveness [15]. So the ultimate goal of nanoencapsulation is to use this nanoshield for EOs to provide effective protection to its components against oxidation to offer physical stability, controlled release, and decreased volatility [15–21]. Various nano-based systems such as chitosan–cinnamic acid nanogel-encapsulated *Mentha piperita* EOs, nanoemulsions loaded with lemongrass, clove, thyme, or palmarosa EOs, nanoencapsulated eucalyptus staigeriana EOs, chitosan NPs-encapsulated *Zataria multiflora* EOs, lemongrass-pectin nanoemulsion, and encapsulated oregano EO with chitosan NPs loaded with *Cinnamomum zeylanicum* EOs have been used to provide effective protection to EO components [15–21].

Thus, various reports have demonstrated that the encapsulation of EOs or their components decreases volatility and improves stability, thereby improving shelf-life and extending the therapeutic effect. OA has prime importance in psycho-aromatherapy where inhalation of EOs promotes calmness, emotional wellness, pleasant memory or rejuvenation of the body, and relaxation. This odor-distinguishing capability of the olfactory system plays an important role in determining psychophysiological behavior including mood, stress, and productivity. Several reports have suggested the importance of EO components in triggering brain activities and cognitive functions. A recent report also demonstrated that inhalation of EOs attenuates stress and depression with improvement in sleep quality. It was found that inhalation of these EOs allows their components to cross physiological barriers to further act at the site of injury where they can exert various antioxidant, antibacterial, antiviral, and anti-inflammatory activities by stimulating immunity. Once inhaled via olfaction, EO components exert various physiological effects by synergistically or independently acting at the site of injury. EOs activate olfaction process by stimulating the limbic system in order to stimulate the emotion center of the brain (limbic system) to control behavioral and emotional responses. Nevertheless, various researchers have also shown that inhalation of EOs considerably increases the levels of the EO components in blood plasma. Inhalation of aromatic compounds stimulate olfactory receptor neurons which can further stimulate highly sensitive cells that relay messages to the brain via the limbic system. Limbic system is the control center for our emotions, blood pressure, breathing, memory, and hormone production. Various reports have evidenced the therapeutic efficacy of EOs in neurological disorders by their anxiolytic, antinociceptive, sedative, hypnotic, mood stabilizer, sedative, analgesic, and anticonvulsive and neuroprotective actions. Anxiety and depression reducing properties ascribed to lavender volatile molecules could be due to an antagonistic effect on the NMDA receptor as well as suppression of serotonin transporter (SERT) receptors [22]. An electroencephalography report obtained after the inhalation of rosemary oil demonstrated its stimulatory effect and provided proof that rosemary EO inhalation impacts the activity of the brain, autonomic nervous system, and mood states [23]. SuHeXiang Wan EO inhalation has been used for the treatment of epileptic disorders in Chinese indigenous systems of medicine. Inhalation of SuHeXiang Wan EO resulted in suppression of the CNS via the GABAergic pathway. It has also extended sleeping duration induced by pentobarbital and reduced lipid peroxidation in brain, which was found to be the main cause anticonvulsive effect [24]. Similar effects of EOs obtained from *Acorus gramineus* on the CNS have been reported [25]. This finding suggests that preinhalation of EOs derived from *Acorus gramineus* delayed convulsion and inhibited the activity of GABA transaminase, a degrading enzyme for GABA [25]. This resulted in increases in GABA level and decreases in glutamate content, which supports the anticonvulsive effect of this AGR oil. Apart from these psychological benefits, OA has also been used in the treatment of respiratory-associated problems such as tuberculosis, cough, bronchitis, asthma, catarrh, and whooping cough. Unlike other natural products, one of the advantages of EOs is that they can be inhaled to reduce acute exacerbation in patients, mainly those associated with respiratory tract diseases (RTDs). RTDs related to viral and bacterial infections, pollutants, inflammation, and other intrinsic or extrinsic factors affect a large number of people globally. Earlier studies suggest the role of OA in the treatment of upper respiratory acute and chronic infections such as common cold, sinusitis, pharyngitis, and chronic obstructive pulmonary disease (COPD). These conditions result in the inflammation of bronchioles, which can be suppressed by EO inhalation. It was also observed that OA can be used to attenuate lung inflammation by reducing IL-1β and Th immune responses in air pollutant-induced acute lung inflammation in mice. OA also resulted in the inhibition of allergic reaction and hyperplasia of mucous cell with inhibition of Muc5b expression as well as T helper 2 cell cytokines in asthmatic rodent. The above reports and studies suggest the significant role of OA in the treatment of various respiratory disorders and mental illnesses.

Coronaviruses have a considerable impact on economies and communities as well as significantly increase mortality and morbidity. These viral agents including severe acute respiratory syndrome (SARS), Middle East respiratory syndrome (MERS), avian infectious bronchitis virus (IBV), and COVID-19 can cause serious illness. The SARS-CoV-2 virus causes COVID-19, and can lead to mild to severe respiratory and systemic illness. This viral infection may progress to severe hypoxemia requiring some form of ventilatory support in suspected and confirmed cases. This highly infectious respiratory disease can lead to respiratory, physical, and psychological dysfunction in patients. Presently (2020) no official therapies or preventative therapeutic approaches are available. Various clinical trials have been conducted with the purpose of finding efficient therapeutics. Plants offer a range of potential phytochemicals with potential antiviral, anti-inflammatory, and immune-boosting therapeutic effects, and therefore could be used as reliable therapeutic agents against coronaviruses. EO inhalation or OA can be effectively used for the treatment of various respiratory illnesses including COPD, asthma, and COVID-19. In contrast to other routes, inhalation of these natural oils has several health benefits. For instance, via the pulmonary route, EOs can be administered directly to the targeted tissue or organ, thus, for example, showing a high level in lungs and low concentration at the systemic level. Thus, inhalation of EOs is normally linked to elevated pulmonary efficiency with minimum side effects at the systemic level. Additionally, various reports claim immunological and psychological benefits of OA. Thus, the inhalation of suitable EOs disinfects lungs, boosts immunity, prevents and treats viral infections, and offers various psychological benefits. These biological properties make OA an ideal treatment strategy to combat COVID-19. So far, the anti-coronaviral potential of only a few EOs has been explored.

8.3 Chemical Composition of EOs

The complex chemical profile of EOs provides distinguished chemical and physical characteristics [26]. Owing to the complex chemical composition, EOs have low density in comparison with water, and therefore, are immiscible with aqueous phase due to density difference. After their separation from different parts of aromatic plants, they can be easily distinguished and identified by their typical odor and flavor. Individual EOs are usually designated by the name of the source (i.e., the aromatic plant from which they are separated) [27]. Flavor and aromatic characteristics are generally attributed to any single active compound present in high proportion or multiple components [28]. Multiple components of EOs are sometimes chemically integrated with each other to provide the unique flavor and aroma to the plant material. These low-molecular-weight chemical components of EOs are lipophilic and highly volatile in nature, which makes them suitable for inhalation to treat various ailments [29]. About 1,340 aromatic plants have been identified for their antimicrobial potential and almost 30,000 active constituents have been explored [30].

EOs usually contain varied number of components (20–60) in different proportions and concentrations; however, their important properties are often controlled by two to three main components, which are comparatively present in high proportion (20%–90%) than other components, which are present in lower amounts [31]. Monoterpenes are present in almost all EOs and contribute to the flavor and aromatic characteristics of the plant from which they are extracted. This class constitutes nearly 90% of the chemical profile of the majority of EOs with diversity in their chemical structures. Monoterpenes are abundantly present in various EOs. Some of the most common monoterpenes include limonene, terpinene, cymene, myrcene, pinene, eucalyptol, citral, menthol, thujene, nerol, thymol, citronellal, phellandrene, and camphene. Based on the arrangement of hydrocarbon skeleton, monoterpenes are classified as acyclic, cyclic, or aromatic monoterpenes. Acyclic monoterpenes are linear acyclic hydrocarbons (e.g., myrcene, citronellol, citronellal, citronellene, citral, geraniol, and ocimene) or their derivatives (e.g., linalool and geraniol). Further, cyclic monoterpenes can be classified on the basis of number of cyclic rings in the structure such as monocyclic (carvone, pulegone, limonene, menthol, α-terpineol), bicyclic (carene, sabinene, thujane, pinane, bornane, iso camphene, α-pinene, camphor, α-pinene), and tricyclic monoterpenes (santonin). These compounds are vulnerable to oxidation as they can quickly react in the presence of air and heat sources [32]. These bioactive compounds are very prone to oxidative, isomerization, cyclization, dehydrogenation, polymerization, and other degradation reactions, which may lead to loss of quality, especially changes in biological properties as well as changes in flavor and aromatic characteristics. These types of chemical transformations due to improper storage conditions with varied temperature, light conditions, or oxygen level can influence EO integrity, which can result in change of physical, chemical, as well as biological properties. Monoterpenes are diversely present among various plants; for example [33,34]:

- Limonene is present in orange and other citrus oils, neroli, lemon, fennel, carrot, and bergamot.
- Pinene is present in pine, oregano, eucalyptus, cypress, coriander, and black pepper.
- Camphene is present in spruce, pine, juniper, and fir.

Antioxidant as well as antibacterial activities are due to the phenolic compounds present in EOs. Some EO components are diversely present among various medicinal plants. For instance, EOs such as oregano, thyme, savory, and cinnamon contain thymol, eugenol, and carvacrol [35]. Next to monoterpenes, sesquiterpenes are considered as the second most diverse and abundant class among various EO-producing plants. Sesquiterpenes are unsaturated compounds, and are classified as linear or acyclic (farnesol), branched, or cyclic sesquiterpenes. Cyclic sesquiterpenes can be classified as monocyclic (zingiberene), bicyclic (cadinene), or tricyclic. Other terpenes such as diterpenes, triterpenes, and tetraterpenes are found at very low levels in EOs. Oxygenated derivatives of hydrocarbon terpenes, known as terpenoids, including acids, alcohols, aldehydes, esters, ethers, and ketones, are a diverse class of bioactive compounds with a wide range of biological activities. Alcohols such as citronellol, farnesol, geraniol, and linalool present in chamomile, rose, geranium, lavender, palmarosa, and other plants are known for their antiseptic and antimicrobial properties [36]. Aldehydes such as citral and citronellal are often present in the lemongrass, orange, lemon, mandarin, eucalyptus, and citronella EOs, and are responsible for very their powerful aromas and properties such as antifungal and anti-inflammatory activity [37]. A vast amount of literature (mainly in vitro findings) is available on the cytotoxicity of EOs against microbial cells, which is mainly attributed to the alcohols, aldehydes, and phenols [38, 39]. As mentioned earlier, the chemical profile of EOs can be influenced by various factors such as type and conditions of extraction procedure, geographical and climatic conditions of plant, plant type, time of collection, and pre-extraction procedure such as plant processing [32]. Different extraction procedures have been employed to separate EOs from various sources such as cold-pressing, enfleurage, solvent extraction, supercritical fluid extraction [32], hydro-distillation [32], microwave-assisted extraction, ultrasound-assisted extraction, and instant controlled pressure drop [32]. After the extraction of EOs, the identification of different chemical compounds present in EOs is done by using various chromatographic methods coupled with different systems [40]. Gas chromatography (GC) analysis is one of the most suitable techniques of separation as well as quantification of the components present in EOs [41]. Gas chromatography coupled with mass spectrometry (GC-MS) facilitates the mass spectrum of each component present in the sample [42]. Moreover, GC-MS can also be employed to determine the chemical composition of EOs both qualitatively and quantitatively. Qualitative analysis is based on matching the mass spectra of sample by means of GC-MS with those present in the spectrum library, and by their retention indexes. Quantitative analysis by using GC-MS is done to determine the amount of each identified component. Depending on the objective of the study, various GC coupled techniques are used such as GC-olfactometry, comprehensive two-dimensional GC, combined with time-of-flight mass spectrometry, heart-cut multidimensional GC-olfactometry. The GC-olfactometry method couples traditional gas chromatographic analysis with sensory detection to investigate complex mixtures of aromatic substances and to identify odor-active compounds. The GC-olfactometry method is extensively employed for the assessment of food aromas [43].

Since monoterpenes are more susceptible to chemical transformation, headspace sampling (HS) is the right approach once EO needs to be selectively presented into a GC. Recently, multidimensional GC has been employed for the separation and identification of EO compounds by using co-elute as in conventional GC, with more accurate qualitative and quantitative characterization of compounds of low abundance [44].

8.4 Sources and Chemical Composition

A number of aromatic plants contain EOs; nevertheless, the rate of biosynthesis or production of EOs may be different in different organs of the plants. Currently, about 3,000 EOs have been identified, out of which around 300 are available commercially. This complex mixture of various polar and nonpolar organic compounds, mainly terpenes/terpenoids, aromatic and aliphatic compounds, is categorized as low-molecular-weight aromatic compounds. Components as well as fragrance of EOs can also be categorized into two classes: oxygenated components as well as terpene hydrocarbons [45]. Generally, EO components are categorized into the following [46]:

- Terpenes: monoterpenes and sesquiterpenes
- Terpenoids: isoprenoids
- Scented components: aldehyde, methoxy alcohol, phenol derivatives

As mentioned earlier, EOs contain two to three main components in comparatively high levels (20%–95%), while other compounds are present in traces. Constituents that are present in high proportion in EOs are as follows:

- *Cinnamomum camphora* EO: 1,8-cineole (50%)
- *Origanum compactum* EO: carvacrol: (30%), thymol: (27%)
- Garlic EO: sulfur-containing compounds allyl methyl trisulfide (7.9%–13.2%), allyl (E)-1-propenyl disulfide (7.9%–12.5%)
- *Anethum graveolens* EO: carvone (58%), d-limonene (37%)
- Citrus peel EO: d-limonene (over 80%)
- *Mentha piperita* E: menthol (59%) and menthone (19%)
- Artemisia EO: α-/β-thujone (57%) and camphor (24%)
- Lavender EO: linalool (20.60%–35.99%)
- Clove EO: eugenol (89%)
- *Ocimum basilicum* EO: methyl chavicol (27.82%) and linalool (25.35%)
- Rosemary EO: camphor (5.0%–21%), 1,8-cineole (15%–55%), and α-pinene (9.0%–26%)
- *Satureja bachtiarica* EO: thymol (65.1%), γ-terpinene (15.0%)
- Thyme EO: thymol (38.1%), p-cymene (29.1%)
- Anethum graveolens EO: α-phellandrene (36%) and limonene (31%)

Various biological assays have shown that the pharmacological properties of active chemical components present in EOs can be assessed against pathogenic microorganisms. Active chemical compounds can synergistically or independently suppress the action of disease- or injury-causing agent. However, sometimes, active chemical compounds cannot restore their biological potential in the presence of disease- or injury-causing agents. For instance, linalool and β-pinene produce an antidepressant-like effect via interaction with the monoaminergic system. It has been reported that WAY 100635 (a 5-HT1A receptor antagonist) can inhibit the antidepressant-like activity of β-pinene as well as linalool. On the contrary, pre-treatment of mice with PCPA (a serotonin synthesis inhibitor) did not cause a decrease in the immobility time provoked by linalool and β-pinene. The yohimbine (a α2 receptor antagonist) altered the antidepressant effect of linalool. Propranolol (a β receptor antagonist) and neurotoxin DSP-4 (a noradrenergic neurotoxin) changed the anti-immobility response of β-pinene; also, SCH23390 (a D1 receptor antagonist) inhibited the antidepressant-like action of β-pinene [47–50]. It was also found that the active compound can follow multiple pathways to exert biological activity; however, some chemical compounds only follow one pathway to show biological activity. As it was demonstrated in the same study, β-pinene induces antidepressant effects by involving dopaminergic, serotoninergic, and noradrenergic pathways, whereas carvacrol only involves dopaminergic pathway to induce antidepressant effects [47–50].

8.4.1 Terpene Hydrocarbons

Hydrocarbons are naturally occurring organic compounds made up of H as well as C atoms positioned in chains. These hydrocarbons can be linear and branched or contain rings, and can be acyclic, alicyclic (monocyclic, bicyclic, or tricyclic), or aromatic. Terpenoids are often found in EOs, comprising a skeleton of two isoprene units (C5) called the "terpene unit." Chemically, EO components primarily contain monoterpenes (C10) and sesquiterpenes (C15), while diterpenes (C20), triterpenes (C30), and tetraterpenes (C40) are present in very low amounts. Terpenoids (isoprenoids, a terpene-containing oxygen) display the most diverse class of chemical compounds present in EOs [51].

8.4.2 Oxygenated Compounds

Oxygenated compounds with terpene backbone known as terpenoidsare present in EOs, offering a wide range of biological activities. Among them, the most extensively investigated and important class present in EOs are alcohols (containing "–OH" as a functional group). Various oxygenated components common in plant EOs are as follows:

- Sesquiterpenes alcohol: bisabolol, nerolidol, α-santalol, elemol
- Phenols: carvacrol, chavicol, thymol, eugenol
- Oxides: bisabolone oxide, linalool oxide, 1,8-cineole, sclareol oxide

TABLE 8.1
Alcohol-Containing EOs and Their Biological Effects

Essential Oil	Major Alcohol Component(s)	Biological Effects	Probable Amount
Basil	Linalool	Improve mood	Almost 80%
Cedarwood	Cedrol		Almost 20%
Clary sage	Linalool		Almost 25%
Coriander	Linalool, geraniol		Almost 30%
Geranium	Citronellol, geraniol		Almost 50%
Jasmine	Phytol, linalool		Almost 45%
Lavender	Linalool		Almost 35%
Marjoram	Linalool, terpineol		Almost 55%
Patchouli	Patchoulol		Almost 25%
Peppermint	Menthol		Almost 50%
Rose	Citronellol, geraniol, nerol		Almost 60%
Sandalwood	Santalol		Almost 90%

- Lactones: psoralen, aesculatine, citropten, bergaptene, nepetalactone
- Ketones: fenchone, camphor, thujone, verbenone, carvone, menthone, pulegone
- Ethers: 1,8-cineole, elemicin, myristicin, anethole
- Esters: citronellyl acetate, geranyl acetate, bomyl acetate, linalyl acetate
- Aldehydes: citral, myrtenal, citronellal, cinnamaldehyde, benzaldehyde, cuminaldehyde
- Monoterpene alcohol: lavandulol, α-terpineol, borneol, isopulegol

Various components in EOs possess variable smells or flavors [51]. Table 8.1 demonstrates alcohol-containing EOs and their biological effects.

8.5 Production of EOs Using Plant Tissue Culture

Aromatic plants are considered as a rich source of a variety of bioactive secondary metabolites present in EOs and offer novel therapeutics to pharmaceutical industries for the formulation of herbal products. Plant tissue culture has been used as an effective tool for large-scale multiplication of EO-producing plants, thus circumventing overexploitation of natural resources [52–76]. Plant cell and organ culture establishes a viable, controllable, and eco-friendly approach for the commercial production of EOs. Moreover, advancement in product secretion, biotransformation, cell line selection, extraction, scale-up, and cell permeabilization help in the improvement of EO yields. Nevertheless, there are still various considerable challenges to the commercial production of high-value chemicals from these sources [52–76]. Advancement in isolation, culturing, and characterization of cambial meristematic cells offer a key platform to avoid many of these possible challenges. Micropropagation-based techniques are independent of climatic and geographical conditions and thus offer a continuous, sustainable, economical, and viable way to produce secondary metabolites [52–76]. Different procedures can be used to improve the yield of EOs in plants and modify their chemical composition [52–76]. One report suggested that 1-deoxy-d-xylulose-5-phosphate synthase (GrDXS) upregulation resulted in an increase in terpenoidal composition of *Pelargonium* spp. (EO) and *Withania somnifera* (withanolides). Upregulation of genes related to precursor pathways in peppermint as well as lavender resulted in an increase in monoterpene level in EOs [77,78]. Jadaun et al. [77] reported that1-deoxy-d-xylulose-5-phosphate synthase (GrDXS) upregulation resulted in an increase in moreaccumulation of terpenoids in *Pelargonium* spp. (EO) and *Withania somnifera* (withanolides). The influence of plant growth regulators (PGRs) on EO composition and in vitro development of *A. alba* shoot cultures has been studied [79], and it was found that morphological development of *A. alba* shoot cultures affects the terpenoid biosynthetic pathway, suggesting the hypothesis for a possible root to shoot signaling. The chemical composition of the EO obtained from the callus and cell suspension cultures of stem and root of *Hypericum triquetrifolium* has been investigated, and it was found that the alkane, aldehyde, and monoterpene levels were higher in EOs [80].

REFERENCES

1. Yim VW, Ng AK, Tsang HW, Leung AY. A review on the effects of aromatherapy for patients with depressive symptoms. *J Altern Complement Med.* 2009;15(2):187–195.
2. Chnaubelt K. *Medical Aromatherapy: Healing with Essential Oils.* Frog Ltd, Berkeley, CA; 1999.
3. Shiina Y, Funabashi N, Lee K, Toyoda T, Sekine T, Honjo S, Hasegawa R, Kawata T, Wakatsuki Y, Hayashi S, Murakami S, Koike K, Daimon M, Komuro I. Relaxation effects of lavender aromatherapy improve coronary flow velocity reserve in healthy men evaluated by transthoracic Doppler echocardiography. *Int J Cardiol.* 2008;129(2):193–197.
4. Smith A. The olfactory process and its effect on human behavior. Biology 202 Second Web Reports On Serendip. 1999.
5. Watt M, Essential oils. Their lack of skin absorption but effectiveness via inhalation. *Aromat Thymes.* 1995;3(2):11–13.
6. Yamada K, Mimaki Y, Sashida Y. Anticonvulsive effects of inhaling lavender oil vapour. *Biol Pharm Bull.* 1994;17(2):359–360.

7. Franz C, Novak J. Effect of essential oils in central nervous system. In: Hu¨snu¨ Can Baser K, Buchbauer G, editors. *Handbook of Essential Oils*. CRC Press, Taylor & Francis Group, Boca Raton, FL; 2010: 345–381.
8. Baldium I, Tonani L, Kress MR, Oliveira W. Lippia sidoides essential oil encapsulated in lipid nanosystem as an antiCandida agent. *Ind Crops Prod*. 2019;127:73–81.
9. Fernandes CC, Rezende JL, Silva EAJ, Silva FG, Stenico L, Crotti AEM, Esperandim VR, Santiago MB, Martins CHG, Miranda MLD. Chemical composition and biological activities of essential oil from flowers of Psidium guajava (Myrtaceae). *Braz J Biol*. 2021;81(3):728–736.
10. Koutsaviti AV, Antonopoulou A, Vlassi S, Antonatos A, Michaelakis D, Papachristos, Tzakou O. Chemical composition and fumigant activity of essential oils from six plants families against Sitophilus oryzaae (col: Curculionidae). *J Pest Sci*. 2018;91(2):873–886.
11. Aziz ZAA, Ahmad A, Setapar SHM, Karakucuk A, Azim MM, Lokhat D, Rafatullah M, Ganash M, Kamal MA, Ashraf GM. Essential oils: Extraction techniques, pharmaceutical and therapeutic potential: A review. *Curr Drug Metab*. 2018;19(13):1100–1110.
12. Benmoussa H, Elfalleh W, Farhat A, Bachoual R, Nasfi Z, Romdhane M. Effect of extraction methods on kinetic, chemical composition and antibacterial activities of Tunisian *Thymus vulgaris* L. essential oil. *Sep Sci Technol*. 2016;51(13):2145–2152.
13. Tongnuanchan P, Benjakul S. Essential oils: Extraction, bioactivities, and their uses for food preservation. *J Food Sci*. 2014;79:R1231–R1249.
14. Chouhan S, Sharma K, Guleria S. Antimicrobial activity of some essential oils-present status and future perspectives. *Medicines (Basel)*. 2017;4(3):58.
15. Beyki M, Mohsenifar A, Abollahi A, et al. Encapsulation of Mentha piperita essential oils in chitosan–cinnamic acid nanogel with enhanced antimicrobial activity against Aspergillus flavus. *Ind Crops Prod*. 2014;54:310–319.
16. Salvia-Trujillo L, Rojas-Graü A, Soliva-Fortuny R, Martín-Belloso O. Physicochemical characterization and antimicrobial activity of foodgrade emulsions and nanoemulsions incorporating essential oils. *Food Hydrocoll*. 2015;43:547–556.
17. Herculano ED, de Paula HCB, de Figueiredo EAT, Dias FGB, de A. Pereira V. Physicochemical and antimicrobial properties of nanoencapsulated *Eucalyptus staigeriana* essential oil. *LWT Food Sci Technol*. 2015;6:484–491.
18. Ali Mohammadi A, Hashemi M, Hosseini SM. Nanoencapsulation of *Zataria multiflora* essential oil preparation and characterization with enhanced antifungal activity for controlling *Botrytis cinerea*, the causal agent of gray mould disease. *Innov Food Sci Emerg Technol*. 2015;28:73–80.
19. Feyzioglu GC, Tornuk F. Development of chitosan nanoparticles loaded with summer savory (*Satureja hortensis L.*) essential oil for antimicrobial and antioxidant delivery applications. *LWT Food Sci Technol*. 2016;70:104–110.
20. Zhang S, Zhang M, Fang Z, Liu Y. Preparation and characterization of blended cloves/cinnamon essential oil nanoemulsions. *LWT Food Sci Technol*. 2017;75:316–322.
21. Mohammadia A, Hashemib M, Masoud SH. Chitosan nanoparticles loaded with *Cinnamomum zeylanicum* essential oil enhance the shelf life of cucumber during cold storage. *Postharvest Biol Technol*. 2015;110:203–213.
22. López V, Nielsen B, Solas M, Ramírez MJ, Jäger AK. Exploring pharmacological mechanisms of lavender (*Lavandula angustifolia*) essential oil on central nervous system targets. *Front Pharmacol*. 2017;8:280.
23. Sayorwan W, Ruangrungsi N, Piriyapunyporn T, Hongratanaworakit T, Kotchabhakdi N, Siripornpanich V. Effects of inhaled rosemary oil on subjective feelings and activities of the nervous system. *Sci Pharm*. 2013;81(2):531–542.
24. Koo BS, Lee SI, Ha JH, Lee DU. Inhibitory effects of the essential oil from SuHeXiang Wan on the central nervous system after inhalation. *Biol Pharm Bull*. 2004;27(4):515–519.
25. Koo BS, Park KS, Ha JH, Park JH, Lim JC, Lee DU. Inhibitory effects of the fragrance inhalation of essential oil from Acorus gramineus on central nervous system. *Biol Pharm Bull*. 2003;26(7):978–982.
26. Falcão SI, Bacem G, Igrejas PJ, Vilas-Boas RM, Amaral JS. Chemical composition and antimicrobial activity of hidrodestilled oil from juniper berries. *Ind Crops Prod*. 2018;124:878–884.
27. Rios JL. Essential oils: What they are and how the terms are used and defined. In: Preddy V. (editor) *Essential Oils in Food Preservation, Flavor and Safety*. Elsevier, London, UK; 2016:3–9.
28. Smeriglio AS, Alloisio FM, Raimondo M, et al., Essential oil of citrus *Lumnia risso*: Phytochemical profile, antioxidant properties and activity on critical reviews in food science and nutrition 9 the central nervous system. *Food Chem Toxicol*. 2018;119:407–416.
29. Turek C, Stintzing F. Stability of essential oils: A review. *Compr Rev Food Sci Food Saf*. 2013;12(1):40–53.
30. Ghabraie, MK. Dang Vu, Tata L, Salmieri S, Lacroix M. Antimicrobial effect of essential oils in combinations against five bacteria and their effect on sensorial quality of ground meat. *LWT Food Sci Technol*. 2016;66:332–339.
31. Solorzano-Santos F, Miranda-Novales M. Essential oils from aromatic herbs as antimicrobial agents. *Curr Opin Biotechnol*. 2012;23(2):136–141.
32. Ju J, Xie Y, Yu H, Guo Y, Cheng Y, Qian H, Yao W. Synergistic interactions of plant essential oils with antimicrobial agents: A new antimicrobial therapy. *Crit Rev Food Sci Nutr*. 2020:1–12. https://pubmed.ncbi.nlm.nih.gov/33207954/
33. Gutierrez J, Barry-Ryan C, Bourke P. The antimicrobial efficacy of plant essential oil combinations and interactions with food ingredients. *Int J Food Microbiol*. 2008;124(1):91–97.
34. Kalemba, D, Kunicka A. Antibacterial and antifungal properties of essential oils. *Curr Med Chem*. 2003;10(10):813–829.
35. Varga, E, Bardocz A, Belak A, Maraz A, Boros B, Felinger A, Böszörmenyi A, Horvath G. Antimicrobial activity and chemical composition of thyme essential oils and the polyphenolic content of different thymus extracts. *Farmacia*. 2015;6(3):357–361.

36. Khan A, Mujeerb FF, Aha F, Farooqui A. Effect of plant growth regulators on growth and essential oil content in Palmarosa (*Cymbopogon martini*). *Asian J Pharm Clin Res.* 2015;8(2):373–376.
37. Qin Z, Feng K, Wang W, Wang W, Wang Y, Lu J, Li E, Niu S, Jiao Y. Comparative study on the essential oils of six hawk tea (Litsea coreana levl. Var. lanuginose) from China: Yields, chemical compositions and biological activities. *Ind Crops Prod.* 2018;124:126–135.
38. Popovici J, Bertrand C, Bagnarol E, Fernandez M, Comte G. Chemical composition of essential oil and headspace-solid microextracts from fruits of *Myrica gale* L. and antifungal activity. *Nat Prod Res.* 2008;22(12):1024–1032.
39. Boukhatem MN, Ferhat MA, Kameli A, Saidi F, Mekarnia M. Liquid and vapour phase antibacterial activity of eucalyptus globulus essential oil ¼ susceptibility of selected respiratory tract pathogens. *Am J Infect Dis.* 2014;10(3):105–117.
40. Feriotto G, Marchetti N, Costa V, Beninati S, Tagliati F, Mischiati C. Chemical composition of essential oils from *Thymus vulgaris*, *Cymbopogon citratus* and *Rosmarinus officinalis*, and their effects on the HIV-1 tat protein function. *Chem Biodivers.* 2018;15:1–10.
41. Hernandez-Molina LR. Purificacion cromatrografica de metabolitos secundarios de origen vegetal. In: Lopez-Olguın JF, Aragon-Garcıa A, Tapia-Rojas AM (editors). *En avances en agroecologıa y ambiente.* Publicacion especial de la Benemerita Universidad Autonoma de Puebla, Puebla, Mexico; 2007;1:173–192. ISBN: 9789689391074.
42. Cserhati T, Forgacs E, Deyl Z, Miksik I. Chromatography in authenticity and traceability tests of vegetable oils and dairy products: A review. *Biomed Chromatogr.* 2005;19(3):183–190.
43. Brattoli M, Cisternino E, Dambruoso PR, de Gennaro G, Giungato P, Mazzone A, Palmisani J, Tutino M. Gas chromatography analysis with olfactometric detection (GC-O) as a useful methodology for chemical characterization of odorous compounds. *Sensors (Basel).* 2013;13(12):16759–16800.
44. Lebanov L, Tedone L, Kaykhaii M. et al. Multidimensional gas chromatography in essential oil analysis. Part 2: Application to characterisation and identification. *Chromatographia.* 2019;82:399–414.
45. Masango P Cleaner production of essential oils by steam distillation. *J Cleaner Prod.* 2005;13:833–839.
46. Bakkali F, Averbeck S, Averbeck D, Idaomar M. Biological effects of essential oils: A review. *Food Chem Toxicol.* 2008;46(2):446–475.
47. Lee KB, Cho E, Kang YS. Changes in 5-hydroxytryptamine and cortisol plasma levels in menopausal women after inhalation of clary sage oil. *Phytother Res.* 2014;28:1599–1605.
48. Lakusić B, Lakusić D, Ristić M, Marcetić M, Slavkovska V. Seasonal variations in the composition of the essential oils of *Lavandula angustifolia* (Lamiacae). *Nat Prod Commun.* 2014;9:859–862.
49. Guzmán-Gutiérrez SL, Bonilla-Jaime H, Gómez-Cansino R, Reyes-Chilpa R. Linalool and β-pinene exert their antidepressant-like activity through the monoaminergic pathway. *Life Sci.* 2015;128:24–29.
50. Melo FH, Moura BA, de Sousa DP, de Vasconcelos SM, Macedo DS, Fonteles MM, Viana GS, de Sousa FC. Antidepressant-like effect of carvacrol (5-Isopropyl-2-methylphenol) in mice: Involvement of dopaminergic system. *Fundam Clin.Pharmacol.* 2011;25:362–367.
51. Burt S. Essential oils: Their antibacterial properties and potential applications in foods: A review. *Int J Food Microbiol.* 2004;94(3):223–253.
52. Bhatia S, Sharma K, Dahiya R, Bera T. Plant tissue culture. In: *Modern Applications of Plant Biotechnology in Pharmaceutical Sciences.* Academic Press, Cambridge, MA; 2015:31–107.
53. Bhatia S, Sharma K, Dahiya R, Bera T. Laboratory organization. In: *Modern Applications of Plant Biotechnology in Pharmaceutical Sciences.* Academic Press, Cambridge, MA; 2015:109–120.
54. Bhatia S, Sharma K, Dahiya R, Bera T. Concepts and techniques of plant tissue culture science. In: *Modern Applications of Plant Biotechnology in Pharmaceutical Sciences.* Academic Press, Cambridge, MA; 2015:121–156.
55. Bhatia S, Sharma K, Dahiya R, Bera T. Application of plant biotechnology. In: *Modern Applications of Plant Biotechnology in Pharmaceutical Sciences.* Academic Press, Cambridge, MA; 2015:157–207.
56. Bhatia S, Sharma K, Dahiya R, Bera T. Somatic embryogenesis and organogenesis. In: *Modern Applications of Plant Biotechnology in Pharmaceutical Sciences.* Academic Press, Cambridge, MA; 2015:209–230.
57. Bhatia S, Sharma K, Dahiya R, Bera T. Classical and non-classical techniques for secondary metabolite production in plant cell culture. In: *Modern Applications of Plant Biotechnology in Pharmaceutical Sciences.* Academic Press, Cambridge, MA; 2015:231–291.
58. Bhatia S, Sharma K, Dahiya R, Bera T. Plant-based biotechnological products with their production host, modes of delivery systems, and stability testing. In: *Modern Applications of Plant Biotechnology in Pharmaceutical Sciences.* Academic Press, Cambridge, MA; 2015:293–331.
59. Bhatia S, Sharma K, Dahiya R, Bera T. Edible vaccines. In: *Modern Applications of Plant Biotechnology in Pharmaceutical Sciences.* Academic Press, Cambridge, MA; 2015: 333–343.
60. Bhatia S, Sharma K, Dahiya R, Bera T. Microenvironmentation in micropropagation. In: *Modern Applications of Plant Biotechnology in Pharmaceutical Sciences.* Academic Press, Cambridge, MA; 2015:345–360.
61. Bhatia S, Sharma K, Dahiya R, Bera T. Micropropagation. In: *Modern Applications of Plant Biotechnology in Pharmaceutical Sciences.* Academic Press, Cambridge, MA; 2015:361–368.
62. Bhatia S, Sharma K, Dahiya R, Bera T. Laws in plant biotechnology. In: *Modern Applications of Plant Biotechnology in Pharmaceutical Sciences.* Academic Press, Cambridge, MA; 2015:369–391.
63. Bhatia S, Sharma K, Dahiya R, Bera T. Technical glitches in micropropagation. In: *Modern Applications of Plant Biotechnology in Pharmaceutical Sciences.* Academic Press, Cambridge, MA; 2015:393–404.
64. Bhatia S, Sharma K, Dahiya R, Bera T. Plant tissue culture-based industries. In: *Modern Applications of Plant Biotechnology in Pharmaceutical Sciences.* Academic Press, Cambridge, MA; 2015:405–417.
65. Bhatia S, Sharma A, Vargas De La Cruz CB, Chaugule B, Al-Harrasi A. Nutraceutical, antioxidant, antimicrobial properties of *Pyropia vietnamensis* (Tanaka et Pham-Hong Ho) J.E. Sutherl. et Monotilla. *Curr Bioact Compd.* 2020;16:1.

66. Bhatia S, Sardana S, Senwar KR, Dhillon A, Sharma A, Naved T. In vitro antioxidant and antinociceptive properties of *Porphyra vietnamensis*. *Biomedicine (Taipei)*. 2019;9(1):3.
67. Bhatia S, Sharma K, Namdeo AG, Chaugule BB, Kavale M, Nanda S. Broad-spectrum sun-protective action of Porphyra-334 derived from *Porphyra vietnamensis*. *Pharmacognosy Res*. 2010;2(1):45–49.
68. Bhatia S, Sharma K, Sharma A, Nagpal K, Bera T. Anti-inflammatory, analgesic and antiulcer properties of *Porphyra vietnamensis*. *Avicenna J Phytomed*. 2015;5(1):69–77.
69. Bhatia S, Sardana S, Sharma A, Vargas De La Cruz CB, Chaugule B, Khodaie L. Development of broad spectrum mycosporine loaded sunscreen formulation from Ulva fasciata delile. *Biomedicine (Taipei)*. 2019;9(3):17.
70. Bhatia S, Garg A, Sharma K, Kumar S, Sharma A, Purohit AP. Mycosporine and mycosporine-like amino acids: A paramount tool against ultra violet irradiation. *Pharmacogn Rev*. 2011;5(10):138–146.
71. Bhatia S, Namdeo AG, Nanda S. Factors effecting the gelling and emulsifying properties of a natural polymer. *SRP*. 2010;1(1):86–92.
72. Bhatia S, Sharma K, Bera T. Structural characterization and pharmaceutical properties of Porphyran. *Asian J Pharm*. 2015;9:93–101.
73. Bhatia S, Sharma A, Sharma K, Kavale M, Chaugule BB, Dhalwal K, Namdeo AG, Mahadik KR. Novel algal polysaccharides from marine source: Porphyran. *Pharmacogn Rev*. 2008;4:271–276.
74. Bhatia S, Sharma K, Nagpal K, Bera T. Investigation of the factors influencing the molecular weight of porphyran and its associated antifungal activity bioact. *Carb Diet Fiber*. 2015;5:153–168.
75. Bhatia S, Kumar V, Sharma K, Nagpal K, Bera T. Significance of algal polymer in designing amphotericin B nanoparticles. *Sci World J*. 2014;2014:564573.
76. Bhatia S, Rathee P, Sharma K, Chaugule BB, Kar N, Bera T. Immuno-modulation effect of sulphated polysaccharide (porphyran) from *Porphyra vietnamensis*. *Int J Biol Macromol*. 2013;57:50–56.
77. Jadaun JS, Sangwan NS, Narnoliya LK, Singh N, Bansal S, Mishra B, Sangwan RS. Over-expression of DXS gene enhances terpenoidal secondary metabolite accumulation in rose-scented geranium and *Withania somnifera*: Active involvement of plastid isoprenogenic pathway in their biosynthesis. *Physiol Plant*. 2017;159(4):381–400.
78. Muñoz-Bertomeu J, Arrillaga I, Ros R, Segura J. Up-regulation of 1-deoxy-D-xylulose-5-phosphate synthase enhances production of essential oils in transgenic spike lavender. *Plant Physiol*. 2006;142(3):890–900. doi: 10.1104/pp.106.086355. Epub 2006 September 15.
79. Danova K, Todorova M, Trendafilova A, Evstatieva L. Cytokinin and auxin effect on the terpenoid profile of the essential oil and morphological characteristics of shoot cultures of *Artemisia alba*. *Nat Prod Commun*. 2012;7(8):1075–1076.
80. Tahir NA, Azeez HA, Muhammad KA, Faqe SA, Omer DA. Exploring of bioactive compounds in essential oil acquired from the stem and root derivatives of *Hypericum triquetrifolium* callus cultures. *Nat Prod Res*. 2019;33(10):1504–1508.

9

Effect of Methods of Extraction on Chemical Composition of Essential Oils

Ahmed Al-Harrasi
Natural and Medical Sciences Research Center, University of Nizwa

Saurabh Bhatia
Natural and Medical Sciences Research Center, University of Nizwa
University of Petroleum and Energy Studies

Md. Tanvir Kabir
BRAC University

Tapan Behl
Chitkara University

Deepak Kaushik
M.D. University

Vineet Mittal
M.D. University

Ajay Sharma
Delhi Pharmaceutical Sciences and Research University

CONTENTS

9.1 Introduction

Essential oils (EOs) are liquid and aromatic extracts composed of volatile chemicals that are obtained from aromatic plants by various conventional and advanced extraction methods. There are various extraction procedures available [1]. The type of extraction method used for extraction determines the biological and physicochemical properties of the finished liquid product. Numerous modern (supercritical fluid extraction (SFE), solvent-free microwave extraction (SFME), subcritical extraction liquid) and conventional (hydrodiffusion, hydrodistillation, solvent extraction, and steam distillation) methods have been used for the extraction of EOs. Modern extraction methods are the most favorable for the extraction of EOs as they offer various advantages such as low energy consumption, low solvent used, less extraction time, and less carbon dioxide emission [1].

DOI: 10.1201/9781003175933-11

9.2 Methods of Extraction

EOs can be isolated from aromatic plants by using various extraction methods. Considering the sensitivity and vulnerability of chemical components of EOs against various degradative conditions such as increased in oxidative environment, isomerization, cyclization, dehydrogenation, polymerization reactions, and to overcome the chemical transformation of EOs, there has been a shift from traditional extraction methods toward advanced techniques to produce quality EOs [2]. Much advancement has been gained in extraction procedures, especially design of the technique, type of solvent system (e.g., supercritical fluid-assisted extraction by using CO_2), and energy sources (e.g., microwaves and ultrasonic waves), with resulting systems having the following advantages [2]:

- Low consumption of energy to make the process cost-effective
- Reduced overall time of extraction process
- Eco-friendly methods, especially in solvent systems
- Quality EOs with minimum exposure to degradation
- Reduced solvent use
- Increases in yield and quality of final products
- Easy to handle and safe
- Less plant material needed and more yield

However, even with continuous advancements in the industries, majority of the industries are facing challenges associated with continuous supply of authenticated material, especially the type of botanical material considered for the extraction. Effective processing such as drying and size reduction and storage of plant material before extraction is another crucial parameter, and can determine the yield of EOs. Substandard extraction methods can result in the production of poor-quality EOs with higher risk of chemical transformation with loss of some important chemical, physical, and biological properties. As described in the following section, various procedures can be used to extract EOs from different plant materials.

9.3 Distillation-Based Extraction

9.3.1 Steam Distillation

Steam distillation is a conventional technique most extensively used to extract EOs from plant material [3,4]. The amount of EOs extracted via steam distillation is 93%, and the residual 7% can be later extracted using other procedures [3,5]. In this process, the plant material to be extracted is heated with boiling water or steam in order to promote cell lysis so that aromatic substances are leached out of the cell sap and released and further separated [3,6]. Recently, various robust steam-assisted extractions with new process designs have been developed to enhance the yield of EOs and to minimize the loss of polar components in water phase [3,5]. In newer systems, the plant material is not treated with boiling water; but instead the steam is passed through packed plant materials to get the EOs. These modifications reduce the proportion of water in the distillate with less of steam and decrease the dissolution of the polar components of EOs in aqueous phase [3,5]. Further, it was also found that distillation time can be used as a crucial parameter to determine the chemical profile of EOs. As has been seen in case of lavender EO, the length of the distillation time influenced the yield as well as chemical composition of when extracted from the same plant material (dried flowers). Findings suggested that out of different distillation times tested during this study, lavender EO showed maximum yield (range 0.5%–6.8%) at 60 minutes' distillation time [7,8]. Further, it was also suggested that the proportion of components was highest at different distillation times such as cineole and fenchol (1.5 minutes), camphor (7.5–15 minutes), and linalool acetate (30 minutes), whereas extending length of the distillation time decreased the yield of EO [7,8]. So it was concluded that distillation time must be optimized before the extraction of EOs. As per the previous report, distillation time modified EO yield, composition, and antioxidant capacity of fennel (*Foeniculum vulgare* Mill) [7,8]. It was found that fennel oils from the 20 and 160 minute distillation times had higher antioxidant potential than the fennel oil derived at 1.25 minutes' distillation time, which could be attributed to its differential composition [7,8].

Recently, a qualitative and quantitative procedure for the determination of the chemical components of jujube volatile oils via coupling steam distillation/drop-by-drop extraction with gas chromatography–mass spectrometry (GC-MS) was developed. It was concluded that the developed procedure was simple, fast, effective, sensitive, and provided a complete profile of the volatile components in jujube extract, and thus, this procedure can be employed to measure the volatile components of extracts [3,9].

Pretreatment of plant material with hydrolytic enzymes before steam or hydrodistillation was also reported to improve the ultimate yield of EO. It was found that pretreatment with hydrolytic enzymes has positive as well as negative effects over the composition of EOs, which can improve or decrease the yield accordingly [10]. Further, it was reported that the antioxidant potential of EOs from steam distillation process was noticeably higher in comparison with the oils extracted using hydrodistillation [3,11].

9.3.2 Hydrodistillation

Hydrodistillation is an old technique for extracting EOs by treating the plant material with boiling water ultimately to isolate non-polar components with high boiling point. This process involves the placement of the plant material in water followed by boiling in order to protect the EOs from the surrounding heat where the water acts as a barrier to avoid it from overheating. Using this process, the plant material can be distilled at a temperature <100°C. Distillation time before hydrodistillation of the plant material must be optimized as it was suggested in the case of steam distillation to further improve EO yield, composition of constituents, and biological activities. As was found in the case of hydrodistillation of *Coriandrum sativum* at different distillation times, *Coriandrum sativum* EO yield was low at the shorter distillation time and yield was improved with increasing distillation time. Variation in the chemical composition was also observed accordingly [12]. Further, advanced techniques such as microwave-assisted hydrodistillation using a microwave oven in the extraction process can be used to save energy, reduce extraction time, and improve the quality of EOs with increase in the level of oxygenated compounds [13]. It was found that hydrodistillation alone is not sufficient enough to extract EOs from certain plant materials like seeds because seeds gain water and swell rapidly, which can further result in the accumulation of seed mass at the bottom. Once the seeds accumulate at the bottom, they can be in direct contact with heated glass material, which can cause the burning of the seeds and can ultimately affect the yield of EOs. This problem can be overcome by using microwave-assisted and supercritical fluid-based hydrodistillation [14]. Considering the cost and sophistication associated with these facilities, the hydrodistillation method with magnetic stirrer and hot plate was developed [14].

A recent study showed the effectiveness of hydrodistillation, hydrodistillation with enzyme-assisted extraction, and SFE in extracting EO from pineapple peels. It was suggested that SFE successfully ruptured the oil gland (observed under the scanning electron microscope) and thus produced EO with better yield than other techniques [15]. The effect of the various extraction methods over the yield and properties of *Rosmarinus officinalis* L. was investigated in the previous study by using hydrodistillation and SFME. It was found that the overall yield obtained from hydrodistillation and SFMEs was 0.31% and 0.39%, respectively. EO obtained from hydrodistillation process showed higher level of monoterpene hydrocarbons, whereas SFMEs showed higher level of oxygenated monoterpenes. In another study, microwave-assisted hydrodistillation and ohmic-assisted hydrodistillation were compared with the efficiency of hydrodistillation extraction alone. In both modified hydrodistillation procedures, overall time period of extraction process was drastically reduced in comparison with traditional hydrodistillation (microwave-assisted: 75 minutes, while HD took 4 hours; ohmic-assisted: 24.75 minutes, while HD took 1 hour) [16]. Several reports suggested that the microwave-assisted hydrodistillation process has now been extensively used to extract *Rosmarinus officinalis*, *Coriander sativum*, *Agrimonia pilosa*, *Mangifera indica*, *Humulus Lupulus*, and *Thymus vulgaris* [17–21]. It was concluded that the microwave-assisted hydrodistillation method offers various advantages over traditional hydrodistillation and did not adversely influence the chemical profile of EOs as this process is robust, green, and fast [17–21]. In the previous report, a microwave turbo hydrodistillation procedure was used to extract EOs from hard dry plant materials such as bark, roots, and seeds. Findings from this study showed that EO extracted from dry *Schinus terebinthifolius* Raddi berries was quantitatively (yield) and qualitatively (aromatic profile) similar to that obtained by turbo hydrodistillation [22]. However, the microwave turbo hydrodistillation procedure was faster than turbo hydrodistillation (30 minutes compared with 180 minutes), so it allows significant savings of time and energy [22].

9.3.3 Hydrodiffusion

Hydrodiffusion is a kind of steam distillation process in which steam is supplied from the bottom to the plant material, which is packed in the column. Developed steam when allowed to pass through column containing the plant material evaporates the volatile components, and then, these volatile components present in vapor phase are directed to a condenser to convert into liquid form. Finally, it is collected in a graduated burette. This process is employed when the plant material is dried and not spoiled at boiling temperature [23]. Hydrodiffusion can be performed under reduced vacuum pressure to decrease steam temperature <100°C. This process is more effective than traditional steam distillation as this process requires less time and less steam provides high yield of EO. An advanced form of hydrodiffusion is microwave-assisted hydrodiffusion and gravity, which is a combination of microwaves for hydrodiffusion of EOs from the inside to the outside of plant material and earth gravity to collect and separate [23].

In previous reports, several researchers equated hydrodiffusion with innovative microwave hydrodiffusion and gravity (MHG) procedure for their efficiency in the isolation of EO from rosemary leaves *(R. officinalis)*, spearmint (*Mentha spicata* L.), pennyroyal (*Mentha pulegium* L.), and lavandin flower [24]. It was found that the MHG method has outstanding advantages over older methods such as shorter isolation times, low energy consumption, eco-friendly, no residue production and no water or solvent consumption, and increased biological activities [25,26]. In an earlier report, researchers investigated the effectiveness of advanced steam diffusion and microwave steam diffusion to extract EOs from the residual material of orange peel. It was found that EOs extracted by microwave steam diffusion take 12 minutes and showed the same yield and aromatic profile as those obtained by advanced steam diffusion for 40 minutes [27,28].

9.4 Solvent-Mediated Extraction

9.4.1 Solvent Extraction

Earlier solvent extraction process has been employed to the plant material to extract the essential oils without using heat. Various polar and non-polar solvents have been used for solvent extraction [3,29]. Usually, during this process, the plant material is treated with solvent followed by heating to extract the EO. Afterward, the solvent is filtered followed by its evaporation to concentrate the final fraction. The concentrated fraction may contain resin (resinoid) or concrete (a combination of wax, fragrance, and EO). To separate the EO fraction, the concentrated fraction is treated with alcohol and distilled at low temperatures. Finally, the alcohol is evaporated to derive the EO. However, one of the major drawbacks of this method is the involvement of hazardous chemicals, residues of which will unavoidably remain in the final product. Additionally, disadvantages like long extraction period, more solvent constraint, and poor reproducibility make this method a secondary choice to extract EOs [3,30]. It was found that solvent residue in the final product can cause allergies and toxicity and affect the immune system [3,31]. A previous study suggested that EO with antioxidant potential derived from *Ptychotis verticillata* contain carvacrol (44.6%) and thymol (3.4%) as the major components [3,32]. Another study demonstrated that EO separated from Thymus praecox by using different solvents showed thymol (40.31%) and o-cymene (13.66%) as the main constituents. Additionally, the water fraction showed the highest total phenolic and flavonoid content and ethanol, methanol, and water fractions possessed substantial antioxidant activity [3,33]. Similarly, another report showed that the water fraction showed high antioxidant activity in comparison with other fractions [3,34]. Recently, solvent-free methods such as SFME have become preferred over conventional solvent-based extraction. SFME produced EO with various advantages such as EOs with more oxygenated compounds and high biological activity. Additionally, microscopic analysis showed that the plant material extracted with SFME undergoes substantial changes in comparison with other methods. SFME showed various advantages such as reduced time period of overall extraction process, faster kinetics, and higher efficiency [35].

SFME is obviously a beneficial process in comparison with old distillation processes in terms of rapidity, productivity, cleanliness, considerable energy savings, and it being eco-friendly [36].

9.4.2 Supercritical Carbon Dioxide

SFE is an effective method of extraction of EOs from various aromatic plants with advantages such as convenience, less time-consuming, clean, solvent-free, higher extraction rate, easy to remove from the extracted materials, and eco-friendliness [37,38]. It is also known that conditions such as pressure, temperature, and co-solvent of SFE can be optimized to improve not only the efficiency of the extraction process but also the yield and chemical profile of the overall physical and chemical properties of EOs. Additionally, supercritical extracts were often identified as being of superior quality in comparison with those obtained by hydrodistillation or liquid–solid extraction. SFE is usually executed with pure CO_2 or using a co-solvent; fractionation of the extract is usually done so as to extract volatile components from other co-extracted substances [37,38].

Old procedures such as solvent extraction and steam distillation have various drawbacks such as prolonged time required and large amount of solvent needed [39]. Additionally, the degradation and loss of a number of volatile compounds, degradation of unsaturated compounds, low extraction efficacy, compromised quality of finished product, and presence of residual toxic solvent in the finished product could be experienced [40]. Thus, supercritical fluids have been recognized as another approach for EO extraction. Because of inertness, easy availability, cost-effectiveness, safety profile, and due to its suitable critical conditions, carbon dioxide (CO_2) is the most commonly used supercritical fluid [41].

Under high-pressure condition, CO_2 turns into liquid, which can be used as a very inert and safe medium to extract the aromatic molecules from raw material. In comparison with other supercritical fluids, CO_2 requires low critical conditions such as pressure to turn into liquid to further extract EO from the plant material, resulting in low energy consumption, which is related to the overall cost of the process. After being in liquid phase, CO_2 can return to gas phase and evaporate under normal atmospheric pressure and temperature conditions. As CO_2 can be recovered and recycled during this process, there is no risk of the presence of residual solvent in the final finished product. In spite of the high solubility of EO components in supercritical CO_2, the rate of extraction can be comparatively slow with pure CO_2 (ca. 80% recovery after 90 minutes) [42]. Nevertheless, certain modifications by initial treatment with methylene chloride (15-minutes static extraction) and then treatment with pure CO_2 (15-minutes dynamic extraction) can result in high recoveries. Extraction efficiency of this modified process was found to be equivalent to HD, which was executed for 4 hours. It is known that SFE is the most suitable for the extraction of volatile compounds such as monoterpenes. Reports also suggest that some organic components that were not extracted by HD can be easily recovered by SFE [42]. Previous reports also suggested that steam distillation in comparison with SFE provides lower yield with higher energy consumption; thus, it has been concluded that SFE is more cost-effective than steam distillation. Old procedures that have been used for the extraction of EOs from plant material present several disadvantages as follows:

- Time-consuming
- High solvent consumption
- Residual solvent present in the finished product
- Low efficiency
- High energy consumption
- Non-eco-friendly
- Influence chemical, physical, and biological properties of EO

Moreover, several EO components are not heat-stable and may degrade during thermal extraction or distillation. High temperature during steam distillation and the presence of a solvent like water can cause chemical changes in EOs. Processes like steam distillation generally can lead to the degradation or loss of highly volatile as well as polar compounds. Additionally, while using solvent extraction, it is usually difficult to get a solvent-free finished product. Additionally, modification of certain adjustable parameters, especially in the case of hydrodistillation, steam distillation, and solvent extraction, to improve the selectivity of the whole process is an additional shortcoming of these procedures [42–46]. The effects of optimized SFE over the chemical composition and yield of EOs in comparison with other extraction processes are given in Table 9.1.

Independent variables such as pressure, temperature, and time were considered as significant parameters affecting extraction yield during SFE. Optimization of SFE conditions plays an important role in improving EO yield. *Cyperus rotundus* EO yield was increased considerably with pressure and CO_2 flow rate (pressure of 294.4 bar and CO_2 flow rate of 20.9 L/h) [78].

Another report showed that under optimized conditions such as pressure of 355 bar, temperature of 65°C, methanol volume of 150 μL, dynamic and static extraction times of 35 and 10 minutes, the main compounds were methyl linoleate (18.2%), camphor (12.32%), cis-thujone (11.3%), and trans-caryophyllene (9.17%). The findings suggested that by using optimum conditions, SFE is more selective than the steam distillation procedure [79].

Based on the Box–Behnken design response surface model, the optimal CO_2 SFE condition of *Rana chensinensis* ovum oil was pressure 29 MPa, flow 82 L/h, temperature 50°C, and time

TABLE 9.1

Effect of Optimized SFE over the Chemical Composition and Yield of EOs in Comparison with Other Extraction Process

EO Source	Comparison with	Merits	Influence of SFE over Yield/Chemical Profile of EO	References
Eucalyptus cinerea	HD	HD offer more EO yield; however, SCE present improved composition	High 1,8-cineole yield	[47]
Eucalyptus citriodora	HD	SCE presented lower amount of EO than HD; but contain more amount of citronellal	Citronellal (79%)	[48]
Nigella sativa	Solvent extraction methods	SFE showed more extraction efficiency	High linoleic acid and thymoquinone level	[49]
Eucalyptus cinerea, Eucalyptus camaldulensis	HD	SCE was superior to HD, regarding shorter extraction times (green approach and present stable components)	*E. camaldulensis*: 8,14-cedranoxide (43.79%), elemol (6.3%); *E. cinerea*: 1 p-menth-1-en-8-ol and 8-cineole (31.87% and 16.1%)	[50]
Curcuma wenyujin	SD	SFE is better than SD in extraction time, power consumption, recovery, and purity	Chemical composition obtained from both processes was found to be the same	[51]
Bupleurum chinense	SD	Increase in yield with decrease in extraction time	Caproaldehyde, saikosaponins	[52]
Curcuma longa	SD	SFE-CO_2 approach is superior than SD, regarding more amount of EO in short duration	Components from both procedures are same, however their level has some variation	[53]
Angelica gigas	SD	Electroencephalographic showed that absolute low beta wave considerably enhanced	-	[54]
Camellia sinensis EO		Showed considerable antioxidant activity than geranium and peppermint EO	59 compounds, including alkanes, esters, ketones, aldehydes, terpenes, acids, alcohols, ethers	[55]
Pineapple peel EO	HD; HD with enzyme-assisted	SFE had successfully extracted the EO and ruptured the oil gland	EO contains propanoic acid ethyl ester, lactic acid ethyl ester, 2-heptanol, propanol, 3-hexanone, butanoic acid ethyl ester	[56]
Pteris multifida	SD	Significant difference in chemical composition	Chemical components of EO extracted by SFE-CO_2 (27) are different from that extracted by SD (45)	[57]
Dalbergia odorifera	SD	SFE is comparatively superior to SD procedure	12 compounds in SFE sample with major compounds: 2-propenoic acid-3(4-methoxyphenyl)-ethyl ester, nerolidol, ageratochromene, and 9 compounds were identified in SD sample	[58]
Schizonepeta tenuifolia	SD	SFE procedure is superior than the SD procedure	54 compounds were identified with main components such as pulegone, menthone, linoleic acid chloride	[59]
Ocimum basilicum	SD	Significant difference in chemical composition	40 and 42 compounds were detected in the SD sample and SFE-CO2 EO sample	[60]
Folium Rhododendri Daurici	SD	Significant difference in chemical composition	52 compounds in SCE-CO2 sample and 48 compounds in SD sample	[61]
Mosla soochowensis	SD and organic solvent (petroleum ether) extraction	SFE is the optimum extraction method	Yield of EO by means of SFE (3.46%) was higher than others with methyleugenol as the main component	[62]
Atractylodes macrocephala	SWE and SD	Extraction rate is higher, and the components are more with the method of SFE-CO2	SFE-CO2 yield: 2.32% (37); SD yield: 1.01% (15); ultrasonic wave yield: 1.6% (20)	[63]
Cymbopogon citronella	HD	Radical scavenging effects of SFE EO were superior than HD derived EO	41 components derived from SFE, whereas 35 components from HD	[64]
Fennel oil	SD as well as solvent based extraction	Sensory assessment demonstrated that the SFE EO was found to be stronger in smell as well as flavor than others	Fennel seeds showed greater EO level (10.0%) than SD (3.0%), hexane fraction (10.6%), and lower yield than alcohol extraction (15.4%)	[65]
Foeniculum vulgare, Thymus vulgaris	Simultaneous distillation extraction (SDE)	Both processes show the same chemical composition; however, SDE showed more level of monoterpenes	SDE as well as SFE demonstrated identical chemical profile. Higher level of monoterpenes derived by SDE	[66]
Schisandra chinensis	SD, ultrasound-assisted extraction (UAE) and Soxhlet extraction (SE)	SFE showed more aromatics and sesquiterpenoidal compounds whereas monoterpenoidal components are low in level	SFE fraction contain 32 components	[67]

(Continued)

TABLE 9.1 (*Continued*)

Effect of Optimized SFE over the Chemical Composition and Yield of EOs in Comparison with Other Extraction Process

EO Source	Comparison with	Merits	Influence of SFE over Yield/Chemical Profile of EO	References
Ligusticum wallichii	MD	SFE combined with MD, a technique better than simple SFE, can be used to extract, separate, and purify the volatile components	45 kinds of chemical constituents from SFE extract, among which 39 were left after distillation by MD	[68]
Satureja Montana	HD	At optimized conditions of SFE, considerable difference in thymoquinone level was found	Thymoquinone level in SFE 1.6-3.0% and 0.2% for HD; variation among other compounds carvacrol, thymol, p-cymene, gamma-terpinene, beta-bisabolene	[69]
Thymus vulgaris	HD	-	Difference in chemical composition (p-cymene, gamma-terpinene, linalool, thymol, carvacrol, carvacryl methyl ether)	[70]
Plumeria rubra	SD	Significant variation among oils derived from SFE as well as SD	53 components in SFE extract	[71]
Elsholtzia fruticosa	HD and headspace (HS)	Significant difference in chemical composition	35 have been detected in HD as well as SFE EOsoils and 14 in the HS; SFE: sesquiterpene hydrocarbons 21.8%; SFE: 3.4% diterpenes; SFE sesquiterpene hydrocarbons : 21.8%	[72]
Pimpinella anisum	HD	At optimized conditions, extraction efficiency significantly increased	SFE (7.5%) is higher than that obtained by HD (3.1%)	[73]
Santolina chamaecyparissus	Hydrodistillation	At optimized SFE conditions, chemical profile of the fractions has been significantly affected by the temperature and pressure	Increased sesquiterpenoidal and volatile components by changing temperature and pressure	[74]
Chamaecyparis obtusa	HD	At optimized SFE conditions	Increased level of 1-muurolol, α-terpinyl acetate and elemol	[75]
Mentha pulegium	HD	At optimized SFE conditions	Menthone (30.3%) and pulegone (52.0%) at optimized SFE conditions	[76]
Perovskia atriplicifolia	SD	Raising the temperature decreased the number of extracted components, but constituents number increased when lower pressure was used	γ-cadinene, 1,8-cineole, β-caryophyllene, α-terpinyl acetate, limonene, camphor, and α-pinene	[77]

SFE, supercritical fluid extraction; SD, steam distillation; SE, Soxhlet extraction; UAE, ultrasound-assisted extraction; MD, molecular distillation; HD, hydrodistillation; and HS, headspace.

132 minutes, and the corresponding predicted optimal yield was 13.61% [80].

Optimal conditions for the SFE of pomegranate (*Punica granatum* L.) peel EO, optimized using a central composite design, were 350 atmospheric pressure, 55°C temperature, 30 minutes extraction time, and 150 μL methanol. Findings from this study suggested that oleic acid, palmitic acid, and (–)-borneol were the main components with extraction yield 1.18% (w/w) [81].

A response surface methodology was applied to optimize the conditions of supercritical CO_2 extraction for extracting *Cymbopogon citronella* EO. The highest EO yield was predicted at extraction time 120 minutes, extraction pressure 25 MPa, extraction temperature 35°C, and CO_2 flow 18 L/h for the SFE processing. Under these experimental conditions, the mean EO yield was found to be 4.40% [82].

In another study, the optimization of independent factors based on the Box–Behnken method was planned, and the extraction yields and overall phenolic levels of *Lavandula angustifolia* flowers were measured for three different variables: pressure, temperature, and extraction time. It was found that highest yield (9.2 wt.%) was attained at a temperature of 60°C under the pressure of 250 bar after 45 minutes. These conditions presented highest total phenolic content (10.17 mg GAE/g extract). Based on the study, these optimal extraction conditions that showed highest total phenolic content from flowers of *Lavandula angustifolia* were at temperature of 54.5°C, pressure of 297.9 bar, and time of 45 minutes. Based on the antioxidant potential of SFE extracts, it was demonstrated that the increase of extraction pressure had a positive influence on the increase of antioxidant activity [83].

9.4.3 Subcritical Water Extraction

Subcritical water extraction (SWE) has been developed as a novel extraction procedure with the following advantages [84,85].

- Eco-friendly process
- Short extraction time
- High efficiency
- Low energy consumption
- Used for the extraction of organic pollutants in ecological samples
- Used for the extraction of active chemical components from various plants

Subcritical water or hot pressured water was obtained after heating water above its boiling point (100°C) and at less than its critical point (374°C). As it is well known that water at high temperature has a lower dielectric constant, which reduces the hydrogen bonding, water in the subcritical region and close to its critical properties presents a decrease in the dielectric constant because of the breakdown of hydrogen bonds between the water molecules [86–88]. This dielectric constant is related to the polarity of water. These changes make subcritical water properties comparable to less polar solvents including methanol and ethanol, which allows the extraction of medium- or non-polar compounds. To avoid evaporation of the solvent as well as to maintain its liquid phase at such a high temperature, high vapor pressure is employed in an enclosed space. SWE is comparatively a unique process for separating less polar components by using water as solvent within a shorter duration of 30 minutes [86–88].

This new form of water system can easily break the cell wall of biomass and solubilize chemical compounds present in the plant material by increasing the extraction process of bioactive compounds. Subcritical water obtained after this has some unique characteristics like high level of ionic strength and a low dielectric constant. Due to these characteristics, it is considered as an outstanding solvent for extracting both hydrophobic and hydrophilic compounds from various medicinal plants [89–92]. Highly ionic characteristics, high temperature, and a low dielectric constant were considered as key for refining the extraction efficiency; nevertheless, the phenomena of conversion and decomposition of mint EO components were observed at higher extraction temperatures and extended extraction times during subcritical water treatment [93,94]. These modified conditions also improve the efficiency of overall extraction process via decreasing viscosity and surface tension as well as improving the self-diffusion of water [10]. Moreover, the subcritical condition increases the ionic level of water to increase the acidity of the medium for promoting hydrolysis reactions [95]. However, these conditions with extended extraction times can cause chemical transformation or degradation of the components present in EOs [93,94].

This chemical transformation as well as degradation can lead to loss of product quality during extraction. Thus, to reduce the effort, to prevent chemical transformation as well as degradation of the components, and to improve extraction efficiency, extraction conditions must be optimized. Extraction conditions such as extraction temperature, extraction time, extraction pressure, the type of entrainers, particle size, solid-to-solvent ratio, and nature of extracted material considerably influence the extraction yield [96].

These factors must be optimized using a response surface method, which is an effective process with the benefits of decreasing costs and optimizing the process conditions, and is extensively used in various areas such as pharmaceuticals, agriculture, biotechnology, and other fields [97].

Temperature is considered as a significant factor that affects the overall extraction process. It is known that factors like viscosity, water dielectric constant, and surface tension decrease with increase in temperature. However, the molecular diffusion rate is increased and decreased with increase in temperature [98].

During this process, a certain level of pressure is utilized to maintain the solvent in the liquid phase as at the high temperature the solvent can evaporate to form steam, which is corrosive, and can damage the equipment. It was also noticed that there is no change in the efficiency of the extraction process even after increasing the pressure [99].

Rise in temperature of subcritical water increased the solubility of certain chemical compounds present in plant material such as polar phenolic compounds. This process is suitable for the extraction of phenolic compounds as it does not require the use of an organic solvent to extract phenolics and flavonoids. Thus, excluding toxic solvent and including less soluble chemical compounds (medium- or nonpolar compounds) can result in the improvement in biological activities.

One investigation showed that continuous SWE is rapid, provides more EO (with high level of oxygenated compounds), good precision, reduces the cost, and improves the efficiency (in terms of volume of EO yield) when compared with hydrodistillation for the extraction of EO from marjoram leaves [99].

In another report, a subcritical extractor was used for performing SWEs in a continuous manner for the isolation of the EO of fennel, and this method was compared with both hydrodistillation and dichloromethane manual extraction. Findings suggested better results in terms of rapidity, efficiency, cleanliness, and possibility of manipulating the composition of the extract [100].

In one publication, it was demonstrated that Japanese mint EO containing (l-menthol, l-menthone, piperitone, and l-menthyl acetate) showed degradation under subcritical water conditions and that extraction conditions must be optimized in order to get quality mint EO using subcritical water [101].

In another report, optimum subcritical fluid extraction conditions of EO from *Cinnamomum camphora* were determined. It was found that the rate of extraction was high (3.54%), which projected the yield of 3.56% with extraction time of 30 minutes at the extraction temperature of 40°C. Forty-seven chemical compounds were identified in the subcritical fluid extract of *Cinnamomum camphora*, out of which the main chemical constituents were eucalyptol, bicyclo[3.1.0]hexan-4-methylene-1-(1-methylethyl), linalool, and caryophyllene. It was concluded that this extraction process is appropriate for the extraction of EO from *Cinnamomum camphora* and the EO also showed good antimicrobial activity [102].

Subcritical fluid coupled with ultrasound-enhanced subcritical fluid extraction was employed to improve the yield of EO from *Nymphaea alba var* (red water lily). It was found that subcritical fluid extraction is appropriate for the extraction of EO from N. alba var, and the EO showed good antioxidant activity. The overall content of EO from *N. alba* was found to be 0.315% with the presence of 47 chemical constituents identified by GC-MS [103].

An earlier study showed that 124 constituents were identified in SWEs, while 94 and 65 signals were gained from hydrodistillation and ultrasonic irradiation extracts of *Lavandula stoechas* EO. The main constituents were found to be fenchone, camphor, myrtenyl acetate, myrtenol, and 1,8-cineol. SWE had a higher level of light oxygenated compounds (responsible for fragrance of the oil) as well as heavy oxygenated compounds. It was also found that oil yield was improved with an increase in temperature. However, more polar constituents including 1,8-cineol, camphor, and fenchone were not effectively extracted by subcritical water. The majority of the constituents were extracted by SWE in shorter duration and also in a rapid manner [104].

Another report showed that subcritical water has been performed at various conditions of pressure, temperature, and water flow rate to extract EO from the Greek oregano. It was found that in comparison with steam distillation, SWE is better in terms of higher yields, less energy consumption, and superior composition/selectivity of the extracts controlled by the extraction parameters [105].

9.4.4 Solvent-Free Microwave Extraction

During the last few decades, there has been growing demand for more robust, cost-effective, and green extraction procedures with improved extraction efficiency in terms of yield of quality of the finished product. Considering these objectives, advancements in microwave extraction have resulted in the development of various procedures including:

- Microwave-assisted solvent extraction
- Vacuum microwave hydrodistillation
- Microwave hydrodistillation
- Compressed air microwave distillation
- Solvent-free microwave hydrodistillation
- Pressurized microwave-assisted extraction

SFME is a green approach for the extraction of EO from aromatic plants by using microwave heating as well as dry distillation executed at atmospheric pressure without the involvement of solvent or water. In this process, volatile compounds are isolated and concentrated at a single stage [106]. One study showed that SFME showed considerably high oregano EO yield (0.054 mL/g), when compared to hydrodistillation (0.048 mL/g). The authors also reported that this process presents significant advantages over conventional approaches including shorter extraction times, improved yield, environmental influence, cleaner features, and high antimicrobial effects. Further, the same authors reported that EO isolated from caraway seeds via microwave dry-diffusion and gravity (MDG) showed comparable yield and aromatic profile to that derived from HD. However, MDG showed better results than HD in terms of shorter process time (45 minutes compared with 300 minutes), energy saving, and cleanliness. Findings obtained from the extraction of EO from aromatic herbs (basil, crispate mint, and thyme) and spices (ajowan, cumin, and star anise) extracted by SFME were similar to those obtained by HD. A high level of oxygenated compounds and lower levels of monoterpenes hydrocarbons were present in the SFME extract in comparison with HD extract.

A recent report also showed that the SFME procedure could be a better approach for the extraction of EO from sweet basil (*Ocimum basilicum* L.) leaves as it can be considered as providing a richer source of natural antioxidants and potential antimicrobial agents for food preservation. In this study, SFME extract when analyzed by GC and GC-MS presented 65 compounds constituting 99.3% of the total oil with major components such as linalool, methyl chavicol, and 1,8-cineole [107].

During SFME, EO is often evaporated by the in situ water in plant materials. It was also suggested that SFME can be further modified by adding microwave absorption solid medium, such as carbonyl iron powders or mixing it directly with the sample, to extract EO from the dried plant materials without any pretreatment. It was found that modified SFME showed improved results over conventional SFME for the extraction of EO from dried *Cuminum cyminum* L. and *Zanthoxylum bungeanum* Maxim [108].

Another report suggested that *Rosmarinus officinalis* EO extracted by SFME in 30 minutes was quantitatively (yield and kinetics profile) and qualitatively (aromatic profile) similar to that obtained using conventional hydrodistillation in 2 hours [109].

One more report showed that SFME-distilled *Calamintha nepeta* oil showed a higher level of lightly oxygenated monoterpenes than HD oil. Additionally, SFME extract showed a higher level of sesquiterpenes and a lower quantity of hydrocarbon monoterpenes [110].

Solvent-free microwave extraction-headspace single-drop microextraction, a further modification of SFME, displayed shorter extraction time and less sample required in comparison with the hydrodistillation for the extraction of EO from *Eugenia caryophyllata* [111].

Recently, the SFME of lemongrass EO was compared with conventional extraction HD. It was found that SFME (15 minutes) is faster than conventional HD (120 minutes). The quality of lemongrass EO obtained from SFME was found to be better than HD as SFME extract contained high levels of citral [112].

Similarly, the results obtained after SFME-based extraction of EO from *Melissa officinalis* L. and *Laurus nobilis* L. suggested that EO obtained with SFME contained considerably high levels of oxygenated compounds and lower amounts of monoterpenes than the oils obtained by conventional methods [113].

Similar findings were demonstrated in another study based on the extraction of EO by SFME [borneol (15.2%–12.8%), α-terpineol (12.3%–10.8%), and trans-sabinene hydrate (11.8%–9.92%)] and hydrodistillation from endemic *Origanum husnucanbaseri*. SFME fraction showed more antibacterial fraction than HD [114].

In another study while comparing SFME results with HD for the extraction of EO from three aromatic herbs: basil, garden mint, and thyme, it was found that EO extracted by SFME for 30 minutes was quantitatively (yield) and qualitatively (aromatic profile) similar to that obtained by HD for 4.5 hours. Additionally, SFME extract presented EO with high level of oxygenated compounds [115].

9.5 Role of Plant Biotechnology in Essential Oil Production

Plant biotechnology facilitates the production of EOs and, thus, decreases overall cost involved in the production of EOs. Certain techniques can be used to produce them in bioreactor facilities mainly to scale up their production [116–141]. This can be done by culturing EO-producing plant cell and tissues or by the use of bacterial and fungal biotransformers. Transgenic plants produce EO, and their genetic trait can be tailored to modify the chemical composition of EOs [116–141]. Other approaches like elicitation as well as precursor feeding can be used to improve the EO-producing capability of established plant cultures. Metabolomics, mainly metabolic engineering of the biosynthetic pathways, can be utilized to synthesize the desired EO compound. EOs usually contain monoterpenoids followed by sesquiterpenoids; in some cases, phenylpropanoids and fatty acids can be components [116–141]. However, it was found that in comparison with the yields from intact plant tissues, the yield of terpenoid from in vitro cultured calli or cell suspensions is much lower. Biotransformations of isolated EO compounds produce mainly hydroxylated, epoxidated, and other catabolic products; some of them, like decalactone, lilac aldehyde, lilac alcohol, phenylethanol, and caryophyllene oxide, being perfume compounds, while others, such as anisic acid, benzyl alcohol, verbenone, and carveol, are also of medicinal value [116–141]. Cineole and pinene EOs can also be extracted from transgenic plants, such as coffee plants with less caffeine, rose geranium with more geraniol, black pepper with altered terpenoid constituency, and eucalyptus with more limonene [116–141].

REFERENCES

1. Aziz ZAA, Ahmad A, Setapar SHM, Karakucuk A, Azim MM, Lokhat D, Rafatullah M, Ganash M, Kamal MA, Ashraf GM. Essential oils: Extraction techniques, pharmaceutical and therapeutic potential: A review. *Curr Drug Metab.* 2018;19(13):1100–1110.
2. Turek C, Stintzing, FC. Stability of essential oils: A Review. *Compr Rev Food Sci Food Saf.* 2013;12:40–53.
3. Tongnuanchan P, Benjakul S. Essential oils: Extraction, bioactivities, and their uses for food preservation. *J Food Sci.* 2014;79(7):R1231–49. doi: 10.1111/1750-3841.12492. Epub 2014 June 2.
4. Reverchon E, Senatore F. Isolation of rosemary oil: Comparison between hydrodistillation and supercritical CO_2 extraction. *Flavour Frag.* 1992;7:227–230.
5. Masango P. Cleaner production of essential oils by steam distillation. *J Cleaner Prod.* 2005;13:833–839.
6. Perineau F, Ganou L, Vilarem G. Studying production of lovage essential oils in a hydrodistillation pilot unit equipped with a cohobation system. *J Chem Technol Biotechnol.* 1992;53:165–171.
7. Zheljazkov VD, Cantrell CL, Astatkie T, Jeliazkova E. Distillation time effect on lavender essential oil yield and composition. *J Oleo Sci.* 2013;62(4):195–199.
8. Zheljazkov VD, Horgan T, Astatkie T, Schlegel V. Distillation time modifies essential oil yield, composition, and antioxidant capacity of fennel (*Foeniculum vulgare* Mill). *J Oleo Sci.* 2013;62(9):665–672.
9. Sun SH, Chai GB, Li P, Xie JP, Su Y. Steam distillation/drop-by-drop extraction with gas chromatography-mass spectrometry for fast determination of volatile components in jujube (*Ziziphus jujuba* Mill.) extract. *Chem Cent J.* 2017;11(1):101.
10. Antoniotti S. Tuning of essential oil properties by enzymatic treatment: Towards sustainable processes for the generation of new fragrance ingredients. *Molecules.* 2014;19(7):9203–9214.
11. Yildirim A, Cakir A, Mavi A, Yalcin M, Fauler G, Taskesenligil Y. The variation of antioxidant activities and chemical composition of essential oils of *Teucrium orientale* L. var. orientale during harvesting stages. *Flavour Frag.* 2004;19:367–372.
12. Zheljazkov VD, Astatkie T, Schlegel V. Hydrodistillation extraction time effect on essential oil yield, composition, and bioactivity of coriander oil. *J Oleo Sci.* 2014;63(9):857–865.
13. Moradi S, Fazlali A, Hamedi H. Microwave-assisted hydro-distillation of essential oil from rosemary: Comparison with traditional distillation. *Avicenna J Med Biotechnol.* 2018;10(1):22–28.
14. Arora R, Singh B, Vig AP, Arora S. Conventional and modified hydrodistillation method for the extraction of glucosinolate hydrolytic products: a comparative account. *Springerplus.* 2016;5:479.
15. Mohamad N, Ramli N, Abd-Aziz S, Ibrahim MF. Comparison of hydro-distillation, hydro-distillation with enzyme-assisted and supercritical fluid for the extraction of essential oil from pineapple peels. *3 Biotech.* 2019;9(6):234.
16. Wang H, Liu Y, Wei S, Yan Z, Jin X. Comparative chemical composition of the essential oils obtained by microwave-assisted hydrodistillation and hydrodistillation from *Agrimonia pilosa* LEDEB. Collected in three different regions of China. *Chem Biodivers.* 2012;9(3):662–668.
17. Wang HW, Liu YQ, Wei SL, Yan ZJ, Lu K. Comparison of microwave-assisted and conventional hydrodistillation in the extraction of essential oils from mango (*Mangifera indica* L.) flowers. *Molecules.* 2010;15(11):7715–7723.
18. Ghazanfari N, Mortazavi SA, Yazdi FT, Mohammadi M. Microwave-assisted hydrodistillation extraction of essential oil from coriander seeds and evaluation of their composition, antioxidant and antimicrobial activity. *Heliyon.* 2020;6(9):e04893.
19. Liu B, Fu J, Zhu Y, Chen P. Optimization of microwave-assisted extraction of essential oil from lavender using response surface methodology. *J Oleo Sci.* 2018;67(10):1327–1337.
20. Tyśkiewicz K, Gieysztor R, Konkol M, Szałas J, Rój E. Essential oils from humulus lupulus $scCO_2$ extract by hydrodistillation and microwave-assisted hydrodistillation. *Molecules.* 2018;23(11):2866.
21. Moradi S, Fazlali A, Hamedi H. Microwave-assisted hydro-distillation of essential oil from rosemary: Comparison with traditional distillation. *Avicenna J Med Biotechnol.* 2018;10(1):22–28.
22. Périno-Issartier S, Abert-Vian M, Petitcolas E et al. Microwave turbo hydrodistillation for rapid extraction of the essential oil from *Schinus terebinthifolius* Raddi Berries. *Chroma.* 2010;72:347–350.
23. Vian MA, Fernandez X, Visinoni F, Chemat F. Microwave hydrodiffusion and gravity, a new technique for extraction of essential oils. *J Chromatogr.* 2008;1190(1–2):14–17.
24. Bousbia, N, Abert Vian M, Ferhat MA, Meklati BY, Chemat F. A new process for extraction of essential oil from Citrus peels: Microwave hydrodiffusion and gravity. *J Food Eng.* 2009;90:409–413.
25. Vian MA, Fernandez X, Visinoni F, Chemat F. Microwave hydrodiffusion and gravity, a new technique for extraction of essential oils. *J Chromatogr A.* 2008;1190(1–2):14–17.

26. Périno-Issartier S, Ginies C, Cravotto G, Chemat F. A comparison of essential oils obtained from lavandin via different extraction processes: Ultrasound, microwave, turbohydrodistillation, steam and hydrodistillation. *J Chromatogr A.* 2013;1305:41–47.
27. Farhat A, Fabiano-Tixier AS, Maataoui M, Maingonnat JF, Romdhane M, Chemat F. Microwave steam diffusion for extraction of essential oil from orange peel: Kinetic data, extract's global yield and mechanism. *Food Chem.* 2011;125:255–261.
28. Golmakani MT, Moayyedi M. Comparison of heat and mass transfer of different microwave-assisted extraction methods of essential oil from *Citrus limon* (*Lisbon variety*) peel. *Food Sci Nutr.* 2015;3(6):506–518.
29. Kosar M, Dorman HJD, Hiltunen R. Effect of an acid treatment on the phytochemical and antioxidant characteristics of extracts from selected Lamiaceae species. *Food Chem.* 2005;91:525–533.
30. Li XM, Tian SL, Pang ZC, Shi JY, Feng ZS, Zhang YM. Extraction of *Cuminumcyminum* essential oil by combination technology of organic solvent with low boiling point and steam distillation. *Food Chem.* 2009;115:1114–1119.
31. Ferhat MA, Tigrine-Kordjani N, Chemat S, Meklati BY, Chemat F. Rapid extraction of volatile compounds using a new simultaneous microwave distillation: Solvent extraction device. *Chromatographia.* 2007;65:217–222.
32. El Ouariachi EM, Tomi P, Bouyanzer A, Hammouti B, Desjobert JM, Costa J, Paolini J. Chemical composition and antioxidant activity of essential oils and solvent extracts of *Ptychotisverticillata* from Morocco. *Food Chem Toxicol.* 2011;49:533–536.
33. Ozen T, Demirtas I, Aksit H. Determination of antioxidant activities of various extracts and essential oil compositions of *Thymus praecox* subsp. skorpilii var. skorpilii. *Food Chem.* 2011;124:58–64.
34. Sarikurkcu C, Arisoy K, Tepe B, Cakir A, Abali G, Mete E. Studies on the antioxidant activity of essential oil and different solvent extracts of *Vitexagnuscastus* L. fruits from Turkey. *Food Chem Toxicol.* 2009;47:2479–2483.
35. Berka-Zougali B, Ferhat MA, Hassani A, Chemat F, Allaf KS. Comparative study of essential oils extracted from Algerian *Myrtus communis* L. leaves using microwaves and hydrodistillation. *Int J Mol Sci.* 2012;13(4):4673–4695.
36. Lucchesi ME, Chemat F, Smadja J. Solvent-free microwave extraction: an innovative tool for rapid extraction of essential oil from aromatic herbs and spices. *J Microw Power Electromagn Energy.* 2004;39(3–4):135–139.
37. Fornari T, Vicente G, Vázquez E, García-Risco MR, Reglero G. Isolation of essential oil from different plants and herbs by supercritical fluid extraction. *J Chromatogr A.* 2012;1250:34–48. doi: 10.1016/j.chroma.2012.04.051. Epub 2012 April 26.
38. Pourmortazavi SM, Hajimirsadeghi SS. Supercritical fluid extraction in plant essential and volatile oil analysis. *J Chromatogr A.* 2007;1163(1–2):2–24. doi: 10.1016/j.chroma.2007.06.021. Epub 2007 June 17.
39. Deng C, Yao N, Wang A, Zhang X. Determination of essential oil in a traditional Chinese medicine, Fructusamomi by pressurized hot water extraction followed by liquid-phase microextraction and gas chromatography-mass spectrometry. *Analytica Chimica Acta.* 2005;536:237–244.
40. Jimenez-Carmona MM, Ubera JL, Luque de Castro MD. Comparison of continuous subcritical water extraction and hydrodistillation of marjoram essential oil. *J Chromatogr A.* 1999;855:625–632.
41. Senorans FJ, Ibanez E, Cavero S, Tabera J, Reglero G. Liquid chromatographic-mass spectrometric analysis of supercritical-fluid extracts of rosemary plants. *J Chromatogr A.* 2000;870:491–499.
42. Hawthorne SB, Rickkola ML, Screnius K, Holm Y, Hiltunen R, Hartonen K. Comparison of hydrodistillation and supercritical fluid extraction for the determination of essential oils in aromatic plants. *J Chromatogr A.* 1993;634:297–308.
43. Langenfeld JJ, Hawthorne SB, Miller DJ, Pawliszyn J. Effects of temperature and pressure on supercritical fluid extraction efficiencies of polycyclic aromatic hydrocarbons and polychlorinated biphenyls. *Anal Chem.* 1993;65(15):338–344.
44. Khajeh M, Yamini Y, Shariati S. Comparison of essential oils compositions of Nepeta persica obtained by supercritical carbon dioxide extraction and steam distillation methods. *Food Bioprod Process.* 2010;88:227–232.
45. Ghasemi E, Raofie F, Najafi NM. Application of response surface methodology and central composite design for the optimisation of supercritical fluid extraction of essential oils from *Myrtus communis L.* leaves. *Food Chem.* 2011;126:1449–1453.
46. Daneshvand B, Ara KM, Raofie F. Comparison of supercritical fluid extraction and ultrasound-assisted extraction of fatty acids from quince (*Cydonia oblonga* Miller) seed using response surface methodology and central composite design. *J Chromatogr A.* 2012;1252:1–7.
47. Mann TS, Kiran Babu GD, Guleria S, Singh B. Comparison of *Eucalyptus cinerea* essential oils produced by hydrodistillation and supercritical carbon dioxide extraction. *Nat Prod Commun.* 2011;6(1):107–110.
48. Mann TS, Babu GD, Guleria S, Singh B. Variation in the volatile oil composition of *Eucalyptus citriodora* produced by hydrodistillation and supercritical fluid extraction techniques. *Nat Prod Res.* 2013;27(7):675–679.
49. Ghahramanloo KH, Kamalidehghan B, Akbari Javar H, Teguh Widodo R, Majidzadeh K, Noordin MI. Comparative analysis of essential oil composition of Iranian and Indian *Nigella sativa* L. extracted using supercritical fluid extraction and solvent extraction. *Drug Des Devel Ther.* 2017;11:2221–2226.
50. Herzi N, Bouajila J, Camy S, Cazaux S, Romdhane M, Condoret JS. Comparison between supercritical CO_2 extraction and hydrodistillation for two species of eucalyptus: Yield, chemical composition, and antioxidant activity. *J Food Sci.* 2013;78(5):C667–72.
51. Li HX, Yang TY, Yang TL, Ge FH, Pan WS, Yang XG, Chen JM. Study on ingredients of essential oils of *Curcuma wenyujin* extracted by supercritical-CO_2 fluid extraction and steam distillation. *Zhongguo Zhong Yao Za Zhi.* 2006;31(17):1445–1446.
52. Ge FH, Li Y, Xie JM, Li Q, Ma GJ, Chen YH, Lin YC, Li XF. Studies on technology of supercritical-CO_2 fluid extraction for volatile oils and saikosaponins in Bupleurum chinense DC. *Zhongguo Zhong Yao Za Zhi.* 2000;25(3):149–153.

53. Ge F, Shi Q, Tan X, Li Z, Jing X. Technological study on the supercritical-CO_2 fluid extraction of Curcuma longa oils. *Zhong Yao Cai*. 1997;20(7):345–350.
54. Sowndhararajan K, Seo M, Kim M, Kim H, Kim S. Effect of essential oil and supercritical carbon dioxide extract from the root of Angelica gigas on human EEG activity. *Complement Ther Clin Pract*. 2017;28:161–168.
55. Chen Z, Mei X, Jin Y, Kim EH, Yang Z, Tu Y. Optimisation of supercritical carbon dioxide extraction of essential oil of flowers of tea (*Camellia sinensis* L.) plants and its antioxidative activity. *J Sci Food Agric*. 2014;94(2):316–321.
56. Mohamad N, Ramli N, Abd-Aziz S, Ibrahim MF. Comparison of hydro-distillation, hydro-distillation with enzyme-assisted and supercritical fluid for the extraction of essential oil from pineapple peels. *3 Biotech*. 2019;9(6):234.
57. Chen F, Chen H, Li SJ, Lin JM, Wang ZY. Comparison of the chemical components of essential oil extracted by supercritical CO_2 fluid and steam distillation from *Pteris multifida*. *Zhong Yao Cai*. 2013;36(8):1270–1274.
58. Song WF, Liao MJ, Luo SY. Analyze on chemical compositions of *Dalbergia odorifera* essential oils extracted by CO_2-supercritical-fluid-extraction and steam distillation extraction. *Zhong Yao Cai*. 2011;34(11):1725–1727. Chinese.
59. Qiu Q, Ling J, Ding Y, Chang H, Wang J, Liu T. Comparison of supercritical fluid extraction and steam distillation methods for the extraction of essential oils from *Schizonepeta tenuifolia* Briq. *Se Pu*. 2005;23(6):646–650.
60. Wang ZY, Zheng JH, Shi SY, Luo ZX, Ni SY, Lin JM. Comparison of chemical components of essential oil from ocimum basilicum var. pilosum extracted by supercritical CO_2 fluid and steam distillation. *Zhong Yao Cai*. 2015;38(11):2327–2330.
61. Jiao SQ, Liu FH. Analysis of the chemical constituents of volatile oil from the Folium Rhododendri Daurici by supercritical CO_2 extraction. *Zhong Yao Cai*. 2009;32(2):213–216.
62. Chen J, Wu Q. Study on extraction methods of volatile oil from *Mosla soochowensis*. *Zhong Yao Cai*. 2005;28(9):823–835.
63. Zhou RB, Wu J, Tong QZ, Liu YM, Liu XD. Studies on volatile oil from *Atractylodes macrocephala* with different distill methods. *Zhong Yao Cai*. 2008;31(2):229–232.
64. Wu H, Li J, Jia Y, Xiao Z, Li P, Xie Y, Zhang A, Liu R, Ren Z, Zhao M, Zeng C, Li C. Essential oil extracted from *Cymbopogon citronella* leaves by supercritical carbon dioxide: antioxidant and antimicrobial activities. *J Anal Methods Chem*. 2019;2019:8192439.
65. Simándi B, Deák A, Rónyai E, Yanxiang G, Veress T, Lemberkovics E, Then M, Sass-Kiss A, Vámos-Falusi Z. Supercritical carbon dioxide extraction and fractionation of fennel oil. *J Agric Food Chem*. 1999;47(4):1635–1640.
66. Díaz-Maroto MC, Díaz-Maroto Hidalgo IJ, Sánchez-Palomo E, Pérez-Coello MS. Volatile components and key odorants of fennel (*Foeniculum vulgare* Mill.) and thyme (*Thymus vulgaris* L.) oil extracts obtained by simultaneous distillation-extraction and supercritical fluid extraction. *J Agric Food Chem*. 2005;53(13):5385–5389.
67. Wang L, Chen Y, Song Y, Chen Y, Liu X. GC-MS of volatile components of *Schisandra chinensis* obtained by supercritical fluid and conventional extraction. *J Sep Sci*. 2008;31(18):3238–3245.
68. Zhou BJ, Zhang ZY, Shi Y, Gu WX, Zhang SY. Analysis with gas chromatography and mass spectrography of volatile components of *Ligusticum wallichii* Franch extracted by CO_2 supercritical fluid extraction in combination with molecular distillation. *Di Yi Jun Yi Da Xue Xue Bao*. 2002;22(7):652–653.
69. Grosso C, Figueiredo AC, Burillo J, Mainar AM, Urieta JS, Barroso JG, Coelho JA, Palavra AM. Enrichment of the thymoquinone content in volatile oil from *Satureja montana* using supercritical fluid extraction. *J Sep Sci*. 2009;32(2):328–334.
70. Grosso C, Figueiredo AC, Burillo J, Mainar AM, Urieta JS, Barroso JG, Coelho JA, Palavra AM. Composition and antioxidant activity of *Thymus vulgaris* volatiles: Comparison between supercritical fluid extraction and hydrodistillation. *J Sep Sci*. 2010;33(14):2211–2218.
71. Xiao XY, Cui LH, Zhou XX, Wu Y, Ge FH. Research of the essential oil of *Plumeria rubra* var. actifolia from Laos by supercritical carbon dioxide extraction. *Zhong Yao Cai*. 2011;34(5):789–794. Chinese.
72. Saini R, Guleria S, Kaul VK, Lal B, Babu GD, Singh B. Comparison of the volatile constituents of *Elsholtzia fruiticosa* extracted by hydrodistillation, supercritical fluid extraction and head space analysis. *Nat Prod Commun*. 2010;5(4):641–644.
73. Yamini Y, Bahramifar N, Sefidkon F, Saharkhiz MJ, Salamifar E. Extraction of essential oil from *Pimpinella anisum* using supercritical carbon dioxide and comparison with hydrodistillation. *Nat Prod Res*. 2008;22(3):212–218.
74. Grosso C, Figueiredo AC, Burillo J, Mainar AM, Urieta JS, Barroso JG, Coelho JA, Palavra AM. Supercritical fluid extraction of the volatile oil from *Santolina chamaecyparissus*. *J Sep Sci*. 2009;32(18):3215–3222. doi: 10.1002/jssc.200900350. Erratum in: *J Sep Sci*. 2009;32(19):3365–3366.
75. Jin Y, Han D, Tian M, Row KH. Supercritical CO_2 extraction of essential oils from *Chamaecyparis obtusa*. *Nat Prod Commun*. 2010;5(3):461–464.
76. Aghel N, Yamini Y, Hadjiakhoondi A, Pourmortazavi SM. Supercritical carbon dioxide extraction of *Mentha pulegium L*. essential oil. *Talanta*. 2004;62(2):407–411.
77. Pourmortazavi SM, Sefidkon F, Hosseini SG. Supercritical carbon dioxide extraction of essential oils from *Perovskia atriplicifolia* Benth. *J Agric Food Chem*. 2003;51(18):5414–5419.
78. Wang H, Liu Y, Wei S, Yan Z. Application of response surface methodology to optimise supercritical carbon dioxide extraction of essential oil from *Cyperus rotundus* Linn. *Food Chem*. 2012;132(1):582–587.
79. Ara KM, Jowkarderis M, Raofie F. Optimization of supercritical fluid extraction of essential oils and fatty acids from flixweed (*Descurainia Sophia* L.) seed using response surface methodology and central composite design. *J Food Sci Technol*. 2015;52(7):4450–4458.
80. Gan Y, Xu D, Zhang J, Wang Z, Wang S, Guo H, Zhang K, Li Y, Wang Y. *Rana chensinensis* ovum oil based on CO_2 supercritical fluid extraction: Response surface methodology optimization and unsaturated fatty acid ingredient analysis. *Molecules*. 2020;25(18):4170.

81. Ara KM, Raofie F. Application of response surface methodology for the optimization of supercritical fluid extraction of essential oil from pomegranate (*Punica granatum* L.) peel. *J Food Sci Technol.* 2016;53(7):3113–3121.
82. Wu H, Li J, Jia Y, Xiao Z, Li P, Xie Y, Zhang A, Liu R, Ren Z, Zhao M, Zeng C, Li C. Essential oil extracted from *Cymbopogon citronella* leaves by supercritical carbon dioxide: Antioxidant and antimicrobial activities. *J Anal Methods Chem.* 2019;2019:8192439.
83. Tyśkiewicz K, Konkol M, Rój E. Supercritical carbon dioxide ($scCO_2$) extraction of phenolic compounds from lavender (*Lavandula angustifolia*) flowers: A box-Behnken experimental optimization. *Molecules.* 2019;24(18):3354.
84. Hawthorne SB, Yang Y, Miller DJ. Extraction of organic pollutants from environmental solids with sub- and supercritical water. *Anal Chem.* 1994;66:2912–2920.
85. Latawiec AE, Reid BJ. Sequential extraction of polycyclic aromatic hydrocarbons using subcritical water. *Chemosphere.* 2010;78(8):1042–1048.
86. Ayala RS, De Castro ML. Continuous subcritical water extraction as a useful tool for isolation of edible essential oils. *Food Chem.* 2001;75:109–113.
87. Ko MJ, Cheigh CI, Chung MS. Relationship analysis between flavonoids structure and subcritical water extraction (SWE). *Food Chem.* 2014;143:147–155.
88. Teo CC, Tan SN, Yong JW, Hew CS, Ong ES. Pressurized hot water extraction (PHWE). *J Chromatogr A.* 2010;1217(16):2484–2494.
89. Marshall WL, Franck EU. Ion product of water substance, 0–1000°C, 1–10,000 bars; new international formulation and its background. *J Phys Chem Ref Data.* 1981;10:295–304.
90. Patrick HR, Griffith K, Liotta CL, Eckert CA, Gläser R. Near-critical water: A benign medium for catalytic reactions. *Ind Eng Chem Res.* 2001;40:6063–6067.
91. Wagner W, Pruß A. The IAPWS formulation 1995 for the thermodynamic properties of ordinary water substance for general and scientific use. *J Phys Chem Ref Data.* 2002;31:387–535.
92. Chiou TY, Neoh TL, Kobayashi T, Adachi S. Antioxidative ability of defatted rice bran extract obtained by subcritical water extraction in bulk oil and aqueous dispersion systems. *Jpn J Food Eng.* 2011;12:147–154.
93. Nomura S, Lee WJ, Konishi M, Saitoh T, Murata M, Ohtsu N, Shimotori Y, Kohari Y, Nagata Y, Chiou TY. Characteristics of Japanese mint extracts obtained by subcritical-water treatment. *Food Sci Technol Res.* 2019;25:695–703.
94. Chiou TY, Konishi M, Nomura S, Shimotori Y, Murata M, Ohtsu N, Kohari Y, Nagata Y, Saitoh T. Recovery of mint essential oil through pressure-releasing distillation during subcritical water treatment. *Food Sci Technol Res.* 2019;25:793–799.
95. Shitu A, Izhar S, Tahir TM. Sub-critical water as a green solvent for production of valuable materials from agricultural waste biomass: A review of recent work. *Global J Environ Sci Manag.* 2015;1:255–264.
96. He L, Zhang X, Xu H, Xu C, Yuan F, Knez Z, Novak Z, Gao Y. Subcritical water extraction of phenolic compounds from pomegranate (*Punica granatum* L.) seed residues and investigation into their antioxidant capacities by HPLC-ABTS·+ assay. *Food Bioprod Process.* 2012;90:215–223.
97. Karacabey E, Mazza G. Optimisation of antioxidant activity of grape cane extracts using response surface methodology. *Food Chem.* 2010;119:343–348.
98. Smith RM. Extractions with superheated water. *J Chromatogr A.* 2002; 975(1):31–46.
99. Jiménez-Carmona MM, Ubera JL, Luque de Castro MD. Comparison of continuous subcritical water extraction and hydrodistillation of marjoram essential oil. *J Chromatogr A.* 1999; 855(2):625–632.
100. Gámiz-Gracia L, Luque de Castro MD. Continuous subcritical water extraction of medicinal plant essential oil: Comparison with conventional techniques. *Talanta.* 2000;51(6):1179–1185.
101. Chiou TY, Nomura S, Konishi M, Liao CS, Shimotori Y, Murata M, Ohtsu N, Kohari Y, Lee WJ, Tsai TY, Nagata Y, Saitoh T. Conversion and hydrothermal decomposition of major components of mint essential oil by small-scale subcritical water treatment. *Molecules.* 2020;25(8):1953.
102. Zhou HX, Li ZH, Fu XJ, Zhang H. Study on subcritical fluid extraction of essential oil from *Cinnamomum camphora* and its antibacterial activity. *Zhong Yao Cai.* 2016;39(6):1357–1360. Chinese.
103. Zhao Y, Fan YY, Yu WG, Wang J, Lu W, Song XQ. Ultrasound-enhanced subcritical fluid extraction of essential oil from *Nymphaea alba* var and its antioxidant activity. *J AOAC Int.* 2019;102(5):1448–1454.
104. Giray ES, Kirici S, Kaya DA, Türk M, Sönmez O, Inan M. Comparing the effect of sub-critical water extraction with conventional extraction methods on the chemical composition of *Lavandula stoechas. Talanta.* 2008;74(4):930–935.
105. Missopolinou D, Tsioptsias C, Lambrou C, Panayiotou C. Selective extraction of oxygenated compounds from oregano with sub-critical water. *J Sci Food Agric.* 2012;92(4):814–820.
106. Lucchesi ME, Chemat F, Smadja J. Solvent-free microwave extraction: An innovative tool for rapid extraction of essential oil from aromatic herbs and spices. *J Microw Power Electromagn Energy.* 2004;39(3–4):135–139.
107. Chenni M, El Abed D, Rakotomanomana N, Fernandez X, Chemat F. Comparative study of essential oils extracted from egyptian basil leaves (*Ocimum basilicum* L.) using hydro-distillation and solvent-free microwave extraction. *Molecules.* 2016;21(1):E113.
108. Wang Z, Ding L, Li T, Zhou X, Wang L, Zhang H, Liu L, Li Y, Liu Z, Wang H, Zeng H, He H. Improved solvent-free microwave extraction of essential oil from dried *Cuminum cyminum* L. and *Zanthoxylum bungeanum* Maxim. *J Chromatogr A.* 2006;1102(1–2):11–17.
109. Filly A, Fernandez X, Minuti M, Visinoni F, Cravotto G, Chemat F. Solvent-free microwave extraction of essential oil from aromatic herbs: From laboratory to pilot and industrial scale. *Food Chem.* 2014;150:193–198.
110. Riela S, Bruno M, Formisano C, Rigano D, Rosselli S, Saladino ML, Senatore F. Effects of solvent-free microwave extraction on the chemical composition of essential oil of *Calamintha nepeta* (L.) Savi compared with the conventional production method. *J Sep Sci.* 2008;31(6–7):1110–1117.
111. Jiang C, Sun Y, Zhu X, Gao Y, Wang L, Wang J, Wu L, Song D. Solvent-free microwave extraction coupled with headspace single-drop microextraction of essential oils from flower of *Eugenia caryophyllata* Thunb. *J Sep Sci.* 2010;33(17–18):2784–2790.

112. Boukhatem MN, Ferhat MA, Rajabi M, Mousa SA. Solvent-free microwave extraction: An eco-friendly and rapid process for green isolation of essential oil from lemongrass. *Nat Prod Res.* 2020:1–4.
113. Uysal B, Sozmen F, Buyuktas BS. Solvent-free microwave extraction of essential oils from *Laurus nobilis* and *Melissa officinalis*: Comparison with conventional hydro-distillation and ultrasound extraction. *Nat Prod Commun.* 2010;5(1):111–114.
114. Uysal B, Sozmen F, Kose EO, Gokhan Deniz I, Oksal BS. Solvent-free microwave extraction and hydrodistillation of essential oils from endemic *Origanum husnucanbaseri* H. Duman, Aytac & A. Duran: Comparison of antibacterial activity and contents. *Nat Prod Res.* 2010;24(17):1654–1663.
115. Lucchesi ME, Chemat F, Smadja J. Solvent-free microwave extraction of essential oil from aromatic herbs: Comparison with conventional hydro-distillation. *J Chromatogr A.* 2004;1043(2):323–327.
116. Bhatia S, Sharma K, Dahiya R, Bera T. Plant tissue culture. In: *Modern Applications of Plant Biotechnology in Pharmaceutical Sciences.* Academic Press, Cambridge, MA; 2015:31–107.
117. Gounaris Y. The role of biotechnology in essential oil production from non-herbaceous plants. In: Malik S. (editor) *Essential Oil Research.* Springer, Cham. 2019: 365–400.
118. Bhatia S, Sharma K, Dahiya R, Bera T. Laboratory organization. In: *Modern Applications of Plant Biotechnology in Pharmaceutical Sciences.* Academic Press, Cambridge, MA; 2015:109–120.
119. Bhatia S, Sharma K, Dahiya R, Bera T. Concepts and techniques of plant tissue culture science. In: *Modern Applications of Plant Biotechnology in Pharmaceutical Sciences.* Academic Press, Cambridge, MA; 2015:121–156.
120. Bhatia S, Sharma K, Dahiya R, Bera T. Application of plant biotechnology. In: *Modern Applications of Plant Biotechnology in Pharmaceutical Sciences.* Academic Press, Cambridge, MA; 2015:157–207.
121. Bhatia S, Sharma K, Dahiya R, Bera T. Somatic embryogenesis and organogenesis. In: *Modern Applications of Plant Biotechnology in Pharmaceutical Sciences.* Academic Press, Cambridge, MA; 2015:209–230.
122. Bhatia S, Sharma K, Dahiya R, Bera T. Classical and non-classical techniques for secondary metabolite production in plant cell culture. In: *Modern Applications of Plant Biotechnology in Pharmaceutical Sciences.* Academic Press, Cambridge, MA; 2015:231–291.
123. Bhatia S, Sharma K, Dahiya R, Bera T. Plant-based biotechnological products with their production host, modes of delivery systems, and stability testing. In: *Modern Applications of Plant Biotechnology in Pharmaceutical Sciences.* Academic Press, Cambridge, MA; 2015:293–331.
124. Bhatia S, Sharma K, Dahiya R, Bera T. Edible vaccines. In: *Modern Applications of Plant Biotechnology in Pharmaceutical Sciences.* Academic Press, Cambridge, MA; 2015:333–343.
125. Bhatia S, Sharma K, Dahiya R, Bera T. Microenvironmentation in micropropagation. In: *Modern Applications of Plant Biotechnology in Pharmaceutical Sciences.* Academic Press, Cambridge, MA; 2015:345–360.
126. Bhatia S, Sharma K, Dahiya R, Bera T. Micropropagation. In: *Modern Applications of Plant Biotechnology in Pharmaceutical Sciences.* Academic Press, Cambridge, MA; 2015:361–368.
127. Bhatia S, Sharma K, Dahiya R, Bera T. Laws in plant biotechnology. In: *Modern Applications of Plant Biotechnology in Pharmaceutical Sciences.* Academic Press, Cambridge, MA; 2015:369–391.
128. Bhatia S, Sharma K, Dahiya R, Bera T. Technical glitches in micropropagation. In: *Modern Applications of Plant Biotechnology in Pharmaceutical Sciences.* Academic Press, Cambridge, MA; 2015:393–404.
129. Bhatia S, Sharma K, Dahiya R, Bera T. Plant tissue culture-based industries. In: *Modern Applications of Plant Biotechnology in Pharmaceutical Sciences.* Academic Press, Cambridge, MA; 2015:405–417.
130. Bhatia S, Sharma A, Vargas De La Cruz CB, Chaugule B, Ahmed Al-Harrasi. Nutraceutical, Antioxidant, Antimicrobial Properties of Pyropia vietnamensis (Tanaka et Pham-Hong Ho) J.E. Sutherl. et Monotilla. *Curr Bioact Compd.* 2020;16:1.
131. Bhatia S, Sardana S, Senwar KR, Dhillon A, Sharma A, Naved T. In vitro antioxidant and antinociceptive properties of *Porphyra vietnamensis. Biomedicine (Taipei).* 2019;9(1):3.
132. Bhatia S, Sharma K, Namdeo AG, Chaugule BB, Kavale M, Nanda S. Broad-spectrum sun-protective action of Porphyra-334 derived from *Porphyra vietnamensis. Pharmacognosy Res.* 2010;2(1):45–49.
133. Bhatia S, Sharma K, Sharma A, Nagpal K, Bera T. Anti-inflammatory, analgesic and antiulcer properties of *Porphyra vietnamensis. Avicenna J Phytomed.* 2015;5(1):69–77.
134. Bhatia S, Sardana S, Sharma A, Vargas De La Cruz CB, Chaugule B, Khodaie L. Development of broad spectrum mycosporine loaded sunscreen formulation from Ulva fasciata delile. *Biomedicine (Taipei).* 2019;9(3):17.
135. Bhatia S, Garg A, Sharma K, Kumar S, Sharma A, Purohit AP. Mycosporine and mycosporine-like amino acids: A paramount tool against ultra violet irradiation. *Pharmacogn Rev.* 2011;5(10):138–146.
136. Bhatia S, Namdeo AG, Nanda S. Factors effecting the gelling and emulsifying properties of a natural polymer. *SRP.* 2010;1(1):86–92.
137. Bhatia S, Sharma K, Bera T. Structural characterization and pharmaceutical properties of porphyran. *Asian J Pharm.* 2015;9:93–101.
138. Bhatia S, Sharma A, Sharma K, Kavale M, Chaugule BB, Dhalwal K, Namdeo AG, Mahadik KR. Novel algal polysaccharides from marine source: Porphyran. *Pharmacogn Rev.* 2008;4:271–276.
139. Bhatia S, Sharma K, Nagpal K, Bera T. Investigation of the factors influencing the molecular weight of porphyran and its associated antifungal activity bioact. *Carb Diet Fiber.* 2015;5:153–168.
140. Bhatia S, Kumar V, Sharma K, Nagpal K, Bera T. Significance of algal polymer in designing amphotericin B nanoparticles. *Sci World J.* 2014;2014:564573.
141. Bhatia S, Rathee P, Sharma K, Chaugule BB, Kar N, Bera T. Immuno-modulation effect of sulphated polysaccharide (porphyran) from *Porphyra vietnamensis. Int J Biol Macromol.* 2013;57:50–56.

10

Essential Oil Stability

Ahmed Al-Harrasi
Natural and Medical Sciences Research Center, University of Nizwa

Saurabh Bhatia
Natural and Medical Sciences Research Center, University of Nizwa
University of Petroleum and Energy Studies

Tapan Behl
Chitkara University

Md. Khalid Anwer
Prince Sattam Bin Abdul Aziz University

CONTENTS

10.1 Introduction

Essential oils (EOs) are made up of non-polar as well as volatile chemical compounds with a molecular mass of <300 Da, which can be extracted from various medicinal plants by using distillation and advanced procedures. EOs are finished products derived from plant-based material by using the following procedures:

- Distillation with steam
- Distillation with water
- Dry distillation
- Mechanical process

Therefore, the majority of EOs present in the market are derived by using hydrodistillation. As there is considerable difference in the conditions of extraction process, each extraction process yields different EOs with different qualities (different physical, chemical, and biological properties). Even optimization or modification of the same extraction method to improve the extraction efficiency often impacts the quality of EO in terms of physical and chemical properties, which can ultimately affect biological properties. Thus, considering this, standards to regulate physical properties of EOs have been given by the ISO and Association Française de Normalisation. Several regulatory bodies have been created to regulate EO quantities as well as other aspects related to the utilization of EOs and their respective compounds including:

- Scientific Committee on Consumer's Safety
- Research Institute for Fragrance Materials
- International Fragrance Association
- Bundesinstitut für Risikobewertung

Moreover, EOs for therapeutic applications must fulfill criteria established by pharmacopoeias. As far as their nutritional consumption is concerned, EOs are usually identified as safe (GRAS) by the US Food and Drug Administration [7]. EOs contain a mixture of various compounds, and the chemical structures of these compounds are often closely related to each other. Aromatic and flavor properties are usually contributed by a single compound; however, these properties are not

DOI: 10.1201/9781003175933-12

exactly dependent on their particular level but instead dependent on the particular aroma or flavor threshold, which is governed by its respective volatile nature and structural features. Thus, a small proportion of compounds obtained from oxidative or deradative reactions could influence the flavor as well as aromatic characteristics of EOs.

10.2 Possible Changes in Chemical Profiles of Essential Oils as well as Likely Effects

Due to the similarity in structure-based features among the different constituents of EOs, various decomposition or degradation reactions (e.g., oxidation, isomerization, cyclization, or dehydrogenation) can lead to chemical transformation. These reactions are often stimulated by enzymes or chemicals. Considering the stability of EOs, it should be always considered that the chemical profiles of EOs are always dependent on the environmental conditions of plant, plant health, plant age, habitat including climate, composition, and nature of soil, harvesting time, post-harvesting storage conditions of plant material, pre-extraction processing conditions, and extraction method type and its conditions [1]. As a result, volatile components present in plant material show natural variations in their chemical composition [1], which should be considered during quality assessment. As mentioned earlier, pre-extraction processing, storage, and extraction conditions of plant material also determine the stability of the volatile and heat-unstable components, as due to their structural characteristics some components are more sensitive to oxidation or hydrolysis reactions [1]. Extraction conditions like duration, temperature, pressure, and type of the solvent affect the chemical composition of EOs [1]. During the extraction, once the plant material is subjected to extraction, EOs present in the shielding compartment are released. EOs released outside the protective compartment are vulnerable to oxidation/polymerization reactions, resulting in chemical changes. These changes can often result in the production of EOs with compromised quality [1]. For instance, change in color, aroma, flavors (unpleasant and pungent flavors), and consistency (resinification) represent the degradation of EOs or single chemical compounds mainly in aged EOs [1]. A recent investigation showed that five main compounds (gamma-terpinene, limonene, alpha as well as beta pinene, and citral) of lemon EO when exposed to copper catalysts as well as air resulted in the considerable gamma-terpinene as well as alpha/beta pinene oxidation. Moreover, the supplementation of antioxidants (BHA and tocopherol) resulted in the suppression of oxidation. γ-terpinene and limonene showed more degradation caused by ultraviolet (UV) in the presence of air. The vulnerability of lemon EO as well as its components to show chemical transformation when exposed to air and temperature conditions has also been established [2].

Another report suggested the change in flavor characteristics of lemon oil due to the acid-mediated exhaustion of citral and chemical transformation of single/double unsaturated monocyclic terpenes due to oxidative dehydrogenation [1]. Apart from these changes in organoleptic characteristics, various earlier stocked EOs showed oxidation of terpenoids, resulting in the induction of hypersensitivity reaction [1].

It is reported that lavender oil failed to prevent autoxidation, which can result in the formation of intense contact allergens after being exposed to air. In this context, the effect of air oxidation on the skin sensitizing potency of the main constituents of lavender oil (monoterpenes: linalyl acetate, linalool, and beta-caryophyllene) was investigated. Based on oxidized products obtained from terpenes it was found that oxidation of pure terpenes occurs at the same rate as those oxidized in lavender EO when they are exposed to air. After exposure to air, the sensitizing power of lavender oil was augmented. A skin patch assessment of lavender EO after being exposed to air revealed a positive allergic reaction. It also showed a positive test when oxidized linalyl acetate was exposed to patients with contact allergic reaction to linalool (oxidized form) [3].

Another report showed that the level of linalyl acetate was reduced once it was exposed to air. Oxidation products of linalyl acetate such as hydroperoxides were identified when exposed to air. Sensitizing test showed that pure linalyl acetate demonstrated less sensitizing potential but the autoxidized form of linalyl acetate improved its sensitizing potential. It was demonstrated that the autoxidized linalyl acetate form further produced several allergenic oxidation products [4]. Lavender EO is obtained from the lavender plant (*Lavandula angustifolia*). The major constituents of lavender EO (linalool and linalyl acetate) in the presence of air were autoxidized to form sensitizing hydroperoxides. Thus, patient allergic reaction (contact dermatitis) when exposed to lavender fragrances could be related to oxidation of lavender oil, mainly oxidized linalool and/or oxidized linalyl acetate [5]. Thus, from these reports, it was found that the allergenic potency of EOs could be related to autoxidation of EO chemical components, which could result in the formation of allergenic oxidation products. Partial production of terpenoid hydroperoxides during the autoxidation process and their non-oxidized components could be the cause of irritation or allergic reactions [1]. This crucial autoxidation reaction that can lead to the deterioration of terpenoidal composition of EO is dependent on various parameters such as:

- Molecular structure of the components
- Level of oxygen
- Energy input
- Influence of further reaction partners

In the presence of oxygen, EO molecules, mainly unsaturated molecules, get oxidized by triggering a free radical chain mechanism with aerial oxygen to produce primary and secondary oxidation products. Various factors such as exposure to heat, light, and redox-reactive metals lead to the production of unstable molecular fragments, namely alkyl radicals having unpaired electrons. These radicals freely react with triplet oxygen to form peroxyl radicals, which can further result in the production of hydroperoxides with alkyl radical, to propagate the chain reaction. Further, hydroperoxides ultimately break down during oxidation, resulting in the formation of additional products such as oxygen-carrying polymers, alcohols (monovalent-polyvalent), peroxides, ketones, acids, aldehydes, and epoxides= or=[1].

Therefore, terpenoids primarily produce oxidation products such as hydroperoxides, which can further decay when exposed to light, high temperature, or high acidic conditions [1]. It was found that even at room temperature, peroxide products that resulted from the terpinolene oxidation deteriorated quickly. Thus, autoxidation is a direct oxidative route that involves the reaction of molecular oxygen with organic compounds in three phases (initiation, propagation, and termination). Propagation reactions include high production of hydroperoxides, and the decomposition of hydroperoxides is reduced. Free radical autoxidation is the addition of oxygen to form unsaturated hydroperoxides and other radicals. Unsaturated hydroperoxides considered as 1° oxidation products react further to form 2° oxidation products. Several structures of secondary oxidation products still remain unidentified. Thus, various degradation reactions such as disproportionation, polymerization reactions, isomerization reaction, oxidation and dehydrogenation reaction can result in oxidation of monoterpenes [1].

10.3 Factors Affecting Stability of EOs

EOs have various advantages, as has been discussed, but they also have disadvantages in terms of chemical instability when exposed to external conditions such as heat, light, air, and moisture. Heat or oxidation sensitive thermal and/or oxidative labile EO components can undergo chemical transformation, resulting in loss of therapeutic effectiveness, stability, and safety profile and also can cause toxic reactions. Some of the common examples of such chemical transformation during the handling, shipping, storage, and use of EOs or EO-based products of are as follows [6–9]:

- Formation of carcinogenic diepoxylimonene by diepoxidation of limonene
- Formation of harmful oxidized derivatives by oxidation of other terpenes (such as pinene) [14,26–27]
- Formation of carcinogenic metabolites by degradation of safrole
- Development of harmful, allergy-causing as well as skin-sensitizing oxygenated byproducts of linalool, caryophyllene, and limonene [29]

The development of such damaging oxygenated derivatives from terpenoidal compounds exposed to varied conditions of oxygen/air/temperature result in loss of physical/chemical/biological properties. Post-extraction degradation of EOs is dependent on various factors, mainly storage conditions including heat, light, and oxygen. Additionally, inherent characteristics of EOs such as chemical profile, structure of chemical components, and the presence of impurities (e.g., presence of residual solvent) can also affect the overall stability [6–9].

10.3.1 Effect of Light

Photooxidation is a complex event that involves chain reactions triggered by the absorption of a photon, which result in the breakdown to free radical products via various oxidative pathways. Photooxidation can be induced by autoxidation (first oxidative pathway) and singlet oxidation (second oxidative pathway). First oxidative pathway to induce oxidation in the presence of light is very common in EOs, whereas the second oxidative pathway to induce oxidation via singlet oxygen in the presence of light is uncommon in EOs. Radiations such as UV as well as visible (Vis) radiations are known to increase the speed of autoxidation by activating the H-atom transfer that leads to the production of alkyl radicals [10]. On storage under light as well as dark conditions, both laurel and fennel oil individually showed the same changes such as drop in trans-anethole, eugenyl acetate, estragole, and numerous monoterpenes with increase in the level of p-cymene, eugenol, and anisaldehyde [11]. Similar findings were obtained in the case of lemon oil. Nevertheless, chemical changes occurred rapidly when light was involved. Particularly, monoterpenes containing EOs showed quick degradation when exposed to light. Chemical transformation was reported when marjoram oil was stored under light conditions, which resulted in the formation of several unknown tracer components. It was also noticed that rapid changes in the composition of EOs occur in the presence of light; nevertheless, EOs from different plant species responded in a different manner (e.g., thyme EO showed fewer changes whereas rosemary oil showed more changes in the presence of light). It was also observed that light-induced autoxidation reactions can lead to the disappearance of old compounds as well as formation of new compounds, which can lead to change in the chemical profile of the respective EO. It was found that light-exposed EO showed a substantial rise in the level of p-cymene, camphor, and caryophyllene oxide, which is related to the degradation of beta-myrcene, alpha-phellandrene, beta-caryophyllene, and alpha-terpinene. Moreover, the formation and disappearance of a minute level of unknown substances takes place when lavender oil is stored under light conditions. These unknown substances that are not naturally found in samples like EO but appear due to the conditions prevailed during study are called artifacts. Artifacts developed in the presence of light such as sunlight or by UV irradiation are called photoartifacts. For example, 4,4′-dimethoxystilbene was discovered to be a photoartifact in anise oil stored for long periods. The formation of this artifact is due to the photocycloaddition between anethole and anisaldehyde. Similarly, the formation of cis-anethole or anisaldehyde via oxidation and isomerization of trans-anethole takes place in sweet fennel EO when stored at room temperature under light for 2 months [12]. Likewise, cis-anethole is formed from trans-anethole (the major chemical compound in sweet and bitter fennel EO) when exposed to UV rays or at high temperatures. It is also known that cis-isomer is more toxic than the trans-form [13]. Based on this information, various photochemical reactions have been described such as isomerization reactions of numerous monoterpenoids that involve trans-to-cis conversion or cycloaddition. The second pathway of inducing oxidation is by non-radical singlet oxygen. Oxidation reactions in EOs can be induced by either diradical triplet oxygen or non-radical singlet oxygen. Singlet oxygen-mediated oxidation of oils happens when nascent oxygen acts as an electrophile to react with double bonds to induce oxidation with more efficiency than atmospheric triplet oxygen oxidation. Singlet oxygen quickly escalates the rate of oxidation of oils at much lower temperatures. Various reports have suggested the formation of new compounds by singlet oxygen oxidation, which are not formed by common triplet oxygen. Several chemicals, enzymes, and photochemical-based reactions can trigger the formation of a highly unstable and reactive state of oxygen (i.e., singlet oxygen). Under the effect of light, various photosensitizers have been reported to form singlet oxygen from triplet oxygen. Relatively, because of the less activation energy, reaction rate of dioxygen with organic components is more than triplet oxygen. In the presence of light, dioxygen usually triggers oxidation of EOs at high rate to form various detrimental components in EOs, mostly while storing as well as processing of EOs. Nevertheless, the addition of antioxidants in EOs can reduce singlet oxygen oxidation and further minimize the production of undesirable substances [14].

Illumination plays an important role in inducing photooxidation by converting triplet oxygen in air to excited singlet oxygen, which can further form hydroperoxide by ene reaction. These hydroperoxides can further break down and yield certain oxidation products in a similar way as via autoxidation.

Nevertheless, this second pathway of inducing oxidation via singlet oxygen in the presence of light is uncommon in EOs as singlet oxygen is basically not present in the usual environmental conditions because of its extreme energy level as well as the violation of Hund's rule of maximum multiplicity. Additionally, the formation of singlet oxygen from airborne ground state by light is nearly impossible. As an alternative, sensitizer molecules such as plant pigments or organic compounds (e.g., chlorophylls or porphyrins) are usually not present in distilled EOs.

A previous investigation showed that storage of *Majorana hortensis* EO in the dark for 1 year was related to minor alterations in the chemical profile of the EO, and its organoleptic features were not influenced. However, storage under light presented significant changes in the chemical profile of the EO, because of the chemical transformation of terpenoids [15].

Similar findings were obtained when *Coriandrum sativum* EO was stored for 1 year in the dark and then stored under light period. Insignificant changes were noticed in the EO chemical profile as well as organoleptic properties when it was stored in dark, whereas EO experienced important chemical transformation of monoterpenes when stored in the light [16].

10.3.2 Effect of Temperature

The stability of EOs must be critically monitored during ambient temperature as onset of temperature-dependent reactions leads to the formation of undesirable products. Usually, an increase in temperature increases the rate of temperature-dependent reactions such as autoxidation and decomposition of hydroperoxides. Thus, increase in temperature can lead to free radical formation. On the other hand, decrease in temperatures improves the aerial oxygen solubility in EO, which in succession can adversely influence EO stability. It was also found that at low or mild temperatures, the rate of formation of hydroperoxide in fatty oil is more than at 50°C. A thermal stability study on *Cinnamomum osmophloeum* EO and its respective components revealed a decrease in trans-cinnamaldehyde level when it was incubated for 8 hours at 100°C. Moreover, the addition of eugenol as antioxidant improved the thermal stability of EO and trans-cinnamaldehyde [17]. A recent study also suggested that heat treatments considerably influence chemical composition and antibacterial activities of EOs extracted from mint species [18].

A recent study suggested that great basil L. EO as well as its beta-cyclodextrin complex provide protection to its chemical components such as linalool and methyl chavicol against the harmful effects of heat or air/oxygen. This complex has been formed by crystallization procedure to attain equilibrium between complexed and free volatile components at 50°C. It was found that this complex form of beta-cyclodextrin with *O. basilicum* EO alters the chemical composition of the volatile principles present in EO (in encapsulated form) [19].

A previous study showed that the level of alpha-pinene and beta-pinene in hydrodistilled and steam distilled oils was high at high temperature, while the level of both compounds was decreased in the EO derived from extraction methods without the involvement of heat [20].

Another report demonstrated that rosemary EO showed improvement in stability at low temperature by preventing onset of oxidation reactions. On the contrary, the stability of pine EO decreased at low temperature (at 5°C) due to the formation of peroxide. Lavender EO at 5°C showed higher rate of formation of peroxides than at room temperature, whereas a slight increase in the temperature (by 38°C) received nearly fully destroyed peroxides in two oils, pine as well as lavender oils. It was found that at different storage temperatures, EOs showed different responses in terms of their vulnerability to autoxidation. Several studies showed that EOs lose their stability when temperature increases from 0°C to 28°C, 4°C to 25°C, and 23°C to 38°C. One report showed considerable changes in chemical composition of EOs from rosemary, clove bud, pine, lavender, and cardamom upon rise in temperature. It was found that increase in temperature reduced the level of terpenoidal compounds including beta-caryophyllene, beta-myrcene, beta-pinene, sabinene, and gamma-terpinene, but the level of para-cymene was found to be increased [21].

Moreover, it was indicated that fennel EO when stored at 25°C (in comparison to low temperature, 4°C) increased the 4-anisaldehyde level. Another report showed that increase in temperature increased the formation of undesirable compounds from myrcene by polymerization reaction [22]. Terpenes and terpenoid aldehydes are unstable at high temperature due to their increase in vulnerability toward rearrangement processes. Terpenes-based chemical transformations at elevated temperature have been reported for isolated components [23] and for EOs. Since the heating of terpenes in the presence of air promotes autoxidation, inert gas such as nitrogen is recommended to overcome autoxidation at elevated temperature. However, an earlier report showed that 2 weeks' storage of EO under inert gas at 50°C showed chemical changes in lemon EO such as depletion of geranial, neral, and other terpenoidal compounds along with increased levels of para-cymene. On the other hand, the storage of lemon and fennel oils at room temperature under nitrogen retained its stability. Fluctuations in *Cuminum cyminum* EO chemical profile were noticed when stored for 6 months under varied temperature conditions [refrigeration (4°C), deep freezing temperature (–20°C), and at room temperature (25°C)]. Findings from this study it was suggested that at room temperature, para-cymene as well as beta-pinene levels were reduced; nevertheless, the level of cumin aldehyde improved during the storage of cumin oil. Moreover, the EO compositions presented minimum changes, and it was also suggested that *C. cyminum* EO almost maintains its chemical composition when stored at low temperatures [24].

Another investigation showed the effect of low-pressure cold plasma treatments on the EO content and composition of lemon verbena leaves. Findings obtained from this study suggested that increasing duration of low-pressure cold plasma treatments decreased EO content from 1.2 to 0.9 (% v/w) with certain changes in chemical profile (high level of monoterpene hydrocarbons as well as oxygenated sesquiterpenes) [25].

10.3.3 Effect of Oxygen Availability

EO stability is mainly determined by the extent of exposure to the oxygen or consumption of oxygen in the presence or absence of other variable factors such as light, humidity, and temperature to induce oxidation reactions ultimately to affect the physicochemical properties of EOs. Oxygen consumption in EOs helps in determining the stability of EOs, especially in the case of monoterpenes enriched EOs. Oxidized EO showed sensitivity, mainly allergic reactions, in the form of allergic contact dermatitis as mentioned earlier. For instance, tea tree EO when stored in containers with or without closures underwent photooxidation in a limited number of days and last up to various months, which resulted in the formation of undesirable products (endoperoxides, epoxides, and peroxides) that are moderate to strong sensitizers. It was found that fresh tea tree EO was found to be a weak sensitizer, while oxidized tea tree EO was three times stronger. Additionally, changes in chemical profile such as detection of degradation products of alpha-terpinene (p-cymene, ascaridole, isoascaridole, a-ketoperoxide) were identified. It was found that oxidation reactions were found to be more dominant in half-loaded EO boxes in comparison to when little or no space was available. A recent review suggested that nanoencapsulation can be used to encapsulate EOs to reduce volatility, improve stability and water solubility, and preserve therapeutic efficacy. To achieve this purpose, nanoparticulate formulations as well as lipid carriers can be made. These nanocarriers can be used to improve not only the stability but also the antimicrobial activity of the EO. Further, polymeric NPs prepared via nanoprecipitation can be utilized to improve the shelf-life of EOs and for controlled and targeted release. Oligosaccharides such as β-cyclodextrin have been recently utilized to make a complex of an oil/β-cyclodextrin supramolecular system to improve the stability of the *Ocimum basilicum* L. EO against oxidation as well as at high temperature. Cyclodextrin-EO complex can be further utilized to improve water solubility, stability, and bioavailability and reduce the volatility of EOs [26,27].

Terpenes are extensively used in cosmetics as well as domestic products. However, it is well known that these compounds on air exposure can easily oxidize due to autoxidation, which can result in the formation of undesirable allergenic oxidation compounds. One investigation suggested that limonene, linalool, and caryophyllene are not responsible for causing allergy on their own but that air exposure readily results in allergenic products, which can increase sensitivity of these compounds toward various biological membranes, especially skin. A previous investigation determined the rate and main features of allergic responses against studied oxidized terpenoidal compounds, except limonene, by using patch test in 1,511 dermatitis patients. It was found that oxidized linalool and its hydroperoxide fraction showed considerable sensitivity. Out of the tested patients, 58% showed fragrance-related contact allergy, 1.3% showed positive test to oxidized linalool, 1.1% to the hydroperoxide fraction, 0.5% to oxidized caryophyllene, and one patient to the oxidized myrcene [28].

Aromatic odors have been reported for their ability to cause allergic contact dermatitis. Several studies have demonstrated that these aromatic or fragrant substances can act as prehaptens or prohaptens. After autoxidation, these substances have the capability to produce substances that can induce allergy more than the parent substance. Frequently used aromatic substances present in EOs often suffer from autoxidation on contact with air, resulting in the formation of weak, moderate, or strong sensitizers, which could be the main cause for contact allergy to aromatic compound products. A number of substances act as prohaptens to cause immunological reactions and can be activated in the skin as well [29].

Linalool is a common perfume chemical due to its fresh, flowery aroma. It was found that due to its unsaturated hydrocarbon nature, on air exposure, linalool in lavender EO autoxidizes and forms allergenic oxidation products. Thus, oxidized linalool can cause contact allergy. The main oxidation products reported from autoxidation of linalool are hydroperoxides, which are reactive components that can be assumed to behave as sensitizers. A report demonstrated that 15% of hydroperoxide 7-hydroperoxy-3,7-dimethylocta-1,5-diene-3-ol was identified in an oil that experienced oxidation. A study has been performed to investigate the sensitizing potential of linalool in pure form, air-treated linalool, as well as oxidized products of linalool. It was found that linalool in pure form presented no sensitizing ability, while linalool (air-exposed form) has given positive responses. Moreover, hydroperoxides showed higher sensitizing potential than others [30].

Similarly, linalyl acetate, the most important compound of lavender EO due to its structural similarities with linalool, is also vulnerable to oxidation reactions when exposed to air, and can form similar oxidation products like linalool. One study demonstrated that allergenic oxidized products formed once slightly allergenic linalyl acetate oxidized [31,32].

A previous study showed that lavandula EO needs inherent protection against autoxidation. Additionally, lavender EO after oxidation produced undesirable compounds (allergenic hydroperoxide) and showed increase in skin sensitizing potency. This was due to the oxidation of terpenes in EOs to produce oxidized products, which are responsible for increasing the sensitizing potency of lavender EO on exposure to air. The rate of oxidation as well as oxidized products was found to be the same as the pure compounds exposed to air. Additionally, a patch test for air-exposed lavender EO as well as oxidized linalyl acetate showed positive reactions in patients with contact allergy to oxidized linalool [33].

In another study, the ability of citronellol with other structurally similar compounds such as linalool and geraniol was compared in terms of its potential to autoxidize as well as its sensitization ability. It was found that the level of citronellol was reduced, whereas the sensitization ability was enhanced in air-exposed citronellol with the formation of hydroperoxides as the main oxidation products and main skin sensitizers. It was also suggested that the chemical transformation of the citronellol can lead to the loss of the 2,3-double bond in the citronellol structure during autoxidation, which could be the reason for the formation of oxidation products [34].

Limonene is another fragrant compound extensively used in cosmetics and scented products. One investigation showed that air-exposed limonene produced various oxidized products such as hydroperoxides. Such products have dominantly shown greater sensitizing effect than pure samples. Findings obtained from patch tests indicated that high rates of considerable reactions were noticed, suggesting that these compounds are the main aromatic allergens. In another study, it was found that linalool and R-limonene once autoxidized increase the sensitivity toward skin. Oxidized R-limonene showed more irritating effect than oxidized linalool. Additionally, non-oxidized terpenes did not show irritating effects at all tested concentrations. It was also noticed that in European countries both oxidized R-(+)- as well as S-(−)-limonene are the frequent sources of contact allergy among dermatitis patients [35].

Another report demonstrated considerable increase in the sensitizing ability of oxidized limonene in comparison with pure limonene when tested by using local lymph node assay. Noticeably, one oxidized product (i.e., limonene-1-hydroperoxide) showed more sensitizing ability than the other hydroperoxides. It was also concluded that oxidized products, mainly hydroperoxides, have a specific reaction, demonstrating that oxygen-derived free radicals are imperative in complex formation such as hapten–protein complex [36–38].

D-Limonene is a fragrance substance that is derived as a residual product from citrus juice and is also used as a solvent that is widely known for inducing contact allergy as its autoxidation readily produces a range of oxygenated monocyclic terpenes that are strong contact allergens [39,40].

Fragrant compound geraniol (trans-3,7-dimethyl-2,6-octadiene-1-ol) is also vulnerable against autoxidation when exposed to air and to cutaneous metabolism. Geraniol is recognized as a weak contact allergen, and just like other monoterpenes (limonene as well as linalool), after autooxidation geraniol also forms serious allergenic products. As per reports, both metabolism and oxidation of geraniol resulted in the formation of isomeric aldehydes (geranial and neral). In another study, it was demonstrated that geraniol is stimulated after being metabolized as well as autoxidized. The formation of allergens like geranial as well as neral via both oxidation mechanisms, play an important role in the sensitization to geraniol [41].

These components (geranial and neral) are also present in citral. Thus, as reported, patients with certain sensitivity responses against citral also showed positive response to geraniol as well as oxidized geraniol. It was found that there is not much cross-reactivity found among citral and geraniol (pure form); nevertheless, simultaneous responses against citral as well as geraniol (oxidized form) were widespread, due to geranial. Patch test results showed that 26% of citral-positive individuals responded positively against geraniol (oxidized form), and 10.5% responded positively to pure geraniol, whereas citral and/or its isomers showed positive response among 25% of those who responded negatively to geraniol [42].

One more study demonstrated a mechanism involved in geraniol autoxidation at room temperature by using lymph node test in rodent. It was found that allylic alcohol geraniol follows different oxidation pathways than limonene as well as linalool, and suffers from autooxidation to form hydroperoxides. The geraniol autoxidation involves different oxidative pathways starting from allylic hydrogen withdrawal close to the two double bonds. Geraniol autooxidation resulted in the formation of hydrogen peroxide along with the formation of aldehydes geranial but hydroxyhydroperoxide has formed from neral. Moreover, traces of hydroperoxide are also formed. It was also found that the autoxidation of geraniol increased sensitizing effect of geraniol. The hydroperoxide along with aldehydes geranial and neral was considered as a major contributor to allergenic effects [43].

10.3.4 Presence of Metal Contaminants

Metal could be an important contaminant found in EOs, and can significantly impact their stability. Metal leaching in EOs can take place at the time of storage in metallic containers or during extraction. These metallic impurities such as heavy metals and copper and ferrous ions can stimulate autoxidation, especially when hydroperoxides are already present [44]. These impurities can induce autoxidation in the same manner as induced by light and heat. By increasing conversion of hydroperoxide into alkoxy and peroxyl radicals, these metallic impurities promote radical oxidation reactions. Furthermore, ferrous ions have been reported for the production of singlet oxygen in the presence of light. Humidity rate and a number of metal contaminants can lead to oxidation reactions, with the prior presence of hydroperoxides in the EO [44].

10.3.5 Presence of Water Content

Water content is recognized as a potential cause for EO contamination. Several extraction procedures that involve water as main or co-solvent such as water distillation at almost 100°C could affect the stability of EOs by changing the compound spectra. Citral has been reported to experience reactions catalyzed by acid mainly in aqueous phase, resulting in the formation of α-p-dimethylstyrene, p-cymene-8-ol, p-cymene, methylacetophenone, and cresols. It has been suggested that dry EO when subjected to distillation after treating it with water-binding compounds showed considerable changes in chemical components of EOs, including decreased level of geraniol as well as linalool and increased level of citronellol and geranyl formate in geranium EO stored at room temperature for 12 months. Nevertheless, changes in chemical shifts can equally contribute via occurrence of 50% air space in the vessel.

10.4 Chemical Composition and Structural Features

Several reports have demonstrated the relationship between molecular structures and degradation, which determine the susceptibility of EOs toward degradation [45]. As oxidized or degraded EO components always show change in molecular structure, which can be detected by comparing parent spectra with spectra of oxidized product, EO components containing allylic hydrogen atoms are more vulnerable to autoxidation than others. These allylic hydrogen atoms are the potential sites for autoxidation. Thus, the removal or abstraction of hydrogen atom can result in resonance-stabilized radicals. Polyunsaturated terpenoid hydrocarbons produce numerous radicals, which are alleviated via conjugated double bonds, or isomerize to 3° radicals, which are thus primarily susceptible to oxidation-mediated degradation [46]. Thus, EOs such as pine and turpentine having unsaturated monoterpenes as well as sesquiterpenes are more vulnerable to oxidation and hence show changes during storage. In addition, EO components comprising additional electron-donating groups and showing more alkyl substitution can easily form stable hydroperoxides. This type of chemical modification occurs via the formation of strong carbon-peroxide bond via hyperconjugation. As is known, hyperconjugation always results in the formation of stabilizing molecules, and increase in number of hyperconjugated structures leads to increase in the stability carbocation. This means that hydroperoxides formed are more stable, whereas other products are not efficiently stabilized and are directly degraded. For instance, caryophyllene hydroperoxides quickly form epoxy caryophyllene, which is more stable. Additionally, when EO compound undergoes any sort of changes in its molecular structure, it may also affect the stability of other molecules, especially those that closely resemble the compound affected [47]. During this process, compounds that are more vulnerable to oxidation get easily oxidized to further initiate autoxidation of other compounds, which are less vulnerable to degradation. However, the addition of antioxidants to the oxidized sample can inhibit this degradation. Phenolic compounds including thymol, carvacrol, or phenolic ether eugenol by antioxidant action (mainly the removal of phenolic hydrogen atom) disrupt or delay oxidative reactions. The removal of hydrogen atom by these phenolic compounds resulted in the formation of free, relatively long-living radicals. These radicals are further isomerized by alkyl-substituted tertiary position or electron-releasing groups. Thus, these free radical scavenging compounds have the ability to search free reactive alkyl, alkoxy, or peroxyl radicals, which result in the formation of more stable products [48]. Thus, it was realized that EO containing more than 80% of phenols generally showed good storage stability. Thus, it was concluded that an individual EO compound can influence the stability of other compounds, in that if one compound oxidizes it affects the chemical integrity of others by promoting the autoxidation reactions by involving its own oxidized products. If oxidized products are strong, they react quickly with other compounds to produce more oxidized products by affecting the chemical integrity of other compounds adversely and vice versa. However, it was demonstrated that lavender EO had no protecting effects on major compounds such as linalyl acetate, linalool, and β-caryophyllene when autoxidation rates in the oil were compared with pure compounds.

Overall, changes seen in EOs or pure compounds could not be due to one particular factor or might be due to multiple related causes. In this context, several of the reports and their respective findings do not corroborate with each other. Previous reports suggested that moisture content has a higher impact over EO spoilage in comparison with light; however, it was not corroborated by the other report, which suggested that it could be due to acid-catalyzed reactions at elevated temperatures. Earlier reports have not advocated to store EOs in the refrigerator due to increase in peroxide value as detected in tea tree EO, whereas other investigations suggested that degradation reaction in EOs was increased at room temperature. It was also found that variation in temperature, light, oxygen level, and water level affects the stability of EOs. However, sometimes, individual factors cannot successfully cause the oxidation or degradation of EO; thus, in such cases, multiple factors influence the stability. Co-existence of multiple factors sometimes creates a unique autoxidation-promoting environment, which can affect the chemical integrity of other compounds. Similarly, the oxidation of a chemical compound of EO triggered by single or multiple factors can also affect other compounds, which belong to the same class or mainly those with similar molecular structure. Light is considered as a key factor that more significantly stimulates storage-induced changes, especially in aromatic or flavoring agents, than temperature rise from 4°C to 20°C. It was also found that cold as well as dark storage of EO in a closed container efficiently stopped autoxidation for a period of 1 year.

10.5 Encapsulation of Essential Oils via Nanoprecipitation Process

Polymeric nanoencapsulation is an effective method to improve the shelf-life of EOs, mainly to preserve EOs for a longer duration. This method has various advantages such as it improves solubility in water, provides an active shield against degradation, avoids evaporation of volatile compounds, and regulates as well as offers site-specific release. Out of various methods polymer-based nanopreparation, specifically nanoprecipitation, has gained considerable focus. EOs have various food and non-food applications such as pharmaceutical applications, which make them attractive from a commercial perspective [48–71]. Nevertheless, their utilization is often challenging due to their high volatile nature and high chances of degradation when exposed to high temperature, humidity, light, or oxygen [48–71]. Using polymer-based nanopreparations, EOs can be encapsulated to protect them by offering improved bioavailability, better stability, targeted as well as controlled delivery, and enhanced therapeutic efficacy [48–71]. Various microbial, mammalian, algal, plant, and synthetic-based polymers have been used to fabricate polymeric nanoparticles (NPs). Merits of some NPs systems such as oil-loaded poly(lactide-co-glycolide) NPs, eugenol into poly-ε-caprolactone NPs, Jasminum officinale L. EO encapsulated in gelatin, and Arabic gum NPs are

TABLE 10.1

EOs Loaded Nano Preparations via Nanoprecipitation Method and Its Merits

EOs	NPs	Merits	References
Cymbopogon citratus	Poly(lactide-co-glycolide)-NP	Superior anti-herpetic activity with a controlled release	[50]
Eugenol	Poly-ε-caprolactone nanoparticles	Improve its stability against light oxidation	[50]
Jasminum officinale L. EO	Gelatin and Arabic gum nanoparticles	Heat resistance of was increased	[50]

listed in Table 10.1. Out of the various procedures employed for the development of polymeric-based NPs, the nanoprecipitation procedure (or solvent displacement) is considered as simple and reproducible [48–71]. To improve shelf-life, overcome stability-associated challenges, and improve oil antimicrobial effects, nanoemulsions and solid-lipid nanopreparations have been suggested [48–71].

REFERENCES

1. Turek C, Stintzing FC. Stability of essential oils: A review. *Compr Rev Food Sci Food Saf.* 2013;12:40–53.
2. Nguyen H, Campi EM, Roy Jackson W, Patti A, Antonio patti effect of oxidative deterioration on flavour and aroma compounds of lemon oil. *Food Chem.* 2009;112(2):388–393.
3. Hagvall L, Sköld M, Bråred-Christensson J, Börje A, Karlberg AT. Lavender oil lacks natural protection against autoxidation, forming strong contact allergens on air exposure. *Contact Derm.* 2008;59(3):143–150.
4. Sköld M, Hagvall L, Karlberg AT. Autoxidation of linalyl acetate, the main component of lavender oil, creates potent contact allergens. *Contact Derma.* 2008;58(1):9–14.
5. Hagvall L, Christensson JB. Patch testing with main sensitizers does not detect all cases of contact allergy to oxidized lavender oil. *Acta Derm Venereol.* 2016;96(5):679–683.
6. Bakkali F, Averbeck S, Averbeck D, Idaomar M. Biological effects of essential oils: A review. *Food Chem Toxicol.* 2008;46(2):446–475.
7. Adams TB, Gavin CL, McGowen MM, Waddell WJ, Cohen SM, Feron VJ, Marnett LJ, Munro IC, Portoghese PS, Rietjens IM, Smith RL. The FEMA GRAS assessment of aliphatic and aromatic terpene hydrocarbons used as flavor ingredients. *Food Chem Toxicol.* 2011;49(10):2471–2494.
8. Sarigiannis DA, Karakitsios SP, Gotti A, Liakos IL, Katsoyiannis A. Exposure to major volatile organic compounds and carbonyls in European indoor environments and associated health risk. *Environ Int.* 2011;37(4):743–765.
9. Sköld M, Karlberg AT, Matura M, Börje A. The fragrance chemical beta-caryophyllene-air oxidation and skin sensitization. *Food Chem Toxicol.* 2006;44(4):538–545.
10. Choe E, Min DB. Mechanisms and factors for edible oil oxidation. *Compr Rev Food Sci Food Saf.* 2006;5:169–186.
11. Misharina TA, Polshkov AN, Ruchkina EL, Medvedeva IB. Changes in the composition of the essential oil of marjoram during storage. *Appl Biochem Microbiol.* 2003;39:311–316.
12. Misharina TA, Polshkov AN. Antioxidant properties of essential oils: Autoxidation of essential oils from laurel and fennel and of their mixtures with essential oil from coriander. *Appl Biochem Microbiol.* 2005;41:610–618.
13. Braun M, Franz G. Quality criteria of bitter fennel oil in the German Pharmacopoeia. *Pharmaceut Pharmacol Lett.* 1999;9:48–51.
14. Choe E, Min DB. Chemistry and reactions of reactive oxygen species in foods. *Crit Rev Food Sci Nutr.* 2006;46(1):1–22.
15. Misharina TA, Polshkov AN, Ruchkina EL, Medvedeva IB. Izmenenie sostava éfirnogo masla maĭorana v protsesse khranenia [Changes in the composition of the essential oil in stored marjoram]. *Prikl Biokhim Mikrobiol.* 2003;39(3):353–358.
16. Misharina TA. Vliianie usloviĭ i srokov khraneniia na sostav komponentov éfirnogo masla semian koriandra [Effect of conditions and duration of storage on composition of essential oil from coriander seeds]. *Prikl Biokhim Mikrobiol.* 2001;37(6):726–732.
17. Yeh HF, Luo CY, Lin CY, Cheng SS, Hsu YR, Chang ST. Methods for thermal stability enhancement of leaf essential oils and their main constituents from indigenous cinnamon (*Cinnamomum osmophloeum*). *J Agric Food Chem.* 2013;61(26):6293–6298.
18. Heydari M, Zanfardino A, Taleei A, et al. Effect of heat stress on yield, monoterpene content and antibacterial activity of essential oils of mentha x piperita var. Mitcham and *Mentha arvensis* var. piperascens. *Molecules.* 2018;23(8):1903.
19. Hădărugă DI, Hădărugă NG, Costescu CI, David I, Gruia AT. Thermal and oxidative stability of the *Ocimum basilicum* L. essential oil/β-cyclodextrin supramolecular system. *Beilstein J Org Chem.* 2014;10:2809–2820.
20. Oztürk M, Tel G, Duru ME, Harmandar M, Topçu G. The effect of temperature on the essential oil components of *Salvia potentillifolia* obtained by various methods. *Nat Prod Commun.* 2009;4(7):1017–1020.
21. Turek C, Stintzing FC. Impact of different storage conditions on the quality of selected essential oils. *Food Res Int.* 2012;46:341–353.
22. Dieckmann RH, Palamand SR. Autoxidation of some constituents of hops. I. The monoterpene hydrocarbon, myrcene. *J Agric Food Chem.* 1974;22:498–503.
23. Ternes W. *Naturwissenschaftliche Grundlagen der Lebensmittelzubereitung,* 3rd ed. Behr's Verlag, Hamburg, Germany; 2008.
24. Mehdizadeh L, Pirbalouti AG, Moghaddam M. Storage stability of essential oil of cumin (*CuminumCyminum* L.) as a function of temperature. *Int J Food Prop.* 2017;20(2):1742–1750.
25. Ebadi MT, Abbasi S, Harouni A, Sefidkon F. Effect of cold plasma on essential oil content and composition of lemon verbena. *Food Sci Nutr.* 2019;7(4):1166–1171.

26. Bilia AR, Guccione C, Isacchi B, Righeschi C, Firenzuoli F, Bergonzi MC. Essential oils loaded in nanosystems: A developing strategy for a successful therapeutic approach. *Evid Based Complement Alternat Med.* 2014;2014:651593.
27. Lammari N, Louaer O, Meniai AH, Elaissari A. Encapsulation of essential oils via nanoprecipitation process: Overview, progress, challenges and prospects. *Pharmaceutics.* 2020;12(5):431.
28. Matura M, Sköld M, Börje A, Andersen KE, Bruze M, Frosch P, Goossens A, Johansen JD, Svedman C, White IR, Karlberg AT. Selected oxidized fragrance terpenes are common contact allergens. *Contact Derm.* 2005;52(6):320–328.
29. Karlberg AT, Börje A, Duus Johansen J, Lidén C, Rastogi S, Roberts D, Uter W, White IR. Activation of non-sensitizing or low-sensitizing fragrance substances into potent sensitizers: Prehaptens and prohaptens. *Contact Derm.* 2013;69(6):323–334.
30. Sköld M, Börje A, Harambasic E, Karlberg AT. Contact allergens formed on air exposure of linalool. Identification and quantification of primary and secondary oxidation products and the effect on skin sensitization. *Chem Res Toxicol.* 2004;17(12):1697–1705.
31. Sköld M, Hagvall L, Karlberg AT. Autoxidation of linalyl acetate, the main component of lavender oil, creates potent contact allergens. *Contact Derm.* 2008;58(1):9–14.
32. Hagvall L, Berglund V, Bråred Christensson J. Air-oxidized linalyl acetate: An emerging fragrance allergen? *Contact Derm.* 2015;72(4):216–223.
33. Hagvall L, Sköld M, Bråred-Christensson J, Börje A, Karlberg AT. Lavender oil lacks natural protection against autoxidation, forming strong contact allergens on air exposure. *Contact Derm.* 2008;59(3):143–150.
34. Rudbäck J, Hagvall L, Börje A, Nilsson U, Karlberg AT. Characterization of skin sensitizers from autoxidized citronellol: Impact of the terpene structure on the autoxidation process. *Contact Derm.* 2014;70(6):329–339.
35. Matura M, Sköld M, Börje A, Andersen KE, Bruze M, Frosch P, Goossens A, Johansen JD, Svedman C, White IR, Karlberg AT. Not only oxidized R-(+)- but also S-(–)-limonene is a common cause of contact allergy in dermatitis patients in Europe. *Contact Derm.* 2006;55(5):274–279.
36. Christensson JB, Johansson S, Hagvall L, Jonsson C, Börje A, Karlberg AT. Limonene hydroperoxide analogues differ in allergenic activity. *Contact Derm.* 2008;59(6):344–352.
37. Bråred Christensson J, Karlberg AT, Andersen KE, Bruze M, Johansen JD, Garcia-Bravo B, Giménez Arnau A, Goh CL, Nixon R, White IR. Oxidized limonene and oxidized linalool: Concomitant contact allergy to common fragrance terpenes. *Contact Derm.* 2016;74(5):273–280.
38. Bråred Christensson J, Forsström P, Wennberg AM, Karlberg AT, Matura M. Air oxidation increases skin irritation from fragrance terpenes. *Contact Derm.* 2009;60(1):32–40.
39. Pesonen M, Suomela S, Kuuliala O, Henriks-Eckerman ML, Aalto-Korte K. Occupational contact dermatitis caused by D-limonene. *Contact Derm.* 2014;71(5):273–279.
40. Karlberg AT, Dooms-Goossens A. Contact allergy to oxidized d-limonene among dermatitis patients. *Contact Derm.* 1997;36(4):201–206.
41. Hagvall L, Baron JM, Börje A, Weidolf L, Merk H, Karlberg AT. Cytochrome P450-mediated activation of the fragrance compound geraniol forms potent contact allergens. *Toxicol Appl Pharmacol.* 2008;233(2):308–313.
42. Hagvall L, Bråred Christensson J. Cross-reactivity between citral and geraniol - can it be attributed to oxidized geraniol? *Contact Derm.* 2014;71(5):280–288.
43. Hagvall L, Bäcktorp C, Svensson S, Nyman G, Börje A, Karlberg AT. Fragrance compound geraniol forms contact allergens on air exposure. Identification and quantification of oxidation products and effect on skin sensitization. *Chem Res Toxicol.* 2007;20(5):807–814.
44. Choe E, Min DB. Mechanisms and factors for edible oil oxidation. *Compr Rev Food Sci Food Saf.* 2006;5:169–186.
45. Treibs W. *E. Gildemeister/Fr. Hoffmann: Die ätherischen Öle Band II*, 4th ed. Akademie-Verlag, Berlin, Germany; 1960.
46. Neuenschwander U, Guignard F, Hermans I. Mechanism of the aerobic oxidation of α-pinene. *ChemSusChem.* 2010;3:75–84.
47. Gopalakrishnan N. Studies on the storage quality of CO_2-extracted cardamom and clove bud oils. *J Agric Food Chem.* 1994;42:796–798.
48. Nanditha B, Prabhasankar P. Antioxidants in bakery products: A review. *Crit Rev Food Sci Nutr.* 2009;49:1–27.
49. Bilia AR, Guccione C, Isacchi B, Righeschi C, Firenzuoli F, Bergonzi MC. Essential oils loaded in nanosystems: A developing strategy for a successful therapeutic approach. *Evid Based Complement Alternat Med.* 2014;2014:651593. doi: 10.1155/2014/651593. Retraction in: *Evid Based Complement Alternat Med.* 2021;2021:7259208.
50. Lammari N, Louaer O, Meniai AH, Elaissari A. Encapsulation of essential oils via nanoprecipitation process: Overview, progress, challenges and prospects. *Pharmaceutics.* 2020;12(5):431.
51. Bhatia S, Namdeo AG, Nanda S. Factors effecting the gelling and emulsifying properties of a natural polymer. *SRP.* 2010;1(1):86–92.
52. Bhatia S, Sharma K, Bera T. Structural characterization and pharmaceutical properties of porphyran. *Asian J Pharm.* 2015;9:93–101.
53. Bhatia S, Sharma A, Sharma K, Kavale M, Chaugule BB, Dhalwal K, Namdeo AG, Mahadik KR. Novel algal polysaccharides from marine source: Porphyran. *Pharmacogn Rev.* 2008;4:271–276.
54. Bhatia S, Sharma K, Nagpal K, Bera T. Investigation of the factors influencing the molecular weight of porphyran and its associated antifungal activity Bioact. *Carb Diet Fiber.* 2015;5:153–168.
55. Bhatia S, Kumar V, Sharma K, Nagpal K, Bera T. Significance of algal polymer in designing amphotericin B nanoparticles. *Sci World J.* 2014;2014:564573.
56. Bhatia S, Rathee P, Sharma K, Chaugule BB, Kar N, Bera T. Immuno-modulation effect of sulphated polysaccharide (porphyran) from *Porphyra vietnamensis. Int J Biol Macromol.* 2013;57:50–56.
57. Bhatia S. *Natural Polymer Drug Delivery Systems: Marine Polysaccharides Based Nano-Materials and Its Applications.* Springer International Publishing, Switzerland; 2016:185–225.

58. Bhatia S. *Natural Polymer Drug Delivery Systems: Plant Derived Polymers, Properties, and Modification & Applications.* Springer International Publishing, Switzerland; 2016:119–184.
59. Bhatia S. *Natural Polymer Drug Delivery Systems: Nanotechnology and Its Drug Delivery Applications.* Springer International Publishing, Switzerland; 2016:1–32.
60. Bhatia S. *Natural Polymer Drug Delivery Systems: Nanoparticles Types, Classification, Characterization, Fabrication Methods and Drug Delivery Applications.* Springer International Publishing, Switzerland; 2016:33–93.
61. Bhatia S. *Natural Polymer Drug Delivery Systems: Natural Polymers vs Synthetic Polymer.* Springer International Publishing, Switzerland; 2016:95–118.
62. Bhatia S. *Systems for Drug Delivery: Mammalian Polysaccharides and Its Nanomaterials.* Springer International Publishing, Switzerland; 2016:1–27.
63. Bhatia S. *Systems for Drug Delivery: Microbial Polysaccharides as Advance Nanomaterials.* Springer International Publishing, Switzerland; 2016:29–54.
64. Bhatia S. *Systems for Drug Delivery: Chitosan Based Nanomaterials and Its Applications.* Springer International Publishing, Switzerland; 2016:55–117.
65. Bhatia S. *Systems for Drug Delivery: Advance Polymers and Its Applications.* Springer International Publishing, Switzerland; 2016:119–146.
66. Bhatia S. *Systems for Drug Delivery: Advanced Application of Natural Polysaccharides.* Springer International Publishing, Switzerland; 2016:147–170.
67. Bhatia S. *Systems for Drug Delivery: Modern Polysaccharides and Its Current Advancements.* Springer International Publishing, Switzerland; 2016:171–188.
68. Bhatia S. *Systems for Drug Delivery: Toxicity of Nanodrug Delivery Systems.* Springer International Publishing, Switzerland; 2016:189–197.
69. Bhatia S. *Nanotechnology in Drug Delivery Fundamentals, Design, and Applications: Part 1: Protein and Peptide-Based Drug Delivery Systems.* Apple Academic Press, Palm Bay, FL; 2016:50–204.
70. Bhatia S. *Nanotechnology in Drug Delivery Fundamentals, Design, and Applications: Part 2: Peptide-Mediated Nanoparticle Drug Delivery System.* Apple Academic Press, Palm Bay, FL; 2016:205–280.
71. Bhatia S. *Nanotechnology in Drug Delivery Fundamentals, Design, and Applications: Part 3: CPP and CTP in Drug Delivery and Cell Targeting.* Apple Academic Press, Palm Bay, FL; 2016:309–312.

11

Quality Control of Essential Oils

Ahmed Al-Harrasi
Natural and Medical Sciences Research Center, University of Nizwa

Saurabh Bhatia
Natural and Medical Sciences Research Center, University of Nizwa
University of Petroleum and Energy Studies

Deepak Kaushik
M. D. University

Mohammed Muqtader Ahmed and Md. Khalid Anwer
Prince Sattam Bin Abdul Aziz University

P.B. Sharma
Amity University Haryana

CONTENTS

11.1 Introduction

Essential oils (EOs) often experience chemical changes upon storage, which can result in the development of undesirable properties such as allergic reactions caused by oxidized EO components. Thus, considering variable storage conditions, the quality of EOs must be monitored by periodically investigating changes in their properties. Usually, the quality of EOs is assessed by comparing the sample with the reference compound (pure or isolated components) during storage where the EOs are experimentally exposed to different conditions such as molecular oxygen, metal catalysts, and photosensitizers [1–3]. Optimization of storage conditions is important in order to achieve appropriate oxidation of the targeted compound up to a certain level. These optimal conditions are sometimes found from previous studies, or new optimal conditions are created to study the behavior of EOs/multiple components/isolated compounds. An experimental simulation chamber for atmospheric smog with ozone, hydroxyl radicals, or nitrous gases has been used for this purpose [4]. These conditions are usually created by targeting two to three compounds present in EOs. However, deep prior understanding related to the behavior of EO components (weakly oxidized, moderately oxidized, strongly oxidized, antioxidant potential, and pro-oxidative properties) must be studied against different experimental conditions in order to target components accordingly [5–7].

EOs contain various volatile compounds; thus, their study requires more advanced techniques. One of the emerging tools used to detect quantitative and qualitative changes in EO components during varied conditions of storage especially in vapor phase is gas chromatography-mass spectrometry (GC-MS). In contrast to high-performance liquid chromatography (HPLC), this method allows the use of buffers and small amounts of solvents. Steam distillation and solvent extraction procedures combined with GC or GC-MS have been used recently for the examination of volatile components. Nevertheless, it is a time-consuming method, and requires a large quantity of samples; thus static headspace GC-MS is a more robust, fast, and effective analytical technique that has been developed for solvent-free fractionation of crude and processed samples. Under

DOI: 10.1201/9781003175933-13

optimized specifications headspace solid-phase microextraction (HS-SPME) combined with GC-MS facilitates quick sampling as well as examination of liquid phase as well as vapor phase components of EOs. HS-SPME is a solvent-free, nondestructive, and easy method for collecting volatile organic compounds produced from plants (Table 11.1). This method could be employed even using living plants without collecting them. Furthermore, the effectiveness of HS-SPME combined with GC has been proven, collecting substantial quantities of volatile compounds (Table 11.1). Several studies have been performed to compare the chemical profile of EOs artificially aged under suitable conditions with genuine EOs, and some studies have been performed to study the compositional variation of EOs under both light and dark conditions [8–11].

TABLE 11.1

Volatile Compounds in Essential Oils

Essential Oils	Volatile Compounds	Technique	References
A. oxymitra leaves	β-pinene, caryophyllene epoxide, α-pinene, caryophyllene, myrtenol, sabinene	GC-MS-FID	[12]
A. oxymitra pericarp	β-pinene, caryophyllene epoxide, myrtenol, trans-pinocarveol, pinocarvone, perillol	GC-MS-FID	[12]
A. oxymitra rhizomes	β-pinene, o-cymene, α-pinene, myrtenol, 1,8-cineole	HP-GC-MS-FID	[12]
A. oxymitra seed oil	Shyobunol, germacrene D, cubebol, 6-epi-shyobunol, germacrene-D4-ol	GC-MS-FID	[12]
Artemisia Annua	1,8 cineole and camphor, artemisia alcohol, α-pinene and pinocarvone	GC/FID and GC/MS	[13]
L. aromatica, B. rotunda	Geraniol, ocimene, d-camphor 1,8-cineole and camphene	GC-MS-FID	[12]
Brassica nigra	Allyl-isothiocyanate	GC-MS-Agilent 5975 C mass spectrometer detector	[14]
C. cambodianum	1,8-cineole, α-terpineol, α-pinene, borneol terpinen-4-ol, β-spathulenol, linalool	GC-MS-FID	[12]
C. lucida oil	Esters, decyl acetate, dodecenyl acetate, carbonylic compounds, sesquiterpenoids, aliphatic alcohols, decanal, caryophyllene epoxide, decan-1-ol	GC-MS-FID	[12]
Centaurium erythraea	α-terpineol, naphthalene, β-caryophyllene, decanal, bornyl acetate	HS-SPME coupled with GC-MS	[15]
Cinnamomum cassia with 8-hydroxyquinoline	Caryophyllene, cinnamyl acetate, bornyl acetate and α-copaene	GC-MS-FID	[16]
Cinnamon	Eugenol, estragole, cinnamaldehyde	SDME-GC-MS	[17]
Cinnamon	β-caryophyllene, eugenol, α-humulene, safrole, linalool, α-phellandrene, and α-pinene	SPME-GC-MS	[18]
Cinnamon bark, clove, peppermint, eucalyptus, and thymeEO	Trans-cinnamaldehyde, 1,8-cineole, thymol, menthol, eugenol	HS-SPME-GC-MS	[19]
Citronella	Citronellal, geraniol, citronellol, and beta-cadinene	GC-MS	[20]
Citronella oil	Citronellal, limonene, and nerol	HS-SPME-GC-MS	[19]
Citronella oils	Citronellal, citronellol, and geraniol	GC-MS	[21]
Citrus limon var pompia	Linalyl acetate, limonene, isomers of citral	HS-SPME/GC-MS	[22]
Eugenia caryophyllus oil	delta-cadinene, alpha- humulene, beta- caryophyllene, eugenol, eugenol acetate, and estragole	SPME-GC-MS	[23]
DaucusEO muricatus L.	alpha-pinene, estragole, terpinolene, myrcene, and limonene	HS-SPME coupled with GC-MS	[24]
Eucalyptus EO	alpha-phellandrene, 1,8-cineole, para-cymene, alpha-pinene, limonene, gamma-terpinene	SPME coupled with GC-MS	[25]
Eucalyptus EO	trans-pinocarveol, alpha-pinene, 1, 8-cineole, globulol	GC apparatus equipped with a polar column HP-5MS	[26]
Garlic	Diallyl disulfide, dithiane, butyric acid, diallyl trisulfide, dihydrodithiine, para-benzoquinone dithiane, and methoxythiophene	GC-MS	[27]
Hertia maroccana	Germanicol, germacrene delta-cadinene, alpha-guaiene, alpha-pinene, beta-pinene,	GC-MS (TRACE TR-5 column)	[28]
Houttuynia cordata	tridecan-2-one, myrcene, geranyl acetate, caryophyllene, beta-ocimene, bornyl acetate, 2-undecanone	GC-MS-FID	[29]
Lavandula×intermedia "Grosso"	Linalyl acetate, 1,8-cineole, terpinenol, linalool	HS-SPME-GC-MS	[30]
Lavender EO	alpha-thujone, eucalyptol, nerol, menthol, and menthone,	SPME coupled with GC/MS	[31]

(*Continued*)

TABLE 11.1 (*Continued*)

Volatile Compounds in Essential Oils

Essential Oils	Volatile Compounds	Technique	References
Lemon Grass (Cymbopogon Citratus)	Geranial, neral	GC-MS-FID	[32]
Litsea citrata	α-citral, β-citral	HS-SPME-GC-MS	[33]
Origanum majorana	Gamma-terpinene, alpha-thujene, beta-caryophyllene, sabinene and alpha-terpinene	SPME coupled with GC/MS	[34]
Melissa officinalis	1-4 cineole, eucalyptol, menthone, and nerol	SPME coupled with GC/MS	[31]
Peppermint oil	alpha-pinene, alpha-thujone, menthol, limonene, myrcene, menthone	SPME coupled with GC/MS	[31]
Peppermint oil	Menthol, beta-pinene, alpha-pinene, alpha-phellandrene, limonene	SPME coupled with GC/MS	[35]
Mentha and rosemary EO	alpha-pinene, methyl salicylate, beta-pinene, eucalyptol	SPME coupled with -GC/MS	[36]
Sweetgale	delta-cadinene, alpha-pinene, 1,8-cineole, para-cymene	HS-SPME coupled with GC/MS	[37]
Origanum vulgare	Carvacrol, camphor, alpha-caryophyllene1,8-cineole	SDME- coupled with GC/MS	[17]
Persicaria odorata	Dodecyl aldehyde, decanoic acid, n-decyl alcohol, 1-dodecanol, alpha-humulene, caryophyllene, and hendecane	GC-MS coupled with FID	[29]
Long pepper EO	alpha-farnesene, eugenol, beta-caryophyllene	HS-SPME coupled with GC/MS	[38]
Piper nigrum	Eugenol, alpha-pinene, 3-carene, -limonene	HS-SPME coupled with GC/MS	[38]
R. dumetorum	Caryophyllene, caryophyllene epoxide, alpha-pinene, humulene-1,2-epoxide,	GC-MS-FID	[12]
S. siamensis oil	β-bourbonene, caryophyllene epoxide, α-pinene, β-spathulenol, and β-pinene, trans-α-bergamotene	GC-MS-FID-DB	[12]
Toothbrush tree	Isothiocyanate	SPME coupled with GC/MS	[39]
Salvia aucheri Boiss. var. mesatlantica Maire	Camphor, 1,8-cineole, viridiflorol, camphene, α-pinene, and p-cymene	GC and GC-MS	[40]
Sage	Alpha-pinene, limonene, camphor, borneol	SPME coupled withGC/MS	[31]
Scots pine oil	alpha-pinene, limonene, beta-pinene,	HS-SPME coupled with GC/MS	[19]
Thyme	Alpha-terpinolene, bornyl acetate, linalool, and limonene	SPME coupled with GC/MS	[17]

A previous report suggested a reduction in the level of unsaturated terpenes of tea tree EO, including γ-terpinene or β-myrcene with increase in the level of p-cymene under light and high temperature. Similar findings were obtained during extended storage of tea tree EO. Furthermore, depending on the chemical nature of EOs, increase in the level of oxidized components during the storage has been reported (e.g., presence of anisaldehyde in fennel oil or linalool oxide as well as caryophyllene oxide in marjoram oil) [41,42]. Stability can also vary with variation in storage conditions; for example, sweet fennel EO was very unstable in the darkness and experienced nearly full degradation in 2 months in the presence of light along with the development of some undesirable and unidentified oxidized products. However, these conditions have only altered the aromatic behavior of laurel EO [41,42].

11.2 Analysis of Essential Oils

To assess the quality and to validate the identity of EO components, various methods have been introduced to assess their physical and chemical properties mainly to determine EO stability upon storage. Various parameters such as viscosity, refractive index, optical rotation, and relative density along with the assessment of organoleptic characters including characteristic odor, color, and flavor (Pudil et al. [43]) have been used to determine the stability of EOs [43].

11.2.1 Chromatographic Characterization of Essential Oils

The composition of EOs mainly to assess certain quality parameters such as identity, likely impurities or possible degradation products, and separation of components can be examined by thin-layer chromatography [44,45]. However, other chromatographic tools have received more attention to assess the stability of volatile components in the liquid phase as well as the gas phase and to study their respective aromatic behavior.

11.2.1.1 Gas Chromatography

The complex chemical composition of oil is dependent on the plant type, its geographical or natural habitat conditions, type of plant organs selected for EOs, season of the harvesting, type of extraction procedure employed, extraction conditions, storage conditions, and most importantly the nature of the EOs (as some get quickly oxidized). GC is often utilized to examine the complex blend of EOs and interactions between their components [46]. GC is suitable for the examination of aromatic compounds due to their volatile nature as GC-based assessment of EOs has been considered by a great number of reports, which have shown effective separation capacity (Table 11.1). The following techniques with diverse applications in the assessment as well as validation of various quality parameters of EOs have been used recently to study compositional analysis more accurately under varied storage conditions [46]:

- GC-olfactometry
- heart-cut multidimensional GC-olfactometry
- HS-SPME couples with GC-MS
- 2-D-GC combination with time-of-flight mass spectrometry
- GC with a flame ionization detector

EOs are complex mixtures of terpenoidal (primarily monoterpenoids and sesquiterpenoids), aromatic as well as aliphatic compounds. Several reports have demonstrated that mass spectral findings of these components are typically close to each other. For this reason, the identification of peak in spectra of complex samples often becomes quite challenging. Thus, it is highly recommended to accurately perform qualitative examination complex composition of oils by using GC-MS. To improve component separation and identification, the 2-D-GC (GC×GC) technique is commonly used in various EO-based studies (Table 11.1). More robust techniques such as multidimensional GC can be used to resolve most of the co-elution difficulties existing with old GC for complex samples, whereas fast-GC leads to raised productivity. GC-olfactometry has been utilized not only for GC-based separation of components but also to execute sensory detection of components, which is used for both the sensory examination and perception of off-flavors [47,48]. GC combined with MS or flame ionization methods has been used recently to evaluate terpenoid composition of EOs. For compositional analysis, GC-MS or GC-flame ionization detector has been used to identify as well as estimate the volatile components present in EOs [49]. However, these procedures are restricted to a comparatively low number of EO components that are having vapor pressures between 350°C and 400°C. EO components that are stable upon vaporization and separation temperatures are more suitable for these techniques. Various reports confirmed structural changes of heat-sensitive or partially volatile compounds with the increased occurrence of artifacts upon GC-based characterization of EOs [50]. Due to elevated injector temperatures and catalytically active column surfaces during GC separation, some EO components experience decomposition and rearrangement reactions [51].

Chiral GC is an experimental and potent method for the validation of EOs and is important for the estimation of contaminants in the EOs. Enantiomers show the same physicochemical properties and different optical behaviors due to which they can show different biological effects; one enantiomer could be safe, whereas the other is harmful and thus suitable, effective investigations are required [52]. In oranges (R)-limonene is responsible for the aroma, whereas (S)-limonene is responsible for the aroma of lemon. (S)-carvone is the main aromatic principle component of the caraway (cumin odor) oil, and (R)-carvone is in spearmint oil (spearmint aroma).

11.2.1.2 High-Performance Liquid Chromatography Profile of Essential Oils

Other than GC, HPLC can also utilized for identifying EO volatiles with the aided advantage of detecting [53] heat-sensitive [54] and less volatile substances [55]. Various validated procedures in terms of linearity, precision, accuracy, and specificity have been demonstrated to determine volatile components of various EOs. Various validated methods must be designed for the instantaneous and quantitative estimation of most potential compounds present in various EOs. However, the majority of EOs are vulnerable to degradation, primarily due to oxidation, hydrolysis, or polymerization on long-term storage. As mentioned earlier, GC techniques have a number of disadvantages for volatile components as structural changes of heat-sensitive components might take place during the study because of the elevated temperature of injector or columns. Thus, there is a serious need for a simple validated liquid chromatographic procedure for simultaneous estimation of all possible compounds found in various EOs. The development of chemical fingerprint by using a rapid technique such as HPLC to assess the chemical quality of EOs could be considered as an effective approach for the quality estimation of EOs. Due to the non-volatile characteristics of some components, investigations based on oxygenated compounds are typically performed by normal or reverse-phase HPLC with fluorescence or ultraviolet detection system. Various validated procedures as options for GC for the determination of carvacrol, thymol, citral in thyme and lemongrass oils were developed by Hajimehdipoor et al. [56] and da S. Rauber et al. [57]. A validated RP-HPLC procedure has been developed for the instantaneous estimation of 22 compounds in various EOs, specifically cardamom, cinnamon, and caraway oils [58]. Five phenolic compounds were found in *Araucaria columnaris* EO by using RP-HPLC-DAD [59]. Only a few reports are available for the analysis of EOs by using HPLC. Usually, HPLC is used for the separation as well as identification of non-volatiles in cold-pressed citrus oils [60]. For volatile components, HPLC utilization is restricted to sample cleanup [61] or prefractionating procedure before GC study [62]. Further, alcohol and its derivatives were identified in EO sample by means of HPLC coupled with mass spectrometry detection. By using a derivatization procedure, a large sensitivity improvement was obtained. Additionally, a HPLC-UV technique was equated to GC with flame ionization detector and GC-MS. It was found that limits of detection received by this method were found to be better in comparison with results received from GC-FID and in the same order as obtained by GC-MS. Thus, the developed method was found to be satisfactory for the determination of alcohols in EOs [63]. A recent investigation showed that a novel validated RP-HPLC method for the determination of cis-trans isomers of citral has been established. The procedure was found to be suitable for citral in between 3 and 100 μg/mL. It was found that this procedure is appropriate for the detection of citral in EOs and aqueous citral based preparations with high resolution of its main constituents neral as well as geranial [64].

A validated HPLC-photodiode array detection procedure (reversed-phase) was recently developed for concurrent determination of β-caryophyllene, alpha-humulene, precocene-I, coumarin, beta and -caryophyllene oxide, in *A. conyzoides* extract as well as oil. The separation of chemical components was completed in 50 minutes. It was demonstrated that the established HPLC-PDA procedure can be effectively used for the detection of the constituents of *A. conyzoides* extracts as well as its oil [65]. Reports that are available suggest multiple volatile hydrocarbon separation in compound preparation, whereas seldom individual terpenoidal compounds have been estimated in EOs by HPLC [66].

Complex chemical components of certain EO chiral components and detection of chiral atoms is essential for the analysis of oil [67]. Recently, polarimetric-based HPLC detection was employed to obtain HPLC-chromatogram for blended oils (lavender/lavandin oils) on various chiral stationary phases. Immobilization of amylose tris-(3,5-dichloro-phenylcarbamate) over silica particles facilitated the finest separation of the many chiral phytoconstituents present in lavender/lavandin EOs [67]. In reversed as well as normal-phase modes, the analysis of different EOs has been accomplished by several researchers [68,69]. HPLC is not extensively employed in EOs; however, it is rather a procedure of preference for characterizing low volatile components. HPLC is more favorable for detecting non-volatile components of EOs [35]. For the detection of EO volatile components, detectors such as UV or photodiode array detectors provide spectral data instantaneously for every peak due to their variability and selectivity.

11.2.1.3 Liquid Chromatography–Mass Spectrometry

Liquid chromatography combined with mass spectrometry is considered as an effective analytical technique for compound identification. In a previous study, simultaneous quantitation of anti-inflammatory components in peppermint oil was achieved by applying a distinctive tandem HPLC column combined with electrospray ionization mass spectrometry. It was found that the developed LC-MS-MS procedure offers an appropriate procedure for the identification of anti-inflammatory components in Mentha spp. [70]. A liquid chromatography-tandem mass spectrometry (LC-MS-MS) analysis in *Zanthoxylum zanthoxyloides* fruit EO has been used to study the coumarins. It was found that the level of coumarins was significantly higher in fruits EO than in other organs of the plant [71].

Other methods such as electrochromatography with LC-MS/MS have been reported recently to detect the chemical profile of *Thymus vulgaris* L. solid oil preparation made up of liquid oil mixed with other solid ingredients. Liquid oil and solid-associated oil have been analyzed via capillary electrochromatography linked to diode array detection and LC-MS/MS methodologies. Thymol and carvacrol along with certain minor components were found during this study [72].

11.3 Characterization of Essential Oils Produced via Plant Tissue Culture

Plant tissue culture has been extensively utilized in the maintenance as well as use of uncommon and threatened medicinal plants, as well as to improve the genetic characteristics of plant material in order to improve their physiological state or manipulate biosynthetic pathways by metabolic engineering to increase the yield of bioactive chemicals. Characterization of these volatile components is usually done by headspace GC-MS procedure coupled with chemometric procedure, which has been used to study and assess the volatile components in wild stock as well as tissue cultures [73–85].

11.4 Chemical Characterization of Essential Oil Encapsulated by Nanoprecipitation Method

Polymeric nanoencapsulation is an efficient procedure to improve the shelf-life of oils mainly to preserve EOs for a longer duration. This method has various advantages such as it improves solubility in water, is effective safeguard against external degradant factors, avoids evaporation of volatile components, and can be controlled targeted release. Of the various methods used for the preparation of polymeric nanoparticles, nanoprecipitation has drawn considerable interest. EOs have various food and non-food applications such as pharmaceutical applications, which make them attractive from a commercial perspective [86–105]. Nevertheless, their utilization is a challenge due to their highly volatile nature and high chance of degradation when exposed to external conditions [86–105]. Using polymeric nanoparticles, EO can be encapsulated to prepare more stable formulations with improved shelf-life, improved bioavailability, better therapeutic effects with targeted as well as controlled release [86–105]. Various microbial, mammalian, algal, plant, and synthetic-based polymers have been used to fabricate polymeric nanoparticles. The characterization of this type of nanoparticles can be done after determining their encapsulation efficiency. Differences in the chemical composition of EOs before and after the encapsulated nanoformulation can be examined by GC-MS. Later, biological assessment can be done between control, pure oil, and EO-loaded nanocapsules. FTIR can be used to reveal the encapsulated EOs into nanoshells, and DSC can also be performed to demonstrate the thermal stability of EOs after encapsulated. The zeta potential of EO-NPs can be determined by using a zeta sizer. GC-MS can also be performed to determine encapsulation of EO into nanocapsules and also to compare the difference chemical profiles of EOs before and after encapsulation.

REFERENCES

1. Blumann A, Ryder L. Autoxidation of α-phellandrene. *J ChemSoc.* 1949;2040–2043. https://pubs.rsc.org/en/Content/ArticleLanding/JR/1949/JR9490002040#!divAbstract.
2. Nilsson U, Bergh M, Shao LP, Karlberg AT. Analysis of contact allergenic compounds in oxidized d-limonene. *Chromatographia.* 1996;42:199–205.
3. Nguyen H, Campi EM, Jackson WR, Patti AF. Effect of oxidative deterioration on flavour and aroma components of lemon oil. *Food Chem.* 2009;112:388–393.
4. Atkinson R, Arey J. Atmospheric chemistry of biogenic organic compounds. *Acc Chem Res.* 1998;31:574–583.
5. Gracza L, Ruff P. The light–stability of trans-isoasarone and related compounds. *Dtsch Apoth Ztg.* 1981;121:2541–2544.
6. Guenther E. Appendix II. Storage of essential oils. In: Guenther E, editor. *The Essential Oils Vol. I: History – Origin in Plants – Production – Analysis.* D. Van Nostrand, Toronto, New York, London;1948:377–379.
7. Gopalakrishnan N. Studies on the storage quality of CO_2-extracted cardamom and clove bud oils. *J Agric Food Chem.* 1994;42:796–798.

8. Fischer R, Still F. Untersuchungen uber genuine ätherische Öle. *Planta Med.* 1967;15:6–16.
9. Toth L. Essential oil of *Foeniculum vulgare.* II. Changes in different fennel oils before and after harvesting. *Planta Med.* 1967;15:371–389.
10. Fincke A, Maurer R. Verhalten von Citronenol bei der Herstellung ünd Lagerung citronenolhaltiger Zuckerwaren. 2. Mitteilung: Lager- und Herstellungsversuche. *Dtsch Lebensm Rdsch.* 1974;70:100–104.
11. Brophy JJ, Davies NW, Southwell IA, Stiff IA, Williams LR. Gas chromatographic quality control for oil of *Melaleuca terpinen*-4-ol type (Australian tea tree). *J Agric Food Chem.* 1989;37:1330–1335.
12. Houdkova M, Urbanova K, Doskocil I, Rondevaldova J, Novy P, Nguon S, Chrun R, Kokoska L. In vitro growth-inhibitory effect of Cambodian essential oils against pneumonia causing bacteria in liquid and vapour phase and their toxicity to lung fibroblasts. *South Afr J Bot.* 2018;118:85–97.
13. Santomauro F, Donato R, Sacco C, Pini G, Flamini G, Bilia AR. Vapour and liquid-phase artemisia annua essential oil activities against several clinical strains of Candida. *Planta Med.* 2016;82(11–12):1016–1020.
14. Mejía-Garibay B, Palou E, López-Malo A. Composition, diffusion, and antifungal activity of black mustard (*Brassica nigra*) essential oil when applied by direct addition or vapor phase contact. *J Food Prot.* 2015;78(4):843–848.
15. Jerkovi I, Gaso-Sokac D, Pavlovic H, Marijanovic Z, Gugic M, Petrovic I, Kovac S. Volatile organic compounds from *Centaurium erythraea* rafn (Croatia) and the antimicrobial potential of its essential oil. *Molecules.* 2012;17(2):2058–2072.
16. Netopilova M, Houdkova M, Urbanova K, Rondevaldova J, van Damme P, Kokoska L. In vitro antimicrobial combinatory effect of Cinnamomum cassia essential oil with 8-hydroxyquinoline against *Staphylococcus aureus* in liquid and vapour phase. *J Appl Microbiol.* 2020. doi: 10.1111/jam.14683.
17. López P, Sánchez C, Batlle R, Nerín C. Solid- and vapor-phase antimicrobial activities of six essential oils: Susceptibility of selected foodborne bacterial and fungal strains. *J Agric Food Chem.* 2005;53(17):6939–6946.
18. Goni P, Lopez P, Sanchez C, Gomez-Lus R, Becerril R, Nerın C. Antimicrobial activity in the vapour phase of a combination of cinnamon and clove essential oils. *Food Chem.* 2009;116 (4):982–989.
19. Ács K, Balázs VL, Kocsis B, et al. Antibacterial activity evaluation of selected essential oils in liquid and vapor phase on respiratory tract pathogens. *BMC Complement Altern Med.* 2018;18:227.
20. Zhang H, Wang J. Constituents of the essential oils of garlic and citronella and their vapor-phase inhibition mechanism against *S. aureus. Food Sci Technol Res.* 2019;25(1):65–74.
21. Timung R, Barik CR, Purohit S, Goud VV. Composition and anti-bacterial activity analysis of citronella oil obtained by hydrodistillation: Process optimization study. *Ind Crops Prod.* 2016;94:178–188.
22. Fancello F, Petretto GL, Marceddu S, Venditti T, Pintore G, Zara G, Mannazzu I, Budroni M, Zara S. Antimicrobial activity of gaseous Citrus limon var pompia leaf essential oil against *Listeria monocytogenes* on ricotta salata cheese. *Food Microbiol.* 2020;87:103386.
23. Goni P, Lopez P, Sanchez C, Gomez-Lus R, Becerril R, Nerın C. Antimicrobial activity in the vapour phase of a combination of cinnamon and clove essential oils. *Food Chem.* 2009;116(4):982–989.
24. Bendiabdellah A, Dib MEA, Djabou N, Allali H, Tabti B, Muselli A, Costa J. Biological activities and volatile constituents of *Daucus muricatus* L. from Algeria. *Chem Cent J.* 2012;6(1):48.
25. Tyagi A, Malik A. Antimicrobial potential and chemical composition of *Eucalyptus globulus* oil in liquid and vapour phase against food spoilage micoorganisms. *Food Chem.* 2011a;126(1):228–235.
26. Mohamed NB, Amine FM, Abdelkrim K, Fairouz S, Maamar M. Liquid and vapour phase antibacterial activity of eucalyptus globulus essential oil susceptibility of selected respiratory tract pathogens. *Am J Infect Dis.* 2014;10:105–117.
27. Zhang H, Wang J. Constituents of the essential oils of garlic and citronella and their vapor-phase inhibition mechanism against *S. aureus. Food Sci Technol Res.* 2019;25(1):65–74.
28. Mohamed B, Bouhlali EDT, Sellam K, Ibijbijen J, El Rhaffari L, Nassiri L. Liquid and vapour-phase bioactivity of *Hertia maroccana* (Batt.) Maire essential oil: An endemic Asteraceae from Morocco. *J Appl Pharm Sci.* 2016;6:131–136.
29. Řebíčková K, Bajer T, Šilha D, Houdková M, Ventura K, Bajerová P. Chemical composition and determination of the antibacterial activity of essential oils in liquid and vapor phases extracted from two different Southeast Asian *Herbs-Houttuynia cordata* (Saururaceae) and *Persicaria odorata* (Polygonaceae). *Molecules.* 2020;25(10):E2432.
30. Garzoli S, Turchetti G, Giacomello P, et al. Liquid and vapour phase of lavandin (lavandula×intermedia) essential oil: Chemical composition and antimicrobial activity. *Molecules (Basel, Switzerland).* 2019;24(15):2701.
31. Adam M, Dobias P, Pavlıkova P, Ventura K. Comparison of solid-phase and single-drop microextractions for headspace analysis of herbal essential oils. *Cent Eur J Chem.* 2009;7(3):303–311.
32. Boukhatem MN, Ferhat MA, Kameli A, Saidi F, Kebir HT. Lemon grass (*Cymbopogon citratus*) essential oil as a potent anti-inflammatory and antifungal drugs. *Libyan J Med.* 2014;9:25431.
33. Feyaerts AF, Mathé L, Luyten W. et al. Essential oils and their components are a class of antifungals with potent vapour-phase-mediated anti-Candida activity. *Sci Rep.* 2018;8:3958.
34. Richter J, Schellenberg I. Comparison of different extraction methods for the determination of essential oils and related compounds from aromatic plants and optimization of solid-phase microextraction/gas chromatography. *Anal Bioanal Chem.* 2007;387(6):2207–2217.
35. Tyagi A, Malik A. Antimicrobial potential and chemical composition of Mentha piperita oil in liquid and vapour phase against food spoiling microorganisms. *Food Control.* 2011b;22(11):1707–1714.
36. Ranger C, Reding M, Oliver J, Shultz P, Moyseenko J, Youssef N. Comparative efficacy of plant-derived essential oils for managing ambrosia beetle (Coleoptera: Curculionidae: Scolytinae) and their corresponding mass spectral characterization. *J Econ Entomol.* 2011;104(5):1665–1673.

37. Popovici J, Bertrand C, Bagnarol E, Fernandez M, Comte G. Chemical composition of essential oil and headspace-solid microextracts from fruits of *Myrica gale* L. and antifungal activity. *Nat Prod Res.* 2008;22(12):1024–1032.
38. Liu L, Song G, Hu Y. GC-MS alanysis of the essential oils of *Piper nigrum* L. and *Piper longum* L. *Chromatographia.* 2007;66(9–10):785–790.
39. Sofrata A, Santangelo E, Azeem M, Borg-Karlson AK, Gustafsson A, Putsep K. Benzyl isothiocyanate, a major component from the roots of *Salvadora persica* is highly active against gram-negative bacteria. *PLoS One.* 2011;6(8): e23045.
40. Laghchimi A, Znini M, Majidi L, et al. Liquid and vapour-phase antifungal activities of essential oil of *Salvia aucheri* Boiss. var. mesatlantica Maire. (Endemic from Morocco) against fungi commonly causing deterioration of apple. *Der Pharma Chemica.* 2014;6(1):370–378.
41. Misharina TA, Polshkov AN, Ruchkina EL, Medvedeva IB. Changes in the composition of the essential oil of marjoram during storage. *Appl Biochem Microbiol.* 2003;39:311–316.
42. Misharina TA, Polshkov AN. Antioxidant properties of essential oils: Autoxidation of essential oils from laurel and fennel and of their mixtures with essential oil from coriander. *Appl Biochem Microbiol.* 2005;41:610–618.
43. Pudil F, Wijaya H, Janda V, Volfova J, Valentov H, Pokorn J. Changes in Citrus hystrix oil during autooxidation. *Dev Food Sci.* 1998;40:707–718.
44. Scott RPW. Essential oils. In: Worsfold P, Townshend A, Poole C, editors. *Encyclopedia of Analytical Science*, 2nd ed. Elsevier, Amsterdam, London, New York; 2005: 554–561.
45. Hefendehl FW. Anforderungen an die Zulassungsunterlagen. In: Carle R, editor. *Atherische Öle – Anspruch und Wirklichkeit.* Wissenschaftliche Verlagsgesellschaft, Stuttgart, Germany; 1993:71–83.
46. Cserhati T. *Chromatography of Aroma Compounds and Fragrances.* Springer-Verlag, Berlin, Heidelberg, Germany; 2010:360.
47. Bonnefille M. Electronic nose technology and applications. In: Goodner K, Rouseff R, editors. *Practical Analysis of Flavor and Fragrance Materials.* Wiley, Hoboken, NJ; 2011:111–154.
48. Mahattanatawee K, Rouseff R. Gas chromatography/olfactometry (GC/O). In: Goodner K, Rouseff R, editors. *Practical Analysis of Flavor and Fragrance Materials.* Wiley, Hoboken, NJ; 2011:69–90.
49. Rastogi SC. Analysis of fragrances in cosmetics by gas chromatography-mass spectrometry. *J High Resol Chromatogr.* 1995;18:653–658.
50. Kallen J, Heilbronner E. Das gas-chromatogramm einer labilen Verbindung (system: A –> B). *Helv Chim Acta.* 1960;43:489–500.
51. Hinshaw JV. Nonlinearity in a chromatographic system. *LCGC North Am.* 2002;20:120–126.
52. Bhatia S, Sharma K, Bera T. Structural characterization and pharmaceutical properties of porphyran. *Asian J Pharm.* 2015;9:93–101.
53. Kovar KA, Friess D. Determination of essential oils in mixtures: HPLC in comparison to GC. *Arch Pharm.* 1980;313:416–428.
54. Hagvall L, Backtorp C, Svensson S, Nyman G, Borje A, Karlberg AT. Fragrance compound geraniol forms contact allergens on air exposure. Identification and quantification of oxidation products and effect on skin sensitization. *Chem Res Toxicol.* 2007;20:807–814.
55. Frerot E, Decorzant E. 2004. Quantification of total furocoumarins in citrus' oils by HPLC coupled with UV, fluorescence, and mass detection. *J Agric Food Chem.* 52:6879–6886.
56. Hajimehdipoor H, Shekarchi M, Khanavi M, Adib N, Amri M. A validated high performance liquid chromatography method for the analysis of thymol and carvacrol in *Thymus vulgaris* L. volatile oil. *Pharmacogn Mag.* 2010;6:154–158.
57. da S Rauber C, Guterres SS, Schapoval EES. LC determination of citral in *Cymbopogon citratus* volatile oil. *J Pharmaceut Biomed Anal.* 2005;37:597–601.
58. Porel A, Sanyal Y, Kundu A. Simultaneous HPLC determination of 22 components of essential oils; method robustness with experimental design. *Indian J Pharm Sci.* 2014;76(1):19–30.
59. Patial PK, Cannoo DS. Evaluation of volatile compounds, phenolic acids, antioxidant potential and DFT study of essential oils from different parts of *Araucaria columnaris* (G. Forst.) Hook from India. *Food Chem Toxicol.* 2020;141:111376.
60. Lockwood GB. Techniques for gas chromatography of volatile terpenoids from a range of matrices. *J Chromatogr A.* 2001;936:23–31.
61. Schieberle P, Maier W, Firl J, Grosch W. HRGC separation of hydroperoxides formed during the photosensitized oxidation of (R)-(+)-limonene. *J High Resol Chromatogr Chromatogr Commun.* 1987;10:588–593.
62. Jones BB, Clark BC Jr, Iacobucci GA. Semipreparative high-performance liquid chromatographic separation of a characterized flavor mixture of monoterpenes. *J Chromatogr A.* 1979;178:575–578.
63. Ródenas-Montano J, Carrasco-Correa EJ, Beneito-Cambra M, Ramis-Ramos G, Herrero-Martínez JM. Determination of alcohols in essential oils by liquid chromatography with ultraviolet detection after chromogenic derivatization. *J Chromatogr A.* 2013;1296:157–163.
64. Gaonkar R, Yallappa S, Dhananjaya BL, Hegde G. Development and validation of reverse phase high performance liquid chromatography for citral analysis from essential oils. *J Chromatogr B Analyt Technol Biomed Life Sci.* 2016;1036–1037:50–56.
65. Shah S, Dhanani T, Sharma S, Singh R, Kumar S, Kumar B, Srivastava S, Ghosh S, Kumar R, Juliet S. Development and validation of a reversed phase high performance liquid chromatography-photodiode array detection method for simultaneous identification and quantification of Coumarin, Precocene-I, β-Caryophyllene Oxide, α-Humulene, and β-Caryophyllene in ageratum conyzoides extracts and essential oils from plants. *J AOAC Int.* 2020;103(3): 857–864.
66. Newbery JE, Lopez de Haddad MP, Charlwood KA. High-performance liquid chromatography of terpenoid alcohols in essential oils. *Anal Chim Acta.* 1983;147:387–391.
67. Lafhal S, Bombarda I, Dupuy N, et al. Chiroptical fingerprints to characterize lavender and lavandin essential oils. *J Chromatogr A.* 2020;1610:460568.

68. Benincasa M, Buiarelli F, Cartoni GP, Coccioli F. 1990. Analysis of lemon and bergamot essential oils by HPLC with microbore columns. *Chromatographia*. 30:271–276.
69. Hudaib M, Bellardi MG, Rubies-Autonell C, Fiori J, Cavrini V. Chromatographic (GC-MS, HPLC) and virological evaluations of *Salvia sclarea* infected by BBWV-I. Il Farm 2001;56:219–227.
70. Shen D, Pan MH, Wu QL, Park CH, Juliani HR, Ho CT, Simon JE. A rapid LC/MS/MS method for the analysis of nonvolatile antiinflammatory agents from *Mentha* spp. *J Food Sci.* 2011;76(6):C900–8.
71. Tine Y, Renucci F, Costa J, Wélé A, Paolini J. A method for LC-MS/MS profiling of Coumarins in *Zanthoxylum zanthoxyloides* (Lam.) B. Zepernich and Timler extracts and essential oils. *Molecules.* 2017;22(1):174.
72. Micucci M, Protti M, Aldini R, et al. *Thymus vulgaris* L. essential oil solid formulation: Chemical profile and spasmolytic and antimicrobial effects. *Biomolecules.* 2020;10(6):860.
73. Bhatia S, Sharma K, Dahiya R, Bera T. Plant tissue culture. In: *Modern Applications of Plant Biotechnology in Pharmaceutical Sciences.* Academic Press, Cambridge, MA; 2015:31–107.
74. Bhatia S, Sharma K, Dahiya R, Bera T. Laboratory organization. In: *Modern Applications of Plant Biotechnology in Pharmaceutical Sciences.* Academic Press, Cambridge, MA; 2015:109–120.
75. Bhatia S, Sharma K, Dahiya R, Bera T. Concepts and techniques of plant tissue culture science. In: *Modern Applications of Plant Biotechnology in Pharmaceutical Sciences.* Academic Press, Cambridge, MA; 2015: 121–156.
76. Bhatia S, Sharma K, Dahiya R, Bera T. Application of plant biotechnology. In: *Modern Applications of Plant Biotechnology in Pharmaceutical Sciences.* Academic Press, Cambridge, MA; 2015:157–207.
77. Bhatia S, Sharma K, Dahiya R, Bera T. Somatic embryogenesis and organogenesis. In: *Modern Applications of Plant Biotechnology in Pharmaceutical Sciences.* Academic Press, Cambridge, MA; 2015:209–230.
78. Bhatia S, Sharma K, Dahiya R, Bera T. Classical and non-classical techniques for secondary metabolite production in plant cell culture. In: *Modern Applications of Plant Biotechnology in Pharmaceutical Sciences.* Academic Press, Cambridge, MA; 2015:231–291.
79. Bhatia S, Sharma K, Dahiya R, Bera T. Plant-based biotechnological products with their production host, modes of delivery systems, and stability testing. In: *Modern Applications of Plant Biotechnology in Pharmaceutical Sciences.* Academic Press, Cambridge, MA; 2015: 293–331.
80. Bhatia S, Sharma K, Dahiya R, Bera T. Edible vaccines. In: *Modern Applications of Plant Biotechnology in Pharmaceutical Sciences.* Academic Press, Cambridge, MA; 2015:333–343.
81. Bhatia S, Sharma K, Dahiya R, Bera T. Microenvironmentation in micropropagation. In: *Modern Applications of Plant Biotechnology in Pharmaceutical Sciences.* Academic Press, Cambridge, MA; 2015:345–360.
82. Bhatia S, Sharma K, Dahiya R, Bera T. Micropropagation. In: *Modern Applications of Plant Biotechnology in Pharmaceutical Sciences.* Academic Press, Cambridge, MA; 2015:361–368.
83. Bhatia S, Sharma K, Dahiya R, Bera T. Laws in plant biotechnology. In: *Modern Applications of Plant Biotechnology in Pharmaceutical Sciences.* Academic Press, Cambridge, MA; 2015:369–391.
84. Bhatia S, Sharma K, Dahiya R, Bera T. Technical glitches in micropropagation. In: *Modern Applications of Plant Biotechnology in Pharmaceutical Sciences.* Academic Press, Cambridge, MA; 2015:393–404.
85. Bhatia S, Sharma K, Dahiya R, Bera T. Plant tissue culture-based industries. In: *Modern Applications of Plant Biotechnology in Pharmaceutical Sciences.* Academic Press, Cambridge, MA; 2015:405–417.
86. Bhatia S, Namdeo AG, Nanda S. Factors effecting the gelling and emulsifying properties of a natural polymer. *SRP.* 2010;1(1):86–92.
87. Bhatia S, Sharma A, Sharma K, Kavale M, Chaugule BB, Dhalwal K, Namdeo AG, Mahadik KR. Novel algal polysaccharides from marine source: Porphyran. *Pharmacogn Rev.* 2008:2:271–276.
88. Bhatia S, Sharma K, Nagpal K, Bera T. Investigation of the factors influencing the molecular weight of porphyran and its associated antifungal activity Bioact. *Carb Diet Fiber* 2015;5:153–168.
89. Bhatia S, Kumar V, Sharma K, Nagpal K, Bera T. Significance of algal polymer in designing amphotericin B nanoparticles. *Sci World J.* 2014;2014:564573.
90. Bhatia S, Rathee P, Sharma K, Chaugule BB, Kar N, Bera T. Immuno-modulation effect of sulphated polysaccharide (porphyran) from Porphyra vietnamensis. *Int J Biol Macromol.* 2013;57:50–56.
91. Bhatia S. *Natural Polymer Drug Delivery Systems: Marine Polysaccharides Based Nano-Materials and Its Applications.* Springer International Publishing, Switzerland; 2016:185–225.
92. Bhatia S. *Natural Polymer Drug Delivery Systems: Plant Derived Polymers, Properties, and Modification & Applications.* Springer International Publishing, Switzerland; 2016:119–184.
93. Bhatia S. *Natural Polymer Drug Delivery Systems: Nanotechnology and Its Drug Delivery Applications.* Springer International Publishing, Switzerland; 2016:1–32.
94. Bhatia S. *Natural Polymer Drug Delivery Systems: Nanoparticles Types, Classification, Characterization, Fabrication Methods and Drug Delivery Applications.* Springer International Publishing, Switzerland; 2016:33–93.
95. Bhatia S. *Natural Polymer Drug Delivery Systems: Natural Polymers vs Synthetic Polymer.* Springer International Publishing, Switzerland; 2016:95–118.
96. Bhatia S. *Systems for Drug Delivery: Mammalian Polysaccharides and Its Nanomaterials.* Springer International Publishing, Switzerland; 2016:1–27.
97. Bhatia S. *Systems for Drug Delivery: Microbial Polysaccharides as Advance Nanomaterials.* Springer International Publishing, Switzerland; 2016:29–54.
98. Bhatia S. *Systems for Drug Delivery: Chitosan Based Nanomaterials and Its Applications.* Springer International Publishing, Switzerland; 2016:55–117.

99. Bhatia S. *Systems for Drug Delivery: Advance Polymers and Its Applications.* Springer International Publishing, Switzerland; 2016:119–146.
100. Bhatia S. *Systems for Drug Delivery: Advanced Application of Natural Polysaccharides.* Springer International Publishing, Switzerland; 2016:147–170.
101. Bhatia S. *Systems for Drug Delivery: Modern Polysaccharides and Its Current Advancements.* Springer International Publishing, Switzerland; 2016:171–188.
102. Bhatia S. *Systems for Drug Delivery: Toxicity of Nanodrug Delivery Systems.* Springer International Publishing, Switzerland; 2016:189–197.
103. Bhatia S. *Nanotechnology in Drug Delivery Fundamentals, Design, and Applications: Part 1: Protein and Peptide-Based Drug Delivery Systems.* Apple Academic Press, Palm Bay, FL; 2016:1–204.
104. Bhatia S. *Nanotechnology in Drug Delivery Fundamentals, Design, and Applications: Part 2: Peptide-Mediated Nanoparticle Drug Delivery System.* Apple Academic Press, Palm Bay, FL; 2016:205–280.
105. Bhatia S. *Nanotechnology in Drug Delivery Fundamentals, Design, and Applications: Part 3: CPP and CTP in Drug Delivery and Cell Targeting.* Apple Academic Press, Palm Bay, FL; 2016:309–312.

12

Mechanism of Action of Essential Oils as well as Its Components

Ahmed Al-Harrasi
Natural and Medical Sciences Research Center, University of Nizwa

Saurabh Bhatia
Natural and Medical Sciences Research Center, University of Nizwa
University of Petroleum and Energy Studies

Deepak Kaushik
M. D. University

Mohammed Muqtader Ahmed and Md. Khalid Anwer
Prince Sattam Bin Abdul Aziz University

P.B. Sharma
Amity University Haryana

CONTENTS

12.1 Introduction

Plant systems act as machines and synthesize secondary metabolites from primary metabolites via various biosynthetic pathways. These metabolites perform a wide range of functions; primary metabolites are necessary for cellular processes, whereas secondary metabolites accumulate in a specific tissue of plant to protect them from unfavorable environmental conditions. At the same time, these secondary metabolites do not determine the survival of the plant. Biosynthetic pathways, sequential metabolic reactions that occur in plants, convert primary metabolites such as amino acids, simple sugars, nucleic acids and lipids, and other compounds into complex molecules in the form of secondary metabolites such as alkaloids, glycosides, terpenes, and phenolic compounds. The rate of this multistep biosynthetic reaction increases several folds when plants are exposed to any biotic or abiotic stress. This exposure against stress stimulates cascades of molecular reactions within the plant system to express genes encodes for the synthesis of enzymes involved in these pathways. Therapeutically active secondary metabolites provide more scientific relevance for the use of medicinal plants in traditional medicine. Terpenes belong to the main class of secondary metabolites and have a five-carbon structure of isoprene (2-methylbuta-1,3-diene) units. They are synthesized in the cytosol of plant cells via mevalonic acid pathway. Terpene hydrocarbons are thermally unstable and easily oxidized to form terpenoids. Terpenes and terpenoids are terms that are often used interchangeably; however, they somewhat different meanings. Terpenes are hydrocarbons or naturally occurring substances that are synthesized in the cytosol of plant cells, and during the processing of plant material, these terpenes get oxidized to form terpenoids. As of 2017, there were more than 80,000 phytochemicals identified as being in the family of terpenoids, which also includes steroids and carotenoids. The structural diversity of this vast class of chemical compounds could be correlated with its biosynthetic pathways. These cellular metabolic reactions that take place in aromatic plants are usually catalyzed by enzymes, namely terpenoid synthases. Among these enzymes, enzymes that are responsible for catalyzing cyclization reactions are called terpenoid cyclases. Terpenoids are cyclic and acyclic organic compounds derived from terpenes with multiple cyclic groups and oxygen. Based on the number of isoprene units, the terpenoids are classified as monoterpenoids (C10), sesquiterpenoids (C15), diterpenoids (C20), sesterterpenoids (C25), triterpenoids (C30), and tetraterpenoids (C40). However, more complex organic compounds like polyterpenoids are present in materials such as natural rubber. The terpenoids also contain the class of active volatile chemical compounds responsible for flavor and fragrance of plants. Such plants are called aromatic plants. Apart from their aromatic and flavor properties, these volatile chemical compounds offer a wide range of biological activities. The diversity of terpenoids ranges from volatile monoterpenoids

DOI: 10.1201/9781003175933-14

to volatile triterpenoids. These low-molecular-weight organic compounds with comprehensive biological activities are considered as important constituents of essential oils (EOs) with a common structural isoprene unit (basic building block) among all classes with the molecular formula (C5H8) [1]. These organic compounds are synthesized and secreted from plant systems in the form of EOs by glandular trichomes and other secretory structures to protect the plant from microbial pathogens and to attract pollinators and seed dispersers. However, these potential organic compounds also perform the following set of functions:

- reduction of abiotic stress
- allelopathic effects
- defense against herbivores
- acts as an interplant signaling molecule
- acts as toxic or antifeedant against herbivorous pests

In addition to performing the above functions, these organic compounds synergistically offer deterrent or toxic effects against herbivorous pests. Aromatherapy uses EOs by inhalation or by application over the skin. The mode of administration of EOs influences their biological properties. Terpenoid structures have a vast range of complexity and present a wide range of biological properties. EOs are widely known for their potential therapeutic, neuroprotective, nephroprotective, cardioprotective, immunomodulatory, antinociceptive, anticancer, anti-inflammatory, antimicrobial, antiviral, and antioxidant effects. Due to the presence of volatile components, EOs have been used for centuries in the treatment of respiratory tract infections. These EOs can be inhaled to treat various respiratory ailments. However, more investigations are required to study the biological properties of other EOs or to explore their mechanisms of action.

12.2 Mechanism of Action of EOs

The complex mixtures of EOs contain various chemical components that create unique multicomponent systems that synergize biological effects in a manner that can suppress the growth and multiplication of a wide range of pathogenic microorganisms. This multicomponent system, mainly comprised of monoterpenes, synchronizes with each other to strengthen their antimicrobial effects against pathogens using the different mechanisms of action offered by individual components. As each component of an EO has its own antimicrobial action that could be similar or different from each other, there may be common or specific microbial targets these components act upon [2].

The majority of the investigations focused on the antimicrobial effects of EO components have involved bacteria. Less information is available on the antimicrobial effects of EO components against molds and yeasts. As has been reported, the antimicrobial effects of EOs mainly rely on chemical composition, characteristics (hydrophilic or hydrophobic), and type of microorganism [3]. The hydrophilic or hydrophobic nature facilitates EO components to change the physiological environment of membrane (e.g., membrane potential) and enter a microorganism's cell wall (lipopolysaccharide-peptidoglycan arrangements) and disturb intracellular structures (Figure 12.1). This event leads to the denaturation of certain key proteins as well as cell membrane destruction of bacteria, resulting in an increase in membrane permeability. Changes in membrane permeability further cause disarrangements of intracellular structures to promote cell leakage or lysis and ultimately microbial death. Certain EO constituents can alter proton motive force and ATP level of the microorganism [4,5]. EO components have the ability to increase membrane permeability causing a "disbalance" in bacteria, which can result in the following events (Figure 12.1):

- Reduction in membrane potential with a loss of ions and other metabolites
- Alteration in proton transport
- Change in intracellular ATP level
- Alteration of membrane fatty acids
- Cytoplasm coagulation
- Denaturation of several enzymes and of cellular proteins

However, in eukaryotic cells, EO components decrease mitochondrial membranes potential by affecting various ionic channels, affecting ionic Caþþ cycling, depolarizing mitochondrial membranes, altering proton transport across the membrane, and affecting intracellular ATP level. Since the outer membrane of Gram-negative bacteria is made up of hydrophilic lipopolysaccharides that act as a strong barrier against EO nonpolar components, Gram-negative microbes are generally less vulnerable to the antimicrobial effects of EOs [6]. Due to the presence of a diverse range of volatile (e.g., alcohols, ethers or oxides, aldehydes, ketones, esters, amines, amides, phenols, heterocycles, and mainly the terpenes) EOs possess considerable antimicrobial effects against pathogens [7]. A recent investigation showed that *Etlingera pavieana* EO containing 22 volatile compounds, mainly t- estragole and anethole, showed antimicrobial effects against food-borne microbes, particularly the Gram-positive bacteria (*L. monocytogenes, B. cereus, and S. aureus*) related to ready-to-eat as well as instant food packs and therefore can be utilized as a natural preservative agent in ready-to-eat food products. Additionally, the main chemical components of EOs act on cell membrane to release and destroy intracellular components such as DNA/nucleic acid and protein [8].

Another investigation reported the effects of *Cinnamomum zeylanicum* bark oil as well as its components in reducing oxidative stress, microbial growth, and prevent the growth of malignant cells. (E)-cinnamaldehyde is considered to be a major chemical compound in *Cinnamomum zeylanicum* bark EO. Notably, EO was demonstrated to possess antibacterial effects via disturbing cell membrane and allowing the release of intracellular components. It was concluded that *C. zeylanicum* EO showed considerable antioxidant, antimicrobial, and antiproliferative effects [9,10].

Cinnamomum verum (cinnamon bark) EO containing nine related compounds of trans-cinnamaldehyde has been reported for potent fumigant antibacterial effects. Based on the findings

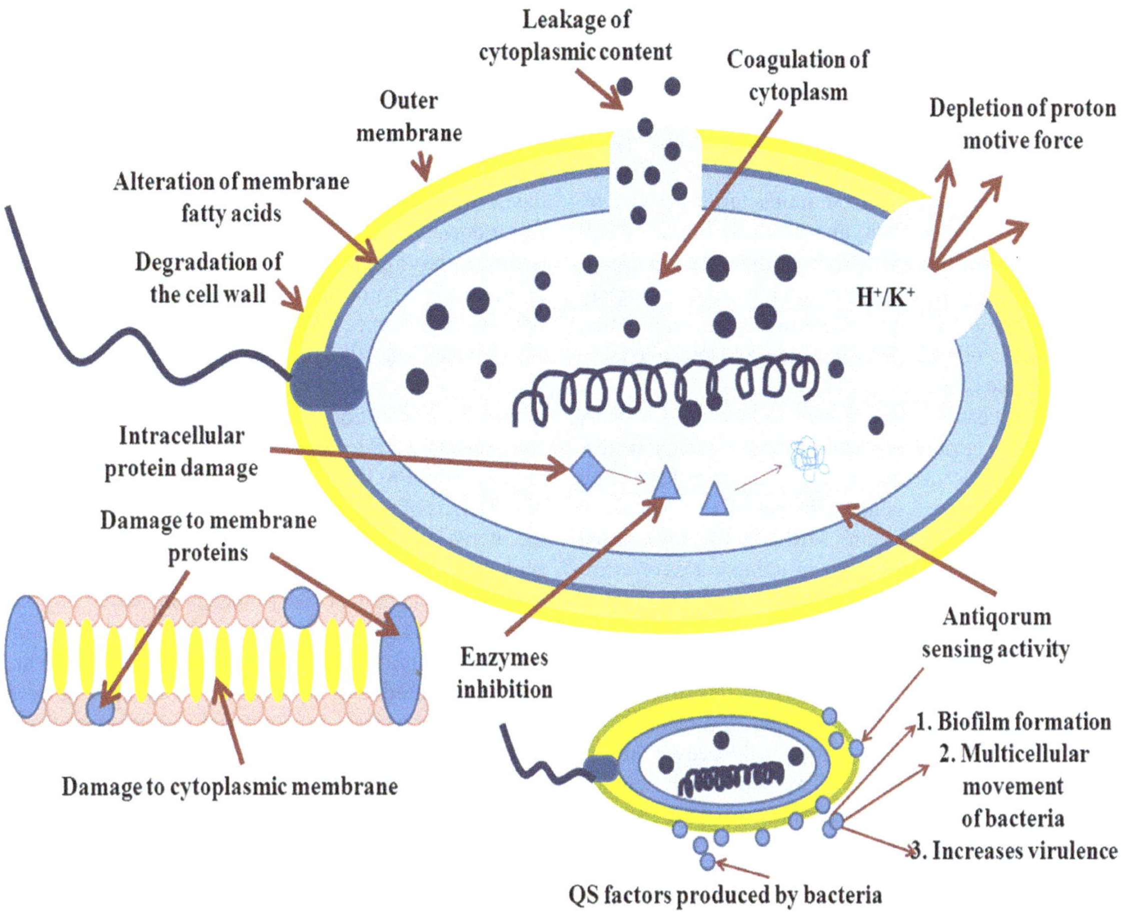

FIGURE 12.1 Antibacterial action of EOs and their components in a bacterial cell.

obtained from intercellular reactive oxygen species production, membrane integrity test, and gene expression, it was concluded that antibacterial activity of salicylaldehyde as well as t-cinnamaldehyde is due to ROS production Additionally, it was revealed that elevated level of ROS impaired the *A. tumefaciens* cell membrane, which caused cell death [11].

The antimicrobial effect of the hydrolate containing traces of *Coridothymus capitatus* EO (enriched with hydrolate and carvacrol) alone and in combination with antimicrobial agents was investigated. It was found that steam-distilled fraction presented a decent antimicrobial effect against different bacterial as well as yeasts strains; with itraconazole, EO demonstrated a synergistic effect against *Candida krusei*, and with tetracycline, showed an additive effect against methicillin-resistant *Staphylococcus aureus* strains. It was also demonstrated that hydrolate altered the membrane permeability of bacteria and yeasts as well as changed mitochondrial function of yeasts [12]. An additional study revealed cellular targets of *Cinnamomum camphora* oil (CCO) containing linalool, camphor, nerolidol, and safrole to possess antibacterial activity against *Escherichia coli*. Findings from this study showed that CCO in vapor phase possessed considerable antibacterial effects at the lowest inhibitory concentration and minimum bactericidal concentration. Vapor-phase CEO treatment of *E. coli* leads to incomplete cell membrane degradation, increase in permeability of the membrane, release of intracellular components, considerable alteration and shrinkage of bacterial cells, and change in bacterial protein structures. Notably, a quantum chemical study revealed that the antibacterial activity of oil is due to the presence of linalool as it contains a reactive center in form of oxygen atom (O10). During antibacterial action, O10 of linalool transferred electrons [13]. The antibacterial potential of *Cinnamomum cassia* oil alone as well as in blend form with several conventional antibiotics against three multidrug-resistant bacterial strains was investigated. It was found that cinnamon oil blend with chloramphenicol or ampicillin showed synergistic effects against *Staphylococcus aureus* and with chloramphenicol also showed synergistic effects against *E. coli* [14].

Antimicrobial and bacterial resistance altering activities of *Nigella sativa* oil and its components (p-cymene, thymoquinone, and carvacrol) against *Listeria monocytogenes* have been investigated recently. Findings showed that *L. monocytogenes* presented considerable sensitivity against *Nigella sativa* oil, carvacrol as well as thymoquinone. A considerable decrease in minimum inhibitory concentrations of ciprofloxacin as well as ethidium bromide has been observed when experimented with in blend form with *N. sativa* oil, reserpine, thymoquinone, and carvacrol. It was also found that oil caused considerable degeneration of membrane integrity, along with an increase in the accumulation of ethidium bromide [15]. Another study based on *N. sativa* demonstrated the bacterial resistance altering as well as antimicrobial effects of *Nigella sativa* oil, p-cymene, thymoquinone, and carvacrol against

MRSA and methicillin-susceptible strains. It was found that all *Staphylococcus aureus* showed high susceptibility against *Nigella sativa* oil as well as its components. Carvacrol as well as p-cymene disturbed membrane integrity of ATCC strain, and all oil components disrupted membrane integrity of MRSA strain [16]. Another study showed that *E. coli* treatment with black pepper EO showed antibacterial activity by causing leakage, disarrangement, and death by breaking cell membrane [17]. Yet another study showed that *Listeria monocytogenes* presented significant sensitivity against *Nigella sativa* oil, carvacrol as well as thymoquinone. In combination with *Nigella sativa* oil, ethylene bromide and ciprofloxacin showed considerable reduction in MIC [18].

Antibacterial mechanisms of various EOs against MRSA (important causative agent of food poisoning and infectious diseases as well as produce several virulence factors) have been demonstrated recently. In this context, the potential of *Amomum villosum* EO has been revealed against MRSA strain. It was found that EO causes cell membrane damage, resulting in loss of membrane integrity and leakage of intracellular components, inhibition of protein, and biofilm synthesis [19]. Additionally, it was found that MRSA treatment with *Amomum villosum* oil showed antibacterial action via metabolome variation. In this study, it was found that EO interrupted TCA cycle, amino acid metabolism, and also prevented ATP and ROS synthesis. Moreover, important enzymes involved in the TCA cycle were inhibited. Elevated ROS proportion might reduce the susceptibility of MRSA against oil, enhancing oil-treated MRSA cell survival. It was concluded that oil triggered metabolic disorder among the microbial strains, resulting in decreased ROS amounts, interference with tricarboxylic acid cycle, suppression of ATP production, and inhibition of important enzymes [20].

A recent investigation showed antimicrobial effect of some commonly used EOs (frankincense, myrtle, thyme, lemon, oregano, and lavender) in aqueous as well as micellar forms against pathogenic bacterial strains (*Staphylococcus aureus, Enterococcus faecalis, Escherichia coli, Klebsiella pneumoniae,* and *Pseudomonas aeruginosa*). The results showed that oregano EO showed up to sixty-four folds low MICs/MBCs in comparison to ethanol, against each microbe. The most vulnerable microbe were the Gram-positive bacteria, such as MRSA, whereas *P. aeruginosa* presented more resistance. Additionally, with several exclusions, micelle suspension of EOs showed the best activity [21].

Another recent investigation showed antifungal effects of thyme oil in affecting growth of *Aspergillus flavus* and aflatoxin B1synthesis, mainly by employing alterations at the molecular level (nuclear condensation, plasma membrane damage, and anti-aflatoxigenic property) causing considerable apoptotic-like cell death [22]. A recent study also suggested that *Cymbopogon khasianus* EO could be possibly considered as safe alternative for the treatment of various pathogenic bacterial strains. This study revealed that concomitant treatment of *Cymbopogon khasianus* EO with streptomycin showed synergistic action in reducing growth of *E. coli* by acting against multiple proteins [23].

In a recent study based on the antibacterial mechanism of limonene against food-borne pathogens, *Listeria monocytogenes* demonstrated that limonene induced the damage to the morphology and integrity of the cell. Limonene treatment increased conductance of the cell wall and the release of intracellular components such as proteins as well as nucleic acids, which established its action on cell membrane permeability. Moreover, limonene treatment also decreases the level of ATP and ATPase action and mitochondrial electron transport chain. This has suggested the role of limonene in delaying ATP production via suppressing the effects of the ATPase as well as respiratory complex. Finally, it was also found that limonene treatment has affected the proteins expression involved in the regulation of respiratory chain, which showed that this oil component can influence energy metabolism and respiratory chain complex activity by suppressing complexes known as respirasomes [24]. Antibacterial effects and its related mechanism of ginger EO containing zingiberene and α-curcumene as main components were recently investigated against *E. coli* and *S. aureus.* SDS-PAGE examination indicated the disappearance of the bands of bacterial proteins bands in electrophoresis with the increase in concentration of ginger EO. Thus, the nucleic acids level in bacterial suspension was increased considerably with a significant decrease in metabolic activity of bacteria. It was concluded that ginger EO mainly acts by disrupting bacterial cell membrane by inhibiting the expression of a number of genes associated with the TCA cycle, metabolism (energy and DNA), and proteins associated with cell membrane [25].

Recently, the inhibitory effects of *Eugenia brejoensis* EO on *Staphylococcus aureus* were investigated. It was found that *Eugenia brejoensis* EO synergistically enhanced the kanamycin, ampicillin, and chloramphenicol effects and suppressed the growth of all *Staphylococcus aureus* strains. Additionally, at sub-inhibitory dose, *Eugenia brejoensis* EO reduced *S. aureus* hemolytic effect and it is potential to survive in human blood as well as significantly decreased the levels of staphyloxanthin [26].

Recently, the antimicrobial activity of citrus oil containing limonene as major compound on an enterotoxin-producing bacteria *Escherichia coli* from pig as well as on *Lactobacillus rhamnosus* was investigated. It was found that commercial citrus EO increased the membrane permeability and disrupted the bacterial cell integrity as shown by the rise in the relative electrical conductance and the release of important cellular components. Noticeably, commercial citrus EO showed more effects against the enterotoxigenic *Escherichia coli* than against *L. rhamnosus*, which was confirmed by electron microscopy. Electron microscopy results indicated considerable morphological damages and disturbances on enterotoxigenic *Escherichia coli* than the *L. rhamnosus* cells [27].

Recently, the antibacterial effect of finger *Citrus medica* EO containing limonene, γ-terpinene, and dodecanoic acid and its action against food-borne microbes have been demonstrated. *In vitro* studies showed moderate antibacterial effects against food-borne microbes. It was found that oil presented better antimicrobial activity against Gram-positive microbes in comparison to Gram-negative bacteria. Further, it was also revealed that with increase in concentration and exposure time, tested microbes were changed and damaged more severely. *Citrus medica* EO treatment also showed a considerable decrease in growth rate, resulting in cell wall damage, release of intracellular component leakage, and, subsequently, death of the cell [28].

Antimicrobial effects of 33 free terpenes usually present in EOs along with the effect on cellular ultrastructure to confirm the likely injury to the membrane of the cell were investigated. Findings from this study showed that only 16 out of 33 components showed antimicrobial effects. Eugenol possessed quick bactericidal effects on *Salmonella enterica* serovar Typhimurium, whereas terpineol presented good bacterial killing effects on *S. aureus* strains. Similarly, geraniol, citronellol, and carveol showed quick bacterial killing activity against *Escherichia coli*. It was found that considerable antimicrobial effects could be associated with the existence of OH groups (alcoholic as well as phenolic compounds), while hydrocarbon presence reduced antimicrobial effects of terpenes such as trans-geraniol, (–)-carveol, carvacrol, and eugenol, and thymol presented considerable antibacterial effects in comparison with sulfanilamide. SEM analysis revealed cellular membrane loss [29].

Another recent investigation showed antibacterial potential of lavender EO alone and in combination with octenidine dihydrochloride (it is an antiseptic that showed bacterial resistance against MRSA strains). Findings demonstrated that lavender EO augmented the octenidine dihydrochloride susceptibility against MRSA strains. Additionally, treatment with octenidine dihydrochloride alone or with lavender EO showed cell wall modifications in MRSA strain [30]. A recent *in vitro* study demonstrated that lemongrass, cinnamon bark, thyme, and oregano EOs showed major zones of inhibition on Gram-positive microbes, while cinnamon bark showed the major diameter on *Pseudomonas aeruginosa*. Cinnamon bark, thyme, and oregano EO showed the major zones of inhibition against Enterobacteriaceae [31]. Another investigation revealed that antimicrobial effects as well as cellular targets of cinnamon oil when used with γ-radiations against *Shewanella putrefaciens*. It was found that γ-radiations enhanced the inhibitory effects on microorganisms of cinnamon EO, and the relative radiation sensitivity of gamma radiation on *S. putrefaciens* was elevated by cinnamon EO. It was found that gamma radiation considerably enhanced the alterations of bacterial morphology, intra-adenosine 5′-triphosphate (intra-ATP) and extra-ATP concentrations, and pH in value of EO-treated *S. putrefaciens*. It was concluded that gamma radiation treatment with cinnamon EO harms the cellular integrity as well as permeability of *S. putrefaciens;* therefore, this type of treatment revealed improved antimicrobial effects in comparison to when they are used alone [32].

Ocimum gratissimum EO containing eugenol with ciprofloxacin and oxacillin showed additive effect for *S. aureus*. Additionally, a considerable decrease in biofilm biomass and cell viability was confirmed for *S. aureus* and *E. coli* [33]. Antimicrobial effects of cuminal containing cumin EO and its cellular targets against *Escherichia coli* and *Listeria innocua* were investigated. Cumin EO showed considerable suppressive effect in β-carotene bleaching assay by neutralizing free radicals. Additionally, cumin EO showed antimicrobial effect in a concentration-dependent manner and triggered a rise in the cellular permeabilization and disruption of membrane integrity [34,35]. The antimicrobial effect of 5-chloroorcylaldehyde containing Allium essential EO extracted via hydrodistillation was assessed on *E. coli, B. cereus, C. albicans S. aureus, B. subtilis, S.pyogenes*, and *P. aeruginosa*. The results obtained from disk diffusion assay revealed that Allium EO considerably inhibited zone diameter in a concentration-dependent manner [36].

A recent study demonstrated chemical composition, antioxidant, anticholinesterase, antimicrobial, and antibiofilm effects of *Anthemis stiparum* EO. GC-MS and GC-FID analysis revealed 72 compounds, whereas germacrene D, t-cadinol, camphor, spathulenol, and isoamyl salicylate were found to be major compounds. In the majority of the assays, methanolic extract showed better activity than *Anthemis stiparum* EO [36]. A previous report showed antibiofilm, antioxidant, and anticholinesterase effects of perillaldehyde, caryophyllene oxide, and β-cadinol containing *Rhanterium suaveolens* EO. The highest antibiofilm effects were reported against *Staphylococcus epidermidis* at 20 μg/mL for EO. However, it was found that EO was not active against acetylcholinesterase and butyrylcholinesterase [37].

The antimicrobial effects of *Carum copticum* EO containing beta-pinene, para cymene, gamma terpinene, and thymol as major compounds have been revealed recently. It was found that EO has been found to be active against the tested microbes especially bacterial as well as yeast strains. Also, EO demonstrated anti-quorum sensing activity against *Chromobacterium violaceum* [38]. Further, antibiofilm effects of *Rosmarinus officinalis* EO (ROEO), containing 8-cineole, camphene, camphor, and β-pinene, have been evaluated recently. EO showed inhibition and bacteria-killing effect against *S.s aureus* and *S. epidermidis*. Moreover, EO showed *S. epidermidis* biofilm inhibition more than 57% at 25 μL/mL, whereas suppression of 67% of the created biofilm was detected at 50 μL/mL of ROEO, while 25 μL/mL separated only 38% of preformed biofilm [39]. Recently, clove, oregano, and garden thyme EOs showed relatively more antimicrobial activity against *Burkholderia cepacia*. It was also found that oils obtained from these plants act at intracellular level by acting on efflux pumps, which can enhance antimicrobial effects [40].

Another report showed antibacterial activity of *Artemisia asiatica* EO containing 1, 8-cineole, para-cymene, piperitone, and (z)-davanone, against respiratory pathogen *Haemophilus influenza*. It was found that EO demonstrated the highest inhibition on growth of *Haemophilus influenzae*. Bacteria treated with the EO resulted in quick reduction in viability of cells. Bacterial culture treated with the EO showed increase in the constituents of the bacterial cells with increase in concentration of EO. Further SEM analysis revealed that bacterial cell treatment with the oil caused cell wall injury, distorted morphology of the cell, and also cause shrinkage to cell [41]. *Taiwania flousiana* EO was recently reported for its algicidal effects, and also has some food applications. The findings suggested that oil extracted from this plant showed antibacterial, antifungal, and anti-algal effects against various microbial strains. SEM analysis showed ultrastructure changes, suggesting main agal cell killing effects by affecting cellular components such as chloroplast as well as cell wall. EO also demonstrated bactericidal as well as antifungal effects on *Rhizoctonia sp., Colletotrichum gloeosporioides, Ralstonia solanacearum*, and *Staphylococcus aureus* [42].

M. leucadendra EO was recently reported on for its capability in inhibiting the growth of microorganisms. Cellular targets of *M. leucadendra* EO is mainly bacteria cell membrane via increasing its permeability. Thus, these recent investigations suggest that EOs and their respective components act in a different manner to possess antimicrobial action by following different pathways. Apart from these mechanisms of action possessed by different EOs, some earlier reports suggested that certain EO components such as carvacrol enhance cell membrane fluidity, resulting in leakage of protons and potassium ions, which can ultimately disrupt membrane potential and suppress ATP production. Other reports suggested antiplasmid effect of a number of EOs or their components (e.g., peppermint EO and menthol evidenced for antiplasmid effect against *E. coli*).

12.3 Nanoparticles vs. Essential Oils (Improved Biological Property) Production by Plants Propagated in in vitro Cultures

EOs contain both volatile as well as non-volatile components; however, the chemical profile of an EO is dependent primarily on the genotype of the plant, environmental factors, age of the plant, and method of extraction of EOs [43–75]. Using plant tissue culture techniques such as elicitation, precursor feeding, metabolic engineering, immobilization, manipulation of plant tissue culture media components, and other techniques, plant chemical composition can be enhanced in such a way that the established culture can represent more yield of chemical compounds than the parent plant. EO produced via this approach could offer a high level of active chemical components that are crucial for biological activity of respective plants. Recently, metallic nanoparticles were used for EO production via *in vitro* culture technique. The investigations by Hatami et al. [43–75] and Ghanati and Bakhtarian [46] demonstrated the use of metal nanoparticles in improving the yield of EOs. These types of approaches can be utilized to improve the yield and enhance the biological activity of EOs [43–75].

REFERENCES

1. Langenheim JH. Higher plant terpenoids: A phytocentric overview of their ecological roles. *J Chem Ecol.* 1994;20(6):1223–1280.
2. Bakkali F, Averbeck S, Averbeck D, Idaomar M. Biological effects of essential oils: A review. *Food Chem Toxicol.* 2008;46:446–475.
3. Reyes-Jurado F, Navarro-Cruz AR, Ochoa-Velasco CE, Palou E, López-Malo A, Ávila-Sosa R. Essential oils in vapor phase as alternative antimicrobials: A review. *Crit Rev Food Sci Nutr.* 2020;60(10):1641–1650.
4. Kalemba D, Kunicka A. Antibacterial and antifungal properties of essential oils. *Curr Med Chem.* 2003;10(10):813–829.
5. Fisher K, Phillips C. Potential antimicrobial uses of essential oils in food: Is citrus the answer? *Trends Food Sci Technol.* 2008;19(3):156–164.
6. Hyldgaard, M, Mygind T, Meyer R. Essential oils in food preservation: Mode of action, synergies, and interactions with food matrix components. *Front Microbiol.* 2012;3(12):12–24.
7. Holley R, Patel D. Improvement in shelf-life and safety of perishable foods by plant essential oils and smoke antimicrobials. *Food Microbiol.* 2005;22(4):273–292.
8. Naksang P, Tongchitpakdee S, Thumanu K, Oruna-Concha MJ, Niranjan K, Rachtanapun C. Assessment of antimicrobial activity, mode of action and volatile compounds of *Etlingera pavieana* essential oil. *Molecules.* 2020;25(14):3245.
9. Alizadeh Behbahani B, Falah F, Lavi Arab F, Vasiee M, Tabatabaee Yazdi F. Chemical composition and antioxidant, antimicrobial, and antiproliferative activities of *Cinnamomum zeylanicum* bark essential oil. *Evid Based Complement Alternat Med.* 2020;2020:5190603.
10. Lee JE, Jung M, Lee SC, Huh MJ, Seo SM, Park IK. Antibacterial mode of action of trans-cinnamaldehyde derived from cinnamon bark (*Cinnamomum verum*) essential oil against *Agrobacterium tumefaciens. Pestic Biochem Physiol.* 2020;165:104546.
11. Lee JE, Jung M, Lee SC, Huh MJ, Seo SM, Park IK. Antibacterial mode of action of trans-cinnamaldehyde derived from cinnamon bark (*Cinnamomum verum*) essential oil against *Agrobacterium tumefaciens. Pestic Biochem Physiol.* 2020;165:104546.
12. Marino A, Nostro A, Mandras N, Roana J, Ginestra G, Miceli N, Taviano MF, Gelmini F, Beretta G, Tullio V. Evaluation of antimicrobial activity of the hydrolate of *Coridothymus capitatus* (L.) Reichenb. fil. (Lamiaceae) alone and in combination with antimicrobial agents. *BMC Complement Med Ther.* 2020;20(1):89.
13. Wu K, Lin Y, Chai X, Duan X, Zhao X, Chun C. Mechanisms of vapor-phase antibacterial action of essential oil from *Cinnamomum camphora* var. linaloofera Fujita against *Escherichia coli. Food Sci Nutr.* 2019;7(8):2546–2555.
14. El Atki Y, Aouam I, El Kamari F, Taroq A, Nayme K, Timinouni M, Lyoussi B, Abdellaoui A. Antibacterial activity of cinnamon essential oils and their synergistic potential with antibiotics. *J Adv Pharm Technol Res.* 2019;10:63–67.
15. Mouwakeh A, Telbisz Á, Spengler G, Mohácsi-Farkas C, Kiskó G. Antibacterial and resistance modifying activities of nigella sativa essential oil and its active compounds against listeria monocytogenes. *In Vivo.* 2018;32(4):737–743.
16. Mouwakeh A, Kincses A, Nové M, Mosolygó T, Mohácsi-Farkas C, Kiskó G, Spengler G. Nigella sativa essential oil and its bioactive compounds as resistance modifiers against *Staphylococcus aureus. Phytother Res.* 2019;33(4):1010–1018.
17. Zhang J, Ye KP, Zhang X, Pan DD, Sun YY, Cao JX. Antibacterial activity and mechanism of action of black pepper essential oil on meat-borne *Escherichia coli. Front Microbiol.* 2017;7:2094.
18. Mouwakeh A, Telbisz Á, Spengler G, Mohácsi-Farkas C, Kiskó G. Antibacterial and resistance modifying activities of nigella sativa essential oil and its active compounds against listeria monocytogenes. *In Vivo.* 2018;32(4):737–743.
19. Tang C, Chen J, Zhang L, Zhang R, Zhang S, Ye S, Zhao Z, Yang D. Exploring the antibacterial mechanism of essential oils by membrane permeability, apoptosis and biofilm formation combination with proteomics analysis against methicillin-resistant *Staphylococcus aureus. Int J Med Microbiol.* 2020;310(5):151435.

20. Tang C, Chen J, Zhou Y, Ding P, He G, Zhang L, Zhao Z, Yang D. Exploring antimicrobial mechanism of essential oil of *Amomum villosum* Lour through metabolomics based on gas chromatography-mass spectrometry in methicillin-resistant *Staphylococcus aureus*. *Microbiol Res.* 2021;242:126608.
21. Man A, Santacroce L, Jacob R, Mare A, Man L. Antimicrobial activity of six essential oils against a group of human pathogens: A comparative study published correction appears in pathogens. *Pathogens.* 2019;8(1):15.
22. Oliveira RC, Carvajal-Moreno M, Correa B, Rojo-Callejas F. Cellular, physiological and molecular approaches to investigate the antifungal and anti-aflatoxigenic effects of thyme essential oil on *Aspergillus flavus*. *Food Chem.* 2020;315:126096.
23. Singh G, Katoch M. Antimicrobial activities and mechanism of action of *Cymbopogon khasianus* (Munro ex Hackel) Bor essential oil. *BMC Complement Med Ther.* 2020;20(1):331.
24. Han Y, Sun Z, Chen W. Antimicrobial susceptibility and antibacterial mechanism of limonene against listeria monocytogenes. *Molecules.* 2019;25(1):33.
25. Wang X, Shen Y, Thakur K, et al. Antibacterial activity and mechanism of ginger essential oil against *Escherichia coli* and *Staphylococcus aureus*. *Molecules.* 2020;25(17):3955.
26. Bezerra Filho CM, da Silva LCN, da Silva MV, et al. Antimicrobial and antivirulence action of *Eugenia brejoensis* essential oil in vitro and in vivo invertebrate models. *Front Microbiol.* 2020;11:424.
27. Ambrosio CMS, Contreras-Castillo CJ, Da Gloria EM. In vitro mechanism of antibacterial action of a citrus essential oil on an enterotoxigenic *Escherichia coli* and *Lactobacillus rhamnosus*. *J Appl Microbiol.* 2020;129(3):541–553.
28. Li ZH, Cai M, Liu YS, Sun PL, Luo SL. Antibacterial activity and mechanisms of essential oil from *Citrus medica* L. var. *Sarcodactylis*. *Molecules.* 2019;24(8):1577.
29. Guimarães AC, Meireles LM, Lemos MF, et al. antibacterial activity of terpenes and terpenoids present in essential oils. *Molecules.* 2019;24(13):2471.
30. Kwiatkowski P, Lopusiewicz L, Kostek M et al. The antibacterial activity of lavender essential oil alone and in combination with octenidine dihydrochloride against MRSA strains. *Molecules (Basel, Switzerland).* 2019;25:95.
31. Patterson JE, McElmeel L, Wiederhold NP. In vitro activity of essential oils against gram-positive and gram-negative clinical isolates, including carbapenem-resistant enterobacteriaceae. *Open Forum Infect Dis.* 2019;6(12):ofz502.
32. Lyu F, Hong YL, Cai JH, et al. Antimicrobial effect and mechanism of cinnamon oil and gamma radiation on *Shewanella putrefaciens*. *J Food Sci Technol.* 2018;55(9):3353–3361.
33. Melo RS, Azevedo AMA, Pereira AMG et al. Chemical composition and antimicrobial effectiveness of *Ocimum gratissimum* L. essential oil against multidrug-resistant isolates of *Staphylococcus aureus* and *Escherichia coli*. *Molecules (Basel, Switzerland)* 2019;24:3864.
34. Alizadeh Behbahani B, Noshad M, Falah F. Cumin essential oil: Phytochemical analysis, antimicrobial activity and investigation of its mechanism of action through scanning electron microscopy. *Microb Pathog.* 2019;136:103716.
35. Alizadeh Behbahani B, Imani Fooladi AA. Evaluation of phytochemical analysis and antimicrobial activities Allium essential oil against the growth of some microbial pathogens. *Microb Pathog.* 2018;114:299–303.
36. Chemsa AE, Zellagui A, Öztürk M, Erol E, Ceylan O, Duru ME, Lahouel M. Chemical composition, antioxidant, anticholinesterase, antimicrobial and antibiofilm activities of essential oil and methanolic extract of *Anthemis stiparum* subsp. sabulicola (Pomel) Oberpr. *Microb Pathog.* 2018;119:233–240.
37. Chemsa AE, Erol E, Öztürk M, Zellagui A, Özgür C, Gherraf N, Duru ME. Chemical constituents of essential oil of endemic Rhanterium suaveolens Desf. growing in Algerian Sahara with antibiofilm, antioxidant and anticholinesterase activities. *Nat Prod Res.* 2016;30(18):2120–2124.
38. Snoussi M, Noumi E, Punchappady-Devasya R, Trabelsi N, Kanekar S, Nazzaro F, Fratianni F, Flamini G, De Feo V, Al-Sieni A. Antioxidant properties and anti-quorum sensing potential of *Carum copticum* essential oil and phenolics against *Chromobacterium violaceum*. *J Food Sci Technol.* 2018;55(8):2824–2832.
39. Jardak M, Elloumi-Mseddi J, Aifa S, Mnif S. Chemical composition, anti-biofilm activity and potential cytotoxic effect on cancer cells of *Rosmarinus officinalis* L. essential oil from Tunisia. *Lipids Health Dis.* 2017;16(1):190.
40. Perrin E, Maggini V, Maida I, Gallo E, Lombardo K, Madarena MP, Buroni S, Scoffone VC, Firenzuoli F, Mengoni A, Fani R. Antimicrobial activity of six essential oils against *Burkholderia cepacia* complex: Insights into mechanism(s) of action. *Future Microbiol.* 2018;13:59–67.
41. Huang J, Qian C, Xu H, Huang Y. Antibacterial activity of *Artemisia asiatica* essential oil against some common respiratory infection causing bacterial strains and its mechanism of action in *Haemophilus influenzae*. *Microb Pathog.* 2018;114:470–475.
42. Liu H, Huang J, Yang S, Li J, Zhou L. Chemical composition, algicidal, antimicrobial, and antioxidant activities of the essential oils of *Taiwania flousiana* Gaussen. *Molecules.* 2020;25(4):967.
43. Bhatia S, Sharma K, Dahiya R, Bera T. Plant tissue culture. In: *Modern Applications of Plant Biotechnology in Pharmaceutical Sciences.* Academic Press, Cambridge, MA; 2015:31–107.
44. Smigielski K, Prusinowska R, Stobiecka A, Kunicka-Styczyñska A, Gruska R. Biological properties and chemical composition of essential oils from flowers and aerial parts of lavender (*Lavandula angustifolia*). *J Essent Oil Bear Pl.* 2018;21:1303–1314.
45. Bhatia S, Sharma K, Dahiya R, Bera T. Laboratory organization. In: *Modern Applications of Plant Biotechnology in Pharmaceutical Sciences.* Academic Press, Cambridge, MA; 2015:109–120.
46. Ghanati, F.; Bakhtiarian, S. Changes of natural compounds of *Artemisia annua* L. by methyl jasmonate and silver nanoparticles. *Adv Envir Biol.* 2013:7:2251–2258.
47. Bhatia S, Sharma K, Dahiya R, Bera T. Concepts and techniques of plant tissue culture science. In: *Modern Applications of Plant Biotechnology in Pharmaceutical Sciences.* Academic Press, Cambridge, MA; 2015:121–156.

48. Wesolowska, A.; Grzeszczuk, M.; Wilas, J.; Kulpa, D. Gas Chromatography-Mass Spectrometry (GC-MS) analysis of indole alkaloids isolated from *Catharanthus roseus* (L.) G. don cultivated conventionally and derived from in vitro cultures. *Not Bot Hort Agrobot Cluj-Napoca.* 2016;44:100–106.
49. Bhatia S, Sharma K, Dahiya R, Bera T. Application of plant biotechnology. In: *Modern Applications of Plant Biotechnology in Pharmaceutical Sciences.* Academic Press, Cambridge, MA; 2015:157–207.
50. Wesolowska A, Grzeszczuk M, Kulpa D. GC-MS analysis of the essential oil from flowers of *Chrysanthemum coronarium* L. propagated conventionally and derived from in vitro cultures. *Acta Chromat.* 2015:27;525–539.
51. Bhatia S, Sharma K, Dahiya R, Bera T. Somatic embryogenesis and organogenesis. In: *Modern Applications of Plant Biotechnology in Pharmaceutical Sciences.* Academic Press, Cambridge, MA; 2015:209–230.
52. Hatami M, Hatamzadeh A, Ghasemnezhad M, Sajidi RH. Variations of the phytochemical compounds in *Rosescented geranium* plant exposed to nanosilver particles. *J Essent Oil Bear Pl.* 2016;19:1747–1753.
53. Bhatia S, Sharma K, Dahiya R, Bera T. Classical and nonclassical techniques for secondary metabolite production in plant cell culture. In: *Modern Applications of Plant Biotechnology in Pharmaceutical Sciences.* Academic Press, Cambridge, MA; 2015:231–291.
54. Bhatia S, Sharma K, Dahiya R, Bera T. Plant-based biotechnological products with their production host, modes of delivery systems, and stability testing. In: *Modern Applications of Plant Biotechnology in Pharmaceutical Sciences.* Academic Press, Cambridge, MA; 2015:293–331.
55. Bhatia S, Sharma K, Dahiya R, Bera T. Edible vaccines. In: *Modern Applications of Plant Biotechnology in Pharmaceutical Sciences.* Academic Press, Cambridge, MA; 2015:333–343.
56. Bhatia S, Sharma K, Dahiya R, Bera T. Microenvironmentation in micropropagation. In: *Modern Applications of Plant Biotechnology in Pharmaceutical Sciences.* Academic Press, Cambridge, MA; 2015:345–360.
57. Bhatia S, Sharma K, Dahiya R, Bera T. Micropropagation. In: *Modern Applications of Plant Biotechnology in Pharmaceutical Sciences.* Academic Press, Cambridge, MA; 2015:361–368.
58. Bhatia S, Sharma K, Dahiya R, Bera T. Laws in plant biotechnology. In: *Modern Applications of Plant Biotechnology in Pharmaceutical Sciences.* Academic Press, Cambridge, MA; 2015:369–391.
59. Bhatia S, Sharma K, Dahiya R, Bera T. Technical glitches in micropropagation. In: *Modern Applications of Plant Biotechnology in Pharmaceutical Sciences.* Academic Press, Cambridge, MA; 2015:393–404.
60. Bhatia S, Sharma K, Dahiya R, Bera T. Plant tissue culture-based industries. In: *Modern Applications of Plant Biotechnology in Pharmaceutical Sciences.* Academic Press, Cambridge, MA; 2015:405–417.
61. Bhatia S. *Natural Polymer Drug Delivery Systems: Marine Polysaccharides Based Nano-Materials and Its Applications.* Springer International Publishing, Switzerland; 2016:185–225.
62. Bhatia S. *Natural Polymer Drug Delivery Systems: Plant Derived Polymers, Properties, and Modification & Applications.* Springer International Publishing, Switzerland; 2016:119–184.
63. Bhatia S. *Natural Polymer Drug Delivery Systems: Nanotechnology and Its Drug Delivery Applications.* Springer International Publishing, Switzerland; 2016:1–32.
64. Bhatia S. *Natural Polymer Drug Delivery Systems: Nanoparticles Types, Classification, Characterization, Fabrication Methods and Drug Delivery Applications.* Springer International Publishing, Switzerland; 2016:33–93.
65. Bhatia S. *Natural Polymer Drug Delivery Systems: Natural Polymers vs Synthetic Polymer.* Springer International Publishing, Switzerland; 2016:95–118.
66. Bhatia S. *Systems for Drug Delivery: Mammalian Polysaccharides and Its Nanomaterials.* Springer International Publishing, Switzerland; 2016:1–27.
67. Bhatia S. *Systems for Drug Delivery: Microbial Polysaccharides as Advance Nanomaterials.* Springer International Publishing, Switzerland; 2016:29–54.
68. Bhatia S. *Systems for Drug Delivery: Chitosan Based Nanomaterials and Its Applications.* Springer International Publishing, Switzerland; 2016:55–117.
69. Bhatia S. *Systems for Drug Delivery: Advance Polymers and Its Applications.* Springer International Publishing, Switzerland; 2016:119–146.
70. Bhatia S. *Systems for Drug Delivery: Advanced Application of Natural Polysaccharides.* Springer International Publishing, Switzerland; 2016:147–170.
71. Bhatia S. *Systems for Drug Delivery: Modern Polysaccharides and Its Current Advancements.* Springer International Publishing, Switzerland; 2016:171–188.
72. Bhatia S. *Systems for Drug Delivery: Toxicity of Nanodrug Delivery Systems.* Springer International Publishing, Switzerland; 2016:189–197.
73. Bhatia S. *Nanotechnology in Drug Delivery Fundamentals, Design, and Applications: Part 1: Protein and peptide-based drug delivery systems.* Apple Academic Press, Palm Bay, FL; 2016:50–204.
74. Bhatia S. *Nanotechnology in Drug Delivery Fundamentals, Design, and Applications: Part 2: Peptide-Mediated Nanoparticle Drug Delivery System.* Apple Academic Press, Palm Bay, FL; 2016:205–280.
75. Bhatia S. *Nanotechnology in Drug Delivery Fundamentals, Design, and Applications: Part 3: CPP and CTP in Drug Delivery and Cell Targeting.* Apple Academic Press, Palm Bay, FL; 2016:309–312.

13

Antimicrobial Activity of Essential Oils in the Vapor Phase

Ahmed Al-Harrasi
Natural and Medical Sciences Research Center, University of Nizwa

Saurabh Bhatia
Natural and Medical Sciences Research Center, University of Nizwa
University of Petroleum and Energy Studies

Tapan Behl
Chitkara University

Deepak Kaushik
M.D. University

Mohammed Muqtader Ahmed and Md. Khalid Anwer
Prince Sattam Bin Abdul Aziz University

P.B. Sharma
Amity University Haryana

CONTENTS

13.1 Introduction

The antimicrobial potential of EOs against various food-borne pathogenic microbes has been widely established. Nevertheless, the antimicrobial effects of the gaseous phase as well as its respective volatile constituents present in EOs have not been studied. The antimicrobial activity of EOs is always determined by its chemical composition. Thus, it is crucial to study the volatility of these compounds and the techniques employed to assess the antimicrobial potential of the components present in gaseous level. This chapter discusses the various approaches to studying the antimicrobial profile of EO components present in the vapor phase.

13.2 Antimicrobial Effects of Essential Oils in the Gaseous Phase

In addition to antimicrobial effects in liquid phase, a number of investigations have evidenced that volatile components produced by oils have significant potential to inhibit the growth of pathogenic microorganisms in comparison with EOs in liquid phase applied by direct contact [1,2]. It has been reported that vapor phase allows free attachment to microorganisms when compared to liquid phase where lipophilic molecules aggregate to form micelles [3]. The antimicrobial potential of EOs in vapor phase has been seen in the case of molds because they grow best on surface, which makes them more

DOI: 10.1201/9781003175933-15

vulnerable to the volatile components of EO [4,5]. As is well known, EOs are mixtures of various chemical components, based on their molecular weight, and each component has different volatility as well as diffusibility, especially when they are released into a non-saturated environment; thus, each component has different stability [6]. Even after attaining different volatility as well as diffusibility, these components still present synergistic or antagonistic interaction with each other or main course medicine in different phases. EOs influence the life cycle of fungi at different phases including germination, hyphae growth, and sporulation. The volatile components of EOs have the ability to inactivate airborne pathogenic conidia that are usually tough to inactivate, when exposed to heat, light, and other chemical compounds [7,8]. The antimicrobial potential of an EO as well as its components is determined by minimum inhibitory concentration (MIC), the minimum concentration of any sample that inhibits microbial growth under standard circumstances (Table 13.1) [9,10]. Additionally, minimum bactericidal concentration (MBC) or minimum fungicidal concentration can be utilized to determine the antimicrobial potential of any sample, which is defined as the minimum dose of any test substance that is bactericidal or kills 99.9% of inoculated microorganisms (i.e., at this concentration no chances of re-growth even after passage into new medium with the same composition (with no test substance)). Furthermore, the antifungal potential of EOs can be examined by determining the capability of EO components to suppress production of fungal spores and toxins (mycotoxin) produced by respective fungal strain [11,12]. Still, MIC is one the most common approaches to determining the antimicrobial potential of EOs; however, the difference between the potential of several EOs cannot be easily determined because often each report is using different units of measurement such as ppm, mg/mL, and g/mL, as well as percentage vol/vol [13,14]. Recently, the antimicrobial properties of EOs as well their components at the gaseous level have been described as MICs in mg per mL of air or ml per L or ll/cm^3 of air [15,16].

13.3 Antibacterial Effects of Essential Oils in Liquid as well as Gaseous Phases

Per the WHO, respiratory tract infections (RTIs) cause significant mortality in both males and females [38]. Furthermore, among all RTIs, pneumonia caused more death mainly among post-neonatal children in 2012 [39]. Various pathogenic microorganisms are responsible for upper/lower RTIs. As per reports available, antibiotic-resistant bacterial strains cause more severe RTIs, mainly *S. pneumoniae, S. mutans,* as well as *S. pyogenes* and the Gram-negative bacteria such as *Moraxella catarrhalis, Haemophilus influenzae,* and *H. parainfluenzae.* RTIs are categorized as acute and chronic respiratory illnesses, which are mainly triggered by bacterial and viral pathogens. For instance, epiglottitis is caused by *H. influenza*; however, this influenza microbe with *M. catarrhalis* as well as *S. pneumoniae* can also cause chronic inflammation of the bronchial tubes [40].

It is well known that lower RTIs are very dangerous infections, and one of the most common examples of this infection is pneumonia, which can easily lead to death. There are different forms of pneumonias: pneumonia acquired outside the hospital (caused by pathogens like *H. influenzae* and *M. catarrhalis*) and nosocomial pneumonia (acquired inside the hospital) (caused by pathogens like *S. pneumonia*) [41]. Apart from their identifications, developing diagnosis tools and main course drugs or lead compounds against these pathogenic microorganisms, it is also important to develop alternative, safe as well as reliable treatments against these pathogenic microorganisms. Among all natural products, EOs are predominantly used to treat various respiratory ailments. However, the antimicrobial effects of EOs are usually investigated via *in vitro* methods, and EOs in liquid form are generally used in such methods in spite of having volatile components in gaseous phase [42]. These in vitro methods involve various parameters, so-called variables such as type of media and its composition, type of microbial strains, and type of procedure used for antimicrobial assessment, and thus findings are always different and comparing such findings is difficult [43]. EO components are lipophilic in nature; consequently, normal microbiological tests must be optimized to this condition (Table 13.1). As EOs contain various volatile compounds, these compounds can pass through the respiratory tract, especially bronchioles, and act directly at the infected site [44].

Thus, it is important to study the potential of EO components in vapor phase to inhibit the growth of pathogenic microbes in the respiratory tract. Various in vitro methods to determine the antimicrobial potential of EO vapors have been evidenced; nevertheless, there is no suitable in vitro vapor-phase method available presently, and also due to the variation between unit of measuring antimicrobial activity/antimicrobial assessment protocol/culture conditions/change in composition of the same EO due to biotic or abiotic factors/change in the type of organism, comparison between findings obtained from each study is very difficult or even not possible [45]. Thus, the antimicrobial effect of EOs might change among various in vitro environments; consequently, the comparable evaluation of this activity in two test systems including liquid medium and vapour phase (VP) must be required to get valuable findings and information for the development of more reliable alternative treatment of RTIs. Agar diffusion and dilution procedures are considered as direct contact tests to determine the antimicrobial potential of EOs in liquid phase due to diffusibility and solubility characteristics of EO components present in liquid phase [46].

In addition, there are many variants such as culture conditions, strains of microorganism, nutrient composition, incubation time, inoculum dose, test sample concentration, type, and quantity of standard compound that determine final results and thus make the study more complicated while comparing results with other studies. Besides this, EOs are lipophilic and highly volatile in nature due to which common antimicrobial screening direct contact assays (disk diffusion, agar absorption) are not suitable for their antimicrobial evaluation. Due to the presence of volatile components in EOs, they can be easily inhaled and are suitable candidates for various respiratory ailments [50]. Among various *in vitro* antimicrobial screening procedures, the vapor-phase test (VPT) has shown the

TABLE 13.1
Antimicrobial Property of EOs and Its Chemical Compounds

Source of EOs/CC	Property	Pathogen	Active CC	Host/Method/Cell	Results	References
Artemisia asiatica	Antibacterial (EO damages cell wall, deforms cell morphology, and shrinks bacterial cells)	*Haemophilus influenzae*	Davanone, 1, 8-cineole, p-menthane monoterpenoid, para-cymene	Disk diffusion method.	Maximum growth inhibition against *Haemophilus influenzae*	[17]
Artemisia capillaris	Antibacterial effect (via causing morphological variations and ions outflow)	*Streptococcus pyogenes, MRSA, MRSA (clinical strain), MGRSA, Streptococcus pneumoniae, Klebsiella pneumoniae, Haemophilus influenzae, and Escherichia coli.*	α-pinene, β-pinene, limonene, 1,8-cineole, piperitone, β-caryophyllene, and capillin 1,8-cineole, alpha pinene, capillin, piperitone, beta-pinene, limonene, and beta-caryophyllene		Most active against MRSA, *Streptococcus pyogenes Klebsiella pneumoniae, Streptococcus pneumoniae, Escherichia coli, Haemophilus influenzae*	[18]
Cinnamon, thyme, and winter savory	Antimicrobial agents (significantly decreased biofilm viability)	*S.suis, A. suis, H. parasuis, A. pleuropneumoniae, P.multocida, B. bronchiseptica,*	Cinnamaldehyde, thymol, and carvacrol	Porcine respiratory infections	Oils showed inhibitory effects against all bacteriawithout any influence on epithelial cells viability	[19]
Coriander EO	Antibacterial against Gram-positive bacteria (combinations of coriander EO/linalool and antibiotics as effective antibacterials)	Gram-positive (methicillin-susceptible and MRSA, S. epidermidis) and Gram-negative bacteria (Pseudomonas aeruginosa, Escherichia coli).	Linalool (70.11%)	MIC method	Synergistic interactions between coriander EO/linalool and antibiotics against MRSA	[20]
Cymbopogon citratus	Antifungal and anti-inflammatory (inhibit the production of pro-inflammatory cytokines and inhibit the production of IL-1β and IL-6)	*Candida albicans*, *C. tropicalis*, and *Aspergillus niger*	Geranial (42.2%) and neral (31.5%)	Ear edema caused by croton oil in rodent	Decreased severe ear edema and showed potential antifungal effects in gassous phase	[21]
Cymbopogon citratus	Anti-asthmatic by reducing the numbers of leukocytes/eosinophils, eosinophil peroxidase, the infiltration of leukocytes in lung tissue	*Bt* (*Blomia tropicalis*) mite extract were administered in rodents	Derivatives of cinnamic acids	A/J mice	Hexane extract modulates allergic asthma by reducing the mucus production, IL-4 level, and NF-κB expression.	[22]
Citral EO	Anti-inflammatory by a significant decrease in TNF-α	*Staphylococcus aureus*	*Citral*	Male mice of BALB/c	Reduced the quantity of microorganisms and showed a significant decrease in TNF-α levels	[23]
E.s citriodora, E. globulus, p eppermint, Origanum syriacum, rosemary oil	To treat upper RTIs	NA		60 indviduals registered in this investigation	Considerable and speedy recovery has been observed	[24]

(*Continued*)

TABLE 13.1 (*Continued*)
Antimicrobial Property of EOs and Its Chemical Compounds

Source of EOs/CC	Property	Pathogen	Active CC	Host/Method/Cell	Results	References
Eucalyptus globulus	Antiviral, anti-inflammatory, antibacterial	*Herpes simplex* virus (antigen types HSV-1 and HSV-2)		Tereticornate A, Cypellocarpin C	Tereticornate (IC_{50}: 0.96 μg/mL) showed the strongest activity in the greater than acyclovir (IC_{50}: 1.92 μg/mL); Cypellocarpin (EC50: 0.73 μg/mL) showed the most potent anti-HSV-2 activity, also more intensive than acyclovir (EC50: 1.75 μg/mL)	[25]
Eucalyptus globulus	Antibacterial and antiviral	*Streptococcus pyogenes, S. pneumoniae, S. agalactiae, Staphylococcus aureus, Haemophilus influenzae, H. parainfluenzae, Klebsiella pneumoniae, Stenotrophomonas maltophilia,* Adenovirus, mumps virus	ND	Vero cells	*H. influenzae, S. maltophilia and H. parainfluenzae* were more sensitive,	[26]
Thyme eucalyptus, tea tree compounds	HSV-1 inhibitory effects via direct inactivation	Herpes simplex virus type 1		Alpha-terpinene, gamma-terpinene, alpha-pinene, p-cymene, terpinen-4-ol, alpha-terpineol, thymol, citral, and 1,8-cineole	Decreased virulence by >96%; the monoterpenoidal components suppressed HSV by about >80%; monoterpene hydrocarbons were slightly superior to monoterpene alcohols in their antiviral activity	[27]
Frankincense, myrtle, thyme, lemon, oregano, lavender EOs	Antibacterial	*Staphylococcus aureus, Enterococcus faecalis, Escherichia coli, Klebsiella pneumoniae,* and *Pseudomonas aeruginosa.*	β-pinene, eucalyptol, limonene, α-pinene, carvacrol, thymol, linalool, linalyl-butyrate	MIC and MBC	Lavender, lemon oregano, and thyme, were found to be more effective, while the myrtle as well as frankincense were the least active. Oregano showed 64 folds decrease MICs/MBCs than ethanol	[28]
Marjoram, clary sage, Anise	Anti-influenza	A/WS/33 virus	Linalool was a common constituent	Madin-Darby canine kidney (MDCK) cells	Anti-influenza A/WS/33 virus activity of >52.8%	[29]
Monarda Punctata EO	Antibacterial (ROS substantially rised in *S. pyogenes* which eventually trigger injury to the membrane)	*H.influenzae, E.coli, S. pneumoniae, S. pyogenes, and* MRSA	Thymol (75.2%), p-cymene (6.7%), limonene (5.4%)	MIC and MBC method	*E. coli, S. pyogenes,* and *S.pneumoniae* were the most vulnerable, and MRSA was the most resistant strain	[30]

(*Continued*)

TABLE 13.1 (*Continued*)

Antimicrobial Property of EOs and Its Chemical Compounds

Source of EOs/CC	Property	Pathogen	Active CC	Host/Method/Cell	Results	References
Ocimum basilicum L. (sweet basil)	Antimicrobial activity (EO could cause the leakage of intracellular ATP and potassium ions leading to cell death)	Gram-positive, Gram-negative bacteria, and fungi	Methyl chavicol, Methyl eugenol		*S. aureus*, *B. subtilis*, *A. fumigatus*, *S. faecalis*, *S. epidermidis*, *P. chrysogenum*, and *A. niger* were found to be more susceptible to the oil *S. faecalis*, *S. epidermidis*, *S. aureus*, *P. chrysogenum*, *B. subtilis*, *A. niger* *A. fumigatus* showed more susceptibility to the oil	[31]
On Guard™	Antiviral	Influenza virus, A/PR8/34 (PR8)	ND	MDCK cells	Viral particles released from MDCK cells were reduced and decreased direct infection of the cells; inhibit viral NP and NS1 protein, but not mRNA expression	[32]
Different EOs	Antibacterial	*S. pyogenes*, *S. agalactiae*, *S. pneumoniae*, *K. pneumoniae*, *S. aureus*, *S. maltophilia*, *H.influenzae*,		Kirby-Bauer paper method, MIC and MBC, cytotoxicity on Vero cells	Thyme as well as cinnamon demonstrated the most potent activity	[33]
Red thyme, common thyme, oregano, and cinnamon	Antimicrobial activity(cinnamon did not show vapor activity, whereas thyme and oregano showed great vapor activity)	20 strains of Streptococcus suis (porcine respiratory infections); EOs were active against including Salmonella, E. coli, S. aureus, as well as various strains of Streptococcus	ND	Disk diffusion test	Considerable effects against Gram-positive and Gram-negative bacterial strains	[34]
Thyme, clove, cinnamon bark	Antibacterial activity	Streptococcus pneumoniae, S. mutans, S. pyogenes, Haemophilus influenzae, H. parainfluenzae, and Moraxella catarrhalis.	Trans-cinnamaldehyde (45.9%), thymol (46.1%), eugenol (66.9%)	Sheep blood agar or chocolate agar	Promising activity against pathogens either in liquid medium or in vapor phase; however, effect is lower than that of the reference antibiotics	[35]
Trachyspermum Ammi EO with conventional antibiotics	Antibacterial against respiratory pathogens	*S.pneumoniae, P. aeruginosa, and S. aureus*	Thymol gamma-terpinene=and para-cymene	MIC method	*S. pneumoniae* showed more sensitivity against ajowan EO, amoxicillin and ciprofloxacin in combination with EO and thymol is effective against these bacteria	[36]
β-santalol	Anti-influenza by the inhibition of viral mRNA synthesis	Influenza A/HK (H3N2) virus that causes influenza (flu)	β-santalol	MDCK cells	Anti-influenza A/HK (H3N2) virus effects without causing any toxicity at cellular level	[37]

antimicrobial effects of volatile components present in vapor phase of EOs. The VPT method involves a disk of the paper impregnated with EO, which is positioned over the inner side of the top lid of a petri dish. During the RTIs, vapors of EOs are passed through airway, which allows EO components to directly interact with infected surface. Thus, it is important to study the antimicrobial properties of EOs in the vapor phase. As the behavior or physical-chemical properties of EO components may change during their transition from liquid phase to vapor phase, it is very important to assess antimicrobial effects in both phases (liquid as well as gaseous phase) such as the assessment of different EOs in in vitro broth macrodilution test and VPT against pathogens. In diffusion methods, the components present in EOs are partitioned through the agar based on their affinity with water, whereas in dilution assays, the hydrophobic nature of EOs has to be overcome by treatment with either emulsifiers or solvents including Tween 80, DMSO, and ethanol. However, this type of treatment may affect the property of EOs. Moreover, various efforts have been made to use the volatile property of EOs, and consequently, a high level of inhibition by EO volatile components in vapor phase has been revealed. Two procedures are often used in VPT. The first procedure is the earlier method in which EO infused paper disk is positioned over the top (inner side) of the petri dish. This procedure has some drawbacks; for example, to express MIC, several researchers divided the dose of EO by volume of the air in the petri dish, which is not correct. EOs are a complex mixture of various volatile components that remain stable in liquid phase; however, each compound has a different level of vapor pressure (i.e., volatility), and when this combination is subjected to non-saturated atmosphere, volatile components attain volatility at different rates, until the point at which the environment becomes saturated with volatiles in the closed environment. Thus, it has been concluded that if an EO is impregnated on a small area such as over paper disk, the zone of inhibition resulting from this would not only represent its antimicrobial property; nevertheless, it also mainly depend on the rate of evaporation of its active components or its vapour phase. Moreover, during the testing of more than one EO, there is always a risk of interference when assessing several EOs on one petri dish. Thus, it is always recommended to use one EO at one concentration per petri dish. Another method is based on the placement of EO as well as microorganisms separately in sealed conditions or facility such as box or jar, with the capacity typically more than one liter. This method has major disadvantages such as with a greater number of samples (EOs) and their testing with different microorganisms always require more amount of EO. Also, standardization of the "box" must be done for every test, which could be challenging. VPT involves a disk of paper that impregnated with EO and positioned over the inner side of the upper cap, whereas the lower lid comprises nutrient medium inoculated with test microbes at a specific inoculum size cfu/mL, which is smeared on the media surface. To avoid leakage of the vapor, the upper lid is prepared last and immediately placed on top of the lower lid. Further, the petri plate is sealed immediately by using semi-transparent and flexible parafilm to avoid any vapor outflow. Once incubated for a certain time period, growth of the microorganisms over the agar medium can be noted to show the antimicrobial activity of the EO. However this technique failed to provide accurate MIC as only a small number of studies estimated the MIC in vapor phase, called MICair. MICair can be estimated in a controlled environment by using airtight containers [46]. Another procedure called inverted plate technique is commonly used in a number of studies, but an airtight container of 1 L volume is often used to improve the vapor intensity of EOs [46].

In 2011, a new modification of disk diffusion method was used involving a four-sectioned petri dish, which offers a more consistent headspace and decreases costs since only 36 petri dishes are needed to assess one oil vapor against 6 microbial strains microorganisms at 6 concentrations in comparison to 108 petri plates used in the disk volatilization procedure. A previous study gave an outline of various antimicrobial screening methods such as airtight box, disk volatilization, divided petri dish, inverted petri dish, and vapor agar contact utilized for the evaluation of the antimicrobial property of oils via gaseous contact procedure [47]. In addition, various parameters such as chemical composition of EO, concentration of EO in VP, evaporation speed of EO, exposure time, growth phase, incubation temperature, and location of microorganism tested, stability of EO, and volatility influence the efficiency of vapor activity of EOs. As discussed above, disk volatilization, a modification of the disk diffusion method, is used for antibiotic susceptibility testing [48,49], and agar vapor methods are frequently used to determine the antimicrobial activity of vapor phase of EOs.

A previous report also demonstrated that due to their antimicrobial potential under optimized conditions, oil might be potentially utilized to disinfect air, mainly to prevent as well as control RTIs. However, only a small number of studies are available in which respiratory pathogenic microorganism pathogens were examined under *in vivo* conditions. In spite of calculating MIC, minimum inhibitory dose (MID) is determined. MID is the lowest vapor concertation to suppress the microbial growth. MID-based assays are usually performed in a closed environment such as sealed container where a sufficient quantity of oil can be put either on the box surface (to cause gentle vaporization) or on a paper disk (rapid vaporization) [50–52]. Several researchers have determined MID by calculating the ratio of the oil dose and air volume in the petri dish, which is comparatively incorrect as EOs contain components with different volatilities. A recent investigation showed that major compounds such as linalool and linalyl acetate, 1,8-cineole, and terpinen-4-ol and minor compounds such as lavandulyl acetate and borneol of lavandin (Lavandula × intermedia) EO maintain the same proportion in both liquid and vapor phases [50–52]. However, EO obtained from Montenegrin *Helichrysum italicum* showed different compositions in liquid phase as well as gaseous phase when analyzed by GC-MS spectrometry study in both liquid and vapor phases. It was found that liquid phase showed the majority of sesquiterpenes with β-eudesmene (21.65%) as well as β-bisabolene (19.90%) and monoterpene fraction [α-pinene (16.90%) and neryl acetate (10.66%)]. However, vapor phase showed mainly monoterpenes with α-pinene (78.76%) [53]. A recent report also demonstrated that EOs derived from *Houttuynia cordata* and *Persicaria odorata* showed similar antimicrobial potential in both vapor and liquid phases at least in the case of one bacterium [54].

Another recent investigation also demonstrated that tea tree oil (TTO) demonstrated strong bactericidal effects against *Staphylococcus aureus*, *Escherichia coli*, *methicillin-resistant S. aureus*, extended-spectrum beta-lactamases producer carbapenem-sensitive Klebsiella pneumonia, carbapenem-resistant *K. pneumonia*, *Acinetobacter baumannii*, *and Pseudomonas aeruginosa*. TTO when blended with other pure antibiotics demonstrated high synergetic effects, especially with oxacillin against methicillin-resistant *Staphylococcus aureus*. The vapor phase test demonstrated strong antimicrobial effects of TTO against *Acinetobacter baumannii* [55].

Volatile components such as thymol as well as carvacrol in liquid phase have been widely reported for their antimicrobial effects alone as well as in blend form with other agents. Nevertheless, standardized method has been established to test its antimicrobial efficacy in vapor phase. Recently, a different broth volatilization chequerboard procedure for assessing the carvacrol/thymol blend and to evaluate antimicrobial effects of oil constituents in both vapor and liquid phases against 12 *Staphylococcus* strains was established. Chequerboard as well as volatilization assays help in the determination of fractional inhibitory concentrations (FICs) (drug in combination divided by the MIC of drug acting alone). FIC is used to determine the interaction between EOs, which could be synergistic, antagonistic, addition, or indifferent. It was concluded that thymol/carvacrol blend showed an additive antimicrobial response against the microorganisms examined. ΣFIC values were found to be <0.6, which represents strong additive interaction. Thus, evaluation as well as assessment of FIC and MIC of test samples in liquid as well as solid media can be used as potential ways for antimicrobial assessment of volatile components at the same time in both vapor and liquid forms [56].

A recent investigation showed that *Artemisia annua* EO in vapor phase represented monoterpene composition of more than 98% of the constituents (α-pinene, 1,8-cineole, and camphene). Additionally, *A. annua* EO in both vapor and liquid phases indicated strong antimicrobial activity toward almost the tested 20 strains of Malassezia (responsible for skin complications in humans and animals). It was found that the MICs obtained by vapor diffusion assay were to be lesser than those found by the liquid technique [57].

Another recent investigation demonstrated that culture conditions like temperature, pH, shaking of cultures, presence of water, or other EO compounds affect antimicrobial activity. Phenolic EO components thymol, menthol, hinokitiol and carvacrol were recently assessed against oral pathogenic microorganisms. It was found that phenolic components present in oil were constant at diverse temperature range; however, at high temperature (>80°C) the effects of thymol reduced, in liquid phase the blend of thymol/carvacrol did not show any synergistic response, the activity of carvacrol and thymol (in vapor phase) were suppressed in water, there was an increase in activity of menthol, and hinokitiol was observed when culture was shaken continuously at different pH as well as temperatures conditions. Hinokitiol when used in liquid and gaseous phases showed stability at various pH and temperatures environmental conditions [58].

A previous investigation demonstrated that the chemical nature of EO determines MID (mg/L in air); for example, thyme (wild/red/geraniol type), cinnamon bark, and lemongrass EOs in gaseous state demonstrated low MID values followed by oils comprising terpene alcohols against *S. aureus*, *H. influenzae*, *S. pyogenes and S. pneumoniae*. Esters (linalyl acetate as well as geranyl) possessed less effects against *S. aureus*, whereas EOs rich in ketone, ether, and hydrocarbon showed high MIDs. Additionally, the antibacterial potential of oils was higher at greater concentration of vapor with little time of exposure. It has also been found that among all EO components studied, cinnamaldehyde and thymol demonstrated the strong effects, followed by other components while linalool, menthol, as well as terpinen-4-ol, demonstrated mild action [1].

Another study based on vapor diffusion and direct contact tests showed the application of a special machine (ST ProTM) to disperse BioScent™ (mixture of vapors of geranium and lemongrass) in a sealed box environment to further test its antimicrobial potential against *Enterococci* strain (resistant to vancomycin) and *S. aureus* strain (resistant to methicillin) [46]. It was found that 20 hours of exposure to BioScent™ vapor reduced the growth of methicillin-resistant *S. aureus* by 38%. It was also found that after 15 hours' exposure, geranium/lemongrass oils showed 89% reduction of airborne bacteria in an office environment, suggesting that this combination can be used as a potential air disinfectant. Another study suggested the airborne anti-tuberculosis potential of Eucalyptus citriodora EO (containing 32 compounds such as β-eudesmol, isopulegol, spatulenol, linalool, α-terpineol, and citronellol) [46] using the most robust technique, biochemometrics (3D rational methodologies including countercurrent chromatography fractionation) along with gas chromatography–mass spectrometry to measure biological effects and to analyze chemometric. Further, an artificial mixture-based procedure was employed to reveal the chemical interaction among oil constituents. It was found that citronellal alone showed weak activity while in combination with citronellol and eucalyptol it demonstrated anti-tuberculosis effects. Thus, it has been observed that it's very important to study different types of interactions between oil components such as synergistic, additive, antagonistic and agonistic in an order to determine its effects on therapeutic properties [46]. The multiple components in EOs form a stable environment by interacting with each other to create the biological activity.

The antimicrobial potential of EOs is widely known as several EOs have shown strong antimicrobial effects in liquid phase under in vitro conditions; however, a greater amount of oils are needed to show a similar response in food systems [59,60].

As mentioned earlier, EOs are comprised of multiple component systems, mainly volatilities with significant antimicrobial effects [59]. Recent studies have revealed that these oils at gaseous phase have high antimicrobial effects in comparison to liquid phases such as thyme, fennel, and lavender EOs [52], *Eucalyptus globulus* EO [52], *Melaleuca alternifolia* EO [52], and lemongrass EO [52]. Because of the lipophilic nature of EO components in the aqueous phase, these lipophilic components self-associate to promote micellization and subsequently prevent the interaction of oil components with microorganism, while EOs in vapor phase interact directly with organisms, which allows free attachment [52]. However, there are only a few reports available on the potential of EOs in vapor phase, mainly because of the challenges related to the non-availability of suitable standardized procedures for antimicrobial assessment.

EOs have been utilized since ancient times via inhalation; however, now various researchers are exploring scientific evidence that support their role in different ailments, especially RTIs caused by different bacterial strains [43].

Conventional antibacterial methods are not designed to assess the antimicrobial potential in vapor phase as they mainly emphasize the effects of oils via direct contact. Presently, major emphasis has been given on VPT and its further modifications, mainly to evaluate the effect of vapors produced by EO or the activity of volatile compounds in gaseous phase so that their actual antimicrobial potential in gaseous phase can be examined [61]. It has been reported that VPT-based antimicrobial assessment can be done by using other pathogens, including fungi and viruses [62,63]. Based on the previous findings related to microbiological assessment of citronella thyme, clove, peppermint, and cinnamon bark EOs, it was found that these oils present effective antimicrobial effects in two phases (liquid and vapor). As per the previous findings during vapor pressure test of EOs, Gram-positive pathogens were less sensitive to treatment with oil than Gram-negative microbes. This multicomponent system can be utilized to offer better effects against bacterial resistance; nevertheless, at the same time, it creates challenges in their standardization, antimicrobial assessment, and when comparing their effects with other EOs [63,64].

Cinnamon bark EO in liquid form was found to be more effective against *S. pneumoniae*, whereas thyme EO displayed the strongest activity against *S. mutans*. Additionally, clove EO was found to be effective against *S. pyogenes* [65].

Another study suggested that eucalyptus fruit EO was more active against *S. pyogenes*. The antimicrobial potential of *Eucalyptus globulus* EO against various isolates of *Streptococcus pyogenes, S. pneumoniae, S. agalactiae, Staphylococcus aureus, Haemophilus influenzae, H. parainfluenzae, Klebsiella pneumoniae, Stenotrophomonas maltophilia* and two viruses, mumps as well as adenovirus strains, received from affected individuals suffering from RTIs was studied. The antibacterial potential of EOs was determined by the disk diffusion procedure, MIC, and MBC. It was found that *S. maltophilia, H. influenzae,* and parainfluenzae were highly vulnerable, followed by *S. pneumoniae.* Viral inhibitory assays findings demonstrated mild effects of EO against mumps virus when tested by plaque reduction neutralization methods (for mumps virus) and end-point dilution (for adenovirus) [65].

Another recent investigation also showed that oil-in-water emulsions prepared with 2% eucalyptus leaves hydroalcoholic extract suppressed A/H1N1 virus (the swine flu) replication completely when the cells were infected by 100 CCID50 as well as reduced HA titer up to four-fold [66,67].

Another study showed that out of all tested EOs, cinnamon bark EOs presented more significant results against all the investigated pathogens (*Pseudomonas aeruginosa* as well as *MRSA*) in the in vitro vapor phase assay; however, in liquid medium, clove EO showed the best inhibition against *MRSA*. Thyme EO also presented antibacterial effects against *MRSA* and the antibiotic-sensitive strain of *P. aeruginosa* in both methods. Peppermint EO at high concentration was found to be effective only in vapor form; however, eucalyptus EO was found to be more effective in liquid medium. Unexpectedly, it was reported by the authors that Scots pine did not show any antimicrobial effect. The authors also concluded that due to the multiple component systems as well as complex mode of action, EOs could be the best solution for the problem of antibiotic resistance but more in vivo investigations are essential to determine the actual safe dose of oils among individual patients [68].

TLC-direct bioautography is a potential technique for rapid chemical and biological screening of natural products [69]. Recently, direct bioautography coupled with TLChas been used as a tool for the identification of oil components with antimicrobial effects. In this context, antimicrobial as well as and antibiofilm effects of different oils as well as their principal constituents against *H. parainfluenzae* as well as *H.s influenzae* were evaluated. Further to increase the solubility of lipophilic components, stable O/W nanopickering emulsions were prepared by using silica-based nanoparticles and EOs. Findings obtained from this study demonstrated that *H. parainfluenzae* is less sensitive to oil than *H. influenzae* (except for cinnamon bark EO). Findings obtained from direct TLC bioautographic detection demonstrated that thyme EO (ethanolic solutions) showed considerable effects against *H. influenzae,* whereas cinnamon EO was found to be more effective against *H. parainfluenzae.* Further, prepared formulation of cinnamon EO effectively suppressed the formation of biofilm by *H. parainfluenzae* in comparison with Tween80 surfactant or absolute ethanol [69].

Similarly, TLC combined with direct bioautographic and DPPH test and *Bacillus subtilis* were used to assess the antibacterial potential of constituents of thyme, cinnamon bark, clove, and rosemary EOs. Later on, by using solid-phase microextraction-gas chromatography-mass spectrometry, seven antibacterial compounds were identified, borneol, eugenol, thymol, cinnamaldehyde, 1,8-cineole, camphor, and α-terpineol, out of which only thymol and eugenol showed a free radical scavenging effect [70].

Recently, the antibacterial effects of oils obtained from *Satureja hortensis* as well as *Thymus daenensis* over the growth of plankton and their capability to form biofilm were studied. Also, the effects of oils over QS of some *S. aureus* were examined. Oils showed considerable inhibition over formation of biofilm and disrupt membranes. It was also found that *Satureja hortensis* EO considerably decreased the expression of hld gene. [71]. Recent reports also showed the significant role played by various EOs such as *Artemisia asiatica* EO against *Haemophilus influenza; Artemisia capillaris* against RTI-causing pathogens *Blumea balsamifera* EO against *Haemophilus parasuis* (Gram-negative organism that colonizes the upper respiratory tract of pigs); clove EO against *Streptococcus iniae, Sardinian Santolina Corsica* EO; nisin and cinnamon, thyme and winter savory against porcine respiratory bacterial pathogens (*Streptococcus suis, Actinobacillus pleuropneumoniae, Actinobacillus suis, Bordetella bronchiseptica, Haemophilus parasuis,* and *Pasteurella multocida*); ajowan EO against S. pneumonia; ajowan EO/thymol and amoxicillin combinations against methicillin-resistant *Staph. aureus;* ajowan EO and ciprofloxacin against *P. aeruginosa, S. aureus* and penicillin (P)-resistant *S. pneumonia; Thymus sipyleus* EO against *S. aureus, Streptococcus pyogenes,* and

Moraxella catarrhalis; Psidium guineense EO Mycobacterium tuberculosis, Allophylus edulis against *Mycobacterium tuberculosis*; thyme EO against *H. influenzae;* and *cinnamon* EO *against H. parainfluenzae* [72].

Recently, anti-inflammatory, antioxidant, and anti-mycobacterial effects of the EO and viridiflorol, the main compound of *Allophylus edulis* EO, were investigated. It was found that EO and viridiflorol showed moderate in vitro activity in the *M. tuberculosis* assay and also presented moderate antioxidant activity compared with reference standards. Both EO and viridiflorol after oral administration showed significant anti-inflammatory effects by inhibiting carrageenan-induced mice paw edema [73].

In addition to antimicrobial effects, especially antibacterial effects, EO-based multicomponent systems offer antioxidant, vasodilatory, and anti-inflammatory effects, which are beneficial for treating various ailments of lungs. Thyme, cinnamon, and lemongrass (Ceylon-type) oils have been extensively utilized for various respiratory ailments. Nevertheless, the mechanism involved in anti-inflammatory effects is not yet clear. Thus, the chemical composition, anti-inflammatory effects along with the mechanism of action of abovementioned EOs were investigated recently in the respiratory performance and acute pneumonitis in rodents. It was found that the abovementioned EOs contain thymol, cinnamaldehyde, and citronellal, respectively. Results showed that thyme and cinnamon EOs attenuated inflammatory airway hyperresponsiveness as well as some cell-based inflammatory processes. Thus, EOs might be used as alternative treatments for various respiratory inflammatory disorders. However, lemongrass (ceylon-type) EO treatment showed irritation (e.g., augmented airway hyperresponsiveness and myeloperoxidase effects) over the inflamed airways and thus would not be recommended [74].

13.4 Antimicrobial Potential of Essential Oil-Based Nanoemulsions

There is an emerging requirement for eco-friendly, safe, effective, as well as reliable approaches to treat various respiratory ailments. One of the natural product classes that have been identified in this context is EOs, which are natural alternatives for replacing synthetic antimicrobials used to treat various respiratory infections. EOs are known for their various biological effects, and their implications in treating various respiratory infections are growing these days. However, due to considerable disadvantages such as low solubility, low bioavailability, low permeability, uncontrolled volatility, and low long-term stability, their utilization is restricted. These limitations can be overcome by the development of stable formulations to encapsulate EOs in the form of nanocapsules, nanoemulsions, etc. There are a number of reports based on the encapsulation of EOs in the form of nanoemulsions by using emulsifier, surfactant, nanocarrier, etc., ultimately to increase solubility, stability, surface area, and overall efficiency of EOs (Table 13.2). Using this approach, EOs can be delivered and encapsulated into nanosized micelles with sizes ranging from 20 to 200 nm (Table 13.2). There are a number of procedures that have been utilized to prepare EOs-based nanoemulsions such as high-pressure homogenization, microfluidizers, ultrasonic homogenization, phase inversion composition, and phase inversion temperature. Nanoemulsion is considered as a reliable approach to encapsulating EOs or their components; however, it still must be optimized to get more fruitful results. Moreover, tools for the characterization of nanoemulsion formulations such as dynamic light scattering, zeta potential, microscopy, and X-ray diffraction have been widely reported. Furthermore, types of nanocarrier (e.g., chitosan), surfactant [nonionic (Tween, polysorbate 80) and ionic surfactants such as cationic surfactant (lauric arginate) and anionic (surfactant lysolecithin) cosurfactant (lecithin)], emulsifiers, and oil phase must be selected and optimized. Additionally, EOs are also encapsulated to mask unpleasant characteristics of oils and enhance biological effects. One of the major objectives of nanoemulsions is a decrease in the size of the of droplets present in emulsions to increase the availability of EO constituents in order to improve the biological effects such as antibacterial, antioxidant, and anti-inflammatory agents at the site of action [75]. Moreover, decrease in the size of the particles improves the physical properties such as physical as well as mechanical features of films [75]. As mentioned above, ultrasound, high-pressure homogenization as well as high-speed mixing are usually employed to create nanoemulsion particle size >200 nm [75]. As per a recent report, one of the most reliable approaches for the preparation of nanoemulsion is ultrasonic emulsification, which involves two mechanisms [75]. Sound wave application generates mechanical vibration and acoustic cavitation. The acoustic and shock waves create high pressure and turbulence, which collapse the droplets. At high frequency (mega Hz), nanoemulsions can even be prepared without using an emulsifier.

The first approach involves the application of acoustic field in generating unstable interfacial waves, and further, oil form might be distributed into particles by erupting in the aqueous layer. The next approach involves ultrasound application using ultrasound waves at less frequency, which can lead to the microbubble development and later on collapse.

Ultrasonic emulsification is extensively used for emulsion preparation [75], modification of protein [75], and reduction of particle size of whey proteins [75]. Furthermore, it has been observed that these days this approach is used to form film with better properties. It was found that wettability as well as tensile strength of *Prosopis chilensis* seed gum as well as *Elaeis guineensis* fruit EO-based emulsion films improved due to even droplet distribution [75].

The emerging trend of formulating EOs in the form of nanoemulsions mainly to overcome poor water solubility of the components as well as to overcome antimicrobial resistant among pathogenic microorganisms has been reported recently (Table 13.2). Additionally, formulating (such as nanoemulsion) and complexing EOs with oligosaccharides improve their stability and biological potential. Recently, *A. maurorum* EO nanoemulsion was formulated by the ionotropic gelation technique using chitosan asbiopolymer. Findings obtained from this investigation demonstrated that nano-emulsion showed suitable morphological characteristics with greater inhibitory effects against antibiotic-resistant pathogenic microorganism when matched with free oil activity. Also, this prepared

TABLE 13.2
Antimicrobial Potential of Essential Oil-Based Nanoemulsions

EO with CC	MI, MOP, Size	Microorganisms	Biological Property and Application	References
Alhagi maurorum (oxygenated sesquiterpenes and hydrocarbons)	Chitosan, ionotropic gelation method, 172±4 nm	*P. aeruginosa, E. coli, S. aureus, K. pneumonia, A. baumannii, B. cereus*	Antibacterial, antibiofilm, plasmid curing effects	[76]
Anise myrtle	Ultrasonication, 10% surfactant, 30.23 nm	*S. aureus, L. monocytogenes, E. coli*	Did not show antibacterial activity	[77]
Cananga odorata EO (linalool and benzyl acetate)	Chitosan, *Cananga odorata* EO and its nanoencapsulated formulation into chitosan nanoemulsion, ionic gelation technique	*Aspergillus flavus*	Antifungal agent to improve the shelf life of the stored food against AFB1 and lipid peroxidation-mediated biodeterioration	[78]
Cedarwood EO	5% surfactant, 135.14±1.1 nm	NF	Exerted higher free radical scavenging activities, iron reducing power, and antibacterial ability	[79]
Cedarwood EO	1% starch, 626.21±6.05 nm	NF	Exerted higher free radical scavenging activities, iron reducing power, and antibacterial ability	[80]
Celery seed oil (extracted from *Apium graveolens*)	Tween 80, ultrasonication technique, 23.4±1.80 nm	S. aureus	Anticancer, antibacterial activity	[81]
Cinnamon bark oil	Lauric arginate and Tween 80, ~100nm	*S. enteritidis, L. monocytogenes E. coli* (O157:H7)	Antimicrobial activities	[82]
Cinnamon EO	Probe ultrasonication, Tween® 80, 65.98 nm	*Aspergillus niger, Rhizopus arrhizus, Penicillium sp., and Colletotrichum gloeosporioides*	Antifungal activity	[83]
Cinnamon oil	Lauric arginate, lysolecithin, Tween, 80 ~100 nm	*F. graminearum*	Antifungal (treatment of mycelium with cinnamon oil NE resulted in the loss of cytoplasm from fungal hyphae and accounted for the antifungal action)	[84]
Citrus sinensis	Sodium alginate, 43.23 nm	Salmonella and Listeria sp.	Edible coating of tomatoes	[85]
Cleome viscosa EO	Tween 80, 7 nm	*MRSA, DR Streptococcus pyogenes, and DR extended-spectrum beta-lactamase-producing E. coli, Klebsiella pneumoniae, Pseudomonas aeruginosa*	Effective against drug-resistant bacteria, by inhibiting the drug efflux mechanism of bacterial strains	[86]
Cleome viscosa EO	Ultrasonic emulsification, Triton-x-100 (polyoxyethylene isooctylphenyl ether), 164 nm	Foodborne pathogenic C. albicans	Antifungal	[87]
Clove EO	Aqueous-phase titration method, Triacetin, Tween 80, Labrasol, 29.1 nm	Bacterial strains	Enhanced antibacterial effects	[88]
Clove EO	Hazelnut meal protein, 160.45 nm	*L. monocytogenes, B. subtilis, S. aureus, P. aeruginosa, E. coli*	To improve mechanical, barrier, and antimicrobial properties of hazelnut meal protein-based edible films	[89]
Clove oil	Purity gum ultra	Gram-positive bacteria *(Listeria monocytogenes, Staphylococcus aureus)*	Antibacterial activity	[90]
Clove oil	Tween 80, BSA, quillaja saponins	*Fusarium mycotoxin contamination*	Antifungal agents	[91]
Clove oil	Corn oil, triacylglycerol, <150 nm	*Fusarium graminearum*	Antifungal, detoxification delivery systems in the food or other industries	[92]

(*Continued*)

TABLE 13.2 (*Continued*)
Antimicrobial Potential of Essential Oil-Based Nanoemulsions

EO with CC	MI, MOP, Size	Microorganisms	Biological Property and Application	References
Copaifera langsdorffii EO	Pluronic F-127	Fungi of the genus Paracoccidioides	Antifungal	[93]
Coriandrum sativum	Chitosan	Aflatoxin, fungal strains	To enhance the shelf life and control the fungal and aflatoxin contamination of the stored rice	[94]
Cumin seed oil	Ultrasonication, Tween 80, 10.4±0.5 nm	*S. aureus*	Anticancer, antibacterial properties	[95]
Cymbopogon flexuosus	Average size <200 nm	*Mycobacterium fortuitum, Mycobacterium massiliense, Mycobacterium abscessus*	Inhibited the formation of mycobacterial biofilm	[96]
Cymbopogon flexuosus	200 nm	*Pseudomonas aeruginosa and Staphylococcus aureus*	Antimicrobial and antibiofilm activities	[96]
EOs (thyme, lemongrass, cinnamon, peppermint, and clove)-in-water NE	Fabricated by microfluidizer under optimized processing conditions (10,000 psi and 2 passes)	*Fusarium graminearum*	Antifungal (long-term physical stability, antifungal activity, and inhibition of mycotoxin production in NE form)	[97]
Eucalyptus globulus	High-energy method of ultrasonication to prepare nanoemulsion-impregnated chitosan film, Tween 80, chitosan film, 9.4 nm	*Staphylococcus aureus*	Wound healing antibacterial film	[98]
Eucalyptus globulus	Ultrasonic emulsification, Tween 80, 3.8 nm	Staphylococcus aureus	Wound healing antibacterial film	[99]
Guava leaves EO (thujene, ***β****-pinene, β-pinene, sabinene, cubenol, P-aucubin and L-scopoletin)*	Chitosan, ionic gelation, 40–96 nm	Multidrug-resistant *K. pneumoniae*	Antibacterial activity against multidrug-resistant K. pneumoniae	[100]
Lemon EO (d-limonene, p-cymene, β-pinene)		Foodborne pathogens (*Staphylococcus aureus, Enterococcus faecalis and Salmonella paratyphi A*)	Natural antimicrobial agent against foodborne pathogen and spoilage bacteria for fish processing industry	[101]
Lemon myrtle	Ultrasonication, 10% surfactant, 16.07 nm	S. aureus, L. monocytogenes, and E. coli	Enhanced antibacterial activity	[102]
Mentha piperita	Spontaneous method, Tween 20, 160±25 nm	S. aureus, E. coli	Antibacterial property	[103]
Myristica fragrans essential oil (MFEO)	Chitosan	15 foodborne molds and aflatoxin B1 secretion by toxigenic Aspergillus flavus LHP R14 strain	Antimicrobial activity, aflatoxin inhibitory potential, safety profiling, and in situ efficacy	[104]
Nanoandi oil	Tween 80, ultrasonification, 88-92 nm	*Leishmania infantum and L. amazonensis.*	Antileishmanial activity	[105]
Nanocopa oil	Tween 80, ultrasonification, 76-80 nm	*Leishmania infantum and L. amazonensis*	Antileishmanial activity	[106]
Ocimum basilicum	Encapsulation by using Polysorbate 80	*Enterococcus faecalis, Staphylococcus aureus, Salmonella paratyphi, Klebsiella pneumonia*	Antibacterial, antioxidants, larvicidal activity, food industry, and drug delivery against the mosquito vector control	[107]
Oregano and clove		*Zygosaccharomyces bailii*	Antifungal (in salad dressings)	[108]
Oregano EO (Thymol)	Sodium alginate by sequential dipping	NA	Shelf life of fresh fruit and vegetables, to develop edible coatings, prolong the tomato shelf life	[109]
Origanum majorana (Terpinen-4-ol)	Chitosan (encapsulated into chitosan nanoemulsion)	*Aspergillus flavus*	Antioxidant, antifungal agent in food preservation	[110]

(*Continued*)

TABLE 13.2 (*Continued*)

Antimicrobial Potential of Essential Oil-Based Nanoemulsions

EO with CC	MI, MOP, Size	Microorganisms	Biological Property and Application	References
Origanum vulgare L (Thymol)	39.54 nm, Pluronic F127, low-energy method	*P. acnes and S. epidermidis*	Anti-acne activity, antibiofilm, antimicrobial	[111]
Peppermint oil	Medium-chain triacylglycerol, modified starch, <200 nm	*Listeria monocytogenes Scott A and Staphylococcus aureus*	Antimicrobial effects for extending shelf life of food products	[112]
Melaleuca alternifolia EO	Carbopol 934, 0.1% adapalene	*Propionibacterium acnes*	Novel carrier for topical delivery of adapalene	[113]
Melaleuca alternifolia EO		*Trichophyton rubrum*	Antifungal activity	[114]
Melaleuca alternifolia EO	Low-energy ultrasonication method, Tea tree oil nanoemulsion loaded with Ag nanoparticles, 17.7 nm	*Escherichia coli, Staphylococcus aureus*	Used against bacterial resistance	[115]
Melaleuca alternifolia EO (nanocapsule)		*Pythium insidiosum*	Antimicrobial activity (pythiosis treatment)	[116]
Tea tree oil with Itraconazole	Thermosensitive gel	*Candida sp.*	Antifungal mainly in vaginal candidiasis	[117]
Thyme	Ultrasound emulsification	Escherichia coli O157:H7	Antibacterial effects	[118]
Thyme and oregano EOs	Cellulose nanocrystals reinforced chitosan-based antifungal films prepared by encapsulating EO nanoemulsion, chitosan, 750 Gy of ionizing radiation, cellulose nanocrystals	*Aspergillus niger, Aspergillus flavus, Aspergillus parasiticus, and Penicillium chrysogenum*	Antifungal effects	[119]
Thyme EO	Layer-by-layer self-assembly of whey protein by high-pressure homogenization, whey protein, chitosan hydrochloride	*E. coli, S. aureus*	Antimicrobial for use in foods	[120]
Thyme oil	Prepared under subcritical water conditions, 184.51 nm	*Staphylococcus aureus, Penicillium digitatum*	High antioxidant activity, high antibacterial and antifungal activities	[121]
Thyme oil	Tween 80, lauric arginate, sodium dodecyl sulfate	Acid-resistant strains (*B. naardenensis, B. bruxellensis, Z. bailii, S. cerevisiae)*	Antifungal activity	[122]
Thymol	Ultrasonication method, 80–150 nm by TEM analysis; thymol and saponin were blended in the ratio of 6:1	*Xanthomonas axonopodis* pv. Glycine that causes bacterial pustule disease in soybean	Antibacterial activity	[123]
Thymol and eugenol	Lauric arginate lecithin mixed with nanoemulsions of thymol and eugenol, <100nm	*Listeria monocytogenes*	Antimicrobial activities	[124]
Thymol based NE	Chitosan, thymol chitosan NE 123.30 nm thyme EO chitosan NE 139.47	*S. aureus, E. coli*	Antibacterial packaging materials for preserving food	[125]
Thymus daenensis	Tween 80, ultrasonication	*Salmonella Typhimurium, Escherichia coli, and Listeria monocytogenes*	Antibacterial effects	[126]
Thymus daenensis	Ultrasound emulsification, 143nm	*Escherichia coli*	Antibacterial activity via disrupting cell membrane	[127]
Thymus daenensis (thymol)	Tween 80 as well as lecithin (0.1%), 131 nm	*S. pneumonia*	Antibacterial effects	[128]
Vitex negundo L.	*Aedes aegypti* L.	Polysorbate80, low-energy method, ultrasound emulsification, 200 nm	Antimicrobial, insecticidal applications, larvicidal activities	[129]
Zataria multiflora	Basil seed gum	Foodborne pathogens	Antimicrobial films were effective against potential foodborne pathogens	[130]
Zataria multiflora	Spontaneous method, Tween 20, 129 ± 12 nm	S. aureus, E. coli	Antibacterial property	[131]

NE, nanoemulsion; MI, major ingredient of formulation (emulsifier/surfactant/nanocarrier); MOP, method of preparation; EOs, essential oils; CC, chemical constituents; and NA, not applicable.

formulation showed considerable antibiofilm effects. This nano-formulation also showed considerable impact in treating R-plasmid of three antibiotic-resistant microbes [132].

Recent TTO nanoemulsions for inhalation treatment of bacterial and fungal pneumonia have been studied, and it was found that inhalation of tree oil nanoemulsions could be an effective treatment against fungal and bacterial pneumonia with no adverse effects [133].

13.4.1 Nanotechnology and Antimicrobial Activity of Essential Oils

Due to the development of various antimicrobial-resistant pathogens demand for effective and safe antimicrobial agent has increased recently. Plant systems also synthesize a wide range of antimicrobial compounds in different forms for their survival in harsh conditions [134–148]. EOs that are produced by plants have been known for their wide range of biological activities. The antimicrobial potential of EOs and metallic nanoparticles represents an effective solution for microbial resistance. Moreover, the use of EOs in combination with metallic nanoparticles may exert synergistic antimicrobial effects and would be a novel approach. Further, these unstable antimicrobial chemical compounds present in EOs can undergo oxidation reactions, resulting in loss or reduction of biological activity [134–148]. Thus, encapsulation of oils in nano forms of using natural polymers has been suggested as a type of delivery system that could improve the efficacy, solubility as well as stability of oil-loaded nanoformulations or nanoencapsulates. This type of delivery system offers sustained release and maintains therapeutic levels of drug in system circulation to exert the maximum biological effects. Additionally, such nanoformulations have also been reported to improve antimicrobial activity [134–148]. Other lipid-based NPs including nanoemulsions, liposomes (mainly phytosomes), and solid lipid nanoparticles can be used in the food industry. More specifically, nanoemulsions effectively improve use of EOs in foods by enhancing their dispersibility in food where microorganisms growth and multiplication rate is reduced by decreasing the impact on the quality attributes of the product, as well as by enhancing their antimicrobial activity [134–148].

13.5 In Vitro Antifungal Effects of EO Vapors

Recently, broth microdilution methods and vapor contact assay have been used to determine the antimicrobial potential of thyme red, fennel, clove, pine, sage, lemon balm, and lavender EOs against three *Candida* strains. It was found that thymol as well as carvacrol demonstrated the greatest response, while linalyl acetate presented the fewest effects and alpha-pinene showed the most superior effects. Additionally, using broth microdilution methods, pine EO showed excellent response against each microbial strain, while sage oil showed weak activity. Furthermore, thyme red EO was the most effective by vapor contact assay, followed by lemon balm, lavender, and sage. Thus, EO components can display different or the same activity with different methods [63].

Reactive oxygen species (ROS)-based fungal inhibitory activity of cinnamon and lemongrass EOs and their respective components against plant pathogenic fungal strains (*Raffaelea quercus-mongolicae* and *Rhizoctonia solani*) have been recently studied. It was found that lemongrass as well as cinnamon bark oils displayed 100% inhibition of both fungal strains. Additionally, it was found that EO components such as hydrocinnamaldehyde, eugenol, and salicylaldehyde demonstrated 100% suppression of *R. quercus-mongolicae*, whereas other components such as geranial, hydrocinnamaldehyde, salicylaldehyde, neral, and trans-cinnamaldehyde demonstrated 100% suppression of *R. solani*. It was also revealed that ROS production as well as and disruption of cell membrane could be the underlying causes behind their antimicrobial potential [149].

Recently, the fumigant antifungal activity of ten EOs was evaluated against two phytopathogenic fungi, *Raffaelea quercus-mongolicae* and *Rhizoctonia solani*. Among all the tested EOs, thyme white (Thymus vulgaris) and summer savory (*Satureja hortensis*) EOs showed the strongest fumigant antifungal activity against the phytopathogenic fungi. Among all the studied compounds, thymol and carvacrol showed fumigant antifungal activity. It was found that EOs cause cell death by ROS production as well as by disruption of fungal cell membranes [150].

Tea tree EO has been reported as a potent antimicrobial, and can be utilized via inhalers (DPIs) in the management of fungal and bacterial pneumonia. Recently, the effect of tea tree EO conjugated with cyclodextrin over the pulmonary system in the management of pneumonia as well as fungal infections was investigated. The results showed that tree oil-β-cyclodextrin powder presented strong and comparable effects on rodents when compared to penicillin as well as fluconazole. It was also found that the antipneumonic effects of tea tree EO-β- cyclodextrin (CD) were greater than tea tree EO alone. It was also found that the underlying mechanisms of action of TTO-β-CD inclusion complexes may be:

- Suppression of neutrophils as well as leucocytes recruitment
- Decreasing microbial load
- Reducing expression of pro-inflammatory cytokines
- Suppressing cyclooxygenase 2 expression
- Preventing lung injury
- It was concluded that TTO-β-CD powder inhalation has the following advantages:
- Compactness
- Convenience of people being able to administer medicine on their own
- High deposition in lungs
- Considerable anti-pneumonic activity

It could be a potential candidate for the management of pneumonia as well fungal infections [151].

Antibacterial, antifungal, as well as antiviral effects of EO blends (cinnamon, wild carrot, eucalyptus, and rosemary) have been investigated recently. It was found that the blend of cinnamon, wild carrot, clove, and oregano EOs showed antifungal effects against Candida strains. Additionally, this blend also showed effectiveness against influenza viruses such as H1N1 and HSV1 viruses as well as better activity against *S. aureus* and *S. pneumonia*. Due to this dual action against influenza A virus and two bacterial strains (*S. pneumoniae and S. aureus*) particularly, this blend could be used as a potential target to deal with viral and post-viral pneumonia infections [152].

Another investigation showed that arborvitae, clove, clary sage, lavender, oregano, and thyme possess significant effects against several pathogenic bacterial and fungal strains. It was also found that thyme, arborvitae, oregano, and clove have potent antibacterial activity and presented different fungistatic and fungicidal effects without causing damage to DNA when tested in HEL 12469 human embryo lung cells. Additionally, it was also reported that both direct contact and the vapor form of certain EOs such as phenol-free arborvitae oil can be utilized as broad-spectrum antimicrobial agents to disinfect indoor settings [153].

The antifungal and antiaflatoxigenic effects of *Thymus vulgaris* EO against *Aspergillus flavus* in vapor and liquid phases have also been investigated recently. It was found that mycelial growth and aflatoxin production were reduced by EO in both vapor and liquid phases. Additionally, EO in vapor phase suppresses the expression of both fungal development-related genes (brlA, abaA, and wetA) and aflatoxin biosynthesis-related genes (aflR, aflD, and aflK). It was also demonstrated that aflatoxin production in brown rice and white rice can be reduced by T. vulgaris EO in vapor phase [154].

Another recent investigation showed that *Eucalyptus citriodora* can be used as a potential antifungal agent against medically important dermatophytes such as *Microsporum canis, Microsporum gypseum, Trichophyton mentagrophytes,* and *Trichophyton rubrum*. It was found that citronellal, citronellol, and isopulegol enriched oil was effective against all strains except *Microsporum gypseum* [155].

Malassezia pachydermatis is a commensal yeast of the skin and also the most isolated pathogenic yeast in canine otitis externa. Recently, lemongrass EO the showed the strongest activity against *M. pachydermatis*. However, other EOs such as cinnamon leaf, clove, manuka, Indian melissa, oregano, palmarosa, and winter savory oil also possessed a strong antifungal activity. These EOs were found to have an active inhibiting effect over *M. pachydermatis* when examined by vapor assay [156].

A recent study also showed that chitosan-based edible films when treated with Mexican oregano or cinnamon EO can enhance the food value by acting over the surface to prevent the molds growth by the volatile compounds. . Thus, antimicrobial agents or EOs can be added into edible films to improve the shelf-life of the product by decreasing the chances of growth of microorganisms over surfaces. Treatment of edible films with EOs offers advantages; for example, very little concentration of EOs can be added, which could be effective in inhibiting the growth of fungal strains. As reported, *Aspergillus niger* and *Penicillium digitatum* were inhibited by using Mexican oregano, cinnamon, lemongrass EOs loaded amaranth, chitosan, or starch edible films [157].

EO derived from lemongrass is enriched with geranial (42.2%), and neral (31.5%) has been widely known for its antifungal effects. Recently, lemongrass EO was assessed for its topical, anti-inflammatory, and antifungal effects against three fungal strains, *Candida albicans, C. tropicalis,* and *Aspergillus niger,* using both liquid and vapor phases. Findings obtained from this study suggest that EO possessed considerable antifungal activity against *Candida albicans, C. tropicalis, and Aspergillus niger.* It was also found that vapor phase showed considerable anti-candida effects. Additionally, it was also revealed that lemongrass EO treatment considerably decreased carrageenan-induced paw edema and also decreased inflammation after oral as well as topical administration [158].

These days various EO-based studies are emphasizing ways to control the early vaporization of EOs, via encapsulation in suitable polymeric materials. Recently, the fungal inhibitory effects of several components of EOs (thymol, cinnamaldehyde, carvacrol, and eugenol l) against the *Aspergillus* strain encapsulated by using Mobil composition of Matter No. 41 (MCM-41) and β-cyclodextrin were evaluated. It was found that carvacrol and thymol in MCM-41 showed significantly more antifungal effects than pure or β-cyclodextrin-loaded EOs. Interestingly, thymol as well as carvacrol maintained its antifungal effects for 30 days [159].

Similarly, the antifungal potential of EOs was improvised in another report by using MCM-41 particles in the form of film containing EOs, which can be used in food packaging or antimicrobial medicine to control the release of EOs from these film nanocomposites. Recently, using zein film and cinnamon oil-encapsulated MCM-41 silica nanoparticles an antibacterial film for food application was fabricated. Findings obtained from this study showed that the film presented an excellent release profile and mechanical properties were enhanced by using MCM-41 nanoparticles. Further, cinnamon oil impregnated in film showed better antibacterial effects, suggesting that the cinnamon oil-based film prepared by modified supercritical carbon dioxide-mediated saturation could be an effective approach [160].

Further application of EOs in remediation of fungal contamination in residential and occupational buildings (mainly for indoor settings) can be utilized as fungal contamination in indoor environments can lead to adverse health effects. Thus, using EOs, fungi present in indoor environments can be removed or EOs can modify the indoor environment to become less favorable to growth. In this context, recently five marketed preparations [vinegar, disinfectant, ethanol (70%) and *Melaleuca alternifolia* EO] were analyzed in vapor as well as liquid form. It was found that *Melaleuca alternifolia* EO showed the greatest inhibitory effect on the growth of two common fungal genera (*Aspergillus fumigatus* and *Penicillium chrysogenum*) when applied in either a liquid or vapor form. Thus, *Melaleuca alternifolia* EO can be used to inhibit the growth of fungal genera found in indoor air environments, mainly remediation of fungal contamination in residential and occupational buildings [161].

A recent study showed that photoactivation of citrus EO enhanced lethal effect on fungal cells (*Candida albicans* and *Trichophyton rubrum*) by 10%–13%. Thus, photoactivation of citrus EO can be used as an effective approach to treat common mucocutaneous fungal infections [162].

Candida strains have been reported for fungal infections called Candidiasis. Among all candida-mediated fungal infections *Candida albicans* is the most widespread. Several new strains emerged recently such as *Candida auris* are linked with multidrug-resistant candidia strain and infection of Candida at a systemic level. Among immune-compromised individuals, *Candida spp.* are frequent causes of infection. Treatment of Candida infections faces several challenges as follows due to which azole and its analogues are considered as reliable treatment:

- availability
- toxicity associated with main course drugs
- resistance offered by Candida strains
- high chances of relapse of infections
- high price of antifungal medications

As EOs are well known for their good antimicrobial potential against filamentous fungi, they have been used as potential antibacterial and/or antifungal agents. A study showed the comparative antifungal potential of *Artemisia annua* EO in both liquid and vapor phases by using vapor contact and microdilution assay. It was found that normal MIC in the liquid phase was 11.88 μL/mL, whereas in the vapor phase, all Candida strains growth evaluated at 2.13 $\mu L/cm^3$ was reduced. Additionally, in comparison to vapor phase of EO, *Candida glabrata* has shown more vulnerability against liquid phase. It has also been reported that against vapor phase, *Candida dubliniensis* and *Candida albicans* showed more susceptibility whereas *Candida parapsilosis* showed more resistance [163].

A recent investigation showed the antifungal effects of EOs (clove, fennel, thyme red, lemon balm, lavender pine, and sage) as well as their components on three *Candida* clinical strains. EOs and components were tested in both vapor and liquid phases against fungal strains. Findings obtained from broth microdilution procedure indicated that pine EO displayed the strongest effects against each fungal strain.. Additionally, EOs, mainly thymus red and pine oils in vapor phase and their components carvacrol, thymol, and α-pinene, showed good activity against Candida spp., including fluconazole-/voriconazole-resistant strains. Thus, vapor forms of EOs might be more beneficial without requiring direct contact, creating easy environmental applications such as in hospitals or schools [63].

Another investigation showed the antifungal activity of lemongrass (*Cymbopogon citratus*) EO, mentha (*Mentha piperita*), and eucalyptus (*Eucalyptus globulus*) EO against Candida albicans in liquid and vapor phase. It was found that lemongrass EO possessed the highest antifungal activity, followed by mentha and eucalyptus EO. Further, it was found that lemongrass EO showed more activity in vapor form against *C. albicans*, resulting in detrimental changes in cell morphology [164].

Recently, the antibacterial effect of *Cymbopogon citratus, Mentha arvensis, Mentha piperita,* and *Eucalyptus globulus* (in both liquid and vapor phases) and negative air ions (NAI) against Pseudomonas fluorescens was investigated. It was found that EOs in liquid form showed more promising results than vapor phase. Moreover, vapor components of EO with negative air ions showed more potent antibacterial effects than vapor components alone [165].

The antifungal potential of cinnamon EO derived from bark as well as leaf were also recently assessed against two Candida species. The findings obtained from direct and vapor diffusion assays revealed that bark CEO showed greater inhibitory effects than leaf CEO. Both EOs showed fungal inhibitory effects at very low dose via damaging membrane of *C. albicans* and *C. auris* as well as inhibiting the formation of hyphae with marked reduction of hemolysin production [166].

Another study also revealed that vapor phase of *Leptospermum petersonii* EO can be potentially utilized in aspergillosis treatment. Findings obtained from the study revealed that *Leptospermum petersonii* in vapor phase showed more potency in inhibiting the growth of fungi with no significant mammalian cell toxicity associated with the volatiles. It was concluded that *L. petersonii* EO (volatiles) treatment significantly reduced the load of fungi in the infected lungs of experimental animals, which was found to be greater than that of conventional antifungal drugs of choice [167]. Similarly, various previous reports suggested that EO vapors of plants such as ginger, basil, clove, and cinnamon are effective against *Penicillium islandicum* as well as *Aspergillus flavus* [46].

Another report showed that vapors of nutmeg, thyme, and sage oil presented better activity against *Penicillium* sp. (environmental isolates) as well as *Aspergillus* sp. (clinical isolates) [168]. However, contrary to the antimicrobial action of lemongrass EO, it does not have effects against *Rhizopus oryzae, Penicillium expansum, Fusarium solani,* and *Aspergillus fumigatus,* while vapors of thyme as well as lavender oil prevent the sporulation of fungal strains just like vapors of bergamot as well as orange oils [169].

The vapor of *M. piperita*, which is considered as a potential antibacterial agent, entirely prevents the growth of yeasts as well as fungal strains such as *Penicillium sp.* and *Aspergillus sp.* in time-kill and disk diffusion methods. Another report showed that vapors of *E. globulus* oil showed similar effects as *M. piperita*. SEM/TEM analysis revealed that lemongrass EO in vapor phase causes the degradation as well as distortion of plasmalemma of *Candida albicans* with extensive internal damage, whereas atomic force microscope results indicated a decrease in roughness. TEM analysis also revealed that treatment with EO makes cytoplasm dense with the presence of liquid globules. Similarly, fungi treatment with EOs vapors such as thyme, fennel, and lavender has also been reported to cause alterations in morphology such as coagulation of cytoplasm, vacuolization, leakage of protoplast, and shrinkage of hyphae among fungal strains [170].

EO vapors have been evidenced for their inhibitory effects on apical growth of *A. fumigatus*. It was found that these inhibitory effects are due to direct accumulation of the vapors on mycelia. Lavender EO and TTO have been known for their fungistatic effect as their components can selectively penetrate into the lipid bilayer and disrupt layer. Lemongrass EO vapors with aldehydes have been reported to cause fungicidal effect by causing permanent changes in cell membrane via cross-linkage reaction [1].

13.6 Evaluation of the Antimicrobial Effects of Vapors of EOs

Recent investigations have shown that vapors of EOs presenting antimicrobial activity are effective for shorter duration when used at high concentrations [171]. Techniques that are employed to assess the antimicrobial potential of vapors of oil EOs have two objectives. The first objective is to generate EO vapor in controlled conditions, and the second objective is to create microenvironmental controlled conditions such as temperature and pressure. So far, no standard or validated procedure has been developed to assess the ability of EO components to inhibit or inactivate microbial growth in vapor phase; however, the following procedures have been developed.

13.6.1 Inverted Petri Dish

In this procedure, a sterile disk made up of paper is saturated with a desirable quantity of oil, which could be earlier mixed with nonpolar solvents such as ethyl acetate. The impregnated disk is positioned in the petri dish inner surface, which is already inoculated with the test microorganism. Later, the petri dish is closed, inverted, and incubated rapidly to check the effect of EO components in vapor phase over the growth of test organisms by determining survival count. A similar procedure is repeated to study the effect of EOs at varied concentrations, incubation temperatures, and incubation time intervals against the same or different test organisms. Thus, air volume between the lid as well as surface of the agar can be measured in order to determine the concentration of EO per L of air. This procedure involves the quick vapor formation of EOs, and thus, volatiles contact the test microorganisms rapidly. This method is primarily utilized to determine the MIC with bacteria, those having faster growth rate in comparison with molds [172].

As is known, each component of an EO has different volatility (different vapor pressure), and thus volatile compounds evaporate at different rates. Therefore, the resulting area of inhibition developed afterward would not be an area of inhibition contributed by all components, because there might be some other components still left in the disk, which have not evaporated because of vapor pressure difference. Another challenge with this method is higher chances of interference if more than one EO is tested on a paper disk.

13.6.2 EO Vapor Phase Development Using Box Made of Glass or Plastic

In this procedure, an airtight box with a transparent lid and about 1 L capacity is used. A predetermined volume of oil is positioned within the airtight container, independently from the inoculated agar. The microenvironment of the box is controlled in such a way to encourage the growth of test organisms as well as to promote the evaporation of EOs. Optimum temperature inside the box is maintained for molds as well as yeasts at 25°C for 72 hours and 37°C for 18 to 24 hours for bacteria [172].

Once optimal conditions are maintained, EOs, mainly volatile components, start evaporating and produce vapors based on their difference in vapor pressure or volatility. These volatile components act against test microorganisms present in the box by inhibiting the growth of microorganisms to produce the zone of inhibition, which represents the antimicrobial potential of volatile components. This procedure can be effectively utilized for both real food and model systems. This hermetically sealed box is mainly used for the multicellular microscopic class of fungi (i.e., molds) as their rate of development is slow. Despite the fact that various microbes can be examined simultaneously, the EO consumption is quite high, and this box-based approach is mostly utilized as a testing strategy. Additionally, standardization of the "box" is challenging [173].

13.6.3 Chamber with Seven Wells

Another screening approach to measure MIC of oil vapors was introduced and fabricated by Seo et al. [174]. This method involves an apparatus made of an upper compartment with seven wells. Each well, out of seven, contains media in solid form on which the desirable microorganism has been inoculated. On the other side, lower compartments containing oils produce vapor. In order to avoid the vapor outflow, seven O-rings are present at the connections of the upper as well as lower compartments. This apparatus is made up of polycarbonate and thus is autoclavable. Also, both chambers are firmly closed. The major benefit of this method is that the antimicrobial effects of vapors at different concentrations can be evaluated, which can reduce the time needed for the whole process.

13.6.4 Agar Plug Vapor-Phase Assay

The agar plug-based vapor-phase method is a new approach reported by Amat et al. [50] that involves a small tube cap with a particular amount of oil (in mL) introduced in a plate of the agar. Afterward, inoculation of agar plug of size 13 mm is done using test organism and then placed over the cap, followed by the incubation (at 37°C for 24 hours). Later, the agar plugs exposed to the EO vapors are studied virtually to look for any growth of test microorganism. Subsequently, the agar plug is carefully collected and then transferred in liquid medium (5 mL) for 10 minutes to recover test organisms. Further liquid medium is vortexed (30 seconds) and then plated for examination. The authors also emphasized sufficient distance between the oil phase and the agar plug to facilitate the vaporization of oil. In the majority of vapor-phase methods, oils are not allowed to come into contact directly with the test organism and thus the efficiency of these procedures is dependent on the volatile components present in the EO samples. Vigilant examination of EOs is essential, from the point of extraction and characterization until utilization as antimicrobial agents. Thus, more emphasis on the stability as well as storage of EOs must be given in order to monitor variation in chemical profile periodically in a vapor phase where the interaction of their components with storage conditions must be studied carefully [175].

13.7 Application of Essential Oil Vapors in Food Industry

These days one of the major concerns in the food industry is microbial contamination, which impacts human health. Studies have shown a number of important causes of food contamination by pathogenic microorganisms such as multidrug-resistant *E. coli* strains, which are listed below [176]:

- animals that produce food
- inappropriate cultivation
- poor sanitation at important phases of food production

Thus, there is an urgent requirement for new safe antimicrobial agents to reduce food contamination and chances of further antimicrobial resistance [177]. In this context, antimicrobials derived from natural resources such as EOs have gained significant attention because in addition to imparting characteristic odor to food, EOs can efficiently deal with microbial contamination, especially resistant strains [178]. As per previous reports, EOs (liquid form) showed high activity against pathogenic foodborne microorganisms; however, their efficacy in food products is often debated as these reported effects are only attained with higher proportion of oils in contrast to the MIC in nutrient media [179]. Thus, the utilization of EOs in food preservation is still not clear because of the harmful effects associated with EOs at such higher concentrations on organoleptic properties [180]. Most recent studies have focused on the utilization of EOs in vapor phase at comparatively lower concentrations to prevent food contamination caused by foodborne pathogens and spoilage bacteria as well as to reduce changes in organoleptic characteristics of food [181]. This alternative approach might be more useful against pathogenic foodborne as well as spoilage microbes at moderately lower dilutions [182] than in liquid form. This approach could be more suitable and effective with the new modified atmospheric packaging [183] and nanoencapsulation technology [184].

Thus, to use EOs for this purpose it is essential to know their chemical profile and component-specific characteristics. It has become clear that not only the liquid phase contributes to the biological effects of EOs but the vapor phase also contributes to their biological properties. Thus, it is important to understand the chemical composition of EOs in vapor phase (gas phase or headspace) and also chemical transformation while movement of molecules from liquid to vapor phase based on their differences in vapor pressure. Movement of these potential vapor components into the headspace is dependent on their affinity with components with liquid phase as well as rate of vaporization of the components. However, a comparative proportion of volatile components in both phases will reach equilibrium, and the partial pressure of each component will be equivalent to the vapor pressure. This directly correlates to the mole fraction in the liquid phase. Thus, volatile components in the headspace are comparative to their proportion in the liquid phase, which could be influenced by multiple factors [39]. So, composition in vapor phase could be dissimilar from liquid phase. Several techniques have been developed for the assessment of the chemical composition of volatile components in headspace at equilibrium with liquid oil [185–187].

The majority of these reports are based on solid-phase microextraction (SPME) by which the volatile components present in headspace are removed via fused silica fiber coated with stationary phase (HS-SPME) [173]. HS-SPME is a sampling method developed with a special emphasis on increasing reproducibility, which allows the absorption of volatile components present in gaseous phase on or into a polymeric material that coats a silica fiber. The stationary phase (SPME) utilized in this process promotes the adsorption of volatile components present in head space on the fiber. These absorbed components are then released by using heat in the GC injector port to execute the qualitative investigation and GC with flame-ionization detection for the quantitative analysis [188–190].

Headspace-solid phase micro-extraction/gas chromatography-mass spectrometry (HS/SPME-GC/MS) is a simple, robust, rapid, effective, and economic technique for the qualitative analysis of EOs. Several other approaches such as high-precision liquid chromatography (HPLC), GC-MS coupled with chemometric resolution technique [15], 2-D gas chromatography [16], and ATR-Fourier transform mid-infrared spectroscopy [38] have also been used for the profiling of volatile components in the liquid phase as well as vapor phase of EOs. Various micropropgation approaches have been also used to improve the level of active chemical compound in essential oils [191–206].

REFERENCES

1. Inouye S, Takizawa T, Yamaguchi H. Antibacterial activity of essential oils and their major constituents against respiratory tract pathogens by gaseous contact. *J Antimicrob Chemother.* 2001;47(5):565–573.
2. Inouye S, Uchida K, Abe S. Vapor activity of 72 essential oils against a *Trichophyton mentagrophytes. J Infect Chemother.* 2006;12(4):210–216.
3. Boukhatem MN, Ferhat MA, Kameli A, Saidi F, Mekarnia M. Liquid and vapour phase antibacterial activity of *Eucalyptus globulus* essential oil ¼ susceptibility of selected respiratory tract pathogens. *Am J Infect Dis.* 2014;10(3):105–117.
4. Edris A, Farrag E. Antifungal activity of peppermint and sweet basil essential oils and their major aroma constituents on some plant pathogenic fungi from the vapor phase. *Mol Nutr Food Res.* 2003;47(2):112–121.
5. Fisher K, Phillips C. Potential antimicrobial uses of essential oils in food: Is citrus the answer? *Trends Food Sci Technol.* 2008;19(3):156–164.
6. Kloucek P, Smid J, Frankova A, Kokoska L, Valterova I, Pavela R. 2012. Fast screening method for assessment of antimicrobial activity of essential oils in vapor phase. *Food Res Int.* 47(2):161–165.
7. Suhr K, Nielsen P Antifungal activity of essential oils evaluated by two different application techniques against rye bread spoilage fungi. *J Appl Microbiol.* 2003;94(4):665–674.

8. Dao T, Bensoussan M, Gervais P, Dantigny P. Inactivation of conidia of *Penicillium chrysogenum*, *P. digitatum* and *P. italicum* by ethanol solutions and vapours. *Int J Food Microbiol.* 2008;122(1–2):68–73.
9. Smith-Palmer A, Stewart J, Fyfe L. Antimicrobial properties of plant essential oils and essences against five important food-borne pathogens. *Lett Appl Microbiol.* 1998;26(2):118–122.
10. Wiegand I, Hilpert K, Hancock R. Agar and broth dilution methods to determine the minimal inhibitory concentration (MIC) of antimicrobial substances. *Nat Proto.* 2008;3(2):163–175.
11. Kalemba D, Kunicka A. Antibacterial and antifungal properties of essential oils. *Curr Med Chem.* 2003;10(10):813–829.
12. Azaiez I, Meca G, Manyes L, Fernandez-Franzon M. Antifungal activity of gaseous allyl, benzyl and phenyl isothiocyanate in vitro and their use for fumonisins reduction in bread. *Food Control.* 2013;32(2):428–434.
13. Gutierrez J, Barry-Ryan C, Bourke P. The antimicrobial efficacy of plant essential oil combinations and interactions with food ingredients. *Int J Food Microbiol.* 2008;124(1):91–97.
14. Oussalah M, Caillet S, Saucier L, Lacroix M. Inhibitory effects of selected plant essential oils on the growth of four pathogenic bacteria: *E. coli* O157:H7, *Salmonella typhimurium*, *Staphylococcus aureus* and *Listeria monocytogenes*. *Food Control.* 2007;18(5):414–420.
15. Aguilar-Gonzalez AE, Palou E, Lopez-Malo A. Response of *Aspergillus niger* inoculated on tomatoes exposed to vapor phase mustard essential oil for short or long periods and sensory evaluation of treated tomatoes. *J Food Qual.* 2017;2017:1–7.
16. Velazquez-Nunez M, Avila-Sosa R, Palou E, opez-Malo AL. Antifungal activity of orange (*Citrus sinensis* var. Valencia) peel essential oil applied by direct addition or vapor contact. *Food Control* 2013;31(1):1–4.
17. Huang J, Qian C, Xu H, Huang Y. Antibacterial activity of Artemisia asiatica essential oil against some common respiratory infection causing bacterial strains and its mechanism of action in Haemophilus influenzae. *Microb Pathog.* 2018;114:470–475.
18. Yang C, Hu DH, Feng Y. Antibacterial activity and mode of action of the Artemisia capillaris essential oil and its constituents against respiratory tract infection-causing pathogens. *Mol Med Rep.* 2015;11(4):2852–2860.
19. LeBel G, Vaillancourt K, Bercier P, Grenier D. Antibacterial activity against porcine respiratory bacterial pathogens and in vitro biocompatibility of essential oils. *Arch Microbiol.* 2019;201(6):833–840.
20. Aelenei P, Rimbu CM, Guguianu E, et al. Coriander essential oil and linalool: Interactions with antibiotics against Gram-positive and Gram-negative bacteria. *Lett Appl Microbiol.* 2019;68(2):156–164.
21. Boukhatem MN, Ferhat MA, Kameli A, Saidi F, Kebir HT. Lemon grass (*Cymbopogon citratus*) essential oil as a potent anti-inflammatory and antifungal drugs. *Libyan J Med.* 2014;9:25431.
22. Santos Serafim Machado M, Ferreira Silva HB, Rios R, et al. The anti-allergic activity of *Cymbopogon citratus* is mediated via inhibition of nuclear factor kappa B (Nf-Kb) activation. *BMC Complement Altern Med.* 2015;15:168.
23. Martins HB, Selis ND, Souza CL, et al. Anti-inflammatory activity of the essential oil citral in experimental infection with *Staphylococcus aureus* in a model air pouch. *Evid Based Complement Altern Med.* 2017;2017:2505610.
24. Ben-Arye E, Dudai N, Eini A, Torem M, Schiff E, Rakover Y. Treatment of upper respiratory tract infections in primary care: A randomized study using aromatic herbs. *Evid Based Complement Altern Med.* 2011;2011:690346.
25. Brezáni V, Leláková V, Hassan STS, et al. Anti-infectivity against herpes simplex virus and selected microbes and anti-inflammatory activities of compounds isolated from *Eucalyptus globulus* Labill. *Viruses.* 2018;10(7):360.
26. Cermelli C, Fabio A, Fabio G, Quaglio P. Effect of eucalyptus essential oil on respiratory bacteria and viruses. *Curr Microbiol.* 2008;56(1):89–92.
27. Astani A, Reichling J, Schnitzler P. Comparative study on the antiviral activity of selected monoterpenes derived from essential oils. *Phytother Res.* 2010;24(5):673–679.
28. Man A, Santacroce L, Jacob R, Mare A, Man L. Antimicrobial activity of six essential oils against a group of human pathogens: A comparative study published correction appears in Pathogens. *Pathogens.* 2019;8(1):15.
29. Choi HJ. Chemical constituents of essential oils possessing anti-influenza A/WS/33 virus activity. *Osong Public Health Res Perspect.* 2018;9(6):348–353.
30. Li H, Yang T, Li FY, Yao Y, Sun ZM. Antibacterial activity and mechanism of action of *Monarda punctata* essential oil and its main components against common bacterial pathogens in respiratory tract. *Int J Clin Exp Pathol.* 2014;7(11):7389–7398.
31. Joshi RK. Chemical composition and antimicrobial activity of the essential oil of *Ocimum basilicum* L. (sweet basil) from Western Ghats of North West Karnataka, India. *Anc Sci Life.* 2014;33(3):151–156.
32. Wu S, Patel KB, Booth LJ, Metcalf JP, Lin HK, Wu W. Protective essential oil attenuates influenza virus infection: An in vitro study in MDCK cells. *BMC Complement Altern Med.* 2010;10:69.
33. Fabio A, Cermelli C, Fabio G, Nicoletti P, Quaglio P. Screening of the antibacterial effects of a variety of essential oils on microorganisms responsible for respiratory infections. *Phytother Res.* 2007;21(4):374–377.
34. de Aguiar FC, Solarte AL, Tarradas C, et al. Antimicrobial activity of selected essential oils against *Streptococcus suis* isolated from pigs. *Microbiologyopen.* 2018;7(6):e00613.
35. Ács K, Balázs VL, Kocsis B, Bencsik T, Böszörményi A, Horváth G. Antibacterial activity evaluation of selected essential oils in liquid and vapor phase on respiratory tract pathogens. *BMC Complement Altern Med.* 2018;18(1):227.
36. Grădinaru AC, Trifan A, Şpac A, Brebu M, Miron A, Aprotosoaie AC. Antibacterial activity of traditional spices against lower respiratory tract pathogens: Combinatorial effects of *Trachyspermum ammi* essential oil with conventional antibiotics. *Lett Appl Microbiol.* 2018;67(5):449–457.
37. Paulpandi M, Kannan S, Thangam R, Kaveri K, Gunasekaran P, Rejeeth C. In vitro anti-viral effect of β-santalol against influenza viral replication. *Phytomedicine.* 2012;19(3–4):231–235.
38. World Health Organization. Causes of death among children under 5 years. Accessed on 03 September 2017. http://apps.who.int/gho/data/view.wrapper.CHILDCOD2v?lang=en.

39. Ács K, Balázs VL, Kocsis B, Bencsik T, Böszörményi A, Horváth G. Antibacterial activity evaluation of selected essential oils in liquid and vapor phase on respiratory tract pathogens. *BMC Complement Altern Med.* 2018;18(1):227.
40. Forbes BA, Sahm DF, Weissfeld AS. *Bailey and Scott's Diagnostic Microbiology*, 12th ed. Mosby Elsevier, St. Louis, MI; 2007.
41. Pauli A, Schilcher H. In vitro antimicrobial activities of essential oils. In: Baser KHC, Buchbauer G, editors. *Handbook of Essential Oils, Science, Technology, and Application.* CRC Press, New York; 2010:353–547.
42. Inouye S, Yamaguchi H, Takizawa T. Screening of the antibacterial effects of a variety of essential oils on respiratory tract pathogens, using a modified dilution assay method. *J Infect Chemother.* 2001;7:251–254.
43. Gy H, Ács K. Essential oils in the treatment of respiratory tract diseases highlighting their role in bacterial infections and their antiinflammatory action: A review. *Flavour Frag J.* 2015;30:331–341.
44. Nedorostova L, Kloucek P, Kokoska L, Stolcova M, Pulkrabek J. Antimicrobial properties of selected essential oils in vapor phase against foodborne bacteria. *Food Control.* 2009;20:157–160.
45. Doran AL, Morden WE, Dunn K, Edwards-Jones V. Vapor-phase activities of essential oils against antibiotic sensitive and resistant bacteria including MRSA. *Lett Appl Microbiol.* 2009;48:387–392.
46. Horváth G, Ács K. Essential oils in the treatment of respiratory tract diseases highlighting their role in bacterial infections and their anti-inflammatory action: A review. *Flavour Fragr J.* 2015;30(5):331–341. https://www.ncbi.nlm.nih.gov/pmc/articles/PMC7163989/#ffj3252-bib-0034
47. Ács K, Bencsik T, Böszörményi A, Kocsis B, Horváth G. Essential oils and their vapors as potential antibacterial agents against respiratory tract pathogens. *Nat Prod Commun.* 2016;11(11):1709–1712.
48. López P, Sánchez C, Batlle R, Nerín C. Solid- and vapor-phase antimicrobial activities of six essential oils: Susceptibility of selected foodborne bacterial and fungal strains. *J Agric Food Chem.* 2005;53(17):6939–6946.
49. Inouye S, Uchida K, Maruyama N, Yamaguchi H, Abe S. A novel method to estimate the contribution of the vapor activity of essential oils in agar diffusion assay. *Nihon Ishinkin Gakkai Zasshi.* 2006;47(2):91–98.
50. Amat S, Baines D, Alexander TW. A vapour phase assay for evaluating the antimicrobial activities of essential oils against bovine respiratory bacterial pathogens. *Lett Appl Microbiol.* 2017;65(6):489–495.
51. Garzoli S, Turchetti G, Giacomello P, Tiezzi A, Laghezza Masci V, Ovidi E. Liquid and vapour phase of lavandin (Lavandula×intermedia) essential oil: Chemical composition and antimicrobial activity. *Molecules.* 2019;24(15):2701.
52. Laird K, Phillips C. Vapour phase: A potential future use for essential oils as antimicrobials? *Lett Appl Microbiol.* 2012;54(3):169–174.
53. Oliva A, Garzoli S, Sabatino M, Tadić V, Costantini S, Ragno R, Božović M. Chemical composition and antimicrobial activity of essential oil of Helichrysum italicum (Roth) G. Don fil. (Asteraceae) from Montenegro. *Nat Prod Res.* 2020;34(3):445–448.
54. Řebíčková K, Bajer T, Šilha D, Houdková M, Ventura K, Bajerová P. Chemical composition and determination of the antibacterial activity of essential oils in liquid and vapor phases extracted from two different southeast asian herbs-houttuynia cordata (saururaceae) and persicaria odorata (polygonaceae). *Molecules.* 2020;25(10):2432.
55. Oliva A, Costantini S, De Angelis M, Garzoli S, Božović M, Mascellino MT, Vullo V, Ragno R. High potency of melaleuca alternifolia essential oil against multi-drug resistant gram-negative bacteria and methicillin-resistant *Staphylococcus aureus. Molecules.* 2018;23(10):2584.
56. Netopilova M, Houdkova M, Rondevaldova J, Kmet V, Kokoska L. Evaluation of in vitro growth-inhibitory effect of carvacrol and thymol combination against *Staphylococcus aureus* in liquid and vapour phase using new broth volatilization chequerboard method. *Fitoterapia.* 2018;129:185–190.
57. Santomauro F, Donato R, Pini G, Sacco C, Ascrizzi R, Bilia AR. Liquid and vapor-phase activity of artemisia annua essential oil against pathogenic *Malassezia* spp. *Planta Med.* 2018;84(3):160–167.
58. Wang TH, Hsia SM, Wu CH, Ko SY, Chen MY, Shih YH, Shieh TM, Chuang LC, Wu CY. Evaluation of the antibacterial potential of liquid and vapor phase phenolic essential oil compounds against oral microorganisms. *PLoS One.* 2016;11(9):e0163147.
59. Burt S. Essential oils: Their antibacterial properties and potential applications in foods--a review. *Int J Food Microbiol.* 2004;94(3):223–253.
60. Bakkali F, Averbeck S, Averbeck D, Idaomar M. Biological effects of essential oils: A review. *Food Chem Toxicol.* 2008;46(2):446–475.
61. Yousef SAA. Essential oils: Their antimicrobial activity and potential application against pathogens by gaseous contact: A review. *Egypt Acad J Biolog Sci.* 2014;6(1):37–54.
62. Usachev EV, Pyankov OV, Usacheva OV, Agranovski IE. Antiviral activity of tea tree and eucalyptus oil aerosol and vapour. *J Aerosol Sci.* 2013;59:22–30.
63. Mandras N, Nostro A, Roana J, et al. Liquid and vapour-phase antifungal activities of essential oils against Candida albicans and non-albicans Candida. *BMC Complem Altern M.* 2016;16:330.
64. Kon KV, Rai MK. Plant essential oils and their constituents in coping with multidrug-resistant bacteria. *Expert Rev Anti-Infect Ther.* 2012;10(7):775–790.
65. Cermelli C, Fabio A, Fabio G, Quaglio P. Effect of eucalyptus essential oil on respiratory bacteria and viruses. *Curr Microbiol.* 2008;56(1):89–92.
66. Sadatrasul MS, Fiezi N, Ghasemian N, Shenagari M, Esmaeili S, Jazaeri EO, Abdoli A, Jamali A. Oil-in-water emulsion formulated with eucalyptus leaves extract inhibit influenza virus binding and replication in vitro. *AIMS Microbiol.* 2017;3(4):899–907.
67. Ács K, Balázs VL, Kocsis B, Bencsik T, Böszörményi A, Horváth G. Antibacterial activity evaluation of selected essential oils in liquid and vapor phase on respiratory tract pathogens. *BMC Complement Altern Med.* 2018;18(1):227.
68. Ács K, Bencsik T, Böszörményi A, Kocsis B, Horváth G. Essential oils and their vapors as potential antibacterial agents against respiratory tract pathogens. *Nat Prod Commun.* 2016;11(11):1709–1712.

69. Balázs VL, Horváth B, Kerekes E, Ács K, Kocsis B, Varga A, Böszörményi A, Nagy DU, Krisch J, Széchenyi A, Horváth G. Anti-haemophilus activity of selected essential oils detected by TLC-direct bioautography and biofilm inhibition. *Molecules.* 2019;24(18):3301.
70. Móricz ÁM, Horváth G, Böszörményi A, Ott PG. Detection and identification of antibacterial and antioxidant components of essential oils by TLC-biodetection and GC-MS. *Nat Prod Commun.* 2016;11(11):1705–1708.
71. Sharifi A, Mohammadzadeh A, Zahraei Salehi T, Mahmoodi P. Antibacterial, antibiofilm and antiquorum sensing effects of *Thymus daenensis* and *Satureja hortensis* essential oils against *Staphylococcus aureus* isolates. *J Appl Microbiol.* 2018;124(2):379–388.
72. Balázs VL, Horváth B, Kerekes E, Ács K, Kocsis B, Varga A, Böszörményi A, Nagy DU, Krisch J, Széchenyi A, Horváth G. Anti-haemophilus activity of selected essential oils detected by TLC-direct bioautography and biofilm inhibition. *Molecules.* 2019;24(18):3301.
73. Trevizan LNF, Nascimento KFD, Santos JA, Kassuya CAL, Cardoso CAL, Vieira MDC, Moreira FMF, Croda J, Formagio ASN. Anti-inflammatory, antioxidant and anti-Mycobacterium tuberculosis activity of viridiflorol: The major constituent of Allophylus edulis (A. St.-Hil, A. Juss. & Cambess.) Radlk. *J Ethnopharmacol.* 2016;192: 510–515.
74. Csikós E, Csekő K, Ashraf AR, Kemény Á, Kereskai L, Kocsis B, Böszörményi A, Helyes Z, Horváth G. Effects of *Thymus vulgaris* L., *Cinnamomum verum* J. Presl and *Cymbopogon nardus* (L.) rendle essential oils in the endotoxin-induced acute airway inflammation mouse model. *Molecules.* 20204;25(15):3553.
75. Gul O, Saricaoglu FT, Besir A, Atalar I, Yazici F. Effect of ultrasound treatment on the properties of nano-emulsion films obtained from hazelnut meal protein and clove essential oil. *Ultrason Sonochem.* 2018;41:466–474.
76. Hassanshahian M, Saadatfar A, Masoumipour F. Formulation and characterization of nanoemulsion from Alhagi maurorum essential oil and study of its antimicrobial, antibiofilm, and plasmid curing activity against antibiotic-resistant pathogenic bacteria. *J Environ Health Sci Eng.* 2020;18(2):1015–1027.
77. Nirmal NP, Mereddy R, Li L, Sultanbawa Y. Formulation, characterisation and antibacterial activity of lemon myrtle and anise myrtle essential oil in water nanoemulsion. *Food Chem.* 2018;254:1–7.
78. Upadhyay N, Singh VK, Dwivedy AK, Chaudhari AK, Dubey NK. Assessment of nanoencapsulated Cananga odorata essential oil in chitosan nanopolymer as a green approach to boost the antifungal, antioxidant and in situ efficacy. *Int J Biol Macromol.* 2021;171:480–490.
79. Huang K, Liu R, Zhang Y, Guan X. Characteristics of two cedarwood essential oil emulsions and their antioxidant and antibacterial activities. *Food Chem.* 2021;346:128970.
80. Huang K, Liu R, Zhang Y, Guan X. Characteristics of two cedarwood essential oil emulsions and their antioxidant and antibacterial activities. *Food Chem.* 2021;346:128970.
81. Nirmala MJ, Durai L, Gopakumar V, Nagarajan R. Preparation of celery essential oil-based nanoemulsion by ultrasonication and evaluation of its potential anticancer and antibacterial activity. *Int J Nanomed.* 2020;15:7651–7666.
82. Hilbig J, Ma Q, Davidson PM, Weiss J, Zhong Q. Physical and antimicrobial properties of cinnamon bark oil co-nanoemulsified by lauric arginate and Tween 80. *Int J Food Microbiol.* 2016;233:52–59.
83. Pongsumpun P, Iwamoto S, Siripatrawan U. Response surface methodology for optimization of cinnamon essential oil nanoemulsion with improved stability and antifungal activity. *Ultrason Sonochem.* 2020;60:104604.
84. Wu D, Lu J, Zhong S, Schwarz P, Chen B, Rao J. Influence of nonionic and ionic surfactants on the antifungal and mycotoxin inhibitory efficacy of cinnamon oil nanoemulsions. *Food Funct.* 2019;10(5):2817–2827.
85. Das S, Vishakha K, Banerjee S, Mondal S, Ganguli A. Sodium alginate-based edible coating containing nanoemulsion of *Citrus* sinensis essential oil eradicates planktonic and sessile cells of food-borne pathogens and increased quality attributes of tomatoes. *Int J Biol Macromol.* 2020;162:1770–1779.
86. Krishnamoorthy R, Athinarayanan J, Periasamy VS, Adisa AR, Al-Shuniaber MA, Gassem MA, Alshatwi AA. Antimicrobial activity of nanoemulsion on drug-resistant bacterial pathogens. *Microb Pathog.* 2018;120:85–96.
87. Krishnamoorthy R, Gassem MA, Athinarayanan J, Periyasamy VS, Prasad S, Alshatwi AA. Antifungal activity of nanoemulsion from Cleome viscosa essential oil against food-borne pathogenic *Candida albicans. Saudi J Biol Sci.* 2021;28(1):286–293.
88. Anwer MK, Jamil S, Ibnouf EO, Shakeel F. Enhanced antibacterial effects of clove essential oil by nanoemulsion. *J Oleo Sci.* 2014;63(4):347–354.
89. Gul O, Saricaoglu FT, Besir A, Atalar I, Yazici F. Effect of ultrasound treatment on the properties of nano-emulsion films obtained from hazelnut meal protein and clove essential oil. *Ultrason Sonochem.* 2018;41:466–474.
90. Majeed H, Liu F, Hategekimana J, Sharif HR, Qi J, Ali B, Bian YY, Ma J, Yokoyama W, Zhong F. Bactericidal action mechanism of negatively charged food grade clove oil nanoemulsions. *Food Chem.* 2016;197(Pt A):75–83.
91. Wan J, Jin Z, Zhong S, Schwarz P, Chen B, Rao J. Clove oil-in-water nanoemulsion: Mitigates growth of *Fusarium graminearum* and trichothecene mycotoxin production during the malting of Fusarium infected barley. *Food Chem.* 202;312:126120.
92. Wan J, Zhong S, Schwarz P, Chen B, Rao J. Influence of oil phase composition on the antifungal and mycotoxin inhibitory activity of clove oil nanoemulsions. *Food Funct.* 2018;9(5):2872–2882.
93. do Carmo Silva L, Miranda MACM, de Freitas JV, Ferreira SFA, de Oliveira Lima EC, de Oliveira CMA, Kato L, Terezan AP, Rodriguez AFR, Faria FSEDV, de Almeida Soares CM, Pereira M. Antifungal activity of *Copaíba resin* oil in solution and nanoemulsion against *Paracoccidioides* spp. *Braz J Microbiol.* 2020;51(1):125–134.
94. Das S, Singh VK, Dwivedy AK, Chaudhari AK, Upadhyay N, Singh P, Sharma S, Dubey NK. Encapsulation in chitosan-based nanomatrix as an efficient green technology to boost the antimicrobial, antioxidant and in situ efficacy of *Coriandrum sativum* essential oil. *Int J Biol Macromol.* 2019;133:294–305.
95. Nirmala MJ, Durai L, Rao KA, Nagarajan R. Ultrasonic nanoemulsification of cuminum cyminum essential oil and its applications in medicine. *Int J Nanomed.* 2020;15:795–807.

96. da Silva Gündel S, de Souza ME, Quatrin PM, Klein B, Wagner R, Gündel A, Vaucher RA, Santos RCV, Ourique AF. Nanoemulsions containing *Cymbopogon flexuosus* essential oil: Development, characterization, stability study and evaluation of antimicrobial and antibiofilm activities. *Microb Pathog.* 2018;118:268–276.
97. Wan J, Zhong S, Schwarz P, Chen B, Rao J. Physical properties, antifungal and mycotoxin inhibitory activities of five essential oil nanoemulsions: Impact of oil compositions and processing parameters. *Food Chem.* 2019;291: 199–206.
98. Sugumar S, Mukherjee A, Chandrasekaran N. Eucalyptus oil nanoemulsion-impregnated chitosan film: Antibacterial effects against a clinical pathogen, *Staphylococcus aureus*, in vitro. *Int J Nanomed.* 2015;10(Suppl 1):67–75.
99. Sugumar S, Ghosh V, Nirmala MJ, Mukherjee A, Chandrasekaran N. Ultrasonic emulsification of eucalyptus oil nanoemulsion: Antibacterial activity against *Staphylococcus aureus* and wound healing activity in Wistar rats. *Ultrason Sonochem.* 2014;21(3):1044–1049.
100. Zhang F, Ramachandran G, Mothana RA, et al. Antibacterial activity of chitosan loaded plant essential oil against multi drug resistant *K. pneumoniae. Saudi J Biol Sci.* 2020;27(12):3449–3455.
101. Yazgan H, Ozogul Y, Kuley E. Antimicrobial influence of nanoemulsified lemon essential oil and pure lemon essential oil on food-borne pathogens and fish spoilage bacteria. *Int J Food Microbiol.* 2019;306:108266.
102. Nirmal NP, Mereddy R, Li L, Sultanbawa Y. Formulation, characterisation and antibacterial activity of lemon myrtle and anise myrtle essential oil in water nanoemulsion. *Food Chem.* 2018;254:1–7.
103. Osanloo M, Abdollahi A, Valizadeh A, Abedinpour N. Antibacterial potential of essential oils of *Zataria multiflora* and *Mentha piperita*, micro- and nano-formulated forms. *Iran J Microbiol.* 2020;12(1):43–51.
104. Das S, Singh VK, Dwivedy AK, Chaudhari AK, Upadhyay N, Singh A, Deepika, Dubey NK. Fabrication, characterization and practical efficacy of *Myristica fragrans* essential oil nanoemulsion delivery system against postharvest biodeterioration. *Ecotoxicol Environ Saf.* 2020;189: 110000.
105. Dhorm Pimentel de Moraes AR, Tavares GD, Soares Rocha FJ, de Paula E, Giorgio S. Effects of nanoemulsions prepared with essential oils of copaiba- and andiroba against *Leishmania infantum* and *Leishmania amazonensis* infections. *Exp Parasitol.* 2018;187:12–21.
106. Dhorm Pimentel de Moraes AR, Tavares GD, Soares Rocha FJ, de Paula E, Giorgio S. Effects of nanoemulsions prepared with essential oils of copaiba- and andiroba against *Leishmania infantum* and *Leishmania amazonensis* infections. *Exp Parasitol.* 2018;187:12–21.
107. Sundararajan B, Moola AK, Vivek K, Kumari BDR. Formulation of nanoemulsion from leaves essential oil of *Ocimum basilicum* L. and its antibacterial, antioxidant and larvicidal activities (Culex quinquefasciatus). *Microb Pathog.* 2018;125:475–485.
108. Ribes S, Fuentes A, Barat JM. Effect of oregano (*Origanum vulgare* L. ssp. hirtum) and clove (*Eugenia* spp.) nanoemulsions on Zygosaccharomyces bailii survival in salad dressings. *Food Chem.* 2019;295:630–636.
109. Pirozzi A, Del Grosso V, Ferrari G, Donsì F. Edible coatings containing oregano essential oil nanoemulsion for improving postharvest quality and shelf life of tomatoes. *Foods.* 2020;9(11):1605.
110. Chaudhari AK, Singh VK, Das S, Deepika, Prasad J, Dwivedy AK, Dubey NK. Improvement of in vitro and in situ antifungal, AFB1 inhibitory and antioxidant activity of *Origanum majorana* L. essential oil through nanoemulsion and recommending as novel food preservative. *Food Chem Toxicol.* 2020;143:111536.
111. Taleb MH, Abdeltawab NF, Shamma RN, Abdelgayed SS, Mohamed SS, Farag MA, Ramadan MA. *Origanum vulgare* L. essential oil as a potential anti-acne topical nanoemulsion-in vitro and in vivo study. *Molecules.* 2018;23 (9):2164.
112. Liang R, Xu S, Shoemaker CF, Li Y, Zhong F, Huang Q. Physical and antimicrobial properties of peppermint oil nanoemulsions. *J Agric Food Chem.* 2012;60(30):7548–7555.
113. Najafi-Taher R, Ghaemi B, Amani A. Delivery of adapalene using a novel topical gel based on tea tree oil nano-emulsion: Permeation, antibacterial and safety assessments. *Eur J Pharm Sci.* 2018;120:142–151.
114. Flores FC, de Lima JA, Ribeiro RF, Alves SH, Rolim CM, Beck RC, da Silva CB. Antifungal activity of nanocapsule suspensions containing tea tree oil on the growth of *Trichophyton rubrum. Mycopathologia.* 2013;175(3–4): 281–286.
115. Najafi-Taher R, Ghaemi B, Kharrazi S, Rasoulikoohi S, Amani A. Promising antibacterial effects of silver nanoparticle-loaded tea tree oil nanoemulsion: A synergistic combination against resistance threat. *AAPS Pharm Sci Tech.* 2018;19(3):1133–1140.
116. de Souza Silveira Valente J, de Oliveira da Silva Fonseca A, Brasil CL, Sagave L, Flores FC, de Bona da Silva C, Sangioni LA, Pötter L, Santurio JM, de Avila Botton S, Pereira DI. In vitro activity of melaleuca alternifolia (Tea Tree) in its free oil and nanoemulsion formulations against pythium insidiosum. *Mycopathologia.* 2016;181(11–12):865–869.
117. Mirza MA, Ahmad S, Mallick MN, Manzoor N, Talegaonkar S, Iqbal Z. Development of a novel synergistic thermosensitive gel for vaginal candidiasis: An in vitro, in vivo evaluation. *Colloids Surf B.* 2013;103:275–282.
118. Guo M, Zhang L, He Q, Arabi SA, Zhao H, Chen W, Ye X, Liu D. Synergistic antibacterial effects of ultrasound and thyme essential oils nanoemulsion against *Escherichia coli* O157:H7. *Ultrason Sonochem.* 2020;66:104988.
119. Hossain F, Follett P, Salmieri S, Vu KD, Fraschini C, Lacroix M. Antifungal activities of combined treatments of irradiation and essential oils (EOs) encapsulated chitosan nanocomposite films in in vitro and in situ conditions. *Int J Food Microbiol.* 2019;295:33–40.
120. Li S, Sun J, Yan J, Zhang S, Shi C, McClements DJ, Liu X, Liu F. Development of antibacterial nanoemulsions incorporating thyme oil: Layer-by-layer self-assembly of whey protein isolate and chitosan hydrochloride. *Food Chem.* 2021;339:128016.
121. Ahmadi O, Jafarizadeh-Malmiri H. Green approach in food nanotechnology based on subcritical water: Effects of thyme oil and saponin on characteristics of the prepared oil in water nanoemulsions. *Food Sci Biotechnol.* 2020;29(6):783–792.

122. Ziani K, Chang Y, McLandsborough L, McClements DJ. Influence of surfactant charge on antimicrobial efficacy of surfactant-stabilized thyme oil nanoemulsions. *J Agric Food Chem.* 2011;59(11):6247–6255.
123. Kumari S, Kumaraswamy RV, Choudhary RC, et al. Thymol nanoemulsion exhibits potential antibacterial activity against bacterial pustule disease and growth promotory effect on soybean. *Sci Rep.* 2018;8(1):6650.
124. Ma Q, Davidson PM, Zhong Q. Nanoemulsions of thymol and eugenol co-emulsified by lauric arginate and lecithin. *Food Chem.* 2016;206:167–173.
125. Liu T, Liu L. Fabrication and characterization of chitosan nanoemulsions loading thymol or thyme essential oil for the preservation of refrigerated pork. *Int J Biol Macromol.* 2020;162:1509–1515.
126. Mansouri S, Pajohi-Alamoti M, Aghajani N, Bazargani-Gilani B, Nourian A. Stability and antibacterial activity of *Thymus daenensis* L. essential oil nanoemulsion in mayonnaise. *J Sci Food Agric.* 2021;101(9):3880–3888.
127. Moghimi R, Ghaderi L, Rafati H, Aliahmadi A, McClements DJ. Superior antibacterial activity of nanoemulsion of *Thymus daenensis* essential oil against *E. coli. Food Chem.* 2016;194:410–415.
128. Ghaderi L, Moghimi R, Aliahmadi A, McClements DJ, Rafati H. Development of antimicrobial nanoemulsion-based delivery systems against selected pathogenic bacteria using a thymol-rich *Thymus daenensis* essential oil. *J Appl Microbiol.* 2017;123(4):832–840.
129. Balasubramani S, Rajendhiran T, Moola AK, Diana RKB. Development of nanoemulsion from *Vitex negundo* L. essential oil and their efficacy of antioxidant, antimicrobial and larvicidal activities (*Aedes aegypti* L.). *Environ Sci Pollut Res Int.* 2017;24(17):15125–15133.
130. Hashemi Gahruie H, Ziaee E, Eskandari MH, Hosseini SM. Characterization of basil seed gum-based edible films incorporated with *Zataria multiflora* essential oil nanoemulsion. *Carbohydr Polym.* 2017;166:93–103.
131. Osanloo M, Abdollahi A, Valizadeh A, Abedinpour N. Antibacterial potential of essential oils of *Zataria multiflora* and *Mentha piperita*, micro- and nano-formulated forms. *Iran J Microbiol.* 2020;12(1):43–51.
132. Hassanshahian M, Saadatfar A, Masoumipour F. Formulation and characterization of nanoemulsion from *Alhagi maurorum* essential oil and study of its antimicrobial, antibiofilm, and plasmid curing activity against antibiotic-resistant pathogenic bacteria. *J Environ Health Sci Eng.* 2020;18(2):1015–1027.
133. Li M, Zhu L, Liu B, Du L, Jia X, Han L, Jin Y. Tea tree oil nanoemulsions for inhalation therapies of bacterial and fungal pneumonia. *Colloids Surf B.* 2016;141:408–416.
134. Bhatia S. *Natural Polymer Drug Delivery Systems: Plant Derived Polymers, Properties, and Modification & Applications.* Springer International Publishing, Switzerland; 2016:119–184.
135. Bhatia S. *Natural Polymer Drug Delivery Systems: Nanotechnology and Its Drug Delivery Applications.* Springer International Publishing, Switzerland; 2016:1–32.
136. Bhatia S. *Natural Polymer Drug Delivery Systems: Nanoparticles Types, Classification, Characterization, Fabrication Methods and Drug Delivery Applications.* Springer International Publishing, Switzerland; 2016:33–93.
137. Bhatia S. *Natural Polymer Drug Delivery Systems: Natural Polymers vs Synthetic Polymer.* Springer International Publishing, Switzerland; 2016:95–118.
138. Bhatia S. *Systems for Drug Delivery: Mammalian Polysaccharides and Its Nanomaterials.* Springer International Publishing, Switzerland; 2016:1–27.
139. Bhatia S. *Systems for Drug Delivery: Microbial Polysaccharides as Advance Nanomaterials.* Springer International Publishing, Switzerland; 2016:29–54.
140. Bhatia S. *Systems for Drug Delivery: Chitosan Based Nanomaterials and Its Applications.* Springer International Publishing, Switzerland; 2016:55–117.
141. Bhatia S. *Systems for Drug Delivery: Advance Polymers and Its Applications.* Springer International Publishing, Switzerland; 2016:119–146.
142. Bhatia S. *Systems for Drug Delivery: Advanced Application of Natural Polysaccharides.* Springer International Publishing, Switzerland; 2016:147–170.
143. Bhatia S. *Systems for Drug Delivery: Modern Polysaccharides and Its Current Advancements.* Springer International Publishing, Switzerland; 2016:171–188.
144. Bhatia S. *Systems for Drug Delivery: Toxicity of Nanodrug Delivery Systems.* Springer International Publishing, Switzerland; 2016:189–197.
145. Bhatia S. *Nanotechnology in Drug Delivery Fundamentals, Design, and Applications: Part 1: Protein and Peptide-Based Drug Delivery Systems.* Apple Academic Press, Palm Bay, FL; 2016:50–204.
146. Bhatia S. *Nanotechnology in Drug Delivery Fundamentals, Design, and Applications: Part 2: Peptide-Mediated Nanoparticle Drug Delivery System.* Apple Academic Press, Palm Bay, FL; 2016:205–280.
147. Bhatia S. *Nanotechnology in Drug Delivery Fundamentals, Design, and Applications: Part 3: CPP and CTP in Drug Delivery and Cell Targeting.* Apple Academic Press, Palm Bay, FL; 2016:309–312.
148. Donsì F, Ferrari G. Essential oil nanoemulsions as antimicrobial agents in food. *J Biotechnol.* 2016;233:106–120.
149. Lee JE, Seo SM, Huh MJ, Lee SC, Park IK. Reactive oxygen species mediated-antifungal activity of cinnamon bark (*Cinnamomum verum*) and lemongrass (*Cymbopogon citratus*) essential oils and their constituents against two phytopathogenic fungi. *Pestic Biochem Physiol.* 2020;168:104644.
150. Kim JE, Lee JE, Huh MJ, Lee SC, Seo SM, Kwon JH, Park IK. Fumigant antifungal activity via reactive oxygen species of *Thymus vulgaris* and *Satureja hortensis* essential oils and constituents against *Raffaelea quercus-mongolicae* and *Rhizoctonia solani. Biomolecules.* 2019; 9(10):561.
151. Li M, Zhu L, Zhang T, Liu B, Du L, Jin Y. Pulmonary delivery of tea tree oil-β-cyclodextrin inclusion complexes for the treatment of fungal and bacterial pneumonia. *J Pharm Pharmacol.* 2017;69(11):1458–1467.
152. Brochot A, Guilbot A, Haddioui L, Roques C. Antibacterial, antifungal, and antiviral effects of three essential oil blends. *Microbiologyopen.* 2017;6(4):e00459.
153. Puškárová A, Bučková M, Kraková L, Pangallo D, Kozics K. The antibacterial and antifungal activity of six essential oils and their cyto/genotoxicity to human HEL 12469 cells. *Sci Rep.* 2017;7(1):8211.

154. Tian F, Lee SY, Chun HS. Comparison of the antifungal and antiaflatoxigenic potential of liquid and vapor phase of *Thymus vulgaris* essential oil against *Aspergillus flavus*. *J Food Prot.* 2019;82(12):2044–2048.
155. Tolba H, Moghrani H, Benelmouffok A, Kellou D, Maachi R. Essential oil of algerian eucalyptus citriodora: Chemical composition, antifungal activity. *J Mycol Med.* 2015;25(4):e128–33.
156. Bismarck D, Dusold A, Heusinger A, Müller E. Antifungal in vitro activity of essential oils against clinical isolates of malassezia pachydermatis from canine ears: A report from a practice laboratory. *Complement Med Res.* 2020;27(3):143–154.
157. Avila-Sosa R, Palou E, Jiménez Munguía MT, Nevárez-Moorillón GV, Navarro Cruz AR, López-Malo A. Antifungal activity by vapor contact of essential oils added to amaranth, chitosan, or starch edible films. *Int J Food Microbiol.* 2012;153(1–2):66–72.
158. Boukhatem MN, Ferhat MA, Kameli A, Saidi F, Kebir HT. Lemon grass (*Cymbopogon citratus*) essential oil as a potent anti-inflammatory and antifungal drugs. *Libyan J Med.* 2014;9(1):25431.
159. Bernardos A, Marina T, Žáček P, Pérez-Esteve É, Martínez-Mañez R, Lhotka M, Kouřimská L, Pulkrábek J, Klou-ek P. Antifungal effect of essential oil components against *Aspergillus niger* when loaded into silica mesoporous supports. *J Sci Food Agric.* 2015;95(14):2824–2831.
160. Liu X, Jia J, Duan S, Zhou X, Xiang A, Lian Z, Ge F. Zein/MCM-41 nanocomposite film incorporated with cinnamon essential oil loaded by modified supercritical CO_2 impregnation for long-term antibacterial packaging. *Pharmaceutics.* 2020;12(2):169.
161. Rogawansamy S, Gaskin S, Taylor M, Pisaniello D. An evaluation of antifungal agents for the treatment of fungal contamination in indoor air environments. *Int J Environ Res Public Health.* 2015;12(6):6319–6332.
162. Fekrazad R, Poorsattar Bejeh Mir A, Ghasemi Barghi V, Shams-Ghahfarokhi M. Eradication of *C. albicans* and *T. rubrum* with photoactivated indocyanine green, *Citrus aurantifolia* essential oil and fluconazole. *Photodiagn Photodyn Ther.* 2015;12(2):289–297.
163. Santomauro F, Donato R, Sacco C, Pini G, Flamini G, Bilia AR. Vapour and liquid-phase artemisia annua essential oil activities against several clinical strains of Candida. *Planta Med.* 2016;82(11–12):1016–1020.
164. Tyagi AK, Malik A. Liquid and vapour-phase antifungal activities of selected essential oils against *Candida albicans*: Microscopic observations and chemical characterization of *Cymbopogon citratus*. *BMC Complement Altern Med.* 2010;10:65.
165. Tyagi AK, Malik A. Antimicrobial action of essential oil vapours and negative air ions against *Pseudomonas fluorescens*. *Int J Food Microbiol.* 2010;143(3):205–210.
166. Tran HNH, Graham L, Adukwu EC. In vitro antifungal activity of *Cinnamomum zeylanicum* bark and leaf essential oils against *Candida albicans* and *Candida auris*. *Appl Microbiol Biotechnol.* 2020;104(20):8911–8924.
167. Hood JR, Burton D, Wilkinson JM, Cavanagh HM. Antifungal activity of *Leptospermum petersonii* oil volatiles against *Aspergillus* spp. in vitro and in vivo. *J Antimicrob Chemother.* 2010;65(2):285–288.
168. Tullio V, Nostro A, Mandras N, Dugo P, Banche G, Cannatelli MA, Cuffini AM, Alonzo V, Carlone NA. Antifungal activity of essential oils against filamentous fungi determined by broth microdilution and vapour contact methods. *J Appl Microbiol.* 2007;102(6):1544–1550.
169. Phillips CA, Laird K, Allen, SC. The use of Citri-V An antimicrobial citrus essential oil vapour for the control of *Penicillium chrysogenum*, *Aspergillus niger* and *Alternaria alternata* in vitro and on food. *Food Res Int.* 2011;47(2):4.
170. Soylu EM, Soylu S, Kurt S. Antimicrobial activities of the essential oils of various plants against tomato late blight disease agent *Phytophthora infestans*. *Mycopathologia.* 2006;161(2):119–128.
171. Dao T, Bensoussan M, Gervais P, Dantigny P. Inactivation of conidia of *Penicillium chrysogenum*, *P. digitatum* and *P. italicum* by ethanol solutions and vapours. *Int J Food Microbiol.* 2008;122(1–2):68–73.
172. Suhr KI, Nielsen PV. Antifungal activity of essential oils evaluated by two different application techniques against rye bread spoilage fungi. *J Appl Microbiol.* 2003;94(4):665–674.
173. Kloucek P, Smid J, Frankova A, Kokoska L, Valterova I, Pavela R. Fast screening method for assessment of antimicrobial activity of essential oils in vapor phase. *Food Res Int.* 2012;47(2):161–165.
174. Seo HS, Beuchat LR, Kim H, Ryu JH. Development of an experimental apparatus and protocol for determining antimicrobial activities of gaseous plant essential oils. *Int J Food Microbiol.* 2015;215:95–100.
175. Kuorwel KK, Cran MJ, Sonneveld K, Miltz J, Bigger SW. Migration of antimicrobial agents from starch-based films into a food simulant. *LWT-Food Sci Technol.* 2013;50 (2):432–438.
176. Martin A, Beutin L. Characteristics of Shiga toxin-producing *Escherichia coli* from meat and milk products of different origins and association with food producing animals as main contamination sources. *Int J Food Microbiol.* 2011;146(1):99–104.
177. Hussain AI, Anwar F, Nigam PS, et al. Antibacterial activity of some Lamiaceae essential oils using resazurin as an indicator of cell growth. *LWT-Food Sci Technol.* 2011;44(4):1199–1206.
178. Weiss J, Gaysinksy S, Davidson M, McClements J. Nanostructured encapsulation systems: Food antimicrobials. In: Barbosa-Cánovas GV, Mortimer A, Lineback D, Spiess W, Buckle K, editors. *IUFoST World Congress Book: Global Issues in Food Science and Technology.* Elsevier, Amsterdam, The Netherlands; 2009:425–479.
179. Hulin V, Mathot AG, Mafart P, Dufossé L. Antimicrobial properties of essential oils and flavour compounds. *Sci Des Aliments.* 1998;18(6):563–582.
180. Nazer AI, Kobilinsky A, Tholozan JL, Dubois-Brissonnet F. Combinations of food antimicrobials at low levels to inhibit the growth of *Salmonella* sv. Typhimurium: A synergistic effect? *Food Microbiol.* 2005;22(5):391–398.
181. Tyagi AK, Malik A. Antimicrobial potential and chemical composition of *Eucalyptus globulus* oil in liquid and vapour phase against food spoilage microorganisms. *Food Chem.* 2011;126(1):228–235.
182. Tyagi AK, Malik A. Antimicrobial potential and chemical composition of *Mentha piperita* oil in liquid and vapour phase against food spoiling microorganisms. *Food Control.* 2011;22(11):1707–1714.

183. López P, Sánchez C, Batlle R, Nerín C. Development of flexible antimicrobial films using essential oils as active agents. *J Agric Food Chem.* 2007;55(21):8814–8824.
184. Donsì F, Annunziata M, Sessa M, Ferrari G. Nanoencapsulation of essential oils to enhance their antimicrobial activity in foods. *LWT-Food Sci Technol.* 2011;44(9): 1908–1914.
185. Popovici J, Bertrand C, Bagnarol E, Fernandez MP, Compte G Chemical composition of essential oil and headspace-solid microextracts from fruits of *Myrica gale* L. and antifungal activity. *Nat Prod Res.* 2008;22:1024–1032.
186. Tranchida PQ, Presti ML, Costa R, Dugo P, Dugo G, Mondello L. High-throughput analysis of bergamot essential oil by fast solid-phase microextraction-capillary gas chromatography-flame ionization detection. *J Chromatogr A.* 2006;1136:162–165.
187. Socaci SA, Tofană M, Socaciu C, Semeniuc C. Optimization of HS/GC–MS method for the determination of volatile compounds from indigenous rosemary. *J Agric Process Technol.* 2009;15:45–49.
188. Baránková E, Dohnal V. Effect of additive on volatility of aroma compounds from dilute aqueous solutions. *Fluid Phase Equilib.* 2016;407:217–223.
189. Herz RS. Aromatherapy facts and fictions: A scientific analysis of olfactory effects on mood, physiology and behavior. *Int J Neurosci.* 2009;119:263–290.
190. Ndao DH, Ladas EJ, Cheng B, Sands SA, Snyder KT, Garvin JH, Kelly KM. Inhalation aromatherapy in children and adolescents undergoing stem cell infusion: Results of a placebo-controlled double-blind trial. *Psychooncology.* 2012;21:247–254.
191. Bhatia S. History and scope of plant biotechnology. In: *Modern Applications of Plant Biotechnology in Pharmaceutical Sciences.* Academic Press; 2015:1–30.
192. Bhatia S. Plant tissue culture. In: *Modern Applications of Plant Biotechnology in Pharmaceutical Sciences.* Academic Press; 2015:31–107.
193. Bhatia S. Laboratory organization. In: *Modern Applications of Plant Biotechnology in Pharmaceutical Sciences.* Academic Press; 2015:109–120.
194. Bhatia S. Concepts and techniques of plant tissue culture science. In: *Modern Applications of Plant Biotechnology in Pharmaceutical Sciences.* Academic Press; 2015:121–156.
195. Bhatia S. Application of plant biotechnology. In: *Modern Applications of Plant Biotechnology in Pharmaceutical Sciences.* Academic Press; 2015:157–207.
196. Bhatia S. Somatic embryogenesis and organogenesis. In: *Modern Applications of Plant Biotechnology in Pharmaceutical Sciences.* Academic Press; 2015:209–230.
197. Bhatia S. Classical and nonclassical techniques for secondary metabolite production in plant cell culture. In: *Modern Applications of Plant Biotechnology in Pharmaceutical Sciences.* Academic Press; 2015:231–291.
198. Bhatia S, Al-Harrasi A, Behl T, Anwer MK, Ahmed MM, Mittal V, Kaushik D, Chigurupati S, Kabir MT, Sharma PB, Chaugule B, Vargas-de-la-Cruz C. Unravelling the photoprotective effects of freshwater alga Nostoc commune Vaucher ex Bornet et Flahault against ultraviolet radiations. *Environ Sci Pollut Res Int.* 2021.
199. Bhatia S. Plant-based biotechnological products with their production host, modes of delivery systems, and stability testing. In: *Modern Applications of Plant Biotechnology in Pharmaceutical Sciences.* Academic Press; 2015:293–331.
200. Bhatia S. Edible vaccines. In: *Modern Applications of Plant Biotechnology in Pharmaceutical Sciences.* Academic Press; 2015:333–343.
201. Bhatia S. Microenvironmentation in micropropagation. In: *Modern Applications of Plant Biotechnology in Pharmaceutical Sciences.* Academic Press; 2015:345–360.
202. Bhatia S. Micropropagation. In: *Modern Applications of Plant Biotechnology in Pharmaceutical Sciences.* Academic Press; 2015:361–368.
203. Bhatia S. Laws in plant biotechnology. In: *Modern Applications of Plant Biotechnology in Pharmaceutical Sciences.* Academic Press; 2015:369–391.
204. Bhatia S. Technical glitches in micropropagation. In: *Modern Applications of Plant Biotechnology in Pharmaceutical Sciences.* Academic Press; 2015:393–404.
205. Bhatia S. Plant tissue culture-based industries. In: *Modern Applications of Plant Biotechnology in Pharmaceutical Sciences.* Academic Press; 2015:405–417.
206. Bhatia S, Al-Harrasi A, Behl T, Anwer MK, Ahmed MM, Mittal V, Kaushik D, Chigurupati S, Kabir MT, Sharma PB, Chaugule B, Vargas-de-la-Cruz C. Anti-migraine activity of freeze dried-latex obtained from *Calotropis Gigantea* Linn. *Environ Sci Pollut Res Int.* 2021.

14

Antibacterial Interactions between EOs and Currently Employed Antibiotics

Ahmed Al-Harrasi
Natural and Medical Sciences Research Center, University of Nizwa

Saurabh Bhatia
Natural and Medical Sciences Research Center, University of Nizwa
University of Petroleum and Energy Studies

Tapan Behl
Chitkara University

Deepak Kaushik
M.D. University

Vineet Mittal
M.D. University

Ajay Sharma
Delhi Pharmaceutical Sciences and Research University

CONTENTS

14.1 Introduction

Due to the development of multidrug-resistant bacteria especially from nosocomial and community sources modern antibiotics are encountering considerable challenges. These major challenges are raising significant health concerns. One of the most threatening classes of drug-resistant microorganisms is *Enterococcus faecium, Staphylococcus aureus, Klebsiella pneumoniae, Acinetobacter baumannii, Pseudomonas aeruginosa, Enterobacter spp.*, and *Escherichia coli* (ESKAPEE). The World Health Organization has designated these microbial pathogens as a high priority for the development of novel therapeutics due to high levels of intrinsic (innate ability) and acquired antimicrobial resistome [1]. As has been reported, due to inaccessibility to safe, effective, and novel antibiotics we are approaching a "post-antibiotic era" where antimicrobials will have completely lost their effectiveness against drug-resistant superbugs. Thus, there is an urgent requirement for safe, effective, and reliable therapeutics from natural resources, which can be considered as safe and effective antimicrobial agents. Recent reports have shown that essential oils (EOs) can offer promising results against antimicrobial-resistant microbes [1]. An EO is a complex mixture of components with broad-spectrum mechanisms of action targeting detrimental factors

DOI: 10.1201/9781003175933-16

that contribute to pathogenicity such as drug resistance. Plants also produce EOs to protect from microbes that are pathogenic to plants. Even an infected plant has an effective antimicrobial system made of EOs against respective microbes, ultimately to sustain or to withstand against harsh microbial conditions. Recent reports have shown that EOs can directly kill pathogenic microorganisms by reactivating failed antibiotics. EOs have also been recently reported to increase antibiotic susceptibility and reverse antibiotic resistance.

Numerous reports are available showing the positive effects of interactions between EOs and currently used antibiotics (Table 14.1). As reported, an interaction between EO and antibiotics could be additive, synergistic, or antagonistic; thus, careful selection as well as optimization is required before its use. The synergistic effect of EOs with current antibiotics could be employed to improve antibiotic susceptibility. Thus, this type of interaction could improve the efficacy of antibiotic to allow its reutilization with EO against resistant bacteria. EO as a multicomponent system with antibiotics acts at various cellular sites of resistant microorganism to counteract its resistance in order to produce effective antimicrobial effects [20]. The checkerboard assay method is often used to determine the antimicrobial synergistic effects by comparing combinations prepared with individual antimicrobial activities. This comparison is then signified as the fractional inhibitory concentration (FIC) index value. Generally, when used with EOs, the checkerboard method is used to quantify the efficacy of an EO or its components in combination with classical antibiotics. However, various types of interactions can be studied by using the checkerboard method such as EO-EO, EO-EO component, EO-antibiotics, EO component-antibiotics, and EO-EO component-antibiotics. The FIC is calculated and interpreted as synergy, addition, indifferent, or antagonism. Based on the FIC value, interaction could be synergistic (FIC=<0.5), antagonistic (FIC=<4), and additive or indifference (FIC=0.5–4). Synergistic effect signifies an increase in the inhibitory activity (decrease in MIC) of one or both components than with the component alone, whereas antagonistic interaction represents the combination of compounds that increases the MIC, or lowers the activity of the compounds. However, the additive effect signifies that the combination that has no increase in inhibitory activity or a slight increase in inhibitory activity due to the additive effect of both compounds considered. Synergy checkerboard assay or synergy time-kill-kinetic assay is usually performed to depict the synergy identified in the microdilution assay. This method can also determine whether the combination has bacteriostatic or bactericidal effects. The objective of this assay is to determine that how the combination of compounds influences the growth of bacteria. This is done by determining the rate of killing of the compounds. Checkerboard tests, isobolograms and time-kill assays can be used to determine antagonistic, synergistic and additive interactions. Isobolographic analysis is also used to determine whether antimicrobial effects are induced by mixtures of compounds that are more, equivalent, or less than individual compound effects and to assess the different interactions. EO interactions with antibiotics against the considered microbial strains can be assessed by microdilution checkerboard assay in combination with chemometric methods (principal components analysis and hierarchical cluster analysis). For instance, using similar protocol interactions of the *Libanotis montana* EO (LMEO) with antimicrobials such as chloramphenicol, tetracycline, and streptomycin and against different microbial strains was assessed. It was found that *L. montana* EO displayed a minor antibacterial effect against the microbial strains *in vitro*; however, their blend with antimicrobials such as LMEO with chloramphenicol and LMEO with tetracycline possessed typically either synergistic or additive actions [21]. These blends help in decreasing the minimum effective dose of the antimicrobials to further reduce any possible toxicities. In contrast, the LMEO blend with streptomycin displayed considerable antagonistic action against *E.coli* [21].

TABLE 14.1

Antimicrobial Interactions between Essential Oils and Antibiotics

EOs	Pathogens	Interaction	References
Ajowan EOthymol and amoxicillin	Methicillin-resistant *Staph. Aureus*	Synergistic effects	[2]
Ajowan EO and ciprofloxacin	*P. aeruginosa, S. pneumoniae* (penicillin resistant), *S. aureus*,	Synergistic effects	[2]
Thymol and ciprofloxacin	*P. aeruginosa* ATCC 27853 and P-resistant *Strep. pneumoniae*	Synergistic effects	[2]
Coriander EO with antibiotics (oxacillin, amoxicillin, gentamicin, ciprofloxacin, tetracycline)	*P. aeruginosa, E. coli,* (methicillin-susceptible and methicillin-resistant) *S. aureus, S. epidermidis)*	Abs resistance reversal activity, Marked decrease in MIC of Abs, Increase in Abs susceptibility	[3]
Blend of eucalyptus, dill, coriander, and cilantro EO	Gram-negative as well as Gram-positive pathogen and Brewer's Yeast	Synergistic, antagonistic, additive, effects	[4]
Pannarin blended with antibiotics	*S. aureus* (methicillin-resistant)	Moderate synergistic action and antagonism	[5]
Tea tree EO with gentamicin	*Acinetobacter baumannii* strain	Synergistic interactions (*Aniba rosaeodoral* gentamicin and *Pelargonium graveolens*/ gentamicin) and improve the antimicrobial effectiveness	[6]
Myrtle EO with ciprofloxacin	Multidrug-resistant *Acinetobacter baumanni*	Synergistic effects	[7]

(*Continued*)

TABLE 14.1 (*Continued*)

Antimicrobial Interactions between Essential Oils and Antibiotics

EOs	Pathogens	Interaction	References
Longbeak eucalyptus EO with polymyxin B, gentamicin, and ciprofloxacin,	*Acinetobacter baumannii* (multidrug-resistant)	Synergistic effects	[8]
Coriander EO with tetracycline, ciprofloxacin, chloramphenicol, and gentamicin	*Acinetobacter baumannii*	Additive effect resensitized *A. baumannii* to the action of chloramphenicol marked decrease in MIC	[9]
Citrus limon & *Cinnamomum zeylanicum* with amikacin, imipenem, meropenem, and gentamicin	Multidrug-resistant Acinetobacter spp	Additive effect marked decrease in MIC synergistic effect	[10]
Lemon EO with Abs	Multidrug-resistant *Acinetobacter spp.*	Marked decrease in MIC of Abs Synergistic effect An additive effect	[10]
Ajwain and Mint EOs mixed with Abs	*Staphylococcus aureus, Enterococcus faecalis, Escherichia coli, Pseudomonas aeruginosa, Staphylococcus epidermidis,* and *Listeria monocytogenes*	Decreased MIC potent synergistic effect	[11]
Salvia sclarea	*Tetracycline*	Synergistic effect against *S. epidermidis*	[12]
Cinnamon (Cinnamomun verum)	*Piperacillin*	Synergistic effect against *E. coli*	[13]
Sage EO	*Tetracycline*	Synergistic effect against *S. epidermidis*	[14]
Eucalyptus EO	*Ciprofloxacin*	Synergistic effect against *A. baumnanii*	[15]
Eugenia jambolana	*Amikacin*	*Antagonistic effect against S. aureus*	[16]
Salvia fruticosa EO	*Tetracycline*	Synergistic effect against *S. epidermidis*	[14]
Lavender (Lavandula officinalis)	*Piperacillin*	Synergistic effect against *E. coli*	[13]
Rosemary (R. officinalis)	*Ciprofloxacin*	Synergistic effect against *K. pneumoniae*	[17]
Savoury (Satureja kitaibelii)	*Chloramphenicol* Chloramphenicol, tetracycline, Chloramphenicol, tetracycline, Chloramphenicol	Synergistic effect against *E. coli, K. pneumonia, P. mirabilis*	[18]
Tea tree (M. alternifolia)	*Ciprofloxacin*	Synergistic effect against *K. pneumoniae*	[17]
Thyme (T. broussonetii)	Cefixime Ciprofloxacin Gentamicin Pristinamycin	Synergistic effect against *B. cereus, B. subtilis, E. cloaceae, E. coli, V. cholera, S. aureus*	[19]
Thyme (T. maroccanus)	Cefixime Ciprofloxacin Gentamicin Pristinamycin	Synergistic effect against *B. cereus, V. cholera, S. aureus, P. aeruginosa, M. leuteus, K. pneumonia, E. coli, E. cloaceae, B. subtilis*	[19]
Thyme (T. vulgaris)	*Ciprofloxacin*	Synergistic effect against *K. pneumoniae*	[17]
Peppermint (M. piperita)	Meropenem, piperacillin, ciprofloxacin	Synergistic effect against *E. coli, K. pneumonia, S. aureus*	[13]

14.2 Role of Essential Oils as Antibacterial Agents

Monocomponent, binary, and tertiary emulsions have been tested, and were used against different microorganisms that cause infections in humans. Recently clove, bergamote, and orange have been used in different combinations as monocomponent, binary, or tertiary emulsions against *Candida albicans, Candida parapsilosis, Escherichia coli, Haemophilus influenzae, Pseudomonas aeruginosa, Salmonella typhimurium, Shigella flexneri, Staphylococcus aureus,* and *Streptococcus pyogenes.*

Findings from this study showed that the monocomponent emulsion had antimicrobial activity, whereas orange and bergamote were not able to prevent the growth of the microorganisms [22]. Among binary or tertiary blends of EOs such as bergamote/clove, clove/orange, and orange/bergamote/clove, clove EO showed more antimicrobial effects owing to the synergistic interactions possessed by the oil's components [22].

Recently, the interaction of norfloxacin with *Cinnamomum zeylanicum, Mentha piperita, Origanum vulgare,* and *Thymus vulgaris* EOs was found to be the most effective in all the tested combinations against the Gram-positive bacteria-forming biofilms. The synergistic effects were tested through the checkerboard microdilution method [23].

Findings obtained from another report showed that *Melaleuca alternifolia, Thymus vulgaris, Mentha piperita,* and *Rosmarinus officinalis* EOs when combined with ciprofloxacin against *Staphylococcus aureus* showed antagonistic effects. Depending on the combined ratio, the same combination against *Klebsiella pneumoniae* showed antagonistic, synergistic, and additive effects. More interestingly, *Rosmarinus officinalis*/ciprofloxacin combination against *K. pneumoniae* showed the most favorable synergistic pattern. *M. alternifolia* (tea tree), *T. vulgaris* (thyme), *M. piperita* (peppermint), and *R. officinalis* (rosemary) EOs with amphotericin B displayed antagonistic effects when tested against *Candida albicans* [17].

It has also been shown that in combination with antimicrobials, EOs comprising chemical components such as thymol, eugenol, cinnamic acid, cinnamaldehyde, and carvacrol showed synergistic effect. Previous reports showed that EOs and antibiotics work together and have synergistic effect against pathogenic microorganism by acting at multiple targets or via physicochemical interactions or by preventing antibacterial-resistant mechanisms. Thus, the broad-spectrum antibacterial activity exhibited by EOs can be utilized to strengthen the efficacy of main-course antibiotics in order to improve the efficacy of the whole therapy [24].

A recent study showed synergistic interactions between coriander EO/linalool and antibiotics against methicillin-resistant *Staphylococcus aureus*, Gram-positive bacteria (*methicillin-susceptible S. aureus, S. epidermidis*), and Gram-negative bacteria (*Pseudomonas aeruginosa, Escherichia coli*). Further increase in antibiotic susceptibility and reversal of antibiotic resistance were also demonstrated. This type of blend of coriander EO/linalool and antibiotics could be considered as one of the most effective antibacterials [25].

A recent report also demonstrated synergistic interactions between coriander EO/linalool and antibiotics against methicillin-resistant *Staphylococcus aureus*, Gram-positive bacteria (methicillin-susceptible *S. aureus, S. epidermidis*), and Gram-negative bacteria (*Pseudomonas aeruginosa, Escherichia coli*). Also, this combination increases antibiotic susceptibility and reverses antibiotic resistance [26].

Additionally, reports also showed that out of all tested combinations, the coriander (linalool)/cumin seed oil (p-coumaric acid) blend demonstrated synergistic interactions in antibacterial as well as antioxidant effects. Moreover, this blend did not show cytotoxic action in brine shrimp lethality bioassays as well as colon cell line (normal) assays [27].

In another report, checkerboard testing and isobolographic analysis showed that combinations of EOs (*Thymus vulgaris, Pinus sylvestris, and Origanum vulgare*) demonstrated synergistic effect against azole-susceptible *Cryptococcusneoformans.* It was also found that itraconazole with *Thymus vulgaris* EO carvacrol showed synergistic effect against azole-non-susceptible *Cryptococcus neoformans* strain. Synergistic interaction between itraconazole and *Origanum vulgare* or *Thymus vulgaris* EO against azole-susceptible *Cryptococcus neoformans* was also established by time-kill kinetics assay. Against azole-non-susceptible *Cryptococcus neoformans* binary blend of itraconazole/thyme EO or carvacrol showed additive interaction [28].

Recently, antibacterial effects of *Petroselinum crispum, Levisticum officinale, Ocimum basilicum*, and *Thymus vulgaris* EOs alone as well as in mixture were evaluated against various foodborne Gram-positive and Gram-negative bacteria. It was found that *Levisticum officinale/Thymus vulgaris* and *Ocimum basilicum/Thymus vulgaris* EOs in combination showed antagonistic activity against all microbes. Similar effects were noticed with a combination of *Petroselinum crispum/Thymus vulgaris* EOs against *Staphylococcus aureus, Escherichia coli, Pseudomonas aeruginosa, and Bacillus cereus* and *Levisticum officinale/Ocimum basilicum* EOs against *Bacillus cereus as well as Escherichia coli.* It was found that *Petroselinum crispum/Levisticum officinale* and *Petroselinum crispum/Ocimum basilicum* EOs possessed poor effects against all microbes. Additionally, thyme EO displayed the highest antimicrobial effects in comparison to other preparations and its blend with *Petroselinum crispum, Levisticum officinale*, and *Ocimum basilicum* showed attenuation in antimicrobial effects. Thus, it's always suggested to use thyme EO only as an antimicrobial agent [29].

Synergic, additive, or antagonist effects were observed with antibacterial activity of *Rosmarinus officinalis, Coriandrum sativum L., Micromeria fruticosa, Cuminum cyminum,* and *Mentha piperita* EOs against *Micrococcus luteus, Bacillus megaterium, Bacillus brevis, Enterococcus faecalis, Pseudomonas pyocyaneus, Mycobacterium smegmatis, Escherichia coli, Aeromonas hydrophila, Yersinia enterocolitica, Staphylococcus aureus, Streptococcus faecalis bacteria, Saccharomyces cerevisiae,* and *Kluyveromyces fragilis* fungi [30].

In another study, flow cytometry results showed that the *Origanum vulgare* EO causes destabilization and rupture of the bacterial cell membrane succeeding in apoptosis of *Acinetobacter baumannii.* Checkerboard assay results showed the synergic interaction between *Origanum vulgare* EO and polymyxin B (FICI: 0.18–0.37). When combined, *Origanum vulgare* EO showed 16-fold reduction of the polymyxin B MIC. Findings showed that *Origanum vulgare* EO used alone or in combination with polymyxin B in the treatment of multidrug-resistant clinical isolates of *Acinetobacter baumannii* infections is promising [31].

Synergistic interaction between more than one EO (EO–EO interaction) was also found, which can ultimately impact the resultant antimicrobial effect of the blend. Recently, a binary combination of two *Moroccan EOs, Pelargonium asperum* EOs, and *Ormenis mixta* EOs against *Staphylococcus aureus* showed a promising synergistic antibacterial interaction calculated by using the FIC index. Furthermore, based on the findings obtained from zones of growth inhibition and the minimum inhibitory concentration values, it was found that *P. asperum* EO was more active than *O. mixta* EO [32].

A recent investigation also showed that cinnamon/clove oil combination showed a synergistic antibacterial activity against foodborne bacteria (*Staphylococcus aureus, Listeria monocytogenes, Salmonella typhimurium,* and *Pseudomonas aeruginosa*) and synergistic antifungal activity against *Aspergillus niger* as well as synergistic antioxidant potential in DPPH radical scavenging model system. Additionally, it was also found that the cinnamon/clove oil combination did not show any cytotoxic potential at the recommended dosage level (IC50 > 2,000 μg/mL) [33].

Melaleuca alternifolia, Mentha piperita, and *Origanum vulgare* EOs displayed antimicrobial activity against *Pythium insidiosum*, which is the etiologic agent of pythiosis, and the greatest activity of *O. vulgare* was reported. Synergistic and/or indifferent effects were found for all combinations; mainly *M. piperita* and *O. vulgare* combination showed 65% synergism [34].

It has been recently reported that *Pistacia lentiscus, Teucrium ramosissimum,* and *Pituranthos chloranthus* alone as well as their mixture with antimicrobial agents effectively reduced the resistance of methicillin-resistant *Staphylococcus aureus* totetracycline, piperacillin, oxacillin, ofloxacin, and amoxicillin. Also, these EOs alone as well as in blend form reduced the resistance of *Acinetobacter baumannii* to amoxicillin as well as ofloxacin by interacting with each other way. In addition, these findings proved the synergistic interaction between EOs and antimicrobial agents novobiocin as well as ofloxacin against the enzymes (extended-spectrum beta-lactamase) produced by *Escherichia coli* [35].

An antibacterial effect of traditional spices (ajowan EO) in combination with conventional antibiotics to treat lower respiratory tract pathogens showed synergistic effects. Ajowan EO/thymol showed synergistic effects with amoxicillin against methicillin-resistant *Staphylococcus aureus* clinical isolates. EO with ciprofloxacin also showed synergistic effects against *P. aeruginosa, Staphylococcus Aureus,* and penicillin (P)-resistant *Streptococcus pneumoniae* bacteria [36].

Laurus nobilis and *Prunus armeniaca* EOs showed considerable antimicrobial effects against Gram-negative bacteria (*Escherichia coli and Pseudomonas aeruginosa*), Gram-positive bacteria (*M. luteus, S. aureus, B. subtilis*), and yeasts (*C. albicans, C. glabrata, C. krusei, and C. parapsilosis*). A recent study showed that the combination of EOs with ciprofloxacin, vancomycin, and fluconazole resulted in a significant decrease in their individual MICs by mainly showing a synergistic effect; however, some showed only partial synergistic effects. *Laurus nobilis* EO possessed the highest synergistic effect with all the antibiotics used, with FIC index values in the range of 0.266–0.75 for bacteria and between 0.258 and 0.266 for yeast [37].

Another study also demonstrated that synergistic interactions between lavender EO and meropenem were noticed, which considerably decreased the inhibitory concentration of both lavender EO and meropenem by 15- and 4-fold, respectively. Further disruption in the bacterial membrane via oxidative stress was observed along with a change in cell surface charge with a considerable increase in membrane permeability when exposed to LVO. Overall, it was found that lavender EO triggered oxidative stress in *K. pneumonia* resulting in outer membrane damage, which may further allow the influx of ROS, lavender EO, and meropenem into the bacterial cells, resulting in damage to the cells and ultimately cell death [38].

A study suggested that MexEF-OprN and mexXY-OprM (efflux pumps) are responsible for resistance of *Pseudomonas aeruginosa* (*P. aeruginosa*) against antibiotics. A recent study demonstrated that *Satureja khuzistanica* EO reduced the expression of efflux pump genes of *P. aeruginosa*. It was also found that *Satureja khuzistanica* EO showed synergistic effects with norfloxacin and gentamicin. Thus, *Satureja khuzistanica* EO reduced the MIC values of norfloxacin and gentamicin *in vitro* [39].

Recently, the antibacterial activity of cinnamon EO alone and in combination with some classical antibiotics against three multidrug-resistant bacteria, *Escherichia coli, Staphylococcus aureus,* and *Pseudomonas aeruginosa*, was investigated by agar disk diffusion and minimum inhibitory concentration assays. EO-chloramphenicol against *E. coli* and EO-ampicillin or chloramphenicol displayed a synergistic interaction against *S. aureus*. Nevertheless, EO-streptomycin showed additive effects against all bacteria stains [40].

Filipendula vulgaris leaf EO consists of salicylaldehyde, which was investigated for its antimicrobial potential by the disk diffusion and microdilution broth assays. It was also found that changing chemical components resulted in synergistic as well as antagonistic interaction. Synergistic effects were found in salicylaldehyde/linalool mixtures with a maximum interaction in the range between 60:40 and 80:20 (mol ratio), whereas an antagonistic relationship was found at a ratio of 40:60 between salicylaldehyde and methyl salicylate [41].

Nepeta nuda EO-antibiotic and 1,8-cineole-antibiotic were found to produce primarily antagonistic interactions as a result of membrane potential/proton motive force dissipation [42].

Dittrichia graveolens EO possessed minor antibacterial effects against the tested bacterial strains *in vitro*; however, *D. graveolens* EO in combination with chloramphenicol and *Dittrichia graveolens* in combination with tetracycline displayed synergistic or additive interactions. Additionally, a minimum effective dose of the antibiotics as well as adverse side effects was reduced using this combination. However, *D. graveolens* EO and streptomycin displayed strong antagonistic interactions against *E. coli, S. aureus*, and *P. aeruginosa* [43].

From the above reports, it's clear that apart from synergistic or partial synergistic effects or addition effects, predominant antagonistic interactions were also reported, which is a major concern. For antagonistic interactions, EOs should be used carefully when combined with antibiotics. For instance, *Melaleuca alternifolia, Thymus vulgaris, Mentha piperita,* and *Rosmarinus officinalis* EOs when combined with ciprofloxacin against *Staphylococcus aureus* showed antagonistic profiles. However, the same combination when tested against *Klebsiella pneumoniae* showed antagonistic, synergistic, and additive interactions depending on the combined ratio. *R. officinalis* EO in combination with ciprofloxacin against *K. pneumoniae* presented the most favorable synergistic effects. *M. alternifolia, T. vulgaris, M. piperita*, and *R. officinalis* EOs with amphotericin B showed antagonistic effects when tested against *Candida albicans* [44].

Combinations of anti-inflammatory drugs, analgesic drugs, and other drugs with EOs have also been reported to induce significant interactions. For instance in traditional medicine, rosemary has been used as mild analgesic for treating renal colic pain and dysmenorrhea. However, some EOs individually at high dose showed more efficacies than in combinations. For instance, rosemary EO in the dose of 20 mg/kg was shown to be more efficient than in the dose of 10 mg/kg, in combinations with both codeine and paracetamol [45].

14.3 Antibacterial Interactions between EO Components and Currently Employed Antibiotics

Inappropriate and disproportionate use of antibiotics is contributing immensely to the development of antibiotic resistance in bacterial or fungal strains. The use of EOs in combination can be a potent alternative strategy to inactivate these pathogens. Recently, various isolated EO components have been studied for antibacterial interactions with antibiotics (Table 14.2). A number of EO components such as eugenol, cinnamaldehyde, and β-caryophyllene, individually as well as in blend form, have been tested against preformed biofilms as well as biofilm formation of *Salmonella typhimurium and Listeria monocytogenes*. It was found that among all EO components tested, cinnamaldehyde as well as eugenol alone showed >50% degradation in biofilm biomass against both bacteria, while β-caryophyllene failed to do so. Additionally, cinnamaldehyde/eugenol combination showed a synergistic antibiofilm efficacy against preformed biofilms of both the studied bacteria, while other tested combinations showed an additive antibiofilm efficacy. It was found that individual EO components alone as well in combination also showed much higher inhibition effect on biofilm formation at the initial stage in comparison with their inhibition effect on preformed biofilms [69].

TABLE 14.2
Biological Interactions between EOs and Drugs

EO/CC	Activity	Drug Name	References
Chenopodium ambrosioides	Antileishmanial effect (synergic) against promastigotes of *Leishmania amazonensis*	Pentamidine	[46]
Peppermint oil	Prolongation of pentobarbitone-induced sleeping time	Pentobarbitone	[47]
Peppermint oil	Increase sedative	Midazolam	[47]
Peppermint oil	Decrease of analgesic effect	Codeine	[47]
Anise (*Pimpinella anisum* L.; Apiaceae)	Considerable rise in analgesic activity	Codeine	[48]
	Augmented effect of drug on motor activity	Diazepam	
	Motor damage induced via midazolam has been increased	Midazolam	
	Considerable decrease in sleeping duration caused by pentobarbital	Pentobarbital	
	Decrease in antidepressant effect has been reduced via prior treatment with oil	Imipramine	
	Decrease in antidepressant effect has been reduced via prior treatment with oil	Fluoxetine	
	Considerable reduction in the level of acetaminophen in the plasma Decrease of total drug exposure following oral administration	Acetaminophen	[49]
	Absorption rate of caffeine administered via oral route considerably reduced following=treatment with EO		
Lavender oil	Increased the static phase in rodent treated with caffeine	Caffeine (for induction of over-agitation)	[50]
Hyssop oil	-	Caffeine (for induction of over-agitation)	[50]
Ginger, thyme, peppermint and *Cupressus sempervirens* oil	Resulted in 5%–22% reduction of immobility	Caffeine (for induction of over-agitation)	[50]
T. eigii EO (0.5 μL)	Antagonistic effect against all bacteria	Vancomycin	[51]
T. eigii EO (0.5 μl)	Antagonistic effect n in all the tested bacteria	Erythromycin	[51]
R. officinalis	Antagonistic effect	Gentamicin	[52]
	Synergic effect against *S. aureus*	Cephalothin antibiotic	[52]
	Additive effect	Ceftriaxone antibiotic	[52]
C. sativum	Antagonistic effect	Gentamicin	[52]
C. sativum	Antagonistic effect	Cephalothin	[52]
C. sativum	Synergistic response against *M. smegmatis* and *S. aureus*	Ceftriaxone	[52]
Cuminum cyminum	Synergistic response against *A. hydrophila* and *P. pyocyaneus*	Gentamicin	[52]
	Synergistic response against *S. aureus, P. pyocyaneus,* and *A. hydrophila*	Cephalothin	[52]
	Synergistic response against *A. hydrophila, P. pyocyaneus, and Y. enterocolitica*	Ceftriaxone	[52]
Micromeria fruticosa	Synergistic response against seen in *M. smegmatis, B. brevis, M. luteus, Y. enterocolitica, and E. faecalis*	Gentamicin	[52]
Micromeria fruticosa	Additive effect was seen in *A. hydrophila*	Gentamicin	[52]
Micromeria fruticosa	Synergistic effect in *M. luteus, S. aureus, Y. enterocolitica,* and *A. hydrophila*	Ceftriaxone	[52]
Cinnamon oil	Additive effects *Escherichia coli, Staphylococcus aureus*, and *Pseudomonas aeruginosa*	Antibiotics	[53]
α-Terpineol	Synergistic properties in colon cancer cells, inhibiting NF-κB expression and resulting in apoptosis	Linalyl acetate	[54]

(Continued)

TABLE 14.2 (*Continued*)

Biological Interactions between EOs and Drugs

EO/CC	Activity	Drug Name	References
Eucalyptol	Synergism (cytotoxic activity)	Geraniol	[55]
β-Caryophyllene	Synergistic antinociceptive interaction	Morphine	[56]
Geophila repens EO	Synergistic effect (*Escherichia coli*)	Streptomycin	[57]
Lemon Beebrush and *Lippia sp.*	Synergistic effect as well as reduced minimum bactericidal concentration	Florfenicol	[58]
Camphor	19-fold increase in penetration through the larval integument (Cabbage Looper)	1,8-Cineole	[59]
Eugenol (EUG), carvacrol (CAR), thymol (TYH), p-cymene (CYM), and γ-terpinene (TER)	Synergistic effect	Tetracycline	[60]
Piperine	Synergic response with rifampicin against *S. aureus*	Piperlongumine	[61]
Piperine	Synergistic effect against *S. aureus*	Tetracycline	[61]
Piperlongumine	Antagonistic interaction against *S. aureus*	Tetracycline	[61]
Piperamide	Antagonistic interaction against *P. aeruginosa*	Rifampicin, tetracycline, and itraconazole	[61]
Piperine	Synergistic interaction against *P. aeruginosa*	Rifampicin	[61]
Cinnamomum tamala	Antibiofilm against *P. aeruginosa* biofilms	DNase (DNaseI) and a DNase (MBD) isolated from a marine bacterium	[62]
Cinnamon bark	Synergistic effect against *Listeria monocytogenes*	Thyme thymol EO gases	[63]
Oregano	Synergistic effect against *Listeria monocytogenes*	Thyme thymol EO gases	[63]
Cinnamon EO loaded chitosan film	Synergic response against *P. digitatum, E.coli, S. aureus, A.oryzae*	Chitosan	[64]
Schinus lentiscifolius EO	Against dermatophytes	Terbinafine and ciclopirox	[65]
Cinnamon bark EO	Additive interaction to disrupt bacterial membrane	Meropenem	[66]
Ocimum basilicum	Synergism effect (antifungal activity)	Fluconazole	[67]
Cinnamon	Synergism effect against *Streptococcus mutans*	Clove, bergamote, and orange	[68]

Recently, antibacterial activity of the blend of thyme, red thyme, oregano as well as cinnamon and their active constituents (thymol, cinnamaldehyde, and carvacrol) with antibiotics (trimethoprim–sulfamethoxazole, penicillin, oxytetracycline, and gentamicin) against Gram-positive bacterium *Streptococcus suis* (swine pathogen) was evaluated. It was found that all the antimicrobials showed a synergistic or additive effect with at least one of the four EOs. Additionally, it was also revealed that the blends of the antimicrobials with the EOs demonstrated good outcomes in comparison to the blends of the antimicrobials with the chemical constituents; however, no antagonist interactions were found. The most definite interaction between antimicrobial agents (oxytetracycline and gentamicin) and oregano, cinnamon, or thyme suggested that this blend can be used as alternative to control *Streptococcus suis* infections [70].

Thyme EO contains carvacrol, thymol, and linalool that show antimicrobial activity. Blends of the carvacrol/linalool and thymol/linalool showed additive antimicrobial effect in a previous study. An increase of the carvacrol oil concentration from one to two times the MIC resulted in considerable acceleration of the kill rate. The antimicrobial activity of thyme EO was partially due to additive effects, which could enhance the rapidity of the antimicrobial action [71].

In an earlier study, *Origanum vulgare* L. EO and its components (carvacrol and thymol) were tested for their capability to modulate antibiotic resistance against *S. aureus* (specifically against tetracycline, erythromycin and norfloxacin). It was revealed that EO and its components when blended with tetracycline modulated its antimicrobial activity, decreased MIC further and via possibly acting as efflux pump inhibitors [72].

Fennel EO and trans-anethole combination has influenced the antibacterial activity of mupirocin (antibiotics used to treat certain skin infections) against *S. aureus*. MIC values for mupirocin combined with fennel EO as well as for mupirocin combined with trans-anethole were reduced in comparison with mupirocin alone, suggesting its efficient antistaphylococcal activity [73].

A recent investigation suggested that *Mikania cordifolia* EO and the isolated component limonene do not have clinically considerable antibacterial effect; nevertheless, it modulates the action of antimicrobial agents against multidrug-resistant strains (*Staphylococcus aureus, Escherichia coli*, and *Pseudomonas aeruginosa*) [74].

Another recent study showed synergistic interaction between blends of terpenes (β-elemene, α-pinene, sabinene, myrcene, bisabolol, (S)-limonene, (R)-limonene) with antibiotics (ethambutol or rifampicin). Findings from this study suggested reduction in MIC of rifampicin by (R)-limonene and isabolol against all selected microbes without any synergistic interaction. Further in vitro cytotoxic studies on normal eukaryotic cells revealed less (bisabolol) or no cytotoxic effect [75].

Citrus fruit extracts blended with EO components (carvacrol and thymol) reduced (positive synergistic effects) the growth of all the pathogenic non-acid-adapted/acid-adapted microbes (*Listeria monocytogenes, Salmonella typhimurium, and Escherichia coli* O157:H7).

Further calamansi in combination with EO components (carvacrol and thymol) totally inactivated even the most resistant pathogen (*E. coli* O157:H7). Also, high citric acid level is likely to contribute to the strong synergistic effect with EO components (carvacrol and thymol) by destructing susceptible bacterial membranes [76].

Other reports demonstrated considerable improvement in the activity of chloramphenicol quinolones and β-lactams when blended with geraniol (derived from *Helichrysum italicumone* EO) [77].

A previous study reported the antibacterial effects of thymol, eugenol, berberine, and cinnamaldehyde against *Listeria monocytogenes* and *Salmonella typhimurium,* either alone or in combination with streptomycin. It was found that a combination of thymol and cinnamaldehyde showed a synergistic effect with streptomycin against *L. monocytogenes,* whereas cinnamaldehyde and eugenol demonstrated synergistic effects against *Salm. Typhimurium.* Additionally, it was found that this synergy was enough to eliminate biofilm-formed microorganisms. Therefore, it was concluded that this type of combination of EO components with streptomycin could be effective for the treatment of food-borne pathogens [78].

Recently, blends of EO components (p-coumaric acid and linalool) with bacteriocin (nisin) have been tested for their antibacterial as well as antibiofilm against *Salmonella typhimurium* and *Bacillus cereus.* The synergistic effect was exhibited by p-coumaric acid and nisin against free-swimming cells of bacteria, while an additive effect (against *S. typhimurium*) and synergistic effect (against *Bacillus cereus*) were seen by nisin and linalool. It was also revealed that nisin alone did not show antibiofilm activity, but when blended with linalool and p-coumaric acid it possessed antibiofilm effectiveness more than 50%. Further findings obtained from FIC values suggested additive antibiofilm effects were seen in nisin and linalool blend while nisin and p-coumaric acid blend presented synergistic antibiofilm effects [79].

Recently, the pro-oxidant effects of EO linalool and vitamin C in combination with copper against *Vibrio fluvialis* and *Salmonella enterica* were studied using (3D) checkerboard microdilution assay. The results showed that the triple combination exerted synergistic antibacterial effects compared with the effects of the components alone. Bactericidal effect and an increase in ROS production were the underlying mechanisms of the enhanced antibacterial potency of this combination (linalool, vitamin C, copper). Furthermore, the combination did not display toxicity to human cells, and it effectively reduced the pathogen levels [80].

Eucalyptus globulus fruit EO containing 1,8-cineole and globulol is known for its antimicrobial activities. A previous study showed that 1,8-cineole in combination with aromadendrene demonstrated synergistic effects. *Eucalyptus globulus* fruit EO showed considerable antimicrobial activity against vancomycin-resistant enterococci, *Enterococcus faecalis* as well as methicillin-resistant *Staphylococcus aureus.* Findings showed that aromadendrene might be responsible for the antimicrobial effects, while other components showed fewer effects. The results obtained from time-kill assay showed a synergistic activity whereas checkerboard assay findings demonstrated an additive effect by the blend of aromadendrene and 1,8-cineole [81].

Ciprofloxacin combination with thyme oil and thymol was found to enhance antibiotic activity and affect the biofilm cell viability. The observed inhibitory/eradication activity on *K. pneumoniae* biofilms was reported. It was concluded that thyme and peppermint EOs, and their active components, are promising antibiofilm agents alone and/or in combination with ciprofloxacin to inhibit/eradicate biofilms of *K. pneumonia* [82].

Trichophyton (*T. erinacei, T. mentagrophytes, T. rubrum, T. schoenleinii,* and *T. soudanense*) susceptibility to ketoconazole was significantly improved by combination with the *Agastache rugosa* EO as well as its main component, estragole [83].

Additionally, checkerboard titer test results demonstrated significant combined effects of streptomycin and *O. koreanum* oil or cresol, one of the main components of this oil, against the two streptomycin-resistant strains of *S. typhimurium,* with FICIs ranging from 0.12 to 0.37 [84].

Cinnamon bark EO or cinnamaldehyde can be considered as adjunctive treatment to treat *P. aeruginosa* infections, and it may potentially have antagonistic effects if combined with antibiotics because of Mex pump activation [85].

Cinnamon bark EO and cinnamaldehyde combined with colistin showed synergistic effects against multidrug-resistant *Pseudomonas aeruginosa* [86].

Another recent investigation showed that *V. arborea* EO and the α-bisabolol had a synergistic effect against *Escherichia coli, Staphylococcus aureus, Candida albicans, Candida krusei, Candida tropicalis,* and multiresistant bacterial strains, except for ampicillin against *S. aureus* 03, which did not show any modifications when combined with the EO [87].

14.4 COVID-19 Treatment with Essential Oils

COVID-19 is a worldwide health threat. Regrettably, only few official medications are present against COVID-19 and its associated complications. With the beginning of New Year 2021, availability of COVID-19 vaccine has become more accessible to all countries as per Geneva/Oslo, December 18, 2020—COVAX the global initiative to ensure rapid and equitable access to COVID-19 vaccines for all countries. Vaccine development for COVID-19 began in 2020, but due to certain factors, it might take time to produce vaccine and to make it accessible to the society. So far various medicines such as remdesivir, chloroquine/hydroxychloroquine, dexamethasone, as well as tocilizumab have been used in various combinations to treat complications caused by COVID-19. EOs are complex multicomponent systems that offer a variety of antiviral, antimicrobial, immunomodulatory, antioxidant, cardioprotective, and anti-inflammatory effects and have proven effective against a broad range of respiratory complications. Recently several EOs have been tested against SARS CoV-2 and its associated complications.

Due to their hydrophobic nature, EOs can easily cross through bacterial as well viral outer membranes resulting in disruption of the membrane. Essential oils are also known to improve the efficacy of main-course medicines. In addition, EOs contain chemical components that can act on various virus target proteins in a synergistic manner to inhibit or prevent viral replication. Additionally, due to their volatile nature and therapeutic effects EOs have been reported for their considerable protective effects on the respiratory tract via reducing oxidative stress, inflammation, and causing mucolytic lytic effects. Presently, only *in silico* approaches such as computer-aided docking via computer simulation and a small number of *in vitro* investigations have been reported for anti-SARS-CoV-2 effects of EOs. Based on previous reports, blends of main course medication and EOs may be considered as a more reliable approach to fighting COVID-19. Only a few studies are available in which the antiviral effect of vapor phase of EOs is studied. Out of these studies, one study showed viral inhibitory effect of vapor phase of tea tree and eucalyptus EOs at different concentrations against influenza A virus. It was found that the vapor phase of both EOs presented significant antiviral activity after 5 to 15 minutes of exposure.

14.5 *In silico* Studies

Recently, 171 EO constituents were screened *in silico* for their binding efficiency with various proteins and enzymes of SARS-Cov-2. It was observed that sesquiterpene hydrocarbon (E)-β-farnesene showed better docking score against SARS-CoV-2 main protease. Additionally, (E, E)-farnesol, (E)-β-farnesene, and (E, E)-α-farnesene have been considered as excellent docking ligands for SARS-CoV-2 endoribonuclease; however, these constituents showed weak docking energies with SARS-CoV-2 targets. These EO constituents can synergistically act to potentiate other antiviral agents to treat COVID-19-associated complications [88].

An *in silico* study was performed to find an effective drug to prevent the binding of the angiotensin-converting enzyme 2 as a receptor for SARS-CoV-2. In this study, natural compound isothymol isolated from the EO of *Ammoides verticillata* demonstrated better docking scores than captopril and chloroquine by forming isothymol-angiotensin-converting enzyme 2 docked complex [89].

Another investigation based on molecular docking technique revealed the possible role of garlic EO in preventing the invasion of coronavirus into the human body. Gas chromatography–mass spectrometry (GC-MS) analysis of garlic EO revealed 17 organosulfur compounds accounting for 99.4% contents of the garlic EO. Based on this molecular docking study, the inhibitory effect of the considered compounds on the host ACE2 receptor was reported. Findings revealed coronavirus resistance of individual compounds on the main protease (PDB6LU7) protein of SARS-CoV-2. Additionally, it was found that with the main protease PDB6LU7 of SARS-CoV-2 as well as the amino acids of the angiotensin-converting enzyme 2, the majority of EO components showed strong binding. Allyl disulfide and allyl trisulfide showed the strongest anticoronavirus activity. The levels of these components were found to be high in the garlic EO (51.3%). Remarkably, docking findings demonstrated the synergistic interactions of the 17 substances, which showed good inhibition of the ACE2 and PDB6LU7 proteins [90].

Docking simulation inhibitory activities of *Melaleuca cajuputi* EO against ACE2 receptor protein in the human body as well as on main protease (PDB6LU7) of the SARS-CoV-2 were recently investigated. It was found that ACE2 and PDB6LU7 proteins were strongly inhibited by 10 out of 24 compounds of *Melaleuca cajuputi* EO. The most dominant anticoronavirus effect was expressed in the order: Terpineol (TA2)≈Guaiol (TA5)≈Linalool (TA19)>Cineol (TA1)>β-Selinenol (TA3)>α-Eudesmol (TA4)>γ-Eudesmol (TA7). Notably, 10 substances of the *Melaleuca cajuputi* EO showed synergistic interactions, and this interaction resulted in excellent inhibition of ACE2 and PDB6LU7 proteins [91].

It's well known that a key enzyme of SARS-CoV (2GTB) plays a crucial role in virus development. Recently, molecular docking and molecular dynamics simulations showed that components from *Mauritia flexuosa* EO 13-cis-β-carotene ligands, 9-cis-β-carotene and mainly α-carotene showed significant interaction with main peptidase of SARS-CoV via formation of the 2GTB peptidase complex [92].

14.6 Effect of Heat Followed by EO Treatment

Further, it was also suggested that the application of optimum heat (to the upper airways can support the immune system by supporting muco-ciliary clearance and inhibiting or deactivating virions where they first lodge) can be utilized to treat and prevent viral infections. This can be further enhanced by the inhalation of steam-containing EOs with antiviral, mucolytic, and anxiolytic properties [93].

14.7 Role of Geranium and Lemon EOs vs. ACE2 Inhibitory Effects

A recent study showed that geranium as well as lemon EOs demonstrated considerable ACE2 inhibitory effects in epithelial cells. Furthermore, it was found that geranium and lemon EOs displayed effective ACE2 inhibitory effects. Moreover, the GC-MS characterization revealed the presence of 22 compounds in geranium EOs (neryl acetate, geraniol, and citronellol as key components) and 9 compounds in lemon EO (limonene as the main chemical compound). Furthermore, it was found that limonene as well as citronellol considerably down-regulated angiotensin-converting enzyme 2 expression. Consequently, these EOs and their derivatives could be act as potential natural antiviral agents, which could be utilized in the prevention of SARS-CoV-2/COVID-19 [94].

There are several reports available demonstrating a virus inhibitory potential of EOs their components particularly against influenza and SARS COV. Various EOs have been evaluated against human respiratory viruses. Cinnamon, bergamot, lemongrass, thyme, and lavender EOs have been evidenced for their effective antiviral activities against Influenza type A virus. *Citrus reshni* EO has been shown to be potent against H5N1 virus. EO derived from *Citrus reshni* demonstrated considerable inhibitory activity against H5N1 virus.

Lippia EO (at 11.1 μg/mL) has been shown to cause complete suppression of yellow fever virus in Vero cells. EOs have shown antiviral effects against coronavirus infectious bronchitis virus.

It has been revealed that components of EO inhibit the development of SARS-CoV in Vero E6 cells. Moreover, viral expansion and capsid disintegration could be the possible mechanism of EO, which ultimately prevents the virus from causing infection in host cell. Additionally, EO components have also been reported on for their inhibitory effects on membrane protein of various viruses such as hemagglutinin, which help the virus enter the host cell. Chemical compounds of EOs can suppress virus development phases via targeting the redox signaling pathway. Certain natural redox modulating agents of EO origin target redox-sensitive pathways to further block both viral development and prevent virus-induced complications. EO derived from *Rosmarinus officinalis, Cymbopogon citratus,* and *Thymus vulgaris* have been reported on for their capability in disintegrating viral membrane and also weaken the complex (Tat/TAR-RNA) of HIV-1 virus, which is crucial for HIV-1 replication [95].

14.7.1 Role of Lemon and Geranium EOs in COVID-19

As mentioned above previous reports have suggested that lemon as well geranium EOs and their respective chemical components downregulate ACE expression to inhibit the entry of virus in epithelial cells [96].

Recently, various reports suggested the significance of EOs in the prevention of COVID-19 infection; however, most of the reports are based on speculations, *in silico* studies, *in vitro* studies, and the role of EOs in the treatment of earlier SARS CoV. Thus, due to lack of evidence, the role of EOs in COVID-19 has not been established.

14.8 Role of EO-Loaded Nanocarrier in COVID-19

Antiviral EOs incorporated into nanocarriers have been proposed recently as a potential approach for prevention of COVID-19 and future infectious pandemics. A number of EOs possess potential antiviral effects with fewer side effects and decent safety profiles. As the utilization of EOs has always been restricted because of poor solubility, solvent toxicity, volatility, and low solubility, nanoformulations of these EOs can be proven as a potential therapy to treat viral and bacterial infections. Numerous nanocarriers, particularly liposomes, dendrimers, nanoparticles, nanoemulsions, microemulsions, etc., can be utilized to overcome the limitations associated with EOs [97].

Nigella sativa (black seed or black cumin) has been known for its medicinal and nutraceutical value from decades. According to their biological potential, the main compounds present in EOs are terpenoids and flavonoids. The possible roles of *Nigella sativa* seed EO in overcoming physiological disturbances related to immune disorder, dysfunction of self-eating mechanism of body to produce new cells, imbalance between the production of free radicals and antioxidant mechanisms, species, decreased perfusion of blood through an organ, and inflammation, in a number of COVID-19 comorbidities such as cardiovascular complications, acute febrile illness, diabetes, and several microbial infections, have been known. Recent findings have strongly suggested the role of *Nigella sativa* seed EO in combating COVID-19 pandemic. Furthermore, *N. sativa* seed EO as nutraceuticals could be enormously utilized to prevent and cure COVID-19 [98].

Recently, an *in silico* structure-based virtual screening approach was used to evaluate the anti-SARS-CoV-2 potential of *Nigella sativa* chemical components against five possible sites of SARS-CoV-2. Out of 20 components studied, 10 compounds showed the best binding affinity against 2 SARS-CoV-2 sites of action, N-terminal RNA binding domain and papain-like protease. Further, drug likeness and toxicity assessment using OSIRIS Data Warrior v5.2.1 software revealed no predicted toxicity. It was concluded that N-terminal RNA binding domain as well as papain-like protease could be the main sites of action for *Nigella sativa* chemical components [99].

Another *in silico* study showed the role of phytochemicals such as α-hederin, thymohydroquinone, and thymoquinone from *N. sativa* against angiotensin-II receptor and key proteins of SARS-CoV-2. Also, these phytochemicals showed efficient binding to angiotensin-II receptor. Additionally, these phytochemicals participate and regulate certain factors and their proteins by involving hypoxia-inducible factor 1, vascular endothelial growth factor, chemokine, interleukin-17, receptor for advanced glycation end products, and calcium signaling pathways, which are involved in elevating oxidative stress, inflammation, and hypoxia. It was concluded that *N. sativa* standardized extract as well as its phytochemicals could be effective in treating COVID-19 and its associated complications [100].

Previously, various EOs have been assessed for their anti-SARS-CoV and anti-HSV-1 activities via inhibiting replication *in vitro*. It was found that out of all EOs, *L. nobilis* EO containing

β-pinene, β-ocimene, α-pinene, and 1,8-cineole as key components exhibited inhibitory effects against SARS-CoV. *J. oxycedrus* EO containing alpha-pinene and beta-myrcene demonstrated antiviral effects against HSV-1 [101].

14.9 Role of Nanotechnology in Antibacterial Potential of EOs

Due to their complex multicomponent composition, EOs possess a wide range of biological effects against multiple pathogenic microorganisms [102–128]. Thus, there are fewer chances that bacteria will develop resistance against EOs in comparison with classical antibiotics.

Thus, possibly there is less scope for pathogenic microorganisms as well as viruses to escape from the strategic action of EO components (e.g., synergistic, additive, modulating multiple pathways by acting at different target proteins of pathogenic host cell, etc.), which reduces chances of developing resistance against components of EOs in comparison to classical antibiotics. However, the physicochemical properties of EOs, especially stability in the presence of various intrinsic and extrinsic factors, is debated. Nanoencapsulated EO or EO-loaded nanop-reparations not only offer physical as well as chemical stability to EOs but also improve biological activity [102–128]. As discussed in previous chapters, EOs can be formulated in the form of nanocapsules or nanoemulsions by nanoprecipitation technique to overcome stability-related problems; thus, there is a possibility to formulate EOs and antibiotics in nanoform as they both have been reported for different types of synergistic, additive, and antagonistic interactions [102–128]. Even pure chemical components of EOs are known for their antimicrobial potential; EOs can be blended with antibiotics to prepare nanoformulations. Moreover, EOs can also be blended with EOs and further encapsulated in nanoforms to improve biological activity. Thus, EOs vs. nanotechnology fall into the following categories [102–128]:

- Synergistic activity of blended EOs (binary or quaternary)
- EOs blended with main course antimicrobial agents
- EOs blended with herbal extracts
- EOs blended with pure phytochemicals
- EO-loadednanopreparations for antimicrobial effects
- EO-loaded nanoformulations for food packaging and biomedical applications

14.10 EO-Based Food Supplement

To achieve this, cow milk yogurt enriched with EOs of basil, lavender, mint, and fennel with high antioxidant and antimicrobial effects encapsulated in sodium alginate were developed for multiple effects in boosting the body's immunity. It was found that antioxidant activity proved to be considerably higher than the control sample. Additionally, the highest antioxidant activity was obtained on the first day of analysis, decreasing onward to measurements taken on days 10 and 20. The cow milk yogurt enriched with volatile basil oil obtained the best results. Thus, such health supplements as well as nutraceuticals can be utilized during the pandemic for the prevention and reduction of the effects caused by pandemic stress in the human body [129].

Based on previous reports it was found that EOs are enriched with high levels of antimicrobial as well as antioxidants components. These phytochemicals present in EOs can be utilized to prepare cow milk yogurt with more nutritional and other desirable characteristics. As per recent reports, EOs namely, fennel, basil, lavender, and mint have been tested to prepare EO-enriched yogurt to further supplement immunity during pandemic. To achieve this, recently cow milk yogurt enriched with these EOs with high antimicrobial and antioxidant effects was prepared by encapsulating in natural food grade polymer, sodium alginate for positive effects in boosting the body's immunity. It was found that antioxidant property of cow milk yogurt enriched with EO was more than control sample. Additionally, antioxidant activity which was found to be high on the first day kept on decreasing for 20 days. Thus, such health supplements as well as nutraceuticals can be utilized during pandemic for the prevention of the ill effects caused by pandemic [129]. Various biotechnological approaches have been utilized to improve the yield of essential oils as well as its components [130–143].

REFERENCES

1. Yu Z, Tang J, Khare T, Kumar V. The alarming antimicrobial resistance in ESKAPEE pathogens: Can essential oils come to the rescue? *Fitoterapia.* 2020;140:104433.
2. Grădinaru AC, Trifan A, Şpac A, Brebu M, Miron A, Aprotosoaie AC. Antibacterial activity of traditional spices against lower respiratory tract pathogens: Combinatorial effects of *Trachyspermum ammi* essential oil with conventional antibiotics. *Lett Appl Microbiol.* 2018;67(5):449–457.
3. Aelenei P, Rimbu CM, Guguianu E, et al. Coriander essential oil and linalool: Interactions with antibiotics against Gram-positive and Gram-negative bacteria. *Lett Appl Microbiol.* 2019;68(2):156–164.
4. Delaquis PJ, Stanich K, Girard B, Mazza G. Antimicrobial activity of individual and mixed fractions of dill, cilantro, coriander and eucalyptus essential oils. *Int J Food Microbiol.* 2002;74(1–2):101–109.
5. Celenza G, Segatore B, Setacci D, Bellio P, Brisdelli F, Piovano M, Garbarino JA, Nicoletti M, Perilli M, Amicosante G. In vitro antimicrobial activity of pannarin alone and in combination with antibiotics against methicillin-resistant *Staphylococcus aureus* clinical isolates. *Phytomedicine.* 2012;19(7):596–602.
6. Rosato A, Piarulli M, Corbo F, Muraglia M, Carone A, Vitali ME, Vitali C. In vitro synergistic antibacterial action of certain combinations of gentamicin and essential oils. *Curr Med Chem.* 2010;17(28):3289–3295.
7. Aleksic V, Mimica-Dukic N, Simin N, Nedeljkovic NS, Knezevic P. Synergistic effect of *Myrtus communis* L. essential oils and conventional antibiotics against multi-drug resistant *Acinetobacter baumannii* wound isolates. *Phytomedicine.* 2014;21(12):1666–1674.
8. Knezevic P, Aleksic V, Simin N, Svircev E, Petrovic A, Mimica-Dukic N. Antimicrobial activity of *Eucalyptus camaldulensis* essential oils and their interactions with conventional antimicrobial agents against multi-drug resistant *Acinetobacter baumannii. J Ethnopharmacol.* 2016;178:125–136.
9. Duarte A, Ferreira S, Silva F, Domingues FC. Synergistic activity of coriander oil and conventional antibiotics against *Acinetobacter baumannii. Phytomedicine.* 2012;19(3–4):236–238.
10. Guerra FQ, Mendes JM, Sousa JP, et al. Increasing antibiotic activity against a multidrug-resistant *Acinetobacter* spp by essential oils of *Citrus limon* and *Cinnamomum zeylanicum. Nat Prod Res.* 2012;26(23):2235–2238.
11. Talei GR, Mohammadi M, Bahmani M, Kopaei MR. Synergistic effect of *Carum copticum* and *Mentha piperita* essential oils with ciprofloxacin, vancomycin, and gentamicin on Gram-negative and Gram-positive bacteria. *Int J Pharm Investig.* 2017;7(2):82–87.

12. Chovanova R, Mezovska J, Vaverkova S, Mikulasova M. The inhibition the Tet(K) efflux pump of tetracycline resistant *Staphylococcus epidermidis* by essential oils from three Salvia species. *Lett Appl Microbiol.* 2015;61:58–62.
13. Yap PS, Krishnan T, Chan KG, Lim SH. Antibacterial mode of action of *Cinnamomum verum* bark essential oil, alone and in combination with Piperacillin, against a multi-drug-resistant *Escherichia coli* strain. *J Microbiol Biotechnol.* 2015;25(8):1299–1306.
14. Chovanová R, Mezovská J, Vaverková Š, Mikulášová M. The inhibition the Tet(K) efflux pump of tetracycline resistant *Staphylococcus epidermidis* by essential oils from three Salvia species. *Lett Appl Microbiol.* 2015;61(1):58–62.
15. Knezevic P, Aleksic V, Simin N, Svircev E, Petrovic A, Mimica-Dukic N. Antimicrobial activity of *Eucalyptus camaldulensis* essential oils and their interactions with conventional antimicrobial agents against multi-drug resistant *Acinetobacter baumannii. J Ethnopharmacol.* 2016;178:125–136.
16. Pereira NLF, Aquino PEA, Júnior JGAS, Cristo JS, Vieira Filho MA, Moura FF, Ferreira NMN, Silva MKN, Nascimento EM, Correia FMA, Cunha FAB, Boligon AA, Coutinho HDM, Ribeiro-Filho J, Matias EFF, Guedes MIF. Antibacterial activity and antibiotic modulating potential of the essential oil obtained from *Eugenia jambolana* in association with led lights. *J Photochem Photobiol B.* 2017;174:144–149.
17. van Vuuren SF, Suliman S, Viljoen AM. The antimicrobial activity of four commercial essential oils in combination with conventional antimicrobials. *Lett Appl Microbiol.* 2009;48(4):440–446.
18. Miladinović DL, Ilić BS, Mihajilov-Krstev TM, Jović JL, Marković MS. In vitro antibacterial activity of *Libanotis montana* essential oil in combination with conventional antibiotics. *Nat Prod Commun.* 2014;9(2):281–286.
19. Fadli M, Saad A, Sayadi S, Chevalier J, Mezrioui NE, Pagès JM, Hassani L. Antibacterial activity of *Thymus maroccanus* and *Thymus broussonetii* essential oils against nosocomial infection: Bacteria and their synergistic potential with antibiotics. *Phytomedicine.* 2012;19(5):464–471.
20. van Vuuren S, Viljoen A. Plant-based antimicrobial studies--methods and approaches to study the interaction between natural products. *Planta Med.* 2011;77(11):1168–1182. doi: 10.1055/s-0030-1250736. Epub 2011 January 31. Erratum in: *Planta Med.* 2012;78(3):302.
21. Miladinović DL, Ilić BS, Mihajilov-Krstev TM, Jović JL, Marković MS. In vitro antibacterial activity of *Libanotis montana* essential oil in combination with conventional antibiotics. *Nat Prod Commun.* 2014;9(2):281–286.
22. Alexa VT, Szuhanek C, Cozma A, Galuscan A, Borcan F, Obistioiu D, Dehelean CA, Jumanca D. Natural preparations based on orange, bergamot and clove essential oils and their chemical compounds as antimicrobial agents. *Molecules.* 2020;25(23):5502.
23. Rosato A, Sblano S, Salvagno L, Carocci A, Clodoveo ML, Corbo F, Fracchiolla G. Anti-biofilm inhibitory synergistic effects of combinations of essential oils and antibiotics. *Antibiotics (Basel).* 2020;9(10):637.
24. Valcourt C, Saulnier P, Umerska A, Zanelli MP, Montagu A, Rossines E, Joly-Guillou ML. Synergistic interactions between doxycycline and terpenic components of essential oils encapsulated within lipid nanocapsules against gram negative bacteria. *Int J Pharm.* 2016;498(1–2):23–31.
25. Scalas D, Mandras N, Roana J, Tardugno R, Cuffini AM, Ghisetti V, Benvenuti S, Tullio V. Use of *Pinus sylvestris* L. (Pinaceae), *Origanum vulgare* L. (Lamiaceae), and *Thymus vulgaris* L. (Lamiaceae) essential oils and their main components to enhance itraconazole activity against azole susceptible/not-susceptible *Cryptococcus neoformans* strains. *BMC Complement Altern Med.* 2018;18(1):143.
26. Aelenei P, Rimbu CM, Guguianu E, Dimitriu G, Aprotosoaie AC, Brebu M, Horhogea CE, Miron A. Coriander essential oil and linalool: Interactions with antibiotics against Gram-positive and Gram-negative bacteria. *Lett Appl Microbiol.* 2019;68(2):156–164.
27. Bag A, Chattopadhyay RR. Evaluation of synergistic antibacterial and antioxidant efficacy of essential oils of spices and herbs in combination. *PLoS One.* 2015;10(7):e0131321.
28. Scalas D, Mandras N, Roana J, Tardugno R, Cuffini AM, Ghisetti V, Benvenuti S, Tullio V. Use of *Pinus sylvestris* L. (Pinaceae), *Origanum vulgare* L. (Lamiaceae), and *Thymus vulgaris* L. (Lamiaceae) essential oils and their main components to enhance itraconazole activity against azole susceptible/not-susceptible *Cryptococcus neoformans* strains. *BMC Complement Altern Med.* 2018;18(1):143.
29. Semeniuc CA, Pop CR, Rotar AM. Antibacterial activity and interactions of plant essential oil combinations against Gram-positive and Gram-negative bacteria. *J Food Drug Anal.* 2017;25(2):403–408.
30. Toroglu S. In-vitro antimicrobial activity and synergistic/antagonistic effect of interactions between antibiotics and some spice essential oils. *J Environ Biol.* 2011;32(1):23–29.
31. Amaral SC, Pruski BB, de Freitas SB, Allend SO, Ferreira MRA, Moreira C Jr, Pereira DIB, Junior ASV, Hartwig DD. *Origanum vulgare* essential oil: Antibacterial activities and synergistic effect with polymyxin B against multidrug-resistant *Acinetobacter baumannii. Mol Biol Rep.* 2020;47(12):9615–9625.
32. Ouedrhiri W, Balouiri M, Bouhdid S, Harki EH, Moja S, Greche H. Antioxidant and antibacterial activities of *Pelargonium asperum* and *Ormenis mixta* essential oils and their synergistic antibacterial effect. *Environ Sci Pollut Res Int.* 2018;25(30):29860–29867.
33. Purkait S, Bhattacharya A, Bag A, Chattopadhyay RR. Synergistic antibacterial, antifungal and antioxidant efficacy of cinnamon and clove essential oils in combination. *Arch Microbiol.* 2020;202(6):1439–1448.
34. de Souza Silveira Valente J, de Oliveira da Silva Fonseca A, Denardi LB, Dal Ben VS, de Souza Maia Filho F, Baptista CT, Braga CQ, Zambrano CG, Alves SH, de Avila Botton S, Pereira DI. In vitro susceptibility of *Pythium insidiosum* to *Melaleuca alternifolia, Mentha piperita* and *Origanum vulgare* essential oils combinations. *Mycopathologia.* 2016;181(7–8):617–622.
35. Lahmar A, Bedoui A, Mokdad-Bzeouich I, Dhaouifi Z, Kalboussi Z, Cheraif I, Ghedira K, Chekir-Ghedira L. Reversal of resistance in bacteria underlies synergistic effect of essential oils with conventional antibiotics. *Microb Pathog.* 2017;106:50–59.
36. Grădinaru AC, Trifan A, Şpac A, Brebu M, Miron A, Aprotosoaie AC. Antibacterial activity of traditional spices against lower respiratory tract pathogens: combinatorial effects of *Trachyspermum ammi* essential oil with conventional antibiotics. *Lett Appl Microbiol.* 2018;67(5):449–457.

37. Nafis A, Kasrati A, Jamali CA, Custódio L, Vitalini S, Iriti M, Hassani L. A comparative study of the in vitro antimicrobial and synergistic effect of essential oils from *Laurus nobilis* L. and *Prunus armeniaca* L. from morocco with antimicrobial drugs: New approach for health promoting products. *Antibiotics (Basel)*. 2020;9(4):140.
38. Yang SK, Yusoff K, Thomas W, Akseer R, Alhosani MS, Abushelaibi A, Lim SH, Lai KS. Lavender essential oil induces oxidative stress which modifies the bacterial membrane permeability of carbapenemase producing *Klebsiella pneumoniae*. *Sci Rep*. 2020;10(1):819.
39. Iman Islamieh D, Goudarzi H, Khaledi A, Afshar D, Esmaeili D. Reduced efflux pumps expression of *Pseudomonas aeruginosa* with *Satureja khuzistanica* essential oil. *Iran J Med Sci*. 2020;45(6):463–468.
40. El Atki Y, Aouam I, El Kamari F, Taroq A, Nayme K, Timinouni M, Lyoussi B, Abdellaoui A. Antibacterial activity of cinnamon essential oils and their synergistic potential with antibiotics. *J Adv Pharm Technol Res*. 2019;10(2):63–67.
41. Radulović N, Misić M, Aleksić J, Doković D, Palić R, Stojanović G. Antimicrobial synergism and antagonism of salicylaldehyde in Filipendula vulgaris essential oil. *Fitoterapia*. 2007;78(7–8):565–570.
42. Miladinović DL, Ilić BS, Kocić BD. Chemoinformatics approach to antibacterial studies of essential oils. *Nat Prod Commun*. 2015;10(6):1063–1066.
43. Miladinović DL, Ilić BS, Kocić BD, Marković MS, Miladinović LC. In vitro trials of *Dittrichia graveolens* essential oil combined with antibiotics. *Nat Prod Commun*. 2016;11(6):865–868.
44. van Vuuren SF, Suliman S, Viljoen AM. The antimicrobial activity of four commercial essential oils in combination with conventional antimicrobials. *Lett Appl Microbiol*. 2009;48(4):440–446.
45. Raskovic A, Milanovic I, Pavlovic N, Milijasevic B, Ubavic M, Mikov M. Analgesic effects of rosemary essential oil and its interactions with codeine and paracetamol in mice. *Eur Rev Med Pharmacol Sci*. 2015;19(1):165–172.
46. Monzote L, Montalvo AM, Scull R, Miranda M, Abreu J. Combined effect of the essential oil from *Chenopodium ambrosioides* and antileishmanial drugs on promastigotes of *Leishmania amazonensis*. *Rev Inst Med Trop Sao Paulo*. 2007;49(4):257–260.
47. Samojlik I, Petković S, Mimica-Dukić N, Božin B. Acute and chronic pretreatment with essential oil of peppermint (Mentha×piperita L., Lamiaceae) influences drug effects. *Phytother Res*. 2012;26(6):820–825.
48. Samojlik I, Mijatović V, Petković S, Skrbić B, Božin B. The influence of essential oil of aniseed (*Pimpinella anisum*, L.) on drug effects on the central nervous system. *Fitoterapia*. 2012;83(8):1466–1473.
49. Samojlik I, Petković S, Stilinović N, Vukmirović S, Mijatović V, Božin B. Pharmacokinetic herb-drug interaction between essential oil of aniseed (*Pimpinella anisum* L., Apiaceae) and acetaminophen and caffeine: A potential risk for clinical practice. *Phytother Res*. 2016;30(2):253–259.
50. Lim WC, Seo JM, Lee CI, Pyo HB, Lee BC. Stimulative and sedative effects of essential oils upon inhalation in mice. *Arch Pharm Res*. 2005;28(7):770–774.
51. Toroglu S. In vitro antimicrobial activity and antagonistic effect of essential oils from plant species. *J Environ Biol*. 2007;28(3):551–559.
52. Toroglu S. In-vitro antimicrobial activity and synergistic/antagonistic effect of interactions between antibiotics and some spice essential oils. *J Environ Biol*. 2011;32(1):23–29.
53. El Atki Y, Aouam I, El Kamari F, et al. Antibacterial activity of cinnamon essential oils and their synergistic potential with antibiotics. *J Adv Pharm Technol Res*. 2019;10(2):63–67.
54. Deeb SJ. Enhancement of cell death by linalyl acetate and [alpha]-terpineol through targeting the nuclear factor-[kappa] B activation pathway in human colon cancer cells. American University of Beirut; 2000.
55. Yang Y, Yue Y, Runwei Y, Guolin Z. Cytotoxic, apoptotic and antioxidant activity of the essential oil of Amomum tsao-ko. *Bioresour Technol*. 2010;101(11):4205–4211.
56. Katsuyama S, Mizoguchi H, Kuwahata H, Komatsu T, Nagaoka K, Nakamura H, Bagetta G, Sakurada T, Sakurada S. Involvement of peripheral cannabinoid and opioid receptors in β-caryophyllene-induced antinociception. *Eur J Pain*. 2013;17(5):664–675.
57. Rao H, Lai P, Gao Y. Chemical composition, antibacterial activity, and synergistic effects with conventional antibiotics and nitric oxide production inhibitory activity of essential oil from *Geophila repens* (L.) I.M. Johnst. *Molecules*. 2017;22(9):1561.
58. de Souza RC, da Costa MM, Baldisserotto B, et al. Antimicrobial and synergistic activity of essential oils of *Aloysia triphylla* and *Lippia alba* against *Aeromonas* spp. *Microb Pathog*. 2017;113:29–33.
59. Tak JH, Isman MB. Penetration-enhancement underlies synergy of plant essential oil terpenoids as insecticides in the cabbage looper, Trichoplusia ni. *Sci Rep*. 2017;7:42432.
60. Miladi H, Zmantar T, Kouidhi B, et al. Synergistic effect of eugenol, carvacrol, thymol, p-cymene and γ-terpinene on inhibition of drug resistance and biofilm formation of oral bacteria. *Microb Pathog*. 2017;112:156–163.
61. Mgbeahuruike EE, Stålnacke M, Vuorela H, Holm Y. Antimicrobial and synergistic effects of commercial piperine and piperlongumine in combination with conventional antimicrobials. *Antibiotics (Basel)*. 2019;8(2):55.
62. Farisa Banu S, Rubini D, Rakshitaa S, et al. Antivirulent properties of underexplored *Cinnamomum tamala* essential oil and its synergistic effects with DNase against *Pseudomonas aeruginosa* biofilms: An in vitro study. *Front Microbiol*. 2017;8:1144.
63. Cho Y, Kim H, Beuchat LR, Ryu JH. Synergistic activities of gaseous oregano and thyme thymol essential oils against *Listeria monocytogenes* on surfaces of a laboratory medium and radish sprouts. *Food Microbiol*. 2020;86:103357.
64. Wang L, Liu F, Jiang Y, et al. Synergistic antimicrobial activities of natural essential oils with chitosan films. *J Agric Food Chem*. 2011;59(23):12411–12419.
65. Danielli LJ, Pippi B, Duarte JA, et al. Antifungal mechanism of action of *Schinus lentiscifolius* Marchand essential oil and its synergistic effect in vitro with terbinafine and ciclopirox against dermatophytes. *J Pharm Pharmacol*. 2018;70(9):1216–1227.

66. Yang SK, Yusoff K, Mai CW, et al. Additivity vs synergism: Investigation of the additive interaction of cinnamon bark oil and meropenem in combinatory therapy. *Molecules.* 2017;22(11):1733.
67. Cardoso NN, Alviano CS, Blank AF, et al. Synergism effect of the essential oil from *Ocimum basilicum* var. Maria bonita and its major components with fluconazole and its influence on Ergosterol biosynthesis. *Evid Based Complement Alternat Med.* 2016;2016:5647182.
68. Alexa VT, Galuscan A, Popescu I, et al. Synergistic/antagonistic potential of natural preparations based on essential oils against *Streptococcus mutans* from the oral cavity. *Molecules.* 2019;24(22):4043.
69. Purkait S, Bhattacharya A, Bag A, Chattopadhyay RR. Evaluation of antibiofilm efficacy of essential oil components β-caryophyllene, cinnamaldehyde and eugenol alone and in combination against biofilm formation and preformed biofilms of *Listeria monocytogenes* and *Salmonella typhimurium. Lett Appl Microbiol.* 2020;71(2):195–202.
70. de Aguiar FC, Solarte AL, Tarradas C, Gómez-Gascón L, Astorga R, Maldonado A, Huerta B. Combined effect of conventional antimicrobials with essential oils and their main components against resistant *Streptococcus suis* strains. *Lett Appl Microbiol.* 2019;68(6):562–572.
71. Iten F, Saller R, Abel G, Reichling J. Additive antimicrobial [corrected] effects of the active components of the essential oil of *Thymus vulgaris*--chemotype carvacrol. *Planta Med.* 2009;75(11):1231–1236. doi: 10.1055/s-0029-1185541. Epub 2009 April 3. Erratum in: *Planta Med.* 2009;75(11):1236.
72. Cirino IC, Menezes-Silva SM, Silva HT, de Souza EL, Siqueira-Júnior JP. The essential oil from *Origanum vulgare* L. and its individual constituents carvacrol and thymol enhance the effect of tetracycline against *Staphylococcus aureus. Chemotherapy.* 2014;60(5–6):290–293.
73. Kwiatkowski P, Pruss A, Masiuk H, Mnichowska-Polanowska M, Kaczmarek M, Giedrys-Kalemba S, Dołęgowska B, Zielińska-Bliźniewska H, Olszewski J, Sienkiewicz M. The effect of fennel essential oil and trans-anethole on antibacterial activity of mupirocin against *Staphylococcus aureus* isolated from asymptomatic carriers. *Postepy Dermatol Alergol.* 2019;36(3):308–314.
74. Justino de Araújo AC, Freitas PR, Rodrigues Dos Santos Barbosa C, Muniz DF, Rocha JE, Albuquerque da Silva AC, Datiane de Morais Oliveira-Tintino C, Ribeiro-Filho J, Everson da Silva L, Confortin C, Amaral WD, Deschamps C, Barbosa-Filho JM, Ramos de Lima NT, Tintino SR, Melo Coutinho HD. GC-MS-FID characterization and antibacterial activity of the *Mikania cordifolia* essential oil and limonene against MDR strains. *Food Chem Toxicol.* 2020;136:111023.
75. Sieniawska E, Sawicki R, Swatko-Ossor M, Napiorkowska A, Przekora A, Ginalska G, Augustynowicz-Kopec E. The effect of combining natural terpenes and antituberculous agents against reference and clinical *Mycobacterium tuberculosis* strains. *Molecules.* 2018;23(1):176.
76. Chung D, Cho TJ, Rhee MS. Citrus fruit extracts with carvacrol and thymol eliminated 7-log acid-adapted *Escherichia coli* O157:H7, *Salmonella typhimurium*, and *Listeria monocytogenes*: A potential of effective natural antibacterial agents. *Food Res Int.* 2018;107:578–588.
77. Lorenzi V, Muselli A, Bernardini AF, Berti L, Pagès JM, Amaral L, Bolla JM. Geraniol restores antibiotic activities against multidrug-resistant isolates from gram-negative species. *Antimicrob Agents Chemother.* 2009;53(5):2209–2211.
78. Liu Q, Niu H, Zhang W, Mu H, Sun C, Duan J. Synergy among thymol, eugenol, berberine, cinnamaldehyde and streptomycin against planktonic and biofilm-associated food-borne pathogens. *Lett Appl Microbiol.* 2015;60(5):421–430.
79. Bag A, Chattopadhyay RR. Synergistic antibacterial and antibiofilm efficacy of nisin in combination with p-coumaric acid against food-borne bacteria *Bacillus cereus* and *Salmonella typhimurium. Lett Appl Microbiol.* 2017;65(5):366–372.
80. Ghosh T, Srivastava SK, Gaurav A, Kumar A, Kumar P, Yadav AS, Pathania R, Navani NK. A combination of linalool, vitamin C, and copper synergistically triggers reactive oxygen species and DNA damage and inhibits *Salmonella enterica* subsp. enterica Serovar Typhi and Vibrio fluvialis. *Appl Environ Microbiol.* 2019;85(4):e02487–18.
81. Mulyaningsih S, Sporer F, Zimmermann S, Reichling J, Wink M. Synergistic properties of the terpenoids aromadendrene and 1,8-cineole from the essential oil of *Eucalyptus globulus* against antibiotic-susceptible and antibiotic-resistant pathogens. *Phytomedicine.* 2010;17(13):1061–1066.
82. Mohamed SH, Mohamed MSM, Khalil MS, Azmy M, Mabrouk MI. Combination of essential oil and ciprofloxacin to inhibit/eradicate biofilms in multidrug-resistant *Klebsiella pneumoniae. J Appl Microbiol.* 2018;125(1):84–95.
83. Shin S. Essential oil compounds from *Agastache rugosa* as antifungal agents against *Trichophyton species. Arch Pharm Res.* 2004;27(3):295–299.
84. Shin S. In vitro effects of essential oils from *Ostericum koreanum* against antibiotic-resistant *Salmonella* spp. *Arch Pharm Res.* 2005;28(7):765–769.
85. Tetard A, Zedet A, Girard C, Plésiat P, Llanes C. Cinnamaldehyde induces expression of efflux pumps and multidrug resistance in *Pseudomonas aeruginosa. Antimicrob Agents Chemother.* 2019;63(10):e01081–19.
86. Utchariyakiat I, Surassmo S, Jaturanpinyo M, Khuntayaporn P, Chomnawang MT. Efficacy of cinnamon bark oil and cinnamaldehyde on anti-multidrug resistant *Pseudomonas aeruginosa* and the synergistic effects in combination with other antimicrobial agents. *BMC Complement Altern Med.* 2016;16:158.
87. Rodrigues FFG, Colares AV, Nonato CFA, Galvão-Rodrigues FF, Mota ML, Moraes Braga MFB, Costa JGMD. In vitro antimicrobial activity of the essential oil from *Vanillosmopsis arborea* Barker (Asteraceae) and its major constituent, α-bisabolol. *Microb Pathog.* 2018;125:144–149.
88. Silva JKRD, Figueiredo PLB, Byler KG, Setzer WN. Essential oils as antiviral agents: Potential of essential oils to treat SARS-CoV-2 infection: An in-silico investigation. *Int J Mol Sci.* 2020;21(10):3426.
89. Abdelli I, Hassani F, Bekkel Brikci S, Ghalem S. In silico study the inhibition of angiotensin converting enzyme 2 receptor of COVID-19 by *Ammoides verticillata* components harvested from Western Algeria. *J Biomol Struct Dyn.* 2020:1–14.

90. Thuy BTP, My TTA, Hai NTT, Hieu LT, Hoa TT, Thi Phuong Loan H, Triet NT, Anh TTV, Quy PT, Tat PV, Hue NV, Quang DT, Trung NT, Tung VT, Huynh LK, Nhung NTA. Investigation into SARS-CoV-2 resistance of compounds in garlic essential oil. *ACS Omega*. 2020;5(14):8312–8320.
91. My TTA, Loan HTP, Hai NTT, Hieu LT, Hoa TT, Thuy BTP, Quang DT, Triet NT, Anh TTV, Dieu NTX, Trung NT, Hue NV, Tat PV, Tung VT, Nhung NTA. Evaluation of the inhibitory activities of COVID-19 of *Melaleuca cajuputi* oil using docking simulation. *Chem Select*. 2020;5(21):6312–6320.
92. Costa AN, de Sá ÉRA, Bezerra RDS, Souza JL, Lima FDCA. Constituents of buriti oil (*Mauritia flexuosa* L.) like inhibitors of the SARS-coronavirus main peptidase: An investigation by docking and molecular dynamics. *J Biomol Struct Dyn*. 2020:1–8. https://pubmed.ncbi.nlm.nih.gov/32567501/
93. Cohen M. Turning up the heat on COVID-19: Heat as a therapeutic intervention. *F1000Res*. 2020;24;9:292.
94. Thuy BTP, My TTA, Hai NTT, Hieu LT, Hoa TT, Thi Phuong Loan H, Triet NT, Anh TTV, Quy PT, Tat PV, Hue NV, Quang DT, Trung NT, Tung VT, Huynh LK, Nhung NTA. Investigation into SARS-CoV-2 resistance of compounds in garlic essential oil. *ACS Omega*. 2020;5(14):8312–8320.
95. Wani AR, Yadav K, Khursheed A, Rather MA. An updated and comprehensive review of the antiviral potential of essential oils and their chemical constituents with special focus on their mechanism of action against various influenza and coronaviruses. *Microb Pathog*. 2020:104620.
96. Senthil Kumar KJ, Gokila Vani M, Wang CS, Chen CC, Chen YC, Lu LP, Huang CH, Lai CS, Wang SY. Geranium and lemon essential oils and their active compounds Downregulate angiotensin-converting enzyme 2 (ACE2), a SARS-CoV-2 spike receptor-binding domain, in epithelial cells. *Plants (Basel)*. 2020;9(6):770.
97. Kaur M, Devi G, Nagpal M, Singh M, Dhingra GA, Aggarwal G. Antiviral essential oils incorporated in nanocarriers: Strategy for prevention from COVID-19 and future infectious pandemics. *Pharm Nanotechnol*. 2020;8(6):437–451.
98. Islam MN, Hossain KS, Sarker PP, Ferdous J, Hannan MA, Rahman MM, Chu DT, Uddin MJ. Revisiting pharmacological potentials of Nigella sativa seed: A promising option for COVID-19 prevention and cure. *Phytother Res*. 2020. doi: 10.1002/ptr.6895.
99. Siddiqui S, Upadhyay S, Ahmad R, Gupta A, Srivastava A, Trivedi A, Husain I, Ahmad B, Ahamed M, Khan MA. Virtual screening of phytoconstituents from miracle herb nigella sativa targeting nucleocapsid protein and papain-like protease of SARS-CoV-2 for COVID-19 treatment. *J Biomol Struct Dyn*. 2020:1–21. doi: 10.1080/07391102.2020.1852117.
100. Jakhmola Mani R, Sehgal N, Dogra N, Saxena S, Pande Katare D. Deciphering underlying mechanism of Sars-CoV-2 infection in humans and revealing the therapeutic potential of bioactive constituents from Nigella sativa to combat COVID19: In-silico study. *J Biomol Struct Dyn*. 2020:1–13. doi: 10.1080/07391102.2020.1839560.
101. Loizzo MR, Saab AM, Tundis R, Statti GA, Menichini F, Lampronti I, Gambari R, Cinatl J, Doerr HW. Phytochemical analysis and in vitro antiviral activities of the essential oils of seven Lebanon species. *Chem Biodivers*. 2008;5(3):461–470.
102. Bhatia S, Sharma A, Vargas De La Cruz CB, Chaugule B, Ahmed Al-Harrasi. Nutraceutical, antioxidant, antimicrobial properties of *Pyropia vietnamensis* (Tanaka et Pham-Hong Ho) J.E. Sutherl. et Monotilla. *Curr Bioact Compd*. 2020;16:1.
103. Bhatia S, Sardana S, Senwar KR, Dhillon A, Sharma A, Naved T. In vitro antioxidant and antinociceptive properties of *Porphyra vietnamensis*. *Biomedicine (Taipei)*. 2019;9(1):3.
104. Bhatia S, Sharma K, Namdeo AG, Chaugule BB, Kavale M, Nanda S. Broad-spectrum sun-protective action of Porphyra-334 derived from *Porphyra vietnamensis*. *Pharmacogn Res*. 2010;2(1):45–49.
105. Bhatia S, Sharma K, Sharma A, Nagpal K, Bera T. Anti-inflammatory, analgesic and antiulcer properties of *Porphyra vietnamensis*. *Avicenna J Phytomed*. 2015;5(1):69–77.
106. Bhatia S, Sardana S, Sharma A, Vargas De La Cruz CB, Chaugule B, Khodaie L. Development of broad spectrum mycosporine loaded sunscreen formulation from Ulva fasciata delile. *Biomedicine (Taipei)*. 2019;9(3):17.
107. Bhatia S, Garg A, Sharma K, Kumar S, Sharma A, Purohit AP. Mycosporine and mycosporine-like amino acids: A paramount tool against ultra violet irradiation. *Pharmacogn Rev*. 2011;5(10):138–146.
108. Bhatia S, Namdeo AG, Nanda S. Factors effecting the gelling and emulsifying properties of a natural polymer. *SRP*. 2010;1(1):86–92.
109. Bhatia S, Sharma K, Bera T. Structural characterization and pharmaceutical properties of porphyran. *Asian J Pharm*. 2015;9:93–101.
110. Bhatia S, Sharma A, Sharma K, Kavale M, Chaugule BB, Dhalwal K, Namdeo AG, Mahadik KR. Novel algal polysaccharides from marine source: Porphyran. *Pharmacogn Rev*. 2008;4:271–276.
111. Bhatia S, Sharma K, Nagpal K, Bera T. Investigation of the factors influencing the molecular weight of porphyran and its associated antifungal activity Bioact. *Carb Diet Fiber*. 2015;5:153–168.
112. Bhatia S, Kumar V, Sharma K, Nagpal K, Bera T. Significance of algal polymer in designing amphotericin B nanoparticles. *Sci World J*. 2014;2014:564573.
113. Bhatia S, Rathee P, Sharma K, Chaugule BB, Kar N, Bera T. Immuno-modulation effect of sulphated polysaccharide (porphyran) from *Porphyra vietnamensis*. *Int J Biol Macromol*. 2013;57:50–56.
114. Bhatia S. *Natural Polymer Drug Delivery Systems: Marine PolysaccharidesBasedNano-MaterialsandItsApplications*. Springer International Publishing, Switzerland; 2016: 185–225.
115. Bhatia S. *Natural Polymer Drug Delivery Systems: Plant Derived Polymers, Properties, and Modification & Applications*. Springer International Publishing, Switzerland; 2016:119–184.
116. Bhatia S. *Natural Polymer Drug Delivery Systems: Nanotechnology and Its Drug Delivery Applications*. Springer International Publishing, Switzerland; 2016:1–32.
117. Bhatia S. *Natural Polymer Drug Delivery Systems: Nanoparticles Types, Classification, Characterization, Fabrication Methods and Drug Delivery Applications*. Springer International Publishing, Switzerland; 2016:33–93.

118. Bhatia S. *Natural Polymer Drug Delivery Systems: Natural Polymers vs Synthetic Polymer.* Springer International Publishing, Switzerland; 2016:95–118.
119. Bhatia S. *Systems for Drug Delivery: Mammalian Polysaccharides and Its Nanomaterials.* Springer International Publishing, Switzerland; 2016:1–27.
120. Bhatia S. *Systems for Drug Delivery: Microbial Polysaccharides as Advance Nanomaterials.* Springer International Publishing, Switzerland; 2016:29–54.
121. Bhatia S. *Systems for Drug Delivery: Chitosan Based Nanomaterials and Its Applications.* Springer International Publishing, Switzerland; 2016:55–117.
122. Bhatia S. *Systems for Drug Delivery: Advance Polymers and Its Applications.* Springer International Publishing, Switzerland; 2016:119–146.
123. Bhatia S. *Systems for Drug Delivery: Advanced Application of Natural Polysaccharides.* Springer International Publishing, Switzerland; 2016:147–170.
124. Bhatia S. *Systems for Drug Delivery: Modern Polysaccharides and Its Current Advancements.* Springer International Publishing, Switzerland; 2016:171–188.
125. Bhatia S. *Systems for Drug Delivery: Toxicity of Nanodrug Delivery Systems.* Springer International Publishing, Switzerland; 2016:189–197.
126. Bhatia S. *Nanotechnology in Drug Delivery Fundamentals, Design, and Applications: Part 1: Protein and Peptide-Based Drug Delivery Systems.* Apple Academic Press, Palm Bay, FL; 2016:50–204.
127. Bhatia S. *Nanotechnology in Drug Delivery Fundamentals, Design, and Applications: Part 2: Peptide-Mediated Nanoparticle Drug Delivery System.* Apple Academic Press, Palm Bay, FL; 2016:205–280.
128. Bhatia S. *Nanotechnology in Drug Delivery Fundamentals, Design, and Applications: Part 3: CPP and CTP in Drug Delivery and Cell Targeting.* Apple Academic Press, Palm Bay, FL; 2016:309–312.
129. Tiţa O, Constantinescu MA, Tiţa MA, Georgescu C. Use of yoghurt enhanced with volatile plant oils encapsulated in sodium alginate to increase the human body's immunity in the present fight against stress. *Int J Environ Res Public Health.* 2020;17(20):7588.
130. Bhatia S. Stem cell culture. In: *Introduction to Pharmaceutical Biotechnology, Volume 3: Animal Tissue Culture and Biopharmaceuticals.* IOP Publishing Ltd, Bristol, UK; 2019:1–24.
131. Bhatia S. Organ culture. In: *Introduction to Pharmaceutical Biotechnology, Volume 3: Introduction to Animal Tissue Culture Science.* IOP Publishing Ltd, Bristol, UK; 2019:1–28.
132. Bhatia S. Animal tissue culture facilities. In: Introduction to Pharmaceutical Biotechnology, Volume 3: *Animal Tissue Culture and Biopharmaceuticals.* IOP Publishing Ltd, Bristol, UK; 2019:1–32.
133. Bhatia S. Characterization of cultured cells. In: *Introduction to Pharmaceutical Biotechnology, Volume 3: Animal Tissue Culture and Biopharmaceuticals.* IOP Publishing Ltd, Bristol, UK; 2019:1–47.
134. Bhatia S. Introduction to genomics. In: *Introduction to Pharmaceutical Biotechnology, Volume 2: Enzymes, Proteins and Bioinformatics.* IOP Publishing Ltd, Bristol, UK; 2018:1–39.
135. Bhatia S. Bioinformatics. In: *Introduction to Pharmaceutical Biotechnology, Volume 2: Enzymes, Proteins and Bioinformatics.* IOP Publishing Ltd, Bristol, UK; 2018:1–16.
136. Bhatia S. Protein and enzyme engineering. In: *Introduction to Pharmaceutical Biotechnology, Volume 2: Enzymes, Proteins and Bioinformatics.* IOP Publishing Ltd, Bristol, UK; 2018:1–15.
137. Bhatia S. Industrial enzymes and their applications. In: *Introduction to Pharmaceutical Biotechnology, Volume 2: Enzymes, Proteins and Bioinformatics.* IOP Publishing Ltd, Bristol, UK; 2018:21.
138. Bhatia S. Introduction to enzymes and their applications. In: *Introduction to Pharmaceutical Biotechnology, Volume 2: Enzymes, Proteins and Bioinformatics.* IOP Publishing Ltd, Bristol, UK; 2018:1–29.
139. Bhatia S. Biotransformation and enzymes. In: *Introduction to Pharmaceutical Biotechnology, Volume 2: Enzymes, Proteins and Bioinformatics.* IOP Publishing Ltd, Bristol, UK; 2018:1–13.
140. Bhatia S. Modern DNA science and its applications. In: *Introduction to Pharmaceutical Biotechnology, Volume 1: Basic Techniques and Concepts.* IOP Publishing Ltd, Bristol, UK; 2018:1–70.
141. Bhatia S. Introduction to genetic engineering. In: *Introduction to Pharmaceutical Biotechnology, Volume 1: Basic Techniques and Concepts.* IOP Publishing Ltd, Bristol, UK; 2018:1–63.
142. Bhatia S. Applications of stem cells in disease and gene therapy. In: *Introduction to Pharmaceutical Biotechnology, Volume 1: Basic Techniques and Concepts.* IOP Publishing Ltd, Bristol, UK; 2018:1–40.
143. Bhatia S. Transgenic animals in biotechnology. In: *Introduction to Pharmaceutical Biotechnology, Volume 1: Basic Techniques and Concepts.* IOP Publishing Ltd, Bristol, UK; 2018:1–67.

15

Antibacterial Mechanism of Action of Essential Oils

Ahmed Al-Harrasi
Natural and Medical Sciences Research Center, University of Nizwa

Saurabh Bhatia
Natural and Medical Sciences Research Center, University of Nizwa
University of Petroleum and Energy Studies

Tapan Behl
Chitkara University

Deepak Kaushik
M.D. University

Mohammed Muqtader Ahmed and Md. Khalid Anwer
Prince Sattam Bin Abdul Aziz University

CONTENTS

15.1 Introduction

Medicinal and aromatic plants synthesize various antimicrobial chemical compounds in order to protect themselves from different microbial infections. Essential oils (EOs) are considered as one of the most important classes of natural products and offer a wide range of antimicrobial effects. The chemical composition of EOs and concentrations of active components often determine their overall antimicrobial potential [1]. When a plant is exposed to any biotic/abiotic stress conditions, these chemical compounds are released via a sequence of molecular interactions. Chemical compounds present in the secretion work in a synergistic manner to prevent microbial attack; however, the mechanism of action of each compound against microbes is different [2]. In addition, the type of microbial pathogen (e.g., bacteria or fungi) and its cellular composition also counteract the antibacterial activity of EOs in a different manner [3]. Based on previous reports, the mechanism of antimicrobial action of EOs is demonstrated in Figure 12.1. Due to their antimicrobial potential, EOs are utilized in different areas, including food packaging, insecticides, pharmaceuticals as well as in the flavor and fragrance industries [4]. Considering these uses, the antibacterial, antifungal, and antiviral properties of EOs derived from medicinal and aromatic plants are broadly discussed in this section.

15.2 Essential Oils vs Antibiotics

Currently, various antibiotics are considered as frontline treatments against microbial infectious diseases. Nevertheless,

DOI: 10.1201/9781003175933-17

antibiotic treatment can also lead to the development of various unfavorable consequences as follows:

- With substantial overuse or abuse of antibiotics, bacteria have now become smarter in terms of developing escape mechanisms to protect themselves against antibiotics. These antimicrobial-resistant bacterial strains can infect the same or different individuals with more severity.
- Some antibiotics cause severe allergic reactions such as penicillin, because of their capability to disrupt the formation of the bacterial cell wall.
- The use of some antibiotics such as aminoglycoside-containing antibiotics increases the chances of acute kidney injury and ototoxicity, because of their capability to block the bacterial 30S ribosome.
- Antibiotics like quinolone derivatives block the bacterial DNA topoisomerase II, and have been linked with an increased possibility of tendinitis.
- It is evidenced that the use of these antibiotics could lead to the production of more ROS from the mitochondria in mammalian cells and *in vivo* in mice, which can result in tissue damage.
- Antibiotics are used to kill pathogenic bacteria. Nevertheless, they occasionally kill the host bacteria, which protect the host from fungal infections. As a result, many people taking antibiotics develop fungal infections. Intestinal microbiomes in response to the antibiotics result in dysbiotic microbiome. These dysbiotic microbiomes cannot carry out essential functions, which are beneficial for the host system such as the production of vitamins, protection from pathogens, and supply of nutrients that could lead to various complications such as metabolic and immunological, in addition to increased propensity for other infections.
- Antibiotic usage can also lead to GIT complications indigestion and diarrhea.
- In addition to their selective toxicity, antibiotics are also responsible for certain adverse drug reactions typically due to malfunctioning of drug metabolism or overuse of antibiotics. Fewer reports are available on antibiotic-induced neurotoxicity, which might be due to change in drug metabolism.
- Use of antimicrobials can lead to potential drug–drug interactions. This kind of drug–drug interaction can be classified as contraindicated (certain drugs are contraindicated for simultaneous use); major (interaction could be dangerous and/or require medical intervention to reduce or avoid serious adverse effects); moderate (interaction could exacerbate patient's condition); or minor (interaction would have limited clinical effects). Manifestations may include an increase in the frequency or severity of adverse effects, but generally would not require a major alteration in therapy. They can interact with other drugs such as anti-psoriasis drugs, blood thinners, oral contraceptives, antihistamines, antacids, nonsteroidal anti-inflammatory drugs, antidiabetic drugs, spasmolytic, tricyclic antidepressants, anti-obesity medication, antifungals, antipsychotic medicines, and steroids.
- Some antibiotics make the skin photosensitive.
- Some antibiotics such as tetracycline cause stains on teeth enamel.

Moreover, the bacterial tendency to create biofilm-associated drug resistance and low immune response of individual could increase the severity of bacterial infections in humans [5].

Due to considerable toxicity, adverse drug reaction, and drug–drug interactions and as antibiotic exposure can lead to the development of multidrug-resistant strains, there is an urgent need for safe, reliable, and effective alternative therapies against different pathogenic microorganisms [6]. In this context, natural EOs as well as their respective active therapeutic components with high antibacterial potential could be considered as an alternative approach to treating a wide range of bacterial infections. Chemical components of an EO work in synergy to offer antibacterial activity; however, blending of different EOs or blending them with medications or their active chemical components could work in both an antagonistic and synergistic manner. EO components act in a manner to either kill (bactericidal) or inhibit the growth (bacteriostatic) of bacterial cells. However, it is quite challenging to determine these effects. As far as the evaluation of antibacterial potential is concerned, MIC (minimum inhibitory concentration) or the MBC (minimum bactericidal concentration) assays are often used to determine the antibacterial potential of EOs [6].

Antibacterial screening of EOs or their individual active components is usually done by means of *in vitro* disk diffusion assay, where EOs are applied on sterile paper disks or added into wells, which are aseptically placed on the inoculated plates [7]. Once kept under suitable incubation period and conditions, the inhibition zones of test and standard samples are compared for bacterial inhibition [8]. The antibacterial potential of EOs is dependent on the form of EO, its chemical composition as well as the type of the targeted bacteria. Sandalwood as well as vetiver EOs were found to be more active against Gram-positive bacteria; however, both have failed to show activity against Gram-negative bacteria [9]. The chemical profile of EOs was also correlated with antibacterial activity and it was found that the antibacterial effects of rosemary, cinnamon, oregano, clove, thyme, and pimento against *Pseudomonas aeruginosa, Salmonella typhimurium*, and *Staphylococcus aureus* could be due to their antibacterial components [10].

Similarly isolated compounds from EOs such as thymol, eugenol, and carvacrol showed higher antibacterial potential against various pathogenic bacteria [11]. It was also observed that some EOs are effective in anaerobic conditions. For example, cinnamic acids, benzoic acids, as well as benzaldehydes showed more antibacterial effect against Gram-positive bacterium in the oxygen free environment [12].

EOs and their application in the meat industry were also explored where oils such as cinnamon, rosemary, clove, and pimento EOs were tested against microbes, which are responsible for meat spoilage, and their antimicrobial activity was correlated with the presence of eugenol and cinnamaldehyde in the EOs [13]. These oils were found to be effective even at a dilution of 1/100. The antibacterial potential of extract derived from spices was also tested against different human pathogenic bacteria, and it was suggested that garlic aqueous extract showed the maximum inhibition (93%) against *S. epidermidis* and *S. typhimurium* [14]. Likewise, the antibacterial potential of clove extracts against the verotoxin-producing *E. coli* bacteria that cause illness in humans was studied, and it was observed that the production of verotoxin was suppressed by the clove extract [15].

The antimicrobial potential of oregano, basil, and coriander plants was found to be effective against pathogenic *P. aeruginosa, S. aureus*, and *Yersinia enterocolitica*. It was suggested that the EOs at greater dose could be more effective against bacterial cells [16]. There are two forms of bacterial lung infections (acute or chronic). The form of bacterial infection depends on the rate at which the disease progresses or possibly the rate at which the disease is resolved by antibiotic treatment. Unlike bacterial infection, viral infection might onset as an acute bronchitis followed by infection, which usually do not resolve even after antibiotic therapy. In contrast to common chronic bacterial infections, chronic infections in lungs progress with the onset of immunologic reaction against bacterial infections that involves inexorable neutrophilic response. Due to this, chronic pulmonary infection is often considered as a persistent infection in which pathogenic bacteria develop escape mechanisms or are trained enough by the treatment used to destroy them, thus remaining permanently in patients in dormant or active stage. An earlier report suggested the effectiveness of *Achillea clavennae* EO containing eucalyptol and camphor as the main chemical components in inhibiting the growth of respiratory disease-causing microorganisms [18]. A previous *in vitro* study suggested the promising antibacterial role of EO obtained from thyme, clove, and cinnamon bark against respiratory tract pathogens either in liquid medium or in vapor phase. Nevertheless, their effect is lower than that of the reference antibiotics. The combination of EOs and antibiotics may be beneficial in the alternative treatment of respiratory tract diseases. It was observed that among all EOs, thyme EO showed the highest inhibition against *S. mutans*, whereas cinnamon and clove oils showed high inhibition in liquid medium against *S. pneumoniae* and *S. pyogenes*. Cinnamon bark EO showed the maximum activity against Gram-negative *Haemophilus influenzae* that can cause infection in the respiratory tract, which can spread to other organs. It was also found that in vapor phase, cinnamon bark showed significant activity against all studied microbial pathogens, whereas unexpectedly, eucalyptus and scots pine presented poor activity against the investigated bacteria in both liquid and vapor phases. Volatile chemical components undergo phase transition from liquid to vapors, and in some cases, oil is absorbed over the solid matrix like cotton wig (to use them in portable inhaler) so it's essential to determine their stability in liquid and vapor phases. Thus, it was concluded from this study that the biological properties of EOs also depend on their stability in all phases (solid, liquid, and vapor phases). As far as the mechanism of action is concerned, EOs mainly disrupt the cellular organization, resulting in membrane damage, which can lead to an increase in membrane permeability. Increase in membrane permeability can disturb various cellular processes such as electron transport system, solute transport, metabolic regulation, energy production (membrane-coupled), the proton motive force, protein translocation, synthesis of cellular components, and transport across the membrane, and other metabolic regulatory functions [17]. However, the mechanism of action of EOs cannot be traceable and unique as it may vary depending on their chemical composition and type of bacterial strain. It was observed that the mechanism of action of EOs against pathogenic bacteria involves a cascade of reactions that involves the entire bacterial cell. Usually, EOs act in a manner to suppress the growth of bacterial cells as well as to prevent the release of toxic products from bacterial cell. The majority of EOs act effectively against Gram-positive and Gram-negative bacteria. Due to the difference in the cell membrane composition of these bacteria, EOs act differently against these bacteria [18].

15.3 Mechanism of Actions of Essential Oils

EOs display various mechanisms to exhibit antibacterial effects against pathogenic bacteria. As suggested above, EOs can affect the integrity of the whole bacterial cell by disrupting the cell wall/membrane as well as the cytoplasm. Due to their lipophilic nature, EOs can easily enter via the bacterial cell membranes (Figure 12.1). After penetration, EOs increase the permeability of bacterial cell membrane, which can affect the various cellular processes of bacteria as mentioned above. Disruption may also affect the osmotic and turgor pressure of bacterial cell [19]. Thus, the effect of EOs on changing membrane organization and integrity could trigger a cascade of events, which are as follows [20] (Figure 12.1):

- Cell wall degradation [21]
- Disruption of the cytoplasmic membrane
- Coagulation of some cytoplasmic components [22]
- Destruction of the membrane proteins
- Increase in cell content leakage [23]
- Decreasing the electrochemical gradient of protons [24]
- Decreasing the intracellular ATP synthesis
- Decreasing the membrane potential through increased membrane permeability [2]
- Change in osmotic pressure

15.4 Essential Oil Composition-Based Mechanism of Action

A previous study demonstrated the effects of various components of EOs on membrane permeability. Cell membrane damage caused by tea tree oil was reported on in a previous study that suggested that cell membrane damage could be the likely cause of a decrease in viability and cell death for all the microorganisms investigated in this study. As a result, the lipophilic nature of these EOs facilitates their penetration into microbial cells and causes significant changes in the organization of membrane structure and its functionality. The lipophilic nature of EOs and their components make them the most suitable and effective candidate against bacteria, except against Gram-positive bacteria. It's also known that capsule of a number of pathogenic bacteria restricts the entry of EOs into the bacterial cytoplasm. EO components are capable enough to interfere with the submerged integral proteins that are responsible for a range of important functions such as transporting molecules across the membrane. Various reports corroborate that EO components act in a different way to perform antimicrobial effects. EO components work in a different manner to destabilize the phospholipid bilayer, resulting in the disruption of the cell membrane. This event may result in the loss of original architecture and function of bacterial cell, which can subsequently lead to the enzymatic inactivation and the loss of key cellular components. A recent study suggested that EOs of *Origanum compactum* disrupt the cell membrane and increase the membrane permeability along with the suppression of quorum-sensing (QS)-mediated phenotypic expression in bacteria. As demonstrated earlier, cellular ATP content acts as an indicator of the physiological state of cells and also indicates the cell viability. EO treatment can change the membrane permeability by causing destruction to the electron transport system [25]. This physiological change allows the entry of EO components, including carvon, thymol, and carvacrol, which can further result in an elevation in the intracellular concentration of ATP. Sudden increase in the level of ATP could be associated with the destruction of the bacterial membrane [13]. These key cellular events such as ATP formation during the bacterial respiration via a sequence of electron transport reactions within the cytoplasmic membrane, which regulates the oxidative phosphorylation of ADP to ATP, are targeted by EO components to kill the bacteria. Thus, sudden changes in physiological processes, listed below, can lead to cell death [26]:

- Inhibition of electron transport system required for generation of energy
- Disruption of the electrochemical gradient of protons
- Interference with translocation of important proteins
- Interference with the production of essential components of bacterial cell

15.5 Effect of Essential Oil on Bacterial Cell Membrane

The bacterial cell membrane plays an important role in determining its survival as it is an important component in the basic biological events that occur at the intracellular level. The bacterial layer stands as an active wall separating the intracellular and extracellular environment, to regulate the transport of the metabolites and ions across that wall, which are required for important cellular events that occur within the cell. In the extracellular presence of antimicrobial compounds, bacteria often respond by modulating the synthesis of fatty acids and changing the arrangement of membrane proteins, ultimately to alter the membrane fluidity [27]. Lipophilicity of the EOs as well as their respective components facilitates their diffusion across the phospholipid bilayer membrane that encloses the bacterial cytoplasm. EOs are known for their capability in changing permeability as well as functional membrane proteins. A number of phenol-enriched oils can effectively penetrate and cross the lipid bilayer of cell walls, where they can efficiently destabilize membrane proteins and change their normal functions (Figure 12.1) [28].

Thus, the bacterial membrane is considered as the primary site of action for EOs. As discussed above, the mechanism of action of EOs involves cascades of events intracellularly as well as extracellularly. Alteration in membrane permeability and disruption of transport mechanism across the membrane disturb the intracellular environment of bacterial cells that results in coagulation of cytoplasm. In addition, these external stress stimuli or rapid extracellular changes can also result in the denaturation of a number of enzymes as well as cellular proteins, which can further lead to the leakage of metabolites and ions [29]. Previous reports also suggested that the EO or antimicrobial-based treatment (at sublethal dose) of bacteria could result in the upregulation of the bacterial stress-response proteins to restore the damage caused to the proteins [30].

In response to the external stress stimuli, bacteria stimulate certain pathways to modulate gene expression eventually to cope up with the stress and to adapt to the prevailing unfavorable conditions. This stress milieu could directly or indirectly influence the regulation of a number of molecular pathways, which control transcription, translation, and stability of transcripts and of proteins. Nevertheless, when the dose of EOs or other antimicrobial substances is higher, these stress stimuli caused by the higher dose are sufficient to cause cell death. In this case, bacterial stress-mediated response would not be sufficient to prevent its cell death as it's more common in Gram-positive bacteria (Figure 12.1). The thin cell wall of Gram-negative bacteria containing peptidoglycan is more resilient to the effects of EOs and their components. Both classes of bacteria, Gram-positive and Gram-negative, are different from each other in terms of their outer membrane architecture. However, both are dependent on diffusion mechanism for transportation of nutrition and release of waste products, which require a selective porous outer membrane to retain the vital components of cell and allow the selective exchange of compounds. Unlike other membrane transport proteins, bacterial membrane contains beta barrel proteins, which act as a pore for the effective diffusion of molecules across a cellular membrane (Figure 12.1). Gram-negative bacteria contain two membranes—outer membrane, more permeable to hydrophilic substances, because of the presence of porins—whereas Gram-positive bacteria is deficient in outer membranes, but contain both types of porins that are bound to specific lipids in the cell walls. The cell wall of Gram-negative bacteria does not allow entry of the effective concentration of EOs and their components to kill the bacterial cell as quickly as Gram-positive bacteria. Thus, EOs cannot efficiently act against Gram-negative bacteria. As the EO, itself, is a mixture of various components, its antimicrobial potential cannot be ascribed to a specific mechanism and follows different ways to act against bacteria, such as (Figure 12.1):

- Structural modification
- Biochemical changes
- Acts over the surface of bacterial cell as well as internal components
- Treatment can modify intracellular components of the bacterial cell
- Treatment can modify shape of the bacterial cell
- Treatment can lead to release of ions or metabolites
- Compromise the microbial metabolism

These changes in bacterial cell can result in lyses or cellular death.

There are various mechanisms of action for an EO and its components to perform an antibacterial action. Cox et al. [31] suggested that the antibacterial effect of tea tree oil over the growth of *S. aureus* and *E. coli* was by escalating the outflow of intracellular K+ ions, interfering with cell respiration, and changing the cell permeability. It was also reported that EOs could efficiently cross cell wall and cytoplasmic membrane barrier that can result in the distortion of the membrane architecture by altering the arrangement of polysaccharide molecules, phospholipid bilayers, and dissimilar fatty acids [32]. These cascades of events can lead to the coagulation of cytoplasmic components and hydrolysis of protein–lipid interactions [2].

Moreover, a change in membrane permeability also affects the intracellular and extracellular ion concentration that can affect intracellular pH and osmotic pressure. This imbalance can lead to cell injury and death. As per earlier reports, the chemical components of EOs showed more antibacterial effects in comparison with the EO. EO can cause various perturbations in cell membrane structure that can lead to the lipid density variation and ultimately influence lyophobic interactions. The antibacterial potential activities of the components present in EO, including thymol, menthol, and linalyl acetate, are reported to cause bacterial membrane lipid perturbation [33].

Perturbation of the peptidoglycan and cytoplasmic membrane can influence the membrane permeability and encourage the leakage of cytoplasmic components. A natural monoterpene derivative of cymene, carvacrol (hydrophobic compound) is reported to cause the perturbation of the lipid fraction of the bacterial membrane. While the actual mechanism of action is not clear yet, it's evidenced that carvacrol affects the membrane permeability by changing the fatty acid composition, which can affect the fluidity of the bacterial membrane [34]. It's also known that typically short-chain fatty acid and elevated level of unsaturated bonds between carbons of fatty acids increase the membrane fluidity. Thus, the effect of EO on structural components of membrane such as fatty acids should be studied carefully. Another report suggested that carvacrol considerably reduces the synthesis of ATP, resulting in a decrease in the intracellular level of ATP [34].

Likewise, carvacrol was also reported to stimulate the ATP release from bacterial cells. Another report suggested the role of the EO components, including thymol, methyl carvacrol, menthol, and citronellol for bacterial cell enlargement, resulting in leakage of ions due to the distortion of phospholipid arrangements [35].

15.6 Microbial Toxins and Membrane Proteins vs Essential Oils

One more report suggested the role of EOs in the inhibition of toxin bacterial metabolite secretion via its respective membranes. This could be due to the change in membrane permeability and because of the effects of EO, which can resist the release of toxic bacterial metabolites in the extracellular matrix. Ultee and Smid [36] suggested that *B. cereus* treatment with carvacrol reduced the toxin production, whereas the treatment of *S. aureus* with oregano EO fully inhibited the production of enterotoxin.

Therefore, the production and the toxin release in an outside environment could be restricted by using EOs or their components as they can efficiently alter the structure of bacterial membrane to influence the transmembrane transport process [37]. Another report suggested the role of natural organic compound, trans-cinnamaldehyde, which penetrates the gel-like matrix (i.e. bacterial periplasm) and disturbs its events [16]. In addition, p-cymene showed higher interaction with cell membranes and consequently could disrupt the membrane structure more efficiently [38]. The outer membrane proteins of bacteria are also influenced by EOs and their constituents such as carvacrol that may disrupt the folding as well as insertion of proteins such as GroEL and DnaK [2]. Many other proteins that are listed below are also affected by the treatment of bacteria with EOs.

- FtsZ: FtsZ is the major cytoskeletal protein that regulates bacterial cell division. Assembly, bundling, and polymerization of FtsZ are inhibited by cinnamaldehyde.
- Misfolded proteins: Many bacterial proteins could be either up-regulated or down-regulated by EOs or its components ultimately to inhibit its growth. Up-regulation of defective (misfolded) outer membrane proteins was reported after the treatment with thymol. This accumulation of misfolded proteins could trigger bacterial envelope stress.
- Suppression of protein participating in the bacterial phosphotransferase system.
- Suppression of the proteins that are responsible for energy metabolism [39]. Similarly, some enzymes are overexpressed after the treatment of *S. typhimurium* with thymol.
- YidC: Proteins that are required for bacterial survival such as *E. coli* protein, YidC, could be considered as excellent targets for EO and its components such as eugenol and carvacrol to inhibit their growth [40].
- Flagellin synthesis: Carvacrol reduces the flagellin synthesis, which is responsible for the motility of bacteria [41].

15.7 Fatty Acid Synthesis vs. Essential Oil

Fatty acid synthesis could be a key target for the development of new antibacterial agents [42]. Because of their lipophilic nature, EOs and their components can easily penetrate, reorganize the proportion of unsaturated fatty acids, and change their structure [43]. EO components such as thymol, carvacrol, and eugenol can elevate the levels of C16 and C18 saturated fatty acids, whereas they reduce the level of C18 unsaturated fatty acids in the outer membrane treatment of *S. typhimurium*. As per reports, EOs and their components also influence the enzymes that are responsible for fatty acid synthesis; for example, desaturase enzyme is required to synthesize saturated fatty acids [44]. EOs are also reported on for their capability in increasing membrane fluidity by increasing the synthesis of saturated fatty acids in the membrane lipid bilayer; however, many reports have also suggested their role in reducing the level of saturated fatty acids, which can lead to a decline in membrane fluidity with an increase in membrane rigidity. Aromatic compounds derived from clove and other sources, were also reported for their capability in altering the fatty acid synthesis and change the bacterial membrane.

15.8 Effect of Essential Oils on Intracellular ATP Production in Microbial Cell

ATP production in bacteria takes place in the cell wall as well as in the cytoplasm via glycolysis. The level of ATP inside and outside the cell is correlated with EOs in some reports. EOs and their components disturb the bacterial membrane, which can cause an imbalance in ATP levels present in intracellular and extracellular environment as most of the ATP is released by the disturbed membrane [45]. In addition, EO also influences various enzymes with ATPase activity such as F1F0 ATPase as well as the ATP-dependent transport proteins. Moreover, EOs can inhibit a variety of enzymes of bacteria, including ATPase, amylase, histidine carboxylase, as well as proteases [46]. Similarly, cinnamaldehyde is evidenced for its role in inhibiting bacterial ATPase enzymes and disturbing the bacterial membrane.

15.9 Effect of Essential Oil on the Production of Metabolites in Microbial Cell

EOs and their components play an important role in affecting the intracellular and extracellular metabolites of bacteria. Bacteria produce a variety of metabolites, whereas each metabolite responds in a different manner against different concentrations of EOs or their components. Some studies have shown that carvacrol at lower concentrations is effective in affecting metabolites. One more study suggested that higher concentration of carvacrol in *E. coli* leads to the accumulation of glucose, and the failure of the cells to use the glucose resulted in a decrease in viability. Earlier reports also suggested that organic acid metabolites except formate showed a considerable decline in concentration at higher dose of carvacrol, whereas formate level initially increased and then considerably declined to almost nil. Sudden initial increase in the level of formate (produced by *E. coli* during fermentation reaction) and then steep decline could suggest likely metabolic change toward fermentation. However, at the higher dose of carvacrol, there would be a permanent loss of cell viability. This could be due to sudden arrest of the cellular metabolism, which may lead to decline in formate level. In addition, the level of aromatic amino acids increased at higher doses of carvacrol, whereas other amino acids remained stable even at the highest doses of the EO. In another report, variable response was reported when bacterial cell was exposed to carvacrol [47]. Gram-negative bacteria exposure to cinnamaldehyde suggested the overproduction of metabolites during the mid-exponential growth phase [47]. It was also suggested that the rate of production of metabolites is somehow dependent on the level of cell stress, extent of treatment against cinnamaldehyde, and density of the bacterial cells.

15.10 Cell Morphology vs. Essential Oils

It was noticed that cell morphology plays a significant role in determining the effect of EOs. EOs and their components showed different activity against different forms of bacteria as rod-shaped bacteria were found to be more sensitive to EOs than spherical-shaped bacteria. For instance, 24-hour exposure of EOs to rod-shaped bacteria (*S. typhimurium* and *E. coli*) and spherical-shaped bacteria (*M. luteus* and *S. aureus*) showed different response as more damage was evidenced in rod-shaped bacteria. Another study suggested that due to their lipophilic nature, cyclic monoterpenes can easily penetrate into the membrane structure and can result in an increase in membrane size, subsequently leading to an increase in membrane fluidity, and leading to the suppression of membrane proteins, especially enzymes [48].

15.11 Anti-Quorum-Sensing Effects of Essential Oils

Another area where the role of EOs has been studied is called quorum-sensing systems. A quorum-sensing (QS) system is a type of bacterial cell–cell communication where bacteria synthesize signaling molecules in response to the cell density and adjust gene expression accordingly. Therefore, bacteria has its own intracellular machinery or setup to synthesize extracellular signaling molecules. Increase in bacterial population density allows the accumulation of more signaling molecules in the extracellular environment. Bacteria always keep a check on these extracellular molecules in order to check a variation in their cell numbers and to modify gene expression accordingly [49]. At the same time, QS systems also regulate activities such as:

- Biofilm formation
- Bioluminescence
- Mating of bacteria

- Spore formation
- Virulence factor expression

Recent reports suggest the role of EO in the inhibition of QS systems to control disease with no development of bacterial-resistant strains. EOs or their components can inhibit QS systems by using various mechanisms such as:

- Direct inhibition of acyl-homoserine lactone production
- Acyl-homoserine lactone transport and/or release inhibition
- Separation of acyl-homoserine lactone
- Antagonistic action
- Inhibition of targets downstream of AHL receptor binding

Various EOs have been reported for their anti-biofilm action against pathogenic bacteria. wherein they can interfere with the development of film. Some of the volatile components of oils were reported on for their direct involvement in the inhibition of the cell–cell contact by acyl-homoserine lactone signaling molecules secreted by different bacteria. It was also suggested that some EOs, including cloves, geraniums, lavender, rosemary, and roses, effectively inhibit QS, whereas orange and juniper EOs didn't show anti-QS properties [50]. A previous report suggested the role of 3,4-dichlorocinnamaldehyde in reducing the growth of *V. vulnificus, V. harveyi,* and *V. anguillarum.* Also, the role of cinnamaldehyde in reducing microbial bioluminescence of *V. harveyi* was also reported on. There are various antimicrobial pathways followed by EOs and their components against different bacterial QS systems. This exploration would be helpful in the identification of key targets to inhibit the growth of the bacteria. Some other investigations have suggested the role of vanillin in blocking several events of bacterial respiration and disturbing the movement of potassium ions and affecting the pH gradient [51].

15.12 Antibacterial Potential of Essential Oil in Vapor Phase

The antibacterial potential of EOs or their components could vary as it depends on the type of microorganisms involved. In addition, thorough examination of the EO components could be useful to gain better knowledge of their mechanism of antibacterial effects. Some other parameters determine the antimicrobial potential of volatile oils such as their stability in the vapor phase and chemical interactions, which could be synergistic or antagonistic. The stability of volatile compounds during their transition from the liquid phase to the vapor phase and while crossing through all physiological barriers to act at the site of infection varies. This variation may impact the chemical and biological integrity of the volatile compound. On the other hand, EO itself is a mixture of multiple components, and often these oils are used in combination or blended with other oils or medications to create a system that promotes the interactions. This interaction could be synergistic or antagonistic. Nedorostova et al. [52] studied the effect of 27 EOs in the vapor phase against different food-borne pathogens by using the disk volatilization method and discovered that *Armoracia rusticana* showed antibacterial activity against all pathogens. An earlier report also suggested that *P. fluorescens*, evidenced for causing acute infections in humans especially in the mouth, stomach, and lungs, was found to be effectively suppressed (reducing cell count up to 65%–80%, 12 hours) by vapors of *Mentha arvensis, Mentha piperita*, and *Cymbopogon citrates.* This effect was further enhanced (up to 100% reduction in cell count, 8 hours) when a combination of EO vapors were used in the presence of negative oxygen ions with *M. arvensis.* In the zone of inhibition test, *Mentha piperita* vapor alone showed antibacterial effects against different bacteria such as *E. coli* isolates, *Pseudomonas sp* (22 mm), *Bacillus subtilis* (35 mm), and *S. aureus* [53]. Findings from time-kill kinetics test assay suggested that the treatment of *B. subtilis* with *Mentha piperita* vapor for almost 8 hours showed 100% reduction, whereas *E. coli* and Pseudomonas sp. showed less reduction in viability (74%–85% in almost 12 hours) [54]. A similar study reported by the same researchers by using *E. globulus* EO vapor suggested that *B. subtilis* showed more sensitivity with 100% decrease in viability after 8 h in comparison with the other bacteria (80% decrease after 12 hours) [55].

As mentioned above, a blend of EOs or EO mixture with medication such as antibiotics shows an antagonistic effect or a synergistic effect, which could be determined by the assessment of the fractional inhibitory concentration index. Mixed vapors of cinnamon and clove EOs represented the antagonistic effect against Gram-negative bacteria *E. coli*, whereas the same blend showed the synergistic effect on various other bacteria, including *L. monocytogenes* and *Yersinia enterolytica* [56].

EO in vapor phase could have a considerable effect on the morphology of bacteria where components cause significant morphological changes. *Cymbopogon citrate* EO vapors were reported for their effect against the complete deformation of *Ps. fluorescens,* whereas *M. piperita* EO vapors were reported for their degradative effect against *B. subtilis.* Citrus EO vapor was reported for causing the following morphological changes against *Enterococcus sp.* such as:

- Decrease in membrane potential
- Increase in cell permeability
- Depletion of intracellular ATP
- Reduction in intracellular pH

Another report suggested that EO vapor (oregano, Chinese cinnamon, and savory)-treated *E. coli* O157 and *L. monocytogenes* showed a reduction in intracellular ATP and pH. However, EOs showed the same effect in the liquid phase [57], which does not essentially mean that the liquid and vapor phases work in the same manner.

15.13 Nanotechnology vs. Antibacterial Activity of EOs

The microbial world, including bacteria, fungi, viruses, parasites, etc., is changing its resistance from less pathogenic to more virulent. Some of the mutated or new strains are causing more death and complications [58–112]. Thus, currently there is an urgent need for safe and effective antimicrobials. Biogenic nanoparticles loaded with EOs are known for their effective antimicrobial activity against multidrug-resistant pathogens. Several investigations have shown the ability of both EOs and metal/metal oxide nanocomposites with a wide range of biological properties [58–112]. Recently using combination therapy, bi- and tri-metallic nanoparticles were used with EOs to offer a wide range of biological activities. Additionally, nanoemulsions and nanocapsules can also improve the antibacterial activity of EOs [58–112].

REFERENCES

1. Rudramurthy GR, Swamy MK, Sinniah UR, Ghasemzadeh A. Nanoparticles: Alternatives against drug-resistant pathogenic microbes. *Molecules*. 2016;21(7):836.
2. Burt S. Essential oils: Their antibacterial properties and potential applications in foods--a review. *Int J Food Microbiol*. 2004;94(3):223–253.
3. Raut JS, Karuppayil SM. A status review on the medicinal properties of essential oils. *Ind Crops Prod*. 2014;62;250–264.
4. Swamy MK, Sinniah UR. A comprehensive review on the phytochemical constituents and pharmacological activities of *Pogostemon cablin* Benth: An aromatic medicinal plant of industrial importance. *Molecules*. 2015;20(5):8521–8547.
5. González JF, Hahn MM, Gunn JS. Chronic biofilm-based infections: Skewing of the immune response. *Pathog Dis*. 2018;76(3):fty023.
6. Mith H, Duré R, Delcenserie V, Zhiri A, Daube G, Clinquart A. Antimicrobial activities of commercial essential oils and their components against food-borne pathogens and food spoilage bacteria. *Food Sci Nutr*. 2014;2(4):403–416.
7. Balouiri M, Sadiki M, Ibnsouda SK. Methods for in vitro evaluating antimicrobial activity: A review. *J Pharm Anal*. 2016;6(2):71–79.
8. Chouhan S, Sharma K, Guleria S. Antimicrobial activity of some essential oils-present status and future perspectives. *Medicines (Basel)*. 2017;4(3):58.
9. Raut JS, Karuppayil SM. A status review on the medicinal properties of essential oils. *Ind Crops Prod*. 2014;62:250–264.
10. Conner DE. Naturally occurring compounds. In: Davidison PM, Branen AL, editors. *Antimicrobials in Foods*. Marcel Dekker, New York; 1993:441–468.
11. Kim J, Marshall MR, Wei CI. Antibacterial activity of some essential oil components against five foodborne pathogens. *J Agric Food Chem*. 1995;43(11):2839–2845.
12. Ramos-Nino ME, Clifford MN, Adams MR. Quantitative structure activity relationship for the effect of benzoic acids, cinnamic acids and benzaldehydes on *Listeria monocytogenes*. *J Appl Bacteriol*. 1996;80(3):303–310.
13. Ouattara B, Simard RE, Holley RA, Piette GJ, Bégin A. Antibacterial activity of selected fatty acids and essential oils against six meat spoilage organisms. *Int J Food Microbiol*. 1997;37(2–3):155–162.
14. Arora DS, Kaur J. Antimicrobial activity of spices. *Int J Antimicrob Agents*. 1999;12(3):257–262.
15. Sakagami Y, Kaikoh S, Kajimura K, Yokoyama H. Inhibitory effect of clove extract on vero-toxin production by enterohemorrhagic *Escherichia coli* O157:H7. *Biocontrol Sci*. 2000;5(1):47–49.
16. Hood JR, Wilkinson JM, Cavanagh HMA. Evaluation of common antibacterial screening methods utilized in essential oil research. *J Essent Oil Res*. 2003;15(6):428–433.
17. Nazzaro F, Fratianni F, De Martino L, Coppola R, De Feo V. Effect of essential oils on pathogenic bacteria. *Pharmaceuticals (Basel)*. 2013;6(12):1451–1474.
18. Marino M, Bersani C, Comi G. Impedance measurements to study the antimicrobial activity of essential oils from Lamiaceae and Compositae. *Int J Food Microbiol*. 2001;67(3):187–195.
19. Poolman B, Driessen AJ, Konings WN. Regulation of solute transport in streptococci by external and internal pH values. *Microbiol Rev*. 1987;51(4):498–508.
20. Uribe S, Ramirez J, Peña A. Effects of beta-pinene on yeast membrane functions. *J Bacteriol*. 1985;161(3):1195–1200.
21. Gill AO, Holley RA. Disruption of *Escherichia coli*, *Listeria monocytogenes* and *Lactobacillus sakei* cellular membranes by plant oil aromatics. *Int J Food Microbiol*. 2006;108(1):1–9.
22. Gustafson JE, Liew YC, Chew S, Markham J, Bell HC, Wyllie SG, Warmington JR. Effects of tea tree oil on *Escherichia coli*. *Lett Appl Microbiol*. 1998;26(3):194–198.
23. Juven BJ, Kanner J, Schved F, Weisslowicz H. Factors that interact with the antibacterial action of thyme essential oil and its active constituents. *J Appl Bacteriol*. 1994;76(6):626–631.
24. Ultee A, Smid EJ Influence of carvacrol on growth and toxin production by *Bacillus cereus*. *Int J Food Microbiol*. 2001;64(3):373–378.
25. Tassou C, Koutsoumanis K, Nychas JE. Inhibition of *Salmonella enteritidis* and *Staphylococcus aureus* in nutrient broth by mint essential oil. *Food Res Int*. 2000;33:273–280.
26. Turina AV, Nolan MV, Zygadlo JA, Perillo MA. Natural terpenes: Self-assembly and membrane partitioning. *Biophys Chem*. 2006;122(2):101–113.
27. Mrozik A, Piotrowska-Seget Z, Łabuzek S. Changes in whole cell-derived fatty acids induced by naphthalene in bacteria from genus Pseudomonas. *Microbiol Res*. 2004;159(1):87–95.
28. Juven BJ, Kanner J, Schved F, Weisslowicz H. Factors that interact with the antibacterial action of thyme essential oil and its active constituents. *J Appl Bacteriol*. 1994;76(6):626–631.
29. Burt SA, Reinders RD. Antibacterial activity of selected plant essential oils against *Escherichia coli* O157:H7. *Lett Appl Microbiol*. 2003;36(3):162–167.
30. Burt SA, van der Zee R, Koets AP, de Graaff AM, van Knapen F, Gaastra W, Haagsman HP, Veldhuizen EJ. Carvacrol induces heat shock protein 60 and inhibits synthesis of flagellin in *Escherichia coli* O157:H7. *Appl Environ Microbiol*. 2007;73(14):4484–4490.
31. Cox SD, Mann CM, Markham JL, Bell HC, Gustafson JE, Warmington JR, Wyllie SG. The mode of antimicrobial action of the essential oil of *Melaleuca alternifolia* (tea tree oil). *J Appl Microbiol*. 2000;88(1):170–175.

32. Longbottom CJ, Carson CF, Hammer KA, Mee BJ, Riley TV. Tolerance of *Pseudomonas aeruginosa* to *Melaleuca alternifolia* (tea tree) oil is associated with the outer membrane and energy-dependent cellular processes. *J Antimicrob Chemother.* 2004;54(2):386–392.
33. Trombetta D, Castelli F, Sarpietro MG, Venuti V, Cristani M, Daniele C, Saija A, Mazzanti G, Bisignano G. Mechanisms of antibacterial action of three monoterpenes. *Antimicrob Agents Chemother.* 2005;49(6):2474–2478.
34. Rudramurthy GR, Swamy MK, Sinniah UR, Ghasemzadeh A. Nanoparticles: Alternatives against drug-resistant pathogenic microbes. *Molecules.* 2016;21(7):836.
35. Ultee A, Bennik MH, Moezelaar R. The phenolic hydroxyl group of carvacrol is essential for action against the foodborne pathogen *Bacillus cereus. Appl Environ Microbiol.* 2002;68(4):1561–1568.
36. Ultee A, Smid EJ. Influence of carvacrol on growth and toxin production by *Bacillus cereus. Int J Food Microbiol.* 2001;64(3):373–378.
37. de Souza EL, de Barros JC, de Oliveira CE, da Conceição ML. Influence of *Origanum vulgare* L. essential oil on enterotoxin production, membrane permeability and surface characteristics of *Staphylococcus aureus. Int J Food Microbiol.* 2010;137(2–3):308–311.
38. Cristani M, D'Arrigo M, Mandalari G, Castelli F, Sarpietro MG, Micieli D, Venuti V, Bisignano G, Saija A, Trombetta D. Interaction of four monoterpenes contained in essential oils with model membranes: Implications for their antibacterial activity. *J Agric Food Chem.* 2007;55(15):6300–6308.
39. Venturi CR, Danielli LJ, Klein F, Apel MA, Montanha JA, Bordignon SA, Roehe PM, Fuentefria AM, Henriques AT. Chemical analysis and in vitro antiviral and antifungal activities of essential oils from *Glechon spathulata* and *Glechon marifolia. Pharm Biol.* 2015;53(5):682–688.
40. Kocevski D, Du M, Kan J, Jing C, Lačanin I, Pavlović H. Antifungal effect of *Allium tuberosum, Cinnamomum cassia*, and *Pogostemon cablin* essential oils and their components against population of Aspergillus species. *J Food Sci.* 2013;78(5):M731–7.
41. Rudramurthy GR, Swamy MK, Sinniah UR, Ghasemzadeh A. Nanoparticles: Alternatives against drug-resistant pathogenic microbes. *Molecules.* 2016;21(7):836.
42. Oke F, Aslim B, Ozturk S, Altundag S. Essential oil composition, antimicrobial and antioxidant activities of *Satureja cuneifolia* Ten. *Food Chem.* 2009;112(4):874–879.
43. Mohamed AA, Ali SI, El-Baz FK. Antioxidant and antibacterial activities of crude extracts and essential oils of *Syzygium cumini* leaves. *PLoS One.* 2013;8(4):e60269.
44. Novy P, Davidova H, Serrano-Rojero CS, Rondevaldova J, Pulkrabek J, Kokoska L. Composition and antimicrobial activity of *Euphrasia rostkoviana* Hayne essential oil. *Evid Based Complement Alternat Med.* 2015;2015:734101.
45. Sinico C, De Logu A, Lai F, Valenti D, Manconi M, Loy G, Bonsignore L, Fadda AM. Liposomal incorporation of *Artemisia arborescens* L. essential oil and in vitro antiviral activity. *Eur J Pharm Biopharm.* 2005;59(1):161–168.
46. Devi KP, Nisha SA, Sakthivel R, Pandian SK. Eugenol (an essential oil of clove) acts as an antibacterial agent against *Salmonella typhi* by disrupting the cellular membrane. *J Ethnopharmacol.* 2010;130(1):107–115.
47. Angioni A, Barra A, Coroneo V, Dessi S, Cabras P. Chemical composition, seasonal variability, and antifungal activity of *Lavandula stoechas* L. ssp. stoechas essential oils from stem/leaves and flowers. *J Agric Food Chem.* 2006;54(12):4364–4370.
48. Trombetta D, Castelli F, Sarpietro MG, Venuti V, Cristani M, Daniele C, Saija A, Mazzanti G, Bisignano G. Mechanisms of antibacterial action of three monoterpenes. *Antimicrob Agents Chemother.* 2005;49(6):2474–2478.
49. Nazzaro F, Fratianni F, Coppola R. Quorum sensing and phytochemicals. *Int J Mol Sci.* 2013;14(6):12607–12619.
50. Brackman G, Celen S, Hillaert U, Van Calenbergh S, Cos P, Maes L, Nelis HJ, Coenye T. Structure-activity relationship of cinnamaldehyde analogs as inhibitors of AI-2 based quorum sensing and their effect on virulence of Vibrio spp. *PLoS One.* 2011;6(1):e16084.
51. Fitzgerald DJ, Stratford M, Gasson MJ, Ueckert J, Bos A, Narbad A. Mode of antimicrobial action of vanillin against *Escherichia coli, Lactobacillus plantarum* and *Listeria innocua. J Appl Microbiol.* 2004;97(1):104–113.
52. Nedorostova, L., Kloucek, P., Kokoska, L., Stolcova, M. Pulkrabek, J. Antimicrobial properties of selected essential oils in vapour phase against foodborne bacteria. *Food Control.* 2009;20:157–160.
53. Shahbazi Y. Chemical composition and in vitro antibacterial activity of *Mentha spicata* essential oil against common food-borne pathogenic bacteria. *J Pathog.* 2015;2015:916305.
54. Tyagi AK, Malik A Antimicrobial potential and chemical composition of *Mentha piperita* oil in liquid and vapour phase against food spoiling microorganisms. *Food Control.* 2011;22(11):1707–1714.
55. Laird K, Phillips C. Vapour phase: A potential future use for essential oils as antimicrobials? *Lett Appl Microbiol.* 2012;54(3):169–174.
56. Gon˜i P, Lo´pez, P, Sa´nchez C, Go´mez-Lus R, Becerril R. Nerı´n C. Antimicrobial activity in the vapour phase of a combination of cinnamon and clove essential oils. *Food Chem.* 2009;116:982–989.
57. Oussalah M, Caillet S, Saucier L, Lacroix M. Inhibitory effects of selected plant essential oils on the growth of four pathogenic bacteria: *E. coli* O157:H7, *Salmonella typhimurium, Staphylococcus aureus* and *Listeria monocytogenes. Food Control.* 2007;18:414–420.
58. Basavegowda N, Patra JK, Baek KH. Essential oils and mono/bi/tri-metallic nanocomposites as alternative sources of antimicrobial agents to combat multidrug-resistant pathogenic microorganisms: An overview. *Molecules.* 2020;25(5):1058.
59. Bhatia S, Sharma A, Vargas De La Cruz CB, Chaugule B, Ahmed Al-Harrasi. Nutraceutical, antioxidant, antimicrobial properties of *Pyropia vietnamensis* (Tanaka et Pham-Hong Ho) J.E. Sutherl. et Monotilla. *Curr Bioact Compd.* 2020;16:1.
60. Bhatia S, Sardana S, Senwar KR, Dhillon A, Sharma A, Naved T. In vitro antioxidant and antinociceptive properties of *Porphyra vietnamensis. Biomedicine (Taipei).* 2019;9(1):3.
61. Bhatia S, Sharma K, Namdeo AG, Chaugule BB, Kavale M, Nanda S. Broad-spectrum sun-protective action of Porphyra-334 derived from *Porphyra vietnamensis. Pharmacogn Res.* 2010;2(1):45–49.

62. Bhatia S, Sharma K, Sharma A, Nagpal K, Bera T. Anti-inflammatory, analgesic and antiulcer properties of *Porphyra vietnamensis*. *Avicenna J Phytomed.* 2015;5(1):69–77.
63. Bhatia S, Sardana S, Sharma A, Vargas De La Cruz CB, Chaugule B, Khodaie L. Development of broad spectrum mycosporine loaded sunscreen formulation from Ulva fasciata delile. *Biomedicine (Taipei).* 2019;9(3):17.
64. Bhatia S, Garg A, Sharma K, Kumar S, Sharma A, Purohit AP. Mycosporine and mycosporine-like amino acids: A paramount tool against ultra violet irradiation. *Pharmacogn Rev.* 2011;5(10):138–146.
65. Bhatia S, Namdeo AG, Nanda S. Factors effecting the gelling and emulsifying properties of a natural polymer. *SRP.* 2010;1(1):86–92.
66. Bhatia S, Sharma K, Bera T. Structural characterization and pharmaceutical properties of porphyran. *Asian J Pharm.* 2015;9:93–101.
67. Bhatia S, Sharma A, Sharma K, Kavale M, Chaugule BB, Dhalwal K, Namdeo AG, Mahadik KR. Novel algal polysaccharides from marine source: Porphyran. *Pharmacogn Rev.* 2008;2:271–276.
68. Bhatia S, Sharma K, Nagpal K, Bera T. Investigation of the factors influencing the molecular weight of porphyran and its associated antifungal activity Bioact. *Carb Diet Fiber.* 2015;5:153–168.
69. Bhatia S, Kumar V, Sharma K, Nagpal K, Bera T. Significance of algal polymer in designing amphotericin B nanoparticles. *Sci World J.* 2014;2014:564573.
70. Bhatia S, Rathee P, Sharma K, Chaugule BB, Kar N, Bera T. Immuno-modulation effect of sulphated polysaccharide (porphyran) from *Porphyra vietnamensis*. *Int J Biol Macromol.* 2013;57:50–56.
71. Bhatia S. *Natural Polymer Drug Delivery Systems: Marine Polysaccharides Based Nano-Materials and Its Applications.* Springer International Publishing, Switzerland; 2016;185–225.
72. Bhatia S. *Natural Polymer Drug Delivery Systems: Plant Derived Polymers, Properties, and Modification & Applications.* Springer International Publishing, Switzerland; 2016;119–184.
73. Bhatia S. *Natural Polymer Drug Delivery Systems: Nanotechnology and Its Drug Delivery Applications.* Springer International Publishing, Switzerland; 2016;1–32.
74. Bhatia S. *Natural Polymer Drug Delivery Systems: Nanoparticles Types, Classification, Characterization, Fabrication Methods and Drug Delivery Applications.* Springer International Publishing, Switzerland; 2016;33–93.
75. Bhatia S. *Natural Polymer Drug Delivery Systems: Natural Polymers vs Synthetic Polymer.* Springer International Publishing, Switzerland; 2016:95–118.
76. Bhatia S. *Systems for Drug Delivery: Mammalian Polysaccharides and Its Nanomaterials.* Springer International Publishing, Switzerland; 2016;1–27.
77. Bhatia S. *Systems for Drug Delivery: Microbial Polysaccharides as Advance Nanomaterials.* Springer International Publishing, Switzerland; 2016;29–54.
78. Bhatia S. *Systems for Drug Delivery: Chitosan Based Nanomaterials and Its Applications.* Springer International Publishing, Switzerland; 2016;55–117.
79. Bhatia S. *Systems for Drug Delivery: Advance Polymers and Its Applications.* Springer International Publishing, Switzerland; 2016;119–146.
80. Bhatia S. *Systems for Drug Delivery: Advanced Application of Natural Polysaccharides.* Springer International Publishing, Switzerland; 2016;147–170.
81. Bhatia S. *Systems for Drug Delivery: Modern Polysaccharides and Its Current Advancements.* Springer International Publishing, Switzerland; 2016;171–188.
82. Bhatia S. *Systems for Drug Delivery: Toxicity of Nanodrug Delivery Systems.* Springer International Publishing, Switzerland; 2016;189–197.
83. Bhatia S. *Nanotechnology in Drug Delivery Fundamentals, Design, and Applications: Part 1: Protein and Peptide-Based Drug Delivery Systems.* Apple Academic Press, Palm Bay, FL;2016;50–204.
84. Bhatia S. Stem cell culture. In: *Introduction to Pharmaceutical Biotechnology, Volume 3: Animal Tissue Culture and Biopharmaceuticals.* IOP Publishing Ltd, Bristol, UK; 2019:1–24.
85. Bhatia S. Organ culture. In: *Introduction to Pharmaceutical Biotechnology, Volume 3: Introduction to Animal Tissue Culture Science.* IOP Publishing Ltd, Bristol, UK; 2019:1–28.
86. Bhatia S. Animal tissue culture facilities. In: *Introduction to Pharmaceutical Biotechnology, Volume 3: Animal Tissue Culture and Biopharmaceuticals.* IOP Publishing Ltd, Bristol, UK; 2019:1–32.
87. Bhatia S. Characterization of cultured cells. In: *Introduction to Pharmaceutical Biotechnology, Volume 3: Animal Tissue Culture and Biopharmaceuticals.* IOP Publishing Ltd, Bristol, UK; 2019:1–47.
88. Bhatia S. Introduction to genomics. In: *Introduction to Pharmaceutical Biotechnology, Volume 2: Enzymes, Proteins and Bioinformatics.* IOP Publishing Ltd, Bristol, UK; 2018:1–39.
89. Bhatia S. Bioinformatics. In: *Introduction to Pharmaceutical Biotechnology, Volume 2: Enzymes, Proteins and Bioinformatics.* IOP Publishing Ltd, Bristol, UK; 2018;3:1–16.
90. Bhatia S. Protein and enzyme engineering. In: *Introduction to Pharmaceutical Biotechnology, Volume 2: Enzymes, Proteins and Bioinformatics.* IOP Publishing Ltd, Bristol, UK; 2018:1–15.
91. Bhatia S. Industrial enzymes and their applications. In: *Introduction to Pharmaceutical Biotechnology, Volume 2: Enzymes, Proteins and Bioinformatics.* IOP Publishing Ltd, Bristol, UK; 2018;2:21.
92. Bhatia S. Introduction to enzymes and their applications. In: *Introduction to Pharmaceutical Biotechnology, Volume 2: Enzymes, Proteins and Bioinformatics.* IOP Publishing Ltd, Bristol, UK; 2018;2:1–29.
93. Bhatia S. Biotransformation and enzymes. In: *Introduction to Pharmaceutical Biotechnology, Volume 2: Enzymes, Proteins and Bioinformatics.* IOP Publishing Ltd, Bristol, UK; 2018:1–13.
94. Bhatia S. Modern DNA science and its applications. In: *Introduction to Pharmaceutical Biotechnology, Volume 1: Basic Techniques and Concepts.* IOP Publishing Ltd, Bristol, UK; 2018:1–70.

95. Bhatia S. Introduction to genetic engineering. In: *Introduction to Pharmaceutical Biotechnology, Volume 1: Basic Techniques and Concepts.* IOP Publishing Ltd, Bristol, UK; 2018:1–63.
96. Bhatia S. Applications of stem cells in disease and gene therapy. In: *Introduction to Pharmaceutical Biotechnology, Volume 1: Basic Techniques and Concepts.* IOP Publishing Ltd, Bristol, UK; 2018:1–40.
97. Bhatia S. Transgenic animals in biotechnology. In: *Introduction to Pharmaceutical Biotechnology, Volume 1: Basic Techniques and Concepts.* IOP Publishing Ltd, Bristol, UK; 2018:1–67.
98. Bhatia S. History and scope of plant biotechnology. In: *Modern Applications of Plant Biotechnology in Pharmaceutical Sciences.* Academic Press, Cambridge, MA; 2015:1–30.
99. Bhatia S. Plant tissue culture. In: *Modern Applications of Plant Biotechnology in Pharmaceutical Sciences.* Academic Press, Cambridge, MA; 2015:31–107.
100. Bhatia S. Laboratory organization. In: *Modern Applications of Plant Biotechnology in Pharmaceutical Sciences.* Academic Press, Cambridge, MA; 2015:109–120.
101. Bhatia S. Concepts and techniques of plant tissue culture science. In: *Modern Applications of Plant Biotechnology in Pharmaceutical Sciences.* Academic Press, Cambridge, MA; 2015:121–156.
102. Bhatia S. Application of plant biotechnology. In: *Modern Applications of Plant Biotechnology in Pharmaceutical Sciences.* Academic Press, Cambridge, MA; 2015:157–207.
103. Bhatia S. Somatic embryogenesis and organogenesis. In: *Modern Applications of Plant Biotechnology in Pharmaceutical Sciences.* Academic Press, Cambridge, MA; 2015:209–230.
104. Bhatia S. Classical and nonclassical techniques for secondary metabolite production in plant cell culture. In: *Modern Applications of Plant Biotechnology in Pharmaceutical Sciences.* Academic Press, Cambridge, MA; 2015:231–291.
105. Bhatia S. Plant-based biotechnological products with their production host, modes of delivery systems, and stability testing. In: *Modern Applications of Plant Biotechnology in Pharmaceutical Sciences.* Academic Press, Cambridge, MA; 2015:293–331.
106. Bhatia S. Edible vaccines. In: *Modern Applications of Plant Biotechnology in Pharmaceutical Sciences.* Academic Press, Cambridge, MA; 2015:333–343.
107. Bhatia S. Microenvironmentation in micropropagation. In: *Modern Applications of Plant Biotechnology in Pharmaceutical Sciences.* Academic Press, Cambridge, MA; 2015:345–360.
108. Bhatia S. Micropropagation. In: *Modern Applications of Plant Biotechnology in Pharmaceutical Sciences.* Academic Press, Cambridge, MA; 2015:361–368.
109. Bhatia S. Laws in plant biotechnology. In: *Modern Applications of Plant Biotechnology in Pharmaceutical Sciences.* Academic Press, Cambridge, MA; 2015:369–391.
110. Bhatia S. Technical glitches in micropropagation. In: *Modern Applications of Plant Biotechnology in Pharmaceutical Sciences.* Academic Press, Cambridge, MA; 2015:393–404.
111. Bhatia S. Plant tissue culture-based industries. In: *Modern Applications of Plant Biotechnology in Pharmaceutical Sciences.* Academic Press, Cambridge, MA; 2015:405–417.
112. Bhatia S, Al-Harrasi A, Behl T, Anwer MK, Ahmed MM, Mittal V, Kaushik D, Chigurupati S, Kabir MT, Sharma PB, Chaugule B, Vargas-de-la-Cruz C. Anti-migraine activity of freeze dried-latex obtained from Calotropis Gigantea Linn. *Environ Sci Pollut Res Int.* 2021.

16

Anti-Inflammatory, Antioxidant, and Immunomodulatory Effects of EOs

Ahmed Al-Harrasi
Natural and Medical Sciences Research Center, University of Nizwa

Saurabh Bhatia
Natural and Medical Sciences Research Center, University of Nizwa
University of Petroleum and Energy Studies

P.B. Sharma
Amity University Haryana

Mohammed Muqtader Ahmed and Md. Khalid Anwer
Prince Sattam Bin Abdul Aziz University

CONTENTS

16.1 Introduction

Inflammation is a host cellular response against internal or external harmful stimuli. Inflammation can progress into a variety of diseases, including cancer and autoimmune diseases. This host response always results in a rise in endothelial lining cell permeability as well as the infiltration of blood leukocytes, oxidative burst, and production of cytokines. Essential oils (EOs) are the reservoir of volatile components derived from aromatic plants. EOs contain a pool of anti-inflammatory compounds that can synergistically act to reduce inflammation. The anti-inflammatory effects possessed by EOs could be due to different mechanisms of action, including antioxidant activities via reducing oxidative stress and via involving inflammation-associated signaling pathways such as cytokines, expression of genes linked to inflammatory pathways. This mediated by the potential of EO components to modulate the process of transcriptional activation of selective pro-inflammatory genes in an order to selective binding of transcription factors such as nuclear factor kappa-light-chain-enhancer of activated B cells to the promoter genes.

EOs can be used solely or in combinations to reduce inflammation. EOs can also be used in combination with main course medication to reduce inflammation. Synthetic antioxidants like butylated hydroxyanisole (BHA) and dibutylated hydroxytoluene (BHT) have recently been studied for their harmful effects on human health. EOs are natural products present in liquid form and known for their potential antioxidant effects. EOs have recently been used in the food industry as natural antioxidants to prevent autoxidation and prolong shelf-life. This can be done by direct treatment of food with EOs or as respective packaging material and edible coatings. This chapter discusses the anti-inflammatory and antioxidant effects of EOs.

DOI: 10.1201/9781003175933-18

16.2 *In vitro* Activity of Essential Oils

EOs modulate immune response by following different mechanisms as they have multiple components, and each component acts through the same or different mechanisms to activate immune reaction in response to pathogenicity caused by the invaded pathogen. To determine the immunomodulatory action of EOs, various *in vitro* studies involving human immune cells, or cell lines obtained from different experimental animals, have been performed. Cultured human monocyte-derived macrophage treatment with eucalyptus oil allowed the stimulation of phagocytic activity without simultaneous treatment of lipopolysaccharide [1]. A previous report suggested the role of lavender and tea tree EOs in inducing non-specific stimulatory response as well as considerably decreasing pro- and anti-inflammatory cytokines [tumor necrosis factor alpha, interleukin (-4 & -6)] after treatment with EOs [1]. Various possible mechanisms such as the involvement of receptors for phagocytosis (complement or Fc-gamma receptors) after the treatment of EOs could explain the augmented phagocytosis, which could be further associated with low level of proinflammatory cytokines. It was also suggested that EO treatment-induced phagocytosis required microtubule lattice integrity in the spindle to form a microtubular network [1]. In one study, the anti-inflammatory potential of eucalyptus EO or 1,8-cineole was evidenced. It was suggested that the treatment of EO and 1,8-cineole showed considerable suppression of interleukin-1β as well as tumor necrosis factor alpha – and downregulated expression of nuclear factor kappa B in leukocytes [2,3]. *In vitro* studies on *Zingiber officinale* oil at a dose of 0.001–10 ng/mL showed a considerable inhibition of T cells proliferation to reduce T cell as well as CD4+ cells in a dose-dependent way; however, treatment with oil elevated the T-regulatory cell to the total T lymphocytes in the mice. Moreover, *Zingiber officinale* oil (0.001–10 ng/mL) also showed the inhibition of interleukin-1alpha release from rodent macrophages that reside in the peritoneal cavity in a dose-dependent manner [4]. Depending on the chemical composition variation among different EOs, there is always a difference in immune response. Further, lymphocytes and activated macrophages culture treatment with *Schinus molle* EO showed an elevation in the levels of nitric oxide as well as tumor necrosis factor alpha, whereas level of interleukin-10 level was decreased, resulting in activation of the immune system [5]. Treatment of isolated bone marrow white blood cells as well as neutrophils with *Ferula iliensis* EO elevated superoxide anion production. Furthermore, *Ferula* EOs stimulated Ca^{2+} influx in TRPV1 channel-transfected HEK293 cells and desensitized the capsaicin-induced response in these cells [6]. EO derived from *Allium sativum* and its organosulfur components stimulated functional responses in isolated human neutrophils, leading to an increase in reactive oxygen species (ROS) production or calcium flux [7]. EO of *Boswellia carterii* demonstrated a strong immunostimulation in the lymphocyte proliferation assay. *Boswellia carterii* EO showed strong immunostimulant activity (90% lymphocyte transformation) due to its strong mitogenic potential, which was almost equivalent to level of immunostimulation caused by levamisole (85%) and *Echinacea purpurea* extract (95%) [8]. Isolated human polymorphonuclear granulocyte treatment with *Thymus vulgaris* EO showed considerable intracellular inhibition of *Candida albicans* [9]. The authors also suggested the role of *Pituranthos tortuosus* EO in the proliferation of splenocytes from naïve mice, which may further demonstrate the stimulation of B cells [10].

The authors suggested that the treatment of non-stimulated mouse peritoneal macrophages with *Syzygium cumini* EO enhanced nitric oxide production against *Leishmania* strains along with the activation of phagocytic response and lysosomal activities [11]. Treatment of human monocyte-derived macrophages with *Lavandula angustifolia* EO resulted in enhanced phagocytic response along with upregulation of genes associated with ROS generation and suppressed interleukins -1 and -6 [12].

16.3 *In vivo* Activity of Essential Oils

Oral administration of EOs derived from clove, sage, and ginger in healthy and cyclophosphamide-immunosuppressed mice was investigated in a previous study. *Syzygium aromaticum* EO administration resulted in an increase in the leukocyte count and delayed-type hypersensitivity response, whereas cellular and humoral immune responses were restored in immunocompromised mice. Similarly, *Zingiber officinale* EO administration resulted in improvement of the humoral immune response among immunocompromised mice [4]. An *in vivo* study demonstrated that treatment with *Zingiber officinale* oil reduced the delayed type of hypersensitivity response to 2,4-dinitro-1-fluorobenzene in the sensitized experimental rodent. This response possessed by the EO suggested that oil components affected cell-mediated immune reactions as well as non-specific T cell proliferation. Also, EO components might possess positive effects in some pathological conditions, such as chronic inflammation. α-pinene and carvacrol treatment (components of *Carum copticum* seeds) enhanced the humoral immunity, primary as well as secondary antibody production, and DTH response in SRBC-immunized group. Also, this treatment stimulated phagocytosis of heat-inactivated *Candida* cells by peritoneal macrophages [13]. Oral administration (in drinking water) of *Eucalyptus globules* EO in immunosuppressed mice (by 5-fluorouracil) considerably augmented the proportion of monocytes as well as their phagocytic ability and reduced myelotoxicity caused by 5-fluorouracil as well as normalized the level of monocytes as well as the phagocytic activity of MDMs (monocyte-derived macrophages) [13]. *Eugenia caryophyllata* EO administration resulted in an increase in primary and secondary antibodies, which suggested the stimulation of humoral response, in contrast to cell-based immune reactions, which was reduced as demonstrated by decrease in foot-pad thickness after treatment with EO [13]. EO derived from *Citrus sinensis* as well as its components (limonene and linalool or citral) considerably augmented the proportion of immunoglobulin A. Limonene considerably augmented the proportion of serum biochemical markers such as immunoglobulins (-A, -G) and interleukin-2, whereas linalool increased immunoglobulins (-A, -G) after intragastric delivery in rodents [14]. Oral administration of Massoia (*Massoia aromatica*) EO and C-10 massoia lactone resulted in an increased phagocytic ability of macrophages. Also, this improved phagocytic response was dependent on the concentration of massoia lactone [15]. Intraperitoneal injection of niaouli (*Melaleuca viridiflora*) in mice immunized with keyhole limpet hemocyanin resulted in the overexpression of CD25, which suggests the stimulation of macrophage activity as well as T lymphocyte-mediated immunity [16].

Inhalation of lavender EO resulted in the inhibition of allergic airway inflammation, as reported by the decreased cell accumulation and mucus production. Lavender EO treatment also decreased IL-5 and IL-13 production and prevented eosinophilic infiltration. As is known, the production of mucus is controlled by the downregulation of the gene MUC5B, which is responsible for the production of the major gel-forming mucin. Various researchers have demonstrated that this downregulation may take place by the suppression of NF-κB (transcription factor) activation by certain compounds of lavender EO, as NF-κB has been found to increase the gene expression of MUC5B. Thus, it was concluded that lavender EO possesses potential immunomodulatory effects and demonstrates great potential as an alternative anti-inflammatory medicine for various respiratory complications.

Eucalyptus oil has been used for decades in folk medicine in the form of inhalation or aromatherapy for the treatment of various respiratory disorders; nevertheless, sufficient information is still not available to corroborate its mechanism of action vs. its chemical profile.

A recent report suggested that eucalyptus oil and its dominant constituent 1,8-cineole (eucalyptol) showed potential anti-inflammatory activity, which was modulated via selective downregulation of the pattern recognition receptor pathways. These pathways included PRR proteins such as TREM-1 and NLRP3 and common downstream signaling cascade partners (NF-κB, MAPKs [mitogen-activated protein kinases], and MKP-1). In conclusion, the role of the anti-inflammatory potential of eucalyptus oil and 1,8-cineol in the modulation of TREM-1 and NLRP3 inflammasome-related genes and the MAPK-negative regulator was clearly established in this study [17].

Previous studies demonstrated the antiviral potential of two EOs – tea tree oil and eucalyptus oil – against the influenza virus (i.e., influenza virus A strain NWS/G70C (H11N9)). Both EOs showed potent viral inhibitory effects and efficiently inactivated captured microorganisms. The viral inhibitory potential of tea tree EO was also effectively experimented in vapor form in the rotational aerosol chamber, and the findings were promising [18]. Oral treatment of red ginseng EO resulted in the augmentation of serum TNF-α level, which suggests the overall stimulating effect when compared to the negative controls [19]. EO obtained from the leaf of *Zanthoxylum rhoifolium* as well as its main constituent, beta-caryophyllene, considerably improved the existence of Ehrlich ascites carcinoma bearing rodent [103]. During this study, it was found that EO and β-caryophyllene considerably augmented the cytotoxicity of natural killer cells against carcinoma cells as well as YAC-1 lymphoma cells [20].

16.4 Effects of Essential Oil on Human Health

There are only a few studies available that examine the direct impacts of oils over the immunological responses of individuals. Komori et al. [21] demonstrated the role of citrus aroma in depressive disorder as well as its effect on the immune system. A blend of lemon EO with *Citrus sinensis* fruit EO, *Citrus bergamia* EO, and cis-4-hexenol has been used to treat individuals suffering from with depression. Aromatherapy of citrus fragrance normalized the level of lymphocytes ratio (CD4/CD8) as well as activity of natural killer cells [21]. Olfactory aromatherapy of healthy male subjects with *Chamaecyparis obtusa* EO augmented NK activity and level of NK cells with considerable increase in antimicrobial immune proteins such as granzyme, perforin, and granulysin in the systemic circulation, whereas T cell count considerably decreased [22]. Aromatherapy massage of *Lavandula angustifolia* oil mixed with almond oil in healthy pregnant women showed a significant increase in salivary IgA, which suggested the possible role of aromatherapy in the enhancement of immune function in pregnant women [23]. Aromatherapy massage in healthy volunteers using blended EOs (orange sweet, true lavender, and marjoram sweet) diluted in carrier oil (macadamia nut) showed a considerable increase in salivary IgA level. In contrast, massage with only carrier EO (which is usually used to dilute EOs) and aromatherapy-based massage did not show considerable variation in level of salivary IgA. Aromatherapy-based topical application of EOs over the skin of healthy volunteers using a blend of lavender, cypress, and *Origanum majorana* EO in *Prunus amygdalus* oil showed a considerable rise in the lymphocytes in peripheral blood and cytotoxic T lymphocytes as well as CD16+ cell counts [24]. Thai massage using ginger EO in coconut oil among colorectal cancer patients registered in a clinical trial showed a considerable increase in mean lymphocyte count with a significant decrease in severity of symptoms such as exhaustion, stress, and pain [25]. Aromatherapy massage using sweet orange, lavender, and sandalwood EOs in jojoba oil among 12 breast cancer patients [26] showed a considerable increase in peripheral blood leukocytes and lymphocyte counts.

16.5 Role of Essential Oils in Reducing Inflammation

Inflammation is a complex defensive immune reaction to protect the body against harmful stimuli such as microbial pathogens, injured tissue, etc. [27]. This inflammatory reaction always leads to certain changes such as:

- Increased permeability of the vascular endothelium.
- Inflows of white blood cells into the interstitium.
- Oxidative burst mechanism in response to harmful stimuli results in the excessive production of ROS in such a manner that the antioxidant system cannot neutralize them, resulting in the damage of cellular molecules.

- Release of small secreted inflammatory proteins in the form of cytokines [interleukins and tumor necrosis factor-±(TNF-±] to regulate and influence immune response.
- Activation of a number of enzymes such as oxygenases, nitric oxide synthases, and peroxidases.
- Arachidonic acid metabolism: Oxygenation of arachidonic acid via two main enzymatic pathways, cyclo-oxygenase and 5-lipoxygenase, leads to the formation of proinflammatory prostanoids and leukotrienes, respectively.
- Upregulation of adhesion molecules: Adhesion molecules play a significant role in the inflammatory process. Onset of inflammation results in increase in the expression of genes regulating the adhesion molecule expression resulting in upregulation of adhesion molecules such as vascular cell adhesion molecule as well as intercellular adhesion molecule in the endothelial and immune cells so as to ease leukocyte adhesion and migration to the sites of inflammation [28].

Besides the antimicrobial action discussed in the above section, EOs are also evidenced for their antioxidant and anti-inflammatory potential. Some oils are important components of traditional medicine and have been used from decades as an anti-inflammatory medicine, such as chamomile EO [29]. Nevertheless, mixed formulations of some EOs such as millefolia, rosemary, eucalyptus, and lavender are mixed with other plants such as myrrh, pine, and clove to exert anti-inflammatory effects [30,31]. So far, little information is available about the exact molecular targets as well as pathways followed by the components of EOs as in the majority of the reports, anti-inflammatory activity is assessed by carrageenan-induced mouse paw edema. The anti-inflammatory potential of EOs and their components is attributed to their antioxidant activities, the way they interact or interfere with signaling proteins such as regulatory transcription factors as well as cytokines and modulate proinflammatory gene expression [31,32].

16.5.1 Effects of Essential Oil on Arachidonic Acid Metabolism

Injury to tissue may cause injury to the cells within such as neutrophils, masses of platelets, endothelial cells, and macrophages. If injury is continuous/repetitive/irreversible, then polyunsaturated fatty acid called arachidonic acid is secreted from the damaged cell by an enzyme known as phospholipase A2. Synthesis of phospholipase A2 is mediated by the intracellular level of the calcium, which accumulates inside the cytoplasm at the time of injury. Influx of calcium elevates the intracellular calcium levels. This may further activate various enzymes inside the cells such as phospholipase A2. Arachidonic acid is generally found in the bound state or esterified to the phospholipid membrane. Stimulation of phospholipase A2 allows the release of arachidonic acid as free allocator. This unbound state of arachidonic acid is rapidly converted to bioactive mediators, and these mediators are called eicosanoids (20-carbon fatty acids). The bioactive mediators metabolized from arachidonic acid are the prostaglandins thromboxane, leukotrienes, and lipoxins in diverse cells and thromboxane A2 in platelets [33].

Arachidonic acid is metabolized by two pathways (cyclo-oxygenase and lipoxygenase pathways). The cyclooxygenase pathway is mediated by cyclooxygenase enzymes (three known COX isoforms, COX-1, COX-2, and COX-3), which are responsible for producing prostaglandins. In particular, cyclooxygenase is responsible for the conversion of arachidonic acid in to PGH2 (prostaglandin H2). The two COX isoforms (COX-1 & 2) showed various biological effects and high expression in the tissues. The same arachidonic acid via 5-lipooxygenase pathway through an intermediate called 5HPETE (5-hydroperoxyeicosatetraenoic acid) is converted to 5HETE (5-hydroxyicosatetraenoic acid), which is further converted to leukotriene B4. This 5HPETE can also be directly converted into leukotriene A4, then subsequently to leukotriene C4, leukotriene D4, and leukotriene E4. This 5HPETE via 12-lipooxygenase pathway can be converted to lipoxin A4 and lipoxin B4. So ultimately, these prostaglandins, leukotrienes, and lipoxins, are the eicosanoids or inflammatory mediators, which are derived from arachidonic acid. Prostaglandins are usually produced by the mast cell, macrophages, endothelial cells, and other cells, whereas leukotrienes and lipoxins are produced by the lipoxygenase pathway. It's not necessarily that arachidonic acid is metabolized by both pathways in each cell; in some cells, one pathway is predominant (cyclooxygenase), whereas in some cells, other pathway (lipoxygenase) is predominant. As far as the role of these mediators in inflammation is concerned, PGD2, PGE2, PGF2, PGI2 (prostacyclin), lipoxin A4, and lipoxin B4 cause vasodilatation, whereas leukotrienes C4, D4, E4, and TXA2 are responsible for vasoconstriction. Apart from vasoconstriction and vasodilation, there are other physiological changes that occur during the inflammation; one among these changes is platelet aggregation. These mediators can inhibit or promote the platelet aggregation: PGI2 inhibits the platelet aggregation, whereas TXA2 promotes the platelet aggregation. Bronchoconstriction is another important effect of inflammation, which is due to the leukotrienes C4, D4, E4, TXA2, and PGF2, whereas bronchodilation is due to the PGD2, PGE2, and PGI2. Another effect, chemotaxis, is an important event of inflammation, which is caused by chemoattractant leukotriene B4 and inhibited by lipoxin A4 and lipoxin B4. Intensification of pain and rise in permeability of the vasculature (regulated by vascular endothelial growth factor) is mediated by prostaglandins, particularly prostaglandin E2, while the leukotrienes cause vasoconstriction, increase permeability of vasculature, as well as regulate several immune reactions responsible for causing allergy and inflammation [34].

Various EOs and their components are reported for their potential in inhibiting various pathways of arachidonic acid metabolism by acting against the mediators or proteins involved in this metabolism to act as potential anti-inflammatory compounds (Table 16.1).

TABLE 16.1

Effects of Essential Oils on Arachidonic Acid Metabolism Pathways

Essential Oils and Its Source	Chemical Components	Mechanism of Action	References
Aloe barbadensis, Illicium verum, Citrus aurantium, Juniperus communis, Thymus vulgaris, Lavandula officinalis, Cananga odorata	1,8-cineole, eugenol, limonene, linalyl acetate, para-cymene, t-caryophyllene, thymol	Inhibition of 5-lipoxygenase	[27]
Salvia essential oils	beta-caryophyllene, 1,8-cineole, alpha-pinene	5-Lipoxygenase inhibitors	[27]
African helichrysum	beta-caryophyllene, 1,8-cineole, alpha-pinene	5-Lipoxygenase inhibitors	[27]
Alpinia murdochii, Alpinia scabra,, Alpinia pahangensis (leaves and rhizomes)	Sabinene and pinene (α- and β-) were key constituents of leaf EO, whereas the alpha-panasinsen, gamma-selinene, alpha-selinene are present in rhizomes EO	5-Lipoxynease inhibitors	[27]
Chamomile essential oil	Chamazulene and α-bisabolol	Inhibition of leukotriene synthesis and 5-lipoxygenase inhibitors	[27]
Zucc (*T. nucifera*), *Musa basjoo* Siebold (*M. basjoo*)	alpha-pinene, limonene, 3-and carene	Inhibit cyclooxygenase-2 selectively and suppressive effects on production of prostaglandin E2	[27]
Present in many essential oils	1,8-Cineole, terpene oxide	Acts on both routes of arachidonic acid metabolism, inhibit leukotrienes and prostaglandins	[27]
Essential oil of *Chamaecyparis obtuse*	α-Terpinyl acetate, sabinene, isobornyl acetate, and limonene	Control the prostaglandin E2 production and expression of TNF-alpha gene via cyclooxygenase-2 pathway	[35]
Mentha longifolia essential oils	Menthone, pulegone, piperitone dihydrocarvone, limonene, 3-terpinolenone, 1,8-cineole, germacrene D, and caryophyllene	Positively affecting COX-2 expression, suppressing inflammatory reactions such as PGE2 and COX-2	[36]
Lindera erythrocarpa essential oil	Nerolidol, caryophyllene, α-humulene, germacrene-D, and α-pinene	Inhibition of the production of NO, PGE2, and other cytokines (e.g., TNF-α and IL-6) via the regulation of the nuclear factor kappa-light-chain-enhancer of activated B cells) and mitogen-activated protein kinase pathway	[37]
Essential oil from blossoms of *Citrus aurantium*	Linalool, α-terpineol, (R)-limonene, and linalyl acetate	Inhibited the production of nitric oxide, interleukin-6, tumor necrosis factor-α, interleukin-1β (IL-1β) (56.09±2.21%), reduced COX-2 gene expression as well as suppressed NF-κB stimulation, inhibited the c-Jun N -terminal kinase and p38 phosphorylation	[38]
Essential oil containing Carvacrol	Carvacrol	Anti-inflammatory potential of this compound due to the inhibition of inducible COX-2 isoform	[39]
Essential oil containing D-limonene	D-Limonene	NF-κB, COX-2 and iNOS repression	[40]
Cassia oil from different parts of *Cinnamomum cassia*	Cinnamaldehyde Cassia oil and cinnamaldehyde	Significantly inhibits the mRNA expression of COX-2 enzymes	[41]
Eugenol-containing oils	Eugenol	Supported downregulation of TNF-alpha, Reduced the IL-6, TNF-α, PGE2, COX, and iNOS levels in another study Decreased expression of IL-1β and COX-2 Decreased TNF-α, NF-κB, and IL-1β, expression	[42]
Apple gum,, Lemongrass, Thyme, *Lindernia anagallis,* and *Pelargonium×fragrans* EO	36 components	5-LOX suppression and downregulation of TNF-α, IL-8, IL-1β, production in Tamm-Horsfall Protein 1 cells	[43]
Sweetgum (leaves and stems)	Leave EO presented pinene (alpha and beta) and d-limonene andstem EO presented α-cadinol, pinene (alpha and beta), germacrene D, and d-limonene	Suppression of PGE2 and 5-LOX	[44]

(Continued)

TABLE 16.1 (*Continued*)

Effects of Essential Oils on Arachidonic Acid Metabolism Pathways

Essential Oils and Its Source	Chemical Components	Mechanism of Action	References
Ocotea quixos, wood EO (leaf and branches); *Callitris intratropica* EO (branches and leaves); *Copaifera reticulata/ langsdorffii* (gum-resin) EO	-	*Ocotea* inhibited LPS-stimulated production of PGE2, LPS-facilitated COX-2 and iNOS production, inhibition of of LPS-mediated production of IL-8 as well as IL-1β	[45]
Hibiscus sabdariffa EO	-	NF-κB signaling pathways and MAPK suppression, decrease in the production of NO, iNOS, COX-2, TNF-α, IL-1, and IL-6,	[46]
Essential oil isolated from the calyx of *Hibiscus sabdariffa*	Fatty acids and ester compounds	NF-κB signaling pathways and MAPK suppression, decrease in the production of NO, iNOS, COX-2, TNF-α, IL-1, and IL-6,	[46]
Teucrium pruinosum Boiss. essential oil	Component (45.53%) followed by caryophyllene (19.35%)	COX-1 and Cox-2 inhibitory activity Significantly ($p<0.05$) prevented the increase of lipid peroxidation, COX-2 and PGE2 levels and liver enzymes. Additionally, the decreased levels of ferric-reducing ability of plasma and glutathione	[47]
Stachys viticina Boiss.	Endo-borneol was the major component, followed by eucalyptol and epizonarene.	Showed high cyclooxygenase inhibitory activity against COX-1 and COX-2	[48]
Chamomile oil	α-Pinene, camphene, β-pinene, sabinene, myrcene, 1,8-cineole, γ-terpinene, caryophyllene, propyl angelate, and butyl angelate	*Aloe vera* oil exhibited the greatest lipoxygenase inhibitory activity (96%)	[49,50]
Zanthoxylum mezoneurispinosum Ake Assi and *Zanthoxylum psammophilum* oil	*Z. psammophilum* contain methyl ketones, thymol, and sesquiterpenoids, Z. *mezoneurispinosum* rich in monoterpenoids and sesquiterpenoids	High lipoxygenase inhibitory activities	[51]
Kadsura longipedunculata	Delta-cadinene, camphene, borneol, cubenol, and delta-cadinol	5-Lipoxygenase inhibition and prostaglandin production inhibition	[52]
Thymus caespititius and *Tillandsia capitata* EOs	Carvacrol/thymol	Suppressed alpha-amylase and LOX	[53]
Thymus caespititius and *Tillandsia capitata* EOs	1,8-Cineole, linalool	alpha-glucosidase inhibition	[54]
Citrus jambhiri Lush. and *C. pyriformis* Hassk	D-Limonene (92.48% and 75.56%, respectively)	Inhibited the activity of 5-lipoxygenase	[55]
Piper miniatum essential oil (chloroform extract)	Caryophyllene oxide (20.3%) and α-cubebene (10.4%)	Highest activity with 94.2% in the lipoxygenase assay	[56]
Galagania fragrantissima and *Origanum tyttanthum* essential oils	-	5-Lipoxygenase (5-LOX) inhibition	[57]
Pistacia integerrima essential oil	Essential oil from galls contains α-pinene, camphene, dl-limonene, 1,8-cineole, α-terpineol, aromadendrene, and caprylic acid	Inhibits 5-lipoxidase enzyme activity	[58]
O. vulgare volatile oil	Carvacrol (81.0%, 78.6%), γ-terpinene (5.5%, 7.1%), and p-cymene (4.9%, 4.1%)	Inhibited soybean lipoxygenase (54.2%).	[58]
Red thyme (*Thymus zygis*), winter thyme (*Thymus hyemalis*) essential oils (EOs)	Thymol, p-cymene, and linalool	Inhibition of lipoxygenase activity	[59]
Oregano (*Thymbra capitata* and *Origanum vulgare*) essential oils	para-cymene, beta-caryophyllene, gamma-terpinene, thymol, and carvacrol	Inhibitory activity on lipoxygenase (LOX) and acetylcholinesterase	[60]
Foeniculum vulgare	Estragole, t-anethole, alpha-pinene, and limonene	Inhibits 5-lipoxygenase	[61]

16.5.2 Protective Effects of Essential Oils on Cytokines Production

Cytokines are small proteins or signaling molecules that are secreted by almost all cells to regulate and control several immune responses. Proinflammatory cytokines (e.g., TNF-α, IL-1β, and IL-6) promote inflammation, whereas anti-inflammatory cytokines (IL-4 and IL-10) suppress inflammation. Nevertheless, these diverse signaling proteins may or may not act in a defined manner; i.e., they can also act as a pro- as well as an anti-inflammatory cytokine. Their action depends on the actual cellular/molecular/immunological situation. Immunoregulatory proinflammatory cytokines are secreted mainly by activated macrophages to stimulate or encourage inflammatory reactions. Various reports are available that corroborate the important role of proinflammatory cytokines (e.g., IL-1, IL-6, and TNF-α) during the process of inflammation. Primary sources of TNF-α are monocyte/macrophage lineage, whereas other cells such as neutrophils, dendritic cells, natural killer cells, T cells, and mastocytes also generate immunoregulatory cytokines. Other inflammatory cytokine, IL-1, is produced by a variety of cells of the innate immune system such as monocytes, macrophages, fibroblasts, and endothelial cells [62]. It's well known that proinflammatory cytokine production can be induced by lipopolysaccharide. Lipopolysaccharide (heat-stable endotoxin), a cell wall component of Gram-negative bacteria that is composed of O-antigen, is used in a variety of *in vivo* and *in vitro* models, to induce inflammatory reaction by stimulating the production of various inflammatory cytokines in various cell types, such as monocytes/macrophages. On the other side, peptidoglycan and lipoteichoic acid, the main components of the cell wall of gram-positive bacteria, are also used to induce a proinflammatory cytokine response, such as the production of TNF-α, interleukin-1 (IL-1), and IL-6 [67]. Several EOs have been reported for their potential in suppressing the production of cytokines (Table 16.2). Apart from the direct role of EOs and their components over the suppression of proinflammatory cytokines, some also act via modulating the expression of the gene related to cytokines. In some of the reports, it has been demonstrated that the EOs as well as their components studied considerably downregulate the mRNA and protein expression of the cytokines in stimulated cells. This suggests the involvement of these EOs at the transcriptional level by inhibiting the expression of the genes responsible for the production of proinflammatory cytokines [68]. In one of the studies, the inhibitory role of thyme EO, consisting of p-cymene and thymol, at high dose considerably downregulated mRNA IL-1β expression in TNBS-treated mouse colon. However, IL-6 expression was not inhibited significantly (Table 16.2). The effects of various EOs on the production of cytokines are given in Table 16.2.

TABLE 16.2
Effect of Essential Oils over the Production of Cytokines

Essential Oils and Its Source	Chemical Components	Mechanism of Action	References
Cheistocalyx operculatus	Not determined	Considerably suppressed IL-1β and TNF-α production	[27]
Tea tree EO	Terpinen-4-ol	Decreased the IL-8, IL-10, PGE2, TNF-α and IL-1β level	[27]
Tea tree EO	Terpinen-4-ol	Suppresses proinflammatory mediators and stimulates the anti-inflammatory mediators	[27]
Taxandria fragrans	alpha-pinene,1,8-cineole, and linalool	Reduced the TNF-α and IL-6 production in mononuclear cells stimulated by PHA from *Phaseolus vulgaris*	[27]
Cinnamomum osmophloeum	1,8-Cineole, santoline, spathulenol, and caryophyllene oxide	Inhibited IL-1β and IL-6 production	[27]
Rosmarinus officinalis	Cymene, pinene,1,8-cineole camphor	Reduced the proinflammatory IL-6 secretion	[27]
Cinnamomum osmophloeum	Cinnamaldehyde	Inhibited the IL-1β and TNF-α secretion	[27]
Cinnamomum osmophloeum	Cinnamaldehyde	Decreased cytokines production	[27]
Erva baleeira	-	Reduced TNF-α levels	[27]
Cordia verbenacea	α-Humulene	Reduced significantly the TNF-α and IL-1β levels in the subcutaneous tissue of the rat paw after LPS treatment	[27]
Cordia verbenacea	α-Humulene, (−)-trans-caryophyllene	Reduced significantly the TNF-α and IL-1β levels in the carrageenan-injected rats, whereas (−)-trans-caryophyllene diminished only TNF-α release	[27]
Cryptomeria japonica	Kaurene, sabinene elemol, gamma-eudesmol	IL-1β, IL-6, and TNF-α supression	[27]
Artemisia fukudo	alpha-Thujone, β-thujone, camphor, and caryophyllene	Inhibited TNF-α, IL-1β, and IL-6 production	[27]
Cymbopogon citratus	Mixture of stereoisomers geranial (E-isomer) and neral (Z-isomer), known as citral,	Suppressed IL-6 as well as IL-1β production	[27]
Syzygium aromaticum	Eugenol	Suppressed IL-6 as well as IL-1β production	[27]
Syzygium aromaticum	Eugenol	Prevented IL-1β, PGE2, and TNF-α production	[27]

(Continued)

TABLE 16.2 (*Continued*)

Effect of Essential Oils over the Production of Cytokines

Essential Oils and Its Source	Chemical Components	Mechanism of Action	References
Lemongrass, geranium, and spearmint essential oils	Main components (citral, geraniol, citronellol, and carvone)	Inhibited the production of proinflammatory cytokines such as TNF-α	[27]
Cinnamomum sp. =	Citral	Inhibited TNF-α production	[27]
Nutmeg oil	Myristicin	Showed liver protective effects via preventing the TNF-α release as well as fragmentation of hepatic DNA	[27]
Pterodon emarginatus	Trans-caryophyllene, β-elemene, and germacrene D	Marked reduction of IL-1 and TNF-α levels after submitted to a single intrapleural injection of carrageenan	[27]
Thyme and oregano	Thyme (thymol and para-cymene and) and oregano (carvacrol)	Decreased the IL-1β and IL-6 levels	[27]
Zanthoxylum coreanum Nakai	β-Ocimene α-pinene, 4-carvomenthenol, sabinene and linalool	Inhibited of NO, IL-6, and TNF-α, as well as decreased of COX-2 and iNOS levels	[65]
Sesame essential oil	Sesamol, sesamolin, and sesaminol	Release of TNF-α, IL-1β, and NO were inhibited	[66]
Geranium essential oil	Citronellol	Prevented the production of TNF-α	[67]
Myristica fragrans seeds with magnesium aluminometasilicate	Sabinene, pinene, camphene, *p*-cymene, phellandrene, terpinene, limonene, and myrcene	Inhibited IL-6 production	[68]
Schizonepeta essential	Pulegone	Downregulated pro-inflammatory mediators expression	[69]
Patchouli essential oil	Pogostone, beta-patchoulene and patchouli alcohol	Suppressed the proinflammatory cytokines	[70]
Alpinia calcarata (Rhizome and leaf)	(Rhizome EO (1,8-cineole, fenchyl acetate, alpha-terpineol); leaves EO (1,8-cineole, camphor alpha-terpineol)	Reduced ear thickness, weight, myeloperoxidase, and cytokines significantly ($p<0.01$) in mouse ear.	[71]
Citrus and bergamot oil	Bergapten (5-methoxysporalen)	Suppression of the expression and production of proinflammatory mediators	[72]
Cinnamomum cassia	Cinnamaldehyde	Inhibited interleukin (IL)-1β-induced IL-6, IL-8, and tumor necrosis factor-α release	[73]
Magnoliae flos essential oil	Camphor and 1,8-cineole	Decreased production of the cytokines TNF-α, IL-6, and IL-12p70 in lipopolysaccharide-stimulated dendritic cells, suppressed the surface markers MHC II, CD80, and CD86 in LPS-stimulated dendritic cells	[74]
Schisandra chinensis	ND	Inhibited TNF-α, IL-6, IL-1β release and reduced levels of nitric oxide and considerably inhibited MAPKs expression	[75]
Peach kernel oil	-	Inhibited the expression of TNF-α-	[76]
Atractylodes macrocephala essential oil combined with *Panax ginseng*	-	Suppressed the 5-fluorouracil-mediated increases in the intestinal inflammatory mediators (IL-17, TNF-α, IL-1β, IFN-γ, and IL-6)	[77]
Hallabong flower [(*Citrus unshiu* Marcov × *Citrus sinensis* Osbeck) × *Citrus reticulata* Blanco]	Sabinene (34.75%), linalool (14.77%), β-ocimene (11.07%), 4-terpineol (9.63%)	Inhibited production as well as expression of PGE2, NO, COX-2 as well as other inflammatory mediators such as IL-6, TNF-α and IL-1β	[78]
Lindera umbellata	Linalool ($C_{10}H_{18}O$)	Suppressed LPS-induced proinflammatory cytokine production such as that of nitric oxide (NO), interleukin-6 (IL-6), and tumor necrosis factor-α (TNF-α). Moreover, iNOS and COX-2 gene expression were downregulated	[79]
Leptospermum scoparium	Calamenene (17.78%), leptospermone (11.86%), α-selinene (7.17%), and α-cadinene (6.40%)	Suppressed UV-B-induced skin inflammation by inhibiting the production of inflammatory cytokines	[80]
Rhizoma curcumae	Curcumol	Inhibited LPS-induced NO production by suppressing iNOS mRNA expression and protein level, inhibited LPS-induced production of TNF-α, IL-1β, and IL-6 at both the transcriptional and translational levels, acted via suppressing JNK-mediated AP-1	[81]
Citrus unshiu flower	y-Terpinene (24.7%), 2-beta-pinene (16.6%), 1-methyl-2-isopropylbenzene (11.5%), L-limonene (5.7%), beta3-ocimene (5.6%), and alpha-pinene (4.7%)	Effective inhibitor of LPS-induced NO and PGE2 production in RAW 264.7 cells, suppressed the production of inflammatory cytokines, including interleukin (IL)-1beta, tumor necrosis factor (TNF)-alpha, and IL-6	[82]

(Continued)

TABLE 16.2 (*Continued*)

Effect of Essential Oils over the Production of Cytokines

Essential Oils and Its Source	Chemical Components	Mechanism of Action	References
Neolitsea sericea	Sericenine (32.3%), sabinene (21.0%), trans-beta-ocimene (13.3%), beta-caryophyllene (4.8%), and 4-terpineol (4.2%)	Dose-dependent inhibitory activities on nitric oxide (NO), prostaglandin E2 (PGE2), tumor necrosis factor (TNF)-alpha, interleukin (IL)-1beta, and IL-6 production in lipopolysaccharide (LPS)-activated RAW 264.7 macrophages; inhibited NF-κB activation by LPS; suppressed the phosphorylation of p38, ERK and JNK	[83]
Perilla frutescens	Isoegomaketone	Inhibited the activation of NF-κB and NO serum levels; downregulation of iNOS gene expression via the blockade of STAT-1 activation	[84]

16.5.3 The Role of Essential Oils and Their Components in Affecting Genes Responsible for the Expression of Proinflammatory Gene

Nitric oxide (NO), prostaglandins, and cytokines are important regulators of the inflammatory process. Production of nitric oxide and products of arachidonic acid metabolism are regulated by nitric oxide synthase and cyclooxygenase enzymes. These enzymes participate in catalyzing the synthesis of prostaglandins and NO. During inflammation, COX-1 acts as a constitutive enzyme, whereas COX-2 and NOS act as inducible enzymes. Lipid inflammatory mediators (prostaglandins) are synthesized by constitutive enzymes such as COX-1 and its inducible isoform COX-2. There are various forms of enzymes participating in the synthesis of inflammatory mediators; some of the enzymes are constitutive (those enzymes whose proportion remains stable during the complete life cycle of the cell), whereas some are inducible (whose production is stimulated when required). In addition, some enzymes are present in their isoforms (i.e., different proteins that have the same enzyme activity) (Table 16.3). Thus, on the basis of the difference in primary amino acid sequences, a manner by which they regulate reaction and distribution among different tissues and cells, there are three main isoforms of nitric oxide synthase:

TABLE 16.3

Effects of Essential Oil over Modulation of Proinflammatory Gene Expression

Essential Oils and Their Source	Chemical Components	Mechanism of Action	References
Teucrium brevifolia Schreber and *Teucrium montbretii*	delta-cadinene and pathulenol in *T.brevifolia;* caryophyllene oxide and carvacrol in *Teucrium montbretia*	Inhibited production of NO	[27]
Teucrium polium, *Teucrium flavum*	*Teucrium flavum* contain 4-vinyl guaiacol caryophyllene and, whereas *Teucrium polium* contain carvacrol and caryophyllene	Suppressed production of NO	[27]
Fortunella japonica (GumGyul) and *Citrus sunki* (JinGyul)		Inhibited LPS-induced NO production	[27]
Origanum EO	*p*-cymene and thymol and	Supressed NO production	[27]
Citrus peel waste essential oil		Supressed NO production	[27]
Distichoselinum tenuifolium	Myrcene	Suppressed NO production	[27]
ND	(−)-Linalool at high concentration	Suppressed PGE2 and NO production	[27]
Cryptomeria japonica essential oil	ND	Suppression of NO production via downregulating expression of iNOS protein/ mRNA iNOS and COX-2 protein/ COX-2 mRNA	[27]
Abies koreana EO	alpha-pinene, bornyl acetate, limonene	Downregulated expression of iNOS mRNA/ protein and COX-2 mRNA/protein	[27]
Farfugium japonicum EO	beta-caryophyllene, undecane, nonene	Suppressed NO and PGE2 release via downregulating the expression of iNOS and COX-2 mRNA	[27]
Essential oil of *Illicium anisatum*	1,8-Cineole	Suppressed NO and PGE2 production via downregulating the expression of iNOS mRNA/proteins and COX-2 mRNA/ proteins	[27]

(*Continued*)

TABLE 16.3 (*Continued*)
Effects of Essential Oil over Modulation of Proinflammatory Gene Expression

Essential Oils and Their Source	Chemical Components	Mechanism of Action	References
Cordia verbenacea	Caryophyllene, alpha-humulene	Downregulated COX-2 and iNOS, expression	[27]
Cordia verbenacea	Systemic treatment with α-humulene and (−)- trans-caryophyllene	Inhibited the LPS-induced NF-kB activation and neutrophil migration in the rat paw	[27]
Pimpinella corymbosa, Pimpinella tragium, Pimpinella rhodantha EOs	4-(2-Propenyl)phenylangelate, 4-(3-methyloxiranyl)phenyl tiglate, 4-methoxy-2-(3-methyloxiranyl)phenyl isobutyrate, 4-methoxy-2-(3-methyloxiranyl)phenylangelate, and epoxypseudoisoeugenol-2-methylbutyrate	Inhibited NF-kB transcription	[27]
	Cinnamaldehyde	Inhibited the cytokine production	[27]
Cinnamomum insularimontanum EO	Citral	Supressed NO production Citral suppressed iNOS protein expression Citral prevented the of IκBα degradation as well as decreased p50 NF-κB levels	[27]
NM	Citral	Inhibited COX-2 mRNA /protein expression	[27]
NM	Citral	Modulated PPARα /PPARγ mRNA expression	[27]
NM	Carvacrol	Inhibited COX-2 mRNA/ protein expression	[27]
Artemisia fukudo EO	Caryophyllene, thujone (alpha and beta), camphor	Inhibited NF-κB and MAPK stimulation	[85]
Artemisia fukudo EO	Caryophyllene, thujone (alpha and beta), camphor	Suppressed the ERK, JNK, and p38 MAPKs phosphorylation	[27]
Syzygium nervosum EO(		Downregulated TNF-α and IL-1β mRNA expression	[27]
Juniper EO (leaves)	alpha-Pinene	Suppression of NO production	[27]
Essential oil of *Curcuma wenyujin*	Sesquiterpenoidal compounds	Suppressed NO production	[86]
Geraniol	Geraniol	Reduced IL-1β, IL-6, TNF-α, and nuclear factor-κB production	[87]
S. ceratophylla essential oil	Linalool	Inhibited NO production and NF-κB activity	[88]
Yarrow EO	ND	Downregulated NF-κB levels, reduced the serum level of IL-6, normalized IL-10 and TNF-α	[89]
Campomanesia phaea EO	Caryophyllene (14%) and caryophyllene oxide (6.9%)	Inhibited the production of intracellular NO and proinflammatory cytokines IL-6 and TNF-α, inhibition of nuclear factor kappa B	[90]
Carvacrol essential oils		Downregulated gene expression levels of TNF-α, IL-1β, IL-6,TLR4, NF-κB p65	[91]
Fructus Alpinia zerumbet (FAZ), a dry and ripe fruit of *Alpinia zerumbet* (Pers.)		Protected against LPS-induced endothelial cell injury and inflammation likely via the inhibition of TLR4-dependent NF-κB signaling	[92]
Rosmarinus officinalis EO	1,8-cineole, α-pinene, and camphor	Inhibited NF-κB transcription and suppression of arachidonic acid cascade	[93]
Curcuma longa	Aromatic turmerone	Decreased NF-κB and COX-2 expression with reduction in TNF-α and IL-6 level	[94]
Pogostemon cablin	beta-Patchoulene	Suppressed the increase of TNF-α, IL-6, and IL-1β	[95]
Zingiber zerumbet	Zerumbone	Decreased secretion of proinflammatory mediators including TNF-α as well as IL-6	[96]

(*Continued*)

TABLE 16.3 (*Continued*)

Effects of Essential Oil over Modulation of Proinflammatory Gene Expression

Essential Oils and Their Source	Chemical Components	Mechanism of Action	References
Liquidambar formosana	Bornyl cinnamate, a cinnamic acid	Suppressed proinflammatory mediators such as NO, PGE-2, TNF- α, IL-1β production Suppression of proinflammatory genes via bornyl cinnamate	[97]
Artemisia capillaries oil		Inhibited the IκB-α phosphorylation, p65 nuclear translocation, and NF-κB stimulation as well as decreased NO as well as PGE-2	[98]
Saffron essential oil	Crocin and safranal	Activation of SAPK/JNK and inhibition of ERK ½ that are related to MAPK pathways	[99]
Cumin essential oil	ND	Suppressed the expressions of mRNA responsible for iNOS, COX-2, IL-1 and IL-6	[100]

NM, Not mentioned; ND, not determined.

- Cytokine-inducible NOS (iNOS)
- Constitutive (cNOS)
- Endothelial (eNOS)

In rodent macrophages (under *in vitro* conditions), inflammatory mediators including interleukin-1, tumor necrosis factor-alpha, and lipopolysaccharide trigger expression of cytokine-inducible NOS. Similarly in an array of mammalian cells, several inflammatory mediators stimulate NO production or iNOS expression, resulting in increased production of NO for an extended period of time. The production of the smallest signaling molecule, nitric oxide, is regulated by nitric oxide synthase during a molecular reaction that involves (Table 16.3):

- Enzyme: cytokine-inducible nitric oxide synthase
- Amino acid: L-arginine
- Substrates: molecular oxygen
- Cofactors: reduced flavin mononucleotide (FMN), flavin adenine dinucleotide (FAD), (6R) 5,6,7,8-tetrahydrobiopterin (BH4), and nicotinamide-adenine-dinucleotide phosphate (NADPH)

When L-arginine is present, molecular oxygen, and cofactors, iNOS produces a large amount of nitric oxide. This reaction is regulated by various signaling proteins such as MAPKs as well as NF-κB. EO as well as its chemical components showed its anti-inflammatory action in the following ways (Table 16.3):

- Direct interference with the expression of signaling proteins responsible for the synthesis of NO/COX-2
- Direct interference with the expression of respective genes responsible for the production of NO/COX-2
- Direct interference with the signaling mechanisms responsible for the production of NO/COX-2
- Direct interference with the expression of NF-κB transcription factors, CRE-binding protein, CCAAT/enhancer-binding protein, and activator protein 1. These factors regulate COX-2 expression

NF-κB as well as MAPK molecular pathways are the common inflammatory signaling pathways. Activation of these inflammatory signaling pathways can result in the production of proinflammatory cytokines such as interleukin-6 (IL-6), IL-8, and TNF-α, which can cause inflammatory response. NF-κB is a transcription factor that directly participates in the progression as well as development of inflammation, which may be considered as a possible target for anti-inflammatory drugs. Once activated, NF-κB can activate the transcription of various genes so as to regulate the inflammatory process. Thus, MAPK and NF-κB both are considered as key targets for anti-inflammatory drugs, to suppress the production of various inflammatory mediators. NF-κB dimers are maintained in the cytoplasm in an inactive form by forming complex with a family of inhibitors, known as IκBs (inhibitor of κB). This transcriptional factor is comprised of homo- and heterodimer proteins such as p50/p105, p52/p100, c-Rel, p65 (aka RelA), and RelB. Activation of NF-κB is mediated by phosphorylation of IκB-α by an enzyme, IκB kinase. This event results in the degradation of IκB via proteasome, which facilitates and promotes NF-κB translocation from the cytoplasm into the nucleoplasm where it interacts with DNA. The extremely common and abundant form of NF-κB dimer is p50/p65 heterodimer. Activation of p50/p65 heterodimer can result in the movement of p65/p50 to the nucleoplasm. This important event ultimately leads to the transcriptional stimulation of multiple proinflammatory genes, linked to cytokines (IL-6, TNF-α, IL-1β) as well as activation of inducible enzymatic pathways (associated with COX-2 as well as iNOS). LPS can trigger the MAPK pathway by stimulating three families of MAPKs [p. 38, extracellular signal-regulated kinase and c-Jun N-terminal kinase (stress-activated kinases)] in a variety of macrophages and other cells. Other transcription factors, such as peroxisome proliferator-activated receptor, are comprised of three subclasses, PPARα, PPARγ, and PPARβ/δ, which are also participating in modulating the expression of inflammatory reactions, in addition to their role in lipid metabolism, cell proliferation, and cell differentiation. The anti-inflammatory effect of PPARs in a variety of mouse models for acute and chronic inflammation is used as a parameter to determine the effectiveness of test drug as PPAR agonist or antagonist effect. The anti-inflammatory activity of PPAR is mediated by the inhibition of NF-κB. Inhibition of NF-κB by PPAR can be done in many ways as follows:

- Obstruction with the transcriptional capacity of NF-κB factor
- Via upregulation of genes that inhibit NF-κB activation
- Weakens/prevents the binding of NF-κB to the DNA by interacting with NF-κB complex to prevent the further activation of inflammatory genes
- Activation of PPARα leads to the augmented expression of the inhibitory protein (IκB), which can avert the translocation of NF-κB to the nucleus

It has also been reported that PPARγ showed anti-inflammatory effects by regulating expression of COX-2 particularly in macrophages via negative feedback loop. Early growth response factor-1 (Erg-1), also known as ZNF268 or NGFI-A, encoded by the EGR1 gene, is another transcription factor that plays an important role in the regulation of the expression of several key genes of inflammation. For EGR1 gene-related studies, human THP-1 cell line is frequently used.

16.6 Nanoencapsulation of Essential Oils

Nanoencapsulation is an interesting approach used for incorporating EOs in food preparations and pharmaceutical formulae. Other EO-loaded nanoforms such as nanoemulsions, nanocapsules, nanocomposites, and nanofilms have been reported. Using synthetic or natural polymers, these nanostructures can be fabricated and utilized with EOs for various biomedical applications [101–127]. It has been found that the transformation of EOs into these nanostructures by selecting the optimized ratio of polymers and other ingredients biological activity, including antioxidant activity, can be improved. These nanoformulations show a better anti-inflammatory profile with improved physical and chemical properties than the pure EO and thus can be effectively utilized against various inflammatory conditions [101–127].

16.7 Antioxidant Proprieties of EO

Damage caused by any external stimuli to mitochondrial electron carriers can result in the generation of reactive oxygen species (ROS). Continuous production of ROS can further cause damage to cellular components such as DNA, lipid, and protein [128]. Thus, free radical scavenging effects of EOs could thus support anticancer properties [128]. The antioxidant potential of EOs could be utilized to prevent the cancer [128]. Eugenol derived from clove oil has a dual effect on oxidative stress, as it can react with ROS to possess an antioxidant effect by scavenging free radicals and can also induce oxidative stress either by the generation of ROS or via the inhibition of antioxidant systems (i.e., antioxidant enzymes) [128]. In addition, eugenol also possesses anticarcinogenic, cytotoxic, and antitumor properties. The anticancer property possessed by eugenol is mediated by increasing the antioxidant enzyme gene expression [128]. Volatile oil from the leaves as well as flowers of *Callistemon citrinus* enriched with phenolic compounds showed significant antioxidant effects [129]. High intracellular antioxidant activity of EO derived from *Wedelia chinensis* further resulted in a considerable decrease in tumor size and an improvement in healing of adjoining healthy tissue [130]. In particular, the glutathione oxidized form (i.e., glutathione disulfide), which is formed during the oxidation of glutathione, acts as an indicator of oxidative stress to measure the level of oxidative stress induced by any external or intrinsic factor. Treatment of EO from *Nigella sativa* modulated the activities of enzymes (i.e., *glutathione-S-transferase*, *glutathione reductase*, and *glutathione peroxidase*) positively against potassium bromate-induced oxidative stress [130]. A recent report also suggested that balsam fir oil treatment reduced proportion of glutathione due to the presence of, γ -caryophyllene, which has further increased ROS [131]. This type of antioxidant treatment can act as a prooxidant by increasing cellular glutathione levels [131]. Thus, EOs and their components following the same antioxidant mechanism can be more useful as anticancer agents for non-tumor tissue. It has been observed that sage EO treatment in co-amoxiclav-induced hepatotoxicity (in rats) decreased glutathione level and further elevated oxidative stress. *Citrus limon* EO treatment was found to considerably reduce the lipid peroxidation level and nitrite content; however, it increased the GSH levels and the SOD, catalase, and GPx activities in the hippocampus of mice. Similarly, chamomile oil has been reported to moderately ameliorate glutathione depletion and decrease the superoxide dismutase activity in the liver of acetaminophen-administered rats [132,133]. Another report suggested that balsam fir oil treatment resulted in decreased glutathione levels. It was observed that a decrease in glutathione levels was due to the presence of α-humulene, whereas an increase in ROS level was due to the presence of gamma-caryophyllene in EO [132,133].

REFERENCES

1. Serafino A, Sinibaldi Vallebona P, Andreola F, Zonfrillo M, Mercuri L, Federici M, Rasi G, Garaci E, Pierimarchi P. Stimulatory effect of Eucalyptus essential oil on innate cell-mediated immune response. *BMC Immunol.* 2008;9:17.
2. Peterfalvi A, Miko E, Nagy T, Reger B, Simon D, Miseta A, Czéh B, Szereday L. Much more than a pleasant scent: A review on essential oils supporting the immune system. *Molecules.* 2019;24(24):4530.
3. Sadlon AE, Lamson DW. Immune-modifying and antimicrobial effects of Eucalyptus oil and simple inhalation devices. *Altern Med Rev.* 2010;15(1):33–47.
4. Zhou HL, Deng YM, Xie QM. The modulatory effects of the volatile oil of ginger on the cellular immune response in vitro and in vivo in mice. *J Ethnopharmacol.* 2006;105(1–2):301–305.

5. Duarte JA, Zambrano LAB, Quintana LD, Rocha MB, Schmitt EG, Boligon AA, Anraku de Campos MM, de Oliveira LFS, Machado MM. Immunotoxicological evaluation of *Schinus molle* L. (Anacardiaceae) essential oil in lymphocytes and macrophages. *Evid Based Complement Alternat Med.* 2018;2018:6541583.
6. Özek G, Schepetkin IA, Utegenova GA, Kirpotina LN, Andrei SR, Özek T, Başer KHC, Abidkulova KT, Kushnarenko SV, Khlebnikov AI, Damron DS, Quinn MT. Chemical composition and phagocyte immunomodulatory activity of *Ferula iliensis* essential oils. *J Leukoc Biol.* 2017;101(6):1361–1371.
7. Schepetkin IA, Kirpotina LN, Khlebnikov AI, Balasubramanian N, Quinn MT. Neutrophil immunomodulatory activity of natural organosulfur compounds. *Molecules.* 2019;24(9):1809.
8. Mikhaeil BR, Maatooq GT, Badria FA, Amer MM. Chemistry and immunomodulatory activity of frankincense oil. *Z Naturforsch C J Biosci.* 2003;58(3–4):230–238.
9. Duarte JA, Zambrano LAB, Quintana LD, Rocha MB, Schmitt EG, Boligon AA, Anraku de Campos MM, de Oliveira LFS, Machado MM. Immunotoxicological evaluation of *Schinus molle* L. (Anacardiaceae) essential oil in lymphocytes and macrophages. *Evid Based Complement Alternat Med.* 2018;2018:6541583.
10. Krifa M, El Mekdad H, Bentouati N, Pizzi A, Ghedira K, Hammami M, El Meshri SE, Chekir-Ghedira L. Immunomodulatory and anticancer effects of *Pituranthos tortuosus* essential oil. *Tumour Biol.* 2015;36(7):5165–5170.
11. Rodrigues KA, Amorim LV, Dias CN, Moraes DF, Carneiro SM, Carvalho FA. *Syzygium cumini* (L.) Skeels essential oil and its major constituent α-pinene exhibit anti-Leishmania activity through immunomodulation in vitro. *J Ethnopharmacol.* 2015;160:32–40.
12. Giovannini D, Gismondi A, Basso A, Canuti L, Braglia R, Canini A, Mariani F, Cappelli G. *Lavandula angustifolia* mill. essential oil exerts antibacterial and anti-inflammatory effect in macrophage mediated immune response to *Staphylococcus aureus. Immunol Invest.* 2016;45(1):11–28.
13. Serafino A, Sinibaldi Vallebona P, Andreola F, Zonfrillo M, Mercuri L, Federici M, Rasi G, Garaci E, Pierimarchi P. Stimulatory effect of Eucalyptus essential oil on innate cell-mediated immune response. *BMC Immunol.* 2008;9:17.
14. Wang L, Zhang Y, Fan G, Ren JN, Zhang LL, Pan SY. Effects of orange essential oil on intestinal microflora in mice. *J Sci Food Agric.* 2019;99(8):4019–4028.
15. Hertiani T, Pratiwi SU, Yuswanto A, Permanasari P. Potency of Massoia bark in combating immunosuppressed-related Infection. *Pharmacogn Mag.* 2016;12(Suppl 3):S363–S370.
16. Nam SY, Chang MH, Do JS, Seo HJ, Oh HK. Essential oil of niaouli preferentially potentiates antigen-specific cellular immunity and cytokine production by macrophages. *Immunopharmacol Immunotoxicol.* 2008;30(3):459–474.
17. Yadav N, Chandra H. Suppression of inflammatory and infection responses in lung macrophages by eucalyptus oil and its constituent 1,8-cineole: Role of pattern recognition receptors TREM-1 and NLRP3, the MAP kinase regulator MKP-1, and NFκB. *PLoS One.* 2017;12(11):e0188232.
18. Pyankov OV, Usachev EV, Pyankova O., Agranovski IE. Inactivation of airborne influenza virus by tea tree and eucalyptus oils. *Aerosol Sci Technol.* 2012;46:1295–1302,
19. Reyes AWB, Hop HT, Arayan LT, Huy TXN, Park SJ, Kim KD, Min W, Lee HJ, Rhee MH, Kwak YS, Kim S. The host immune enhancing agent Korean red ginseng oil successfully attenuates *Brucella abortus* infection in a murine model. *J Ethnopharmacol.* 2017;198:5–14.
20. da Silva SL, Figueiredo PM, Yano T. Chemotherapeutic potential of the volatile oils from *Zanthoxylum rhoifolium* Lam leaves. *Eur J Pharmacol.* 2007;576(1–3):180–188.
21. Komori T, Fujiwara R, Tanida M, Nomura J, Yokoyama MM. Effects of citrus fragrance on immune function and depressive states. *Neuroimmunomodulation.* 1995;2(3): 174–180.
22. Li Q, Kobayashi M, Wakayama Y, Inagaki H, Katsumata M, Hirata Y, Hirata K, Shimizu T, Kawada T, Park BJ, Ohira T, Kagawa T, Miyazaki Y. Effect of phytoncide from trees on human natural killer cell function. *Int J Immunopathol Pharmacol.* 2009;22(4): 951–959.
23. Chen PJ, Chou CC, Yang L, Tsai YL, Chang YC, Liaw JJ. Effects of aromatherapy massage on pregnant women's stress and immune function: A longitudinal, prospective, randomized controlled trial. *J Altern Complement Med.* 2017;23(10):778–786.
24. Kuriyama H, Watanabe S, Nakaya T, Shigemori I, Kita M, Yoshida N, Masaki D, Tadai T, Ozasa K, Fukui K, Imanishi J. Immunological and psychological benefits of aromatherapy massage. *Evid Based Complement Alternat Med.* 2005;2(2):179–184.
25. Khiewkhern S, Promthet S, Sukprasert A, Eunhpinitpong W, Bradshaw P. Effectiveness of aromatherapy with light than massage for cellular immunity improvement in colorectal cancer patients receiving chemotherapy. *Asian Pac J Cancer Prev.* 2013;14(6):3903–3907.
26. Imanishi J, Kuriyama H, Shigemori I, Watanabe S, Aihara Y, Kita M, Sawai K, Nakajima H, Yoshida N, Kunisawa M, Kawase M, Fukui K. Anxiolytic effect of aromatherapy massage in patients with breast cancer. *Evid Based Complement Alternat Med.* 2009;6(1):123–128.
27. Miguel MG. Antioxidant and anti-inflammatory activities of essential oils: A short review. *Molecules.* 2010;15(12): 9252–9287.
28. Gomes A, Fernandes E, Lima JL, Mira L, Corvo ML. Molecular mechanisms of anti-inflammatory activity mediated by flavonoids. *Curr Med Chem.* 2008;15(16): 1586–1605.
29. Kamatou GPP, Viljoen AM. A review of the application and pharmacological properties of α-bisabolol and α-bisabolol-rich oils. *J Am Oil Chem Soc.* 2010;87:1–7.
30. Darshan S, Doreswamy R. Patented antiinflammatory plant drug development from traditional medicine. *Phytother Res.* 2004;18(5):343–357.
31. Santos FA, Rao VS. Antiinflammatory and antinociceptive effects of 1,8-cineole a terpenoid oxide present in many plant essential oils. *Phytother Res.* 2000;14(4):240–244.
32. Lino CS, Gomes PB, Lucetti DL, Diógenes JP, Sousa FC, Silva MG, Viana GS. Evaluation of antinociceptive and antiinflammatory activities of the essential oil (EO) of *Ocimum micranthum* Willd. from Northeastern Brazil. *Phytother Res.* 2005;19(8):708–712.
33. Gomes A, Fernandes E, Lima JL, Mira L, Corvo ML. Molecular mechanisms of anti-inflammatory activity mediated by flavonoids. *Curr Med Chem.* 2008;15(16):1586–1605.

34. González SB, Houghton PJ, Hoult JR. The activity against leukocyte eicosanoid generation of essential oil and polar fractions of *Adesmia boronioides* Hook. *Phytother Res.* 2003;17(3):290–293.
85. Yoon WJ, Moon JY, Song G, Lee YK, Han MS, Lee JS, Ihm BS, Lee WJ, Lee NH, Hyun CG. *Artemisia fukudo* essential oil attenuates LPS-induced inflammation by suppressing NF-κB and MAPK activation in RAW 264.7 macrophages. *Food Chem Toxicol.* 2010;48(5): 1222–1229.
35. An BS, Kang JH, Yang H, Jung EM, Kang HS, Choi IG, Park MJ, Jeung EB. Anti-inflammatory effects of essential oils from *Chamaecyparis obtusa* via the cyclooxygenase-2 pathway in rats. *Mol Med Rep.* 2013;8(1):255–259.
36. Dadkhah A, Fatemi F, Rasooli A, Mohammadi Malayeri MR, Torabi F. Assessing the effect of *Mentha longifolia* essential oils on COX-2 expression in animal model of sepsis induced by caecal ligation and puncture. *Pharm Biol.* 2018;56(1):495–504.
37. Ko YJ, Ahn G, Ham YM, et al. Anti-inflammatory effect and mechanism of action of *Lindera erythrocarpa* essential oil in lipopolysaccharide-stimulated RAW264.7 cells. *EXCLI J.* 2017;16:1103–1113.
38. Shen CY, Jiang JG, Zhu W, Ou-Yang Q. Anti-inflammatory effect of essential oil from *Citrus aurantium* L. var. amara. *Engl J Agric Food Chem.* 2017;65(39):8586–8594.
39. Landa P, Kokoska L, Pribylova M, Vanek T, Marsik P. In vitro anti-inflammatory activity of carvacrol: Inhibitory effect on COX-2 catalyzed prostaglandin E(2) biosynthesis. *Arch Pharm Res.* 2009;32(1):75–78.
40. Rehman MU, Tahir M, Khan AQ, et al. D-limonene suppresses doxorubicin-induced oxidative stress and inflammation via repression of COX-2, iNOS, and NFκB in kidneys of Wistar rats. *Exp Biol Med.* 2014;239:465.
41. Pannee C, Chandhanee I, Wacharee L. Antiinflammatory effects of essential oil from the leaves of *Cinnamomum cassia* and cinnamaldehyde on lipopolysaccharide-stimulated J774A.1 cells. *J Adv Pharm Technol Res.* 2014;5(4):164–170.
42. Barboza JN, da Silva Maia Bezerra Filho C, Silva RO, Medeiros JVR, de Sousa DP. An Overview on the anti-inflammatory potential and antioxidant profile of Eugenol. *Oxid Med Cell Longev.* 2018;2018:3957262.
43. Tsai ML, Lin CC, Lin WC, Yang CH. Antimicrobial, antioxidant, and anti-inflammatory activities of essential oils from five selected herbs. *Biosci Biotechnol Biochem.* 2011;75(10):1977–1983.
44. El-Readi MZ, Eid HH, Ashour ML, Eid SY, Labib RM, Sporer F, Wink M. Variations of the chemical composition and bioactivity of essential oils from leaves and stems of *Liquidambar styraciflua* (Altingiaceae). *J Pharm Pharmacol.* 2013;65(11):1653–1663.
45. Destryana RA, Young DG, Woolley CL, Huang TC, Wu HY, Shih WL. Antioxidant and anti-inflammation activities of Ocotea, Copaiba and Blue Cypress essential oils in vitro and in vivo. *J Am Oil Chem Soc.* 2014;91(9):1531–1542.
46. Shen CY, Zhang TT, Zhang WL, Jiang JG. Anti-inflammatory activities of essential oil isolated from the calyx of *Hibiscus sabdariffa* L. *Food Funct.* 2016;7(10):4451–4459.
47. Jaradat N, Al-Lahham S, Abualhasan MN, et al. Chemical constituents, antioxidant, cyclooxygenase inhibitor, and cytotoxic activities of *Teucrium pruinosum* Boiss Essential Oil. *Biomed Res Int.* 2018;2018:4034689.
48. Rasooli A, Fatemi F, Hajihosseini R, Vaziri A, Akbarzadeh K, Mohammadi Malayeri MR, Dini S, Foroutanrad M. Synergistic effects of deuterium depleted water and *Mentha longifolia* L. essential oils on sepsis-induced liver injuries through regulation of cyclooxygenase-2. *Pharm Biol.* 2019;57(1):125–132.
49. Jaradat N, Al-Maharik N. Fingerprinting, antimicrobial, antioxidant, anticancer, cyclooxygenase and metabolic enzymes inhibitory characteristic evaluations of *Stachys viticina* Boiss essential oil. *Molecules.* 2019;24(21):3880.
50. Wei A, Shibamoto T. Antioxidant/lipoxygenase inhibitory activities and chemical compositions of selected essential oils. *J Agric Food Chem.* 2010;58(12):7218–7225.
51. Tanoh EA, Nea F, Kemene TK, Genva M, Saive M, Tonzibo FZ, Fauconnier ML. Antioxidant and lipoxygenase inhibitory activities of essential oils from endemic plants of Côte d'Ivoire: Zanthoxylum mezoneurispinosum Ake Assi and Zanthoxylum psammophilum Ake Assi. *Molecules.* 2019;24(13):2445.
52. Mulyaningsih S, Youns M, El-Readi MZ, Ashour ML, Nibret E, Sporer F, Herrmann F, Reichling J, Wink M. Biological activity of the essential oil of *Kadsura longipedunculata* (Schisandraceae) and its major components. *J Pharm Pharmacol.* 2010;62(8):1037–1044.
53. Aazza S, El-Guendouz S, Miguel MG, Antunes MD, Faleiro ML, Correia AI, Figueiredo AC. Antioxidant, anti-inflammatory and anti-hyperglycaemic activities of essential oils from *Thymbra capitata*, *Thymus albicans*, *Thymus caespititius*, *Thymus carnosus*, *Thymus lotocephalus* and *Thymus mastichina* from Portugal. *Nat Prod Commun.* 2016;11(7):1029–1038.
54. Hamdan D, El-Readi MZ, Nibret E, Sporer F, Farrag N, El-Shazly A, Wink M. Chemical composition of the essential oils of two Citrus species and their biological activities. *Pharmazie.* 2010;65(2):141–147.
55. Salleh WM, Kammil MF, Ahmad F, Sirat HM. Antioxidant and anti-inflammatory activities of essential oil and extracts of Piper miniatum. *Nat Prod Commun.* 2015;10(11): 2005–2008.
56. Sharopov F, Braun MS, Gulmurodov I, Khalifaev D, Isupov S, Wink M. Antimicrobial, antioxidant, and anti-inflammatory activities of essential oils of selected aromatic plants from Tajikistan. *Foods.* 2015;4(4):645–653.
57. Shirole RL, Shirole NL, Kshatriya AA, Kulkarni R, Saraf MN. Investigation into the mechanism of action of essential oil of *Pistacia integerrima* for its s antiasthmatic activity. *J Ethnopharmacol.* 2014;153(3):541–551.
58. Hodaj-Çeliku E, Tsiftsoglou O, Shuka L, Abazi S, Hadjipavlou-Litina D, Lazari D. Antioxidant activity and chemical composition of essential oils of some aromatic and medicinal plants from Albania. *Nat Prod Commun.* 2017;12(5):785–790.
59. Cutillas AB, Carrasco A, Martinez-Gutierrez R, Tomas V, Tudela J. Thyme essential oils from Spain: Aromatic profile ascertained by GC-MS, and their antioxidant, anti-lipoxygenase and antimicrobial activities. *J Food Drug Anal.* 2018;26(2):529–544.
60. Carrasco A, Perez E, Cutillas AB, Martinez-Gutierrez R, Tomas V, Tudela J. *Origanum vulgare* and *Thymbra capitata* essential oils from Spain: Determination of aromatic profile and bioactivities. *Nat Prod Commun.* 2016;11(1):113–120.

61. Miguel MG, Cruz C, Faleiro L, Simões MT, Figueiredo AC, Barroso JG, Pedro LG. *Foeniculum vulgare* essential oils: Chemical composition, antioxidant and antimicrobial activities. *Nat Prod Commun.* 2010;5(2):319–328.
62. Dung NT, Bajpai VK, Yoon JI, Kang SC. Anti-inflammatory effects of essential oil isolated from the buds of *Cleistocalyx operculatus* (Roxb.) Merr and Perry. *Food Chem Toxicol.* 2009;47(2):449–453.
63. Schröder NW, Morath S, Alexander C, Hamann L, Hartung T, Zähringer U, Göbel UB, Weber JR, Schumann RR. Lipoteichoic acid (LTA) of *Streptococcus pneumoniae* and *Staphylococcus aureus* activates immune cells via Toll-like receptor (TLR)-2, lipopolysaccharide-binding protein (LBP), and CD14, whereas TLR-4 and MD-2 are not involved. *J Biol Chem.* 2003;278(18):15587–15594.
64. Bukovská A, Cikos S, Juhás S, Il'ková G, Rehák P, Koppel J. Effects of a combination of thyme and oregano essential oils on TNBS-induced colitis in mice. *Mediators Inflamm.* 2007;2007:23296.
65. Guo RH, Park JU, Jo SJ, et al. Anti-allergic inflammatory effects of the essential oil from fruits of *Zanthoxylum coreanum* Nakai. *Front Pharmacol.* 2018;9:1441.
66. Khorrami S, Daneshmandi S, Mosayeb G. Sesame seeds essential oil and Sesamol modulate the pro-inflammatory function of macrophages and dendritic cells and promote Th2 response. *Med J Islam Repub Iran.* 2018;32:98.
67. Yuko Kobayashi, Harumi Sato, Mika Yorita, Hiroto Nakayama, Hironari Miyazato, Keiichiro Sugimoto & Tomoko Jippo Inhibitory effects of geranium essential oil and its major component, citronellol, on degranulation and cytokine production by mast cells. *Biosci Biotechnol Biochem.* 2016;80:1172–1178.
68. Matulyte I, Jekabsone A, Jankauskaite L, et al. The essential oil and hydrolats from *Myristica fragrans* seeds with Magnesium Aluminometasilicate as excipient: Antioxidant, antibacterial, and anti-inflammatory activity. *Foods.* 2020;9(1):37.
69. Yang Q, Luo J, Lv H, Wen T, Shi B, Liu X, Zeng N. Pulegone inhibits inflammation via suppression of NLRP3 inflammasome and reducing cytokine production in mice. *Immunopharmacol Immunotoxicol.* 2019;41(3):420–427.
70. Leong W, Huang G, Khan I, et al. Patchouli essential oil and its derived compounds revealed prebiotic-like effects in C57BL/6J mice. *Front Pharmacol.* 2019;10:1229.
71. Chandrakanthan M, Handunnetti SM, Premakumara GSA, Kathirgamanathar S. Topical anti-inflammatory activity of essential oils of *Alpinia calcarata* Rosc., its main constituents, and possible mechanism of action. *Evid Based Complement Alternat Med.* 2020;2020:2035671.
72. Adakudugu EA, Ameyaw EO, Obese E, Biney RP, Henneh IT, Aidoo DB, Oge EN, Attah IY, Obiri DD. Protective effect of bergapten in acetic acid-induced colitis in rats. *Heliyon.* 2020;6(8):e04710.
73. Cheng WX, Zhong S, Meng XB, Zheng NY, Zhang P, Wang Y, Qin L, Wang XL. Cinnamaldehyde inhibits inflammation of human Synoviocyte cells through regulation of Jak/Stat pathway and ameliorates collagen-induced arthritis in rats. *J Pharmacol Exp Ther.* 2020;373(2):302–310.
74. Chen CH, Chen HC, Chang WT, Lee MS, Liu YC, Lin MK. *Magnoliae Flos* essential oil as an immunosuppressant in dendritic cell activation and contact hypersensitivity responses. *Am J Chin Med.* 2020;48(3):597–613.
75. Xu M, Zhang X, Ren F, Yan T, Wu B, Bi K, Bi W, Jia Y. Essential oil of *Schisandra chinensis* ameliorates cognitive decline in mice by alleviating inflammation. *Food Funct.* 2019;10(9):5827–5842.
76. Hao E, Pang G, Du Z, Lai YH, Chen JR, Xie J, Zhou K, Hou X, Hsiao CD, Deng J. Peach Kernel oil Downregulates expression of tissue factor and reduces atherosclerosis in ApoE knockout Mice. *Int J Mol Sci.* 2019;20(2):405.
77. Wang J, Feng W, Zhang S, Chen L, Sheng Y, Tang F, He J, Xu X, Ao H, Peng C. Ameliorative effect of *Atractylodes macrocephala* essential oil combined with Panax ginseng total saponins on 5-fluorouracil induced diarrhea is associated with gut microbial modulation. *J Ethnopharmacol.* 2019;238:111887.
78. Kim MJ, Yang KW, Kim SS, Park SM, Park KJ, Kim KS, Choi YH, Cho KK, Lee NH, Hyun CG. Chemical composition and anti-inflammatory effects of essential oil from Hallabong flower. *EXCLI J.* 2013;12:933–942.
79. Maeda H, Yamazaki M, Katagata Y. Kuromoji (*Lindera umbellata*) essential oil inhibits LPS-induced inflammation in RAW 264.7 cells. *Biosci Biotechnol Biochem.* 2013;77(3):482–486.
80. Kwon OS, Jung SH, Yang BS. Topical administration of Manuka oil prevents UV-B irradiation-induced cutaneous photoaging in mice. *Evid Based Complement Alternat Med.* 2013;2013:930857.
81. Chen X, Zong C, Gao Y, Cai R, Fang L, Lu J, Liu F, Qi Y. Curcumol exhibits anti-inflammatory properties by interfering with the JNK-mediated AP-1 pathway in lipopolysaccharide-activated RAW264.7 cells. *Eur J Pharmacol.* 2014;723:339–345.
82. Kim MJ, Yang KW, Kim SS, Park SM, Park KJ, Kim KS, Choi YH, Cho KK, Hyun CG. Chemical composition and anti-inflammation activity of essential oils from Citrus unshiu flower. *Nat Prod Commun.* 2014;9(5):727–730.
83. Yoon WJ, Moon JY, Kang JY, Kim GO, Lee NH, Hyun CG. *Neolitsea sericea* essential oil attenuates LPS-induced inflammation in RAW 264.7 macrophages by suppressing NF-κB and MAPK activation. *Nat Prod Commun.* 2010;5(8):1311–1316.
84. Jin CH, Lee HJ, Park YD, Choi DS, Kim DS, Kang SY, Seo KI, Jeong IY. Isoegomaketone inhibits lipopolysaccharide-induced nitric oxide production in RAW 264.7 macrophages through the heme oxygenase-1 induction and inhibition of the interferon-beta-STAT-1 pathway. *J Agric Food Chem.* 2010;58(2):860–867.
86. Xia G, Zhou L, Ma J, Wang Y, Ding L, Zhao F, Chen L, Qiu F. Sesquiterpenes from the essential oil of *Curcuma wenyujin* and their inhibitory effects on nitric oxide production. *Fitoterapia.* 2015;103:143–148.
87. Younis NS, Abduldaium MS, Mohamed ME. Protective effect of geraniol on oxidative, inflammatory and apoptotic alterations in isoproterenol-induced cardiotoxicity: Role of the Keap1/Nrf2/HO-1 and PI3K/Akt/mTOR pathways. *Antioxidants (Basel).* 2020;9(10):E977.
88. Abu-Darwish MS, Cabral C, Ali Z, Wang M, Khan SI, Jacob MR, Jain SK, Tekwani BL, Zulfiqar F, Khan IA, Taifour H, Salgueiro L, Efferth T. *Salvia ceratophylla* L. from South of Jordan: New insights on chemical composition and biological activities. *Nat Prod Bioprospect.* 2020;10(5):307–316.

89. Mohamed ME, Elsayed SA, Madkor HR, Eldien HMS, Mohafez OM. Yarrow oil ameliorates ulcerative colitis in mice model via regulating the NF-κB and PPAR-γ pathways. *Intest Res.* 2021;19(2):194–205.
90. Lorençoni MF, Figueira MM, Toledo E Silva MV, Pimentel Schmitt EF, Endringer DC, Scherer R, Barth T, Vilela Bertolucci SK, Fronza M. Chemical composition and anti-inflammatory activity of essential oil and ethanolic extract of *Campomanesia phaea* (O. Berg.) Landrum leaves. *J Ethnopharmacol.* 2020;252:112562.
91. Liu SD, Song MH, Yun W, Lee JH, Kim HB, Cho JH. Effect of carvacrol essential oils on immune response and inflammation-related genes expression in broilers challenged by lipopolysaccharide. *Poult Sci.* 2019;98(5):2026–2033.
92. Ji YP, Shi TY, Zhang YY, Lin D, Linghu KG, Xu YN, Tao L, Lu Q, Shen XC. Essential oil from *Fructus Alpinia zerumbet* (fruit of *Alpinia zerumbet* (Pers.) Burtt.et Smith) protected against aortic endothelial cell injury and inflammation in vitro and in vivo. *J Ethnopharmacol.* 2019;237:149–158.
93. Borges RS, Ortiz BLS, Pereira ACM, Keita H, Carvalho JCT. *Rosmarinus officinalis* essential oil: A review of its phytochemistry, anti-inflammatory activity, and mechanisms of action involved. *J Ethnopharmacol.* 2019;229:29–45.
94. Li YL, Du ZY, Li PH, Yan L, Zhou W, Tang YD, Liu GR, Fang YX, Zhang K, Dong CZ, Chen HX. Aromatic-turmerone ameliorates imiquimod-induced psoriasis-like inflammation of BALB/c mice. *Int Immunopharmacol.* 2018;64:319–325.
95. Chen XY, Dou YX, Luo DD, Zhang ZB, Li CL, Zeng HF, Su ZR, Xie JH, Lai XP, Li YC. β-Patchoulene from patchouli oil protects against LPS-induced acute lung injury via suppressing NF-κB and activating Nrf2 pathways. *Int Immunopharmacol.* 2017;50:270–278.
96. Ho YC, Lee SS, Yang ML, Huang-Liu R, Lee CY, Li YC, Kuan YH. Zerumbone reduced the inflammatory response of acute lung injury in endotoxin-treated mice via Akt-NFκB pathway. *Chem Biol Interact.* 2017;271:9–14.
97. Kumar KJ, Li J, Vani MG, Hsieh YH, Kuo YH, Wang SY. Bornyl cinnamate inhibits inflammation-associated gene expression in macrophage cells through suppression of nuclear factor-κB signaling pathway. *Planta Med.* 2015;81(1):39–45.
98. Cha JD, Moon SE, Kim HY, Lee JC, Lee KY. The essential oil isolated from Artemisia capillaris prevents LPS-induced production of NO and PGE(2) by inhibiting MAPK-mediated pathways in RAW 264.7 macrophages. *Immunol Invest.* 2009;38(6):483–497.
99. Rahiman N, Akaberi M, Sahebkar A, Emami SA, Tayarani-Najaran Z. Protective effects of saffron and its active components against oxidative stress and apoptosis in endothelial cells. *Microvasc Res.* 2018;118:82–89.
100. Wei J, Zhang X, Bi Y, Miao R, Zhang Z, Su H. Anti-inflammatory effects of cumin essential oil by blocking JNK, ERK, and NF-κB signaling pathways in LPS-stimulated RAW 264.7 cells. *Evid Based Complement Alternat Med.* 2015;2015:474509.
101. Bhatia S, Sharma A, Vargas De La Cruz CB, Chaugule B, Ahmed Al-Harrasi. Nutraceutical, antioxidant, antimicrobial properties of *Pyropia vietnamensis* (Tanaka et Pham-Hong Ho) J.E. Sutherl. et Monotilla. *Curr Bioact Compd.* 2020;16:1.
102. Bhatia S, Sardana S, Senwar KR, Dhillon A, Sharma A, Naved T. In vitro antioxidant and antinociceptive properties of *Porphyra vietnamensis. Biomedicine (Taipei).* 2019;9(1):3.
103. Bhatia S, Sharma K, Namdeo AG, Chaugule BB, Kavale M, Nanda S. Broad-spectrum sun-protective action of Porphyra-334 derived from *Porphyra vietnamensis. Pharmacognosy Res.* 2010;2(1):45–49.
104. Bhatia S, Sharma K, Sharma A, Nagpal K, Bera T. Anti-inflammatory, analgesic and antiulcer properties of *Porphyra vietnamensis. Avicenna J Phytomed.* 2015; 5(1):69–77.
105. Bhatia S, Sardana S, Sharma A, Vargas De La Cruz CB, Chaugule B, Khodaie L. Development of broad spectrum mycosporine loaded sunscreen formulation from Ulva fasciata delile. *Biomedicine (Taipei).* 2019;9(3):17.
106. Bhatia S, Garg A, Sharma K, Kumar S, Sharma A, Purohit AP. Mycosporine and mycosporine-like amino acids: A paramount tool against ultra violet irradiation. *Pharmacogn Rev.* 2011;5(10):138–146.
107. Bhatia S, Namdeo AG, Nanda S. Factors effecting the gelling and emulsifying properties of a natural polymer. *SRP.* 2010;1(1):86–92.
108. Bhatia S, Sharma K, Bera T. Structural characterization and pharmaceutical properties of porphyran. *Asian J Pharm.* 2015;9:93–101.
109. Bhatia S, Sharma A, Sharma K, Kavale M, Chaugule BB, Dhalwal K, Namdeo AG, Mahadik KR. Novel algal polysaccharides from marine source: Porphyran. *Pharmacogn Rev.* 2008;2:271–276.
110. Bhatia S, Sharma K, Nagpal K, Bera T. Investigation of the factors influencing the molecular weight of porphyran and its associated antifungal activity Bioact. *Carb Diet Fiber.* 2015;5:153–168.
111. Bhatia S, Kumar V, Sharma K, Nagpal K, Bera T. Significance of algal polymer in designing amphotericin B nanoparticles. *Sci World J.* 2014;2014:564573.
112. Bhatia S, Rathee P, Sharma K, Chaugule BB, Kar N, Bera T. Immuno-modulation effect of sulphated polysaccharide (porphyran) from Porphyra vietnamensis. *Int J Biol Macromol.* 2013;57:50–56.
113. Bhatia S. *Natural Polymer Drug Delivery Systems: Marine Polysaccharides Based Nano-Materials and Its Applications.* Springer International Publishing, Switzerland; 2016:185–225.
114. Bhatia S. *Natural Polymer Drug Delivery Systems: Plant Derived Polymers, Properties, and Modification & Applications.* Springer International Publishing, Switzerland; 2016:119–184.
115. Bhatia S. *Natural Polymer Drug Delivery Systems: Nanotechnology and Its Drug Delivery Applications.* Springer International Publishing, Switzerland; 2016:1–32.
116. Bhatia S. *Natural Polymer Drug Delivery Systems: Nanoparticles Types, Classification, Characterization, Fabrication Methods and Drug Delivery Applications.* Springer International Publishing, Switzerland; 2016:33–93.
117. Bhatia S. *Natural Polymer Drug Delivery Systems: Natural Polymers vs Synthetic Polymer.* Springer International Publishing, Switzerland; 2016:95–118.
118. Bhatia S. *Systems for Drug Delivery: Mammalian Polysaccharides and Its Nanomaterials.* Springer International Publishing, Switzerland; 2016:1–27.

119. Bhatia S. *Systems for Drug Delivery: Microbial Polysaccharides as Advance Nanomaterials.* Springer International Publishing, Switzerland; 2016:29–54.
120. Bhatia S. *Systems for Drug Delivery: Chitosan Based Nanomaterials and Its Applications.* Springer International Publishing, Switzerland; 2016:55–117.
121. Bhatia S. *Systems for Drug Delivery: Advance Polymers and Its Applications.* Springer International Publishing, Switzerland; 2016:119–146.
122. Bhatia S. *Systems for Drug Delivery: Advanced Application of Natural Polysaccharides.* Springer International Publishing, Switzerland; 2016:147–170.
123. Bhatia S. *Systems for Drug Delivery: Modern Polysaccharides and Its Current Advancements.* Springer International Publishing, Switzerland; 2016:171–188.
124. Bhatia S. *Systems for Drug Delivery: Toxicity of Nanodrug Delivery Systems.* Springer International Publishing, Switzerland; 2016:189–197.
125. Bhatia S. *Nanotechnology in Drug Delivery Fundamentals, Design, and Applications: Part 1: Protein and Peptide-Based Drug Delivery Systems.* Apple Academic Press, Palm Bay, FL; 2016:50–204.
126. Bhatia S. *Nanotechnology in Drug Delivery Fundamentals, Design, and Applications: Part 2: Peptide-Mediated Nanoparticle Drug Delivery System.* Apple Academic Press, Palm Bay, FL; 2016:205–280.
127. Bhatia S. *Nanotechnology in Drug Delivery Fundamentals, Design, and Applications: Part 3: CPP and CTP in Drug Delivery and Cell Targeting.* Apple Academic Press, Palm Bay, FL; 2016:309–312.
128. Bezerra DP, Militão GCG, de Morais MC, de Sousa DP. The dual antioxidant/Prooxidant effect of Eugenol and its action in cancer development and treatment. *Nutrients.* 2017;9(12):1367.
129. Larayetan RA, Okoh OO, Sadimenko A, Okoh AI. Terpene constituents of the aerial parts, phenolic content, antibacterial potential, free radical scavenging and antioxidant activity of *Callistemon citrinus* (Curtis) Skeels (Myrtaceae) from Eastern Cape Province of South Africa. *BMC Complement Altern Med.* 2017;17(1):292.
130. Sultan MT, Butt MS, Karim R, Ahmed W, Kaka U, Ahmad S, Dewanjee S, Jaafar HZ, Zia-Ul-Haq M. Nigella sativa fixed and essential oil modulates glutathione redox enzymes in potassium bromate induced oxidative stress. *BMC Complement Altern Med.* 2015;15:330.
131. El-Hosseiny LS, Alqurashy NN, Sheweita SA. Oxidative stress alleviation by Sage essential oil in co-amoxiclav induced hepatotoxicity in rats. *Int J Biomed Sci.* 2016;12(2):71–78.
132. Ebada ME. Essential oils of green cumin and chamomile partially protect against acute acetaminophen hepatotoxicity in rats. *An Acad Bras Cienc.* 2018;90(Suppl 1):2347–2358.
133. Campêlo LM, Gonçalves FC, Feitosa CM, de Freitas RM. Antioxidant activity of *Citrus limon* essential oil in mouse hippocampus. *Pharm Biol.* 2011;49(7):709–715.

17

Anticancer Properties of Essential Oils

Ahmed Al-Harrasi
Natural and Medical Sciences Research Center, University of Nizwa

Saurabh Bhatia
Natural and Medical Sciences Research Center, University of Nizwa
University of Petroleum and Energy Studies

Md. Tanvir Kabir
BRAC University

Tapan Behl
Chitkara University

Deepak Kaushik
M.D. University

Vineet Mittal
M.D. University

Ajay Sharma
Delhi Pharmaceutical Sciences and Research University

CONTENTS

17.1 Introduction

Limited information is available on the molecular targets of essential oil (EO) components in the treatment of cancer. EOs as well as their components offer various antitumor, cytotoxic, antioxidant, and antimutagenic biological activities as well as detoxification abilities by modulating on a variety of pathways of the biochemicals or proteins involved in the development of cancerous cells. EOs can directly act on mutagen and prevent its invasion in the cell. EOs and their components act as chemo-preventive agents by enhancing the detoxification process. The detoxification process is mediated by modulating the activity of phase I and phase II enzymes. EO components reduce the activity of enzyme (phase I such as Cytochrome c) in order to prevent the development of mutagen. Also, these components enhance the phase II detoxification process by improving the activity of phase II enzymes. Another way EOs and their components neutralize the deleterious effects of ROS is by activating antioxidative enzymes (GSH, CAT, GPx, and SOD) that control the first line of defense by preventing cell/tissue against ROS- mediated injury. Increases in the production of antioxidative enzymes can further avert oxidative stress to prevent cancer onset. On the other hand, some EOs are known for their potential in increasing the production of ROS by disturbing mitochondrial membrane, to reduce the production of antioxidative enzymes such as GSH. EOs as well as their components have been used in a number of investigations (*in vitro*) to act against cancerous cells, with no or noticeably

DOI: 10.1201/9781003175933-19

TABLE 17.1
Anticancer Properties of EOs

Name of EO	Chemical Component	Targeted Cells	Mechanism	References
Datura stramonium	Phytol acetate, beta-damascenone, and beta-eudesmol	Human lymphocytes were treated to destroy cancerous cells HCT-116 and SW620	Stimulated lymph cells triggered cell death via ROS and via disturbing membrane potential of mitochondria	[1]
Curcuma wenyujin	Curcumol	Hep3B cells	Activation of transcription-(3) via JAK-1, JAK-2, and Src mediated pathways and suppressed hypoxia-inducible factor-1α	[2]
Origanum majorana	Marjoram	P70S6K in colorectal cancer cells	Triggers p38 MAPK-mediated protective self-eating of cell, programmed cell death, and caspase-mediated cleavage of P70S6K	[3]
Rhizoma Curcumae	Curcumol	MDA-MB-231 cells & TNBC cells	Enhances the doxorubicin sensitivity against breast cancerous cells	[4]
Cedrus deodara	2-(tert-Buyl)-6-methyl-3-(2-(trifluoromethyl) benzyl)imidazo [1,2-a]pyridine; 9-octadecenoic acid; copaene; 2-(4-methoxy-2,6-dimethylphenyl)-3-methyl-2H-benzo[g]indazole, 9(E),11(E)-conjugated linoleic acid	Colon cancer cell lines of HCT-116 and SW-620	Induces apoptosis in human colon cancer cells by inhibiting nuclear factor kappa B	[5]
Clove essential oil	Eugenol (Eu)	MCF10A human breast epithelial cells	Inhibits phosphorylation (oxidative) as well as oxidation of fatty acid	[6]
Foeniculum vulgare	*trans*-Anethole (36.8%); α-ethyl-*p*-methoxy-benzyl alcohol (9.1%); *p*-anisaldehyde (7.7%); carvone (4.9%)	HeLa, Caco-2, MCF-7 , CCRF-CEM, CEM/ADR5000	Exhibited low cytotoxicity as compared to cytotoxic reference compounds	[7]
Artemisia herba alba	Viridiflorol and longiverbenone	P815 mastocytoma and BSR kidney carcinoma cell lines	P815 cells are the most sensitive to the cytotoxic effect, and no cytotoxic effect was observed on the peripheral blood mononuclear cells	[8]
Curcuma zedoaria	ND	SKOV3 cells	EO with wipaclitaxel synergistically enhance suppression of SKOV3 cells proliferation as well as promote apoptosis	[53]
Mustard essential oil	Allyl isothiocyanate	Bladder transitional carcinoma cell lines (RT4, TP53 (wild-type); and T24, mutated TP53 gene)	DNA damage, apoptosis, and necrosis rates in the TP53 (wild-type)	[9]
Monarda citriodora	para-cymene, thymol, carvacrol, terpinen-4-ol, beta-myrcene	Human promyelocytic leukemia HL-60 cells	Disruption of the PI3K/AKT/mTOR signaling cascade and induction of apoptosis	[10]
Boswellia sacra	Boswellic acids	MCF10-2A, MDA-MB-231, T47D, MCF7 cell lines	Triggered apoptosis as well as suppress tumor growth	[58]
Curcuma wenyujin		Human HepG2 cells	Antiproliferative effect by inducing apoptosis, associated with cell cycle arrest,	[11]
Cymbopogon flexuosus	Isointermedeol	Human leukemia HL-60 cells	Induce apoptosis via increasing mitochondrial cytochrome-c as well as apical death proteins expression	[12]

minimum toxicity against the cells (normal) by using various pathways and by acting at different sites (Tables 17.1 and 17.2). This may further lead to a decrease in the release of small membrane protein, cytochrome complex, involving the onset of the following set of sequential events that may lead to apoptotic cell death:

- Imbalance in Bcl/Bax ratio or dysregulation of BCL-2 family proteins or inhibition of the Bcl-2 gene expression. BCL-2 family proteins are membrane-associated antiapoptotic proteins that regulate apoptosis by the regulation of outer mitochondrial membrane permeabilization. These proteins protect

TABLE 17.2
In vitro Antiproliferative Effects of EOs

Phytochemicals	Pharmacological Activity	Lung Cell Type	Mechanism	References
Camphene and geraniol	Offer protection to rodent alveolar macrophages against oxidative stress induced by t-BHP-	Rat alveolar macrophages	Reduce lipid peroxidation, suppress NO as well as ROS production	[13]
Cymbopogon citratus EO	Programmed cell death with cell cycle detention, antiproliferative effect	A549 cell line	Via changing apoptic proteins including (caspase-3, Bax, Bcl-2)	[14]
β-Caryophyllene in the essential oil from *Chrysanthemum boreale*	Induces G 1 phase cell cycle arrest in human lung cancer cells, antiproliferative effect (cytotoxic activity)	A549 and NCI-H358 cells	Essential oil reduced the membrane potential of mitochondria disturbed the equilibrium among anti-apoptotic and pro-apoptotic Bcl-2 proteins, and stimulated caspases (-3, -8, -9). Moreoverbeta-Caryophyllene caused G1 cell cycle detention	[39]
Vapor of *Litsea cubeba* seed oil	Caused cell cycle detention and programmed cell death	Non-small-cell lung cancerous cells	Apoptosis occurred due to a significant decline in the mTOR expression	[60]
Seed oil of *Brucea javanica*	Antitumor effect	Non-small-cell lung cancer, A549 cells (NSCLC) and H446 cells (SCLC)	Cell cycle arrest and apoptosis of cancerous cells	[16]
α-Terpineol	-	Small-cell lung carcinoma cells(NCI-H69)	Downregulate the transcription of NF-κB	[63]
Lemongrass essential oil (LG-EO) and its major constituent, citral	Antiproliferative effect	LU135 SCLC cell line (LU135-wt-src)	Prevented Src-TK from phosphorylating Stat-3 lead tp downregulating expression of Bcl(xL) and Mcl-(1)	[16]
Alpinia officinarum	Antilung cancer activity	Five lung cancer cell lines	Inhibits the cell viability and the colony formation capacity via downregulating Bcl (2) as well as Mcl (1)	[46]
Citrus reticulata EO	-	Non-small-cell lung cancer cell line (A549)	Cell cycle cessation (in G0/G1 phase)	[17]
Plectranthus amboinicus (Lour)		Melanoma cell line (B16F (10))	Chemo-preventive effect	[18]
Myrica gale		Colon adenocarcinoma as well as human lung carcinoma cell line	Cytotoxicity	[19]

neoplastic cells from DNA damage-induced apoptosis. Antiproliferative effects of bergamot EO by modulating Bcl-2 and Bax signaling pathways have been reported. Similarly, the anticancer potential of frankincense oil via suppressing melanoma cancer by decreasing the expression of Bcl-2 Bax genes is also evidenced. Likewise, the anticancer potential of three *Lebanese salvia* species EOs is reported via downregulation of Bax and Bcl-2 to induce apoptosis [20–22].

- Caspase-mediated apoptotic cell death: Augmentation of caspase 3 and caspase 9 activities can cause the destruction of cellular components such as DNA fragmentation or degradation of cytoskeletal proteins. Caspase-mediated apoptosis involves various molecular events to degrade a number of proteins that are required for cellular functioning and survival.
- PARP cleavage: Increase in the activity of caspase can result in an increase in PARP cleavage, which may further result in caspase-mediated apoptotic cell death. PARP-1 is an enzyme that is encoded by the PARP1 gene. There are several reports that suggest EOs induce cleavage of PARP-1 via caspases to cause apoptotic cell death. The anticancer property of *Teucrium alopecurus* oil was recently reported on, and it was suggested that this oil can increase the cleavage of PARP and increase the expression of caspases-3-, -8-, and -9-dependent pathways to induce apoptosis [23].
- EOs are also reported on for their suppressing effect on PDK1/mTOR signaling, resulting in the dephosphorylation of protein kinase B (PKB), suggesting its significant role in various cellular tasks such as apoptosis. Dephosphorylation of PKB activates the caspase activity and deactivates the expression of mouse double minute 2 gene, which is a p53 tumor suppressor gene found to be upregulated in tumors. This suppressive effect over PDK1/mTOR signaling subsequently leads to the upregulation of gene (p21), which regulates cell cycle

development (G1/S phases), to further activate the caspase activity resulting in apoptosis. This occurs via the inhibition of the cyclin-dependent protein kinase (CDK1)/cyclin complex activity to arrest the cell cycle. EOs and their components follow various pathways in the treatment and prevention of cancer as follows:

- Cell cycle arrest
- Apoptosis
- DNA repair mechanisms
- Reduces cancer cell proliferation
- Reduces cancer cell metastasis
- Reduces cancer cell MDR
- As a potential candidate toward adjuvant anticancer therapeutic agents
- Elevates RNS and ROS to prevent the cancer cell proliferation and metastasis

17.2 Antimutagenic Properties of the Essential Oils

Direct inhibition of mutagen by EOs to prevent its entry into the host cell has been evidenced; however, the principal mechanism is still unclear [24]. Various other anticancer mechanisms followed by EOs and their components include:

- Antioxidant-quenching reaction
- Induction of phase II detoxification enzymes. These enzymes are mainly comprised of transferases [25].
- Inhibition of phase I enzymes involved in drug metabolism such as CYP450 [26]

Antimutagenicity caused by ginger EOs as well as their potential to alter expression of enzymes (phase I) involved in carcinogen metabolism has been reported. *In vitro* as well as *in vivo* findings suggested that EO components inhibit cytochrome P-450 (A1, A2, and B1/2), aniline hydroxylase, and aminopyrine-N-demethylase. In addition, ginger EO considerably enhanced the proportion of phase II enzymes (glutathione transferase and UDP-glucuronosyltransferases), which have been involved in the metabolism of cancer-causing agents, suggesting its role as antimutagen and as a potential chemopreventive agent [27]. Sulfur-containing EO derived from garlic and onions [66–71] showed a considerable increase in the activity of quinone reductase, uridine 5′-diphospho-glucuronosyltransferase, glutathione S-transferase, and epoxide hydrolase [28]. Likewise, the induction of phase II enzymes via EO component, citral, derived from lemongrass due to its isoform (geranial), was also reported [29]. This monoterpene was also reported for its potential in inhibiting tumor progression as well as proliferation of cell by elevating ROS inside the cancerous cells to increase oxidative stress. Induction of oxidative stress by citral decreased cancer cell proliferation, which eventually led to cell death [30].

17.3 Antiproliferative Properties of Essential Oils

Important characteristics of cancer cells include [31]:

- Resisting cell death: Cancer cells are resistant to apoptosis or apoptosis inducers.
- Sustaining proliferative signaling: One of the most prominent characteristics of a cancer cell is its ability to proliferate constantly and in the absence of external stimuli.
- Cancer cells have escape mechanisms against growth suppressors [31].
- Induction of angiogenesis: Cancer cells always encourage the formation of new blood vessels to get a continuous supply of nutrients and oxygen, to dispose their metabolic wastes, and to encourage hematogenous spread.
- Activate invasion and metastasis: Cancer cells can follow invasion–metastasis cascade, which includes various biological changes. This facilitates cancerous cells to enter and interfere with normal physiological environment of noncancerous tissues to further affect or spread via lymphatic/blood tissues.
- Facilitating replicative immortality: In comparison with normal cells, which have limited replication potential, cancerous cells show nearly unlimited replication.

Thus, considering these characteristics, various approaches have been considered to induce apoptosis and cellular arrest. EOs and their components have been proven to cause apoptosis via both the mitochondria (intrinsic) and receptor (extrinsic) pathways. *Pamburus missionis* EO, which contains beta-caryophyllene, phytol, aromadendrene oxide, and eudesmadiene, induced apoptosis via mitochondrial pathway and extrinsic pathway of apoptosis in squamous carcinoma and immortalized human keratinocytes cells. It was found that EO-induced apoptosis could be due to the loss of membrane potential of mitochondria mitochondrial, Bax/Bcl-2 ratio enhancement, mitochondrial Cyt c release, and caspases stimulation [separated type (I, II, III)]) via poly(ADP-ribose) polymerase separation [32]. Treatment of male Wistar rats with linalool resulted in modulation of the expression of Nrf2 dependent as well as oxidative stress markers (NADPH, CAT, MDA, SOD, GSH). Additionally, linalool treatment improved the cytotoxic effect of cisplatin when studied on prostate cancer, and HeLa cells and PC3 human cancer cell lines alleviated level of markers of apoptosis induced by cisplatin including caspase (3,9), expression of BAX gene as well as anti-apoptotic Bcl2, [33].

EO derived from *Vitex agnus* has been found to induce apoptosis via activation of caspase-mediated apoptotic pathway in multidrug-resistant lung cancer cell line. This was mediated by both extrinsic as well as intrinsic pathways. *Vitex agnus* castus EO induced caspase 3/7 activation and apoptosis via the activation of both extrinsic and intrinsic pathways. It was reported that *Vitex agnus* EO modulates the expression of apoptosis regulators such as TNF-related apoptosis-inducing ligand, caspases, Bcl-2, Fas-associated protein with death domain (Fas for extrinsic apoptosis pathway) [34]. *C. tiglium* EO showed significant antitumor activity on A549 cancer cells by inhibiting the migration as well as growth and division of these adenocarcinomic alveolar epithelial cells. This was mediated by disruption of cell cycle of the cancer cells as well as downregulating the expression of markers, especially CDK1 and cyclin (A,B). *C. tiglium* EO has been reported on for its ability to induce apoptosis by altering membrane potential of mitochondria and activating the caspase mediated pathway [35]. *In vitro* findings indicated that the treatment of cells with *Zataria multiflora* EO resulted in considerable suppression growth and division of breast and cervical cancer cells. Also, EO has been reported on for its ability to induce apoptosis as well as trigger immune reactions in breast as well as cervical cancer cell lines [36]. Other *in vitro* findings suggested that *C. zeylanicum* EO showed considerable anticancer effects against breast cancer cells by suppressing their viability and didn't show any cytotoxicity against normal cells. These effects were found to be mediated by poly(ADP-ribose) polymerase, Bcl-2, tumor-associated protein (annexin), and membrane potential of mitochondria [37]. Germacrone, the active chemical component present in *Rhizoma curcumae* EOs, stopped the cell cycle in the G2/M stage suggesting damage of intracellular DNA with no chances of repair. This treatment has considerably modulated the expression of cyclin-dependent kinase as well as G2/mitotic-specific cyclin-B. Moreover, this type of treatment also caused cleavage of nuclear enzyme [poly(ADP-ribose) polymerase] with activation of caspase protein-3 [38].

β-Caryophyllene isolated from the *Chrysanthemum boreale* EO induced arrest of cell cycle (G1 phase) lung cancer cell line via the downregulation of cyclin-(D1, E) and cyclin-dependent kinases (2,4,6) and phosphorylation of retinoblastoma via upregulation of cyclin-dependent kinase inhibitors [39]. *Liriodendron tulipifera* EO was recently reported to induce apoptotic death in grade IV astrocytoma. Additionally, this EO has been also reported for its potency in inducing cytotoxicity against human glioblastoma, colon carcinoma, and malignant melanoma [40]. Alpha-hederin, the main ingredient of the *Nigella sativa* EO, induced apoptosis by decreasing the mitochondrial membrane potential, inactivating anti-apoptotic protein B-cell lymphoma 2 gene, as well as activating caspase-9, -3, and -7. Moreover, in this study, human ovarian cancer cell treatment with alpha-hederin caused the cessation of the cell cycle arrest in G0/G1 phase [41]. *Ferula asafoetida* EO, which contains a high level of dithiolane, showed antiproliferative activity in human liver carcinoma cell lines (HepG2 and SK-Hep1) via the induction of apoptosis and alteration of NF-κB and TGF-β signaling with an increase in caspase-3 and TNF-α expression [42]. It was recently reported that frankincense EO suppressed skin cancer by decreasing the expression Bcl-2/Bax ratio as well as by enhancing toxicity of liver cells via modulating the action of phase (I & II) enzymes [43]. Out of all the EOs, carvacrol showed the maximum cellular toxicity against cancerous cells. Also, in human prostate cancer cells (*in vitro*) 4-terpineole, 1,8-cineole, and carvacrol showed upregulation of the expression of caspase proteins, cleaved peroxisome proliferator-activated receptor, and Bax protein [44]. It was reported that EO from *Carpesium abrotanoides* induced cell cycle arrest at synthesis and Mitotic G2 phases, via mitochondria-mediated intrinsic apoptotic pathway. This is done by downregulating Bcl-2/Bax protein ratio as well as caspase (-3 &-9) stimulation [45]. Volatile oil from *Alpinia officinarum* showed anticancer effects via downregulation of B-cell lymphoma 2 gene and Mcl-1 and caspase-3 activation, and it also triggered dysfunction of the mitochondrial membrane potential to induce lung cancer cells apoptosis [46].

β-caryophyllene with aromadendrene oxide 2 and phytol from *Pamburus missionis* showed synergistic effects by inducing apoptotic death on the squamous cell carcinoma cells. Synergistic response was due to the upregulation of Bax/Bcl-2 ratio, change in membrane potential of mitochondria, cyt c release from mitochondria, and caspases activation of caspases (caspase-3, -8, -9) resulting in cleavage of nuclear proteins such as PARP [47]. 6,7-Dehydroroyleanone present in the EO of *Plectranthus madagascariensis* showed the possible caspase (-3 & -9) stimulation to induce apoptic death by stimulating the intrinsic cell death pathway [48]. It was found that the treatment with *Salvia* EO enriched with caryophyllene oxide reduced the f prostate cancer cell growth via triggering an apoptosis as well as elevating ROS production generation [49]. EOs from *Siegesbeckia pubescens* were reported to induce apoptic death via mitochondrial mediated apoptosis pathway in human liver cancer cells (*in vitro*). It was found that this mitochondrial mediated apoptosis resulted in the modulation of the expression of apoptotic proteins such as upregulation of caspase (-3-9) as well as Bax and downregulation of bcl-2 expression [50]. The EO of *Decatropis bicolor* containing the major components 1-(3-methyl-cyclopent-2-enyl)-cyclohexene, 3-(methyl-2)propenyl, 1,5-cyclooctadiene, and β-terpineol showed potential cytotoxic and antitumoral effects against breast cancer cells. It was also found that EO of *Decatropis bicolor* induced apoptosis in the breast cancer cells via stimulation of apoptic proteins caspases (-9 & -3) and Bax [51]. EO of *Chenopodium ambrosioides* could considerably inhibit the cell proliferation of SMMC-7721 cells by arresting cell cycle in G0/G1phase and induced apoptosis the apoptotic rate in a dose-dependent way [52]. It was found that *Curcuma zedoaria* (Berg.) Rosc. EO and paclitaxel synergistically enhance the apoptosis and cell cycle arrest of SKOV3 cells via enhancing caspase-3 expression [53]. β-bisabolene present in *Commiphora guidottii* is reported to increase apoptosis of human breast cancer cells via the activation of caspase-3/7 activity [54]. *Acori graminei* oil has been reported to induce apoptosis via activation of both caspase-dependent as well as -independent pathways in p53 wild-type A172 as well as mutant U251 cells. It was also found that treatment of both types of cells with oil displayed autophagic cell death. Oil-induced autophagy in U251 cells was mediated via mTOR-independent signaling pathway, whereas in A172 cells it was induced by the activation of p53/AMPK/mTOR signaling pathway [55]. Recently, camphene induced apoptosis via the intrinsic pathway in melanoma cells primarily via inducing endoplasmic reticulum stress. Camphene exerted an antitumor activity by decreasing the mitochondrial membrane potential and increasing the caspase-3 activity [56]. One more study suggested that carvacrol, mainly present in thyme and oregano EOs, induced apoptosis in metastatic breast adenocarcinoma cells via permeabilization of mitochondria membrane. This change in permeability of mitochondria led to release of cyt. C protein as well as activation of caspases. Furthermore, caspases activation caused DNA fragmentation as well as PARP cleavage [57]. Another report suggested that extracts obtained from *Boswellia sacra* induced apoptosis via PARP cleavage in MDA-MB-231 cells [58]. Citral, abundantly present in lemongrass oil, increases the caspase activity for apoptosis induction in a number of cancer cell lines such as colorectal cancer and glioblastoma [58]. Various other reports suggest that citral treatment can result in a decrease in the expression of prosurvival proteins in cancerous cells [59]. PKB, also known as Akt, is an important messenger that regulates proliferation, metabolism as well as cellular apoptic death. Additionally, it also regulates transcription factors. Gaseous phase of *Litsea cubeba* EO arrested the cell cycle and caused apoptotic death of non-small cell lung cancer cells via a considerable decrease in the expression of mTOR protein and phosphorylating ability of PPDK1, resulting in PKB dephosphorylation. PKB dephosphorylation initiated a caspase-mediated apoptotic death and inactivated expression of MDM2. This event resulted in an increase in the expression of p21 with successive caspase activation after the G1/S phase arrest [60]. These events support antiproliferative as well as antioxidant effects of *Litsea cubeba* seed oil in the vapor phase. A recent report also suggested the role of organosulfur components derived from garlic in considerably reducing cell viability in hepatic cellular carcinoma J5 cells via stopping G2/M cycle, resulting in apoptosis. This is mainly due to the downregulation of CDK-activating kinase 7 as well as suppression of CDK-activating kinasel/cyclin. [61]. As it's well known, in cancer cells there is an unusual upregulation of nuclear factor-κB, which is associated with the onset and progression of cancer [62]. It's reported that α-terpineol decreased expression of nuclear factor-κB in several cancerous cells, with the main suppressive activity on NCI-H69 [63]. Also, in colon cancer cells, α-terpineol in combination with linalyl acetate synergistically act via downregulating the expression of nuclear factor-κB leading to apoptic death.

17.4 Radical Scavenging Activity of EO

At cellular level, injury caused by any external stimuli to mitochondrial electron transport chain can result in ROS generation. Continuous production of ROS can further cause damage to cellular components such as DNA, lipid, and protein [90]. Thus, due to the presence of abundant reservoirs of antioxidants, EOs possess free radical scavenging activity to reduce the cellular oxidate stress, which can further prevent cellular injury. This pathway prevents metastatic growth of the cell and thus prevents progression of cancer [64]. Thus, the antioxidant potential of EOs can be utilized to prevent cancer [64]. Eugenol derived from clove oil has a dual effect on oxidative stress, as it can react with ROS to possess an antioxidant effect by scavenging free radicals and also can induce oxidative stress either by the generation of ROS or via the inhibition of antioxidant systems (i.e., antioxidant enzymes) [65,66]. In addition, eugenol also possesses anticarcinogenic, cytotoxic, and antitumor properties. The anticancer property possessed by eugenol is mediated by increasing the expression of antioxidant enzymes [66]. *Callistemon citrinus* leaves EO contains eucalyptol and α-terpineol, whereas EO obtained from the flower of the same plant contains eucalyptol, caryophyllene, α-eudesmol, and (–)-bornyl-acetate. It was found that both EOs (leaves and flowers) contain phenolic compounds that are potentially accountable for high antioxidant activity [67]. High intracellular antioxidant activity showed by EO derived from *Wedelia chinensis* containing 96% of the components, carvacrol and trans-caryophyllene, further resulted in a considerable decrease in tumor size and an improvement in healing of the adjoining healthy tissue [68]. Nevertheless, another report suggested that augmentation in antioxidant properties inside cell can result in an increase in survival of the cancerous cell [68]. In particular, the oxidized form of glutathione (i.e., glutathione disulfide), which is formed during the oxidation of glutathione, acts as an indicator of oxidative stress to measure the level of oxidative stress induced by any external or intrinsic factor. Treatment of EO from *Nigella sativa* modulated the activities of enzymes (i.e., glutathione-S-transferase, glutathione reductase, and glutathione peroxidase) positively against potassium bromate-induced oxidative stress [69]. A recent report also suggested that balsam fir oil treatment reduced glutathione activity. It was also found that this activity was due to the presence of the component, γ -caryophyllene, which has further increased ROS [70]. This type of antioxidant treatment can act as a prooxidant by increasing cellular glutathione levels [71]. Thus, EO and its components following the same antioxidant mechanism can be more useful as anticancer agents for non-tumor tissues. It has been observed that sage EO treatment in co-amoxiclav-induced hepatotoxicity (in rats) decreased glutathione level and further elevated oxidative stress [71]. *Citrus limon* EO treatment has been found to considerably reduce lipid peroxidation as well as nitrite levels; however, it enhanced the activities of superoxide dismutase, catalase, and glutathione peroxidase in the rodent hippocampal region. Similarly, chamomile oil was reported to moderately ameliorate the glutathione depletion and the decrease in superoxide dismutase activity in the liver of acetaminophen-administered rats [72,73]. Another report suggested that balsam fir oil treatment resulted in decreased glutathione levels. It was observed that the decrease in glutathione levels is due to the presence of α-humulene, whereas an increase in ROS level is due to the presence of gamma-caryophyllene in EO.

17.5 Cancerous Cells vs. Essential Oils

EOs as well as their components have been used in a number of *in vitro* investigations to suppress the growth of cancerous cells, with no or noticeably less toxicity at cellular level against the normal cells (Tables 17.1 and 17.2). Various EOs derived from *Thymus fallax, Boswellia sacra, Amomum tsaoko, Lippia alba, Casearia sylvestris, Zanthoxylum rhoifolum,*

Commiphora gileadensis, and *Aniba rosaeodora* have been tested for their anticancer effects against various cancer and non-cancer cell lines. The results obtained from these studies showed that EO components have various antioxidative, antiproliferative, and cytotoxic pathways to express these anticancer effects.

17.6 Nanoencapsulation of Essential Oil Extracts Using Natural Polymers

Nanoencapsulation is an interesting approach used for incorporating EOs in food preparations and pharmaceutical formulae [74–129]. Other EO-loaded nanoforms such as nanoemulsions, nanocapsules, nanocomposites, and nanofilms have been reported. It has been found by transforming these EOs into these nanostructures via selecting optimized ratio of polymers and other ingredients biological activity, including antioxidant activity, can be improved. These nanoformulations show better antioxidant profile with improved physical and chemical properties than the pure EOs, and thus, these nanoformulations can be effectively utilized for food processing and packaging applications [91–129].

REFERENCES

1. Chandan G, Kumar C, Verma MK, Satti NK, Saini AK, Saini RV. *Datura stramonium* essential oil composition and it's immunostimulatory potential against colon cancer cells. *3 Biotech.* 2020;10(10):451.
2. Zuo HX, Jin Y, Wang Z, Li MY, Zhang ZH, Wang JY, Xing Y, Ri MH, Jin CH, Xu GH, Piao LX, Ma J, Jin X. Curcumol inhibits the expression of programmed cell death-ligand 1 through crosstalk between hypoxia-inducible factor-1α and STAT3 (T705) signaling pathways in hepatic cancer. *J Ethnopharmacol.* 2020;257:112835.
3. Athamneh K, Alneyadi A, Alsamri H, Alrashedi A, Palakott A, El-Tarabily KA, Eid AH, Al Dhaheri Y, Iratni R. *Origanum majorana* essential oil triggers p38 MAPK-mediated protective autophagy, apoptosis, and caspase-dependent cleavage of P70S6K in colorectal cancer cells. *Biomolecules.* 2020;10(3):412.
4. Zeng C, Fan D, Xu Y, Li X, Yuan J, Yang Q, Zhou X, Lu J, Zhang C, Han J, Gu J, Gao Y, Sun L, Wang S. Curcumol enhances the sensitivity of doxorubicin in triple-negative breast cancer via regulating the miR-181b-2–3p-ABCC3 axis. *Biochem Pharmacol.* 2020;174:113795.
5. Bhagat M, Kumar A, Suravajhala R. *Cedrus deodara* (Bark) essential oil induces apoptosis in human colon cancer cells by inhibiting nuclear factor kappa B. *Curr Top Med Chem.* 2020;20(22):1981–1992.
6. Yan X, Zhang G, Bie F, Lv Y, Ma Y, Ma M, Wang Y, Hao X, Yuan N, Jiang X. Eugenol inhibits oxidative phosphorylation and fatty acid oxidation via downregulation of c-Myc/PGC-1β/ERRα signaling pathway in MCF10A-ras cells. *Sci Rep.* 2017;7(1):12920.
7. Sharopov F, Valiev A, Satyal P, Gulmurodov I, Yusufi S, Setzer WN, Wink M. Cytotoxicity of the essential oil of fennel (*Foeniculum vulgare*) from Tajikistan. *Foods.* 2017;6(9):73.
8. Tilaoui M, Ait Mouse H, Jaafari A, Zyad A. Comparative phytochemical analysis of essential oils from different biological parts of *Artemisia herba* alba and their cytotoxic effect on cancer cells. *PLoS One.* 2015;10(7):e0131799.
9. Savio AL, da Silva GN, de Camargo EA, Salvadori DM. Cell cycle kinetics, apoptosis rates, DNA damage and TP53 gene expression in bladder cancer cells treated with allyl isothiocyanate (mustard essential oil). *Mutat Res.* 2014;762:40–46.
10. Pathania AS, Guru SK, Verma MK, Sharma C, Abdullah ST, Malik F, Chandra S, Katoch M, Bhushan S. Disruption of the PI3K/AKT/mTOR signaling cascade and induction of apoptosis in HL-60 cells by an essential oil from *Monarda citriodora. Food Chem Toxicol.* 2013;62:246–254.
11. Xiao Y, Yang FQ, Li SP, Hu G, Lee SM, Wang YT. Essential oil of *Curcuma wenyujin* induces apoptosis in human hepatoma cells. *World J Gastroenterol.* 2008;14(27):4309–4318.
12. Kumar A, Malik F, Bhushan S, Sethi VK, Shahi AK, Kaur J, Taneja SC, Qazi GN, Singh J. An essential oil and its major constituent isointermedeol induce apoptosis by increased expression of mitochondrial cytochrome c and apical death receptors in human leukaemia HL-60 cells. *Chem Biol Interact.* 2008;171(3):332–347.
13. Tiwari M, Kakkar P. Plant derived antioxidants: Geraniol and camphene protect rat alveolar macrophages against t-BHP induced oxidative stress. *Toxicol in Vitro.* 2009;23(2):295–301.
14. Trang DT, Hoang TKV, Nguyen TTM, et al. Essential oils of lemongrass (*Cymbopogon citratus* Stapf) induces apoptosis and cell cycle arrest in A549 lung cancer cells. *Biomed Res Int.* 2020;2020:5924856.
15. Wang D, Qu X, Zhuang X, et al. Seed oil of *Brucea javanicaInduces* cell cycle arrest and apoptosis via reactive oxygen species-mediated mitochondrial dysfunction in human lung cancer cells. *Nutr Cancer.* 2016;68(8):1394–1403.
16. Maruoka T, Kitanaka A, Kubota Y, et al. Lemongrass essential oil and citral inhibit SRC/Stat3 activity and suppress the proliferation/survival of small-cell lung cancer cells, alone or in combination with chemotherapeutic agents. *Int J Oncol.* 2018;52(5):1738–1748.
17. Castro MA, Rodenak-Kladniew B, Massone A, Polo M, García de Bravo M, Crespo R. Citrus reticulata peel oil inhibits non-small cell lung cancer cell proliferation in culture and implanted in nude mice. *Food Funct.* 2018;9(4):2290–2299.
18. Manjamalai A, Grace VM. The chemotherapeutic effect of essential oil of *Plectranthus amboinicus* (Lour) on lung metastasis developed by B16F-10 cell line in C57BL/6 mice. *Cancer Invest.* 2013;31(1):74–82.
19. Sylvestre M, Legault J, Dufour D, Pichette A. Chemical composition and anticancer activity of leaf essential oil of *Myrica gale* L. *Phytomedicine.* 2005;12(4):299–304.
20. Navarra M, Ferlazzo N, Cirmi S, Trapasso E, Bramanti P, Lombardo GE, Minciullo PL, Calapai G, Gangemi S. Effects of bergamot essential oil and its extractive fractions on SH-SY5Y human neuroblastoma cell growth. *J Pharm Pharmacol.* 2015;67(8):1042–1053.
21. Russo A, Cardile V, Graziano ACE, Avola R, Bruno M, Rigano D. Involvement of Bax and Bcl-2 in induction of apoptosis by essential oils of three lebanese salvia species in human prostate cancer cells. *Int J Mol Sci.* 2018;19(1):292.

22. Hakkim FL, Bakshi HA, Khan S, et al. Frankincense essential oil suppresses melanoma cancer through down regulation of Bcl-2/Bax cascade signaling and ameliorates heptotoxicity via phase I and II drug metabolizing enzymes. *Oncotarget.* 2019;10:3472–3490.
23. Guesmi F, Tyagi AK, Prasad S, Landoulsi A. Terpenes from essential oils and hydrolate of *Teucrium alopecurus* triggered apoptotic events dependent on caspases activation and PARP cleavage in human colon cancer cells through decreased protein expressions. *Oncotarget.* 2018;9(64):32305–32320.
24. Kada T, Shimoi K. Desmutagens and bio-antimutagens--their modes of action. *Bioessays.* 1987;7(3):113–116.
25. Jancova P, Anzenbacher P, Anzenbacherova E. Phase II drug metabolizing enzymes. *Biomed Pap Med Fac Univ Palacky Olomouc Czech Repub.* 2010;154(2):103–116.
26. De Flora S, Ramel C. Mechanisms of inhibitors of mutagenesis and carcinogenesis. *Classif Overview. Mutat Res.* 1988;202(2):285–306.
27. Jeena K, Liju VB, Viswanathan R, Kuttan R. Antimutagenic potential and modulation of carcinogen-metabolizing enzymes by ginger essential oil. *Phytother. Res.* 2014;28:849–855.
28. Wattenberg LW, Hanley AB, Barany G, Sparnins VL, Lam LK, Fenwick GR. Inhibition of carcinogenesis by some minor dietary constituents. *Princess Takamatsu Symp.* 1985;16:193–203.
29. Nakamura Y, Miyamoto M, Murakami A, Ohigashi H, Osawa T, Uchida K. A phase II detoxification enzyme inducer from lemongrass: Identification of citral and involvement of electrophilic reaction in the enzyme induction. *Biochem Biophys Res Commun.* 2003;302(3):593–600.
30. Sanches LJ, Marinello PC, Panis C, Fagundes TR, Morgado-Díaz JA, de-Freitas-Junior JC, Cecchini R, Cecchini AL, Luiz RC. Cytotoxicity of citral against melanoma cells: The involvement of oxidative stress generation and cell growth protein reduction. *Tumour Biol.* 2017;39(3). doi: 1010428317695914.
31. Gutschner T, Diederichs S. The hallmarks of cancer: A long non-coding RNA point of view. *RNA Biol.* 2012;9(6):703–719.
32. Pavithra PS, Mehta A, Verma RS. Induction of apoptosis by essential oil from *P. missionis* in skin epidermoid cancer cells. *Phytomedicine.* 2018;50:184–195.
33. Mohamed ME, Abduldaium YS, Younis NS. Ameliorative effect of linalool in cisplatin-induced nephrotoxicity: The role of HMGB1/TLR4/NF-κB and Nrf2/HO1 pathways. *Biomolecules.* 2020;10(11):E1488.
34. Ilhan S. Essential oils from *Vitex agnus* castus L. leaves induces caspase-dependent apoptosis of human multidrug-resistant lung carcinoma cells through intrinsic and extrinsic pathways. *Nutr Cancer.* 2021;73(4):1–9.
35. Niu QL, Sun H, Liu C, Li J, Liang CX, Zhang RR, Ge FR, Liu W. Croton tiglium essential oil compounds have anti-proliferative and pro-apoptotic effects in A549 lung cancer cell lines. *PLoS One.* 2020;15(5):e0231437.
36. Azadi M, Jamali T, Kianmehr Z, Kavoosi G, Ardestani SK. In-vitro (2D and 3D cultures) and in-vivo cytotoxic properties of *Zataria multiflora* essential oil (ZEO) emulsion in breast and cervical cancer cells along with the investigation of immunomodulatory potential. *J Ethnopharmacol.* 2020;257:112865.
37. Kubatka P, Kello M, Kajo K, Samec M, Jasek K, Vybohova D, Uramova S, Liskova A, Sadlonova V, Koklesova L, Murin R, Adamkov M, Smejkal K, Svajdlenka E, Solar P, Samuel SM, Kassayova M, Kwon TK, Zubor P, Pec M, Danko J, Büsselberg D, Mojzis J. Chemopreventive and therapeutic efficacy of *Cinnamomum zeylanicum* L. bark in experimental breast carcinoma: Mechanistic in vivo and in vitro analyses. *Molecules.* 2020;25(6):1399.
38. Wu L, Wang L, Tian X, Zhang J, Feng H. Germacrone exerts anti-cancer effects on gastric cancer through induction of cell cycle arrest and promotion of apoptosis. *BMC Complement Med Ther.* 2020;20(1):21.
39. Chung KS, Hong JY, Lee JH, Lee HJ, Park JY, Choi JH, Park HJ, Hong J, Lee KT. β-caryophyllene in the essential oil from chrysanthemum Boreale induces G1 phase cell cycle arrest in human lung cancer cells. *Molecules.* 2019;24(20):3754.
40. Quassinti L, Maggi F, Ortolani F, Lupidi G, Petrelli D, Vitali LA, Miano A, Bramucci M. Exploring new applications of tulip tree (*Liriodendron tulipifera* L.): Leaf essential oil as apoptotic agent for human glioblastoma. *Environ Sci Pollut Res Int.* 2019;26(29):30485–30497.
41. Adamska A, Stefanowicz-Hajduk J, Ochocka JR. Alpha-Hederin, the active Saponin of nigella sativa, as an anticancer agent inducing apoptosis in the SKOV-3 cell line. *Molecules.* 2019;24(16):2958.
42. Verma S, Khambhala P, Joshi S, Kothari V, Patel T, Seshadri S. Evaluating the role of dithiolane rich fraction of *Ferula asafoetida* (apiaceae) for its antiproliferative and apoptotic properties: In vitro studies. *Exp Oncol.* 2019;41(2):90–94.
43. Hakkim FL, Bakshi HA, Khan S, Nasef M, Farzand R, Sam S, Rashan L, Al-Baloshi MS, Abdo Hasson SSA, Jabri AA, McCarron PA, Tambuwala MM. Frankincense essential oil suppresses melanoma cancer through down regulation of Bcl-2/Bax cascade signaling and ameliorates heptotoxicity via phase I and II drug metabolizing enzymes. *Oncotarget.* 2019;10(37):3472–3490.
44. Tayarani-Najaran Z, Akaberi M, Hassanzadeh B, Shirazi N, Asili J, Al-Najjar H, Sahebkar A, Emami SA. Analysis of the essential oils of five artemisia species and evaluation of their cytotoxic and proapoptotic effects. *Mini Rev Med Chem.* 2019;19(11):902–912.
45. Wang Q, Pan LH, Lin L, Zhang R, Du YC, Chen H, Huang M, Guo KW, Yang XZ. Essential oil from *Carpesium abrotanoides* L. induces apoptosis via activating mitochondrial pathway in hepatocellular carcinoma cells. *Curr Med Sci.* 2018;38(6):1045–1053.
46. Li N, Zhang Q, Jia Z, Yang X, Zhang H, Luo H. Volatile oil from alpinia officinarum promotes lung cancer regression in vitro and in vivo. *Food Funct.* 2018;9(9):4998–5006.
47. Pavithra PS, Mehta A, Verma RS. Synergistic interaction of β-caryophyllene with aromadendrene oxide 2 and phytol induces apoptosis on skin epidermoid cancer cells. *Phytomedicine.* 2018;47:121–134.
48. Garcia C, Silva CO, Monteiro CM, Nicolai M, Viana A, Andrade JM, Barasoain I, Stankovic T, Quintana J, Hernández I, González I, Estévez F, Díaz-Lanza AM, Reis CP, Afonso CA, Pesic M, Rijo P. Anticancer properties of the abietane diterpene 6,7-dehydroroyleanone obtained by optimized extraction. *Future Med Chem.* 2018;10(10):1177–1189.

49. Russo A, Cardile V, Graziano ACE, Avola R, Bruno M, Rigano D. Involvement of Bax and Bcl-2 in induction of apoptosis by essential oils of three lebanese salvia species in human prostate cancer cells. *Int J Mol Sci.* 2018;19(1):292.
50. Lv D, Guo KW, Xu C, Huang M, Zheng SJ, Ma XH, Pan LH, Wang Q, Yang XZ. Essential oil from *Siegesbeckia pubescens* induces apoptosis through the mitochondrial pathway in human HepG2 cells. *J Huazhong Univ Sci Technolog Med Sci.* 2017;37(1):87–92.
51. Estanislao Gómez CC, Aquino Carreño A, Pérez Ishiwara DG, San Martín Martínez E, Morales López J, Pérez Hernández N, Gómez García MC. Decatropis bicolor (Zucc.) Radlk essential oil induces apoptosis of the MDA-MB-231 breast cancer cell line. *BMC Complement Altern Med.* 2016;16:266.
52. Wang YN, Zhu XH, Ma H, Du RY, Li DR, Ma DW. Essential oil of *Chenopodium ambrosioides* induced caspase-dependent apoptosis in SMMC-7721 cells. *Zhong Yao Cai.* 2016;39(5):1124–1128.
53. Zhou Y, Shen J, Xia L, Wang Y. *Curcuma zedoaria* (Berg.) Rosc. essential oil and paclitaxel synergistically enhance the apoptosis of SKOV3 cells. *Mol Med Rep.* 2015;12(1):1253–1257.
54. Yeo SK, Ali AY, Hayward OA, Turnham D, Jackson T, Bowen ID, Clarkson R. β-Bisabolene, a Sesquiterpene from the essential oil extract of opoponax (*Commiphora guidottii*), exhibits cytotoxicity in breast cancer cell lines. *Phytother Res.* 2016;30(3):418–425.
55. Chen L, Jiang Z, Ma H, Ning L, Chen H, Li L, Qi H. Volatile oil of acori graminei rhizoma-induced apoptosis and autophagy are dependent on p53 status in human Glioma cells. *Sci Rep.* 2016;6:21148.
56. Girola N, Figueiredo CR, Farias CF, Azevedo RA, Ferreira AK, Teixeira SF, Capello TM, Martins EG, Matsuo AL, Travassos LR, Lago JH. Camphene isolated from essential oil of *Piper cernuum* (Piperaceae) induces intrinsic apoptosis in melanoma cells and displays antitumor activity in vivo. *Biochem Biophys Res Commun.* 2015;467(4):928–934.
57. Arunasree KM. Anti-proliferative effects of carvacrol on a human metastatic breast cancer cell line, MDA-MB 231. *Phytomedicine.* 2010;17(8–9):581–588.
58. Suhail MM, Wu W, Cao A, Mondalek FG, Fung KM, Shih PT, Fang YT, Woolley C, Young G, Lin HK. Boswellia sacra essential oil induces tumor cell-specific apoptosis and suppresses tumor aggressiveness in cultured human breast cancer cells. *BMC Complement Altern Med.* 2011;11:129.
59. Naz F, Khan FI, Mohammad T, Khan P, Manzoor S, Hasan GM, Lobb KA, Luqman S, Islam A, Ahmad F, Hassan MI. Investigation of molecular mechanism of recognition between citral and MARK4: A newer therapeutic approach to attenuate cancer cell progression. *Int J Biol Macromol.* 2018;107(Pt B):2580–2589.
60. Seal S, Chatterjee P, Bhattacharya S, Pal D, Dasgupta S, Kundu R, Mukherjee S, Bhattacharya S, Bhuyan M, Bhattacharyya PR, Baishya G, Barua NC, Baruah PK, Rao PG, Bhattacharya S. Vapor of volatile oils from *Litsea cubeba* seed induces apoptosis and causes cell cycle arrest in lung cancer cells. *PLoS One.* 2012;7(10):e47014.
61. Wu CC, Chung JG, Tsai SJ, Yang JH, Sheen LY. Differential effects of allyl sulfides from garlic essential oil on cell cycle regulation in human liver tumor cells. *Food Chem Toxicol.* 2004;42(12):1937–1947.
62. Hoesel B, Schmid JA. The complexity of NF-κB signaling in inflammation and cancer. *Mol Cancer.* 2013;12:86.
63. Hassan SB, Gali-Muhtasib H, Göransson H, Larsson R. Alpha terpineol: A potential anticancer agent which acts through suppressing NF-κB signalling. *Anticancer Res.* 2010;30(6):1911–1919.
64. Fitsiou E, Anestopoulos I, Chlichlia K, Galanis A, Kourkoutas I, Panayiotidis MI, Pappa A. Antioxidant and antiproliferative properties of the essential oils of *Satureja thymbra* and *Satureja parnassica* and their major constituents. *Anticancer Res.* 2016;36(11):5757–5763.
65. Blowman K, Magalhães M, Lemos MFL, Cabral C, Pires IM. Anticancer properties of essential oils and other natural products. *Evid Based Complement Alternat Med.* 2018;2018:3149362.
66. Bezerra DP, Militão GCG, de Morais MC, de Sousa DP. The dual antioxidant/prooxidant effect of Eugenol and its action in cancer development and treatment. *Nutrients.* 2017;9(12):1367.
67. Larayetan RA, Okoh OO, Sadimenko A, Okoh AI. Terpene constituents of the aerial parts, phenolic content, antibacterial potential, free radical scavenging and antioxidant activity of *Callistemon citrinus* (Curtis) Skeels (Myrtaceae) from eastern cape province of South Africa. *BMC Complement Altern Med.* 2017;17(1):292.
68. Manjamalai A, Berlin Grace VM. Antioxidant activity of essential oils from *Wedelia chinensis* (Osbeck) in vitro and in vivo lung cancer bearing C57BL/6 mice. *Asian Pac J Cancer Prev.* 2012;13(7):3065–3071.
69. Sultan MT, Butt MS, Karim R, et al. Nigella sativa fixed and essential oil modulates glutathione redox enzymes in potassium bromate induced oxidative stress. *BMC Complement Altern Med* 2015;15:330.
70. Legault J, Dahl W, Debiton E, Pichette A, Madelmont JC. Antitumor activity of balsam fir oil: Production of reactive oxygen species induced by alpha-humulene as possible mechanism of action. *Planta Med.* 2003;69(5):402–407.
71. El-Hosseiny LS, Alqurashy NN, Sheweita SA. Oxidative stress alleviation by Sage essential oil in Co-amoxiclav induced hepatotoxicity in rats. *Int J Biomed Sci.* 2016;12(2): 71–78.
72. Ebada ME. Essential oils of green cumin and chamomile partially protect against acute acetaminophen hepatotoxicity in rats. *An Acad Bras Cienc.* 2018;90(2 suppl 1): 2347–2358.
73. Campêlo LML, Gonçalves FCM, Feitosa CM, de Freitas RM. Antioxidant activity of *Citrus limon* essential oil in mouse hippocampus. *Pharmaceutical Biol.* 2011;49:709–715.
74. Bhatia S, Sharma A, Vargas De La Cruz CB, Chaugule B, Ahmed Al-Harrasi. Nutraceutical, Antioxidant, Antimicrobial properties of *Pyropia vietnamensis* (Tanaka et Pham-Hong Ho) J.E. Sutherl. et Monotilla. *Curr Bioact Compd.* 2020;16:1.
75. Bhatia S, Sardana S, Senwar KR, Dhillon A, Sharma A, Naved T. In vitro antioxidant and antinociceptive properties of Porphyra vietnamensis. *Biomedicine (Taipei).* 2019;9(1):3.
76. Bhatia S, Sharma K, Namdeo AG, Chaugule BB, Kavale M, Nanda S. Broad-spectrum sun-protective action of porphyra-334 derived from Porphyra vietnamensis. *Pharmacognosy Res.* 2010;2(1):45–49.

77. Bhatia S, Sharma K, Sharma A, Nagpal K, Bera T. Anti-inflammatory, analgesic and antiulcer properties of Porphyra vietnamensis. *Avicenna J Phytomed.* 2015;5(1):69–77.
78. Bhatia S, Sardana S, Sharma A, Vargas De La Cruz CB, Chaugule B, Khodaie L. Development of broad spectrum mycosporine loaded sunscreen formulation from Ulva fasciata delile. *Biomedicine (Taipei).* 2019;9(3):17.
79. Bhatia S, Garg A, Sharma K, Kumar S, Sharma A, Purohit AP. Mycosporine and mycosporine-like amino acids: A paramount tool against ultra violet irradiation. *Pharmacogn Rev.* 2011;5(10):138–146.
80. Bhatia S, Namdeo AG, Nanda S. Factors effecting the gelling and emulsifying properties of a natural polymer. *SRP.* 2010;1(1):86–92.
81. Bhatia S, Sharma K, Bera T. Structural characterization and pharmaceutical properties of porphyran. *Asian J Pharm* 2015:9;93–101.
82. Bhatia S, Sharma A, Sharma K, Kavale M, Chaugule BB, Dhalwal K, Namdeo AG, Mahadik KR. Novel algal polysaccharides from marine source: Porphyran. *Pharmacogn Rev.* 2008;2(4):271–276.
83. Bhatia S, Sharma K, Nagpal K, Bera T. Investigation of the factors influencing the molecular weight of porphyran and its associated antifungal activity Bioact. *Carb Diet Fiber.* 2015;5:153–168.
84. Bhatia S, Kumar V, Sharma K, Nagpal K, Bera T. Significance of algal polymer in designing amphotericin B nanoparticles. *Sci World J.* 2014;2014:564573.
85. Bhatia S, Rathee P, Sharma K, Chaugule BB, Kar N, Bera T. Immuno-modulation effect of sulphated polysaccharide (porphyran) from Porphyra vietnamensis. *Int J Biol Macromol.* 2013;57:50–56.
86. Bhatia S. *Natural Polymer Drug Delivery Systems: Marine Polysaccharides Based Nano-Materials and Its Applications.* Springer International Publishing, Switzerland; 2016:185–225.
87. Bhatia S. *Natural Polymer Drug Delivery Systems: Plant Derived Polymers, Properties, and Modification & Applications.* Springer International Publishing, Switzerland; 2016:119–184.
88. Bhatia S. *Natural Polymer Drug Delivery Systems: Nanotechnology and Its Drug Delivery Applications.* Springer International Publishing, Switzerland; 2016:1–32.
89. Bhatia S. *Natural Polymer Drug Delivery Systems: Nanoparticles Types, Classification, Characterization, Fabrication Methods and Drug Delivery Applications.* Springer International Publishing, Switzerland; 2016:33–93.
90. Bhatia S. *Natural Polymer Drug Delivery Systems: Natural Polymers vs Synthetic Polymer.* Springer International Publishing, Switzerland; 2016:95–118.
91. Bhatia S. *Systems for Drug Delivery: Mammalian Polysaccharides and Its Nanomaterials.* Springer International Publishing, Switzerland; 2016:1–27.
92. Bhatia S. *Systems for Drug Delivery: Microbial Polysaccharides as Advance Nanomaterials.* Springer International Publishing, Switzerland; 2016:29–54.
93. Bhatia S. *Systems for Drug Delivery: Chitosan Based Nanomaterials and Its Applications.* Springer International Publishing, Switzerland; 2016:55–117.
94. Bhatia S. *Systems for Drug Delivery: Advance Polymers and Its Applications.* Springer International Publishing, Switzerland; 2016:119–146.
95. Bhatia S. *Systems for Drug Delivery: Advanced Application of Natural Polysaccharides.* Springer International Publishing, Switzerland; 2016:147–170.
96. Bhatia S. *Systems for Drug Delivery: Modern Polysaccharides and Its Current Advancements.* Springer International Publishing, Switzerland; 2016:171–188.
97. Bhatia S. *Systems for Drug Delivery: Toxicity of Nanodrug Delivery Systems.* Springer International Publishing, Switzerland; 2016:189–197.
98. Bhatia S. *Nanotechnology in Drug Delivery Fundamentals, Design, and Applications: Part 1: Protein and peptide-based drug delivery systems.* Apple Academic Press, Palm Bay, FL; 2016:50–204.
99. Bhatia S. *Nanotechnology in Drug Delivery Fundamentals, Design, and Applications: Part 2: Peptide-Mediated Nanoparticle Drug Delivery System.* Apple Academic Press, Palm Bay, FL; 2016:205–280.
100. Bhatia S. *Nanotechnology in Drug Delivery Fundamentals, Design, and Applications: Part 3: CPP and CTP in Drug Delivery and Cell Targeting.* Apple Academic Press, Palm Bay, FL; 2016:309–312.
101. Bhatia S. Stem cell culture. In: *Introduction to Pharmaceutical Biotechnology, Volume 3: Animal Tissue Culture and Biopharmaceuticals.* IOP Publishing Ltd, Bristol, UK; 2019:1–24.
102. Bhatia S. Organ culture. In: *Introduction to Pharmaceutical Biotechnology, Volume 3: Introduction to Animal Tissue Culture Science.* IOP Publishing Ltd, Bristol, UK; 2019:1–28.
103. Bhatia S. Animal tissue culture facilities. In: *Introduction to Pharmaceutical Biotechnology, Volume 3: Animal Tissue Culture and Biopharmaceuticals.* IOP Publishing Ltd, Bristol, UK; 2019:1–32.
104. Bhatia S. Characterization of cultured cells. In: *Introduction to Pharmaceutical Biotechnology, Volume 3: Animal Tissue Culture and Biopharmaceuticals.* IOP Publishing Ltd, Bristol, UK; 2019:1–47.
105. Bhatia S. Introduction to genomics. In: *Introduction to Pharmaceutical Biotechnology, Volume 2: Enzymes, Proteins and Bioinformatics.* IOP Publishing Ltd, Bristol, UK; 2018:1–39.
106. Bhatia S. Bioinformatics. In: *Introduction to Pharmaceutical Biotechnology, Volume 2: Enzymes, Proteins and Bioinformatics.* IOP Publishing Ltd, Bristol, UK; 2018:1–16.
107. Bhatia S. Protein and enzyme engineering. In: *Introduction to Pharmaceutical Biotechnology, Volume 2: Enzymes, Proteins and Bioinformatics.* IOP Publishing Ltd, Bristol, UK; 2018:1–15.
108. Bhatia S. Industrial enzymes and their applications. In: *Introduction to Pharmaceutical Biotechnology, Volume 2: Enzymes, Proteins and Bioinformatics.* IOP Publishing Ltd, Bristol, UK; 2018:21.
109. Bhatia S. Introduction to enzymes and their applications. In: *Introduction to Pharmaceutical Biotechnology, Volume 2: Enzymes, Proteins and Bioinformatics.* IOP Publishing Ltd, Bristol, UK; 2018:1–29.

110. Bhatia S. Biotransformation and enzymes. In: *Introduction to Pharmaceutical Biotechnology, Volume 2: Enzymes, Proteins and Bioinformatics.* IOP Publishing Ltd, Bristol, UK; 2018:1–13.
111. Bhatia S. Modern DNA science and its applications. In: *Introduction to Pharmaceutical Biotechnology, Volume 1 Basic Techniques and Concepts.* IOP Publishing Ltd, Bristol, UK; 2018:1–70.
112. Bhatia S. Introduction to genetic engineering. In: *Introduction to Pharmaceutical Biotechnology, Volume 1 Basic Techniques and Concepts.* IOP Publishing Ltd, Bristol, UK; 2018:1–63.
113. Bhatia S. Applications of stem cells in disease and gene therapy. In: *Introduction to Pharmaceutical Biotechnology, Volume 1 Basic Techniques and Concepts.* IOP Publishing Ltd, Bristol, UK; 2018:1–40.
114. Bhatia S. Transgenic animals in biotechnology. In: *Introduction to Pharmaceutical Biotechnology, Volume 1 Basic Techniques and Concepts.* IOP Publishing Ltd, Bristol, UK; 2018:1–67.
115. Bhatia S. History and scope of plant biotechnology. In: *Modern Applications of Plant Biotechnology in Pharmaceutical Sciences.* Academic Press, Cambridge, MA; 2015:1–30.
116. Bhatia S. Plant tissue culture. In: *Modern Applications of Plant Biotechnology in Pharmaceutical Sciences.* Academic Press, Cambridge, MA; 2015: 31–107.
117. Bhatia S. Laboratory organization. In: *Modern Applications of Plant Biotechnology in Pharmaceutical Sciences.* Academic Press, Cambridge, MA; 2015:109–120.
118. Bhatia S. Concepts and techniques of plant tissue culture science. In: *Modern Applications of Plant Biotechnology in Pharmaceutical Sciences.* Academic Press, Cambridge, MA; 2015:121–156.
119. Bhatia S. Application of plant biotechnology. In: *Modern Applications of Plant Biotechnology in Pharmaceutical Sciences.* Academic Press, Cambridge, MA; 2015:157–207.
120. Bhatia S. Somatic embryogenesis and organogenesis. In: *Modern Applications of Plant Biotechnology in Pharmaceutical Sciences.* Academic Press, Cambridge, MA; 2015:209–230.
121. Bhatia S. Classical and nonclassical techniques for secondary metabolite production in plant cell culture. In: *Modern Applications of Plant Biotechnology in Pharmaceutical Sciences.* Academic Press, Cambridge, MA; 2015:231–291.
122. Bhatia S. Plant-based biotechnological products with their production host, modes of delivery systems, and stability testing. In: *Modern Applications of Plant Biotechnology in Pharmaceutical Sciences.* Academic Press, Cambridge, MA; 2015:293–331.
123. Bhatia S. Edible vaccines. In: *Modern Applications of Plant Biotechnology in Pharmaceutical Sciences.* Academic Press, Cambridge, MA; 2015:333–343.
124. Bhatia S. Microenvironmentation in micropropagation. In: *Modern Applications of Plant Biotechnology in Pharmaceutical Sciences.* Academic Press, Cambridge, MA; 2015:345–360.
125. Bhatia S. Micropropagation. In: *Modern Applications of Plant Biotechnology in Pharmaceutical Sciences.* Academic Press, Cambridge, MA; 2015:361–368.
126. Bhatia S. Laws in plant biotechnology. In: *Modern Applications of Plant Biotechnology in Pharmaceutical Sciences.* Academic Press, Cambridge, MA; 2015:369–391.
127. Bhatia S. Technical glitches in micropropagation. In: *Modern Applications of Plant Biotechnology in Pharmaceutical Sciences.* Academic Press, Cambridge, MA; 2015:393–404.
128. Bhatia S. Plant tissue culture-based industries. In: *Modern Applications of Plant Biotechnology in Pharmaceutical Sciences.* Academic Press, Cambridge, MA; 2015:405–417.
129. Bhatia S, Al-Harrasi A, Behl T, Anwer MK, Ahmed MM, Mittal V, Kaushik D, Chigurupati S, Kabir MT, Sharma PB, Chaugule B, Vargas-de-la-Cruz C. Anti-migraine activity of freeze dried-latex obtained from *Calotropis Gigantea* Linn. *Environ Sci Pollut Res Int.* 2021.

18

Effects of Essential Oils on CNS

Ahmed Al-Harrasi
Natural and Medical Sciences Research Center, University of Nizwa

Saurabh Bhatia
Natural and Medical Sciences Research Center, University of Nizwa
University of Petroleum and Energy Studies

Tapan Behl
Chitkara University

Deepak Kaushik
M.D. University

CONTENTS

DOI: 10.1201/9781003175933-20

18.1 Introduction

CNS-associated complications mainly due to poor lifestyle and general aging process have caused a significant impact in the world. Anxiety as well as stress are complications that can trigger other psychological complications such as insomnia or depression. Various psychological complications and psychological imbalances in the form of mental stress, anxiety, depression, posttraumatic stress disorder, frustration, and uncertainty during COVID-19 pandemic developed at high rates. Psychological complications associated with the COVID-19 pandemic could worsen these preexisting conditions and can badly influence treatment outcomes [1]. When an individual suffering from psychological complications becomes COVID-19-positive, antiviral drugs should be used with psychotropic drugs, including antipsychotic, antidepressant, and antianxiety drugs. Antidepressant drugs like selective serotonin reuptake inhibitors (such as fluoxetine, paroxetine, citalopram) that act by selectively blocking the serotonin transporter and benzodiazepines (diazepam, lorazepam, or alprazolam) that act via binding to γ-aminobutyric acid (GABAA) receptors are more commonly recommended to treat anxiety and depression-related disorders. However, both classifications have considerable adverse/side effects such as somnolence, cognitive impairment, sexual dysfunction, and neuropsychiatric complications, including suicidal tendencies and sleep-related complications. Both classes cause various problems such as discontinuation syndrome, re-emergence of symptoms, dependency, diversion, driving impairment, misuse, mortality, and morbidity related to overdose and withdrawal. Thus, essential oil (EO)-based olfactory aromatherapy therapies have been considered at alternative treatment options. Among the various types of EOs, volatile oils have been used for centuries to treat various mental disorders via olfactory aromatherapy; however, their neuroprotective effects have not yet been explained. EOs are mixtures of hydrophobic volatile aromatic substances (with molecular weights >300 Daltons) that create the fragrances of certain plants. EOs possess various neuropharmacological properties and are alternatively utilized to treat various complications such as anxiety, attention deficit hyperactivity disorder, bipolar disorder, depression, and pain [2,3]. Various investigations have shown that EOs were effectively utilized in relieving stress, anxiety, and pain in experimental animal models and individuals with various CNS complications [2,3]. EOs are categorized into two classes based on their chemical profiles:

- Terpenoids (monoterpenes and sesquiterpenes)
- Phenylpropanoid derivatives

Depending on the properties of EOs, their safety, and their biological significance, EOs can be used orally and topically and also via inhalation. Certain EOs are used as anxiolytic remedies, orally but also by inhalation or combined with massage. Olfactory aromatherapy is an emerging therapy used to stimulate the olfaction process or olfactory nerve, which is directly connected to the brain. Olfactory chemoreceptors are molecular signaling proteins that are expressed in the cilia of olfactory sensory neurons. It's known that each olfactory sensory neuron in the nasal mucosa expresses a single type of olfactory receptor gene. This expression stimulates olfaction, mainly to detect as well as distinguish odorants and accordingly affect emotion, behaviors, and physiological functions [4].

The olfactory system involves the insular cortex, amygdala, thalamus, orbitofrontal cortex, hippocampus, and hypothalamus. Various reports supported the role of EOs in aromatherapy to stimulate the olfactory response in order to affect emotion, behaviors, and physiological functions. After inhalation, an interaction between volatile oil components and olfactory chemoreceptors in the nasal mucosa occurs to stimulate the primary olfactory regions located in the central nervous system. Thus, through this process, impulse or olfactory information is transmitted to the limbic system, which controls the emotions and autonomic nervous system [5]. Various EOs as well as their components are used as aromatherapy agents to attenuate stress, anxiety, and depression [6]. Inhalation of lavender oil can result in the prevention of stress, anxiety, and postpartum depression. Likewise, bergamot EO inhalation attenuates behavior-linked depressive disorder [7]. Similarly, there are various reports available on psychological benefits of inhaling rose, lavender, bergamot, lemon, and sandalwood EOs. Umezu T. [8] compared psychotropic effects of various EOs by discrete shuttle-type conditioned avoidance task in mice. It was found that mint and camomile EOs had CNS stimulant-like effects in a dose-dependent manner; they ameliorated rate of the response of the avoidance response rate. In another study, however, rate of response was not dependent on dose. In contrast, *Cupressus sempervirens, Citrus paradisi,* and *Citrus sinensis* EOs demonstrated depressant effects as these EOs reduced the rate of the response of the avoidance response rate. Rose and *Eucalyptus globulus* EOs reduced the avoidance rate with no impact on the rate of the response demonstrating its effects on the CNS. Moreover, the rest of the EOs derived from plants such as clary sage, ylang-ylang, vetivert, patchouli, niaouli, neroli, lemon, lavender, juniper, jasmine, geranium, and frankincense didn't show any effect on the avoidance response in mice. To assess the effects of EOs on the CNS, the following strategies can be utilized:

- Expression of Fos protein in CNS: Fos protein is a marker of neuronal activity and also a useful tool in the study of the mechanism of action of natural products with analgesic activity. It was found that seizure activity results in increased c-fos gene expression. It was also found that an increase in brain inflammation elevated the expression of c-fos gene to synthesize more Fos protein. Seizure activity increased a rapid and transient expression of c-fos protein in the hippocampal structures. Likewise, a transient activation of c-fos can result in cortical brain injury in a way that looks like that of spreading depression. Thus, studying the effects of EO over the expression of Fos protein would be a worthy strategy to assess its CNS-related protective effects [1,9].
- Shuttling response or avoidance response: In this model, rodents are trained to a high level of act of a trained avoidance response in a shuttlebox to test the effects of EO or any test compound [10].
- Open-field test (locomotor activity): This test can be used to instantaneously measure locomotion (ambulatory activity), exploration, and anxiety (emotionality). This model can be used in the evaluation of behavioral performance of the test animals and also useful in studying neurobiological mechanism-mediating behaviors [11].
- Miscellaneous models: hole board behavioral test, acetic acid-induced writhing test, elevated cross maze, rotarod performance test, formalin-induced pain test, pentobarbital-induced sleep duration, pentylenetetrazol-induced seizure
- Tail suspension and forced swimming test (FST) tests (depression): Extensively used in the screening of antidepressant drugs. The FST is used to assess the experimental model response against stress.
- EOs vs. GABAergic System act as GABA receptor agonists: It was found that EO components interact with GABA receptor and Na+channels and alter their function in order to exert biological effects.
- Action of EOs on muscarinic and opioids receptors.
- Biochemical assays such as acetylcholinesterase, superoxide dismutase, glutathione peroxidase, and malondialdehyde.
- Scopolamine-treated mice: For determining the neuroprotective effects in Alzheimer's disease model *in vivo* (scopolamine-treated mice).
- *In vitro* assays (H_2O_2-induced PC_{12} cells): To measure the effect of EOs in modulating oxidative stress and acetylcholinesterase activity.
- Rotarod performance test: The rotarod test was used for evaluating the motor coordination and presence of any muscle relaxation effects of EOs.
- Hole board tests and EPM test: In this test, EPM apparatus was used for evaluating anxiolytic-like effects of EOs.
- Marble-burying test: It was used for evaluating anxiolytic-like effects of EOs.

- Apomorphine-induced stereotypy: Potential of EOs to attenuate apomorphine-induced stereotyped behavior in an animal model to check for the presence of any psychoactive principles, which could be either sedative or neuroleptic in nature.
- Behavioral tests: During these tests, experimental animals (induced with fibromyalgia) were assessed for von Frey (mechanical hyperalgesia), Grip Strength Metter (muscle strength), and rotarod (motor coordination) [12].
- Sleeping time/sleep-prolonging effects: Effect of EOs over pentobarbital- and ethyl ether-induced sleep duration is a parameter to test the effectiveness of EOs over various sleeping disorders such as insomnia. Sleep-prolonging effect or decreasing the sleep latency ability of various EOs can be evaluated. This type of model can also be related to the effectiveness of EOs in sleep-promoting neurotransmitter [13].
- Haloperidol-induced catalepsy: Effect of EOs (antiparkinsonian activity) over several neurodegenerative movement disorders like Parkinson's due to the loss of dopamine neurons in midbrain dopaminergic nucleus can be studied via this model. Anticataleptic effect of EOs can be evaluated by haloperidol-induced catalepsy in experimental models [14].
- Stress-induced biomarkers: Effect of EO on the level of fast nerve growth factor receptor and activity-regulated cytoskeletal-associated protein (Arc) gene expression, and brain-derived neurotrophic factor and galactokinase 1 protein expression.
- Ketamine-induced hyperkinesia: It is evident that ketamine at low dose (30 mg/kg) increased the locomotor activity, while at greater concentration (150 mg/kg), it suppressed the locomotion. The effect of EOs on decreasing ketamine-induced hyperkinesia can be tested. It has been reported that ketamine at low dose increased the dopamine (DA) turnover to initiate and regulate the locomotor activity, while at high dose ketamine not only increased the DA level although also increased noradrenaline as well as and 5-hydroxytryptamine production in several areas of the brain. It was also reported that the locomotor activity caused at both concentrations of ketamine was found to be suppressed by antipsychotic drug, haloperidol (0.10 mg/kg, IP) [15].
- Anxiolytic-like effects: Several EOs demonstrated the anxiolytic effects; however, still there is no clarity on its action. Neurotransmitter analysis in the hippocampus, striatum, and hypothalamus is a possible way to reveal the mechanism of action. EOs components have been reported for their interaction with dopamine (D1), serotonin receptor (5-HT) to modulate dopaminergic/serotoninergic/GABAergic pathways to exert anxiolytic-like effects [16].

The most important studies reported on the neuropharmacological effects of EOs have included some of the important findings related to the mechanism of action of EOs (Tables 18.1–18.3):

- Effect on the transcription of NF-kB.
- Effect on inflammatory mediators: proinflammatory cytokines (IL-1, IL-6, and TNF-α), inducible nitric oxide synthase, and cyclooxygenase-2, expressions of proteins as well as cytokine genes such as Ccl2, Il6, Cxcl10, Ccl19, and Il1rl in the hippocampus of rats.
- Effect of EOs on corticotrophin-releasing-hormone: Increased glucocorticoids (cortisol in humans and corticosterone in rodents) in the adrenal glands.
- Indirect or direct effect of EOs on neurotransmission: EOs can modulate dopaminergic system (D1 receptor), serotoninergic (5-HT(1A) receptors), and GABAergic pathways to exert anxiolytic effects [47].
- Effect of EOs on Na(+) and Ca(+2) channels, recombinant T-type calcium channel [47].
- Effect of EOs on proteins such as N-methyl-D-aspartate, monoamine oxidase A, γ-Aminobutyric acid type A, and serotonin transporter [47].
- Effect of EOs on tauopathies, oxidative stress, cholinergic deficit, Nrf2/HO-1 pathway proteins, deposition of amyloid, synaptic transmission, and expression of Fos protein [47–49].
- Effect of EOs on enzymes (glutathione peroxidase, catalase, and superoxide dismutase) that control anti-oxidant mechanism and level of malondialdehyde.
- Effect of EOs on p-CaMKII, TrkB, brain-derived neurotrophic factor, calcium-calmodulin-dependent protein kinase II, nuclear factor erythroid-derived 2-like 2, synapse plasticity-related proteins, heme oxygenase-1 pathway, activity-regulated cytoskeletal-associated protein gene, and galactokinase 1 protein, a fast nerve growth factor receptor [47–49].
- Effect of EOs on EO components interaction with M2, M3, and M4 (muscarinic) as well as delta and mu (opioids) receptors.
- Effect of EOs on the acetylcholinesterase activity.
- Effect on stress inducers → ↑ corticotrophin-releasing-hormone → ↑ adrenocorticotropin (via pituitary gland) → ↑ glucocorticosteroids (hydrocortisone in humans and 17-deoxycortisol and 11β,21-dihydroxyprogesterone in rodents) in the adrenal glands → ↑ anti-inflammatory response.
- ↑Hypothalamic–pituitary– ↑ adrenal activation → ↑ corticosteroids → ↓ serotonin and DA levels in the brain → ↑ anxiety disorders or depression.
- Sympathetic nervous system stimulation → ↑ noradrenaline and adrenaline → ↑ nuclear factor kappa-light-chain-enhancer → ↑ transcription and release of proinflammatory cytokines (IL-1, IL-6 and TNF-α) → ↑ stimulation of the afferent vagus nerve → ↑ Infiltration of inflammatory mediators via crossing the blood–brain-barrier → ↑ Interaction with numerous neurotransmitter systems (serotonergic and DA nergic neurotransmission) → ↑ alterations in cognitive, emotional, and behavior [47–49].

TABLE 18.1

CNS Effects of Various Essential Oils

EO	Route of Administration	Biological Effects	Mechanism of Actions	References
Achillea wilhelmsii	Intraperitoneal	Reduce anxiety	Without the involvement of opioid as well as GABA receptors	[17]
Acorus gramineus Rhizoma	Oral and via inhlataion	Reduce the seizures caused via Pentylenetetrazol	Enhanced GABA expression; reduced expression of *GABA transaminase*	[18]
Acorus tatarinowii		Pain reducing effects	Suppressed sodium channels	[19]
Lemon verbena	*In vitro effect*	Reduce free radicals and offer protection to nerve cells	Suppressed binding of [3H]nicotine	[20]
White wormwood	*In vitro*	Reduce inflammation and showed fungal inhibitory effects	NA	[21]
White sagebrush	Intraperitoneal	Antinociceptive effects	Somewhat facilitated via opioid receptors	[22]
Judean Wormwood	*In vitro*	Reduce inflammation and showed fungal inhibitory effects	NA	[23]
Tarragon	Intraperitoneal	Nocioception effects	NA	[24]
Wild ginger (Chinese)	Inhalation	Reduced depression-like effects	NA	[25]
Tea plant	Inhalation	Sleeping duration is increased	Improved the expression of GABA-typeA receptors	[26]
Bitter orange	Oral	Reduce anxiety-like effects	Via serotonergic pathway (5-HT1(A))	[27]
Bergamot		Reduced anxiety triggered by stress	Tune the changes that occurs at synapses	[28]
Sweet orange	Inhalation	Reduce anxiety related effects	NA	[29]
Coriander	Inhalation	Reduced anxiety as well as depression	NA	[30]
West Indian lemon grass	Oral	Reduce anxiety	Mediated via GABA-A receptor	[31]
Java Citronella	Intraperitoneal	Prevent seizures activities	GABAergic pathway	[32]
Fetid Goosefoot.	Oral	Prevent convulsions	NA	[33]
Tropical bushmint	Oral	Induce calmness and sleep	Without participation of the GABA(A)	[34]
English lavender	Inhalation	Reduce anxiety	Via 5-HTergic	[35]
Bushy matgrass	Oral	Anesthetic effect (Central)	Mediated via GABAergic pathway	[36]
Citrus limon EO		Reduce anxiety and depression	Suppression of dopamine effects	[37]
Lemon balm	Oral	Reduce depression as well as agitation	Supressed GABA-mediated neuro-transmission	[38]
Fennel flower	Oral	Increase in anticonvulsant activity caused by valproate	Enhanced GABAergic activity	[39]
Scent and phytoncide	*In vitro*	Reduce anxiety, convulsions, and induce sedation	Increasing GABA(A) activity	[40]
Climbing black pepper	Inhalation	Cause sedation and reduce anxiety	NA	[3]
Crab's claw	*In vitro*	Cause vasorelaxation	Viabeta-adrenoceptors and Ca $^{+2}$ channels	[41]
Clary sage	Intraperitoneal, inhalation	Reduce depression	Via altering DA nergic system	[42]
Clove		Local anesthetic	Supressing Na+ channels	[43]
Southern cone marigold	Subcutaneous	Panicogenic -like activity	GABAergic pathway (negative modulation)	[44]
Mediterranean wild thyme	Oral	Antinociception	Peripheral nerve blockage	[45]
Valerian officinalis L	Oral	Sedatives	NA	[46]

Source: Wang ZJ, Heinbockel T, Molecules, 2018, 23(5), 1061, https://doi.org/10.3390/molecules23051061. With permission.
NA: not available

TABLE 18.2

Effect of Various EOs on Sodium Channels and GABA-ergic Pathway

Chemical Components	Biological Effects	Mechanism of Actions	References
Eucalyptol	Potentiate nerve activity	Enhance neurotransmission (hyper response)and sharp waves associated with epilepsy in neurons neurons via suppressing inhibiting K^+ channels	[50]
1-Nitro-2-phenylethene	Vasodilation in intact aortic rings	Suppression of contraction without involvement of calcium Ca^{2+} inflow	[51,52]

(*Continued*)

TABLE 18.2 (*Continued*)

Effect of Various EOs on Sodium Channels and GABA-ergic Pathway

Chemical Components	Biological Effects	Mechanism of Actions	References
Borneol	Reduce pain	Via positive altering GABA-AR response	[53]
Borneol	Improved hyperalgesia (mechanical)	Increased GABA-AR-associated GABA-ergic neurotransmission	[54]
Dehydrofukinone	Cause sedation as well as anesthesia-like responses	Via GABAergic pathway to suppress ; a nerve hyper neurotransmission	[55]
Dehydrofukinone	Showed sedative effect, reduced seizures, and also showed aneshetic effects	Improved GABA-A expression	[55]
Limonene	Reduce anxiety	NA	[56]
(S)-Limonene	Reduce stress	Via the involvement of GABA receptors	[57]
1,8-Cineole	Cause muscle relaxation (smooth muscle) antinociception effects	Decrease of nerve (peripheral) excitation via inhibiting voltage-mediated sodium channel	[58]
Nitro-phenylethane	Reduce hypnosis, convulsion and anxiety effects	NA	[59]
Methyl eugenol	Anticonvulsant	Blocked Na^+ channel, potentiated GABAA receptors	[47]
alpha-Bisabolol	Antinociception induction	Reduced excitability of nerve (peripheral) possibly via inhibition of voltage-dependent sodium channels	[60]
alpha-Asarone	Reduce seizures	Increased GABAergic supression	[61]
alpha-Asarone	Reduce seizures	Inhibition of sodium channels as wellas GABA-(A) receptors stimulation	[47]

Source: Wang ZJ, Heinbockel T, *Molecules*, 2018, 23(5), 1061, https://doi.org/10.3390/molecules23051061. With permission.

TABLE 18.3

Effect of EO Inhalation on CNS

Essential Oils	Biological Affects	Mechanism of Actions	References
Piper guineense	Sedative and anxiolytic-like effects		[3]
Salvia sclarea	Antidepressant-like effect	Modulating DAnergic pathway	[42]
English lavender	Reduce anxiety-like symptoms	Via 5-HTergic pathway	[35,62]
Coriander	Reduce anxiety as well as depression-like symptoms	-	[30]
Citrus sinensis	Acute anxiolytic activity	-	[29]
Tea plant	Enhanced sleeping duration	Increased the expression of GABA-(A) receptors	[26]
Asarum heterotropoides	Decreased depression-like behaviors		[63]
Acorus gramineus Rhizoma	Reduced seizures caused by pentylenetetrazol and also induce sedation CNS inhibitory effects	Enhanced the activity of GABAergic system and decreased the level of *GABA transaminase*	[18]
Anshen EO	Caused sedation and hypnosis	Rise in the level of 5-HT and GABA	[64]
Lavandula hybrida Reverchon	Analgesic activity	-	[65]
Lavandula angustifolia	Improve sleep quality in patients with ischemic heart disease	-	[66]
SuHeXiang Wan (Storax pill)	Anticonvulsive effect	Level of GABA was significantly enhanced and level of glutamate content was decreased after the EO inhalation Prolonged the sleeping duration caused by pentobarbital, with reduction in lipid peroxidation	[67]
Acori graminei Rhizoma	Sedative effect, anticonvulsive effect	Suppressed level of GABA transaminase Prolonged the sleeping duration caused by pentobarbital as the duration of EO inhalation was extended	[18]
Different EOs	Lessen central fatigue	Via boosting physical strength, decreasing anxiety as well as depression-like activity	[68]
Sweet orange lemon lavender sage and rosemary Lavender, rosemary, sage, sweet orange, lemon	Free radical scavenging effects	EOs ameliorated memory impairment (antiamnesia effect) caused by scopolamine via normalization of cholinergic pathway as well as antioxidant activity in the brain	[69]
Different EOs	Showed anti-inflammatory, antioxidant, and anxiolytic effects	-	[70]

(*Continued*)

TABLE 18.3 (*Continued*)
Effect of EO Inhalation on CNS

Essential Oils	Biological Affects	Mechanism of Actions	References
Pimpinella peregrina	Inhibited memory loss caused by scopolamine-induced, anxiolytic. and antidepression effects	Considerably enhanced memory and reduced anxiety and depression	[71]
Anthriscus nemorosa	Inhibited memory loss caused by scopolamine-and anxiolytic and antidepression	Considerable enhamcement in memory	[72]
Anshen EO	Induced sedation as well as hypnosis Sedative and hypnotic effects	Decrease spontaneous activity of rodent, and extend sleeping duration Probably increase the content of 5-HT as well as GABA	[64]
Roman chamomile essential oil	Improved the depression-reducing action of clomipramine	Via enhancing new neurons formation in hippocampus and alter levels of corticosterone among individuals with treatment-resistant depression	[73]
Cang-ai EO	Reduced depression-like symptoms	Via regulating dopamine as well as 5-HT metabolism	[74]
Chrysanthemum indicum Linné (*C. indicum* Linné)	Decreased blood pressure	EEG findings showed the appearance of theta and alpha waves, (while relaxation), reduction in beta and gamma waves (during extreme attention)	[75]
Rosmarinus officinalis	Decreased in stress as well as stimulation of nerve cell differentiation	Promoted nerve cell differentiation via alteration of acetylcholine, choline, and Gap43 gene inside the cell.	[76]
Angelica gigas	Enhanced capability of human brain to learn the language	Considerable differences in the absolute low beta wave response	[77]
Roman chamomile EO	Decreased depression-like symptoms	Antidepressant effect could be due to the presence of alpha-pinene	[78]
Polianthes tuberosa	Effective in reducing test anxiety	-	[79]
Vetiveria zizanioides	Cool effects of EO on EEG brain activity	EO inhalation reduced α and β waves in frontal and parietal cortices and enhanced γ waves in the frontal cortex.	[80]
Binasal and uninasal of Abies koreana Twigs	Changes in electrical brain activity after inhalation of EO could be due to increase in relaxation (binasal inhalation) and alertness (right uninasal inhalation) states of brain	Absolute α(left frontal and right parietal) and absolute fast α (right parietal) activities considerably enhanced through the binasal inhalation while in the uninasal inhalation, absolute βand θ activities reduced considerably in the right frontal and parietal areas (left and right)	[81]
t- cinnamaldehyde, benzylacetone, and 1-phenyl-2-butanone	Highly potent in the treatment of anorexia among aged group individuals	In the hypothalamus region, expression of neuropeptide (Y mRNA) considerably increased	[82]
Bergamot EO	Inhalation of EO reduced behavior-associated depressive disorder	Decreased the immobility time forced swimming test	[83]
Chamaecyparis obtuse	Anxiolytic-like effect	Owing to the greater level of alpha-pinene in the brain rise in in locomotor activity was observed	[84]
Ferulago angulata	Antiamnesic and antioxidants effects	Many treatment with EO improve spatial memory damage caused by scopolamine via reduction of the oxidative stress	[85]
Asarum Heterotropoides	Suppressed depression-like symptoms	Expression of corticotropin-releasing factor as well as tyrosine hydroxylase enhanced while serotonin level reduced	[25]
Juniper volatile oil	Reduced oxidative stress as well as acetylcholinesterase activity in Alzheimer's associated experimental model	Anti-acetylcholinesterase and antioxidant activities	[30]
Vetiver essential oil	Anxiolytic properties	Alteration of neuronal activation in central amygdaloid nucleus via increasing the expression of c-fos	[86]
Rose and orange EO	Caused physiological and psychological relaxation	Considerable reduction in oxy-Hb levels in the right prefrontal cortex	[87]
Coriander EO	Reduced anxiety as well as depression-like symptoms via reducing oxidative stress	Reduced activity of catalase and enhanced level of glutathione in the hippocampal region with decline in locomotor activity	[30]
Chamaecyparis obtusa	Antianxiety	Downregulated the expressions of cytokine genes (altered cytokines expression in the hippocampal region)	[88]
Lavender	Neuro-protective effects	Antioxidant and antiapoptotic effects	[89]
Rosemary EO	Stimulatory effect on ANS, as well as mood states	Rise in β activity in the brain (anterior region)	[90]

(*Continued*)

TABLE 18.3 (*Continued*)
Effect of EO Inhalation on CNS

Essential Oils	Biological Affects	Mechanism of Actions	References
Blend of EOs	-	Blend enhanced physical strength, reduced negative emotion via reducing anxiety/depression associated symptoms	[91]
Lavender, ylangylang, and bergamot	-	Decreased mental stress with decrease in cortisol as well as BP level	[92]
Lavender essential oil	-	Decreased systolic blood pressure	[93]
Lavender essential oil	-	Decreased anxiety level	[94]
Lavender essential oil	-	Decrease in blood cortisol & anxiety	[95]
Lavender fleur EO and odorless EO	-	Lowered anxiety	[96]
Rose essential oil	-	Rose EO failed in reducing anxiety significantly	[97]
Aromatherapy	-	Decreased anxiety, pain, and HR	[98]
EO enriched with beta-pinene, beta-caryophyllene, 1,8-cineole, 3-carene, and carnosic acid	-	Reduced stress and improves sleep quality	[99]
Zingiber zerumbet oil	-	Increased the weight gain	[100]
Cymbopogon nardus L. (Citronella oil)	-	Decreased body weight by decreasing appetite	[101]

18.2 Influence of EOs on Voltage-Gated Na^+ Channels as well as GABAergic Pathway

To treat various neurological disorders, it's important to maintain an equilibrium between excitability and inhibitory activities of neurons. To maintain equilibrium the stimulation of the neuronal voltage-gated sodium channels as well as GABA receptor is required. This action potential or electrical signal-based neuron activities are important for the functioning of the brain under normal conditions and also important for understanding the pathophysiology of CNS-related complications. Various reports have suggested that EO components act via involving the GABAergic system and blocking Na^+ channels (Tables 18.2 and 18.3).

It is well known that GABA, an inhibitory neurotransmitter, is required for normal functioning of the brain, in neuronal activity and neuronal plasticity, and is involved in various other aspects of CNS. Impairment associated with the GABAergic system could result in manifestations like epilepsy, pain, and anxiety (Table 18.2). On the other hand, voltage-gated Na^+ channels regulated excitability in neuronal plasticity, via propagating action potentials in neurons, and thus are considered as important targets of anticonvulsant drugs. As reported, anesthetics and analgesics act via inhibiting the transmission of nerve impulses or interfering with the action potential via interacting with Na^+ channels. Tetrodotoxin (TTX) is a neurotoxin that acts via blocking the sodium channel to inhibit the neuron excitability activity by interfering with action potential. TTX is widely employed to explore the role of specific voltage-gated sodium channel subtypes during various neurobiological and neuropathophysiological events. Na^+ currents are categorized based on their response against TTX (i.e., TTX-sensitive and TTX-resistant sodium channels). These channels are located in posterior root ganglion [102–105]. Previous reports suggested that Nav1.7 encodes for expression of TTX-sensitive Na^+ channels mainly in the sympathetic nerve cells of PNS (peripheral nervous system). These channels have been reported in regulating inflammatory pain [102–105] and pain sensation [102–105]. Several reports showed that EOs as well as their components can be utilized in the management of anxiety, convulsion, and pain in various subjects/models with their respective underlying mechanisms. Based on the mechanism of action, EOs act via involving voltage-gated sodium channels and GABAergic pathway in different ways (Tables 18.2 and 18.3):

- Several EOs showed anxiolytic effects via modulating GABAergic system [31,53,67,106].
- Many EOs showed antinociceptive and antiseizure effects via blocking neuronal voltage-gated Na^+ channels [67].
- A number of EOs modulated both GABAergic system and voltage-gated Na^+ channels (Table 18.2) [106,107].

18.3 Antiepileptic Effects of EOs

Because of advantages such as fewer side effects, various modes of administration, and potential biological activities, EOs remain as the first choice for treating various neurological complications such as epilepsy. Various EOs have been evidenced for their anticonvulsant effects and could be beneficial for patients suffering from epilepsy. Clove, dill, lavender, lemongrass, and other EOs contain therapeutic active compounds such as linalool, citral, eugenol, asarone, and carvone, which must be evaluated for their antiepileptic effects. In contrast, a number of EOs have been reported to exacerbate convulsant effects and could promote seizures in both epileptic and healthy individuals. It has been reported that various compounds such as thuja, sage, rosemary, pennyroyal, hyssop, fennel, eucalyptus, cedar, and camphor are responsible for aggravating epileptic seizures as chemically they constitute camphor, pinocamphone, 1,8-cineole, and thujone, which have been considered as convulsive agents. However, more understanding is necessary to investigate the molecular targets of EOs [108,109]. It's also known that the convulsant or anticonvulsant effects of EOs are possibly due to their potential in modulating neurotransmission in neurons as well as their ability to change ionic transport via ion channels. As reported, anticonvulsant EOs have been mainly reported from the Apiaceae and Lamiaceae family. As far as chemical components are concerned, β-caryophyllene, nerolidol, eugenol, and borneol have been evidenced for their ability in reducing the oxidative stress that triggers convulsion. Their potential in attenuating oxidative stress could contribute to their role in treating various other neurological conditions [108,109].

18.4 Anxiolytic Effects of Essential Oils

EOs are widely used as anxiolytics to relieve anxiety symptoms due to the presence of terpenoids and other potential compounds. From earlier times, EOs have also been utilized in relieving nervousness and depression and as mood boosters. In contrast to modern medicine, EOs have fewer less side effects and more specialized application options, such as topical as well as via inhalation. Various studies based on the anxiolytic effects of EOs have been reported. In the majority of the clinical studies, EOs are administered via inhalation and the oral route to induce anxiolytic effects. Some clinical studies also showed topical application as well as intraperitoneal administration of EO to induce anxiolytic effects. There are almost 20 organic compounds obtained from EOs, reported for their anxiolytic activity in various experimental animals, and two-thirds of them are terpenoids and alcohols. It was also found that the anxiolytic effect of EOs is mediated by monoamines (adrenaline, noradrenaline, serotonin, dopamine), amino acid (GABA, glutamate, glycine), and the HPA axis. *In vivo* investigations demonstrated the anxiolytic effects of EOs and the interactions of their respective active components with CNS receptors [110]. It was reported that the alteration of the GABAergic system and glutamatergic pathway could be the possible sites of action of EOs to induce sedative, anxiolytic, and anticonvulsant effects. It was found that EOs efficient in reducing anxiety are usually enriched with terpene alcohols such as dihydrogeraniol, geraniol, as well as linalool and monoterpenoidal compounds such as limonene and citral [110]. Thus, EO preparations comprising these compounds as main compounds could serve as possible treatment for relieving anxiety, depression, and convulsions [111].

EOs are extensively used for the prevention of anxiety, insomnia, convulsion, pain, and cognitive deficit symptoms via inhalation, oral administration, and aromatherapy. It has been reported that the effects of EOs are mediated via the modulation of the GABAergic system and sodium ion channels (Table 18.3). It is evidenced that a number of compounds target transient receptor potential (TRP) channels to possess analgesic effects [112].

18.5 Role of Essential Oils in Neurodegenerative Disorders

EOs as well as their components have been used in conventional medication and used as effective aroma therapeutics for the treatment of neurodegenerative disorders. Numerous reports have suggested neuroprotective and antiaging effects of EOs. Various EOs as their components derived from *Rosmarinus officinalis, Piper nigrum, Nigella sativa, Mentha piperita, Lavandula angustifolia, Jasminum sambac, Eucalyptus globulus*, and *Acorus gramineus* are evidenced for neuroprotective effects. Based on previous reports, the mechanism of action of EOs in the management of Alzheimer's disease and dementia involves targeting (Table 18.1) [113].

- Oxidative stress
- Neurofibrillary tangles
- Glutamatergic abnormalities
- Cholinergic hypofunction
- Amyloid deposition.

Additionally, anxiolytic, antiamyloid efficiency, antioxidant, anticholinesterase, antidepression, antiepilepsy, antiaging, anticonvulsion, and potential effects on dementia contribute to the neuroprotective effects of EOs. As it is known, amyloid, a key pathological marker of Alzheimer's disease, can easily self-aggregate, which can result in the clump formation of insoluble fibrils in the brain. This event of clump formation can further result in the formation of senile plaques. This pathological event further causes apoptosis in neurons via oxidative or nitrosative stress. A previous study suggested the role of 6-gingerol in providing protection against amyloid beta-peptide 25–35 peptide-induced toxicity and programmed cell death. Cellular protection was provided by

- Suppressing increased Bax/Bcl-2 ratio
- Interfering with mitochondrial membrane potential
- Inhibiting DNA fragmentation
- Inhibiting the activation of caspase-3

The neuroprotective effects of 6-gingerol were mediated by the inhibition of amyloid beta-peptide 25–35 peptide-induced production of reactive nitrogen species as well as reactive oxygen species inside the cell. Other EO components such as thymol and carvacrol have also been reported for their antiamyloid potential. Oxidative stress resulting from too much generation of free radicals can lead to oxidative injury and diseased state. This excessive production of free radicals is mainly due to the

- Progression of Alzheimer's disease (event of β-amyloid deposition is a powerful initiator of ROS/RNS)
- Free radical/ROS/RNS involvement in aged brain
- Mitochondrial dysfunction
- Cyclooxygenase also mediates neuroinflammation by the production of proinflammatory prostaglandins.

These events cause excessive production of oxidizing free radicals followed by pathological abnormalities such as damage to neural, microglial, cerebrovascular cells, and tissues. Neuroprotective effects of various EOs can also be mediated via reducing oxidative stress. Various EOs such as basil, chamomile, cinnamon leaf, clove, coriander, cumin, eucalyptus, juniper, and thyme have been demonstrated to have potent antioxidant properties and can be proficiently utilized for oxidative stress-tempted complications such as age-related disorders as well as neurological complications [114].

Numerous EOs have also been assessed for the management of psychomotor agitation-related disorders and various complications associated with dementia. In 2007, *Lavandula angustifolia* and *Melissa officinalis* were used for the treatment of agitation in subjects suffering from acute dementia. Both oils were reported for their ability in inhibiting ligand interaction with M1(muscarinic), 5-HT2A (subtype of the 5-HT_2 serotonin receptor), H3 (histamine receptors), and GABA (GABAA receptor). It was also reported that Lavandula EO prevented the interaction between GABAA receptors and GABA receptor antagonist, t-butyl bicyclophosphorothionate in rodent brain [115]. The anxiolytic-like effects of several EOs have been demonstrated in many reports; however, the molecular targets responsible for this biological effects are still not known (Table 18.1). Neurotransmitter analysis in the hippocampus, striatum, and hypothalamus is a possible way to reveal the mechanism of action. Serotoninergic, GABAergic as well as dopaminergic have been reported for their possible role in contributing the anxiolytic-like of EOs. Anxiolytic agents such as benzodiazepines have various side effects such as sedation, drug abuse as well as drug tolerance. As a result, treatment with psychostimulant EOs could be more valuable treatment to cure episodes of anxiety [116]. Numerous EOs have been evidenced for their strong anxiolytic potentials such as *Anthemis nobilis, Citrus bergamia, Citrus sinensis, L. angustifolia, Pelargonium species, Rosa damascene, Salvia sclarea,* and *Santalum album* [117,118].

A number of reports are available on the anticonvulsant and antiepileptic effects of EOs as well as their components potentially treat epilepsy. Numerous EOs such as *Ocimum basilicum*, *Myristica fragrans*, *Crocus sativus* (terpinen-4-ol considerably decreased convulsions and spontaneous motor activity), *Cymbopogon proximus,* and *Pimpinella anisum* have been reported for their antiepileptic and depressant-like effects via GABAergic pathway [113,119,120].

The anticonvulsant effects of several EOs as well as their components such as dill, lemongrass, clove, lavender, and linalool, citral, carvone, eugenol, and asarone could be beneficial for epileptic patients. However, the same EOs have also been reported for depressant as well as convulsant effects and can cause seizures in both epileptic and healthy subjects. EOs such as camphor, cedar, eucalyptus, fennel, hyssop, pennyroyal, rosemary, sage, and thuja trigger epileptic seizures in both epileptic and healthy subjects as they contain thujone, 1,8-cineole, camphor, or pinocamphone, which have been reported as agents to cause convulsions. It was observed that convulsant as well as anticonvulsant activities of EOs are usually mediated via modulating the GABAergic system or to alter ionic currents via ion channels [108].

The inhibitory activities of various EOs such as *Polygonum hydropiper, Rumex hastatus, Marlierea racemosa, Salvia lerifolia, Narcissus poeticus*, and *Cistus salvifolius* over acetylcholinesterase and butyrylcholinesterase have been reported. It is well known that acetylcholinesterase and butyrylcholinesterase enzymes are responsible for the degradation of acetylcholine; thus, EOs with inhibitory effects on these enzymes could be further be utilized in the symptomatic management of Alzheimer's disease [113].

Cognitive impairment that affects learning and memory is considered as the common causes of Alzheimer's disease, which can result in the selective degeneration of cognitive skills. Cognitive impairment involves the degeneration of cholinergic neurons that have been identified in the cognitive deficits of Alzheimer's disease patients. Several reports based on the psychophysiological potencies of EOs have been identified, via an improvement in cognitive functions. Various EOs have been proven for their effects on memory and attention; for example, *Salvia lavandulifolia, M. piperita,* and *R. officinalis* have been used memory-boosting effects in rodents and dogs mice and dogs and *L. angustifolia* has been reported for improving attention in a vigilance task [121–124].

18.6 Effects of Essential Oils on T-type Calcium Channels

Based on their activation threshold, voltage-activated calcium channels are categorized as low-voltage-activated and high-voltage-activated. Several reports have suggested the role of EOs in modulating T-type calcium channels, which actively participate in various physiological and pathophysiological processes, and are available, suggesting that these channels could be the possible targets for EOs [125]. T-type calcium channels are usually inactivated in a resting membrane; however, events like neuronal excitability considerably affect T-type calcium channels [125].

Recently, it was reported that the major chemical compounds of lavender and rosemary (rosmarinic acid as well as linalool) alter the electrical responses of T-type calcium channels (recombinant) expressed in HEK-293T cells. It was found that LEO as well rosemary EO suppressed channel current and was dose-dependent. The authors concluded that T-type calcium channels are considered as primary molecular targets for LEO as well as rosemary compounds. These findings evidenced by authors demonstrated that T-type calcium channel inhibition by EO components might contribute to its neuroprotective and anxiolytic properties [126].

Earlier investigations have suggested that voltage-gated Na^+ channels and high-voltage-activated Ca^{2+} channels are expressed in neurons detecting dental pain and thus are considered as potential targets of EO compounds such as eugenol for their pain-relieving effects. Recent investigation showed that other than that voltage-gated Na^+ channels, eugenol also affects neuronal T-type calcium channels. This study suggested that T-type Ca^{2+} channels can also be molecular targets for the analgesic effects of eugenol; however, analgesia effects are mainly mediated by the suppression of Na^+ current

[127,128]. It was also found that α-terpineol reduced calcium influx, which takes place via the voltage-sensitive CavL channels. This inhibitory effect of α-terpineol over calcium influx can reduce vascular resistance, which results in hypotension induction [129].

18.7 Essential Oils Acting on CNS

The following EO-containing plants have been reported for their effects on the CNS.

18.7.1 *Lavandula angustifolia*

EO derived from *Lavandula angustifolia* (LEO) is frequently used to treat mental disorders, and that from lavender (*Lavandula angustifolia Miller or Lavandula officinalis Chaix*) is used to treat anxiety. LEO has been widely utilized to treat anxiety, stress, and depression. Various studies have revealed that LEO is enriched with linalool and linalyl acetate. LEO has been officially accepted for its capability to alleviate anxiety, stress, and restlessness by the WHO and European Scientific Cooperative on Phytotherapy. López et al. (2017) showed pharmacological mechanisms of LEO on CNS targets such as MAO-A, SERT, GABAA, and NMDA receptors as well as *in vitro* models of neurotoxicity. Findings from this investigation showed that LEO as well as its active components possess high affinity for the NMDA(N-methyl-D-aspartate) glutamate receptor, and this affinity was dependent on concentration-of LEO [118]. Moreover, it was found that lavender and linalool did not show affinity for GABAA-benzodiazepine receptor, whereas both showed their ability to bind to the serotonin transporter. The authors also investigated the effects of LEO on SH-SY5Y cells, and it was observed that lavender did not elevate the neurotoxic insult and promote the viability of hydrogen peroxide-treated SH-SY5Y cells. Thus, it was concluded by the authors that the anxiolytic and antidepressant properties of LEO could be because of the inhibitory effects on the N-methyl-D-aspartate receptor and suppression of the protein known as sodium-dependent serotonin transporter, showing that LEO has biological potential via altering the expression of NMDA receptor and SERT protein [118].

Another report showed that LEO ameliorates the cognitive effects of scopolamine-induced mice in behavioral tests. Also, LEO considerably reduced the acetylcholinesterase activity, level of malondialdehyde, and ameliorated the activity of antioxidant enzymes (superoxide dismutase and glutathione peroxidase). Additionally, LEO reduced cytotoxicity caused by H_2O_2 to PC_{12} cells via decreasing lactate dehydrogenase, nitric oxide producton, accumulation of ROS inside the cells, and loss of mitochondrial membrane potential. Thus, it was concluded by the authors that LEO provides neuroprotection in Alzheimer's disease model *in vivo* (scopolamine-treated mice) and *in vitro* (H_2O_2 induced PC_{12} cells) via modulating oxidative stress and acetylcholinesterase activity [130].

One more report demonstrated a key role for the serotonergic system in the anxiolytic-like effect of lavender EO. As per this report, the treatment of male Swiss mice with LEO (1% to 5%) reduced marble burying-locomotor activity, increased plus maze, and did not alter the binding of GABA-A receptors agonist, flunitrazepam, to the GABAA receptor benzodiazepine-site. In addition, pretreatment with picrotoxin did not have the behavioral effect of LEO in the marble-burying test, whereas pretreatment with the WAY100635 suppressed the anxiolytic-like effect of LEO. Concomitant treatment of LEO with 5-HT1A receptor agonist 8-hydroxy-2-(di-n-propylamino) tetralin decreased the number of marbles buried. LEO treatment was also reported to reduce serotonin syndrome triggered by fluoxetine as well as 5-hydroxytryptophan. These findings reported by the authors demonstrate the anxiolytic-like effects of LEO when administered by inhalation in experimental animals via the involvement of serotonergic neurotransmission [62]. Another report on LEO inhalation demonstrated that stimulation of olfaction has no correlation with efficiency of LEO in reducing anxiety anxiolytic-like effect. It was found that anosmia did not contribute to the anxiolytic-like effect of LEO inhalation in the marble-burying test [35]. One more report suggested that linalyl acetate and linalool chemical components of LEO work synergistically to cause antianxiety effects (i.e., the presence of both chemical components is required during the inhalation to cause anti-anxiety effects) [131].

As per reports, it's clearly evident that the inhalation of LEO causes behavioral changes as a result of a multifarious centrally coordinated response. However, it's also important to understand the molecular mechanisms of action of LEO involved in triggering the emotional responses against varied levels of stress. Takahashi et al. [132] demonstrated that LEO inhalation causes dual alterations in the CNS, either by reducing the effects of stress or by acting as a stressor, depending on the state of the subject.

Takahashi et al. [133] reported that LEO inhalation showed considerable increase in anxiety-associated response, which could be olfactory system dependent or with no involvement of olfactory system, suggesting that activation is not essential for the biological action of LEO. LEO considerably elevated the 5-HT levels in the striatal and hippocampal region, which corroborates the assumption that the anxiolytic effect of LEO is mediated via serotonergic neurotransmission.

Further effects of LEO inhalation on behavior of the small rodent in the EPM test by involving both sex of rodents were investigated, and it was found that lavender inhalation produced anxiolytic effects in gerbils in the same manner as is seen in case of diazepam-treated gerbils. Moreover, LEO inhalation for a longer period enhanced probing behavior in females signifying a reduction in the level of anxiety in this sex [134]. Further, silexan is derived from *Lavandula angustifolia* EO and has been found to be effective in treating various anxiety-related disorders. A previous investigation showed considerable anxiolytic effects of silexan in experimental models, and the effects were equivalent to those of lorazepam [135]. Recently, the effects of LEO and linalool against aluminum chloride as well as D-galactose induced cognitive disorder in the experimental model along with its mechanisms were investigated. It was found that LEO and linalool both showed the following ways to reduce cholinergic activity, oxidative stress, modulation of synaptic plasticity as well as nuclear factor erythroid 2/heme oxygenase-1 axis.

- Considerably improved the level of antioxidant enzymes such as glutathione peroxidase and superoxide dismutase
- Reduced the level of AChE as well as MDA
- Reduced level of proteins involved in the activation of synapse plasticity
- Reduced expression of proteins (calcium/calmodulin-activated protein kinase) responsible for intracellular accumulation of Ca^{+2}
- Reduced expression of another calcium/calmodulin-activated protein kinase (p-CaMKII)
- Reduced expression of abrineurin

It was concluded that LEO and linalool both might be possible candidates for treating cognitive impairment in Alzheimer's disease [136].

Shanzhizi (*Gardenia jasminoides* Ellis) based study revealed that *G. jasminoides* EO inhalation considerably decreased 5-HIAA/5-HT in the prefrontal cortex and decreased 5-HIAA level in the hippocampus. The author concluded that *G. jasminoides* EO inhalation showed an anxiolytic effect, which is mediated by the involvement of monoamine neurotransmitters mainly the serotonergic system [137]. An additional report demonstrated that LEO inhibited the activity of GABA receptor antagonist, TBPS (tert-butylbicyclophosphorothionate)-binding gamma-aminobutyric acid (A) receptor channel in the rat forebrain. It was also evidenced that *Melissa officinalis* EO as well as LEO in 50:50 ratio suppressed [3H] flunitrazepam binding, while the individual EO had no considerable activity. The authors reported that LEO and MEO both suppressed GABA-induced currents and this effect was dependent on dose and provoked a considerable concentration-dependent decrease in electrical signaling (inhibitory as well as excitatory transmission), with an overall depressant activity over neurotransmission. It was indicated that antiagitation as well as antidepressant effects of LEO in neural membranes was unlikely to represent a sedative interaction with ionotropic receptors [138]. Another recent investigation showed the ability of lavender and rosemary in modulating T-type calcium channels as they play significant roles in:

- Neuronal excitability
- Neuroprotection
- Sensory processes
- Sleep
- Involved in epilepsy and pain

18.7.2 *Achillea wilhelmsii*

Various plants belonging to genus Achillea demonstrated analgesic, sedative, and antiinflammatory effects. p-Ocimen, 1,8-cineole, and carvone were identified as the main components of *Achillea wilhelmsii*. It was found that the anxiolytic effects of *A. wilhelmsii* EO were possibly not mediated via GABA and opioid receptors in rats [17].

18.7.3 *Acorus gramineus*

Acorus gramineus EO inhalation has been reported for its sedative, anticonvulsant, and antioxidant effects [18]. β-Asarone, euasarone, and α-euasarone [102] were identified as the main constituents of *A. gramineus* EO. A previous report showed a considerable sedative effect of *A. gramineus* EO via involving the GABAergic system. It has been evidenced that pre-inhalation or oral administration of EO considerably postponed the appearance of PTZ-induced seizure in the experimental animal model. Further inhalation of EO remarkably protracted the pentobarbital-induced sleeping time in the experimental animal model. It was found that anticonvulsive effects could be due to the inhibitory effects of EO on lipid peroxidation.

18.7.4 Agarwood

For decades, agarwood EO has been used as a tranquilizer; however, molecular targets have not been explored yet. A recent investigation revealed the capability of agarwood EO in causing hypnotic as well as sedative effects. It was found that agarwood EO showed considerable calming effect by suppressing locomotor behavior. Additionally, agarwood EO was found to have no considerable influence over the expression of gamma-aminobutyric acid as well as glutamic acid in the brain. GABAA receptor antagonists like bicuculline and flumazenil have inhibited sedative-hypnotic effects of agarwood EO. Moreover, in human neuroblastoma cells, agarwood EO enhanced chlorine ion influx via GABAA receptors. Thus, it was concluded by the authors that agarwood EO possesses hypnotic and sedative activities via modulating of GABA-A expression as well as increasing activity of GABA-A [139].

18.7.5 *Aloysia citrodora*

Limonene, geranial, neral, 1,8-cineole, curcumene, spathulenol, and caryophyllene oxide were identified as the main chemical compounds of *Aloysia citrodora* EOs. EO from *A. citrodora* has been reported for its capability to suppress binding of [3H] nicotine to the rat forebrain membranes and remove the excess iron from the brain (which can progress or cause neuro degenerative disorder) by ameliorating iron chelation [20]. EO obtained from *A. citrodora* showed potential neuroprotective and antioxidant effects [20].

18.7.6 *Alpinia zerumbet*

de Araújo et al. [140] reported the depressant and possible antipsychotic effects of *A. zerumbet* EOs as they can reverse the stereotypy induced by apomorphine, which suggests their response is the same as it is after haloperidol treatment. Findings from this study suggested that treatment with EO decreases the locomotor activity and apomorphine-induced stereotypy in a dose-dependent manner. Further treatment with EO reduced grooming response and augmented cataleptic activity as well as the immobility period in the FST and tail suspension test. Decrease in locomotor activity, augmentation in cataleptic activity, and immobility period were observed after pretreatment with haloperidol.

18.7.7 Artemisia EO

EOs obtained from various Artemisia species have been reported for their antinociceptive and anti-inflammatory effects. In Iranian folk medicine, *Artemisia dracunculus* has been used to treat pain and GIT complications [24]. *Artemisia dracunculus* or tarragon EO has also been reported for its potential antinociceptive effect [24]. Another report suggested that the antinociceptive effects of *Artemisia ludoviciana* EO are mediated via opioid receptors [22]. One more report suggested anti-inflammatory effects exhibited by *Artemisia herba-alba* [21]. In the same study, the authors investigated the chemical profile of *Artemisia herba-alba* and found that α-thujone and β-thujone were the major chemical compounds. In another study, the antifungal and anti-inflammatory effects of *Artemisia judaica* were demonstrated. Also, it has been revealed that *A. judaica* EO contains piperitone, camphor, and ethyl cinnamate as the major compounds [23].

18.7.8 *Asarum heterotropoides* (Wild Ginger)

Asarum heterotropoides has been known for reducing anxiety and inflammation [25]. In 2015, *A. heterotropoides* EO noticeably suppressed antidepression-like effect via elevating the expression of brain corticotropin-releasing factor and tyrosine hydroxylase and reducing the expression of serotonin in mice induced with stress.

18.7.9 *Cananga odorata* (Ylang-Ylang Essential Oil)

Zhang et al. [141] suggested the anxiolytic effects of *Cananga odorata* EOs on the experimental animals and revealed the main chemical compound responsible for a change in neurotransmitters after exposure against its odor. It was found that the treatment of male mice with *Cananga odorata* EOs showed considerable anxiolytic effect. The major chemical compounds of the EO were found to be benzyl benzoate, linalool, and benzyl alcohol. Each chemical compound showed an anxiolytic effect on the male mice. Exposure of *Cananga odorata* EOs also indicated more changes in neurotransmitter levels in the male mice than in the female mice. The authors also found that EO treatment attenuated DA level in the striatum and elevated the 5-hydroxytryptamine level in the hippocampus of the male mice. In addition, EO treatment also attenuated 5-HIAA/5-HT level in the hippocampus region. It was concluded by the authors that benzyl benzoate-enriched *Cananga odorata* EO presented an anxiolytic activity on the rodent, whereas benzyl benzoate action might be possibly mediated by 5-HTnergic and DAnergic pathways.

18.7.10 *Chamaecyparis obtuse*

A previous report demonstrated significant anxiolytic-like and stress-reducing effects of *Chamaecyparis obtuse* EO [142]. Researchers demonstrated the effect of EOs over level as well as the expression of stress-induced biomarkers within the brain such as fast nerve growth factor receptor, activity-regulated cytoskeletal-associated protein gene, brain-derived neurotrophic factor, and galactokinase 1 protein. It was found that EO inhalation considerably increased the expression of fast nerve growth factor receptor, which demonstrates anxiolytic-like and stress-reducing effects of EO [142]. Another report suggested that *Chamaecyparis obtuse* EO inhalation protected spatial learning and memory from the damages caused by Aβ(1–40) administration [143]. Moreover, the behavioral deficits associated with Aβ(1–40)-induced Alzheimer's disease were reduced by *Chamaecyparis obtuse* EO inhalation. Also, EO inhalation significantly inhibited acetylcholinesterase activity and neuronal apoptosis in rats treated with Aβ(1–40) and EOCO. Thus, the authors concluded that *Chamaecyparis obtuse* EO inhibited both Alzheimer's disease-associated neuronal cell apoptosis and Alzheimer's disease-associated dysfunction of the memory system [143]. Another report revealed the analgesic and anti-inflammatory effects of *Chamaecyparis obtuse* EO. It was reported that *Chamaecyparis obtuse* EO administration considerably attenuates acetic acid-induced writhing and paw-licking time in late response of the formalin tests. Further EO treatment decreased the expression of tumor necrosis factor-α, interleukin-1β, inducible nitric oxide synthase, and cyclooxygenase-2 in the formalin-injected paws of mice. The analgesic effect could be due to the suppression of peripheral pain linked to inflammatory response [63]. One more report showed that *Chamaecyparis obtusa* EO-treated maternal separated rats showed a decrease in anxiety-linked response in the EPM test. Further, it was also indicated that *Chamaecyparis obtusa* EO decreased the expressions of proteins as well as cytokine genes such as Ccl2, Il6, Cxcl10, Ccl19, and Il1rl in the hippocampus of rats [88]. The authors concluded that EO attenuated maternal separated-induced anxiety-linked responses and down-regulated cytokines, mainly Ccl2 and Il6, in the hippocampus of rats. Additionally, it was reported that *Chamaecyparis obtuse* EO inhalation increased the level of α-pinene in the brain more specifically in the striatum and the hippocampus regions, which contributed to an increase in the locomotor activity [84].

18.7.11 *Citrus aurantium* (Lemon Oil)

Citrus aurantium EOs have been reported for their traditional usage in treating sleeping disorders as well, and they have been used as alternatives to antidepressant medications in previous investigations. In 2013, the possible mechanism involved its antidepressant and its potential in reducing anxiety along with its capability in causing neurochemical alterations in certain regions of the brain was investigated. It was found that acute *Citrus aurantium* EO treatment showed anxiolytic-like effects during the light/dark box method, which was mediated by the serotonin 1A receptor [27]. In addition, treatment with *Citrus aurantium* EO didn't present any effects in the FST, no changes in neurotransmitter levels as well as no locomotor damage or variations in biochemical profile, apart from attenuation in levels of cholesterol [27]. In 2006, antistress effects of lavender, rose, and lemon EOs were evaluated, and it was found that lemon oil comparatively showed significant antistress effects [37]. Komiya et al. demonstrated anxiolytic and antidepressant-like effects of lemon oil by inhibiting DA pathways and stimulating serotonergic (5-HT) activity. Plants belonging to Citrus genus are the main source of lemon oil.

Another report indicated the anxiolytic property of *Citrus sinensis* EO at all doses in the light/dark box as well as in EPM tests.

18.7.12 *Citrus bergamia* (Bergamot)

EOs derived from *Citrus bergamia* have been reported for antinociceptive and anti-inflammatory effects, mainly to treat stress-induced anxiety, mood disorders, and pain associated with cancer [144]. An earlier investigation revealed the effect of bergamot EO or linalool on the nociceptive response to formalin and capsaicin. Findings from the effects of bergamot EO on nociceptive effects caused by formalin in rodents suggested the involvement of opioid receptors in peripheral tissue in nocioception caused by EO and linalool. It was also suggested that the stimulation of peripheral opioid receptors could play a significant role in attenuating formalin-induced nociception [144]. Bergamot EO after intraplantar administration considerably reduced capsaicin-induced nociceptive response. It was also found that *Salvia sclarea* EO, thyme EO, Lavandula hybrid EO, and *Lavandula angustifolia* EO showed the same antinociceptive activity against nociceptive effects caused by capsaicin. Bergamot EOs contain volatile compounds (monoterpenes), including β-pinene, limonene, γ-terpinene, and oxygenated terpenes, such as linalyl acetate and linalool. It was also reported that after intraperitoneal administration of linalool antihyperalgesic as well as antinociceptive properties were seen [145]. Additionally, the inhalation of linalool-enriched EOs has been reported for their relaxation effects and ability to reduce anxiety [146].

18.7.13 Coriander Volatile Oil

It has been indicated that *Coriander sativum* EO inhalation augmented antidepressant as well as anxiolytic effects and reduced oxidative stress in β-amyloid induced Alzheimer's in experimental animals. Additionally, *Coriander sativum* EO treatment also reduced the catalase level and augmented the glutathione activity in the hippocampus [30]. Chemical analysis of EO revealed that linalool was determined to be the main component of EO along with other constituents such as α-pinene and γ-terpinene [30]. It was also suggested that linalool could be the likely cause for anxiolytic- and antidepressant-like effects. Another report confirmed these findings that the inhalation of linalool-rich EOs can be utilized to reduce anxiety [30].

18.7.14 *Croton conduplicatus*

Croton conduplicatus EO treatment of experimental animals showed considerable antinociceptive effects. Also, pretreatment of *Croton conduplicatus* EO in combination with atropine/naloxone hydrochloride changed the antinociception, which suggests the association of opioid and muscarinic receptors. The authors also reported the presence of the main chemical compounds in EO [eucalyptol, cymene, and bicyclic sesquiterpenes (caryophyllene oxide), tricyclic sesquiterpene compound (spathulenol)]. Molecular docking findings showed the positive interaction of major components with various M (2, 3, 4) muscarinic receptors and opioids receptors (δ and μ). Sedative anxiolytic effects in mice shown by EO were reversed by flumazenil, which suggests the likely involvement of GABAA receptors [147]. In this study, the authors concluded that *Croton conduplicatus* EO is a multi-target plant-based product that can be used as natural analgesic with promising dose-dependent pharmacological effects such as antinociceptive effect, anxiolytic, and sedative [147]. A recent report showed the neuropharmacological effects of Croton EO in treating anxiety, pain, and sleeping disorder. It was found that *Croton conduplicatus* EO showed considerable antinociceptive effects in all experimental models. During this study, antinociceptive effects were reversed with the pretreatment of atropine or naloxone demonstrating that the antinociceptive effects of EO were mediated by muscarinic as well as opioid receptors. Further molecular modeling studies revealed the possible interaction between EO components (eucalyptol, spathulenol, p-cymene, and caryophyllene oxide) with opioids and muscarinic receptors. Anxiolytic and sedative properties of EO in mice were also reported [147]. It was also observed that the treatment with flumazenil reversed the pharmacological activities of EO, suggesting the likely involvement of GABAA receptors. The authors also concluded that EO can be used as a natural way to relieve pain and proposed that EO as multitarget plant-based product, demonstrating dose-dependent antinociceptive, anxiolytic, and sedative effects [147].

18.7.15 *Cymbopogon citratus*

Cymbopogon citratus EOs have been reported for an array of pharmacological activities mainly for treating various neurological disturbances. Citral, geranial and neral, or β-myrcene T were identified as the main constituents. In 2011, the authors reported anxiolytic-like effects of the EO, and it was found that these responses were changed by benzodiazepine antagonist (i.e., flumazenil). These reported findings suggested that an anxiolytic-like effect of the EO was mediated via the GABA(A) receptor–benzodiazepine complex. Further, simultaneous treatment of ineffective doses of diazepam with EO enhanced duration passed inside the light chamber, showing its synergistic effect [31]. One more report demonstrated that this *Cymbopogon citratus* EO contains geraniol and citronellol as the major compounds and *Cymbopogon winterianus* EO is considered as a major source for citronellal. It was found that both EOs showed anticonvulsant effects via attenuating strychnine-induced convulsion and pilocarpine-induced convulsion. Further, *C. citratus* was found to be more efficient in potentiating barbiturate-induced sleeping time. Both EOs have myeloperoxidase release from human neutrophils, whereas they didn't show any effect on DPPH. The authors concluded that the antioxidant effects of EOs haven't contributed to anticonvulsant effect of the EOs, which was mediated by GABAergic pathways and their suppressive effect on inflammatory biomarkers [32]. Another report showed that *Cymbopogon citratus* EO enhanced the duration of sleeping, the number of submissions, as well as the period passed in the open arms of the EPM test and amount of time spent in the light section of light/dark box. Moreover, *Cymbopogon citratus*

EO postponed clonic seizures and inhibited tonic extensions, representing increases in seizure threshold. Thus, the authors demonstrated anxiolytic, sedative, or anticonvulsive effects of *Cymbopogon citratus* in this study [148]. One more report showed that *Cymbopogon citratus* leaf EO contains citral as a major compound that is then derived from culm. It was found that *Cymbopogon citratus* leaf EO showed significant effects on lung cancer cell lines. Additionally, it was observed that Kim Duc culm EO possessed high cytotoxic activity against H1650 cells. Further, *Cymbopogon citratus* leaf EO-induced apoptosis and cycle arrest in A549 cells, which was mediated by caspase-3, Bcl-2, and Bax [149]. Further, an antinociceptive effect of *Cymbopogon citratus* was evidenced in the rodent model based on CNS activity [149].

18.7.16 *Dennettia tripetala*

In 2013, the anxiolytic, antiepileptic, and hypnotic activities of aromatic nitro compound (1-nitro-2-phenylethane) derived from the *Dennettia tripetala* EO along with their mechanisms of action were investigated. The compound 1-nitro-2-phenylethane, the main constituent of *Aniba canelilla*, is the main nitro-based aromatic component derived from plants and is supposed to be responsible for the plant's cinnamon aroma [12]. Further, EO showed concentration-dependent protection against PTZ- and strychnine-induced convulsions, and flumazenil inhibited the hypnotic and anticonvulsant activities of EO and 1-nitro-2-phenylethane. It was concluded that this aromatic nitro compound exhibited a concentration-dependent considerable anxiolytic, antiepileptic, and hypnotic activities and 1-nitro-2-phenylethane is mainly responsible for these effects [59].

18.7.17 *Dysphania graveolens*

Dysphania graveolens is known for its various biological effects mainly to treat various gastric complications. *D. graveolens* EO has been reported for antinociceptive effects in a mouse model.

18.7.18 *Eugenia uniflora*

In 2013, various researchers have investigated the antidepressant-like effect of *E. uniflora* EO using the tail suspension test via the involvement of serotoninergic and adrenergic systems. One study revealed that the oral administration of *E. uniflora* in mice showed an antidepressant-like effect, whereas these effects were inhibited after the pretreatment of mice with prazosin, ketanserin, and yohimbine. The authors also revealed the potential antioxidant activity of EO [150].

18.7.19 *German chamomile*

Bisabolol, a sesquiterpene, is derived from various EO-producing plants such as *German chamomile.* A recent report revealed the anxiolytic-like effects of bisabolol, mainly behavioral effects by using EPM, open-field, and rotarod tasks. It was demonstrated that bisabolol could mediate anxiolytic-like and sedative effects via involving GABAA receptors [151].

18.7.20 *Hyptis martiusii*

A recent study showed *Hyptis martiusii* EO containing 1,8-cineole demonstrated CNS activity. Findings obtained from open-field test showed that the treatment of animals with *Hyptis martiusii* EO and 1,8-cineole decreased animal motility. Also, this treatment enhanced sleeping duration induced by ethyl ether and pentobarbital. Furthermore this treatment also enhanced death latency of animals pre-treated with pentylenetetrazole. Nevertheless, the authors also reported that *Hyptis martiusii* EO and 1,8-cineole didn't show anxiolytic-like and myorelaxant effects [152]. Moreover, *Hyptis martiusii* EO and 1,8-cineole increased catalepsy caused by haloperidol and decreased hyperkinesia caused by ketamine. Thus, it was concluded by the authors that the treatment with *Hyptis martiusii* EO showed hypnotic–sedative and antipsychotic-like effects due to the presence of its major compound 1,8-cineole [152]. A previous report also demonstrated that *Hyptis mutabilis* EO and its chemical components [(+)-1-terpinen-4-ol and (–)-globulol] showed anesthetic and sedative properties in silver catfish. It was found that both the EO and the chemical components displayed dose-dependent sedative and anesthetic effects [153].

18.7.21 *Juniperus virginiana*

Juniperus virginiana EO is widely known for its relaxing effects over the mind and providing comfort; however, less research is available on its anxiolytic effect in animal models. A recent investigation showed that *Juniperus virginiana* EOs contain (–)-α-cedrene, (+)-β-cedrene, (–)-thujopsene, and (+)-cedrol. It was observed that among these chemical compounds, cedrol has the capability to reduce anxiety in light/dark box and elevated plus maze tests. After the treatment of mice with *Juniperus virginiana* EO, cedrol showed an increase in locomotor activity. Also, it was found that *Juniperus virginiana* EO treatment augmented the 5-hydroxytryptamine level. In addition, it also altered the ratio of 5-hydroxyindoleacetic acid to 5-hydroxytryptamine as well as 3, 4-dihydroxyphenyl acetic acid/dopamine. Thus, it was concluded that *Juniperus virginiana* EO and cedrol possibly showed anxiolytic activity via 5-HTnergic and DAnergic pathways [154].

18.7.22 *Lantana camara*

A recent report demonstrated the sedative effects of monoterpene-enriched *Lantana camara* EO in mice by the administration through the inhalation route. It was found that the chemical profile of EO is dominated by sabinene and 1,8-cineole. Treatment of mice with *Lantana camara* EO mice considerably attenuated the locomotor activity in a dose-dependent manner [155]. The authors concluded that *Lantana camara* EO as well as sabinene and 1,8-cineole might be used as possible candidates for the treatment of dementia, insomnia, attention deficit hyperactivity disorder, and other CNS-associated diseases [155].

18.7.23 Lavender-Based Perfumes and EOs

Likewise, the inhalation of perfume and EOs, which are made up of a blend of several EOs, mainly lavender, affected GABAA receptors expressed in *Xenopus* oocytes [40]. Chemical analysis showed that perfume contains hinokitiol, pinene, eugenol, citronellol, and citronellals which possibly potentiated the GABAA receptor expression in *Xenopus* oocytes [40].

18.7.24 *Lippia alba* (False-Melissa)

Lippia alba is known for its sedative effects in some experimental animal models [36,156]. Citral, carvone, and linalool have been identified as constituents of *L. alba* EO [36,156]. An earlier report indicated anesthetic properties of *Lippia alba* EO via the involvement of GABAergic pathway in silver catfish. It has been suggested that *L. alba* EO can be used as an antistress agent in fish to decrease commercial losses in fish culture [36,156]. Additionally, *L. alba* EO repeated treatment showed anxiolytic activity in elevated T-maze mouse model [36,156].

18.7.25 *Melissa officinalis*

In 2008, the antiagitation effects of *Melissa officinalis* EO focusing on ligand-gated channels were demonstrated, and it was revealed that *Melissa officinalis* EO inhibited the binding of GABA receptor antagonist, [35S] t-butylbicyclophosp horothionate, to the gamma-aminobutyric acid (A) receptor channel in the rat forebrain. Further measurements of voltage changes or electric current in primary cultures of rat cortical neurons showed that *Melissa officinalis* EO reversibly suppressed GABA-induced currents [38]. It was also reported that *Melissa officinalis* EO increased substantial concentration-dependent decrease in both inhibitory (inhibits the generation of an electrical signal) and excitatory transmission (promotes the generation of an electrical signal), with an overall depressant effect on neurotransmission. Thus, the authors concluded depressant as well as antiagitation effects of *Melissa officinalis* EO in *in vitro* [38].

18.7.26 *Nigella sativa*

Nigella sativa seed EO containing thymoquinone, α-pinene, and p-cymene showed antiepileptic effects in PTZ and maximal electroshock-induced convulsion animal models [117]. *Nigella sativa* seed EO protected experimental animal efficiently against PTZ-induced convulsions, which could be due to the presence of thymoquinone and p-cymene. Additionally, EO constituent p-cymene efficiently reduced convulsions induced by MES. The authors concluded that these protective effects were probably due to the involvement of opioid receptor to further upsurge GABAergic tone. Further, thymoquinone, the main chemical compound derived from *Nigella sativa* seeds EO, showed anticonvulsant effects in the PTZ-induced seizure experimental animal model [157]. These effects were possibly due to the opioid receptor-facilitated GABAergic transmission. It was also found that an antianxiety effect of thymoquinone was due to the involvement of GABAergic and nitrergic pathways [157]. Treatment with thymoquinone has been reported for its efficacy in reducing anxiety with a substantial reduction in nitrite level in plasma and the restored reduced GABA content in the brain of stressed mice [157].

18.7.27 *O. basilicum*

Monoterpene-enriched *O. basilicum* EO (OBEO) has limitations such as short half-life and water insolubility due to which most of the biological applications are not being explored. Nascimento et al. [12] used β-cyclodextrin to improve the biological potential (mainly antihyperalgesic activity) of OBEO in an animal model for fibromyalgia. Since the EOs attained volatility at room temperature and easily oxidized in the presence of oxygen it's important to encapsulate EO by using a non-toxic, bridgeable, inert carrier. Due to its easy recovery, economical production, capability to form polar civility to encapsulate molecules of interest and low solubility, protect molecules against external unfavorable conditions and decrease the volatility of the molecules entrapped, β-cyclodextrin has been considered as a suitable delivery agent. It has been revealed that OBEO was encapsulated by β-CD and forms a stable complex with reduced volatality. The authors reported that the oral administration of mice with OBEO or OBEO-Bcd (at all tested doses) resulted in considerable decrease in mechanical hyperalgesia and also considerably improved Fos protein expression. Thus, the authors concluded that OBEO alone as well as in complex form (with β-CD) offers analgesic property in an animal model for fibromyalgia [12].

18.7.28 *P. guineense*

P. guineense has been used traditionally as anticonvulsant in African traditional medicine [3]. It was found that *P. guineense* EO inhalation showed considerable sedative and anxiolytic properties. Due to these effects, *P. guineense* EO can be used as a tranquilizer. Further chemical analysis revealed that EOs contain linalool and 3,5-dimethoxytoluene as the main constituents, which can contribute to their sedative effects [3]. Additionally, the sedative property was partially mediated by GABAergic pathway [3].

18.7.29 *Pelargonium roseum*

A recent study demonstrated that *Pelargonium roseum* EO showed antidepressant and anxiolytic properties in male rodents by EPM, FST, and open-field tests. GC-MS studies revealed that *P. roseum* EOs contain citronellol and geraniol (18.5%) as major compounds. Pretreatment of male Swiss albino mice with *P. roseum* EO reversed the anxiolytic effects of the EO, suggesting that its activity is mediated via the serotonergic transmission [158].

18.7.30 Peppermint (*Mentha piperita*)

Based on various reports, the available roles of EOs in modulating mood and cognitive behaviors in humans are possibly linked to their overall effects on cholinergic and GABAergic neurotransmission. Recently, *Mentha spicata* (spearmint) and *Mentha piperita* (peppermint) EOs were investigated for their cognitive and mood effects. This study revealed that EOs at highest dose ameliorated response on the cognitively demanding rapid visual information processing task as well as reduced fatigue. The authors also concluded that peppermint EO enriched with menthol/menthone improved performance on demanding cognitive tasks and reduced mental fatigue in healthy adults. Previous reports also suggested *in vitro* cholinergic inhibitory, calcium regulatory, and GABAA/nicotinic receptor binding properties of peppermint EO [159]. Earlier reports demonstrated that *Salvia officinalis* and *Salvia lavandulaefolia* can be used as memory-enhancing agents coupled with cholinergic activities, which could be associated with the improvement of the cognitive deficits linked with Alzheimer's disease. It was reported that *S. lavandulaefolia* EO (with cholinesterase–inhibiting activity) is efficient in modulating cognition and mood performance of adults [160]. As per this study, oral administration of *S. lavandulaefolia* resulted in the improvement of performance of secondary memory, attention tasks, and attenuated mental fatigue as well as ameliorated alertness in healthy participants. *Salvia* is capable of acute modulation of mood and cognition in healthy young adults.

18.7.31 *Piper guineense*

Tankam and Ito [3] demonstrated mild tranquilizing effect of *Piper guineense* EO inhalation. The authors reported that *P. guineense* EO demonstrated noticeable sedative and anxiolytic effects. Also, it was found that sedative activity might be due to the presence of the major compounds, linalool and 3,5-dimethoxytoluene.

18.7.32 *Pistacia integerrima*

Pistacia integerrima is widely known for its sedative and spasmolytic effects. *Pistacia integerrima* displayed antispasmodic and myorelaxant effects, which were possibly facilitated via Ca^{+2} channels and β-adrenergic receptors [41].

18.7.33 *Salvia sclarea* (clary)

There are various EOs such as *Anthemis nobilis, Lavandula angustifolia, Rosa damascene, Rosmarinus officinalis,* and *Salvia sclarea* known for their anxiolytic effects [42]. These EOs have been used for decades in the form of herbal tea preparations to relieve depressive effects and cause mild sedation. By means of FST in rats, the antidepressant activity of these EOs was investigated, and it was found that clary oil showed a significant antistressor effect [42]. These effects might be due to the modulation of the dopaminergic system [42].

18.7.34 *Spiranthera odoratissima*

In 2013, an anxiolytic-like effect of *Spiranthera odoratissima* EO as well as its main component, β-caryophyllene, was investigated. It was demonstrated that *Spiranthera odoratissima* EO reduced anxiety and this response was mediated by serotonin 1A receptor without changing motor performance. Moreover, beta-caryophyllene has been reported for its efficacy in reducing anxiety [161].

18.7.35 SuHeXiang Wan (Storax pill)

In addition to CNS effects of EO alone, a blend of different EOs in the form of SuHeXiang Wan (Storax pill) has been studied for their possible inhibitory effects on the CNS. SuHeXiang Wan is a Chinese folk medicine that uses aromatherapy with a mixture of 15 crude drugs such as *Aquilaria agallocha, Boswellia carterii, Cyperus rotundus, Dryobalanops aromatica, Eugenia caryophyllata, Liquidambar orientalis, Santalum album, Saussurea lappa*, and *Styrax benzoin*. An earlier report demonstrated the inhibitory effects of the SuHeXiang Wan EO on the CNS via involving the GABAergic system [67]. It was observed that SuHeXiang Wan EO inhalation significantly increased the sleep duration induced by pentobarbital and attenuated lipid peroxidation in brain homogenate [67]. In addition, it was found that anticonvulsant effects could be due to antilipid peroxidation effects exhibited by EO.

18.7.36 *Tugetes minute*

Tugetes minutu EO showed panicogenic substance-like response on behavioral tests (tonic immobility response as well as T-maze) in chickens possibly via modulation of GABAergic system [44].

18.7.37 *Valerian officinalis*

Valerian (*Valerian officinalis* L) EO has been evidenced for its sedative effects [46]. Besides other sesquiterpenes, valerenic acid as well as bornyl acetate were identified as the main components of EOs. In 1966, nonvolatile triesters of a monoterpene alcohol, valepotriates, were isolated. These nonvolatile compounds have been known for their sedative effects on the CNS [46].

18.7.38 Sideritis Flowering Plants

Sideritis flowering plants have been evidenced for their sedative, anxiolytic, and anticonvulsant effects. It was reported that aromatic compounds derived from sideritis tea extracts showed significant modulation of GABAA receptors present at synaptic compartment (including or with no γ2 subunits) [162]. Volatile aromatic compounds such as pinene (isomeric terpenes) derived from Siderites extracts and its metabolites such as verbenol and myrtenol were reported for their efficacy in binding the GABAA receptor of α1β2 and α1β2γ2 subunits at a different (allosteric) binding site [162]. Further, it was suggested that verbenol as well as myrtenol act to bind GABAA receptors present at synaptic as well as extrasynaptic compartments GABAA receptors, thus ameliorating tonic and phasic GABAergic suppression [162].

18.8 Effect of EO Components on CNS

18.8.1 (+)-Limonene and s-Limonene

(+)-Limonene is a chemical compound present in various EOs, mainly isolated from *Citrus aurantifolia* as well as *C. bergamia* EO [57,163]. A recent study showed that the anxiolytic-like effects of *C. aurantium L.* in rodent models could be associated with (+)-limonene. Another report showed that (+)-limonene was also reported for anxiolytic-like effects in mice. s-Limonene is a monoterpenoid chemical compound, isolated from lemon EO. A previous investigation showed an antistress property of s-limonene; this property was mediated via GABAergic receptors [57,163].

18.8.2 (+)-Dehydrofukinone

(+)-Dehydrofukinone, a sesquiterpenoid ketone, is a major chemical component of *Nectandra grandiflora* Ness EO. An earlier study showed sedative and anesthetic effects of dehydrofukinone in fish via modulating GABAergic pathway [55,164]. Similarly, dehydrofukinone caused sedative and anesthetic effects via involving GABAA receptors in a rodent model [55,164]. These findings suggested that (+)-dehydrofukinone has inhibitory effects on neuronal excitability.

18.8.3 1,8-Cineole

1,8-Cineole (eucalyptol), a monoterpenoid found in various aromatic as well as medicinal plants, has diverse therapeutic properties such as antinociceptive, spasmolytic, and ion channel modulator. Moreover, 1,8-cineole inhibited electrical impulses cross a neuron's membrane, thus attenuating the excitability of peripheral nerve cells [50,58,165]. A previous report showed that 1,8-cineole modulates sodium currents of the SCG (superior cervical ganglion) neurons by influencing a number of ion channels that may be the main cause of excitability obstruction [50,58,165]. 1,8-cineole is also known for its ability to decrease the neuronal membrane excitability (via rapidly changing membrane potential) of SCG nerve cells and rat sciatic nerve [50,58,165]. In contrast, one more report demonstrated that 1,8-cineole caused epileptiform discharges on EEG and neuronal hyperexcitability in the nerve cells of snail, possibly facilitated via blocking potassium channels [50,58,165]. Thus, in conclusion, 1,8-cineole showed analgesic effects via modulating Na^+ and TRP channels.

18.8.4 Alpha(α)-Asarone

Alpha(α)-asarone from *Acorus tatarinowii* has been to have anticonvulsant activity in the CNS via stimulating GABAergic suppression. *In vitro* and *in vivo* studies revealed that alpha-asarone can inhibit neuronal excitability in hippocampus of rats (*in vitro*) and showed antiepileptic effects. Further, α-asarone was evidenced for inhibiting the impulsive firing caused by mitral cells (neurons that are part of the olfactory bulb brain) [47,48]. Alpha-asarone relieves convulsions by altering expression of GABAA receptor as well as suppressing voltage-gated sodium channels [47,48]. A previous study showed that α-asarone was considered as a GABA-positive allosteric modulator (i.e., agonist, ccompounds that modulate the expression of the GABAA receptor protein in the CNS) and neuronal voltage-gated Na^+ channel blocker [47,48]. However, other EOs such as borneol were reported to be only positive allosteric GABAA receptor agonist to reduce anxiety.

18.8.5 Bicyclic Ethers 1,8- and 1,4-Cineole

A recent report suggested the anxiolytic and antidepressant-like effects of 1,8-cineole and 1,4-cineole (its structural isomer) in mice via inhalation or administration. The authors found that 1,8-cineole considerably ameliorated duration spent by mice in the light box and the number of entries in the light box in the light–dark box test along with decreased number of marbles buried, revealing its anxiolytic activity [166]. Likewise, 1,8-cineole considerably decreased immobility times in the FST and tail suspension test, revealing its antidepressant effects. It was also demonstrated that 1,8-cineole affects the GABAA/benzodiazepine receptors. The authors concluded that the inhalation of 1,8- and 1,4-cineole reduced anxiety and depressive-like symptoms in experimental animals [166].

18.8.6 Bisabolol

Bisabolol or levomenol, chemically a sesquiterpene alcohol, is mainly derived from *Matricaria chamomilla* [60] and known for various pharmacological properties. Previous investigations showed an antinociceptive-like effect of bisabolol, which might be linked with the reduced peripheral nerve hyperexcitability [60]. The reduced peripheral nerve hyperexcitability caused by levomenol could be due to its irreversible inhibitory action on voltage-gated sodium channels [60].

18.8.7 Carvacrol

Carvacrol is a monoterpenoidal phenolic analgesic compound found in thyme as well as oregano EOs. [167,168]. Gonçalves et al. explored the chemical profile of *Thymus capitatus* EO and assessed its antinociceptive effects [167,168]. It was found that *Thymus capitatus* EO contains a high level of carvacrol. It was also revealed that *Thymus capitatus* EO reduced compound action potential in a concentration manner by mediating voltage-dependent sodium channels [167,168].

18.8.8 Carvacryl Acetate

In 2013, the anxiolytic-like activities of carvacryl acetate were evidenced. It was indicated that carvacryl acetate effectively reduced anxiety, possibly via GABAergic agonist activity [169].

18.8.9 Carvone

Carvone volatile monoterpene isolated from *Carum carvi* as well as *Mentha spicata* EOs showed various neuropharmacological effects, including antiepilepsy [170,171], antinociceptive

[170,171], and anxiolytic-like effects [35]. The effect of enantiomers of carvone [(S)-(+)-carvone and (R)-(–)-carvone] on the CNS was investigated, and it was found that both have a depressant effect on the CNS. Further, (S)-(+)-carvone showed anticonvulsant-like effects against PTZ- and picrotoxin-induced seizures [170,171]. Both enantiomers of carvone reduced the peripheral nerve activity, possibly via the inhibition of voltage-gated Na^+ channels [170,171]. Both enantiomers were reported for their mood-stabilizing effects in an experimental rodent model [170,171]. Further, it was indicated that both enantiomers trigger transient receptor potential vanilloid 1 and ankyrin 1 channels, leading to an enhancement in impulsive release of the L-glutamate [170,171].

18.8.10 Cedrol

Cedrol, the major chemical compound of *Juniperus virginiana* L.EO, has been recently reported to have an anxiolytic effect. Zhang et al. [16] demonstrated that cedrol attenuated the levels of DA and NE in the hippocampus, striatum, and hypothalamus. It was found that rather the involvement of serotoninergic or GABAergic, dopaminergic system (D1 receptor) is involved in the alteration of anxiolytic-like effects induced by cedrol- in rodents.

18.8.11 Methyl Jasmonate/cis-Jasmone

A previous investigation indicated the effect of aromatic compounds present in oolong tea on GABAergic system expressed in *Xenopus oocytes.* It was found that phytochemicals of the EO considerably enhanced the reaction to GABA. Furthermore, the sleeping time of mice induced by pentobarbital was considerably increased after inhalation of methyl jasmonate or cis-jasmone. Findings from this study also suggested that these aromatic compounds can enter the brain to possibly potentiate the GABAergic system and to cause a tranquilizing effect on the brain [26].

18.8.12 Dihydrocarvone and Thujone (Non-Terpene Constituents) as GABAA Receptor Antagonists

The majority of EOs components act by stimulating GABA receptors; however, few EO components have shown antagonistic effects against GABAA receptor. Thujone derived from wormwood oil and other plants [172] showed antagonistic effects specifically against GABAA receptor, resulting in muscle spasms and convulsions [172]. Likewise, dihydrocarvone derived from caraway EO showed a negative allosteric modulator of this GABAA receptor [172].

18.8.13 Estragole

Estragole, a phenylpropene, is found in the *Artemisia dracunculus* EO. Estragole has been reported to have various antioxidant, anxiolytic, and antimicrobial biological properties [34]. The neuronal excitability potential of estragole due to its ability to rapidly change membrane potential was studied in an earlier investigation. Findings from this study showed that the estragole inhibited the excitability of neurons via blocking Na^+ channels conductance activation.

18.8.14 Eugenol

Eugenol (4-allyl-2-methoxyphenol) chemically belongs to a class called phenylpropanoids, and is a main volatile phenolic component of *Syzygium aromaticum* EO, which is known for its analgesic and anesthetic effects [19,43]. A previous report demonstrated the analgesic effects of eugenol, which may be associated with the blockage of Na^+ channels or the stimulation of TRPV1 receptors or both. Another report suggested the inhibitory action of eugenol via modifying electrical stimuli or action potential of neurons [19,43]. Further, it was also suggested that eugenol influences electrical impulses and neurotransmitters via the synergistic blocking effect of Na^+ currents in order to attenuate firing of neuronal action potentials and hyperexcitability [19,43]. Likewise, Vatanparast et al. demonstrated dose-dependent suppressant and excitatory actions of eugenol over the neuronal membrane excitability of snail. It was indicated that eugenol could have antiepileptic effects at low dose, whereas at a high dose, eugenol can cause epileptiform activity. Eugenol showed concentration-dependent inhibition of the Na^+ currents, which could be an underlying cause of the variation in action potential, which is further associated with its suppressant and excitatory effects.

18.8.15 Isopulegol

Isopulegol, a monoterpene alcohol, can be isolated from the EOs of various aromatic plants, including *Eucalyptus citriodora* and *Zanthoxylum schinifolium* [173]. As per a previous report, isopulegol considerably extended the seizure latency and rodent mortality injected with PTZ, a GABA-A receptor antagonist, used to induce convulsion in mice [173]. These findings suggest that antiepileptic property of isopulegol against seizures caused by PTZ could be due to alteration of GABAA receptors sensitive to benzodiazepines [173].

18.8.16 Linalool

EO components of Lavandula genus such as linalyl acetate, eucalyptol, and linalool have been known for their various effects on the CNS. EOs that contain these components such as lavender, lavandin, and bergamot were reported on for their neuropharmacological effects. Linalyl acetate and linalool-enriched EO showed antinociceptive activity; however, these isolated compounds showed more potency than the bergamot EO or other EOs (used in the study) in suppressing the short-lived licking/biting response induced by capsaicin [28,131,141]. Various reports corroborate that the anxiolytic activity of lavender is possibly because of the presence of linalool [28,131,141]. Additionally, one more report demonstrated that the linalool-induced anxiolytic activity in mice is enhanced by linalyl acetate [28,131,141]. Other reports demonstrated the depressant effects of linalool on the CNS and olfactory receptors [28,131,141]. It was found that linalool affects the neuronal excitability of the somatosensory cortex via inhibiting the membrane voltage potential by directly interacting with voltage-gated sodium channels [28,131,141].

18.8.17 Menthol

Menthol derived from *Mentha piperita* has been reported for its analgesic effects via stimulating ion channels such as TRP and melastatin-8 channels [154]. Menthol is known as a transient receptor potential vanilloid 1 (TRPV1) ion channel agonist as at higher dose it prevents action potential conduction in the neurons to induce local anesthetic effect. In 2013, a report showed that menthol-related chemicals such as (–), (+)-menthone, -menthone, (–), (+)–carvone, (+)-pulegone and (+)-carveol inhibited compound action potentials of frog sciatic nerve (by using the air-gap method) in a similar manner as menthol to possess local anesthetic effects. These effects were found to be equivalent to lidocaine and cocaine. It was also found that the activity of the menthol wasn't facilitated via transient receptor potential cation channels [174].

18.8.18 Methyleugenol

Methyleugenol (allylveratrol) is a natural chemical compound belonging to the phenylpropanoid class and derived from the EOs of numerous aromatic plants. Methyleugenol is known for its various anticonvulsant, antinociceptive, and anesthetic neuropharmacological effects. Methyleugenol showed anesthetic effects via disappearance of the labyrinthine head righting reflex as well as reduced response to a pinching of the tail of the rodents as well as the disappearance of the corneal reflex in rabbits [48,175]. It was also found that methyleugenol showed antinociceptive and anesthetic effects via blocking peripheral voltage-gated Na^+ channels [48,175]. Another report suggested that methyleugenol showed antinociceptive activity (during the second phase) against formalin-induced pain in mice, which could be because of the blockage of NMDA receptor-facilitated hyperalgesia by involving GABAAergic signaling. *In vitro* studies revealed that methyleugenol (at low dose) considerably enhanced GABA-stimulated action potential in hippocampal neurons in vitro [48,175]. Also, methyleugenol (at low dose) considerably enhanced GABA-mediated neuronal currents facilitated via recombinant GABAARs ($\alpha1\beta2\gamma2$ or $\alpha5\beta2\gamma2$). Besides the effects of methyleugenol over the inhibition of Na^+ channels [48,175], this report also demonstrated that methyleugenol triggers GABAAR in human embryonic kidney cells [48,175].

18.8.19 Natural Borneol [(+)-Borneol]

(+)-Borneol, a monoterpene found in the EOs of several plants, such as lavandula valerian, and german chamomile, is traditionally utilized for its analgesic and anesthetic effects [54]. A previous report showed that borneol presented antihyperalgesic effects on inflammatory nociceptive as well as neuropathic pain [54]. It was found that (+)-borneol can enhance mechanical hyperalgesia of the cervical spine via ameliorating GABA type A receptor-mediated GABAergic transmission [54]. Another report demonstrated that both enantiomers [(+)-borneol and (–)-borneol] enhance the expression of human recombinant $\alpha1\beta2\gamma2L$ GABAA receptors in *Xenopus laevis* oocytes [53]. Further, it was found that both enantiomers showed high activity in positively modulating action at GABAA receptors [53]. (+)-Borneol showed notable antinociceptive activity during *in vivo* experimental animal models of chronic pain without causing damage to motor skills or movement. The authors concluded that borneol can enhance mechanical hyperalgesia by potentiating spinal GABA type A receptor-mediated GABAergic transmission.

18.8.20 Nerolidol

Nerolidol (synonyms: peruviol, penetrol) is a sesquiterpenoidal component of numerous EOs including *Burchardia umbellata* and *Piper claussenianum* [38]. The antinociceptive effects of nerolidol were evaluated and it was found that nerolidol demonstrated antinociceptive effects in animal models of nociception induced by chemical (formalin as well as acetic acid-induced writhing tests), but not in the nociception animal model using thermal stimuli (hot-plate test) [38]. It has also been found that the pain-relieving activity of nerolidol could be mediated by GABAergic pathway without the involvement of Adenosine triphosphate-sensitive potassium channels or opioidergic pathway [176].

18.8.21 Pine EO

Pine EO contains terpinene, 3-carene, pinenes (both alpha and beta), and limonene [177]. Inhalation of α-pinene has been reported on for its ability to induce anxiolytic and hypnotic effects. Moreover, these effects with sleep-inducing properties were found to be modulated via direct binding to GABAA receptors [177].

18.8.22 Terpinen-4-ol

Terpinen-4-ol is a volatile component mainly isolated from tea tree oil and other aromatic plants. An earlier investigation showed anticonvulsant effects of terpinen-4-ol against seizures caused by PTZ in rodents [178,179]. Further, it was found that terpinen-4-ol demonstrated these effects by involving the GABAergic system [178,179]. Moreover, terpinen-4-ol has been reported on for its potential in inhibiting voltage-gated Na+ channels to further reduce sodium current. Therefore, its antiepileptic activity could be associated with its direct effect on neuronal excitability via involving GABAergic system and Na^+ channels [178,179].

18.8.23 Thymol

Thymol is a phenolic monoterpene isolated from the EO of *Thymus vulgaris*. Thymol is known for its various properties such as antimicrobial, antinociception, and its inhibitory effect over fast nerve conduction [180]. Thymol has been found to trigger cell membrane-embedded ion channels known as TRP in heterologous cells. Also, thymol therapeutically acts as a positive allosteric modulator molecule to enhance human GABAA activity in the CNS as well as homo-oligomeric

GABA receptor from *Drosophila melanogaster* [180]. This study showed GABA-modulating and GABA-mimetic activities of the thymol on human GABAA and *Drosophila melanogaster* homomeric RDLac GABA receptors expressed in *Xenopus laevis* oocytes. As per a previous report, thymol showed an inhibitory effect on glutamatergic transmission in rodent neurons of substantia gelatinosa. This finding suggests that thymol improves the level of L-glutamate in the nerve cells via stimulating transient receptor potential channels (A1) channels without TRP activation [180]. Thus, these effects of thymol on substantia gelatinosa via modulating nociceptive transmission could partially contribute to antinociceptive effects [180].

18.9 Essential Oils Loaded in Nano- and Cyclodextrin-Based Systems

Natural compounds might not be able to enter the brain while circulating in the blood because of the presence of the blood–brain barrier that restricts its entry into the brain and protects it from infections or harmful substances. The barrier inhibits the diffusion of even small molecules into the brain [181–206]. The inability of phytochemicals to cross the blood–brain barrier represents the requirement for developing NP-based strategies targeted toward drug delivery. Volatile chemical compounds present in EOs offer a wide range of biological activities. Developing nanoformulations of these EOs can increase bioavailability and enhance their ability to target the CNS from the bloodstream (geraniol with 2% (w/w) of chitosan oleate). Furthermore, nanoformulations can also increase the availability of these chemicals in the CNS following nasal administration at low doses [181–239]. Apart from the considerable pharmacological effects attributed to EO, water insolubility is one of the major constraints to the use of the majority of EOs for pharmacological applications. Recently, it was found that the preparation formed by encapsulating EOs as well as its components in cyclodextrin especially beta-cyclodextrin (cyclodextrin-complexed *Ocimum basilicum* EO) prevents volatility and improves biological activity, overall stability, and water solubility and enhances bioavailability [12,207–239].

REFERENCES

1. Herrera DG, Robertson HA. Activation of c-fos in the brain. *Prog Neurobiol.* 1996;50(2–3):83–107.
2. Lee YL, Wu Y, Tsang HW, Leung AY, Cheung WM. A systematic review on the anxiolytic effects of aromatherapy in people with anxiety symptoms. *J Altern Complement Med.* 2011;17(2):101–108.
3. Tankam JM, Ito M. Inhalation of the essential oil of *Piper guineense* from Cameroon shows sedative and anxiolytic-like effects in mice. *Biol Pharm Bull.* 2013;36(10): 1608–1614.
4. Liu Y, Lieberwirth C, Jia X, Curtis JT, Meredith M, Wang ZX. Chemosensory cues affect amygdaloid neurogenesis and alter behaviors in the socially monogamous prairie vole. *Eur J Neurosci.* 2014;39(10):1632–1641.
5. McCabe C, Rolls ET. Umami: A delicious flavor formed by convergence of taste and olfactory pathways in the human brain. *Eur J Neurosci.* 2007;25(6):1855–1864.
6. Mannucci C, Navarra M, Calapai F, Squeri R, Gangemi S, Calapai G. Clinical pharmacology of citrus bergamia: A systematic review. *Phytother Res.* 2017;31(1):27–39.
7. Kianpour M, Mansouri A, Mehrabi T, Asghari G. Effect of lavender scent inhalation on prevention of stress, anxiety and depression in the postpartum period. *Iran J Nurs Midwifery Res.* 2016;21(2):197–201.
8. Umezu T. Evaluation of the effects of plant-derived essential oils on central nervous system function using discrete shuttle-type conditioned avoidance response in mice. *Phytother Res.* 2012;26(6):884–891.
9. Laudanna A, Nogueira MI, Mariano M. Expression of Fos protein in the rat central nervous system in response to noxious stimulation: Effects of chronic inflammation of the superior cervical ganglion. *Braz J Med Biol Res.* 1998;31(6):847–850.
10. Davis WM, Hatoum HT. Comparison of stimulants and hallucinogens on shuttle avoidance in rats. *Gen Pharmacol.* 1987;18(2):123–128.
11. Koofreh GD, Christopher EOG, Atim A, et al. Locomotor and exploratory behaviour in mice treated with oral artesunate. *Br J Sci.* 2013;8:43–57.
12. Nascimento SS, Araújo AA, Brito RG, et al. Cyclodextrin-complexed *Ocimum basilicum* leaves essential oil increases Fos protein expression in the central nervous system and produce an antihyperalgesic effect in animal models for fibromyalgia. *Int J Mol Sci.* 2014;16(1):547–563.
13. Ghorbani A, Rakhshandeh H, Sadeghnia HR. Potentiating effects of *Lactuca sativa* on pentobarbital-induced sleep. *Iran J Pharm Res.* 2013;12(2):401–406.
14. Nishchal BS, Rai S, Prabhu MN, Ullal SD, Rajeswari S, Gopalakrishna HN. Effect of *Tribulus terrestris* on haloperidol-induced catalepsy in mice. *Indian J Pharm Sci.* 2014;76(6):564–567.
15. Irifune M, Shimizu T, Nomoto M. Ketamine-induced hyperlocomotion associated with alteration of presynaptic components of dopamine neurons in the nucleus accumbens of mice. *Pharmacol Biochem Behav.* 1991;40(2):399–407.
16. Zhang K, Lu J, Yao L. Involvement of the dopamine D1 receptor system in the anxiolytic effect of cedrol in the elevated plus maze and light-dark box tests. *J Pharmacol Sci.* 2020;142(1):26–33.
17. Majnooni MB, Mohammadi-Farani A, Gholivand MB, Nikbakht MR, Bahrami GR. Chemical composition and anxiolytic evaluation of Achillea Wilhelmsii C. Koch essential oil in rat. *Res Pharm Sci.* 2013;8(4):269–275.
18. Koo BS, Park KS, Ha JH, Park JH, Lim JC, Lee DU. Inhibitory effects of the fragrance inhalation of essential oil from *Acorus gramineus* on central nervous system. *Biol Pharm Bull.* 2003;26(7):978–982.
19. Moreira-Lobo DC, Linhares-Siqueira ED, Cruz GM, Cruz JS, Carvalho-de-Souza JL, Lahlou S, Coelho-de-Souza AN, Barbosa R, Magalhães PJ, Leal-Cardoso JH. Eugenol modifies the excitability of rat sciatic nerve and superior cervical ganglion neurons. *Neurosci Lett.* 2010;472(3):220–224.
20. Abuhamdah S, Abuhamdah R, Howes MJ, Al-Olimat S, Ennaceur A, Chazot PL. Pharmacological and neuroprotective profile of an essential oil derived from leaves of *Aloysia citrodora* Palau. *J Pharm Pharmacol.* 2015;67(9):1306–1315.

21. Abu-Darwish MS, Cabral C, Gonçalves MJ, Cavaleiro C, Cruz MT, Efferth T, Salgueiro L. Artemisia herba-alba essential oil from Buseirah (South Jordan): Chemical characterization and assessment of safe antifungal and anti-inflammatory doses. *J Ethnopharmacol.* 2015;174:153–160.
22. Anaya-Eugenio GD, Rivero-Cruz I, Bye R, Linares E, Mata R. Antinociceptive activity of the essential oil from *Artemisia ludoviciana. J Ethnopharmacol.* 2016;179:403–411.
23. Abu-Darwish MS, Cabral C, Gonçalves MJ, Cavaleiro C, Cruz MT, Zulfiqar A, Khan IA, Efferth T, Salgueiro L. Chemical composition and biological activities of *Artemisia judaica* essential oil from southern desert of Jordan. *J Ethnopharmacol.* 2016;191:161–168.
24. Maham M, Moslemzadeh H, Jalilzadeh-Amin G. Antinociceptive effect of the essential oil of tarragon (*Artemisia dracunculus*). *Pharm Biol.* 2014;52(2):208–212.
25. Park HJ, Lim EJ, Zhao RJ, Oh SR, Jung JW, Ahn EM, Lee ES, Koo JS, Kim HY, Chang S, Shim HS, Kim KJ, Gwak YS, Yang CH. Effect of the fragrance inhalation of essential oil from *Asarum heterotropoides* on depression-like behaviors in mice. *BMC Complement Altern Med.* 2015;15:43.
26. Hossain SJ, Aoshima H, Koda H, Kiso Y. Fragrances in oolong tea that enhance the response of GABAA receptors. *Biosci Biotechnol Biochem.* 2004;68(9):1842–1848.
27. Costa CA, Cury TC, Cassettari BO, Takahira RK, Flório JC, Costa M. *Citrus aurantium* L. essential oil exhibits anxiolytic-like activity mediated by 5-HT(1A)-receptors and reduces cholesterol after repeated oral treatment. *BMC Complement Altern Med.* 2013;13:42.
28. Bagetta G, Morrone LA, Rombolà L, Amantea D, Russo R, Berliocchi L, Sakurada S, Sakurada T, Rotiroti D, Corasaniti MT. Neuropharmacology of the essential oil of bergamot. *Fitoterapia.* 2010;81(6):453–461.
29. Faturi CB, Leite JR, Alves PB, Canton AC, Teixeira-Silva F. Anxiolytic-like effect of sweet orange aroma in Wistar rats. *Prog Neuropsychopharmacol Biol Psychiatry.* 2010;34(4):605–609.
30. Cioanca O, Hritcu L, Mihasan M, Trifan A, Hancianu M. Inhalation of coriander volatile oil increased anxiolytic-antidepressant-like behaviors and decreased oxidative status in beta-amyloid (1–42) rat model of Alzheimer's disease. *Physiol Behav.* 2014;131:68–74.
31. Costa CA, Kohn DO, de Lima VM, Gargano AC, Flório JC, Costa M. The GABAergic system contributes to the anxiolytic-like effect of essential oil from *Cymbopogon citratus* (lemongrass). *J Ethnopharmacol.* 2011;137(1):828–836.
32. Silva MR, Ximenes RM, da Costa JG, Leal LK, de Lopes AA, Viana GS. Comparative anticonvulsant activities of the essential oils (EOs) from Cymbopogon winterianus Jowitt and Cymbopogon citratus (DC) Stapf. in mice. *Naunyn Schmiedebergs Arch Pharmacol.* 2010;381(5):415–426.
33. Déciga-Campos M, Mata R, Rivero-Cruz I. Antinociceptive pharmacological profile of *Dysphania graveolens* in mouse. *Biomed Pharmacother.* 2017;89:933–938.
34. Silva-Alves KS, Ferreira-da-Silva FW, Peixoto-Neves D, Viana-Cardoso KV, Moreira-Júnior L, Oquendo MB, Oliveira-Abreu K, Albuquerque AA, Coelho-de-Souza AN, Leal-Cardoso JH. Estragole blocks neuronal excitability by direct inhibition of Na^+ channels. *Braz J Med Biol Res.* 2013;46(12):1056–1063.
35. Chioca LR, Antunes VD, Ferro MM, Losso EM, Andreatini R. Anosmia does not impair the anxiolytic-like effect of lavender essential oil inhalation in mice. *Life Sci.* 2013;92(20–21):971–975.
36. Heldwein CG, Silva LL, Reckziegel P, Barros FM, Bürger ME, Baldisserotto B, Mallmann CA, Schmidt D, Caron BO, Heinzmann BM. Participation of the GABAergic system in the anesthetic effect of *Lippia alba* (Mill.) N.E. Brown essential oil. *Braz J Med Biol Res.* 2012;45(5):436–443.
37. Komiya M, Takeuchi T, Harada E. Lemon oil vapor causes an anti-stress effect via modulating the 5-HT and DA activities in mice. *Behav Brain Res.* 2006;172:240–249.
38. Abuhamdah S, Huang L, Elliott MS, Howes MJ, Ballard C, Holmes C, Burns A, Perry EK, Francis PT, Lees G, Chazot PL. Pharmacological profile of an essential oil derived from Melissa officinalis with anti-agitation properties: Focus on ligand-gated channels. *J Pharm Pharmacol.* 2008;60(3):377–384.
39. Raza M, Alghasham AA, Alorainy MS, El-Hadiyah TM. Potentiation of valproate-induced anticonvulsant response by *Nigella sativa* seed constituents: The role of GABA receptors. *Int J Health Sci (Qassim).* 2008;2(1):15–25.
40. Aoshima H, Hamamoto K. Potentiation of GABAA receptors expressed in *Xenopus oocytes* by perfume and phytoncid. *Biosci Biotechnol Biochem.* 1999;63:743–748.
41. Shirole RL, Shirole NL, Saraf MN. In vitro relaxant and spasmolytic effects of essential oil of *Pistacia integerrima* Stewart ex Brandis Galls. *J Ethnopharmacol.* 2015;168:61–65.
42. Seol GH, Shim HS, Kim PJ, Moon HK, Lee KH, Shim I, Suh SH, Min SS. Antidepressant-like effect of *Salvia sclarea* is explained by modulation of dopamine activities in rats. *J Ethnopharmacol.* 2010;130(1):187–190.
43. Huang CW, Chow JC, Tsai JJ, Wu SN. Characterizing the effects of Eugenol on neuronal ionic currents and hyperexcitability. *Psychopharmacology (Berl).* 2012;221(4):575–587.
44. Marin RH, Garcia DA, Martijena ID, Zygadlo JA, Arce A, Perillo MA. Anxiogenic-like effects of *Tagetes minuta* L essential oil on T-maze and tonic immobility behaviour in domestic chicks. *Fundam Clin Pharmacol.* 1998;12(4):426–432.
45. Gonçalves JC, de Meneses DA, de Vasconcelos AP, Piauilino CA, Almeida FR, Napoli EM, Ruberto G, de Araújo DA. Essential oil composition and antinociceptive activity of *Thymus capitatus. Pharm Biol.* 2017;55(1):782–786.
46. Houghton PJ. The scientific basis for the reputed activity of Valerian. *J Pharm Pharmacol.* 1999;51(5):505–512.
47. Wang ZJ, Levinson SR, Sun L, Heinbockel T. Identification of both GABAA receptors and voltage-activated Na(+) channels as molecular targets of anticonvulsant α-asarone. *Front Pharmacol.* 2014;5:40.
48. Wang ZJ, Tabakoff B, Levinson SR, Heinbockel T. Inhibition of Nav1.7 channels by methyl eugenol as a mechanism underlying its antinociceptive and anesthetic actions. *Acta Pharmacol Sin.* 2015;36(7):791–799.
49. Elliott AA, Elliott JR. Characterization of TTX-sensitive and TTX-resistant sodium currents in small cells from adult rat dorsal root ganglia. *J Physiol.* 1993;463:39–56.
50. Zeraatpisheh Z, Vatanparast J. Eucalyptol induces hyperexcitability and epileptiform activity in snail neurons by inhibiting potassium channels. *Eur J Pharmacol.* 2015;764:70–78.

51. Arruda-Barbosa L, Rodrigues KM, Souza-Neto Fd, Duarte GP, Borges RS, Magalhães PJ, Lahlou S. Vasorelaxant effects of 1-nitro-2-phenylethene in rat isolated aortic rings. *Vascul Pharmacol.* 2014;63(2):55–62.
52. Interaminense Lde F, dos Ramos-Alves FE, de Siqueira RJ, Xavier FE, Duarte GP, Magalhães PJ, Maia JG, Sousa PJ, Lahlou S. Vasorelaxant effects of 1-nitro-2-phenylethane, the main constituent of the essential oil of *Aniba canelilla*, in superior mesenteric arteries from spontaneously hypertensive rats. *Eur J Pharm Sci.* 2013;48(4–5):709–716.
53. Granger RE, Campbell EL, Johnston GA. (+)- and (−)-borneol: Efficacious positive modulators of GABA action at human recombinant alpha1beta2gamma2L GABA(A) receptors. *Biochem Pharmacol.* 2005;69(7):1101–1111.
54. Jiang J, Shen YY, Li J, Lin YH, Luo CX, Zhu DY. (+)-Borneol alleviates mechanical hyperalgesia in models of chronic inflammatory and neuropathic pain in mice. *Eur J Pharmacol.* 2015;757:53–58.
55. Garlet QI, Pires LC, Silva DT, Spall S, Gressler LT, Bürger ME, Baldisserotto B, Heinzmann BM. Effect of (+)-dehydrofukinone on GABAA receptors and stress response in fish model. *Braz J Med Biol Res.* 2016;49(1):e4872.
56. Lima NG, De Sousa DP, Pimenta FC, Alves MF, De Souza FS, Macedo RO, Cardoso RB, de Morais LC, Melo Diniz Mde F, de Almeida RN. Anxiolytic-like activity and GC-MS analysis of (R)-(+)-limonene fragrance, a natural compound found in foods and plants. *Pharmacol Biochem Behav.* 2013;103(3):450–454.
57. Zhou W, Yoshioka M, Yokogoshi H. Sub-chronic effects of s-limonene on brain neurotransmitter levels and behavior of rats. *J Nutr Sci Vitaminol (Tokyo).* 2009;55(4):367–373.
58. Ferreira-da-Silva FW, da Silva-Alves KS, Alves-Fernandes TA, Coelho-de-Souza AN, Leal-Cardoso JH. Effects of 1,8-cineole on Na(+) currents of dissociated superior cervical ganglia neurons. *Neurosci Lett.* 2015;595:45–49.
59. Oyemitan IA, Elusiyan CA, Akanmu MA, Olugbade TA. Hypnotic, anticonvulsant and anxiolytic effects of 1-nitro-2-phenylethane isolated from the essential oil of *Dennettia tripetala* in mice. *Phytomedicine.* 2013;20(14): 1315–1322.
60. Alves Ade M, Gonçalves JC, Cruz JS, Araújo DA. Evaluation of the sesquiterpene (−)-alpha-bisabolol as a novel peripheral nervous blocker. *Neurosci Lett.* 2010;472(1):11–15.
61. Huang C, Li WG, Zhang XB, Wang L, Xu TL, Wu D, Li Y. α-asarone from *Acorus gramineus* alleviates epilepsy by modulating A-type GABA receptors. *Neuropharmacology.* 2013;65:1–11.
62. Chioca LR, Ferro MM, Baretta IP, Oliveira SM, Silva CR, Ferreira J, Losso EM, Andreatini R. Anxiolytic-like effect of lavender essential oil inhalation in mice: Participation of serotonergic but not GABAA/benzodiazepine neurotransmission. *J Ethnopharmacol.* 2013;147(2):412–418.
63. Park Y, Jung SM, Yoo SA, Kim WU, Cho CS, Park BJ, Woo JM, Yoon CH. Antinociceptive and anti-inflammatory effects of essential oil extracted from *Chamaecyparis obtusa* in mice. *Int Immunopharmacol.* 2015;29(2): 320–325.
64. Zhong Y, Zheng Q, Hu P, et al. Sedative and hypnotic effects of compound Anshen essential oil inhalation for insomnia. *BMC Complement Altern Med.* 2019;19(1):306.
65. Barocelli E, Calcina F, Chiavarini M, et al. Antinociceptive and gastroprotective effects of inhaled and orally administered Lavandula hybrida Reverchon "Grosso" essential oil. *Life Sci.* 2004;76(2):213–223.
66. Moeini M, Khadibi M, Bekhradi R, Mohmoudian SA, Nazari F. Effect of aromatherapy on the quality of sleep in ischemic heart disease patients hospitalized in intensive care units of heart hospitals of the Isfahan University of Medical Sciences. *Iran J Nurs Midwifery Res.* 2010;15(4):234–239.
67. Koo BS, Lee SI, Ha JH, Lee DU. Inhibitory effects of the essential oil from SuHeXiang Wan on the central nervous system after inhalation. *Biol Pharm Bull.* 2004;27(4):515–519.
68. Yamada K, Mimaki Y, Sashida Y. Anticonvulsive effects of inhaling lavender oil vapour. *Biol Pharm Bull.* 1994;17(2):359–360.
69. Boiangiu RS, Brinza I, Hancianu M, et al. Cognitive facilitation and antioxidant effects of an essential oil mix on scopolamine-induced amnesia in rats: Molecular modeling of in vitro and in vivo approaches. *Molecules.* 2020;25(7):1519.
70. Aponso M, Patti A, Bennett LE. Dose-related effects of inhaled essential oils on behavioural measures of anxiety and depression and biomarkers of oxidative stress. *J Ethnopharmacol.* 2020;250:112469.
71. Aydin E, Hritcu L, Dogan G, Hayta S, Bagci E. The effects of inhaled *Pimpinella peregrina* essential oil on scopolamine-induced memory impairment, anxiety, and depression in laboratory rats. *Mol Neurobiol.* 2016;53(9):6557–6567.
72. Bagci E, Aydin E, Ungureanu E, Hritcu L. Anthriscus nemorosa essential oil inhalation prevents memory impairment, anxiety and depression in scopolamine-treated rats. *Biomed Pharmacother.* 2016;84:1313–1320.
73. Hashikawa-Hobara N, Otsuka A, Ishikawa R, Hashikawa N. Roman chamomile inhalation combined with clomipramine treatment improves treatment-resistant depression-like behavior in mice. *Biomed Pharmacother.* 2019;118:109263.
74. Chen B, Li J, Xie Y, et al. Cang-ai volatile oil improves depressive-like behaviors and regulates DA and 5-HT metabolism in the brains of CUMS-induced rats. *J Ethnopharmacol.* 2019;244:112088.
75. Kim DS, Goo YM, Cho J, et al. Effect of volatile organic chemicals in *Chrysanthemum indicum* linné on blood pressure and electroencephalogram. *Molecules.* 2018;23(8):2063.
76. Villareal MO, Ikeya A, Sasaki K, Arfa AB, Neffati M, Isoda H. Anti-stress and neuronal cell differentiation induction effects of *Rosmarinus officinalis* L. essential oil. *BMC Complement Altern Med.* 2017;17(1):549.
77. Sowndhararajan K, Seo M, Kim M, Kim H, Kim S. Effect of essential oil and supercritical carbon dioxide extract from the root of *Angelica gigas* on human EEG activity. *Complement Ther Clin Pract.* 2017;28:161–168.
78. Kong Y, Wang T, Wang R, et al. Inhalation of *Roman chamomile* essential oil attenuates depressive-like behaviors in Wistar Kyoto rats. *Sci China Life Sci.* 2017;60(6):647–655.
79. Ghorat F, Shahrestani S, Tagabadi Z, Bazghandi M. The effect of inhalation of essential oils of polianthes tuberosa on test anxiety in students: A clinical trial. *Iran J Med Sci.* 2016;41(3 Suppl):S13.
80. Cheaha D, Issuriya A, Manor R, Kwangjai J, Rujiralai T, Kumarnsit E. Modification of sleep-waking and electroencephalogram induced by vetiver essential oil inhalation. *J Intercult Ethnopharmacol.* 2016;5(1):72–78.

81. Seo M, Sowndhararajan K, Kim S. Influence of binasal and uninasal inhalations of essential oil of *Abies koreana* twigs on electroencephalographic activity of human. *Behav Neurol.* 2016;2016:9250935.
82. Ogawa K, Ito M. Appetite-enhancing effects of trans-Cinnamaldehyde, benzylacetone and 1-phenyl-2-butanone by inhalation. *Planta Med.* 2016;82(1–2):84–88.
83. Saiyudthong S, Mekseepralard C. Effect of inhaling bergamot oil on depression-related behaviors in chronic stressed rats. *J Med Assoc Thai.* 2015;98(Suppl 9):S152–S159.
84. Kasuya H, Iida S, Ono K, Satou T, Koike K. Intracerebral distribution of a-pinene and the anxiolytic-like effect in mice following inhaled administration of essential oil from *Chamaecyparis obtuse. Nat Prod Commun.* 2015;10(8): 1479–1482.
85. Hritcu L, Bagci E, Aydin E, Mihasan M. Antiamnesic and antioxidants effects of *Ferulago angulata* essential oil against scopolamine-induced memory impairment in laboratory rats. *Neurochem Res.* 2015;40(9):1799–1809.
86. Saiyudthong S, Pongmayteegul S, Marsden CA, Phansuwan-Pujito P. Anxiety-like behaviour and c-fos expression in rats that inhaled vetiver essential oil. *Nat Prod Res.* 2015;29(22):2141–2144.
87. Igarashi M, Ikei H, Song C, Miyazaki Y. Effects of olfactory stimulation with rose and orange oil on prefrontal cortex activity. *Complement Ther Med.* 2014;22(6):1027–1031.
88. Park HJ, Kim SK, Kang WS, Woo JM, Kim JW. Effects of essential oil from *Chamaecyparis obtusa* on cytokine genes in the hippocampus of maternal separation rats. *Can J Physiol Pharmacol.* 2014;92(2):95–101.
89. Hancianu M, Cioanca O, Mihasan M, Hritcu L. Neuroprotective effects of inhaled lavender oil on scopolamine-induced dementia via anti-oxidative activities in rats. *Phytomedicine.* 2013;20(5):446–452.
90. Sayorwan W, Ruangrungsi N, Piriyapunyporn T, Hongratanaworakit T, Kotchabhakdi N, Siripornpanich V. Effects of inhaled rosemary oil on subjective feelings and activities of the nervous system. *Sci Pharm.* 2013;81(2):531–542.
91. Han C, Li F, Tian S, et al. Beneficial effect of compound essential oil inhalation on central fatigue. *BMC Complement Altern Med.* 2018;18(1):309.
92. Hwang JH. The effects of the inhalation method using essential oils on blood pressure and stress responses of clients with essential hypertension. *JKAN.* 2006;36(7):1123–1134.
93. Bikmoradi A, Seifi Z, Poorolajal J, Araghchian M, Safiaryan R, Oshvandi K. Effect of inhalation aromatherapy with lavender essential oil on stress and vital signs in patients undergoing coronary artery bypass surgery: A single-blinded randomized clinical trial. *Complement Ther Med.* 2015;23(3):331–338.
94. Seifi Z, Beikmoradi A, Oshvandi K, Poorolajal J, Araghchian M, Safiaryan R. The effect of lavender essential oil on anxiety level in patients undergoing coronary artery bypass graft surgery: A double-blinded randomized clinical trial. *Iran J Nurs Midwifery Res.* 2014;19(6):574–580.
95. Hosseini S, Heydari A, Vakili M, Moghadam S, Tazyky S. Effect of lavender essence inhalation on the level of anxiety and blood cortisol in candidates for open-heart surgery. *Iran J Nurs Midwifery Res.* 2016;21(4):397–401.
96. Franco L, Blanck TJ, Dugan K, et al. Both lavender fleur oil and unscented oil aromatherapy reduce preoperative anxiety in breast surgery patients: A randomized trial. *J Clin Anesth.* 2016;33:243–249.
97. Fazlollahpour-Rokni F, Shorofi SA, Mousavinasab N, Ghafari R, Esmaeili R. The effect of inhalation aromatherapy with rose essential oil on the anxiety of patients undergoing coronary artery bypass graft surgery. *Complement Ther Clin Pract.* 2019;34:201–207.
98. Abdelhakim AM, Hussein AS, Doheim MF, Sayed AK. The effect of inhalation aromatherapy in patients undergoing cardiac surgery: A systematic review and meta-analysis of randomized controlled trials. *Complement Ther Med.* 2020;48:102256.
99. Liu J, Cai S, Chen D, et al. Behavioral and neural changes induced by a blended essential oil on human selective attention. *Behav Neurol.* 2019;2019:5842132.
100. Batubara I, Suparto IH, Sadiah S, Matsuoka R, Mitsunaga T. Effect of *Zingiber zerumbet* essential oils and zerumbone inhalation on body weight of Sprague Dawley rat. *Pak J Biol Sci.* 2013;16(19):1028–1033.
101. Batubara I, Suparto IH, Sa'diah S, Matsuoka R, Mitsunaga T. Effects of inhaled citronella oil and related compounds on rat body weight and brown adipose tissue sympathetic nerve. *Nutrients.* 2015;7(3):1859–1870.
102. Toledo-Aral JJ, Moss BL, He ZJ, Koszowski AG, Whisenand T, Levinson SR, Wolf JJ, Silos-Santiago I, Halegoua S, Mandel G. Identification of PN1, a predominant voltage-dependent sodium channel expressed principally in peripheral neurons. *Proc Natl Acad Sci U S A.* 1997;94(4):1527–1532.
103. Black JA, Liu S, Tanaka M, Cummins TR, Waxman SG. Changes in the expression of tetrodotoxin-sensitive sodium channels within dorsal root ganglia neurons in inflammatory pain. *Pain.* 2004;108(3):237–247.
104. Nassar MA, Stirling LC, Forlani G, Baker MD, Matthews EA, Dickenson AH, Wood JN. Nociceptor-specific gene deletion reveals a major role for Nav1.7 (PN1) in acute and inflammatory pain. *Proc Natl Acad Sci U S A.* 2004;101(34):12706–12711.
105. Cox JJ, Reimann F, Nicholas AK, Thornton G, Roberts E, Springell K, Karbani G, Jafri H, Mannan J, Raashid Y, Al-Gazali L, Hamamy H, Valente EM, Gorman S, Williams R, McHale DP, Wood JN, Gribble FM, Woods CG. An SCN9A channelopathy causes congenital inability to experience pain. *Nature.* 2006;444(7121):894–898.
106. van Brederode J, Atak S, Kessler A, Pischetsrieder M, Villmann C, Alzheimer C. The terpenoids myrtenol and verbenol act on δ subunit-containing GABAA receptors and enhance tonic inhibition in dentate gyrus granule cells. *Neurosci Lett.* 2016;628:91–97.
107. Manayi A, Nabavi SM, Daglia M, Jafari S. Natural terpenoids as a promising source for modulation of GABAergic system and treatment of neurological diseases. *Pharmacol Rep.* 2016;68(4):671–679.
108. Bahr TA, Rodriguez D, Beaumont C, Allred K. The effects of various essential oils on epilepsy and acute seizure: A systematic review. *Evid Based Complement Alternat Med.* 2019;2019:6216745.

109. da Fonsêca DV, da Silva Maia Bezerra Filho C, Lima TC, de Almeida RN, de Sousa DP. Anticonvulsant essential oils and their relationship with oxidative stress in epilepsy. *Biomolecules.* 2019;9(12):835.
110. Zhang N, Yao L. Anxiolytic effect of essential oils and their constituents: A review. *J Agric Food Chem.* 2019;67(50): 13790–13808.
111. Agatonovic-Kustrin S, Kustrin E, Gegechkori V, Morton DW. Anxiolytic terpenoids and aromatherapy for anxiety and depression. *Adv Exp Med Biol.* 2020;1260:283–296.
112. Wang ZJ, Heinbockel T. Essential oils and their constituents targeting the GABAergic system and sodium channels as treatment of neurological diseases. *Molecules.* 2018;23(5):1061.
113. Ayaz M, Sadiq A, Junaid M, Ullah F, Subhan F, Ahmed J. Neuroprotective and anti-aging potentials of essential oils from aromatic and medicinal plants. *Front Aging Neurosci.* 2017;9:168.
114. Wei A, Shibamoto T. Antioxidant/lipoxygenase inhibitory activities and chemical compositions of selected essential oils. *J Agric Food Chem.* 2010;58(12):7218–7225.
115. Elliott M, Abuhamdah S, Howes M, Lees G, Ballard C, Holmes C. The essential oils from *Melissa officinalis* L. and *Lavandula angustifolia* Mill. as potential treatment for agitation in people with severe dementia. *Int J Essent Oil Ther* 2007;1:143–152.
116. Woelk H, Schläfke S. A multi-center, double-blind, randomised study of the lavender oil preparation Silexan in comparison to Lorazepam for generalized anxiety disorder. *Phytomedicine.* 2010;17(2):94–99.
117. Setzer WN. Essential oils and anxiolytic aromatherapy. *Nat Prod Commun.* 2009;4(9):1305–1316.
118. López V, Nielsen B, Solas M, Ramírez MJ, Jäger AK. Exploring pharmacological mechanisms of lavender (*Lavandula angustifolia*) essential oil on central nervous system targets. *Front Pharmacol.* 2017;8:280.
119. Oliveira JS, Porto LA, Estevam CDS, et al. Phytochemical screening and anticonvulsant property of *Ocimum basilicum* leaf essential oil. *Bol Latinoam Caribe Plant Med Aromat.* 2009;8;195–202.
120. Pathan S, Zaidi S, Jain G, Vohora D, Ahmad F, Khar R. Anticonvulsant evaluation of safranal in pentylenetetrazole-induced status epilepticus in mice. *Int J Essent Oil Ther.* 2009;3;106–108.
121. Shimizu K, Gyokusen M, Kitamura S, Kawabe T, Kozaki T, Ishibashi K, Izumi R, Mizunoya W, Ohnuki K, Essential oil of lavender inhibited the decreased attention during a long-term task in humans. *Kondo R Biosci Biotechnol Biochem.* 2008;72(7):1944–1947.
122. Hongratanaworakit T. Simultaneous aromatherapy massage with rosemary oil on humans. *Sci Pharm.* 2009;77:375–387.
123. Robbins G, Broughan C. The effects of manipulating participant expectations of an essential oil on memory through verbal suggestion. *Int J Essent Oil Ther.* 2007;1:56–60.
124. Schliebs R, Arendt T. The cholinergic system in aging and neuronal degeneration. *Behav Brain Res.* 2011;221(2):555–563.
125. Lambert RC, Bessaih T, Leresche N. Modulation of neuronal T-type calcium channels. *CNS Neurol Disord Drug Targets.* 2006;5(6):611–627.
126. El Alaoui C, Chemin J, Fechtali T, Lory P. Modulation of T-type Ca^{2+} channels by lavender and rosemary extracts. *PLoS One.* 2017;12(10):e0186864.
127. Seo H, Li HY, Perez-Reyes E, Lee JH. Effects of eugenol on T-type Ca^{2+} channel isoforms. *J Pharmacol Exp Ther.* 2013;347(2):310–317.
128. Cho JS, Kim TH, Lim JM, Song JH. Effects of eugenol on Na+ currents in rat dorsal root ganglion neurons. *Brain Res.* 2008;1243:53–62.
129. Sabino CK, Ferreria-Filho ES, Mendes MB, Da Silva-Filho JC. Cardiovascular effects induced by α-terpineol in hypertensive rats. *Flavour Frag. J* 2013;28(5):333–339.
130. Xu P, Wang K, Lu C, Dong L, Gao L, Yan M, Aibai S, Liu X. Protective effect of lavender oil on scopolamine induced cognitive deficits in mice and H_2O_2 induced cytotoxicity in PC_{12} cells. *J Ethnopharmacol.* 2016;193:408–415.
131. Takahashi M, Satou T, Ohashi M, Hayashi S, Sadamoto K, Koike K. Interspecies comparison of chemical composition and anxiolytic-like effects of lavender oils upon inhalation. *Nat Prod Commun.* 2011;6(11):1769–1774.
132. Takahashi M, Yoshino A, Yamanaka A, Asanuma C, Satou T, Hayashi S, Masuo Y, Sadamoto K, Koike K. Effects of inhaled lavender essential oil on stress-loaded animals: Changes in anxiety-related behavior and expression levels of selected mRNAs and proteins. *Nat Prod Commun.* 2012;7(11):1539–1544.
133. Takahashi M, Yamanaka A, Asanuma C, Asano H, Satou T, Koike K. Anxiolytic-like effect of inhalation of essential oil from Lavandula officinalis: Investigation of changes in 5-HT turnover and involvement of olfactory stimulation. *Nat Prod Commun.* 2014;9(7):1023–1026.
134. Bradley BF, Starkey NJ, Brown SL, Lea RW. Anxiolytic effects of *Lavandula angustifolia* odour on the Mongolian gerbil elevated plus maze. *J Ethnopharmacol.* 2007;111(3):517–525.
135. Kumar V. Characterization of anxiolytic and neuropharmacological activities of Silexan. *Wien Med Wochenschr.* 2013;163(3–4):89–94.
136. Xu P, Wang K, Lu C, Dong L, Gao L, Yan M, Aibai S, Yang Y, Liu X. The protective effect of lavender essential oil and its main component linalool against the cognitive deficits induced by d-galactose and aluminum trichloride in mice. *Evid Based Complement Alternat Med.* 2017;2017:7426538.
137. Zhang N, Luo M, He L, Yao L. Chemical composition of essential oil from flower of 'Shanzhizi' (*Gardenia jasminoides* Ellis) and involvement of serotonergic system in its anxiolytic effect. *Molecules.* 2020;25(20):4702.
138. Huang L, Abuhamdah S, Howes MJ, Dixon CL, Elliot MS, Ballard C, Holmes C, Burns A, Perry EK, Francis PT, Lees G, Chazot PL. Pharmacological profile of essential oils derived from Lavandula angustifolia and *Melissa officinalis* with anti-agitation properties: Focus on ligand-gated channels. *J Pharm Pharmacol.* 2008;60(11):1515–1522. doi: 10.1211/jpp/60.11.0013. Erratum in: *J Pharm Pharmacol.* 2009;61(2):267.
139. Wang S, Wang C, Peng D, Liu X, Wu C, Guo P, Wei J. Agarwood essential oil displays sedative-hypnotic effects through the GABAergic system. *Molecules.* 2017;22:2190.

140. de Araújo FY, Silva MI, Moura BA, et al. Central nervous system effects of the essential oil of the leaves of *Alpinia zerumbet* in mice. *J Pharm Pharmacol.* 2009;61(11):1521–1527.
141. Zhang N, Zhang L, Feng L, Yao L. The anxiolytic effect of essential oil of Cananga odorata exposure on mice and determination of its major active constituents. *Phytomedicine.* 2016;23(14):1727–1734.
142. Kasuya H, Hata E, Satou T, Yoshikawa M, Hayashi S, Masuo Y, Koike K. Effect on emotional behavior and stress by inhalation of the essential oil from *Chamaecyparis obtusa. Nat Prod Commun.* 2013;8(4):515–518.
143. Bae D, Seol H, Yoon HG, Na JR, Oh K, Choi CY, Lee DW, Jun W, Youl Lee K, Lee J, Hwang K, Lee YH, Kim S. Inhaled essential oil from *Chamaecyparis obtuse* ameliorates the impairments of cognitive function induced by injection of β-amyloid in rats. *Pharm Biol.* 2012;50(7):900–910.
144. Katsuyama S, Otowa A, Kamio S, Sato K, Yagi T, Kishikawa Y, Komatsu T, Bagetta G, Sakurada T, Nakamura H. Effect of plantar subcutaneous administration of bergamot essential oil and linalool on formalin-induced nociceptive behavior in mice. *Biomed Res.* 2015;36(1):47–54.
145. Sakurada T, Kuwahata H, Katsuyama S, Komatsu T, Morrone LA, Corasaniti MT, Bagetta G, Sakurada S. Intraplantar injection of bergamot essential oil into the mouse hindpaw: Effects on capsaicin-induced nociceptive behaviors. *Int Rev Neurobiol.* 2009;85:237–248.
146. Linck VM, da Silva AL, Figueiró M, Caramão EB, Moreno PR, Elisabetsky E. Effects of inhaled Linalool in anxiety, social interaction and aggressive behavior in mice. *Phytomedicine.* 2010;17(8–9):679–683.
147. Oliveira Júnior RG, Ferraz CAA, Silva JC, et al. Neuropharmacological effects of essential oil from the leaves of *Croton conduplicatus* Kunth and possible mechanisms of action involved. *J Ethnopharmacol.* 2018;221:65–76.
148. Blanco MM, Costa CA, Freire AO, Santos JG Jr, Costa M. Neurobehavioral effect of essential oil of *Cymbopogon citratus* in mice. *Phytomedicine.* 2009;16(2–3):265–270.
149. Trang DT, Hoang TKV, Nguyen TTM, Van Cuong P, Dang NH, Dang HD, Nguyen Quang T, Dat NT. Essential oils of lemongrass (*Cymbopogon citratus* Stapf) induces apoptosis and cell cycle arrest in A549 lung cancer cells. *Biomed Res Int.* 2020;2020:5924856.
150. Victoria FN, de Siqueira Brahm A, Savegnago L, Lenardão EJ. Involvement of serotoninergic and adrenergic systems on the antidepressant-like effect of *E. uniflora* L. leaves essential oil and further analysis of its antioxidant activity. *Neurosci Lett.* 2013;544:105–109.
151. Tabari MA, Tehrani MAB. Evidence for the involvement of the GABAergic, but not serotonergic transmission in the anxiolytic-like effect of bisabolol in the mouse elevated plus maze. *Naunyn Schmiedebergs Arch Pharmacol.* 2017;390(10):1041–1046.
152. de Figuêiredo FR, Monteiro ÁB, Alencar de Menezes IR, et al. Effects of the *Hyptis martiusii* benth. leaf essential oil and 1,8-cineole (eucalyptol) on the central nervous system of mice. *Food Chem Toxicol.* 2019;133:110802.
153. Silva LL, Garlet QI, Benovit SC, Dolci G, Mallmann CA, Bürger ME, Baldisserotto B, Longhi SJ, Heinzmann BM. Sedative and anesthetic activities of the essential oils of *Hyptis mutabilis* (Rich.) Briq. and their isolated components in silver catfish (Rhamdia quelen). *Braz J Med Biol Res.* 2013;46(9):771–779.
154. Zhang K, Yao L. The anxiolytic effect of *Juniperus virginiana* L. essential oil and determination of its active constituents. *Physiol Behav.* 2018;189:50–58.
155. Dougnon G, Ito M. Sedative effects of the essential oil from the leaves of *Lantana camara* occurring in the republic of Benin via inhalation in mice. *J Nat Med.* 2020;74(1): 159–169.
156. Vale TG, Matos FJ, de Lima TC, Viana GS. Behavioral effects of essential oils from *Lippia alba* (Mill.) N.E. Brown chemotypes. *J Ethnopharmacol.* 1999;67(2):127–133.
157. Hosseinzadeh H, Parvardeh S. Anticonvulsant effects of thymoquinone, the major constituent of *Nigella sativa* seeds, in mice. *Phytomedicine.* 2004;11(1):56–64.
158. Abouhosseini Tabari M, Hajizadeh Moghaddam A, Maggi F, Benelli G. Anxiolytic and antidepressant activities of *Pelargonium roseum* essential oil on *Swiss albino* mice: Possible involvement of serotonergic transmission. *Phytother Res.* 2018;32(6):1014–1022.
159. Kennedy D, Okello E, Chazot P, Howes MJ, Ohiomokhare S, Jackson P, Haskell-Ramsay C, Khan J, Forster J, Wightman E. Volatile terpenes and brain function: Investigation of the cognitive and mood effects of mentha×piperita L. essential oil with in vitro properties relevant to central nervous system function. *Nutrients.* 2018;10(8):1029.
160. Tildesley NT, Kennedy DO, Perry EK, Ballard CG, Wesnes KA, Scholey AB. Positive modulation of mood and cognitive performance following administration of acute doses of Salvia lavandulaefolia essential oil to healthy young volunteers. *Physiol Behav.* 2005;83(5):699–709.
161. Galdino PM, Nascimento MV, Florentino IF, Lino RC, Fajemiroye JO, Chaibub BA, de Paula JR, de Lima TC, Costa EA. The anxiolytic-like effect of an essential oil derived from *Spiranthera odoratissima* A. St. Hil. leaves and its major component, β-caryophyllene, in male mice. *Prog Neuropsychopharmacol Biol Psychiatry.* 2012;38(2): 276–284.
162. Kessler A, Sahin-Nadeem H, Lummis SC, Weigel I, Pischetsrieder M, Buettner A, Villmann C. GABA(A) receptor modulation by terpenoids from Sideritis extracts. *Mol Nutr Food Res.* 2014;58(4):851–862.
163. Spadaro F, Costa R, Circosta C, Occhiuto F. Volatile composition and biological activity of key lime *Citrus aurantifolia* essential oil. *Nat Prod Commun.* 2012;7(11):1523–1526.
164. Garlet QI, Pires LDC, Milanesi LH, Marafiga JR, Baldisserotto B, Mello CF, Heinzmann BM. (+)-Dehydrofukinone modulates membrane potential and delays seizure onset by GABAa receptor-mediated mechanism in mice. *Toxicol Appl Pharmacol.* 2017;332:52–63.
165. Lima-Accioly PM, Lavor-Porto PR, Cavalcante FS, Magalhães PJ, Lahlou S, Morais SM, Leal-Cardoso JH. Essential oil of croton nepetaefolius and its main constituent, 1,8-cineole, block excitability of rat sciatic nerve in vitro. *Clin Exp Pharmacol Physiol.* 2006;33(12): 1158–1163.
166. Dougnon G, Ito M. Inhalation administration of the bicyclic ethers 1,8- and 1,4-cineole prevent anxiety and depressive-like behaviours in mice. *Molecules.* 2020;25(8):1884.
167. Joca HC, Vieira DC, Vasconcelos AP, Araújo DA, Cruz JS. Carvacrol modulates voltage-gated sodium channels kinetics in dorsal root ganglia. *Eur J Pharmacol.* 2015;756: 22–29.

168. Melo FH, Venâncio ET, de Sousa DP, de França Fonteles MM, de Vasconcelos SM, Viana GS, de Sousa FC. Anxiolytic-like effect of carvacrol (5-isopropyl-2-methylphenol) in mice: Involvement with GABAergic transmission. *Fundam Clin Pharmacol.* 2010;24(4):437–443.
169. Pires LF, Costa LM, Silva OA, de Almeida AA, Cerqueira GS, de Sousa DP, de Freitas RM. Anxiolytic-like effects of carvacryl acetate, a derivative of carvacrol, in mice. *Pharmacol Biochem Behav.* 2013;112:42–48.
170. Nogoceke FP, Barcaro IM, de Sousa DP, Andreatini R. Antimanic-like effects of (R)-(–)-carvone and (S)-(+)-carvone in mice. *Neurosci Lett.* 2016;619:43–48.
171. de Sousa DP, de Farias Nóbrega FF, de Almeida RN. Influence of the chirality of (R)-(–)- and (S)-(+)-carvone in the central nervous system: A comparative study. *Chirality.* 2007;19(4):264–268.
172. Mariani ME, Sánchez-Borzone ME, García DA. Effects of bioactive monoterpenic ketones on membrane organization. A langmuir film study. *Chem Phys Lipids.* 2016;198: 39–45.
173. Silva MI, Silva MA, de Aquino Neto MR, Moura BA, de Sousa HL, de Lavor EP, de Vasconcelos PF, Macêdo DS, de Sousa DP, Vasconcelos SM, de Sousa FC. Effects of isopulegol on pentylenetetrazol-induced convulsions in mice: Possible involvement of GABAergic system and antioxidant activity. *Fitoterapia.* 2009;80(8):506–513.
174. Kawasaki H, Mizuta K, Fujita T, Kumamoto E. Inhibition by menthol and its related chemicals of compound action potentials in frog sciatic nerves. *Life Sci.* 2013;92(6–7):359–367.
175. Ding J, Huang C, Peng Z, Xie Y, Deng S, Nie YZ, Xu TL, Ge WH, Li WG, Li F. Electrophysiological characterization of methyleugenol: A novel agonist of GABA(A) receptors. *ACS Chem Neurosci.* 2014;5(9):803–811.
176. da Fonsêca DV, Salgado PR, de Carvalho FL, Salvadori MG, Penha AR, Leite FC, Borges CJ, Piuvezam MR, Pordeus LC, Sousa DP, Almeida RN. Nerolidol exhibits antinociceptive and anti-inflammatory activity: Involvement of the GABAergic system and proinflammatory cytokines. *Fundam Clin Pharmacol.* 2016;30(1):14–22.
177. Yang H, Woo J, Pae AN, Um MY, Cho NC, Park KD, Yoon M, Kim J, Lee CJ, Cho S. α-Pinene, a major constituent of pine tree oils, enhances non-rapid eye movement sleep in mice through GABAA-benzodiazepine receptors. *Mol Pharmacol.* 2016;90(5):530–539.
178. Gonçalves JC, Oliveira Fde S, Benedito RB, de Sousa DP, de Almeida RN, de Araújo DA. Antinociceptive activity of (–)-carvone: Evidence of association with decreased peripheral nerve excitability. *Biol Pharm Bull.* 2008;31(5): 1017–1020.
179. Nóbrega FF, Salvadori MG, Masson CJ, Mello CF, Nascimento TS, Leal-Cardoso JH, de Sousa DP, Almeida RN. Monoterpenoid terpinen-4-ol exhibits anticonvulsant activity in behavioural and electrophysiological studies. *Oxid Med Cell Longev.* 2014;2014:703848.
180. Xu ZH, Wang C, Fujita T, Jiang CY, Kumamoto E. Action of thymol on spontaneous excitatory transmission in adult rat spinal substantia gelatinosa neurons. *Neurosci Lett.* 2015;606:94–99.
181. Bhatia S, Sardana S, Senwar KR, Dhillon A, Sharma A, Naved T. In vitro antioxidant and antinociceptive properties of Porphyra vietnamensis. *Biomedicine (Taipei).* 2019;9(1):3.
182. Bhatia S, Sharma K, Namdeo AG, Chaugule BB, Kavale M, Nanda S. Broad-spectrum sun-protective action of Porphyra-334 derived from Porphyra vietnamensis. *Pharmacogn Res.* 2010;2(1):45–49.
183. Bhatia S, Sharma K, Sharma A, Nagpal K, Bera T. Anti-inflammatory, analgesic and antiulcer properties of Porphyra vietnamensis. *Avicenna J Phytomed.* 2015;5(1): 69–77.
184. Bhatia S, Sardana S, Sharma A, Vargas De La Cruz CB, Chaugule B, Khodaie L. Development of broad spectrum mycosporine loaded sunscreen formulation from Ulva fasciata delile. *Biomedicine (Taipei).* 2019;9(3):17.
185. Bhatia S, Garg A, Sharma K, Kumar S, Sharma A, Purohit AP. Mycosporine and mycosporine-like amino acids: A paramount tool against ultra violet irradiation. *Pharmacogn Rev.* 2011;5(10):138–146.
186. Bhatia S, Namdeo AG, Nanda S. Factors effecting the gelling and emulsifying properties of a natural polymer. *SRP.* 2010;1(1):86–92.
187. Bhatia S, Sharma K, Bera T. Structural characterization and pharmaceutical properties of porphyran. *Asian J Pharm.* 2015;9:93–101.
188. Bhatia S, Sharma A, Sharma K, Kavale M, Chaugule BB, Dhalwal K, Namdeo AG, Mahadik KR. Novel algal polysaccharides from marine source: Porphyran. *Pharmacogn Rev.* 2008;2(4):271–276.
189. Bhatia S, Sharma K, Nagpal K, Bera T. Investigation of the factors influencing the molecular weight of porphyran and its associated antifungal activity Bioact. *Carb Diet Fiber.* 2015;5:153–168.
190. Bhatia S, Kumar V, Sharma K, Nagpal K, Bera T. Significance of algal polymer in designing amphotericin B nanoparticles. *Sci World J.* 2014;2014:564573.
191. Bhatia S, Rathee P, Sharma K, Chaugule BB, Kar N, Bera T. Immuno-modulation effect of sulphated polysaccharide (porphyran) from Porphyra vietnamensis. *Int J Biol Macromol.* 2013;57:50–56.
192. Bhatia S. *Natural Polymer Drug Delivery Systems: Marine Polysaccharides Based Nano-Materials and Its Applications.* Springer International Publishing, Switzerland; 2016:185–225.
193. Bhatia S. *Natural Polymer Drug Delivery Systems: Plant Derived Polymers, Properties, and Modification & Applications.* Springer International Publishing, Switzerland; 2016:119–184.
194. Bhatia S. *Natural Polymer Drug Delivery Systems: Nanotechnology and Its Drug Delivery Applications.* Springer International Publishing, Switzerland; 2016:1–32.
195. Bhatia S. *Natural Polymer Drug Delivery Systems: Nanoparticles Types, Classification, Characterization, Fabrication Methods and Drug Delivery Applications.* Springer International Publishing, Switzerland; 2016:33–93.
196. Bhatia S. *Natural Polymer Drug Delivery Systems: Natural Polymers vs Synthetic Polymer.* Springer International Publishing, Switzerland; 2016:95–118.
197. Bhatia S. *Systems for Drug Delivery: Mammalian Polysaccharides and Its Nanomaterials.* Springer International Publishing, Switzerland; 2016:1–27.
198. Bhatia S. *Systems for Drug Delivery: Microbial Polysaccharides as Advance Nanomaterials.* Springer International Publishing, Switzerland; 2016:29–54.

199. Bhatia S. *Systems for Drug Delivery: Chitosan Based Nanomaterials and Its Applications.* Springer International Publishing, Switzerland; 2016:55–117.
200. Bhatia S. *Systems for Drug Delivery: Advance Polymers and Its Applications.* Springer International Publishing, Switzerland; 2016:119–146.
201. Bhatia S. *Systems for Drug Delivery: Advanced Application of Natural Polysaccharides.* Springer International Publishing, Switzerland; 2016:147–170.
202. Bhatia S. *Systems for Drug Delivery: Modern Polysaccharides and Its Current Advancements.* Springer International Publishing, Switzerland; 2016:171–188.
203. Bhatia S. *Systems for Drug Delivery: Toxicity of Nanodrug Delivery Systems.* Springer International Publishing, Switzerland; 2016:189–197.
204. Bhatia S. *Nanotechnology in Drug Delivery Fundamentals, Design, and Applications: Part 1: Protein and Peptide-Based Drug Delivery Systems.* Apple Academic Press, Palm Bay, FL; 2016:50–204.
205. Bhatia S. *Nanotechnology in Drug Delivery Fundamentals, Design, and Applications: Part 2: Peptide-Mediated Nanoparticle Drug Delivery System.* Apple Academic Press, Palm Bay, FL; 2016:205–280.
206. Bhatia S. *Nanotechnology in Drug Delivery Fundamentals, Design, and Applications: Part 3: CPP and CTP in Drug Delivery and Cell Targeting.* Apple Academic Press, Palm Bay, FL; 2016:309–312.
207. Bonferoni MC, Ferraro L, Pavan B, Beggiato S, Cavalieri E, Giunchedi P, Dalpiaz A. Uptake in the central nervous system of geraniol oil encapsulated in chitosan oleate following nasal and oral administration. *Pharmaceutics.* 2019;11(3):106.
208. Bhatia S, Sharma A, Vargas De La Cruz CB, Chaugule B, Ahmed Al-Harrasi. Nutraceutical, antioxidant, antimicrobial properties of *Pyropia vietnamensis* (Tanaka et Pham-Hong Ho) J.E. Sutherl. et Monotilla. *Curr Bioact Compd.* 2020;16:1.
209. Kennedy DO, Dodd FL, Robertson BC, Okello EJ, Reay JL, Scholey AB, Haskell CF. Monoterpenoid extract of sage (*Salvia lavandulaefolia*) with cholinesterase inhibiting properties improves cognitive performance and mood in healthy adults. *J Psychopharmacol.* 2011;25(8):1088–1100.
210. Bhatia S. *Systems for Drug Delivery: Safety, Animal, and Microbial Polysaccharides.* Springer Nature, Basingstoke, UK; 2016:122–127.
211. Bhatia S. Stem cell culture. In: *Introduction to Pharmaceutical Biotechnology, Volume 3: Animal Tissue Culture and Biopharmaceuticals.* IOP Publishing Ltd, Bristol, UK; 2019:1–24.
212. Bhatia S. Organ culture. In: *Introduction to Pharmaceutical Biotechnology, Volume 3: Introduction to Animal Tissue Culture Science.* IOP Publishing Ltd, Bristol, UK; 2019:1–28.
213. Bhatia S. Animal tissue culture facilities. In: *Introduction to Pharmaceutical Biotechnology, Volume 3: Animal Tissue Culture and Biopharmaceuticals.* IOP Publishing Ltd, Bristol, UK; 2019:1–32.
214. Bhatia S. Characterization of cultured cells. In: *Introduction to Pharmaceutical Biotechnology, Volume 3: Animal Tissue Culture and Biopharmaceuticals.* IOP Publishing Ltd, Bristol, UK; 2019:1–47.
215. Bhatia S. Introduction to genomics. In: *Introduction to Pharmaceutical Biotechnology, Volume 2: Enzymes, Proteins and Bioinformatics.* IOP Publishing Ltd, Bristol, UK; 2018:1–39.
216. Bhatia S. Bioinformatics. In: *Introduction to Pharmaceutical Biotechnology, Volume 2: Enzymes, Proteins and Bioinformatics.* IOP Publishing Ltd, Bristol, UK; 2018:1–16.
217. Bhatia S. Protein and enzyme engineering. In: *Introduction to Pharmaceutical Biotechnology, Volume 2: Enzymes, Proteins and Bioinformatics.* IOP Publishing Ltd, Bristol, UK; 2018:1–15.
218. Bhatia S. Industrial enzymes and their applications. In: *Introduction to Pharmaceutical Biotechnology, Volume 2: Enzymes, Proteins and Bioinformatics.* IOP Publishing Ltd, Bristol, UK; 2018:21.
219. Bhatia S. Introduction to enzymes and their applications. In: *Introduction to Pharmaceutical Biotechnology, Volume 2: Enzymes, Proteins and Bioinformatics.* IOP Publishing Ltd, Bristol, UK; 2018:1–29.
220. Bhatia S. Biotransformation and enzymes. In: *Introduction to Pharmaceutical Biotechnology, Volume 2: Enzymes, Proteins and Bioinformatics.* IOP Publishing Ltd, Bristol, UK; 2018:1–13.
221. Bhatia S. Modern DNA science and its applications. In: *Introduction to Pharmaceutical Biotechnology, Volume 1: Basic Techniques and Concepts.* IOP Publishing Ltd, Bristol, UK; 2018:1–70.
222. Bhatia S. Introduction to genetic engineering. In: *Introduction to Pharmaceutical Biotechnology, Volume 1: Basic Techniques and Concepts.* IOP Publishing Ltd, Bristol, UK; 2018:1–63.
223. Bhatia S. Applications of stem cells in disease and gene therapy. In: *Introduction to Pharmaceutical Biotechnology, Volume 1: Basic Techniques and Concepts.* IOP Publishing Ltd, Bristol, UK; 2018:1–40.
224. Bhatia S. Transgenic animals in biotechnology. In: *Introduction to Pharmaceutical Biotechnology, Volume 1: Basic Techniques and Concepts.* IOP Publishing Ltd, Bristol, UK; 2018:1–67.
225. Bhatia S. History and scope of plant biotechnology. In: *Modern Applications of Plant Biotechnology in Pharmaceutical Sciences.* Academic Press, Cambridge, MA; 2015:1–30.
226. Bhatia S. Plant tissue culture. In: *Modern Applications of Plant Biotechnology in Pharmaceutical Sciences.* Academic Press, Cambridge, MA; 2015:31–107.
227. Bhatia S. Laboratory organization. In: *Modern Applications of Plant Biotechnology in Pharmaceutical Sciences.* Academic Press, Cambridge, MA; 2015:109–120.
228. Bhatia S. Concepts and techniques of plant tissue culture science. In: *Modern Applications of Plant Biotechnology in Pharmaceutical Sciences.* Academic Press, Cambridge, MA; 2015:121–156.
229. Bhatia S. Application of plant biotechnology. In: *Modern Applications of Plant Biotechnology in Pharmaceutical Sciences.* Academic Press, Cambridge, MA; 2015:157–207.
230. Bhatia S. Somatic embryogenesis and organogenesis. In: *Modern Applications of Plant Biotechnology in Pharmaceutical Sciences.* Academic Press, Cambridge, MA; 2015:209–230.

231. Bhatia S. Classical and nonclassical techniques for secondary metabolite production in plant cell culture. In: *Modern Applications of Plant Biotechnology in Pharmaceutical Sciences.* Academic Press, Cambridge, MA; 2015:231–291.
232. Bhatia S. Plant-based biotechnological products with their production host, modes of delivery systems, and stability testing. In: *Modern Applications of Plant Biotechnology in Pharmaceutical Sciences.* Academic Press, Cambridge, MA; 2015:293–331.
233. Bhatia S. Edible vaccines. In: *Modern Applications of Plant Biotechnology in Pharmaceutical Sciences.* Academic Press, Cambridge, MA; 2015:333–343.
234. Bhatia S. Microenvironmentation in micropropagation. In: *Modern Applications of Plant Biotechnology in Pharmaceutical Sciences.* Academic Press, Cambridge, MA; 2015:345–360.
235. Bhatia S. Micropropagation. In: *Modern Applications of Plant Biotechnology in Pharmaceutical Sciences.* Academic Press, Cambridge, MA; 2015:361–368.
236. Bhatia S. Laws in plant biotechnology. In: *Modern Applications of Plant Biotechnology in Pharmaceutical Sciences.* Academic Press, Cambridge, MA; 2015:369–391.
237. Bhatia S. Technical glitches in micropropagation. In: *Modern Applications of Plant Biotechnology in Pharmaceutical Sciences.* Academic Press, Cambridge, MA; 2015:393–404.
238. Bhatia S. Plant tissue culture-based industries. In: *Modern Applications of Plant Biotechnology in Pharmaceutical Sciences.* Academic Press, Cambridge, MA; 2015:405–417.
239. Bhatia S, Al-Harrasi A, Behl T, Anwer MK, Ahmed MM, Mittal V, Kaushik D, Chigurupati S, Kabir MT, Sharma PB, Chaugule B, Vargas-de-la-Cruz C. Anti-migraine activity of freeze dried-latex obtained from *Calotropis Gigantea* Linn. *Environ Sci Pollut Res Int.* 2021.

19

Olfactory Aromatherapy vs. Human Psychophysiological Activity

Ahmed Al-Harrasi
Natural and Medical Sciences Research Center, University of Nizwa

Saurabh Bhatia
Natural and Medical Sciences Research Center, University of Nizwa
University of Petroleum and Energy Studies

Tapan Behl
Chitkara University

Deepak Kaushik
M.D. University

CONTENTS

19.1 Introduction

An essential oil (EO) contains a variety of aromatic substances with distinguished aromatic characteristics. These aromatic substances have been evidenced for their psychophysiological effects in humans for centuries. The majority of aromatic compounds (ACs) present in EOs are volatile in nature with mol. wt. <300 Da. Once inhaled, these volatile substances are identified by the olfactory system. The olfactory system accordingly responds against the stimuli by activating olfactory receptor-associated genes to generate impulse or signal for regulating emotion, cognition, and behavior (Figure 19.1). Aromatic compound-induced emotional and behavior changes can be examined via various electrophysiological techniques including the following [1–5]:

- Contingent negative variation
- Electroencephalograph (EEG)
- Functional magnetic resonance imaging
- Near-infrared spectroscopy

19.2 Olfactory Aromatherapy and Psychological Interventions

Electrophysiological and behavioral analysis of several volatile aromatic substances on EO-treated animal models has been reported. Various findings (EEG) from the electrophysiological study of EO-treated experimental animals indicated how EO components can influence spontaneous brain activities and cognitive functions. An EEG is an excellent means to study electrical properties, mainly electrical transmission in cells and tissues of the central nervous system (CNS) to further study the functional condition of the brain in both healthy as well as diseased states. The EEG can also be used to examine the effectiveness and safety profile of therapeutic agents in psychiatry. EEG spectral analysis is categorized into various bands of frequency including the following:

- Δ waves (0.5 to 4 hertz)
- θ waves (4 to 8 hertz)

DOI: 10.1201/9781003175933-21

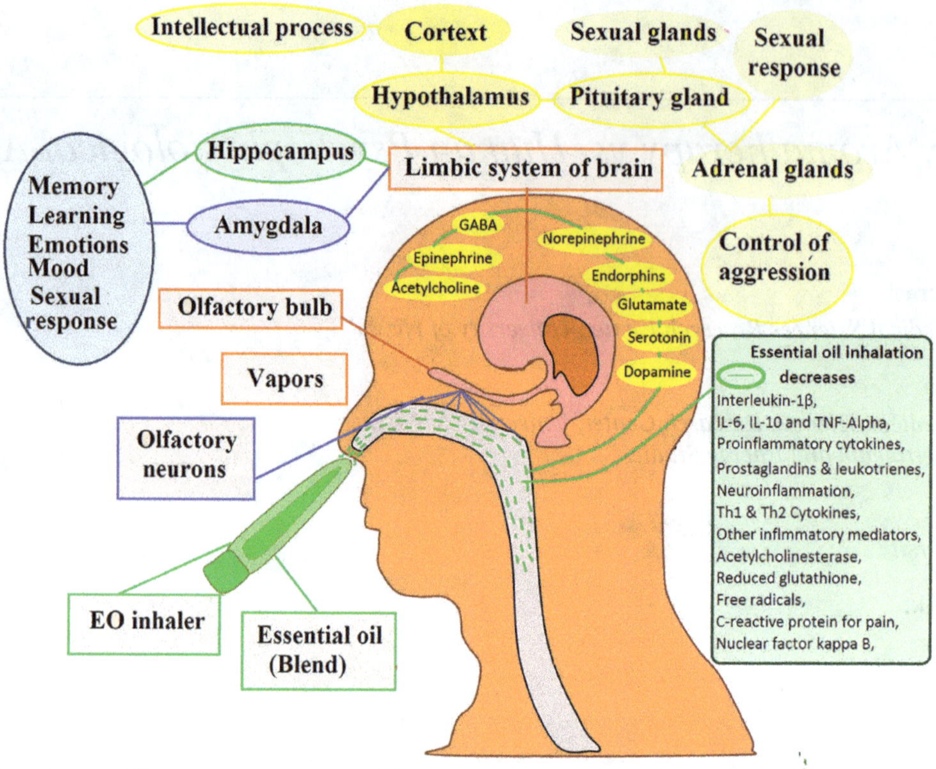

FIGURE 19.1 Olfaction process stimulation via inhalation of EOs via involving olfactory receptor cells in the nasal epithelium connected to the olfactory bulb.

- α waves (8 to 13 hertz)
- β waves (13 to 30 hertz)
- γ waves (30 to 50 hertz)

These different frequency ranges are correlated with different brain activities that help in understanding the physiological state of the brain. This computer-aided process provides the topographical surveys of the neuroanatomy as well as various other features of the brain such as neural movements and responses. A quantitative EEG uses a computational tool based on complex mathematical algorithms to understand spatial relations between cells. It has been reported that decline in alpha and beta signals with increase in delta as well as theta signals is linked with pathological conditions of the brain and with deterioration in cognitive behavior. EEG spectrum analysis can be assessed using Fourier analysis, which facilitates the quantifiable investigation of electrical signal. This complex signaling resulting from postsynaptic potentials of pyramidal neurons (located in the cerebral cortex of the brain) is measured by small metal discs (electrodes) on the scalp [5]. Several reports corroborate that after inhalation of aromatic compounds present in EOs can influence the electrophysiology of the brain via stimulating the olfactory system to alter neurological-based responses in terms of cognition, mood, and social behavior. EOs contain a wide range of ACs which are responsible for distinguishing the aromatic character. These ACs present in EOs have potential physical as well as mental effects on the human brain. The physical impact of EOs shows its direct action on the individual systems, whereas the mental impact on the senses or their processes such as olfaction can ultimately impact a physical effect. It is well known that EO inhalation-based aromatherapy has physiological and psychological effects on the human brain [6]. Additionally, it is also known that these AC stimulations are induced by both pharmacological and psychological mechanisms. Both mechanisms are different from each other, although they usually ensue at the same time [7]. To understand the effects of these ACs, researchers have studied the fluctuations in the neuronal as well as electromagnetic patterns in the brain and assessed various functional factors (pulse rate, galvanic skin response, blood pressure, muscle rigidity, temperature as well as conductance response of the skin).

19.3 EO vs. Human Psychophysiological Activity

For decades, EOs have been used in the management of complications associated with mental and physical health [8]. It has been shown that the activation of olfaction via inhalation of EO triggers many effects on mind and body in individuals [9]. Earlier investigations showed that inhalation of ACs present in an EO can induce positive and negative effects via stimulating the olfactory system. Thus, these small ACs are very critical in directing human behavior [10]. During the olfaction process, volatile and aromatic EO components present in the air interface bind to the olfactory cilia located in the olfactory epithelium. Afterward, activation of glycoprotein-mediated receptors, mainly G protein, allows the generation of electrical signals, which creates a small voltage difference. These electrical impulses are transmitted via olfactory nerves to the brain (Figure 19.1). As a result, these electrical transmissions influence brain activity such as memory, thoughts, and emotions. These aromatic organic compounds of EOs present in systemic circulation can easily pass the blood–brain barrier to bind with the receptors present in the CNS to further change physical or mental response [9]. It was also found that olfactory stimulation caused by these active ACs can further lead to instantaneous changes in physical parameters including the following [11]:

- Blood pressure
- Brain activity
- Muscle tension
- Pulse rate
- Pupil dilation
- Skin temperature

However, various studies also showed that some ACs do not act via stimulating olfactory receptors.

19.4 Human Olfaction Process

The olfactory system involves interaction between the olfactory epithelium (sensory organ) and olfactory bulb as well as the higher olfactory cortex (definite olfactory brain regions). The olfactory mucosa located in the nasal cavity detects ACs [12] by activating the respective olfactory receptor to generate impulse via onset of sensory transduction [13].

Binding of the AC to the cilia of olfactory receptor protein (G-protein-coupled receptor) present in the olfactory epithelium involves the following two G-protein-coupled transduction mechanisms:

- formation of adenosine monophosphate via triggering adenylyl cyclase
- formation of inositol trisphosphate via triggering phospholipase C

Activation of cell membrane channels allows the transport of ions (Cl^{-1}, Na^{+1}, Ca^{+2}) across the cellular membrane → membrane depolarization → generation of membrane voltage potential in the form of electrical signals → transmission of electrical signals via olfactory bulb → via glomeruli → via mitral cells → via cerebral cortex (olfaction) → transmission of olfactory information to chemosensory area of the cortical amygdala, the part of the primary olfactory cortex, and lateral entorhinal cortex → transmission of olfactory information to other cortical and subcortical areas → decoding of the signaling process → olfactory interpretation → passing this olfactory information to the tertiary olfactory structures such as hippocampus as well as amygdala → generate response [14–16] (Figure 19.1). In humans, expressions of olfactory-receptor proteins are regulated via active olfactory receptor genes (around 350) and olfactory receptor pseudogenes (almost 560). It has been found that the olfactory system can directly influence various regions (frontal cortex, thalamus, as well as hippocampus) in the brain that are involved in the regulation of memory and emotion.

Olfactory information is processed by neurons in the human cortex via generating electrical signals. Recording of these electrical signals can be performed by the electroencephalogram (EEG). These electrical signals could be excitatory or inhibitory depending on the involvement of the type of neurotransmitters (excitatory and inhibitory). Activation of excitatory and inhibitory pathways mediated via binding of neurotransmitters to postsynaptic receptors results in the opening or closing of ion channels in the postsynaptic cell. This event results in the generation of postsynaptic action potentials across nerve fibers. The EEG signal is considered as a sum of enormous excitatory (depolarizing) and inhibitory (hyperpolarizing) postsynaptic potentials produced in pyramidal neurons present in the cerebral cortex. Recording of these fluctuating electrical signals via the EEG is a modest, reliable, and noninvasive way to study the effects of ACs over electrophysiology of the brain [17]. These investigations are critical in understanding AC-mediated change in the EEG, which can be directly or indirectly correlated with psychophysiological activities of the subject. Various neurological complications, such as injury or death of the brain, cerebrovascular injuries, structural brain abnormalities, dementia, and disorder of consciousness, epilepsy as well as other psychological complications, can be diagnosed by using the EEG.

19.5 EO Delivery Systems

There are a number of effective delivery methods available for administration of EOs to study the effects on brain function. Usually, delivery of EOs is done by administering the given dose of EO using a filter paper placed in front of the subject's nose to allow effective inhalation [18–20]. EOs could also be delivered to a subject at a specific flow rate (oil/min) by using a cone-modeled provider set up over the rib cage [18–20]. A sterilized toothette in a perforated metallic vessel can be used for infants (kept at a distance of 15 cm away from the infant's head) [18–20]. A sample chamber containing a filter paper soaked/spotted with EOs can be used by placing it 5 cm away from the front of the nose, and later at a specific flow rate (e.g., 1 L/min), fragrance-free air is supplied into the vessel [18–20]. A number of researchers have used this odorant delivery system using a constant flow-olfactometer (flow rate at 1.0 L/min) to deliver EOs. For safe and effective delivery of EOs, it is important to predetermine the flow rate. The odorant delivery system transmits air from the chamber air via stainless tubing to an advanced respiratory mask restrained at 15 cm away from the nasal cavity of an individual [18–20]. One more report showed that EOs can be delivered by adding oil to a poly bag or pouch and presented via mask. Furthermore, a nebulizer can be used for the administration of EOs in such a way so that EOs can be inhaled via nebulization using mask of the nebulizer at a gap of about 10 cm away from the nasal cavity.

19.6 Neuroprotective Effects of EO Inhalation on Brain EEG Activity and Psychological Abilities

Various EOs are known for their antioxidant effects as well as neuroprotective effects. These EOs have the ability to improve cognitive function and prevent brain injury. In this regard, EOs can influence various psychological abilities such as speech, reasoning, planning, memory, language, judgment decision-making, and attention span [21]. Cognitive dysfunction can result from impairment of cholinergic neurons, which can result in serious cognitive deficits, mainly in the case of neurodegenerative disorders. A vast amount of literature shows the significant physiological effects of EOs in humans including on respiratory rate, heart rate, corticosteroid serum levels, blood pressure, and alpha and beta brain waves. Moreover, various behavioral perception tests have been performed in humans, which have also evidenced the psychological effects of EOs [22]. Additionally, to study the psychological effects of EOs, a variety of behavioral perception examinations have been conducted in humans. Like psychotropic drugs, EOs have the ability to affect the brain function via interacting with a variety of neurotransmitter pathways such as noradrenergic, serotonergic, GABAergic, and DAergic systems [23]. A number of investigations have shown that due to the intrinsic ability of ACs to interact and influence the CNS, inhalation of EOs can affect the mood, physiology, and behavior of an individual. Inhalation of EOs can cause positive/negative psychological changes, which can be seen in EEG spectra (activation of alpha wave). It has been reported that inhalation of lavender EO considerably reduced alpha wave 1 activity at posterior temporal as well as parietal lobes. Similarly, inhalation of eugenol or chamomile also caused considerable changes of alpha wave 1 activity. These considerable changes in EEG amplitude (alpha or beta waves) after inhalation of EOs could have a positive or negative effect on brain functioning. A previous report suggested that a drop in brain α-1-adrenergic neurotransmission is mainly associated with the cognitive state of individuals [20]. Another report suggested that the administration of neroli and grapefruit oil considerably promotes slowing of α(8 to 10 hertz) and θ brain waves indicating EOs can decrease the inactivation of cortical to further promote the relaxation state of mind [24]. To understand the influence of binasal and uninasal inhalations, the effect of *Abies koreana* EOs on EEG activity was investigated, and it was found that the alpha activity in parietal cortices was considerably improved in the course of inhalation via binasal mode whereas inhalation of EOs via uninasal mode considerably decreased brain waves (absolute β as well as θ values), particularly in the frontal and parietal lobes of the brain. These findings suggest that inhalation of the *Abies koreana* EO could be responsible for augmentation of relaxation when administered via binasal route and improves attentiveness/awareness when delivered via the right uninasal route [25].

Further changes in the theta wave activity modify mind or mental load (drop in theta wave represents decrease in attention). It was found that chocolate as well as *Mentha spicata* EO odors considerably decreased the theta wave in comparison with no-odor control [19]. Similarly, EO obtained from *Betula alba, Jasminun officinale, Lavandula angustifolia,* and *Citrus limon* considerably augmented the brain theta rhythms [26]. Additionally, inhalation of the *Vetiveria zizanioides* EO caused decrease in the alpha and betal activity in both frontal and parietal cortices and increased gamma activity in the frontal cortex. Moreover, the effects of inhalation of the cannabis EO on the central-nervous-system in subjects were investigated, and it was found that EEG spectra showed considerable enhancement in the overall α wave (8 to 13 hertz) and a substantial drop in beta 2 activity. It was concluded that the activity of brain wave and autonomic nervous system (ANS) were influenced by inhalation of the EO, demonstrating neuromodulation in cases of nervousness, depression, and stress [27]. A recent investigation showed that inhalation of the undiluted tangerine EO (*Citrus tangerina*) decreased αwave activities (slow as well as fast) and enhanced β wave activities (low as well as mid waves), whereas dilution of subthreshold as well as threshold demonstrated the reverse outcome in the brain [28]. Another recent study showed that inhalation of *Michelia alba* EO could decrease alertness level, which was observed by decrease in beta wave and increase in fast alpha wave activity. On the other hand, inhalation of pure linalool showed the same responses as inhalation of *Michelia alba* EO [29]. Another study showed sedative (lemon, lavender, and sandalwood) and awakening effects (jasmine, ylang-ylang, rose, and peppermint) of ACs on visual display terminal task activities. Another study showed sedative (lemon, lavender, and sandalwood) and awakening effects (peppermint, rose, ylang-ylang, and jasmine) of EO components on activities of visual display terminal task. It was found that EO components influenced concentration of individuals involved in the study and emotionally calmed them then control group [30]. Inhalation of *Abies sibirica* EO showed enhanced θ brain activity and visual display terminal work showed that the *Abies sibirica* EO considerably decreased arousal levels [31].

It was revealed that isomers of the same ACs present in EOs can also present dissimilar smell characteristics for humans, and due to this variation in their structural configuration, their medicinal as well as biological effects also varied considerably. For instance, the sedative effects of various forms of linalool showed variation among different isomers. It was reported that (RS)-(±)-linalool and (R)-(−)-linalool considerably decreased beta wave activity whereas (S)-(+)-linalool reversed this effect. Another study demonstrated the consequences of linalools (optically active) inhalation on humans, and it was found that stereoisomer-based specificity of linalool caused different smell sensitivity as well as reactions that were dependent on chiral and task [32–34]. One more study based on olfactory stimulation caused by the aromatic isomeric components of EOs [(+)-limonene and terpinolene] suggested that female subjects reacted equally to these components via substantial enhancement of absolute fast brain α activity [32–34]. Investigation on the effect of listening to music on the activity of autonomic nervous system with/without inhalation of the *Citrus bergamia* EO revealed that soft music listening with inhalation of *Citrus bergamia* EO enhanced the relaxation state of the brain. Except the control group, all groups (music, the aroma, and the combined) showed negative variation of the ratio of low frequency to high frequency [32–34]. One more report studied the soothing effects of the fragrance of the yuzu EO from the perspective of the autonomic nervous system activity. It was concluded that yuzu's (*Citrus junos*) aromatic effects could be used to partially relieve negative emotional stress and improve parasympathetic nervous system activity [32–34]. A previous investigation showed that *Chamaemelum nobile* or α-pinene (its major component) inhalation showed antidepressant-like effects among Wistar–Kyoto rodents in the rodent behavioral test (FST). Findings from this study demonstrated that inhalation of α-pinene augmented protein expression that mediates oxidative phosphorylation including acyl carrier protein, adenosine triphosphate (ATP) synthase subunit e, hippocampal ATPase inhibitor, cytochrome b-c1 complex subunit 6, cytochrome c oxidase subunit 6C-2, and cytochrome c oxidase subunit 7A2, in the prefrontal cortex. Moreover, the treatment of Wistar–Kyoto rats with α-pinene–augmented expression of parvalbumin (calcium-binding protein) mRNA level in the hippocampal region. It was also concluded that inhalation of α-pinene showed an antidepressant effect via involving mitochondrial functions and parvalbumin-associated signaling [35]. Another report investigated the effect of music therapy and aromatherapy with chamomile–lavender EO on the anxiety of clinical nurses. It was found that involvement of music therapy and aromatherapy with chamomile–lavender EO can decrease anxiety [36]. One more report investigated the effect of aromatherapy massage (using aromatic oils of lavender and chamomile) on the anxiety and sleep quality of patients with burn injuries. It was found that massage with oils of patients with burn injuries is effective in promoting quality of sleep as well as reducing anxiety [37]. A study based on the effect of inhalation of rose aroma and Benson showed that this combination has a synergistic effect and more effects in the reduction of pain anxiety in patients with burns than a single intervention [38]. A study based on aromatherapy (inhalation and topical treatment) with blend of almond and lavender EOs in treating patients with burns showed better results in terms of in decreasing pain as well as anxiety [39].

A recent meta-analysis based on randomized controlled trials as well as nonrandomized studies that examined the effectiveness of lavender, in any form and way of administration, on patients with anxiety were identified by using electronic database searches. It was concluded that oral administration of lavender EO is effective in the management of anxiety, whereas for inhalation, there is only suggestion of an effect of rational size, owing to the heterogeneity of existing reports. There is so much misperception related to the effective mode of administration of EOs mainly between inhalation and massage of EOs.

EO blend-based back massage and foot bath treatment effects on psychological and physiological state of stroke patients were investigated recently, and it was found these treatments decreased mood state as well as stress and enhanced satisfaction with sleep as well as body temperature among stroke patients [40]. Lavender EO applied via massage seems to be effective; nevertheless, existing investigations are not satisfactory to conclude whether the effectiveness is because of a specific effect of lavender. It was also found that lavender EO-based treatment seems to be safe, as well as simple and cost-effective [41]. The psychophysiological effects of inhalation of lavender EO have recently been studied in various investigations. Earlier reports showed various neuroprotective effects of inhalation of lavender EO such as anxiolytic, mood stabilizer, sedative, and analgesic effects. Chemically, lavender EO contains various components such as camphor, β-ocimene, geraniol, terpinen-4-ol, linalyl acetate, β-caryophyllene, and linalool [42].

Lavender EO-based aromatherapy involves administration of EO via topical or inhalation route or while bathing. Lavender EO is usually obtained from *L. latifolia, L. intermedia, L. stoechas,* and *L. angustifolia* [42].

A previous investigation demonstrated the effects of rosemary and lavender on brain activity, mood as well as attentiveness [43]. It was found that treatment with lavender EO increased drowsiness via increasing beta activity whereas treatment with rosemary EO improved alertness via reducing frontal alpha and beta activity [43].

Moreover, both EOs could cause EEG changes in the left frontal region among infants as well as adults [44]. Furthermore, a study based on determining the impact of lavender or rosemary treatment on the activity of the brain demonstrated that kids of nondepressed as well as depressed moms react in a different manner to aromas [44]. One more report investigated the impact of lavender oil on the EEG activity of females with sleeping complaints, and it was found that the EO reduced alpha activity in the parietal as well as occipital parts of the brain among individuals with improved sleep condition. Additionally, it was shown that the EO elicited β as well as θ brain activities in the occipital and frontal parts of the brain among individuals with great sleep condition. In contrast, inhalation of *L. angustifolia* elicited the θ rhythm throughout the cranial areas among individuals with disturbed sleep. The authors also concluded that aromatic components of *L. angustifolia* could be useful for female adults with sleep complications. A recent investigation showed that inhalation of citrus ginger aroma during sleep may increase sympathetic nervous and endocrine system activity while alleviating psychological tension and anxiety [44]. A recent report demonstrated that Citrus sinensis EO inhalation can be a possible agent to treat anxiety, apparently without involvement of melatonin and corticosterone physiological levels [45].

Another report suggested that inhalation of lavender EO leads to more relaxed, energetic, as well as joyful individuals in comparison to base oil. When compared with base oil, lavender EO efficiently elicited the β as well as θ rhythms. Neuronal mapping revealed that the lavender EO-treated group showed additional scattering effects mainly in the central, temporal as well as bilateral regions for α brainwaves. These findings demonstrate the relaxing property of lavender EO-mediated inhalation [4]. A previous investigation showed the effects of inhalation of Bergamot orange as well as English lavender EO on brain activity, and it was found that inhalation of the EO considerably augmented the absolute θ activity in the prefrontal (right lateral) cortex of the brain [4]. Additionally, inhalation of the EO resulted in considerable variations in the α activity (relative fast as well as slow) in comparison with the control group. Moreover, it was found that a blend of orange bergamot as well as English lavender EO showed greater efficacy than the English lavender EO alone. It is clear that *L. angustifolia*

EO could be potentially used in the management of various mental and physical health-related complications.

One more report indicated that *Zizyphus jujuba* EO considerably reduced the θ rhythm of the brain and elicited electroencephalographic spectral edge frequency and relative power of α as well as γ bands by 50%. Inhalation of the *Z. jujuba* EO resulted in a considerable increase in comparative fast α rhythm i. These findings show that this Jujube EO enhances the relaxation as well as awareness conditions of the brain [46]. An additional study by Cho et al. demonstrated the effect of ACs from the Mentha arvensis EO on EEG activity [46]. It was revealed that inhalation of *M. arvensis* EO considerably increased relative fast α wave whereas γ wave activities as well as electroencephalographic spectral edge frequency 90% were considerably reduced. It was concluded that changes in EEG activity could be linked with a decrease in mental stress. Furthermore, inhalation of jasmine EO has been found to augment the β rhythm in the left posterior as well as anterior center locations of the brain. These fluctuations in EEG activity were linked with intensification of certain feelings including feelings of well-being or feeling active, fresh, and romantic [47].

Another report indicated that inhalation of Kouju (pan-fired Japanese green tea) stimulated positive emotion and influenced the β-1 wave of brain (right frontal area) as well as enhanced memory=[48]. Furthermore, it was found that inhalation of lemon, peppermint, and vanilla showed considerable variation in theta wave activity, which suggested that stimulation of the olfactory system due can influence electrical activity of the brain [48]. Effects of inhalation of Inula helenium EO on human EEG activity was investigated, and it was found that there was a considerable decrease in absolute theta, beta and midβ, and relative θ wave rhythms for the duration of the EO inhalation [48]. Thus, it has been suggested that inhalation of the *I. helenium* EO can increase the alertness state of the brain.

In addition to the effects of inhalation of the EO on brain electrical activity (EEG), other factors such as gender difference also play a significant role in EEG analysis. Earlier reports showed different laterization patterns among the brains of both genders (male and female) in the context of cerebral function [49]. Wood, used for home interior design, showed relaxation of mind and body due to release of volatile organic compounds from wood chips. It was reported that inhalation of isomeric organic compounds [terpinolene as well as (+)-limonene] considerably changed the absolute and relative beta activities in males than in females. Furthermore, female subjects showed considerable increase in absolute fast α wave than males throughout the isomer inhalation [50]. A recent study revealed the effects of VOCs released from inner wood blocks in both male as well as female subjects. It was found that wooden based inside architecture showed positive effects on female's health.

A recent investigation also showed the effects of Japanese cedar wood EO on the regaining condition of woman subjects once they accomplished tedious effort. It was demonstrated that stimulation of olfaction by aromatic components (in vapor phase) of EO isolated from cedar wood (Japanese) changed frame of mind and may reduce the activity of sympathetic nerves. The authors concluded that olfaction caused by these volatile components might be beneficial for providing better mental condition with females.

19.7 Effect of Inhalation of EOs on Sympathetic as well as Parasympathetic Nerves

Several reports confirm that ACs present in EOs modulate function of sympathetic as well as parasympathetic nerves and neurophysiological brain activity. Additionally, these potential compounds independently or synergistically act on neuroendocrine system, neurotransmitters, and neuromodulators, via affecting mental behavior and body function. Inhalation of these ACs can influence various physiological pathways, and in a number of circumstances, can also affect skin function; however, the underlying mechanism behind this is still unclear [51]. These findings suggest that besides regulating smell, the olfactory system (olfaction) in the CNS also regulates other parameters. In this regard, the ACs present in EOs can affect the cutaneous barrier, cutaneous immune system, dehydroepiandrosterone, dopamine, estradiol, oxidative stress, sebum secretion, and stress biomarkers in humans. ACs affecting skin function directly or indirectly could modulate various biochemical parameters via various pathways [51]. It is known that fragrances can positively or negatively affect human behavior via involving psychophysiological activity. Previous reports suggested that fragrances can directly stimulate the olfaction process and affect CNS functions to possess a physiological effect [51]. It was found that inhalation of an EO as well as EO constituents (linalool and its enantiomers) alone causes physiological effects such as changes in verbal as well as nonverbal expressions. Furthermore, it was also found that inhalation of an EO can affect mood and odor in humans. Inhalation of geranium and rosemary has been reported for its anxiolytic effects. Another study revealed the psychophysiological effects of ylang-ylang, orange, geranium, cypress, bergamot, spearmint, and juniper. It was found that inhalation of cypress post-physical activity showed more promising results, and inhalation of juniper after mental work produced favorable impression. Inhalation of orange has been found to decrease nervousness as well as enhance positive mood and stillness among females [52]. A recent study suggested that inhalation of sweet orange EO seemed more effective than inhalation of lavender EO in subjective sleep measures. In addition, inhalation of lavender EO seemed to be more effective than that of sweet orange EO in objective measures, especially in improving sleep latency.

Another report on the effects of inhalation of rose, jasmine, and lavender fragrances of preference revealed that inhalation of preferred aromas decreased muscle sympathetic vasoconstrictor activity. It was also found that black pepper, grapefruit, *Foeniculum vulgare*, and tarragon EOs enhanced sympathetic nerve activities whereas rose or patchouli EOs reduced sympathetic activity [53]. Moreover, chemical components of these oils also influence the autonomic nervous system activity. Generally, the behavior of human beings is mainly connected to attention processes. It has been shown that inhalation of *Mentha piperita*, *Jasminun officinale*, *Cananga odorata*, and

EO constituents (1,8-cineole and menthol) alone considerably affect attention behavior [54]. Further effects of carvone as well as limonene (and their respective enantiomers) inhalation on the ANS and on self-assessment capability were investigated, and it was found that inhalation of EOs for an extended period influenced ANS parameters. Additionally, it was indicated that chirality of ACs could be a major parameter that determines its biological activity.

Psychophysiological effects of lavender oils were investigated, and it was found that inhalation of lavender aroma considerably decreased stress, increased the arousal states of the brain, decreased fatigue (with rosemary), and can be used in the management of disturbing behavior among advanced dementia patients [55]. Recently, EOs from nine aromatic plants (*Santalum album, Citrus aurantium, Citrus limonum, Styrax benzoin, Citrus paradisi, Mentha piperata, Acori tatarinowii* rhizoma, *Rhodiolae crenulatae* radix et rhizoma, and *Camellia sinensis*) were extracted to create a compound EO and were assessed for their therapeutic effect of central fatigue by daily aerial diffusion. It was found that these EOs could reduce fatigue on rats and could be possibly used in the treatment of insomnia, depression, and other disorders [56]. A randomized controlled investigation based on the effect of inhalation of an EO on healthy adults suggested that inhalation of an EO decreased perceived stress and depression and improved sleep quality but did not affect physiological parameters, such as the stress index or immune state. A study on the impacts of Lavandula (soothing effect) and orange blossom (cause olfactory stimulation) on feelings showed relaxation effects by lavender (reduced heart rate as well as conductance of the skin) and stimulating effects by neroli (opposite effects). Additionally, lavender has also been reported on for its ability to relieve pain, to act as a mild sedative, and to improve deep sleep [57]. A randomized controlled trial was performed to study the effect of aromatherapy-based and normal massage on the sleeping patterns of patients with cardiac complications, and it was found that there was considerable variation between sleeping quality patterns assessed by Pittsburgh sleep quality indexes. It was concluded that aromatherapy-based and normal massage may enhance sleep in patients with heart-related problems [58]. It was also suggested that lavender EO improved the condition of sleep and decreased anxiety in patients suffering from coronary heart disease [59]. Randomized controlled investigations revealed that inhalation of lavender EO and sleep hygiene together, and sleep hygiene alone to a lesser degree, improved sleep quality for college students with self-reported sleep issues, with an effect remaining at follow-up [60]. One more study on orange and lavender EOs revealed that lavender decreased anxiety and improved mood [61]. A recent study also showed that aromatherapy with lavender and orange EOs can decrease fatigue in patients who have undergone hemodialysis. Another report demonstrated that aromatherapy based on Lavandula can be used as an efficient treatment to alleviate tiredness as well as nervousness among patients with renal complications such as hemodialysis and chronic kidney failure. However, another report did not find that lavender EO could reduce tiredness among hemodialysis patients [62,63]. Lavender-scented bath oil was used in another study and showed positive relaxation effects with positive improvement in behavioral and cognitive changes on mothers and their infants. One more report demonstrated that aromatherapy-based treatment (massage) with Lavandula EO successfully reduced pain in patients suffering from joint osteoarthritis [64]. An additional study suggested that lavender considerably reduced levels of stress as well as pain. It has been reported that exposure to lavender EO influences work performance by considerably enhancing concentration levels. A recent study compared the efficacy of aromatherapy (English lavender EO alone and blended EO: English lavender, clary sage, and Marjoram) and acupressure on the condition of the sleep as well as well-being in professional females. It was found that the blended EO possessed better dual benefits of improving both quality of life and sleep quality in comparison with the lavender EO alone and acupressure massage in career women [65]. Additionally, a previous study also suggested that massage with lavender, rosemary, lemon, and chamomile EOs decreased anxiety in Korean elderly women [66]. Peppermint odor has been reported for its ability to considerably enhance athletic task performance; nevertheless, it had no effect on skill-related tasks. A recent study showed that lavender aromatherapy had positive effects on peripheral venous cannulation pain, anxiety, and the satisfaction level of patients undergoing surgery [67]. The effects of dimethyl sulfide, *Jasminun officinale* EO, and *Mentha piperita* EO on the physical performance of athletes were investigated in a previous report. It was observed that aromatic components from peppermint induced a slower wave phase of sleep (indicated by delta waves) with improvement in overall sleep and showed variation in response among different genders [68]. Moreover, peppermint oil was also evidenced for its ability to improve exercise performance among young male students [68]. A recent report showed the effect of inhalation of peppermint as well as lavender EOs on the sleep condition of patients suffering from cancer. It was found that mean Pittsburgh sleep quality inventory scores were lower in peppermint as well as lavender treated patients, suggesting that this inhalation treatment can enhance sleep quality among such patients. Another study suggested that peppermint oil considerably improved performance among different subjects [69]. Another report indicated that peppermint oil reduced sleep in a dark room in comparison with a group with a no-odor condition. One more report suggested that peppermint oil enhances memory as well as alertness while ylang-ylang impaired memory and augmented calmness [70]. A recent study showed that *Lavandula angustifolia* as well as *Rosmarinus officinalis* EOs can considerably improve visual perception. It was found that inhalation of *Rosmarinus officinalis* EO enhanced image memory, especially the capability of the brain to memorize numbers while *Lavandula angustifolia* EO deteriorated this response. A recent report showed that exposure to lavender EO reduced anxiety in a fear-conditioned animal test of anxiety [71]. A recent study revealed that inhalation of *Lavandula angustifolia* EO increased memory extinction and, therefore, prevented memory revising among rodents undergoing Pavlovian conditioning protocol [72]. A study based on ylang-ylang oil revealed that oil caused a considerable reduction of blood pressure along with a substantial rise in skin temperature. Additionally, the group treated with ylang-ylang oil was found to be calmer and more relaxed than controls [73]. A previous report based on the effects of *Chamaemelum nobile* EO on mood as well as perception among healthy subjects showed that subjective alertness was linked to sedative effect, and subjective stillness was linked to sedation caused by aroma [74]. A recent investigation also showed that inhalation of Roman chamomile EO can increase the antidepressant property of clomipramine via ameliorating hippocampal neurogenesis and altering corticosterone levels in patients with treatment-resistant depression.

The effects of AC heliotropin on sleep quality were investigated, and it was found that heliotropin effectively improves sleep. An earlier investigation established the relationship between cognitive performance and plasma 1,8-cineole when exposed to *Rosmarinus officinalis* EO volatile components. It was found that 1,8-cineole absorbed from rosemary aroma influenced cognition and subjective state independently via various neurochemical mechanisms. Furthermore, the previous study suggested that inhalation of eucalyptus EO considerably reduced patient's pain and blood pressure after total knee replacement surgery. One more study investigated the effects of bergamot EO in reducing stress associated with work in Taiwan school instructors [75]. Findings from this study revealed that treatment with bergamot EO demonstrated less impact on young instructors with more workload. The psychophysiological effects of inhalation of various EOs were investigated, and it was concluded that EOs may have versatile psychophysiological effects.

Recent systematic reviews have been performed to examine the effects of aromatherapy on the psychophysiological health of postpartum women. The majority of the investigations showed that aromatherapy improved postpartum physiological and psychological health, with positive effects shown on stress, sleep quality, postepisiotomy recovery, postepisiotomy pain, postcesarean-delivery pain, postcesarean-delivery nausea, physical pain, nipple fissure pain, mood, fatigue, distress, depression, and anxiety with no serious intervention-related side effects [76].

19.8 Brain vs. Biotechnology and Nanotechnology

Recent advancements in molecular biology, informatics, and nanoscience facilitate the screening of the effects of CNS-altering drugs. Stem-cell and gene therapies help in treating a wide variety of inherited and acquired human diseases (e.g., inborn error genetic diseases and cancer). Additionally, nanotechnology has the potential to allow the development of new therapeutics for various CNS-related disorders. The libraries of screened nanotherapeutics can be established in neuropharmacological centers for future studies [77–119]. So far, there are limited therapeutics available for many patients with CNS disorders. Nanotechnology can be used to treat neurological disease via screening various CNS-targeted nanotherapeutics. These therapeutics are nanoengineered to cross the blood–brain barrier, act as vehicles for gene delivery and as a matrix to promote axon elongation, respond to endogenous stimuli, support cell survival, and target specific cell or signaling systems [77–119]. EOs have been potentially used to treat different neurological complications; however, low bioavailability and stability-related factors always affect their therapeutic profiles. Encapsulation of EOs in polymeric matrix and surface functionalization of nanomaterials allows for more specific targeted delivery of EOs. This can significantly enhance the bioavailability of EOs both in vitro and in vivo conditions, provide target-specific delivery of EOs, and control the release of EOs [77–119].

19.9 Role of Inhalation of EOs in Depression

Depression is one of the most common psychiatric conditions and can adversely affect quality of life. Antidepressant drugs (first generation: tricyclic antidepressants; second generation: selective serotonin reuptake inhibitors, selective serotonin noradrenaline reuptake inhibitors) primarily increase the accessibility of neurotransmitters such as serotonin so that nerve cells restore these chemicals to pass on signals that were lost along the nerves during depression. There are various antidepressants available for treating depression; however, it is quite challenging to predict in what way these particular drugs will help an individual. Antidepressant medications mainly work by enhancing the amount of the monoamine at the synaptic gap by the following:

- Inhibiting monoamine transporter to eliminate free transmitters
- Monoamine oxidases inhibition to degrade monoamine neurotransmitters
- Binding to pre- or postsynaptic proteins to control the release of monoamine neurotransmitter [120]

Antidepressants can cause various side effects and the most common are due to rapid increase in monoamine level at the receptor sites. Due to the side effects and lack of effectiveness of these drugs along with noncompliance of some patients with treatment, alternative approaches to treating depression are needed. Aromatherapy is an economical and noninvasive therapeutic approach to using plant-derived EOs for various ailments [121]. Recently, aromatherapy has been employed to promote mental health as well as relaxation [122]. EOs comprise an array of aromatic volatile components with a wide range of pharmacological effects. These components can be administered via oral, topical (aromatherapy massage) [123], or olfactory administration (inhalation aromatherapy) [124]. Normally, EOs are administered at varied dose depending on their mode of delivery:

- Delivery via topical application: 1 to 5% EO is required
- Delivery via oral route: 8 to 50% EO is required
- Olfactory administration: A concentrated EO is utilized via inhalation aromatherapy

Nevertheless, the amount as well as concentration of EOs used in practice is not standardized. As EOs are lipophilic, they can easily cross biological membranes organs in the body. Oral administration of EOs is the most effective procedure as via oral administration, components of EOs can reach the bloodstream. On the other hand, olfactory aromatherapy involves the inhalation of EOs that can not only reach the systemic circulation via the rich vascular capillary bed present in the nasal mucosa and the bronchi in the lungs but also trigger various regions of the brain directly via the olfactory epithelium. The olfactory system activation by EOs to further stimulate various regions of the brain involves various mechanisms. Olfactory stimulation via inhalation of EOs involves activation of the olfactory proteins present in the olfactory epithelium, which are connected to the olfactory bulb (Figure 19.1). Once receptors are stimulated, they allow the exchange of ions to generate an impulse in the form of a signal to transmit this olfactory information to the limbic system via the olfactory bulb as well as olfactory afferent nerve fibers. The olfactory cortex receives the signals to release neurotransmitters such as serotonin [125] (Figure 19.1). Composition of EOs usually presents volatile as well non-volatile components, which makes their chemical profiles more complex. Various reports have shown that EOs can be used by topical application (massage), inhalation, or oral route, thus supplementing pharmacodynamic interventions. A vast amount of literature supports the idea that EOs can be used to treat major depressive disorders and associated complications, such as anxiety disorders [126].

19.10 Antidepressant-Like Effects of EOs

Various studies have been performed to study the impact of EOs on human mental health, mainly disorders like depression, anxiety, etc. [127,128]. A recent study showed that cinnamon EO can be used as an alternative therapy in improving symptoms of depressive and anxiety disorders, and it was found that trans-cinnamaldehyde (TCA) could be accountable for the positive effects.

Another recent study showed the antidepressant-like effects of Citrus sinensis EO and its main component, limonene, using the chronic unpredictable mild stress model mice as well its likely mechanisms. The findings suggested that *Citrus sinensis* EO showed antidepressant effects among mice in a chronic unpredictable stress model with decline in body weight, sucrose preference, curiosity, and mobility as well as reduced immobile time as well as dyslipidemia. The limonene level was found to be rich in the inhaling *Citrus sinensis* EO setting as well as the brain of the mice after exposure to inhalation. It was also found that limonene was not metabolized directly in the mice brain. Moreover, inhalation of limonene considerably retained chronic unpredictable mild stress-induced depressive performance, stimulated interaction between hypothalamus, pituitary, and adrenal glands, and reduced monoamine levels with the attenuated pleiotropic protein (brain-derived neurotrophic factor) and expression of its receptor in the hippocampus. The authors concluded that EO treatment improved neuroendocrine, neurotrophic, and monoaminergic systems, which could contribute to the antidepressant activity of limonene [129].

Lavender-based formulations such as lavender EO capsules have been assessed for their effectiveness in treating depression among patients under main course medication treatment [130]. The findings showed that lavender EO decreased some anxiety-associated indications, motor restlessness as well as mental tension, and sleeping disorders among patients suffering from depression, therefore demonstrating considerable recovery in contrast to conventional antidepressant medication alone [130]. The effects of acute inhalation of lavender EO were also investigated on moods among healthy males, and it was found that subjects showed elevated β waves, reported feeling more relaxed, and had fewer depressive moods. The results obtained from this study demonstrated that lavandula EO can boost mood. A recent study also showed that treatment with lavender EO increased depression-like behavior induced by corticosterone. Additionally, it also showed the effect of lavender EO on neuroplasticity and neurogenesis. Treatment with lavender EO inhibited the corticosterone-induced reduction in the number of BrdU positive cells and increased dendritic complexity of immature neurons suggesting the neurogenic property as well as the restorative effect of lavender EO in the presence of high corticosterone. Additionally, it was found that lavender EO treatment increased the brain-derived neurotrophic factor and oxytocin level in male Sprague–Dawley rats [131].

Treatment with garlic EO containing organosulfur (diallyl disulfide [DADS]) as a major component showed antidepressant-like effects. It was found that oral administration of garlic EO considerably reduced immobility time in the FST and, along with DADS, considerably reversed the sucrose preference index decrease induced by unpredictable chronic mild stress. Treatment with garlic EO efficiently reduced the frontal cortex turnover ratio of serotonin as well as dopamine and consequently elevated the serotonin and dopamine levels. The chronic garlic EO was found to elevate the cyclic AMP response element-binding protein, protein kinase B expression, and brain-derived neurotrophic factor in the hippocampus, which showed its potential via modulation of monoamine neurotransmitter and pathways related with brain-derived neurotrophic factor [132].

A recent study showed the antidepressant property of *T. ciliate* EO (containing estragole, β-elemene, β-cubebene, and γ-elemene) by open field test, tail suspension test (TST), and FST. The findings demonstrated that immobility time was considerably decreased by the EO, and no changes were observed in ambulation. Moreover, dopamine, norepinephrine and 5-hydroxytryptamine, and level of hippocampal proteins (brain-derived neurotrophic factor) of chronic mild stress rodents could be elevated by EO treatment [124]. Recent report results demonstrated that the pepper-rosmarin EO as well as thymol showed an antidepressant-like effect similar to fluoxetine [133].

SuHeXiang is known for its potential in treating various CNS-related ailments. A recent study showed that repeated exposure of acute stress-induced mice to inhalation of SuHeXiang considerably produced antidepressant and anxiolytic effects and also decreased levels of tumor necrosis factor-α, thrombopoietin, angiogenin, and interleukin 6 in the serum. Additionally, inhalation of SuHeXiang reversed the depressive and anxiety-like behaviors and decreased the levels of angiogenin and thrombopoietin in the serum of mice exposed to chronic mild stress. These effects could be associated with the ability of SuHeXiang to alter inflammatory pathways and decrease clot formation in blood vessels as well as angiogenesis [134]. A previous investigation showed the antidepressant property of *Acorus tatarinowii* EO as well as asarones (its major components) by using the FST, TST, and open field test. It was found that immobility time was reduced by the EO as well as its component, α-asarone, without any change in ambulation, suggesting its antidepressant-like effects [135]. Another investigation was performed to study the antidepressant property of *Origanum majorana* EO on rodent by using the FST, and it was found that *Origanum majorana* treatment considerably decreased immobility time and enhanced swimming and climbing times. It was also suggested that Origanum majorana EO displayed antidepressant-like effects via involving dopaminergic (Dl and D2), serotonergic (5HT1A, 5-HT2A receptors), and noradrenergic (α1 and α2 adrenoceptors) pathways [136]. In accordance with a recent study, oregano EO could have antidepressant-like effects but had no effect on stress-induced TLR-2/4 upregulation [137]. Inhalation of Cang-ai volatile oil has been used for centuries to treat some depressive and emotive disorders. A recent investigation showed that Cang-ai volatile oil can improve depressive-like behaviors concomitant with the regulation of serotonin and dopamine metabolism in the brains of chronic unpredictable mild stress-induced rats [138]. A recent report revealed that agarwood EO considerably reduced the gene expression of the corticotropin-releasing factor and considerably prevented the transcription of gene as well as expression of protein its receptor CRFR (corticotropin-releasing factor and its receptor) in the hippocampus and cerebral cortex. Moreover, agarwood EO decreased the level of corticosterone as well as adrenocorticotropic hormone with downregulation of hypothalamic–pituitary–adrenal activity in a dose-dependent manner. The authors concluded that agarwood EO reduced anxiety as well as depression, which could be associated with the suppression of corticotropin-releasing factor and hyperstimulation of hypothalamic–pituitary–adrenal activity [139]. A recent study showed the anxiolytic, sedative, antiepileptic, and antidepressant effects of *Annona vepretorum* EO. Findings from this study suggested that EO acute treatment showed anxiolytic, sedative, antiepileptic, and antidepressant effects [139]. In addition, anxiolytic and anticonvulsant effects were possibly mediated by the GABAergic system whereas the antidepressant effect was possibly mediated by serotonergic receptors. Furthermore, it was observed that the EO when complexed with β-cyclodextrin improved various behavior parameters [140]. One more report showed the effectiveness of *Onosma bracteatum* EO in reducing anxiety as well as depression by using the elevated plus-maze, open field FST, and TST tests. Findings from this study suggested that the EO in the FST reduced immobility time and prolonged mobility time in a dose-dependent manner. Similarly, in the TST, the EO extended the time span of mobility and reduced immobility time in a dosage-dependent manner. A recent study indicated antidepression-like effects of *Satureja bachtiarica* EO against reserpine-induced depression in a rat model. The results obtained from this study demonstrated that *Satureja bachtiarica* EO considerably enhanced the immobility time of rats in the FST and improved the reserpine-induced changes. The authors concluded that the Marze EO could prevent depression induced by reserpine probably via its antioxidant activity [141]. *Rosmarinus officinalis* EO has been known to have various pharmacological properties. A recent investigation showed that *Rosmarinus officinalis* EO has antidepressant-like effects, acts as cognitive enhancer, and prevents oxidative stress in the brain as well as prevents changes in acetylcholinesterase activity in the zebrafish model. Findings suggested that *Rosmarinus officinalis* EO possessed antidepressant-like effects and cognitive-enhancing action. Additionally, *Rosmarinus officinalis* EO was able to stop acetylcholinesterase change and brain oxidative stress induced by scopolamine [142].

In another study, the ability of *Thymus vulgaris* EO to ameliorate cognitive function via action on cholinergic neurons by means of the scopolamine-induced zebrafish model of memory impairments was investigated. It was revealed that *Thymus vulgaris* EO improved scopolamine-induced increasing AChE (Acetylcholinesterase) activity, memory loss, and anxiety and decreased brain antioxidant ability. The findings suggested that *Thymus vulgaris* EO could be used in the treatment of memory deficits through the inhibition of AChE activity and brain oxidative stress in scopolamine-treated zebrafish with amnesia [143]. A recent report revealed that *Schinus terebinthifolius* EO could be used in the treatment of memory deficits through the inhibition of AChE activity and brain oxidative stress in scopolamine-treated zebrafish with amnesia [144]. It was also reported that Ferulago angulata EO improved scopolamine-induced spatial memory impairment by reducing oxidative stress in rat hippocampus [145].

A recent study based on monoterpene-enriched Tetraclinis articulata EO showed its ability in reversing the Aβ1–42-induced decline of the spontaneous alternation in the Y-maze test and the Aβ1–42-induced increase of the working and reference memory errors in the radial arm maze test. These findings suggested that Tetraclinis articulata EO can be effectively used against dementia by modulating cholinergic activity and stimulating antioxidant property in rat hippocampus [146]. Similarly, *Pinus halepensis* EO has been demonstrated for its nootropic and neuroprotective effect, which could be considered as a therapeutic tool for reducing Aβ toxicity and neuronal dysfunction [147]. An additional report also suggested that inhalation of coriander volatile oil improves Aβ(1–42)-induced spatial memory impairment by reducing the oxidative stress in rat hippocampus [148]. Later, it was show that many treatments with coriander EO can reduce oxidative stress, depression, and anxiety in Alzheimer's. It was found that coriander volatile oil exposure to beta-amyloid (1–42)–treated rats improved complications caused by beta-amyloid, demonstrating its effectiveness in reducing anxiety and depression. Additionally, in β-amyloid treated rodents, coriander EO reduced catalase level and augmented the level of glutathione in the hippocampal region [149]. The study also suggested that *Juniperus communis* EO can be potentially utilized to reduce oxidative damage linked to Alzheimer's via acting as acetylcholinesterase inhibitor as well as antioxidant [150]. Another report suggested that cardamom EO treatment considerably improves behavioral parameters, inhibits AChE activity, and decreases oxidative stress in the brain. Histopathological studies showed that cardamom oil treatment inhibits neuronal damage and amyloid β plaque formation. An immunohistochemistry analysis showed that cardamom EO prevented amyloid β expression and increased the brain-derived neurotrophic factor level. It was found that cardamom EO provides a neuroprotective effect in aluminum chloride-induced neurotoxicity associated with suppression of the AChE level and decrease in oxidative injury. It was also concluded that cardamom EO could be useful as a potential agent to manage the symptoms of Alzheimer's disease [151].

A recent report also suggested the neuroprotective property of sesame oil in the modulation of the diverse molecular pathways responsible for causing oxidative stress and neuroinflammation. Additionally, it was also found that sesame oil can possibly influence various molecular mechanisms involved in pathogenesis of Alzheimer's disease via modulation of NF-κB/p38MAPK/BDNF/PPAR-γ signaling, and these effects could be due to the synergistic effect of the active compounds present in it [152]. Aniba rosaeodora (pau-rosa), Aniba parviflora (macacaporanga), and Aeollanthus suaveolens (catinga-de-mulata) EOs contain linalool as the main component and have been used in Brazil for its various CNS-related effects including sedative, anticonvulsant, and antidepressant effects. Findings from this study suggested that possibly due to the presence of linalool or via synergistic action of other constituents, *Aniba rosaeodora*, *Aniba parviflora*, and *Aeollanthus suaveolens* EOs have antidepressant effects with no compromise of spontaneous locomotion and memory retention in rodents [153]. A recent study showed antidepressant-like and sedative-like activity effects of the *Listea glaucescens* EO, which contains β-pinene and linalool as the main components whereas chemical components eucalyptol, limonene, and α-pinene did not show antidepressant-like effects [154]. A recent study showed that the *Piper guineense* EO, which contains β-sesquiphellandrene as a major component, exhibited CNS depressant, hypothermic, sedative, muscle relaxant, antipsychotic, and anticonvulsant effects [155]. *Ocimum basilicum* EO increased the chronic unpredictable mild stress-induced depressive status and considerably deceased corticosterone level and increased gene as well as protein expressions of glucocorticoid receptors and brain-derived neurotropic factor. *Ocimum basilicum* EO decreased chronic unpredictable mild stress-induced hippocampal neuron atrophy and apoptosis, as well as elevated number of astrocytes and new nerve cells. *Ocimum basilicum* EO considerably ameliorated glial fibrillary acidic protein (GFAP)-positive cells along with the expression of the hippocampal glucocorticoid proteins as well as brain-derived neurotropic factor [156].

Ocimum basilicum EO reduced symptoms associated with depression and diminished short-term memory linked with degeneration of nerves triggered in rodents when exposed to chronic erratic moderate stress [157]. Furthermore, *Ocimum basilicum* EO increased the corticosterone level in serum, the level of brain-derived neurotropic factor protein as well as glucocorticoid protein in the hippocampus. In addition, *Ocimum basilicum* EO decreased the degeneration of nerves and any changes at tissue level triggered in the hippocampus when exposed to chronic unpredictable mild stress [157]. Thus, it was concluded by the authors that *Ocimum basilicum* EO can be used as an effective natural agent to treat Alzheimer's disease.

An earlier study suggested that concomitant treatment of rats with scopolamine and *Anthriscus nemorosa* showed substantial enhancement of memory formation as well as possessed anxiolytic- and antidepressant-like effects. The results obtained from this study demonstrated that inhalation of *Anthriscus nemorosa* EO can inhibit scopolamine-mediated depression, memory impairment, and anxiety [158]. A previous report suggested that inhalation of P. peregrina EO improves scopolamine-induced memory impairment, anxiety, and depression. In addition, P. peregrina EO may be used as a possible therapeutic agent to treat neurological complications associated with Alzheimer's disease [159].

Silexan is an EO obtained from *Lavandula angustifolia* and has been used to treat various anxiety disorders. Recently, the antidepressant-like effects of Silexan using *in vivo* and *in vitro* assays models were studied. It was found that the antidepressant property of Silexan in the FST were equivalent to the tricyclic antidepressant imipramine. In addition, silexan has been reported to activate neurite outgrowth and synaptogenesis in neuronal cell models and considerably alleviated synaptogenesis in primary hippocampal neurons. Furthermore, silexan has also been reported to increase phosphorylation of protein kinase A and succeeding CREB (cAMP response element-binding protein) phosphorylation [160].

A recent report also supports the antidepressant-like effects of Silexan® among anxious patients, especially those suffering from comorbid depressive symptoms and in patients with mixed anxiety–depression disorder. A possible molecular mechanism followed by Silexan® is similar to pregabalin (i.e., suppression of voltage-dependent calcium channels). Nevertheless, pregabalin primarily suppresses P/Q-type channels via binding to a modulatory subunit, whereas Silexan® reasonably suppresses primarily T-type and N-type channels and slightly P/Q-type channels. In comparison with pregabalin, Silexan® did not cause hypnotic or sedative side effects and does not have abuse potential. As far as antidepressant effects are concerned, Silexan® improves numerous aspects of neuroplasticity via activation of the transcription factor CREB, intracellular signaling kinases (protein kinase and the mitogen-activated protein kinase), which is considered as the ultimate mechanism of all antidepressant drugs. It was concluded by the authors that Silexan® modulates intracellular signaling kinases expression via intracellular signaling cascade resulting in voltage-dependent calcium channel modulation, CREB activation, and improved neuroplasticity [161].

A previous study showed the antidepressant-like effects of *Asarum heterotropoides* EO in mice [31]. GC analysis revealed main compounds such as methyl 2,3,5-trimethoxytoluene pentadecane and eugenol. Acute inhalation of *Asarum heterotropoides* EO showed antidepressant-like effects in behavioral despair assays in mice. Antidepressant-like effects could be due to the prevalence of methyl eugenol [162]. Treatment with the EO upregulated the expression of corticotropin-releasing factor level as well as tyrosine hydroxylase and downregulated the expression of serotonin in brain. Also, EO administration considerably decreased serotonin in mouse dorsal raphe after FST. It was also found that inhalation of the *Asarum heterotropoides* EO normalized the level of 5-HT, corticotropin-releasing factor, as well as tyrosine hydroxylase. Thus, this EO suppressed depression-like effects among mice exposed to stress [163].

Acute inhalation treatment of *Citrus limon* EO decreased immobility time in the FST in rodents (rats as well as mice) [164]. Nevertheless, a similar study demonstrated that lemon EO decreased locomotion and exploration in the open field, suggesting its sedative action [164]. In another report, the antidepressant, anxiolytic, and sedative properties of lemon EO were investigated by open field, elevated plus-maze, rotarod, pentobarbital-induced sleeping time, and FSTs in mice. It was revealed that the EO possibly showed sedative and anxiolytic effects via involving benzodiazepine-type receptors and antidepressant effect via noradrenergic and serotoninergic pathways. It was suggested by Lopes et al. that *Citrus limon* EO contains various monoterpenes such as limonene, geranyl acetate, and trans-limonene oxide.

On the other hand, limonene showed the opposite effects on mood states in the rat model. Acute treatment with limonene was found to be inactive in the mouse FST. Nevertheless, after continued administration, limonene reversed augmented immobility time in the FST caused by neuropathic pain in the rodent model. It was suggested that 5-HT and dopamine mediate the antidepressant-like effects of lemon EO. The antidepressant action of *Citrus limon* EO was inhibited by pretreatment with buspirone, DOI (5-HT2A receptor agonist), miaserin, apomorphin, and haloperidol [164]. In addition, the acute administration of *Citrus limon* EO considerably augmented the hippocampal dopamine level and prefrontal cortex as well as hippocampal 5-HT level [164]. Because dopamine and 5-HT mediate mood states, the prefrontal cortex as well as hippocampal region are the primary sites of action. It was concluded that the antidepressant-like effects of *Citrus limon* EO could be due to the presence of limonene.

Acute *Eugenia uniflora* EO treatment of mice showed antidepressant-like activities in the TST in a concentration-dependent manner [165]. Gas chromatography–mass spectrometry (GC–MS) analysis showed that *Eugenia uniflora* EO contains selina-1,3,7-trien-8-one-oxide, selina-1,3,7-trien-8-one, β-caryophyllene, germacrene A, B & D, and curzerene.

It was also found that acute treatment of mice with β-caryophyllene caused strong antidepressant-like effects in the FST and the TST and novelty-suppressed feeding behavior. AM630 (CB2 receptor antagonist) inhibited the antidepressant effects of β-caryophyllene, suggesting that β-caryophyllene activates CB 2 cannabinoid receptors. Cannabinoid CB2 receptors are involved in brain function and in neuropsychiatric disorders. A previous study suggested that genetically induced low function of the CB2Rs intensifies vulnerability to depression, thus these receptors' modulation of anxiety and depressive states. It was also demonstrated that Eugenia uniflora EO-induced antidepressant effects were mediated via involvement of monoamines neurotransmission [165]. It was found that inhibition of α1- as well as α2-receptors and serotonin 5-HT2A suppressed the antidepressant action of *Eugenia uniflora* EO in the rodent TST.

Two different groups of researchers from China have evidenced the antidepressant-like activity of *Perilla frutescens* EO. In both reports, the EO reversed behavioral, neurochemical, and immunological changes induced by stress in chronic unpredictable mild stress mice [122]. The first report demonstrated that *Perilla frutescens* EO administration in mice was found to restore the chronic unpredictable mild stress-induced reduced sucrose preference and enhanced immobility time, without affecting body weight gain and locomotor activity. Also, EO treatment increased the reduced level of behaviors and brain-derived neurotrophic factor mRNA and protein expression in the hippocampus of mice.

The second report demonstrated that chronic administration resulted in restoration of sucrose-preference in stressed mice. Additionally, treatment with the EO also restored the augmented immobility time in the FST and the TST in chronic unpredictable mild stress mice, therefore corroborating the strong antidepressant-like effects [122]. Furthermore, both studies showed changes in the level of 5-HT and the brain-derived neurotrophic factor, suggesting its antidepressant effects. Treatment with the EO efficiently restored the decreased hippocampal level of 5-HT as well 5-HIAA, brain-derived neurotrophic factor, and mRNA [122]. Several reports suggested that proinflammatory cytokines, mainly interleukin-1 beta (IL-1β), interleukin 6 (IL-6), and tumor necrosis factor α (TNF-α), have been found to be increased in major depression [51]. Treatment with the *Perilla frutescens* EO reduced the serum level of TNF-α, IL-1β, and IL-6 among chronic unpredictable mild stress mice. A previous report revealed the chemical profile of an EO containing β-caryophyllene, selinene, santalene, perillaldehyde, limonene, and bergamotene [52].

Administration of L-perillaldehyde also showed an antidepressant-like property in mice [166]. Continuous treatment (oral and inhaled) with L-perillaldehyde reversed depressant-like effects caused by chronic unpredictable mild stress and lipopolysaccharide [166]. The antidepressant effects of L-perillaldehyde are mediated by noradrenaline as well as serotonin as EO treatment restored the 5-HT and noradrenaline level in the prefrontal cortex in lipopolysaccharide-treated mice as well as reduced lipopolysaccharide-induced surge of TNF-α and IL-6 levels [166]. The *Perilla frutescens* EO also contains limonene and beta-caryophyllene, which have been reported on for their antidepressant-like effects [43,49].

A recent study showed that *S. terebinthifolius* EO as well as its components, including (R)-(+)-limonene and α-phellandrene, exhibit antihyperalgesic effects against mechanical hyperalgesia and are antidepressive, while only α-phellandrene inhibited cold hyperalgesia in spared nerve injury rats [167].

An earlier report showed that acute exposure of *Salvia sclarea* EO (contains linalyl acetate, linalool, and geraniol) rats in the FST reduced immobility time, which has been found to be similar to conventional antidepressant drugs [166]. It was found that the antidepressant effect of this EO was inhibited by pretreatment with haloperidol, SCH-23390, and buspirone. Acute administration of linalool and geraniol has demonstrated to have consistent antidepressant effects in experimental animal models [168]. The antidepressant effects of linalool were inhibited by WAY100635 and yohimbine, suggesting that these effects were mediated via monoaminergic neurotransmission [168,169]. Finally, it was concluded that *Salvia sclarea L.* EO possessed antidepressant action due to the synergistic effects of chemical compounds present in the EO. A new report indicated that *Salvia multicaulis* EO possesses considerable antiamnesic activity and anxiolytic- and antidepressant-like effects in scopolamine-treated rats. It was also concluded that *Salvia multicaulis* EO could be used as a promising agent for improving dementia-related abnormalities.

Another report showed that the safety of *S. aromaticum* EO as well as its effectiveness in exhibiting antidepressant-like effects could be due to improvement in the hippocampal pERK1/2-pCREB-BDNF pathway in the rodent model when exposed to chronic unpredictable mild stress [170]. Earlier findings revealed the chemical profile of *S. aromaticum* EO, which contains major compounds such as eugenol, β-caryophyllene, and eugenyl acetate [170].

Previous reports corroborated the effectiveness of β-caryophyllene as well as eugenol in reducing depression-like effects [171], which might be synergistically contributing to the antidepressant properties of *S. aromaticum* EO. It was observed that repetitive treatment with eugenol decreased immobility in the FST and TST [171]. The antidepressant effects of eugenol could be due to its inhibitory effects over the level of monoamine oxidase A as well as elevated hippocampal brain-derived neurotrophic factor [171]. The results obtained from this study demonstrated that not only β but both caryophyllene as well as eugenol may perhaps mediate the antidepressant-like effects of *S. aromaticum* EO by ameliorating monoamine neurotransmission and neuroplastic properties.

Treatment of mice in the FST and TST with the *Toona ciliata* EO (containing estragole, β-elemene, γ-elemene, and β-cubebene) suggested antidepressant-like effects in a dose-dependent way [124]. Moreover, *Toona ciliata* EO administration in mice augmented brain-derived neurotrophic factor level and hippocampal monoamines (5-HT, noradrenaline, and dopamine) among rats exposed to unpredictable mild stress [124].The *Valeriana wallichii* EO showed different antidepressant responses as acute or chronic treatment. Acute treatment with *Valeriana wallichii* EO decreased time of immobility in mice in the FST. Chronic treatment with *Valeriana wallichii* EO increased serotonin as well as norepinephrine levels in rodent brain [171]. It was also demonstrated that these acute antidepressant-like effects of *V. wallichii* EO are mediated via involvement of the nitric oxide (NO) signaling pathway. Chronic treatment of mouse indicated elevated brain serotonin as well as norepinephrine levels [171]. Additional reports showed involvement of NO-mediated path in the antidepressant-like actions of *V. wallichii* EO. It was also found that the antidepressant effect was inhibited when the mouse was pretreated with L-arginine and sildenafil; however, the effect was increased with L-NAME and methylene blue. The results obtained from this study corroborated earlier reports that showed decrease of NO levels in the brain resulting in improvement of antidepressant-like effects. GC–MS analysis showed that oil contains patchouli alcohol as the main component. Additionally, it also contains other components such as δ-guaiene, virdiflorol, seychellene, and 8-acetoxyl patchouli alcohol [171].

19.11 Antidepressant Effects of EO Components

The antidepressant effects of isolated EO components along with their possible mechanism of action are described in this section.

Several reports are available that corroborate the antidepressant-like effects of eugenol confirmed by FST and TSTs. The primary target of eugenol is monoamine oxidase inhibitors enzyme [172], to metabolize monoamines, including serotonin, norepinephrine, and dopamine. Eugenol showed its antidepressant-like effects via specifically inhibiting MAOA (Monoamine oxidase A) activity. In addition, chronic treatment with eugenol elevates the brain-derived neurotrophic factor level, a protein that plays a significant role in the maintenance and survival of neurons and in synaptic plasticity. The level of brain-derived neurotrophic factor is found to be decreased in depressed patients, which can be reversed by eugenol.

Linalool, mainly isolated from lavender and Salvia sclarea EOs [173], showed antidepressant effects via stimulation of monoamine 5-HT1A and α2-receptors during acute administration [168]. A previous report demonstrated that linalool and β-pinene produce an antidepressant-like effect via interaction with the monoaminergic system. It was found that WAY-100635 (a 5-HT1A receptor antagonist) inhibited the antidepressant-like effect of linalool and β-pinene. In contrast, pretreatment of mice with PCPA (a serotonin synthesis inhibitor) did not affect decrease in the immobility time provoked by linalool and β-pinene. The yohimbine (an α2 receptor antagonist) altered the antidepressant effect of linalool. Propranolol (a β receptor antagonist) and neurotoxin DSP-4 (a noradrenergic neurotoxin) reversed the anti-immobility effect of β-pinene; also, SCH23390 (a D1 receptor antagonist) inhibited the antidepressant-like action of β-pinene.

On the other hand, pretreatment with prazosin, yohimbine, and PCPA did not modify the antidepressant effects induced by carvacrol. These findings suggest that β-pinene appears to induce antidepressant effects via involving dopaminergic, serotoninergic, and noradrenergic pathways whereas carvacrol only involves dopaminergic pathway to induce antidepressant effects.

EO components including L-menthone, perillaldehyde, thymol, and thymoquinone possibly show antidepressant-like effects via involving monoamines neurotransmission. These EO components elevate the level of monoamines in the brain. Various reports showed that carvacrol and β-pinene potentiate antidepressant-like effects in the TST and the TST [174]. It was found that acute administration with these EO components reduced the immobility time, and this response was changed via dopamine D1 antagonist pretreatment [174].

A previous report showed antidepressant-like effects of thymol, monoterpene isolated from *Thymus vulgaris,* among mice exposed to chronic unpredictable mild stress. Thymol treatment considerably changed the reduction of sucrose intake, decrease in weight of the body, and the decrease of immobile time in the TSTs and FSTs caused by chronic unpredictable mild stress paradigm. Chronic treatments with thymol considerably normalized the chronic unpredictable mild stress-induced changes of the monoamine level in the hippocampus. Findings from this report also showed treatment with thymol decreased the level of proinflammatory cytokines such as interleukin (IL)-1β, IL-6 and tumor necrosis factor-α in chronic unpredictable mild stress-induced mice. Additionally, thymol also suppressed the stimulation of inflammasome (NLRP3) and its adaptor and afterward reduced the caspase-1 expression [175]. Similar findings have been reported in the case of geraniol, which is known for its neuroprotective and anti-inflammatory effects, and is frequently found in the EOs of rose, ginger, lemon, orange, lavender, etc. Findings from this report suggested that geraniol treatment considerably relieved the depression-related effects of chronic unpredictable mild stress-induced mice, as shown by restoring reduced sucrose liking as well as reduced immobile time in the FSTs and TSTs. These actions of geraniol were mediated via altering CUMS (chronic unpredictable mild stress)-induced proinflammatory cytokine IL-1β associated neuroinflammation. It was also discovered by the researchers that treatment with geraniol reversed CUMS-induced IL-1β raise, probably via blocking transcription factor (NF-κB) route stimulation as well as via regulating expression of NLRP3 inflammasome [176].

Various other EO components such as L-menthone, the main chemical compound of mint (has been considered as safe and healthy natural component by the FDA, USA), have been reported for their potential antidepressant-like effects in rodents L-menthone [177]. L-menthone produced antidepressant-like effects in the FST in mice, which were mediated by the modification of 5-HTergic, GABAergic, and DAergic pathways.

Another report demonstrated that L-menthone, from Mentha species (which has been extensively utilized as a cooling agent as well as analgesic), has been reported for its antidepressant-like effects. The results obtained from this study demonstrated the potential antidepressant-like action of L-menthone in rodents exposed to unpredictable chronic mild stress via regulating the NLRP3 inflammasome, mediating inflammatory cytokines (TNF-α, (IL)-1β and IL-6) and central neurotransmitters (norepinephrine and serotonin) in the hippocampus [178].

Natural anti-inflammatory agents from EOs have been evidenced for their antidepressant-like effects as their capability in reducing inflammation could be possibly related to their antidepressant-like effects. Several reports showed a relation between the level of proinflammatory cytokines [such as interleukin (IL)-1β, IL-6, and tumor necrosis factor-α] and depressive symptoms. A simultaneous decrease in both proinflammatory cytokine level and depressive symptoms after treatment with anti-inflammatory agents has been observed [73]. In this context, proinflammatory mediators and as well as intracellular signaling proteins such as TLR4, NF-κB-1, p-p65, TNF-α, NLRP3, ASC, and caspase-1 usually increased by stress inhibited by L-menthone, thymol, geraniol, and trans-cinnamaldehyde [179].

As is known TCA is a cyclooxygenase-2 (COX-2) inhibitor and is also known for its inhibitory effects over depression-like behavior in chronic unexpected mild stress, plus maze test, and open field test. A recent study demonstrated the molecular mechanism of TCA-induced antidepression effect by using the FST in male BALB/c mice. Findings from this study showed that TCA produced a substantial effect on reduced immobility in the FST, which showed that TCA inhibited depression-like behavior. Furthermore, TCA increased the 5-HT level with reduction in the Glu/GABA level in the hippocampus of mice. TCA considerably reduced the level of COX-2, TRPV1, and CB1 protein in mice hippocampus. These results demonstrated that treatment with TCA possessed an antidepressive effect and regulated neurotransmitters in the FST [180]. Various biotechnological approaches can be utilized to improve the yield of CNS acting phytochemicals present in EOs [181–195].

REFERENCES

1. Chandra SR, Asheeb A, Dash S, Retna N, Ravi Teja KV, Issac TG. Role of electroencephalography in the diagnosis and treatment of neuropsychiatric border zone syndromes. *Indian J Psychol Med.* 2017;39(3):243–249.
2. Angelucci FL, Silva VV, Dal Pizzol C, Spir LG, Praes CE, Maibach H. Physiological effect of olfactory stimuli inhalation in humans: An overview. *Int J Cosmet Sci.* 2014;36(2):117–123.
3. Grabenhorst F, Rolls ET, Margot C. A hedonically complex odor mixture produces an attentional capture effect in the brain. *Neuroimage.* 2011;55(2):832–843.
4. Sayorwan W, Siripornpanich V, Piriyapunyaporn T, Hongratanaworakit T, Kotchabhakdi N, Ruangrungsi N. The effects of lavender oil inhalation on emotional states, autonomic nervous system, and brain electrical activity. *J Med Assoc Thai.* 2012;95(4):598–606.
5. Achermann P. EEG analysis applied to sleep. *Epileptologie.* 2009;26:28–33.
6. Tisserand R. *The Art of Aromatherapy.* C.W. Daniel, Essex; 1977.
7. Jellinek JS. Psychodynamic odor effects and their mechanisms. *Cosmet Toiletr.* 1997;112:61–71.
8. Kako H, Fukumoto S, Kobayashi Y, Yokogoshi H. Effects of direct exposure of green odour components on dopamine release from rat brain striatal slices and PC12 cells. *Brain Res Bull.* 2008;75(5):706–712.
9. Herz RS. Aromatherapy facts and fictions: A scientific analysis of olfactory effects on mood, physiology and behavior. *Int J Neurosci.* 2009;119(2):263–290.
10. Touhara K, Vosshall LB. Sensing odorants and pheromones with chemosensory receptors. *Annu Rev Physiol.* 2009;71:307–332.
11. Field T, Diego M, Hernandez-Reif M, Cisneros W, Feijo L, Vera Y, Gil K, Grina D, Claire He Q. Lavender fragrance cleansing gel effects on relaxation. *Int J Neurosci.* 2005;115(2):207–222.
12. Féron F, Perry C, McGrath JJ, Mackay-Sim A. New techniques for biopsy and culture of human olfactory epithelial neurons. *Arch Otolaryngol Head Neck Surg.* 1998; 124(8):861–866.
13. Alan MS, Royet JP. Structure and function of the olfactory system. In: Brewer WJ, Castle D, Pantelis C, editors. *Olfaction and the Brain.* Cambridge University Press, Cambridge, UK; 2006:3–27.
14. Breer H. Sense of smell: Recognition and transduction of olfactory signals. *Biochem Soc Trans.* 2003;31(Pt 1): 113–116.

15. Benarroch EE. Olfactory system: Functional organization and involvement in neurodegenerative disease. *Neurology.* 2010;75(12):1104–1109.
16. Dade LA, Zatorre RJ, Jones-Gotman M. Olfactory learning: Convergent findings from lesion and brain imaging studies in humans. *Brain.* 2002;125(Pt 1):86–101.
17. Krbot Skorić M, Adamec I, Jerbić AB, Gabelić T, Hajnšek S, Habek M. Electroencephalographic response to different odors in healthy individuals: A promising tool for objective assessment of olfactory disorders. *Clin EEG Neurosci.* 2015;46(4):370–376.
18. Iijima M, Osawa M, Nishitani N, Iwata M. Effects of incense on brain function: Evaluation using electroencephalograms and event-related potentials. *Neuropsychobiology.* 2009;59(2):80–86.
19. Martin GN. Human electroencephalographic (EEG) response to olfactory stimulation: Two experiments using the aroma of food. *Int J Psychophysiol.* 1998;30(3):287–302.
20. Masago R, Matsuda T, Kikuchi Y, Miyazaki Y, Iwanaga K, Harada H, Katsuura T. Effects of inhalation of essential oils on EEG activity and sensory evaluation. *J Physiol Anthropol Appl Human Sci.* 2000;19(1):35–42.
21. Fisher GG, Chacon M, Chaffee DS. Theories of cognitive aging and work. In: Baltes B, Rudolph C, Zacher H (editors). *Work Across the Lifespan.* Elsevier, Amsterdam; 2019;17–45.
22. Lizarraga-Valderrama LR. Effects of essential oils on central nervous system: Focus on mental health. *Phytother Res.* 2020;35(6):1–23.
23. Perry N, Perry E. Aromatherapy in the management of psychiatric disorders. *CNS Drugs.* 2006;20:257–280.
24. Iijima M, Nio E, Nashimoto E, Iwata M. Effects of aroma on the autonomic nervous system and brain activity under stress conditions. *Auton Neurosci.* 2007;135:97–98.
25. Seo M, Sowndhararajan K, Kim S. Influence of binasal and uninasal inhalations of essential oil of *Abies koreana* twigs on electroencephalographic activity of human. *Behav Neurol.* 2016;2016:9250935.
26. Cheaha D, Issuriya A, Manor R, Kwangjai J, Rujiralai T, Kumarnsit E. Modification of sleep-waking and electroencephalogram induced by vetiver essential oil inhalation. *J Intercult Ethnopharmacol.* 2016;5(1):72–78.
27. Gulluni N, Re T, Loiacono I, Lanzo G, Gori L, Macchi C, Epifani F, Bragazzi N, Firenzuoli F. Cannabis essential oil: A preliminary study for the evaluation of the brain effects. *Evid Based Complement Alternat Med.* 2018;2018:1709182.
28. Chandharakool S, Koomhin P, Sinlapasorn J, et al. Effects of tangerine essential oil on brain waves, moods, and sleep onset latency. *Molecules.* 2020;25(20):4865.
29. Koomhin P, Sattayakhom A, Chandharakool S, et al. Michelia essential oil inhalation increases fast alpha wave activity. *Sci Pharm.* 2020;88:23.
30. Kawakami M, Aoki S, Ohkubo T. A study of "fragrance" on working environment characteristics in VDT work activities. *Int J Prod Econ.* 1999;60–61:575–581.
31. Matsubara E, Fukagawa M, Okamoto T, Ohnuki K, Shimizu K, Kondo R. The essential oil of *Abies sibirica* (pinaceae) reduces arousal levels after visual display terminal work. *Flavour Frag J.* 2011;26:204–210.
32. Laska M, Teubner P. Olfactory discrimination ability of human subjects for ten pairs of enantiomers. *Chem Senses.* 1999;24(2):161–170.
33. Sugawara Y, Hara C, Aoki T, Sugimoto N, Masujima T. Odor distinctiveness between enantiomers of linalool: Difference in perception and responses elicited by sensory test and forehead surface potential wave measurement. *Chem Senses.* 2000;25(1):77–84.
34. Peng SM, Koo M, Yu ZR. Effects of music and essential oil inhalation on cardiac autonomic balance in healthy individuals. *J Altern Complement Med.* 2009;15(1):53–57.
35. Kong Y, Wang T, Wang R, Ma Y, Song S, Liu J, Hu W, Li S. Inhalation of roman chamomile essential oil attenuates depressive-like behaviors in Wistar Kyoto rats. *Sci China Life Sci.* 2017;60(6):647–655.
36. Zamanifar S, Bagheri-Saveh MI, Nezakati A, Mohammadi R, Seidi J. The effect of music therapy and aromatherapy with chamomile-lavender essential oil on the anxiety of clinical nurses: A randomized and double-blind clinical trial. *J Med Life.* 2020;13(1):87–93.
37. Rafii F, Ameri F, Haghani H, Ghobadi A. The effect of aromatherapy massage with lavender and chamomile oil on anxiety and sleep quality of patients with burns. *Burns.* 2020;46(1):164–171.
38. Daneshpajooh L, Najafi Ghezeljeh T, Haghani H. Comparison of the effects of inhalation aromatherapy using Damask rose aroma and the Benson relaxation technique in burn patients: A randomized clinical trial. *Burns.* 2019;45(5):1205–1214.
39. Seyyed-Rasooli A, Salehi F, Mohammadpoorasl A, Goljaryan S, Seyyedi Z, Thomson B. Comparing the effects of aromatherapy massage and inhalation aromatherapy on anxiety and pain in burn patients: A single-blind randomized clinical trial. *Burns.* 2016;42(8):1774–1780.
40. Lee JH, Seo EK, Shim JS, Chung SP. The effects of aroma massage and foot bath on psychophysiological response in stroke patients. *J Phys Ther Sci.* 2017;29(8):1292–1296.
41. Donelli D, Antonelli M, Bellinazzi C, Gensini GF, Firenzuoli F. Effects of lavender on anxiety: A systematic review and meta-analysis. *Phytomedicine.* 2019;65:153099.
42. Woronuk G, Demissie Z, Rheault M, Mahmoud S. Biosynthesis and therapeutic properties of Lavandula essential oil constituents. *Planta Med.* 2011;77(1):7–15.
43. Diego MA, Jones NA, Field T, Hernandez-Reif M, Schanberg S, Kuhn C, McAdam V, Galamaga R, Galamaga M. Aromatherapy positively affects mood, EEG patterns of alertness and math computations. *Int J Neurosci.* 1998;96(3–4):217–224.
44. Sanders C, Diego M, Fernandez M, Field T, Hernandez-Reif M, Roca A. EEG asymmetry responses to lavender and rosemary aromas in adults and infants. *Int J Neurosci.* 2002;112(11):1305–1320.
45. Wolffenbüttel AN, Zamboni A, Becker G, Dos Santos MK, Borille BT, de Cássia Mariotti K, Fagundes AC, de Oliveira Salomón JL, Coelho VR, Ruiz LV, de Moura Linck V, Dallegrave E, Cano P, Esquifino AI, Leal MB, Limberger RP. Citrus essential oils inhalation by mice: Behavioral testing, GCMS plasma analysis, corticosterone, and melatonin levels evaluation. *Phytother Res.* 2018;32(1):160–169.
46. Cho H, Sowndhararajan K, Jung JW, Jhoo JW, Kim S. Fragrant chemicals in the supercritical carbon dioxide extract of Magnolia Kobus DC. Flower buds increase the concentration state of brain function. *J Essent Oil Bear Plants.* 2015;18:1059–1069.

47. Sayowan W, Siripornpanich V, Hongratanaworakit T, Kotchabhakdi N, Ruangrungsi N. The effects of jasmine oil inhalation on brain wave activities and emotions. *J. Health Res.* 2013;27:73–77.
48. Krbot Skorić M, Adamec I, Jerbić AB, Gabelić T, Hajnšek S, Habek M. Electroencephalographic response to different odors in healthy individuals: A promising tool for objective assessment of olfactory disorders. *Clin EEG Neurosci.* 2015;46(4):370–376.
49. Matsubara E, Kawai S. Gender differences in the psychophysiological effects induced by VOCs emitted from Japanese cedar (*Cryptomeria japonica*). *Environ Health Prev Med.* 2018;23(1):10.
50. Sowndhararajan K, Cho H, Yu B, Kim S. Effect of olfactory stimulation of isomeric aroma compounds, (+)-limonene and terpinolene on human electroencephalographic activity. *Eur J Integr Med.* 2015;7:561–566.
51. Angelucci FL, Silva VV, Dal Pizzol C, Spir LG, Praes CE, Maibach H. Physiological effect of olfactory stimuli inhalation in humans: An overview. *Int J Cosmet Sci.* 2014;36(2):117–123.
52. Lehrner J, Eckersberger C, Walla P, Pötsch G, Deecke L. Ambient odor of orange in a dental office reduces anxiety and improves mood in female patients. *Physiol Behav.* 2000;71(1–2):83–86.
53. Haze S, Sakai K, Gozu Y. Effects of fragrance inhalation on sympathetic activity in normal adults. *Jpn J Pharmacol.* 2002;90(3):247–253.
54. Ilmberger J, Heuberger E, Mahrhofer C, Dessovic H, Kowarik D, Buchbauer G. The influence of essential oils on human attention. I: Alertness. *Chem Senses.* 2001;26(3):239–245.
55. Motomura N, Sakurai A, Yotsuya Y. Reduction of mental stress with lavender odorant. *Percept Mot Skills.* 2001;93(3):713–718.
56. Han C, Li F, Tian S, Liu Y, Xiao H, Wu X, Zhang W, Zhang W, Mao M. Beneficial effect of compound essential oil inhalation on central fatigue. *BMC Complement Altern Med.* 2018;18(1):309.
57. Gedney JJ, Glover TL, Fillingim RB. Sensory and affective pain discrimination after inhalation of essential oils. *Psychosom Med.* 2004;66:599–606.
58. Cheraghbeigi N, Modarresi M, Rezaei M, Khatony A. Comparing the effects of massage and aromatherapy massage with lavender oil on sleep quality of cardiac patients: A randomized controlled trial. *Complement Ther Clin Pract.* 2019;35:253–258.
59. Karadag E, Samancioglu S, Ozden D, Bakir E. Effects of aromatherapy on sleep quality and anxiety of patients. *Nurs Crit Care.* 2017;22(2):105–112.
60. Lillehei AS, Halcón LL, Savik K, Reis R. Effect of inhaled lavender and sleep hygiene on self-reported sleep issues: A randomized controlled trial. *J Altern Complement Med.* 2015;21(7):430–438.
61. Karadag E, Samancioglu Baglama S. The effect of aromatherapy on fatigue and anxiety in patients undergoing hemodialysis treatment: A randomized controlled study. *Holist Nurs Pract.* 2019;33(4):222–229.
62. Ahmady S, Rezaei M, Khatony A. Comparing effects of aromatherapy with lavender essential oil and orange essential oil on fatigue of hemodialysis patients: A randomized trial. *Complement Ther Clin Pract.* 2019;36:64–68.
63. Bagheri-Nesami M, Shorofi SA, Nikkhah A, Espahbodi F, Ghaderi Koolaee FS. The effects of aromatherapy with lavender essential oil on fatigue levels in haemodialysis patients: A randomized clinical trial. *Complement Ther Clin Pract.* 2016;22:33–37.
64. Nasiri A, Mahmodi MA, Nobakht Z. Effect of aromatherapy massage with lavender essential oil on pain in patients with osteoarthritis of the knee: A randomized controlled clinical trial. *Complement Ther Clin Pract.* 2016;25:75–80.
65. Kao YH, Huang YC, Chung UL, Hsu WN, Tang YT, Liao YH. Comparisons for effectiveness of aromatherapy and acupressure massage on quality of life in career women: A randomized controlled trial. *J Altern Complement Med.* 2017;23(6):451–460.
66. Rho KH, Han SH, Kim KS, Lee MS. Effects of aromatherapy massage on anxiety and self–esteem in Korean elderly women: A pilot study. *Int J Neurosci.* 2006;116:1447–1455.
67. Karaman T, Karaman S, Dogru S, Tapar H, Sahin A, Suren M, Arici S, Kaya Z. Evaluating the efficacy of lavender aromatherapy on peripheral venous cannulation pain and anxiety: A prospective, randomized study. *Complement Ther Clin Pract.* 2016;23:64–68.
68. Hamzeh S, Safari-Faramani R, Khatony A. Effects of aromatherapy with lavender and peppermint essential oils on the sleep quality of cancer patients: A randomized controlled trial. *Evid Based Complement Alternat Med.* 2020;2020:7480204.
69. Ho C, Spence C. Olfactory facilitation of dual-task performance. *Neurosci Lett.* 2005;389(1):35–40.
70. Moss M, Hewitt S, Moss L, Wesnes K. Modulation of cognitive performance and mood by aromas of peppermint and ylang-ylang. *Int J Neurosci.* 2008;118(1):59–77.
71. Coelho LS, Correa-Netto NF, Masukawa MY, Lima AC, Maluf S, Linardi A, Santos-Junior JG. Inhaled *Lavandula angustifolia* essential oil inhibits consolidation of contextual- but not tone-fear conditioning in rats. *J Ethnopharmacol.* 2018;215:34–41.
72. Manganiello-Terra FA, Correa-Netto NF, Masukawa MY, Ruzzi A, Linardi A, Santos-Junior JG. Inhaled *Lavandula angustifolia* essential oil enhances extinction learning and inhibits memory updating in mice submitted to the contextual fear conditioning. *J Ethnopharmacol.* 2020;260:113048.
73. Hongratanaworakit T, Buchbauer G. Relaxing effect of ylang ylang oil on humans after transdermal absorption. *Phytother Res.* 2006;20(9):758–763.
74. Hashikawa-Hobara N, Otsuka A, Ishikawa R, Hashikawa N. Roman chamomile inhalation combined with clomipramine treatment improves treatment-resistant depression-like behavior in mice. *Biomed Pharmacother.* 2019;118:109263.
75. Liu SH, Lin TH, Chang KM. The physical effects of aromatherapy in alleviating work-related stress on elementary school teachers in Taiwan. *Evid Based Complement Alternat Med.* 2013;2013:853809.
76. Tsai SS, Wang HH, Chou FH. The effects of aromatherapy on postpartum women: A systematic review. *J Nurs Res.* 2020;28(3):e96.
77. Bhatia S. Bioinformatics. In: *Introduction to Pharmaceutical Biotechnology, Enzymes, Proteins and Bioinformatics.* IOP Publishing Ltd, Bristol, UK, Volume 2; 2018:1–16.

78. Bhatia S. Protein and enzyme engineering. In: *Introduction to Pharmaceutical Biotechnology, Enzymes, Proteins and Bioinformatics*. IOP Publishing Ltd, Bristol, UK, Volume 2; 2018:1–15.
79. Bhatia S. Introduction to genomics. In: *Introduction to Pharmaceutical Biotechnology, Enzymes, Proteins and Bioinformatics*. IOP Publishing Ltd, Bristol, UK, Volume 2; 2018:1–39.
80. Bhatia S. Characterization of cultured cells: Animal tissue culture and biopharmaceuticals. In: *Introduction to Pharmaceutical Biotechnology*. IOP Publishing Ltd, Bristol, UK; Volume 3; 2019;3:1–47.
81. Bhatia S. Industrial enzymes and their applications. In: *Introduction to Pharmaceutical Biotechnology, Enzymes, Proteins and Bioinformatics*. IOP Publishing Ltd, Bristol, UK, Volume 2; 2018:1–21.
82. Bhatia S. Introduction to enzymes and their applications. In: *Introduction to Pharmaceutical Biotechnology, Enzymes, Proteins and Bioinformatics*. IOP Publishing Ltd, Bristol, UK, Volume 2; 2018:1–29.
83. Bhatia S. Biotransformation and enzymes. In: *Introduction to Pharmaceutical Biotechnology, Enzymes, Proteins and Bioinformatics*. IOP Publishing Ltd, Bristol, UK, Volume 2; 2018:1–13.
84. Bhatia S. Transgenic animals in biotechnology. In: *Introduction to Pharmaceutical Biotechnology, Volume 1 Basic Techniques and Concepts*. IOP Publishing Ltd, Bristol, UK; 2018:1–67.
85. Bhatia S. Applications of stem cells in disease and gene therapy. In: *Introduction to Pharmaceutical Biotechnology, Volume 1 Basic Techniques and Concepts*. IOP Publishing Ltd, Bristol, UK; 2018:1–40.
86. Bhatia S. Introduction to genetic engineering. In: *Introduction to Pharmaceutical Biotechnology, Volume 1 Basic Techniques and Concepts*. IOP Publishing Ltd, Bristol, UK; 2018:1–63.
87. Bhatia S. Modern DNA science and its applications. In: *Introduction to Pharmaceutical Biotechnology, Volume 1 Basic Techniques and Concepts*. IOP Publishing Ltd, Bristol, UK, 2018:1–70.
88. Bhatia S. Animal tissue culture facilities: Animal tissue culture and biopharmaceuticals. In: *Introduction to Pharmaceutical Biotechnology*. IOP Publishing Ltd, Bristol, UK, Volume 3; 2019:1–32.
89. Bhatia S. Culture media for animal cells: Animal tissue culture and biopharmaceuticals. In: *Introduction to Pharmaceutical Biotechnology*. IOP Publishing Ltd, Bristol, UK, Volume 3; 2019;1–33.
90. Bhatia S. Stem cell culture: Animal tissue culture and biopharmaceuticals. In: *Introduction to Pharmaceutical Biotechnology*. IOP Publishing Ltd, Bristol, UK, Volume 3; 2019:1–24.
91. Bhatia S. Organ culture: Introduction to animal tissue culture science. In: *Introduction to Pharmaceutical Biotechnology*. IOP Publishing Ltd, Bristol, UK, Volume 3; 2019:1–28.
92. Watkins R, Wu L, Zhang C, Davis RM, Xu B. Natural product-based nanomedicine: Recent advances and issues. *Int J Nanomed*. 2015;10:6055–6074.
93. Srikanth M, Kessler JA. Nanotechnology-novel therapeutics for CNS disorders. *Nat Rev Neurol*. 2012;8(6):307–318.
94. Bhatia S, Sharma A, Vargas De La Cruz CB, Chaugule B, Ahmed Al-Harrasi. Nutraceutical, antioxidant, antimicrobial properties of *Pyropia vietnamensis* (Tanaka et Pham-Hong Ho) J.E. Sutherl. et Monotilla. *Curr Bioact Compd*. 2020;16:1.
95. Bhatia S, Sardana S, Senwar KR, Dhillon A, Sharma A, Naved T. In vitro antioxidant and antinociceptive properties of Porphyra vietnamensis. *Biomedicine (Taipei)*. 2019;9(1):3.
96. Bhatia S, Sharma K, Namdeo AG, Chaugule BB, Kavale M, Nanda S. Broad-spectrum sun-protective action of Porphyra-334 derived from Porphyra vietnamensis. *Pharmacogn Res*. 2010;2(1):45–49.
97. Bhatia S, Sardana S, Sharma A, Vargas De La Cruz CB, Chaugule B, Khodaie L. Development of broad spectrum mycosporine loaded sunscreen formulation from Ulva fasciata delile. *Biomedicine (Taipei)*. 2019;9(3):17.
98. Bhatia S, Garg A, Sharma K, Kumar S, Sharma A, Purohit AP. Mycosporine and mycosporine-like amino acids: A paramount tool against ultra violet irradiation. *Pharmacogn Rev*. 2011;5(10):138–146.
99. Bhatia S, Namdeo AG, Nanda S. Factors effecting the gelling and emulsifying properties of a natural polymer. *SRP*. 2010;1(1):86–92.
100. Bhatia S, Sharma K, Bera T. Structural characterization and pharmaceutical properties of porphyran. *Asian J Pharm*. 2015;9:93–101.
101. Bhatia S, Sharma A, Sharma K, Kavale M, Chaugule BB, Dhalwal K, Namdeo AG, Mahadik KR. Novel algal polysaccharides from marine source: Porphyran. *Pharmacogn Rev*. 2008; 2(4):271–276.
102. Bhatia S, Sharma K, Nagpal K, Bera T. Investigation of the factors influencing the molecular weight of porphyran and its associated antifungal activity Bioact. *Carb Diet Fiber*. 2015;5:153–168.
103. Bhatia S, Kumar V, Sharma K, Nagpal K, Bera T. Significance of algal polymer in designing amphotericin B nanoparticles. *Sci World J*. 2014;2014:564573.
104. Bhatia S, Rathee P, Sharma K, Chaugule BB, Kar N, Bera T. Immuno-modulation effect of sulphated polysaccharide (porphyran) from Porphyra vietnamensis. *Int J Biol Macromol*. 2013;57:50–56.
105. Bhatia S. *Natural Polymer Drug Delivery Systems: Marine Polysaccharides Based Nano-Materials and Its Applications*. Springer International Publishing, Switzerland; 2016:185–225.
106. Bhatia S. *Natural Polymer Drug Delivery Systems: Plant Derived Polymers, Properties, and Modification & Applications*. Springer International Publishing, Switzerland; 2016:119–184.
107. Bhatia S. *Natural Polymer Drug Delivery Systems: Nanotechnology and Its Drug Delivery Applications*. Springer International Publishing, Switzerland; 2016: 1–32.
108. Bhatia S. *Natural Polymer Drug Delivery Systems: Nanoparticles Types, Classification, Characterization, Fabrication Methods and Drug Delivery Applications*. Springer International Publishing, Switzerland; 2016:33–93.
109. Bhatia S. *Natural Polymer Drug Delivery Systems: Natural Polymers vs Synthetic Polymer*. Springer International Publishing, Switzerland; 2016:95–118.

110. Bhatia S. *Systems for Drug Delivery: Mammalian Polysaccharides and Its Nanomaterials.* Springer International Publishing, Switzerland; 2016:1–27.
111. Bhatia S. *Systems for Drug Delivery: Microbial Polysaccharides as Advance Nanomaterials.* Springer International Publishing, Switzerland; 2016:29–54.
112. Bhatia S. *Systems for Drug Delivery: Chitosan Based Nanomaterials and Its Applications.* Springer International Publishing, Switzerland; 2016:55–117.
113. Bhatia S. *Systems for Drug Delivery: Advance Polymers and Its Applications.* Springer International Publishing, Switzerland; 2016:119–146.
114. Bhatia S. *Systems for Drug Delivery: Advanced Application of Natural Polysaccharides.* Springer International Publishing, Switzerland; 2016:147–170.
115. Bhatia S. *Systems for Drug Delivery: Modern Polysaccharides and Its Current Advancements.* Springer International Publishing, Switzerland; 2016:171–188.
116. Bhatia S. *Systems for Drug Delivery: Toxicity of Nanodrug Delivery Systems.* Springer International Publishing, Switzerland; 2016:189–197.
117. Bhatia S. *Nanotechnology in Drug Delivery Fundamentals, Design, and Applications: Part 1: Protein and Peptide-Based Drug Delivery Systems.* Apple Academic Press, Palm Bay, FL; 2016:50–204.
118. Bhatia S. *Nanotechnology in Drug Delivery Fundamentals, Design, and Applications: Part 2: Peptide-Mediated Nanoparticle Drug Delivery System.* Apple Academic Press, Palm Bay, FL; 2016:205–280.
119. Bhatia S. *Nanotechnology in Drug Delivery Fundamentals, Design, and Applications: Part 3: CPP and CTP in Drug Delivery and Cell Targeting.* Apple Academic Press, Palm Bay, FL; 2016:309–312.
120. Nemeroff CB, Owens MJ. Treatment of mood disorders. *Nat Neurosci.* 2002;5:1068–1070.
121. Seol GH, Shim HS, Kim PJ, Moon HK, Lee KH, Shim I, Suh SH, Min SS. Antidepressant-like effect of *Salvia sclarea* is explained by modulation of dopamine activities in rats. *J Ethnopharmacol.* 2010;130(1):187–190.
122. Yi LT, Li J, Geng D, Liu BB, Fu Y, Tu JQ, Liu Y, Weng LJ. Essential oil of Perilla frutescens-induced change in hippocampal expression of brain-derived neurotrophic factor in chronic unpredictable mild stress in mice. *J Ethnopharmacol.* 2013;147(1):245–253.
123. Viana CC, de Oliveira PA, Brum LF, Picada JN, Pereira P. Gamma-decanolactone effect on behavioral and genotoxic parameters. *Life Sci.* 2007;80(11):1014–1019.
124. Duan D, Chen L, Yang X, Tu Y, Jiao S. Antidepressant-like effect of essential oil isolated from *Toona ciliata* Roem. var. yunnanensis. *J Nat Med.* 2015;69(2):191–197.
125. Sah SP, Mathela CS, Chopra K. Involvement of nitric oxide (NO) signalling pathway in the antidepressant activity of essential oil of Valeriana wallichii Patchouli alcohol chemotype. *Phytomedicine.* 2011;18(14):1269–1275.
126. Lee YL, Wu Y, Tsang HW, Leung AY, Cheung WM. A systematic review on the anxiolytic effects of aromatherapy in people with anxiety symptoms. *J Altern Complement Med.* 2011;17(2):101–108.
127. Sohrabi R, Pazgoohan N, Seresht HR, Amin B. Repeated systemic administration of the cinnamon essential oil possesses anti-anxiety and anti-depressant activities in mice. *Iran J Basic Med Sci.* 2017;20(6):708–714.
128. Sowndhararajan K, Kim S. Influence of fragrances on human psychophysiological activity: with special reference to human electroencephalographic response. *Sci Pharm.* 2016;84(4):724–751. doi: 10.3390/scipharm84040724. PMID: 27916830; PMCID: PMC5198031.
129. Kasper S, Anghelescu I, Dienel A. Efficacy of orally administered Silexan in patients with anxiety-related restlessness and disturbed sleep: A randomized, placebo-controlled trial. *Eur Neuropsychopharmacol.* 2015;25(11):1960–1967.
130. Fißler M, Quante A. A case series on the use of lavendula oil capsules in patients suffering from major depressive disorder and symptoms of psychomotor agitation, insomnia and anxiety. *Complement Ther Med.* 2014;22(1):63–69.
131. Sánchez-Vidaña DI, Po KK, Fung TK, Chow JK, Lau WK, So PK, Lau BW, Tsang HW. Lavender essential oil ameliorates depression-like behavior and increases neurogenesis and dendritic complexity in rats. *Neurosci Lett.* 2019;701:180–192.
132. Huang YJ, Lu KH, Lin YE, Panyod S, Wu HY, Chang WT, Sheen LY. Garlic essential oil mediates acute and chronic mild stress-induced depression in rats via modulation of monoaminergic neurotransmission and brain-derived neurotrophic factor levels. *Food Funct.* 2019;10(12):8094–8105.
133. Parente MSR, Custódio FR, Cardoso NA, Lima MJA, Melo TS, Linhares MI, Siqueira RMP, Nascimento AÁD, Catunda Júnior FEA, Melo CTV. Antidepressant-like effect of *Lippia sidoides* CHAM (verbenaceae) essential oil and its major compound thymol in mice. *Sci Pharm.* 2018;86(3):E27.
134. Liang M, Du Y, Li W, Yin X, Yang N, Qie A, Lebaron TW, Zhang J, Chen H, Shi H. SuHeXiang essential oil inhalation produces antidepressant- and anxiolytic-like effects in adult mice. *Biol Pharm Bull.* 2018;41(7):1040–1048.
135. Han P, Han T, Peng W, Wang XR. Antidepressant-like effects of essential oil and asarone, a major essential oil component from the rhizome of *Acorus tatarinowii. Pharm Biol.* 2013;51(5):589–594.
136. Abbasi-Maleki S, Kadkhoda Z, Taghizad-Farid R. The antidepressant-like effects of *Origanum majorana* essential oil on mice through monoaminergic modulation using the forced swimming test. *J Tradit Complement Med.* 2019;10(4):327–335.
137. Amiresmaeili A, Roohollahi S, Mostafavi A, Askari N. Effects of oregano essential oil on brain TLR4 and TLR2 gene expression and depressive-like behavior in a rat model. *Res Pharm Sci.* 2018;13(2):130–141.
138. Chen B, Li J, Xie Y, Ming X, Li G, Wang J, Li M, Li X, Xiong L. Cang-ai volatile oil improves depressive-like behaviors and regulates DA and 5-HT metabolism in the brains of CUMS-induced rats. *J Ethnopharmacol.* 2019;244:112088.
139. Wang S, Wang C, Yu Z, Wu C, Peng D, Liu X, Liu Y, Yang Y, Guo P, Wei J. Agarwood essential oil ameliorates restrain stress-induced anxiety and depression by inhibiting HPA axis hyperactivity. *Int J Mol Sci.* 2018;19(11):3468.
140. Diniz TC, de Oliveira Júnior RG, Miranda Bezerra Medeiros MA, Gama E Silva M, de Andrade Teles RB, Dos Passos Menezes P, de Sousa BMH, Abrahão Frank L, de Souza Araújo AA, Russo Serafini M, Stanisçuaski Guterres S, Pereira Nunes CE, Salvador MJ, da Silva Almeida JRG. Anticonvulsant, sedative, anxiolytic and antidepressant activities of the essential oil of Annona vepretorum in mice: Involvement of GABAergic and serotonergic systems. *Biomed Pharmacother.* 2019;111:1074–1087.

141. Bakhtiarpoor M, Setorki M, Kaffashian MR. Effects of essential oil of *Satureja bachtiarica* bunge in a rat model of reserpine-induced depression. *Iran J Med Sci.* 2018;43(4):409–415.
142. Capatina L, Boiangiu RS, Dumitru G, Napoli EM, Ruberto G, Hritcu L, Todirascu-Ciornea E. *Rosmarinus officinalis* essential oil improves scopolamine-induced neurobehavioral changes via restoration of cholinergic function and brain antioxidant status in Zebrafish (Danio rerio). *Antioxidants (Basel).* 2020;9(1):62.
143. Capatina L, Todirascu-Ciornea E, Napoli EM, Ruberto G, Hritcu L, Dumitru G. *Thymus vulgaris* essential oil protects Zebrafish against cognitive dysfunction by regulating cholinergic and antioxidants systems. *Antioxidants (Basel).* 2020;9(11):1083.
144. Todirascu-Ciornea E, El-Nashar HAS, Mostafa NM, Eldahshan OA, Boiangiu RS, Dumitru G, Hritcu L, Singab ANB. *Schinus terebinthifolius* essential oil attenuates scopolamine-induced memory deficits via cholinergic modulation and antioxidant properties in a Zebrafish model. *Evid Based Complement Alternat Med.* 2019; 2019:5256781.
145. Hritcu L, Bagci E, Aydin E, Mihasan M. Antiamnesic and antioxidants effects of *Ferulago angulata* essential oil against scopolamine-induced memory impairment in laboratory rats. *Neurochem Res.* 2015;40(9):1799–1809.
146. Sadiki FZ, Idrissi ME, Cioanca O, Trifan A, Hancianu M, Hritcu L, Postu PA. Tetraclinis articulata essential oil mitigates cognitive deficits and brain oxidative stress in an Alzheimer's disease amyloidosis model. *Phytomedicine.* 2019;56:57–63.
147. Postu PA, Sadiki FZ, El Idrissi M, Cioanca O, Trifan A, Hancianu M, Hritcu L. Pinus halepensis essential oil attenuates the toxic Alzheimer's amyloid beta (1–42)-induced memory impairment and oxidative stress in the rat hippocampus. *Biomed Pharmacother.* 2019;112:108673.
148. Cioanca O, Hritcu L, Mihasan M, Hancianu M. Cognitive-enhancing and antioxidant activities of inhaled coriander volatile oil in amyloid β(1–42) rat model of Alzheimer's disease. *Physiol Behav.* 2013 15;120:193–202.
149. Cioanca O, Hritcu L, Mihasan M, Trifan A, Hancianu M. Inhalation of coriander volatile oil increased anxiolytic-antidepressant-like behaviors and decreased oxidative status in beta-amyloid (1–42) rat model of Alzheimer's disease. *Physiol Behav.* 2014;131:68–74.
150. Cioanca O, Hancianu M, Mihasan M, Hritcu L. Anti-acetylcholinesterase and antioxidant activities of inhaled juniper oil on amyloid beta (1–42)-induced oxidative stress in the rat hippocampus. *Neurochem Res.* 2015;40(5): 952–960.
151. Auti ST, Kulkarni YA. Neuroprotective effect of cardamom oil against aluminum induced neurotoxicity in rats. *Front Neurol.* 2019;10:399.
152. Mohamed EA, Ahmed HI, Zaky HS, Badr AM. Sesame oil mitigates memory impairment, oxidative stress, and neurodegeneration in a rat model of Alzheimer's disease. A pivotal role of NF-κB/p38MAPK/BDNF/PPAR-γ pathways. *J Ethnopharmacol.* 2020;276:113468.
153. Dos Santos ÉRQ, Maia CSF, Fontes Junior EA, Melo AS, Pinheiro BG, Maia JGS. Linalool-rich essential oils from the Amazon display antidepressant-type effect in rodents. *J Ethnopharmacol.* 2018;212:43–49.
154. Guzmán-Gutiérrez SL, Gómez-Cansino R, García-Zebadúa JC, Jiménez-Pérez NC, Reyes-Chilpa R. Antidepressant activity of *Litsea glaucescens* essential oil: Identification of β-pinene and linalool as active principles. *J Ethnopharmacol.* 2012;143(2):673–679.
155. Oyemitan IA, Olayera OA, Alabi A, Abass LA, Elusiyan CA, Oyedeji AO, Akanmu MA. Psychoneuropharmacological activities and chemical composition of essential oil of fresh fruits of *Piper guineense* (piperaceae) in mice. *J Ethnopharmacol.* 2015;166:240–249.
156. Ali SS, Abd El Wahab MG, Ayuob NN, Suliaman M. The antidepressant-like effect of *Ocimum basilicum* in an animal model of depression. *Biotech Histochem.* 2017;92(6):390–401.
157. Ayuob NN, El Wahab MGA, Ali SS, Abdel-Tawab HS. Ocimum basilicum improve chronic stress-induced neurodegenerative changes in mice hippocampus. *Metab Brain Dis.* 2018;33(3):795–804.
158. Bagci E, Aydin E, Ungureanu E, Hritcu L. Anthriscus nemorosa essential oil inhalation prevents memory impairment, anxiety and depression in scopolamine-treated rats. *Biomed Pharmacother.* 2016;84:1313–1320.
159. Aydin E, Hritcu L, Dogan G, Hayta S, Bagci E. The effects of inhaled *Pimpinella peregrina* essential oil on scopolamine-induced memory impairment, anxiety, and depression in laboratory rats. *Mol Neurobiol.* 2016;53(9):6557–6567.
160. Friedland K, Silani G, Schuwald A, Stockburger C, Koch E, Nöldner M, Müller WE. Neurotrophic properties of Silexan, an essential oil from the flowers of lavender-preclinical evidence for antidepressant-like properties. *Pharmacopsychiatry.* 2020;54(1):37–46.
161. Müller WE, Sillani G, Schuwald A, Friedland K. Pharmacological basis of the anxiolytic and antidepressant properties of Silexan®, an essential oil from the flowers of lavender. *Neurochem Int.* 2020;143:104899.
162. Norte MC, Cosentino RM, Lazarini CA. Effects of methyl-eugenol administration on behavioral models related to depression and anxiety, in rats. *Phytomedicine.* 2005;12(4):294–298.
163. Waters RP, Rivalan M, Bangasser DA, Deussing JM, Ising M, Wood SK, Holsboer F, Summers CH. Evidence for the role of corticotropin-releasing factor in major depressive disorder. *Neurosci Biobehav Rev.* 2015;58:63–78.
164. Komori T, Fujiwara R, Tanida M, Nomura J. Potential antidepressant effects of lemon odor in rats. *Eur Neuropsychopharmacol.* 1995;5(4):477–480.
165. Victoria FN, de Siqueira Brahm A, Savegnago L, Lenardão EJ. Involvement of serotoninergic and adrenergic systems on the antidepressant-like effect of *E. uniflora* L. leaves essential oil and further analysis of its antioxidant activity. *Neurosci Lett.* 2013;544:105–109.
166. Ji WW, Li RP, Li M, Wang SY, Zhang X, Niu XX, Li W, Yan L, Wang Y, Fu Q, Ma SP. Antidepressant-like effect of essential oil of *Perilla frutescens* in a chronic, unpredictable, mild stress-induced depression model mice. *Chin J Nat Med.* 2014;12(10):753–759.
167. Piccinelli AC, Santos JA, Konkiewitz EC, Oesterreich SA, Formagio AS, Croda J, Ziff EB, Kassuya CA. Antihyperalgesic and antidepressive actions of (R)-(+)-limonene, α-phellandrene, and essential oil from *Schinus terebinthifolius* fruits in a neuropathic pain model. *Nutr Neurosci.* 2015;18(5):217–224.

168. Guzmán-Gutiérrez SL, Bonilla-Jaime H, Gómez-Cansino R, Reyes-Chilpa R. Linalool and β-pinene exert their antidepressant-like activity through the monoaminergic pathway. *Life Sci.* 2015;128:24–29.
169. Bagci E, Akbaba E, Maniu C, Ungureanu E, Hritcu L. Evaluation of antiamnesic activity of *Salvia multicaulis* essential oil on scopolamine-induced amnesia in rats: In vivo and in silico approaches. *Heliyon.* 2019;5(8):e02223.
170. Liu BB, Luo L, Liu XL, Geng D, Li CF, Chen SM, Chen XM, Yi LT, Liu Q. Essential oil of *Syzygium aromaticum* reverses the deficits of stress-induced behaviors and hippocampal p-ERK/p-CREB/brain-derived neurotrophic factor expression. *Planta Med.* 2015;81(3):185–192.
171. Irie Y, Itokazu N, Anjiki N, Ishige A, Watanabe K, Keung WM. Eugenol exhibits antidepressant-like activity in mice and induces expression of metallothionein-III in the hippocampus. *Brain Res.* 2004;1011(2):243–246.
172. Tao G, Irie Y, Li DJ, Keung WM. Eugenol and its structural analogs inhibit monoamine oxidase A and exhibit antidepressant-like activity. *Bioorg Med Chem.* 2005;13(15):4777–4788.
173. Lakusić B, Lakusić D, Ristić M, Marcetić M, Slavkovska V. Seasonal variations in the composition of the essential oils of *Lavandula angustifolia* (Lamiacae). *Nat Prod Commun.* 2014;9(6):859–862.
174. Melo FH, Moura BA, de Sousa DP, de Vasconcelos SM, Macedo DS, Fonteles MM, Viana GS, de Sousa FC. Antidepressant-like effect of carvacrol (5-Isopropyl-2-methylphenol) in mice: Involvement of dopaminergic system. *Fundam Clin Pharmacol.* 2011;25(3):362–367.
175. Deng XY, Li HY, Chen JJ, Li RP, Qu R, Fu Q, Ma SP. Thymol produces an antidepressant-like effect in a chronic unpredictable mild stress model of depression in mice. *Behav Brain Res.* 2015;291:12–19.
176. Deng XY, Xue JS, Li HY, Ma ZQ, Fu Q, Qu R, Ma SP. Geraniol produces antidepressant-like effects in a chronic unpredictable mild stress mice model. *Physiol Behav.* 2015;152(Pt A):264–271.
177. Wang W, Jiang Y, Cai E, et al. L-menthol exhibits antidepressive-like effects mediated by the modification of 5-HTergic, GABAergic and DAergic systems. *Cogn Neurodyn.* 2019;13(2):191–200.
178. Xue J, Li H, Deng X, Ma Z, Fu Q, Ma S. L-Menthone confers antidepressant-like effects in an unpredictable chronic mild stress mouse model via NLRP3 inflammasome-mediated inflammatory cytokines and central neurotransmitters. *Pharmacol Biochem Behav.* 2015;134:42–48.
179. Meng W, Yan S, Zhou Y, Xie P. trans-Cinnamaldehyde reverses depressive-like behaviors in chronic unpredictable mild stress rats by inhibiting NF-κB/NLRP3 inflammasome pathway. *Evid Based Complement Alternat Med.* 2020;17: 2020.
180. Lin J, Song Z, Chen X, Zhao R, Chen J, Chen H, Yang X, Wu Z. trans-Cinnamaldehyde shows anti-depression effect in the forced swimming test and possible involvement of the endocannabinoid system. *Biochem Biophys Res Commun.* 2019;518(2):351–356.
181. Bhatia S. History and scope of plant biotechnology. In: *Modern Applications of Plant Biotechnology in Pharmaceutical Sciences.* Academic Press, Cambridge, MA; 2015:1–30.
182. Bhatia S. Plant tissue culture. In: *Modern Applications of Plant Biotechnology in Pharmaceutical Sciences.* Academic Press, Cambridge, MA; 2015:31–107.
183. Bhatia S. Laboratory organization. In: *Modern Applications of Plant Biotechnology in Pharmaceutical Sciences.* Academic Press, Cambridge, MA; 2015:109–120.
184. Bhatia S. Concepts and techniques of plant tissue culture science. In: *Modern Applications of Plant Biotechnology in Pharmaceutical Sciences.* Academic Press, Cambridge, MA; 2015:121–156.
185. Bhatia S. Application of plant biotechnology. In: *Modern Applications of Plant Biotechnology in Pharmaceutical Sciences.* Academic Press, Cambridge, MA; 2015:157–207.
186. Bhatia S. Somatic embryogenesis and organogenesis. In: *Modern Applications of Plant Biotechnology in Pharmaceutical Sciences.* Academic Press, Cambridge, MA; 2015:209–230.
187. Bhatia S. Classical and nonclassical techniques for secondary metabolite production in plant cell culture. In: *Modern Applications of Plant Biotechnology in Pharmaceutical Sciences.* Academic Press, Cambridge, MA; 2015: 231–291.
188. Bhatia S. Plant-based biotechnological products with their production host, modes of delivery systems, and stability testing. In: *Modern Applications of Plant Biotechnology in Pharmaceutical Sciences.* Academic Press, Cambridge, MA; 2015:293–331.
189. Bhatia S. Edible vaccines. In: *Modern Applications of Plant Biotechnology in Pharmaceutical Sciences.* Academic Press, Cambridge, MA; 2015:333–343.
190. Bhatia S. Microenvironmentation in micropropagation. In: *Modern Applications of Plant Biotechnology in Pharmaceutical Sciences.* Academic Press, Cambridge, MA; 2015:345–360.
191. Bhatia S. Micropropagation. In: *Modern Applications of Plant Biotechnology in Pharmaceutical Sciences.* Academic Press, Cambridge, MA; 2015:361–368.
192. Bhatia S. Laws in plant biotechnology. In: *Modern Applications of Plant Biotechnology in Pharmaceutical Sciences.* Academic Press, Cambridge, MA; 2015:369–391.
193. Bhatia S. Technical glitches in micropropagation. In: *Modern Applications of Plant Biotechnology in Pharmaceutical Sciences.* Academic Press, Cambridge, MA; 2015:393–404.
194. Bhatia S. Plant tissue culture-based industries. In: *Modern Applications of Plant Biotechnology in Pharmaceutical Sciences.* Academic Press, Cambridge, MA; 2015:405–417.
195. Bhatia S, Al-Harrasi A, Behl T, Anwer MK, Ahmed MM, Mittal V, Kaushik D, Chigurupati S, Kabir MT, Sharma PB, Chaugule B, Vargas-de-la-Cruz C. Anti-migraine activity of freeze dried-latex obtained from *Calotropis Gigantea* Linn. *Environ Sci Pollut Res Int.* 2021.

20

Essential Oils in the Treatment of Respiratory Tract Infections

Ahmed Al-Harrasi
Natural and Medical Sciences Research Center, University of Nizwa

Saurabh Bhatia
Natural and Medical Sciences Research Center, University of Nizwa
University of Petroleum and Energy Studies

Tapan Behl
Chitkara University

Deepak Kaushik
M.D. University

CONTENTS

20.1 Introduction

A recent trial conducted by the World Health Organization (WHO) (Solidarity Therapeutics trial, the world's largest ongoing randomized control trial of potential coronavirus disease 2019 [COVID-19] therapeutics) that involved a large number of adult patients (n=11,266) in 405 hospitals across 30 countries found that remdesivir, hydroxychloroquine, HIV drug, and interferon were ineffective in treating COVID-19 [1]. Thus, this small number of repurposed drugs that were earlier found to be useful in COVID-19 treatment have since been determined to be ineffective against SARS-CoV-2. Therefore, there is an urgent need for safe and effective alternate treatments. Essential oils (EOs) contain various biologically active volatile compounds that can be inhaled to treat various respiratory infections. The chemical profiles of these EOs are usually affected by various factors such as environmental conditions of plant, the type of chemovar, isolation process, storage conditions, etc. All these factors can directly influence the proportion of active volatile compounds, which can indirectly influence the pharmacological properties of an EO. Due to the development of more pathogenic microbes and their emerging resistance against many antibiotics as well as antineoplastic agents and also their tendency to interfere with therapeutic effects of other medications, this is the time when more reliable alternative treatments such as natural products should be tested and explored. Multidrug resistance is a phenomenon in which microbial strains become resistant to different antibiotics by the following two mechanisms. Primarily, these microorganisms once exposed to antibiotics accumulate certain genes that encode for the development of various antibiotic-resistant proteins against a specific class of antibiotics. This accumulation usually takes place at resistance plasmids called R plasmids. Secondly, overexpression of these genes induced by mutation that code for multidrug efflux pumps lead to increased resistance against multiple antibiotics. The most suggested way to deal with multidrug-resistant bacterial strains is with the use of natural antimicrobial compounds in the form of EOs (single or blend) or their components for the treatment of various infections. There has been an exponential increase in the number of reports on the antimicrobial potential of EOs. A diverse class of natural compounds called terpenes that are usually present in EOs are obtained from various herbs containing fragrant and active antimicrobial compounds [2–4]. It is widely known that terpenoids, which are oxygenated derivatives of hydrocarbon terpenes such as aldehydes, ketones, alcohols, acids, ethers, and esters, possess high antimicrobial potential [2–4].

DOI: 10.1201/9781003175933-22

20.2 Advantages of EOs for Respiratory Infections

The potential roles of various EOs as well their components in respiratory tract infections are listed in Tables 20.1 and 20.2. EOs are suitable for use as treatments for various respiratory infections due to the following properties:

- Therapeutic effects: EO components have been reported for their broad antimicrobial, free radical scavenging, anti-inflammatory, immunomodulatory, antitumor, etc., medicinal properties.
- Easy to use: As they are available in liquid form, they can be directly used in any dispenser or inhaler for various respiratory ailments.

TABLE 20.1

Effect of EOs on Lungs

EOs	Pulmonary Effects	Mechanism	References
Citrus sinensis flower and *Mentha spicata*	Improvement in lung function and exercise performance	Considerable rise in level of air that can be forcibly exhaled from lungs	[5]
Calamintha nepeta	Lung protective effect	Suppression of NF-κB pathway, increase in alveolar volume suppression of iNOS and COX	[6]
Turmeric volatile oil	Treatment of respiratory diseases	inconsiderable improvement in symptoms such as removal of sputum, reducing cough as well as inhibiting asthmatic attacks	[7]
Mentha spicata and *Citrus sinensis*	-	Rise in the forced expiratory volume of lungs	[5]
Peppermint, eucalyptus, picea, and boswellia	-	Suppress PM2.5-caused severe inflammation of lungs with decrease in the release of IL-1β	[8]
Peppermint oil	For respiratory diseases such as coughs and colds	-	[38]
Thyme oil	For several Respiratory complications such as bronchial catarrh	-	
(−)-menthol	Reduced cough formation in guinea pigs	-	[9]
=menthol and =1,8-cineole blend	Considerably decreased cough formation among healthy individuals	-	[10]
Menthol	Decreased cough formation in the respiratory tract	-	[11]
Lavender EO	Reduced the number of eosinophils and theover all level of leukocytes in bronchoalveolar lavage fluid, reduced numbers of IL-4, 5, and 13 in lung tissue, and reduced Muc5b expression in the lung tissue	-	[12]
EOs	Suppression of severe respiratory illness and relief from rhinitis	Resulted in a 42.5% decrease of acute respiratory diseases with no side effects	[13]
Eucalyptus oil	Immune-modifying and antimicrobial effects	-	[14]
Lavandula latifolia, Thymus mastichina Balsam abies, Mentha x piperita	In the treatment of respiratory viral infections	-	[15]
Lavandula latifolia	Expectorant	-	[16]
1,8-cineol (eucalyptol)	Suppression of 1 cytokine production	-	[17]
Menthol	Inhalation of menthol reduced cough formation	-	[10]
Menthol	Reduces cough response against capsaicin after inhiation inhaled	-	[18]
l-menthol	l-menthol inhalation inhibits cough and has been shown to reduce respiratory discomfort associated with loaded breathing	Menthol caused a considerable rise of the peak respiratory flow decreased sensation of dyspnea	[19]
Soy oil - 69.18%; coconut oil - 20.00%; orange oil - 4.90%; aloe vera oil - 4.90%; peppermint oil - 0.75%; vitamin E - 0.27%	Antioxidant and anti-inflammatory activity	Aerosolized pretreatment with the mixed oil preparation significantly attenuated ozone-induced nasal inflammation, decrease oxidant stress, upregulate expression of antioxidant enzymes	[20]
1,8-cineole	1,8-cineole–adjuvanted vaccine provide better cross-protective immunity to infection with influenza than an inactivated vaccine only	Elevated production of Ig-G2a and s-IgA	[21]
Peppermint EO		Improvement in the spirometric measurements because of the direct impact over tonicity of bronchial smooth muscle	[22]

TABLE 20.2
***In vitro* Therapeutic Potential of EOs**

EO Components	Pharmacological Activity	Lung Cell Type	Mechanism	References
Camphene and geraniol	Provide protection to rodent macrophages (alveolar) against oxidative stress	Rat alveolar macrophages	Suppressed lipid peroxidationas well as NO and and ROS production	[23]
Lemongrass	Programmed cell death as cell cycle cessation	Lung cancer cell line (A549)	Via modulating the apoptic proteins (regulatory) including caspase-3, Bax, and BCL-2	[24]
β-Caryophyllene in the EO from *Chrysanthemum boreale*	Induces G1 phase cell cycle arrest in human lung cancer cells, antiproliferative effect (cytotoxic activity)	A549 and NCI-H358 cells	EO reduced mitochondrial membrane potential (MMP), disrupted the balance between proapoptotic and antiapoptotic BCL- proteins, as well as stimulated caspase (-8, -3, -9) - β-caryophyllene with cell cycle cessation (G1)	[25]
Vapor of *Litsea cubeba* EO (seed)	Induced cell cycle cessation and apoptosis of human NSCLC cells, (A549)	Apoptosis occurred because of a significant decline in the mTOR protein expression	Nonsmall cell lung carcinoma cells	[26]
Brucea javanica	Antitumor effect	Cell cycle cessation as well as induction of programmed cell death	Nonsmall cell lung cancer cell lines	[27]
α-terpineol	-	Downregulation of NFκB in a variety of cancerous cells	NCI-H69	[28]
Lemongrass EO (LG-EO) and its major constituent, citral	Antiproliferative effect	Reduced expression of BCL-xL and MCL-1	LU135 SCLC cell line (LU135-wt-src)	[29]
Alpinia officinarum	Antilung cancer activity	Inhibits the cell viability via suppressing expression of BCL-2 and MCL-1, inducing apoptic death via activating caspase-3	Different lung cancer cells	[30]
Citrus reticulata EO	-	Cell cycle cessation (at the G0/G1)	Nonsmall cell lung cancer (A549)	[31]
Plectranthus amboinicus	Chemotherapeutic/ chemopreventive effect	-	B16F-10 melanoma cell line	[32]
Myrica gale	Cytotoxicity	-	Human lung carcinoma (A549) and colon adenocarcinoma (DLD-1)	[33]

- Stability: Some EOs contain volatile antimicrobial compounds that remain stable in both liquid and vapor phases.
- Synergistic and antagonistic effects: EOs contain multiple components that can act synergistically to suppress infections. In addition, these EOs can be used as an adjuvant therapy to create a perfect blend with main course medications such as antimicrobials, analgesics, anti-inflammatories, and others to suppress or antagonize detrimental or side effects or toxicities induced by them.
- Shelf-life: If stored properly, these EOs usually have longer shelf-life than medications.
- Volatile compounds: EOs evaporate at room temperature because of the presence of volatile antimicrobial components. Inhalation of these volatile principles allows them to spontaneously present the maximum therapeutic effects. Once inhaled, they can directly act at the site of infection to show their antimicrobial or other effects.
- Side effects: EOs may be safe for most people to inhale, as long as dilution of the EO is performed properly as per the prescription.
- Fragrance: EOs are blend of volatile organic components found in plants containing fragrant compounds and are generally responsible for their unique fragrance or characteristic odor with an array of biological activities. These oils are lipophilic in nature as they can easily solubilize in alcoholic solution, ether, or vegetable oil, but are not soluble in water. At room temperature, the volatile components present in EOs remain in liquid phase with neutral color. Because of the presence of aromatic compounds, these oils are extensively used in topical preparations, perfumes, and also as aromatherapeutics for massage.
- Respiratory benefits: Apart from their known antimicrobial potential, EOs are also beneficial for the respiratory system due to their anti-inflammatory, analgesic, antitussive, bronchodilating, mucolytic,

ciliary transporting, and lung function improvement properties, which can reduce the complications caused by the pathogen.

- Lipophilic and high penetration property: Their lipophilic property makes them suitable to cross the membrane of the host cell to bind with intracellular targets where they can prevent intracellular multiplication of bacteria.
- Inhibition of angiotensin-converting enzyme 2 via EOs as well as their components: The ACE2 is a key protein that facilitates entry of SARS-CoV-2 in the host cell. Thus, inhibitors as well as blockers of ACE2 receptor prevent virus entry and thus this approach could be considered as effective antiviral therapy. Downregulation of ACE2 protein expression by EO treatment in airway epithelial cells (enriched with ACE2 receptors) has been reported. As a result, EOs and their components could be alternatively used an anti-SARS-CoV-2 agents of natural origin that can restrict virus invasion into the host cell and offer relief from COVID symptoms.

20.3 *In vitro* Antimicrobial effects of EOs

For evaluation of the *in vitro* antimicrobial effects of EOs, the following procedures have been used:

- Agar diffusion assay
- Broth dilution assay
- Disc diffusion assay

These assays may vary depending on the type of strains (bacterial or fungal), time of incubation, solvents, and nutritional composition of media. Therefore, it is quite challenging to compare them, which is the reason their usefulness has been debated. Due to the lipophilic and volatile characteristics of EOs, the most common screening procedures such as disc diffusion are not suitable for the evaluation of their antimicrobial potential. Various researchers have compared the findings obtained after the antimicrobial assessment of same EOs using different methods and found that their results are different. The results obtained from antimicrobial assessment of EOs using different assays were compared by Hood et al. [34]. This study demonstrated using the disc diffusion method that the lipophilic components of EOs could not uniformly distribute (because of solubility issues, which can directly influence the diffusion of EO components) into the agar medium. As a result, this assay does not present factual findings as only hydrophilic components diffused into the agar medium and showed antimicrobial activity. Another procedure based on broth dilution is generally suitable; however, the concentration of Tween used for increasing the solubility of EOs should be carefully considered, as it may enhance bacterial growth or change membrane permeability of the bacterial cell. In addition, Tween can interact with EO components to either cause antagonistic or synergistic effects, which may change the original antimicrobial potential of EOs. Thus, optimization of various parameters of antimicrobial assays must be carefully carried out to produce factual or real antimicrobial results of EOs.

20.4 Antiviral Effects of EOs

Previous studies have shown the promising role of EOs against some pathogenic viruses [35]. However, recently, a molecular docking study was performed by means of 171 EO components against severe acute respiratory syndrome coronavirus 2 (SARS-CoV-2) targets such as the following [35] (Figure 20.1):

- Human angiotensin–converting enzyme
- SARS-CoV-2 Adenosine diphosphate (ADP)-ribose-1″-phosphatase (SARS-CoV-2 ADRP)
- SARS-CoV-2 endoribonuclease
- SARS-CoV-2 main protease (SARS-CoV-2 Mpro)
- SARS-CoV-2 RNA-dependent RNA polymerase
- SARS-CoV-2 spike protein

It was found that the EO as well as its components can directly interact and bind with certain important SARS-CoV-2 proteins to prevent its pathogenicity. The sesquiterpene hydrocarbon, (E)-β-farnesene, showed a better docking score against main protease of SARS-CoV-2 whereas as per molecular modeling α and β farnesene were found to be finest complementary ligands for Nsp15 endoribonuclease of SARS-CoV. trans-farnesol demonstrated the best exothermic energy against ADP-ribose phosphatase of SARS-CoV-2. Thus, for this reason, their interaction with the SARS-CoV-2 targets is still doubtful. But there is a possibility that the EO and its components can act efficiently in a synergistic manner, can potentiate other antiviral agents, or can also be used in reliving COVID-19 symptoms [35]. For respiratory infections, EOs such as peppermint, menthol, eucalyptus, or frankincense can be used by means of vaporizers, diffusers, humidifiers, steam/portable inhalers, and nasal sticks. Inhalers and vaporizers can be applied with decongestants or EOs. However, there are no or few scientific reports that support the role of home remedies in eliminating coronaviruses.

20.5 The Role of EOs in Respiratory Infections

The potential roles of various EOs as well their components in respiratory tract infections are listed in Tables 20.1 and 20.2. The possible role of EOs and their components on infected lungs, infected alveolar sacs, and alveolar epithelial cell by SARS-CoV-2 is demonstrated in Figure 20.2. Based on a WHO report (2017), lower respiratory tract infections and pneumonia are two of the leading causes of death, accounting for more than 4 million deaths per year. There are almost 25 EOs officially listed in the European Pharmacopoeia [36]. Out of these oils, tea tree, thyme, fennel fruit, eucalyptus, anise, and peppermint are often employed in the management of respiratory illness. Thus, it is very important to discuss these oils separately [36].

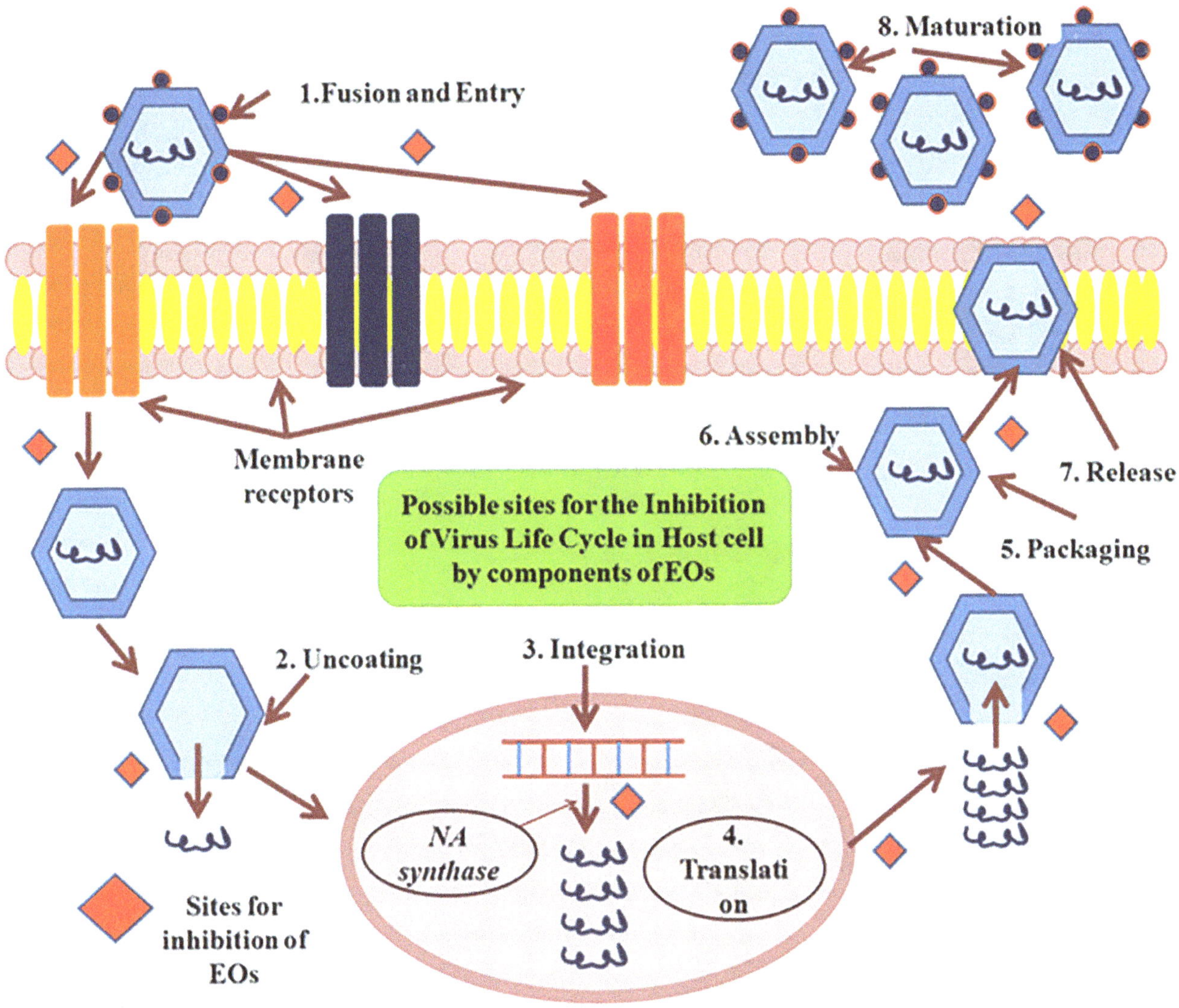

FIGURE 20.1 Antiviral action of EOs and their components in bacterial cell (1-8); possible sites for the inhibition of viral life cycle in host cell by EO are highlighted in red.

Anise oil or *Anisi aetheroleum* (derived from *Pimpinella anisum* L., via steam distillation) contains trans-anethole (80%–95%) whereas star anise oil (*Illicium verum*) contains trans-anethole and methyl-cavicol. Anethole is also present in large quantities in fennel oil (~60%) and a number of other plants from the Apiaceae, Myrtaceae, and Fabaceae families [37,38].

Anise oil can be used to treat various respiratory complications and principally acts as a mucolytic to clear the cough associated with the common cold [37,38]. Due to its contraindications and the presence of a natural organic compound phenylpropene, estragole, its use should be avoided in children and adolescents <18 years of age. Estragole is present in various plants and their related products and is responsible for various toxicities such as genotoxicity and carcinogenicity. Individuals who experience allergic reactions when exposed to the vapor phase of anethole should only use anise as well as its respective formulations under physician recommendations. Due to the reported estrogenic and antifertility effects in rat model, anethole is not recommended for pregnant/lactating females [39,40]. The use of anise oil can also cause topical allergy or allergy to lungs; thus, individuals use should be considered carefully.

Pelargonium graveolens (geranium) EO has been widely used in cosmetic products and is also considered as a component of aromatherapy to improve health and well-being. Usually, this oil is used to treat both physiological and psychological complications. Lemongrass oil obtained from *Cymbopogon citratus* (DC.) is widely used in folk medicine for the treatment of various ailments. The angiotensin-converting enzyme 2 (ACE2) inhibitory effects of geranium and lemon EOs as well as their main components were evaluated recently. This study suggested that *Pelargonium graveolens* as well as *Cymbopogon citratus* EOs showed considerable inhibition against ACE2 receptors present in HT-29 colon adenocarcinoma cell line cells. Moreover, western blotting and real-time polymerase chain reaction results also suggested that *Pelargonium graveolens* as well as *Cymbopogon citratus* EOs exhibit significant inhibition against ACE2. Furthermore, GC–MS analysis revealed that geranium oil contains neryl acetate, geraniol, and citronellol as the main chemical components whereas limonene is the main chemical compound of

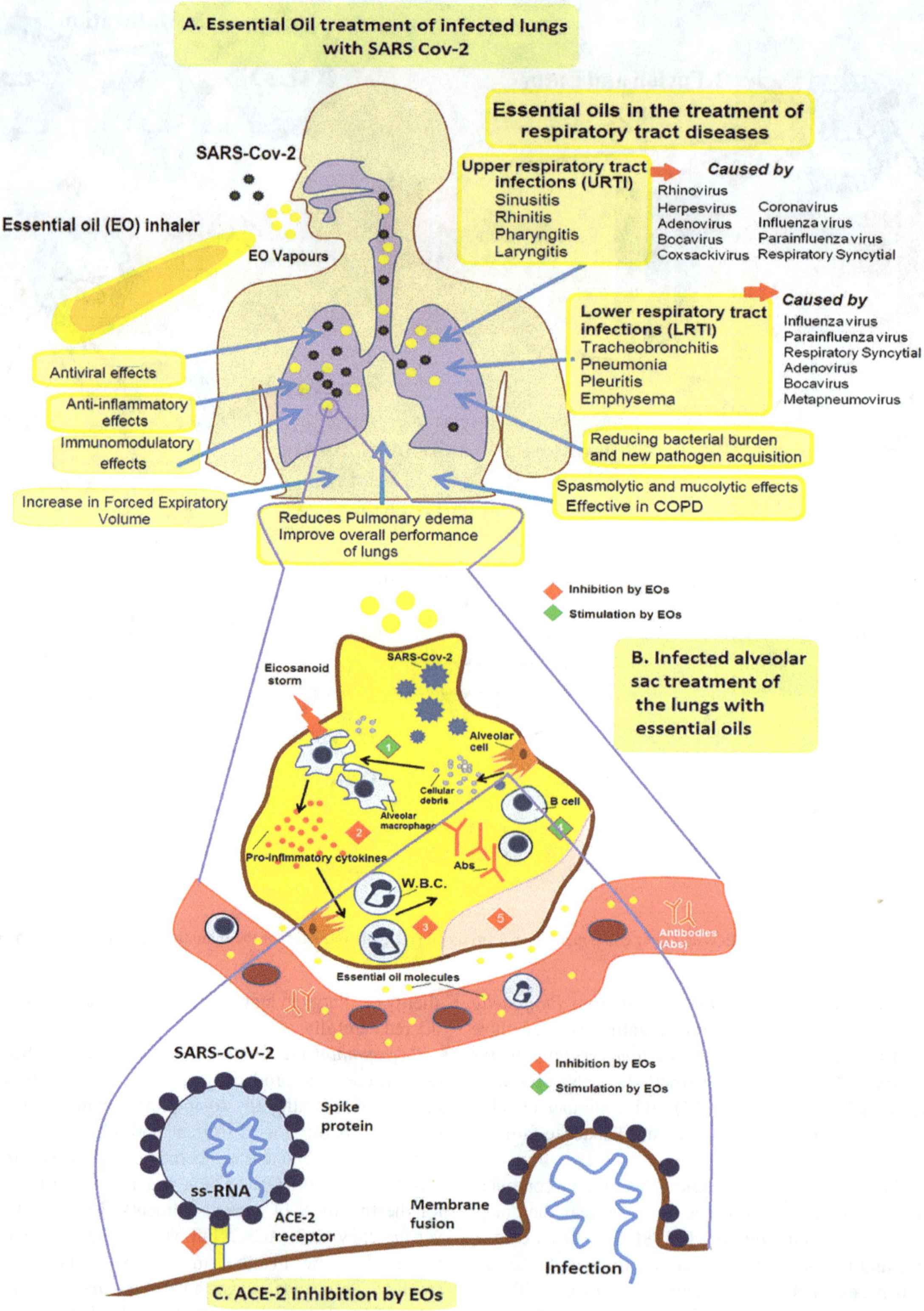

FIGURE 20.2 Possible mechanism of the specific action of the EO and its components on infected lungs (a), infected alveolar sacs, (b) alveolar epithelial cell, and (c) by SARS-CoV-2.

lemon oil. It was also discovered that citronellol and limonene treatment considerably downregulate ACE2 expression in epithelial cells. These findings draw a clear correlation between the chemical components of EOs with inhibitory effects against different viruses mainly against SARS-CoV-2; thus, these natural antiviral agents could play an important role in the inhibition of the invasion of SARS-CoV-2 [41].

Garlic (*Allium sativum* L.) is a spice, herbaceous plant, and traditional medicine that has been used for centuries for various ailments such as for the treatment of common viral infection, seasonal flu, as well as other respiratory illness [42]. Studies suggest that garlic EO contains a large number of organosulfur compounds. These organosulfur compounds, which contribute more than 99% of the garlic EO content, are responsible for various pharmacological activities such as reducing oxidative stress and causing antimicrobial anti-inflammatory effects, and are considered as natural chemotherapeutic agents [42]. Recently, 17 organosulfur compounds were detected by gas chromatography–mass spectrometry analysis of garlic EO. Molecular docking results suggest that these 17 sulfur components, mainly diallyl disulfide and trisulfide, showed strong interactions with ACE2 protein and the main protease, PDB6LU7, of SARS-CoV-2 [42]. Allyl disulfide and allyl trisulfide form 51.3% of garlic EO. Findings from this study also suggest these 17 substances synergistically act together and have potent inhibitory effects against proteins ACE2 as well as PDB6LU7. These findings indicate that *Allium sativum* EO components could be considered as important antiviral lead compounds to effectively prevent SARS-CoV-2 entry into cells. [42].

Bitter fennel fruit oil is derived from *Foeniculum vulgare* (family: Apiaceae) and contains fenchone and trans-anethole [43]. Traditionally, *Foeniculum vulgare* EO has been used as an mucoactive agent to relieve chest congestion due to mucus production in response to respiratory illness. Just like anise oil, it contains estragole and thus should not be used in treatment of children and adolescents. Bitter fennel fruit oil contains a high amount of lipophilic chemical compounds, which can freely diffuse through cell membranes. Oil components contain a high amount of carbonyl functional moieties which are highly reactive in nature and could possibly form Schiff's bases after interacting with the free amino moiety of amino acid present in nucleic acid or proteins. As discussed above, fennel EO also contains a high level of 4-anisaldehyde, which can interact with the amino acid of cellular proteins or nucleic acid to upregulate or downregulate their expression to affect their associated pathways. Trans-anethole present in fennel possesses estrogenic activity, which can cause allergic reaction [43].

Eucalyptus EO is obtained by steam distillation and rectification from the fresh leaves or fresh terminal branchlets of various species of eucalyptus rich in 1,8-cineole. The most frequently used species are *Eucalyptus globulus* Labill., *E. polybractea* R.T. Baker, and *E. smithii* R.T. Baker.

Eucalyptus EO, mainly *Eucalypti aetheroleum,* is derived from the crude as well as steam distillation of aerial parts of various plants (*E. smithii, E. globules,* and *E. polybractea*) belonging to genus eucalyptus that contain high levels of eucalyptol [44]. Eucalyptus oil (*Eucalypti aetheroleum*) is derived from the fresh leaves of *E. globules, E. polybractea*, and *E. smithii* by steam distillation process; it contains 1,8-cineole (>70%), also known as cineole or eucalyptol, as major components whereas α-pinene (2%–8%) and camphor (<0.1%) are minor components [44]. Eucalyptus oil is used in various types of respiratory ailments such as respiratory infections (both viral and bacterial), lung inflammation, and respiratory congestion. Eucalyptol, also known as 1,8-cineole, is the main component of eucalyptus, and has been used for centuries to treat colds, flu, and respiratory inflammation. A recent study suggested that normal use of eucalyptol can stimulate the immune system of the respiratory system as well as increase overall immunity, but could be having a harmful effect at larger dose, which is associated with alteration of phagocytosis and phagocyte migration and action of cytotoxic T lymphocytes and decreasing the level of B lymphocytes, natural killer cells, and immunoglobulin A. Recently, among 14 EOs, cinnamon bark, lemongrass, and thyme oils showed the lowest minimal inhibitory dose whereas EOs comprising hydrocarbon, ether, and, terpene ketone showed high MIC against *Staphylococcus aureus, Streptococcus pneumoniae, Streptococcus pyogenes,* and *Haemophilus influenzae.* In addition, eucalyptus oil showed minimum antibacterial activity against *E. coli.* Findings from this study suggest that the antibacterial property of EOs is more significant at high vapor concentration for a short duration [44]. As sufficient human trial data is not available, eucalyptus oil should always be used with medical advice, especially during pregnancy and lactation [44].

Mentha piperita EO (peppermint EO) is derived by steam distillation of peppermint aerial parts [45], and is mainly comprised of menthol and menthon. However, it also contains other components such as limonene, eucalyptol, isomenthone, and menthyl acetate. In addition, it contains certain chemical components in low amount such as carvone, pulegone, etc. Due to its various medicinal properties, especially in treating respiratory as well as GIT complications, *Mentha piperita* EO has gained attention for its possible use against viral infections. However, its use is not recommended in kids (<2 years of age) as its chemical component, mainly menthol, can cause hyperactivation of laryngeal chemoreflex resulting in temporary vocal cord contraction, which can cause difficulty in speaking or breathing [45]. Thus, application of mentha EO-based formulations directly over the necks, nasal cavities, and chests of infants and children (<2 years of age) must be avoided. Among individuals that are allergic or more vulnerable, menthol inhalation can lead to cessation of breathing and laryngospasm. Menthol application to neonates that are deficient in glucose-6-phosphate dehydrogenase can result in jaundice [46]. Use of mentha EO has not been recommended during the pregnancy without medical supervision.

Tea tree EO is derived from *M. alternifolia, M. linariifolia,* and *M. dissitiflora* (family: Melaleuca) via steam distillation process, and contains monoterpenoids including γ-terpinene, terpineol, and eucalyptol. Tea tree oil can be used in the management of various pulmonary infections such as common influenza and inflammation and irritation of the bronchioles.

Recently, a docking-based study revealed that natural *Melaleuca cajuputi* EO can be used to prevent entry of SARS-CoV-2 into cells. In this study, 24 main chemical compounds were identified by using GC–MS analysis, out of which 10 chemical compounds synergistically showed strong inhibition against SARS-CoV-2 ACE2 protein as well as its key protease (PDB6LU7). Terpineol, guaiol, linalool, α-eudesmol, cineol, γ-eudesmol, and β-selinenol were identified as the most potential compounds against ACE2 and PDB6LU7 proteins [47].

Thyme oil (reminiscent of thymol) is derived from the *Thymus vulgaris* and *Thymus zygis,* or a blend of oil obtained from both plants by steam distillation containing phenolic compounds, mainly p-cymene (thymol) and/or carvacrol and other terpenes. Thymol and carvacrol are known to suppress growth and biofilm formation of *Streptococcus mutans.* Also, they are known for stimulating autolysis (self-digestion of the cell wall by peptidoglycan hydrolases) and stress in bacterials cell. Thyme oil has been used therapeutically for the treatment of various respiratory ailments such as asthma and bronchitis. Thyme has also been used for the treatment of other ailments because of its considerably wide range of antiviral, antioxidative, antifungal, antitussive, antimicrobial, antispasmodic, and antiseptic properties. It was also reported that thyme oil did not show activity against *Staphylococcus aureus, Salmonella choleraesuis,* or *Klebsilela pneumoniae* but suppressed the growth of *Pseudomonas aeruginosa* and *Candida albicans.*

20.6 The Role of EO-Loaded Nanoparticles against Multidrug-Resistant Bacterial Strains

Metallic nanoparticles are known for their potential antimicrobial effects. Nanofabrication of silver enhances the antibacterial activity even at low concentrations, and because of the changes in the surface-to-volume ratio, silver nanoparticles offer drastic improvement in physical, chemical, and biological properties [48–65]. The lipophilic components of EOs showed antibacterial effects by disrupting cell membrane, causing cytoplasmic modifications, disturbing cellular pH, enhancing cell permeability, interfering in adenosine triphosphate (ATP) and protein synthesis, and interfering with quorum sensing.

EOs/nanoparticles in one system can be used to cause cell membrane disruption, decrease the synthesis of ATP, improve cell surface permeability, induce DNA damage, and inhibit bacterial enzymes and other antigenic proteins with increased free radical generation. Silver nanoparticles alone have shown significant antimicrobial effects; however, microorganisms exposed to silver-resistant microorganisms rapidly develop resistance to silver nanoparticles by genetic changes [48–65]. Thus, EOs coupled with silver nanoparticles could be a reliable solution to suppress the development of antibiotic-resistant microorganisms. Previous reports showed that the additive or synergistic antimicrobial effects of silver nanoparticles combined with volatile components of EOs and it was found that this preparation showed better results classical.

REFERENCES

1. Bright B, Babalola CP, Sam-Agudu NA, Onyeaghala AA, Olatunji A, Aduh U, Sobande PO, Crowell TA, Tebeje YK, Phillip S, Ndembi N, Folayan MO. COVID-19 preparedness: Capacity to manufacture vaccines, therapeutics and diagnostics in sub-Saharan Africa. *Global Health.* 2021;17(1):24.
2. Chouhan S, Sharma K, Guleria S. Antimicrobial activity of some essential oils-present status and future perspectives. *Medicines (Basel).* 2017;4(3):58.
3. Swamy MK, Akhtar MS, Sinniah UR. Antimicrobial properties of plant essential oils against human pathogens and their mode of action: An updated review. *Evid Based Complement Alternat Med.* 2016;2016:3012462.
4. Horváth G, Ács K. Essential oils in the treatment of respiratory tract diseases highlighting their role in bacterial infections and their anti-inflammatory action: A review. *Flavour Fragr J.* 2015;30(5):331–341.
5. Jaradat NA, Al Zabadi H, Rahhal B, et al. The effect of inhalation of *Citrus sinensis* flowers and *Mentha spicata* leave essential oils on lung function and exercise performance: A quasi-experimental uncontrolled before-and-after study. *J Int Soc Sports Nutr.* 2016;13:36.
6. Raha S, Kim SM, Lee HJ, et al. Essential oil from Korean *Chamaecyparis obtusa* leaf ameliorates respiratory activity in Sprague Dawley rats and exhibits protection from NF-κB-induced inflammation in WI38 fibroblast cells. *Int J Mol Med.* 2019;43(1):393–403.
7. Li C, Li L, Luo J, Huang N. Effect of turmeric volatile oil on the respiratory tract. *Zhongguo Zhong Yao Za Zhi.* 1998;23(10):624–625.
8. Wang, H., Song L, Ju W, et al. The acute airway inflammation induced by PM2.5 exposure and the treatment of essential oils in Balb/c mice. *Sci Rep.* 2017;7:44256.
9. Laude EA, Morice AH, Grattan TJ. The antitussive effects of menthol, camphor and cineole in conscious guinea-pigs. *Pulm Pharmacol.* 1994;7:179.
10. Morice AH, Marshall AE, Higgins KS, Grattan TJ. Effect of inhaled menthol on citric acid induced cough in normal subjects. *Thorax.* 1994;49(10):1024–1026.
11. Plevkova J, Kollarik M, Poliacek I, et al. The role of trigeminal nasal TRPM8-expressing afferent neurons in the antitussive effects of menthol. *J Appl Physiol.* 2013;115(2):268–274.
12. Ueno-Iio T, Shibakura M, Yokota K, et al. Lavender essential oil inhalation suppresses allergic airway inflammation and mucous cell hyperplasia in a murine model of asthma. *Life Sci.* 2014;108(2):109–115.
13. Kilina AV, Kolesnikova MB. The efficacy of the application of essential oils for the prevention of acute respiratory diseases in organized groups of children. *Vestn Otorinolaringol.* 2011;(5):51–54.
14. Sadlon AE, Lamson DW. Immune-modifying and antimicrobial effects of Eucalyptus oil and simple inhalation devices. *Altern Med Rev.* 2010;15(1):33–43.
15. Rivera DG, Hernández I, Merino N, et al. *Mangifera indica* L. extract (Vimang) and mangiferin reduce the airway inflammation and Th2 cytokines in murine model of allergic asthma. *J Pharm Pharmacol.* 2011;63(10):1336–1345.
16. Charron JM. Use of *Lavandula latifolia* as an expectorant. *J Altern Complement Med.* 1997;3:211.
17. Juergens UR, Engelen T, Racke K, et al. Inhibitory activity of 1,8- cineol (eucalyptol) on cytokine production in cultured human lymphocytes and monocytes. *Pulm Pharmacol Ther.* 2004;17:281–287.
18. Millqvist E, Ternesten-Hasséus E, Bende M. Inhalation of menthol reduces capsaicin cough sensitivity and influences inspiratory flows in chronic cough. *Respir Med.* 2013;107(3):433–438.
19. Haidl P, Kemper P, Butnarasu SJ, Klauke M, Wehde H, Köhler D. Beeinflusst die inhalation von 1%-iger L-Menthol-Lösung die Hustenhäufigkeit und die Dyspnoeempfindung bei der Fiberbronchoskopie? Does the inhalation of a 1% L-menthol solution in the premedication of fiberoptic bronchoscopy affect coughing and the sensation of dyspnea? *Pneumologie.* 2001;55(3):115–119.

20. Gao M, Singh A, Macri K, et al. Antioxidant components of naturally-occurring oils exhibit marked anti-inflammatory activity in epithelial cells of the human upper respiratory system. *Respir Res.* 2011;12(1):92.
21. Li Y, Xu YL, Lai YN, Liao SH, Liu N, Xu PP. Intranasal co-administration of 1,8-cineole with influenza vaccine provide cross-protection against influenza virus infection. *Phytomedicine.* 2017;34:127–135.
22. Meamarbashi A. Instant effects of peppermint essential oil on the physiological parameters and exercise performance. *Avicenna J Phytomed.* 2014;4(1):72–78.
23. Tiwari M, Kakkar P. Plant derived antioxidants: Geraniol and camphene protect rat alveolar macrophages against t-BHP induced oxidative stress. *Toxicol In Vitro.* 2009;23(2):295–301.
24. Trang DT, Hoang TKV, Nguyen TTM, et al. Essential oils of lemongrass (*Cymbopogon citratus* Stapf) induces apoptosis and cell cycle arrest in A549 lung cancer cells. *Biomed Res Int.* 2020;2020:5924856.
25. Chung KS, Hong JY, Lee JH, et al. β-caryophyllene in the essential oil from *Chrysanthemum boreale* induces G1 phase cell cycle arrest in human lung cancer cells. *Molecules.* 2019;24(20):3754.
26. Seal S, Chatterjee P, Bhattacharya S, et al. Vapor of volatile oils from *Litsea cubeba* seed induces apoptosis and causes cell cycle arrest in lung cancer cells. *PLoS One.* 2012;7(10):e47014.
27. Wang D, Qu X, Zhuang X, et al. Seed oil of *Brucea javanicaInduces* cell cycle arrest and apoptosis via reactive oxygen species-mediated mitochondrial dysfunction in human lung cancer cells. *Nutr Cancer.* 2016;68(8):1394–1403.
28. Hassan SB, Gali-Muhtasib H, Göransson H, Larsson R. Alpha terpineol: A potential anticancer agent which acts through suppressing NF-κB signaling. *Anticancer Res.* 2010;30(6):1911–1919.
29. Maruoka T, Kitanaka A, Kubota Y, et al. Lemongrass essential oil and citral inhibit SRC/Stat3 activity and suppress the proliferation/survival of small-cell lung cancer cells, alone or in combination with chemotherapeutic agents. *Int J Oncol.* 2018;52(5):1738–1748.
30. Li N, Zhang Q, Jia Z, Yang X, Zhang H, Luo H. Volatile oil from alpinia officinarum promotes lung cancer regression in vitro and in vivo. *Food Funct.* 2018;9(9):4998–5006.
31. Castro MA, Rodenak-Kladniew B, Massone A, Polo M, García de Bravo M, Crespo R. *Citrus reticulata* peel oil inhibits non-small cell lung cancer cell proliferation in culture and implanted in nude mice. *Food Funct.* 2018;9(4):2290–2299.
32. Manjamalai A, Grace VM. The chemotherapeutic effect of essential oil of *Plectranthus amboinicus* (Lour) on lung metastasis developed by B16F-10 cell line in C57BL/6 mice. *Cancer Invest.* 2013;31(1):74–82.
33. Sylvestre M, Legault J, Dufour D, Pichette A. Chemical composition and anticancer activity of leaf essential oil of *Myrica gale* L. *Phytomedicine.* 2005;12(4):299–304.
34. Hood JR, Wilkinson JM, Cavanagh HMA. Evaluation of common antibacterial screening methods utilized in essential oil research. *J Essent Oil Res.* 2003;15(6):428–433.
35. Silva JKRD, Figueiredo PLB, Byler KG, Setzer WN. Essential oils as antiviral agents. Potential of essential oils to treat SARS-CoV-2 infection: An in-silico investigation. *Int J Mol Sci.* 2020;21(10):3426.
36. GBD. LRI collaborators. Estimates of the global, regional, and national morbidity, mortality, and aetiologies of lower respiratory tract infections in 195 countries: A systematic analysis for the global burden of disease study 2015. *Lancet Infect Dis.* 2017;17(11):1133–1161.
37. Kulkarni SA, Nagarajan SK, Ramesh V, Palaniyandi V, Selvam SP, Madhavan T. Computational evaluation of major components from plant essential oils as potent inhibitors of SARS-CoV-2 spike protein. *J Mol Struct.* 2020;1221:128823.
38. Ernst E. *ESCOP Monographs: The Scientific Foundation for Herbal Medicinal Products*, 2nd edn. Thieme, Stuttgart, New York; 2003.
39. Dhar SK. Anti-fertility activity and hormonal profile of trans-anethole in rats. *Indian J Physiol Pharmacol.* 1995;39(1):63–7.
40. Dosoky NS, Setzer WN. Maternal reproductive toxicity of some essential oils and their constituents. *Int J Mol Sci.* 2021;22(5):2380.
41. Senthil Kumar KJ, Gokila Vani M, Wang CS, Chen CC, Chen YC, Lu LP, Huang CH, Lai CS, Wang SY. Geranium and lemon essential oils and their active compounds down-regulate angiotensin-converting enzyme 2 (ACE2), a SARS-CoV-2 spike receptor-binding domain, in epithelial cells. *Plants (Basel).* 2020;9(6):770.
42. Thuy BTP, My TTA, Hai NTT, et al. Investigation into SARS-CoV-2 resistance of compounds in garlic essential oil published correction appears in ACS omega. *ACS Omega.* 2020;5(14):8312–8320.
43. Zhang S, Chen X, Devshilt I, Yun Q, Huang C, An L, Dorjbat S, He X. Fennel main constituent, trans-anethole treatment against LPS-induced acute lung injury by regulation of Th17/Treg function. *Mol Med Rep.* 2018;18(2):1369–1376.
44. Inouye S, Takizawa T, Yamaguchi H. Antibacterial activity of essential oils and their major constituents against respiratory tract pathogens by gaseous contact, *J Antimicrob Chemother.* 2001;47(5):565–573.
45. European Medicines Agency. European Union herbal monograph on *Mentha×piperita* L., aetheroleum. https://www.ema.europa.eu/en/documents/herbal-monograph/european-union-herbal-monograph-mentha-x-piperita-l-aetheroleum-revision-1_en.pdf.
46. Olowe SA, Ransome-Kuti O. The risk of jaundice in glucose-6-phosphate dehydrogenase deficient babies exposed to menthol. *Acta Pædiatrica.* 1980;69:341–345.
47. My TTA, Loan HTP, Hai NTT, et al. Evaluation of the inhibitory activities of COVID-19 of *Melaleuca cajuputi* oil using docking simulation. *Chem Sel.* 2020;5(21):6312–6320.
48. Bhatia S, Kumar V, Sharma K, Nagpal K, Bera T. Significance of algal polymer in designing amphotericin B nanoparticles. *Sci World J.* 2014;2014:564573.
49. Bhatia S, Rathee P, Sharma K, Chaugule BB, Kar N, Bera T. Immuno-modulation effect of sulphated polysaccharide (porphyran) from *Porphyra vietnamensis. Int J Biol Macromol.* 2013;57:50–56.
50. Bhatia S. *Natural Polymer Drug Delivery Systems: Marine Polysaccharides Based Nano-Materials and Its Applications.* Springer International Publishing, Switzerland; 2016:185–225.
51. Bhatia S. *Natural Polymer Drug Delivery Systems: Plant Derived Polymers, Properties, and Modification & Applications.* Springer International Publishing, Switzerland; 2016:119–184.

52. Bhatia S. *Natural Polymer Drug Delivery Systems: Nanotechnology and Its Drug Delivery Applications.* Springer International Publishing, Switzerland; 2016:1–32.
53. Bhatia S. *Natural Polymer Drug Delivery Systems: Nanoparticles Types, Classification, Characterization, Fabrication Methods and Drug Delivery Applications.* Springer International Publishing, Switzerland; 2016:33–93.
54. Bhatia S. *Natural Polymer Drug Delivery Systems: Natural Polymers vs Synthetic Polymer.* Springer International Publishing, Switzerland; 2016:95–118.
55. Bhatia S. *Systems for Drug Delivery: Mammalian Polysaccharides and Its Nanomaterials.* Springer International Publishing, Switzerland; 2016:1–27.
56. Bhatia S. *Systems for Drug Delivery: Microbial Polysaccharides as Advance Nanomaterials.* Springer International Publishing, Switzerland; 2016:29–54.
57. Bhatia S. *Systems for Drug Delivery: Chitosan Based Nanomaterials and Its Applications.* Springer International Publishing, Switzerland; 2016:55–117.
58. Bhatia S. *Systems for Drug Delivery: Advance Polymers and Its Applications.* Springer International Publishing, Switzerland; 2016:119–146.
59. Bhatia S. *Systems for Drug Delivery: Advanced Application of Natural Polysaccharides.* Springer International Publishing, Switzerland; 2016:147–170.
60. Bhatia S. *Systems for Drug Delivery: Modern Polysaccharides and Its Current Advancements.* Springer International Publishing, Switzerland; 2016:171–188.
61. Bhatia S. *Systems for Drug Delivery: Toxicity of Nanodrug Delivery Systems.* Springer International Publishing, Switzerland; 2016:189–197.
62. Bhatia S. *Nanotechnology in Drug Delivery Fundamentals, Design, and Applications: Part 1: Protein and Peptide-Based Drug Delivery Systems.* Apple Academic Press, Palm Bay, FL; 2016:50–204.
63. Bhatia S. *Nanotechnology in Drug Delivery Fundamentals, Design, and Applications: Part 2: Peptide-Mediated Nanoparticle Drug Delivery System.* Apple Academic Press, Palm Bay, FL; 2016:205–280.
64. Bhatia S. *Nanotechnology in Drug Delivery Fundamentals, Design, and Applications: Part 3: CPP and CTP in Drug Delivery and Cell Targeting.* Apple Academic Press, Palm Bay, FL; 2016:309–312.
65. Scandorieiro S, de Camargo LC, Lancheros CA, Yamada-Ogatta SF, Nakamura CV, de Oliveira AG, Andrade CG, Duran N, Nakazato G, Kobayashi RK. Synergistic and additive effect of oregano essential oil and biological silver nanoparticles against multidrug-resistant bacterial strains. *Front Microbiol.* 2016;7:760.

21

The Cardioprotective Effects of Essential Oils

Ahmed Al-Harrasi
Natural and Medical Sciences Research Center, University of Nizwa

Saurabh Bhatia
Natural and Medical Sciences Research Center, University of Nizwa
University of Petroleum and Energy Studies

Tapan Behl
Chitkara University

Deepak Kaushik
M.D. University

CONTENTS

DOI: 10.1201/9781003175933-23

21.1 Introduction

Cardiovascular diseases (CVDs) are the main cause of death in developed countries and considered as leading causes of disease burden in developing countries. CVDs are classified into two broad ranges of disorders:

- Diseases associated with the cardiac muscle.
- Diseases associated with the vascular system that supplies blood to the heart, brain, and other vital organs.

This chapter focuses on the most common causes of CVD morbidity and mortality. However, both conditions can result in ischemic heart disease, stroke, and congestive heart failure [1]. Myocardial infarction, colloquially known as "heart attack," is the most common cause of heart disease. The root cause of this heart-associated abnormality is sudden decline or complete cessation of blood supply to a part of the cardiac muscle. Myocardial infarction can remain undetected or undiagnosed or cause a terrible episode resulting in hemodynamic worsening and sudden death [1]. In the United States, the majority of myocardial infarction episodes occurs because of primary coronary artery disease. Several vascular complications, such as cerebrovascular and coronary heart diseases, can result in cardiac injury in the form of atherosclerosis and thromboembolism. Atherosclerosis is characterized by deposition of fat, bad cholesterol such as low-density lipoprotein along with high triglycerides, and other organic matter over the wall of the artery resulting in the formation of plaque, which can ultimately cause obstruction in the blood flow. Several investigations have shown that increase in low-density lipoprotein in various susceptible regions called atherosclerosis-prone areas of arteries such as intima of human arteries can result in oxidation of low-density lipoprotein. This type of oxidative reaction is a complex event that can result in the formation of complex products such as fatty streaks. This event can further elevate inflammatory responses, which can subsequently cause the development of advanced atherosclerotic injuries. High-density lipoprotein, called "good" cholesterol, removes bad cholesterol from the atherosclerotic plaque and other parts of the human body back to the liver, mainly hepatocytes. For the excretion, sterol, mainly cholesterol, is metabolized to bile acids as end products in liver cells. This route of transporting sterol from the site of their deposition (i.e., sclerotic plaque to liver cells) somewhat elucidates the antiatherogenic property of high-density lipoproteins. Herbal medicine use as an alternative treatment is considered as a reliable approach to treating several diseases including CVDs. Recently, there has been increased use of natural products especially in the treatment of CVDs. Due to the possible synergistic and adverse side effects of herb-drug interactions, it is essential to study the effect of natural products more deeply before their inclusion in the mainstream of healthcare [2].

Antioxidants derived from medicinal plants are being used in the treatment of various cardiovascular complications. Cardioprotective effects exhibited by various antioxidants and other phytochemicals via different mechanisms have been explored. Essential oils (EOs) obtained from various plants are considered as diverse antioxidants and other components that can synergistically or antagonistically act on the cardiovascular system to exhibit therapeutic effects at the site of injury. These components are known to possess various cardioprotective effects via influencing vasodilatation, inducing hypotension, and decreasing heart rate (HR) ultimately to promote the health of the circulatory system.

Certain EOs as well as their chemical components have shown beneficial effects on the cardiovascular system via widening of blood vessels, reducing the HR, and showing hypotensive effects. So far numerous molecular pathways have been explored to establish for the role of EOs and components in improving the cardiovascular system. In the myocardial infarction-induced rat model, the EO of lavender (*Lavandula angustifolia*) showed cardioprotective effect via suppressing oxidative stress and inflammatory pathway. Lavender oil treatment via inhalation showed decrease in cholesterol plaques in cholesterol-fed rabbits (to induce atherosclerotic plaques in rabbits); however, it did not show any effect on serum cholesterol levels [3,4]. Lavender oil treatment is also reported on for its hypolipidemic effect in rats [5]. Moreover, lavender treatment showed increase in coronary circulation and vasorelaxation effects in humans [6]. The aqueous extract derived from the flowers of *Lavandula angustifolia* showed cardioprotective effect against ischemic reperfusion injury in isolated rat hearts. Earlier reports demonstrated the protective action of Lavender EO on isoproterenol-induced myocardial infarction in rats [5]. It was found that *Lavandula angustifolia* EO treatment normalized electrocardiogram, reduced hemodynamic damage, decreased lipid peroxidation as well as expression of proinflammatory mediators, and promoted the radical scavenging activity of various enzymes. Additionally, lavender EO reduced heart tissue injury and improved cardiac function via increasing strength of cardiac muscles and maintained cardiac cells architecture [5]. The cardioprotective effects of several EOs and their components are listed in Table 21.1.

TABLE 21.1
Cardioprotective Effects of EOs and Their Components

EOs or Chemical Component	Biological Effects	Mechanism of Action (MOA)	References
1,8-cineole	*In vivo* cardioprotective effects	Reduced hypertension via regulating NO as well as oxidative stress among rodents	[7]
1-nitro-phenylethane	*In vivo* cardioprotective effects	Decreased heart rate as well as blood pressure	[8]
4-chloro-m-cresol	Caffeine-like responses in ferret cardiac muscle; contractile response in saponin-skinned but not intact fibers	Ca^{2+} release via the ryanodine receptor	[9]
Seseli pallasii Besser (Aerial parts) [α-pinene (42.7%–48.2%)]	Vasorelaxant effects	Vasorelaxing and ACE inhibitory effects	[10]
Alpinia zerumbet Terpinen-4-ol (57.4%)	Blood pressure reduction, vasorelaxation	Prevented Ca^{+2} entry via VOCC and ROC channels	[11]
Alpinia zerumbet (1,8-cineole)	Vasorelaxant effects	Endothelium-dependent vasorelaxant effects	[12]
Alpinia zerumbet (1,8-cineole)	Vasorelaxant effects	Antihypertensive effect and vasorelaxant effects Prevented Ca^{+2} entry via VOCC and ROC channels with prevention of calcium movement from calcium- store inside cell	[13]
Alpinia zerumbet (leaves)	Induced an immediate and significant hypotension	Vasorelaxant effects due to terpinen-4-ol	[14]
Aniba Canelilla Bark	Hypotensive activity, and cause vasodilation	Showed direct action over smooth muscles of vasculature via endothelial L-arginine/NO pathway	[15]
Aniba rosaeodora Linalool (87.7%)	Blood pressure reduction and vasorelaxation	Causes vagovagal reflex controls in rodents	[16]

(*Continued*)

TABLE 21.1 (*Continued*)
Cardioprotective Effects of EOs and Their Components

EOs or Chemical Component	Biological Effects	Mechanism of Action (MOA)	References
Artemisia campestris (spathulenol, *β*-eudesmol, and p-cymene)	Vasorelaxation	Vasodilation effects were facilitated via suppression of L-type Ca^{2+} receptors	[17]
Auraptene	*In vivo* cardioprotective effects	Reduce blood pressure (dose as well as time based)	[18]
Bergamot EO	Via modulating Ca^{+2} levels intracellularly	Obstruction of Ca^{2+} entry	[19]
Bisabolol	*In vitro* cardioprotective effects	Cause vasorelaxation via modulating Ca^{2+} voltage-dependent channel	[20]
Borneol	*In vitro* cardioprotective effects	Vasorelaxation with and without endothelium Vasorelaxation perhaps due to stimulation of potassium channels, prevention of calcium inflow along with suppression calcium movement from calcium stores inside the cell	[21]
Borneol	*In vivo* cardioprotective effects	Decrease of proinflammatory mediators with reduction in oxidative stress.	[22]
Carvacrol	*In vitro* cardioprotective effects	Vasodilation via antioxidant effects with stimulation of NOS Vaso relaxation via rise in calcium inflow, via stimulating TRPV3 receptor Vasodilation via suppressing calcium inflow via the L-type Cav, ROC, and SOC channels Negative inotropic and chronotropic effect	[23]
Carvacrol	*In vivo* cardiovascular effects	Decrease in blood pressure as well as heart rate (dependent on dose)	[24]
Carvone	*In vitro* cardioprotective effects	Vasorelaxant effect Vasorelaxation via suppressing Ca^{2+} inflow as well as its production Vasodilation via suppressing Ca^{2+} sensitivity as well as Ca^{2+} inflow Vasorelaxation effect via suppressing L-type Ca^{2+} receptors	[25,26]
Cinnamaldehyde	*In vitro* cardioprotective effects	Prevents endothelial dysfunction by attenuating ROS generation and	[27]
Cinnamaldehyde	*In vivo* cardioprotective effects	Reduce cardiac damage and proinflammatory mediators with rise in NO as well as SOD levels	[28]
Cinnamic acid	*In vitro* cardioprotective effects	Vasorelaxation via the NO–cGMP-PKG pathway, after stimulating Ca^{2+}-triggered K^+ channels	[29]
Cinnamic acid	*In vivo* cardioprotective effects	Antioxidant effects with modulation of biochemical markers and rise in levels of NO	
Cinnamyl alcohol	*In vitro* cardioprotective effects	Vasorelaxation via stimulation of K^+ release and suppression of Rho-kinase	[30]
Citral	*In vitro* cardioprotective effects	Vasodilation via restricting calcium entry by inhibiting voltage-mediated L-type Ca^{2+} channels	[30]
Citronellal	*In vivo* cardioprotective effects	Decrease heart rate as well as blood pressure among normotensive rodents.	[31]
Citrus bergamia	Vasorelaxant activity	Vasodilation (endothelium-independent) via modulating the smooth muscle tone as well as K^+ channels stimulation	[32]
Inhalation of lavender EO with cold treatment	Reduced pain and anxiety associated with postcoronary artery bypass grafting and postsurgical chest tube removal	Reduced intensity of the pain as well as anxiety	[33]
Crocus sativus aq.fraction and safranal	Cardioprotective effect in isoproterenol-triggered myocardial infarction	Decreased the serum LDH and creatine kinase-muscle and myocardial lipid peroxidation, preserved nearly normal tissue architecture, reduction of oxidative stress	[34]
Croton nepetaefolius (Methyleugenol and alpha-terpineol)	Vasodilatory effects	Stimulation of endothelium–NO pathway in the mediation of vasodilatory effects	[35]
Croton zambesicus	Vasorelaxant activity	Vasorelaxant activity	[36]
Croton zehntneri EO	Hypotensive and vasoconstrictive action	Decrease in blood pressure (phase I) is facilitated via cholinergic pathway with simultaneous induction of bradycardia	[37]
Curcuma longa L. Ar-turmerone (20.5%)	eNOS expression, antiplatelet, lipid improvement, liver function improvement, vasorelaxation	Antihyperlipidaemic effect and reduced lipid-stimulated oxidative stress, platelet activation and dysfunction in vasculature	[38]

(*Continued*)

TABLE 21.1 (*Continued*)

Cardioprotective Effects of EOs and Their Components

EOs or Chemical Component	Biological Effects	Mechanism of Action (MOA)	References
Cymbopogon citrates	Cardioprotective and antilipid peroxidative	Decreased level of biochemical markers associated with heart in serum	[39]
Cymbopogon citrates (Citronellol)	Vasodilation	Decreased blood via acting directly over vascular smooth muscle resulting in vasorelaxation	[40]
Cymbopogon proximus EO	Pretreatment confers cardioprotective effects	Downregulated expression of hypertrophy markers	[41]
D-Limonene	Protective effect against myocardial infraction	Decreased level of myocardial enzymes, normalize blood pressure indices, reduced Bax expression and increased Bcl-2 expression and decreased myocardial injury	[42]
Eugenol	Reduced ATP concentration	Activation of the cardiac thin filaments by strongly attached cross-bridges	[43]
Eugenol	Muscle contraction	Two pathways of calcium secretion from the SR is mediated via heparin-sensitive pathway or the ryanodine receptors activation	[44]
Eugenol	Reduces the force produced by electrically paced intact papillary muscles	L-type calcium channel inhibition	[45]
Farnesene	In vitro cardiovascular effects	Vasodilatation by inhibiting calcium influx	[46]
Ferula asafetida	Vasodilatory effect	Vasodilatory effect was facilitated via potassium channels stimulation as well as decreased release of calcium from intracellular stores	[47]
Foeniculum vulgare Anethole (75.8%)	Antiplatelet, antithrombosis, vasorelaxation	Broad spectrum antiplatelet activity, clot destabilizing effect and vasorelaxant action	[48]
Garlic EO	Increases serum fibrinolytic activity in patients with coronary artery disease.	Vasodilation, and fibrinolytic effects	[49]
Garlic EO (diallyl disulfide and diallyl trisulfide)	Reduces blood lipids and increases fibribolytic activity in patients with coronary artery disease	Considerable decrease in overall serum cholesterol and triglycerides level and improved HDL-cholesterol as well as fibrinolytic effects	[50]
Garlic EO	Antiobesity effects	Reduces triglycerides, cholesterol in serum with rise increases fibrinolytic effects and reduced adhesion of platelets	[51]
Garlic and onion EO	Antiobesity effects	Improved lipid profile via reducing TG, TC, and LDL-C and elevating the HDL-C in serum	[52]
Geraniol	Protective effect against myocardial infraction	Via improving the activity of antioxidant enzymes, stimulate Keap1/Nrf2 pathway, modulate the PI3K/Akt/mTOR pathway, resulting in decrease in inflammation, apoptotic death and myocardial autophagy)	[53]
Hinoki EOs	Systolic blood pressure, HR, and parasympathetic nervous system were decreased	Sympathetic nervous activity was increased with increased HR variability	[54]
Hyptis fruticosa Salzm 1,8-cineole (16.9%)	Blood pressure reduction vasorelaxation	Induced hypotension associated with tachycardia	[55]
Lavandula angustifolia	Cardioprotective effects	Protects myocardium due to its antioxidant properties	[5]
Lavandula angustifolia	Cardioprotective effect	Decreased cardiac damage via reducing oxidative stress as well as tumor necrosis factor-alpha	[56]
Lavandula angustifolia	Cardioprotective effects	Decreased plaques made via cholesterolin experimental animals, however demonstrated no effect on cholesterol levels in serum	[57]
Lavandula angustifolia	Cardioprotective effects	Neuroprotective effects as well as antioxidant effects in an experimental model of stroke	[58]
Lavandula angustifolia	Cardioprotective effects	Vasorelaxation and increased coronary blood flow	[59]
Lavender roman chamomile, and neroli	Decrease anxiety, and increase sleeping condition of percutaneous coronary intervention patients	Significantly decreased the level of anxiety and improved the sleeping condition of coronary angioplasty patients	[60]
Lavender and grapefruit oil	Reduces diastolic blood pressure and anxiety	Suppress the diastolic blood pressure among stroke patients with greater levels of anxiety	[61]
Lavender EO (linalyl acetate)	Vasorelaxant effect	Cause vasorelaxation of vascular smooth muscle via partly stimulation of NO/cGMP pathway	[62]

(*Continued*)

TABLE 21.1 (*Continued*)

Cardioprotective Effects of EOs and Their Components

EOs or Chemical Component	Biological Effects	Mechanism of Action (MOA)	References
Lavender oil	Decreased HR	Considerably decreased heart rate, anxiety, and pain among patients underwent cardiac surgery	[63]
Lemon (Limon Citrus)	Reduce blood pressure	Lemon inhalation in acute myocardial infarction decreased anxiety, systolic blood pressure, and proportion of ST-part and T wave adjustments	[64]
Linalool	*In vivo* cardioprotective effects	Stimulates hypotension (biphasic) as well as bradycardia via cholinergic pathway as well as vagal reflex stimulation	[65]
Linalyl acetate	*In vitro* cardioprotective effects	Increase the intracellular K^+ levels	[19]
Linum usitatissimum α-Linolenic acid	Lipid profile improvement	Blood pressure reduction, lipid improvement	[66]
Lippia alba myrcenone (30.4%)	Lipid profile improvement	Lipid improvement via inhibition of mevalonate pathway	[67]
Lippia alba [geranial (48.58%) and neral (35.42%)]	Vasorelaxant effect	Caused vasodilation, which is not mediated via endothelium, partially via inhibiting Ca^{2+} inflow via voltage-based Ca^{2+} channels	[68]
Lippia alba (Citral)	Vasorelaxant effect	Relieved vasocontractions caused by BAY-K 8644 and phorbol 12,13-dibutyrate	[69]
Meniki EOs	Reduced heart rate as well as systolic BP while diastolic BP elevated	Activity sympathetic nerves considerably reduced with rise in parasympathetic effects	[54]
Mentha×villosa Piperitenone oxide (95.9%)	Hypotensive action	Blood pressure reduction and vasorelaxation via involvement of NO	[70]
Mentha×villosa	Vasorelaxant effect	Endothelium-dependent hypotensive and vasorelaxant effects	[71]
Menthol	*In vitro* cardioprotective effects	Vasodilation via suppressing Ca^{2+} inflow through Ca^{2+} channels (nifedipine-sensitive)	[72]
Nardostachyos radix	Vasorelaxation via increase in release of NO	Activation of phosphorylation of endothelial NO synthase; increased phosphorylation level of Akt kinase; elevated the intracellular Ca^{2+} level	[73]
Nardostachys jatamasi Calarene (38%)	Vasorelaxant effect	Vasorelaxation and NO production increase	[73]
N-Butylidenephtalide	*In vitro* cardioprotective effects	Antiangiogenic effects via activating apoptotic death	[74]
Nepeta cataria	Vasorelaxant effect	Spasmolytic and myorelaxant activities facilitated possibly via calcium channels and phosphodiesterase inhibition	[75]
Nigella sativa Thymol (32.0%)	Lipid improvement, antioxidation	*Hyper lipidemia*	[76]
Ocimum gratissimum	Hypotensive activity	Vasodilatory effects directly upon vascular smooth muscle	[77]
Ocimum gratissimum Eugenol (43.7%)	Hyper tension	Blood pressure reduction, vasorelaxation	[78]
Ocimum gratissimum leaves	Increased hypotension and bradycardia	Smooth muscle-relaxant activity	[79]
Ocimum micranthum (Methyl cinnamate	Vasorelaxant effect	Caused vasodiation, which is not dependent on endothelium and possibly facilitated via suppression of Ca^{2+} inflow via voltage-mediated Ca^{2+} channels	[80]
Ocotea quixos Trans-cinnamaldehyde (27.8%)	Vasorelaxant effect	Antiplatelet, antithrombosis, vasorelaxation in pulmonary thromboembolism	[81]
Oenothera biennis	Antioxidation, antiplatelet, antithrombosis, lipid improvement	Atherosclerosis	[82]
Olive oil, oleic acid	Decrease in BP, antioxidation, increase in endothelial function	Decrease in serum asymmetric dimethylarginine, oxidized low-density lipoprotein, and plasma C-reactive protein	[83]
Origanum vulgare	Cardioprotective effect	Normalized CK-MB, LDH, and troponin I levels to protect myocardium and improved antioxidant level and reduced malondialdehyde level	[84]
Pectis brevipedunculata	Vasorelaxant effect	EO and citral caused vasodilation via modulating NO/cyclic GMP pathway and the calcium inflow via voltage-mediated L-type Ca^{2+} channels	[85]
Pinus koraiensis Camphene (21.1%)	Antioxidation, lipid improvement	Increase in the expression of low-density lipoprotein receptor as well as acyl-coenzyme A suppression	[86]

(*Continued*)

TABLE 21.1 (*Continued*)
Cardioprotective Effects of EOs and Their Components

EOs or Chemical Component	Biological Effects	Mechanism of Action (MOA)	References
Pogostemon elsholtzioides (Curzerene, benzophenone, α-cadinol and germacrone)	Vasorelaxant effect	Vasorelaxant effect caused decrease in systolic as well as diastolic blood pressure, heart rate and mean arterial pressure via NO-dependent pathway	[87]
Psidium guajava	Vasorelaxant	Antispasmodic effects facilitated via calcium channel suppression	[88]
Angelica sinensis 3-Carene (32.1%)	Angiogenesis inhibition	-	[74]
Chrysopogon zizanioides (Roots)	Vasorelaxant	Vasodilation effect via stimulation of muscarinic receptor and inhibition of as calcium channels b	[89]
Rosa indica L.	-	Vasorelaxation	[90]
Rosa indica L. Petals	Vasorelaxant and antispasmodic	Inhibition of calcium channel	[90]
Rotundifolone	*In vitro* cardioprotective effects	Vasodilation via stimulation of BKCa proteins as well as suppression of Ca^{2+} inflow via L-type Ca^{2+} channels	[91]
Schisandra chinensis (Borneol)	Antioxidation, anti-inflammatory effects, inhibition formation of new blood vessels	Prevent TNF-α induced injury	[92]
Syringa pinnatifolia	Antioxidation and antiplatelet	Myocardial infarction, hypoxia damage due to the presence of α-cadinol	[93]
Syzygium aromaticum	Lipid improvement	Role of eugenolin in dyslipidemia	[94]
Thymol and carvacrol	-	Caused vasodilation without involvement of an endothelium- Thymol and carvacrol, effectively inhibit Ca^{2+} entry	[95]
Thymoquinone	*In vivo* cardioprotective effects	Pretreatment with thymoquinone decreased, IL-6 production, leukocytes and increase SOD activity; decreased numbers of platelets; showed cardioprotective and antioxidant effects Antioxidant and cardioprotective effects Decrease in oxidative stress and prevent histopathologic damage in different tissues	[96]
Trachyspermum ammi	Vasorelaxation	Vasorelaxation due to thymol in the thoracic aorta of Wistar albino rats	[97]
Trachyspermum ammi seeds	Vasorelaxation	Vasodilation induced via EO, without the involvement of endothelium and EO also suppressed Ca^{2+} entry	[97]
Ylang-Ylang aroma	Sedative effect	Caused a reduction of the HR and blood pressure	[98]
α-Terpineol	*In vivo* cardioprotective effects	Cardio-protective property via decreasing blood pressure and activating antioxidant enzymes	[99]
β-caryophyllene	Cardioprotective effect against myocardial infarction	Via suppressing HSP-60/TLR/MyD88/NFκB signaling pathways	[100]

21.2 Role of EOs in Hypertension

Various positive implications of EOs on the heart and its vasculature such as reducing clot formation, preventing endothelial dysfunction, causing vasorelaxation and antiaggregant effect, and lowering blood pressure as seen in Table 21.1. Various investigations have demonstrated the key role of vascular endothelium in maintaining vascular homeostasis, as well as the function of vascular endothelial via the production of vasoactive substances, stimulation/inhibition of receptors, and increase/decrease in neural excitability via various terpenoids. Various classes of secondary metabolites such as monoterpenes and phenylpropanoids have shown protective effects on the cardiovascular system via various pathways. To discuss the cardioprotective effect exhibited by EOs as well as their components, it is important to know their effect on vascular function, mainly vasoconstriction and vasorelaxation cellular events and pathways, as discussed below.

21.2.1 Vasoconstriction Effects and Underlying Cellular Mechanisms

Vascular structure and function are regulated by various cellular mechanisms. These mechanisms are mediated by the involvement of vascular endothelial cells, stromal cells of the vascular wall, and the outer layer of connective tissue that surrounds vessel with inflammatory cells, autonomic nervous system, and network of small blood vessels. Vascular smooth muscle cell contraction via a calcium-dependent pathway is demonstrated in Figure 21.1. Normally, the rate of blood flow via vessels in a tissue is governed by the equilibrium among two physiological processes, vasodilation as well as

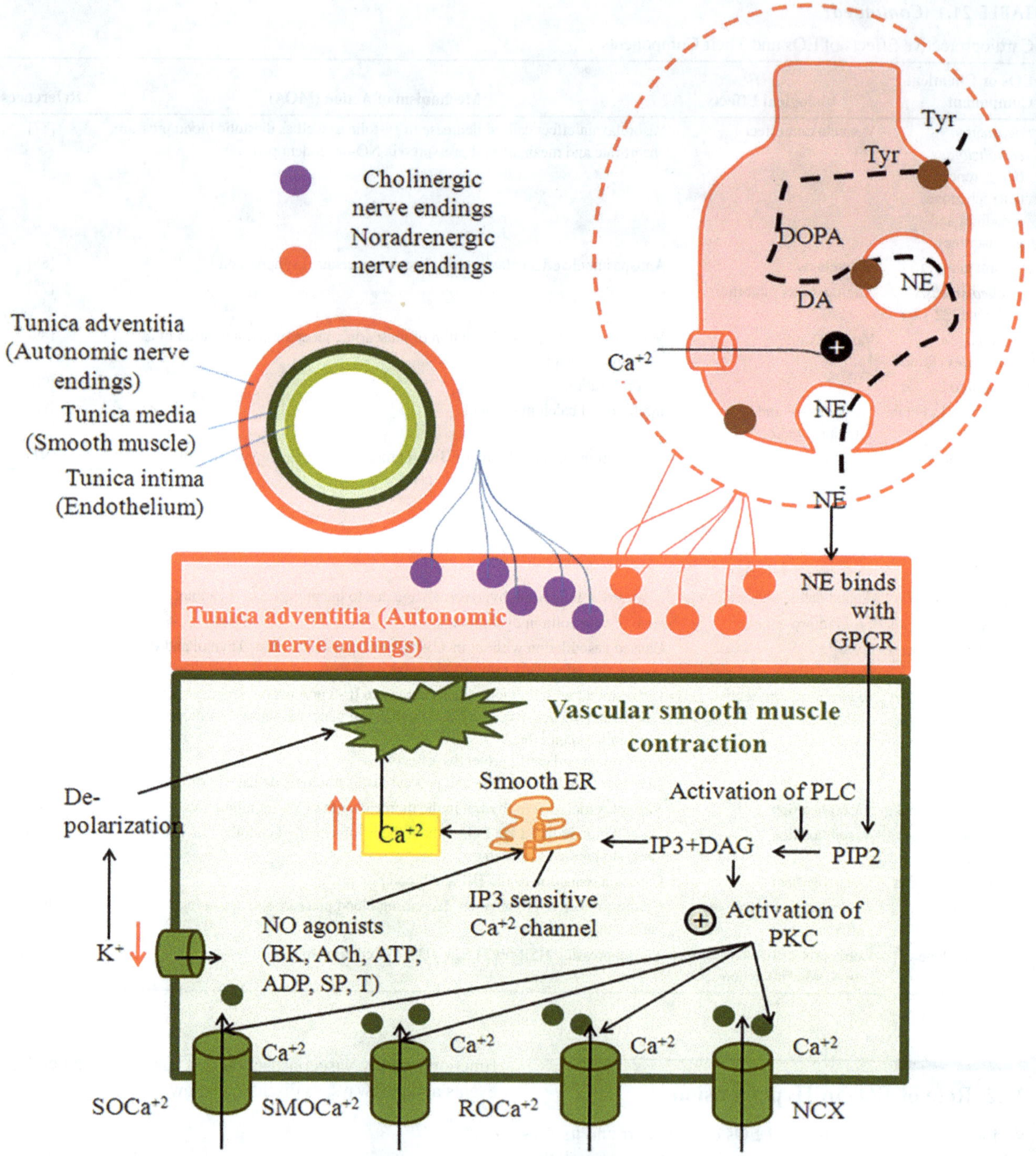

FIGURE 21.1 Vascular smooth muscle cell contraction via calcium-dependent pathway. ITP: inositol trisphosphate, DAG: diacylglycerol, GPCR: G protein-coupled receptors, ER: endoplasmic reticulum, PLC: phospholipase c, PIP2: phosphatidylinositol 4,5-bisphosphate, $SOCa^{2+}$: store-operated Ca^{2+} channel, ER: endoplasmic reticulum, SR: sarcoplasmic reticulum, SOC: store-operated Ca^{2+} channel, SMOC: second messenger–operated Ca^{2+} channel, ROC: receptor-operated Ca^{2+} channel, VOC: voltage-gated Ca^{2+} channel, NCX: Na^{1+}–Ca^{2+} exchanger, RyR: ryanodine Ca^{2+} channel, PKC: protein kinase C, Tyr: tyrosine, DOPA: dihydroxyphenylalanine, NE: norepinephrine, Ach: acetylcholine, BK: bradykinin, ATP: adenosine triphosphate, ADP: adenosine diphosphate, SP: substance P.

vasoconstriction. Vasoconstriction in most cases is caused by activation of sympathetic neurons via the synthesis of norepinephrine (NE) and its involvement with α-adrenoreceptors. NE mainly binds to α1 receptors to cause smooth muscle contraction and vasoconstriction. This results in calcium release from calcium-gated channels present over sarcoplasmic reticulum cell membrane to induce smooth muscle contraction. On the other hand, stimulation of parasympathetic and sympathetic cholinergic nerves allows nerves to release ACh, which binds to muscarinic receptors to inhibit contraction and to induce relaxation. Nitric oxide plays an important role in smooth muscle relaxation via the inositol triphosphate (IP3) pathway as illustrated in Figure 21.1. Endothelial cells that form the inner layer of the vasculature present on the intima regulate the vascular function via reacting against a variety of hormones, neurotransmitters, and vasoactive factors, which have an effect on blood clot formation, contraction–relaxation of vasculature, and inflammation. It was found that contraction of smooth muscles is stimulated by the neurochemical messenger, resulting in increase in the level of Ca^{+2} via facilitating its entry out of the voltage-dependent Ca^{+2} channel as well as released Ca^{+2} sarcoplasmic reticulum stores into the cytosol.

Change in action potential due to the sequential opening and closing of voltage-gated cation channels can further stimulate the motor neuron. Stimulation of the motor neuron at the synaptic cleft results in the activation of voltage-gated Ca^{2+} channel, which can further stimulate the inflow of Ca^{2+} ions in the cytoplasm. Increase in the level of Ca^{2+} in the sympathetic nerve terminal allows the release of the noradrenaline from interstitial sites where NE binds to the G protein-coupled receptors present over the smooth muscle to activate phospholipase C (Figure 21.1). Activation of phospholipase C allows the breakdown of phospholipids into IP3s and diacylglycerols (DAGs). IP3 binds to the IP receptor Ca^{+2} channel and stimulates the release of Ca^{+2} from the sarcoplasmic reticulum (SR) into the cytoplasm. DAG activates protein kinase C (PKC), which can affect voltage-gated calcium (Ca^{2+}) channels including sodium–calcium exchanger (NCX), receptor-operated calcium channel (ROC), second messenger-operated calcium channel (SMOC), store-operated calcium channel (SOC), as well as voltage-gated calcium channel (VOC).

DAG acts by binding to the plasma membraneCa^{2+} receptors to allow Ca^{2+}entry. The IP3 also binds to the sarcoplasmic reticulum receptors (such as ryanodine receptors), also called Ca2+ release channels, resulting in Ca^{2+} release from the sarcoplasmic reticulum into the cytosol. Thus, vascular smooth muscle contraction occurs as long as the high level of intracellular free-calcium concentration is present to promote cross-bridging between actin and myosin. Several reports suggest that vascular smooth muscle contraction is also facilitated through calcium-independent ways such as the following:

- Stimulation of immune or inflammatory pathways
- Noncoding RNAs stimulation
- Mitogen-activated protein kinase signaling
- Protein kinase C
- Reactive oxygen species
- Reorganization of the actin cytoskeleton
- RhoA-Rho kinase

These all are considered as key regulators of the vascular function.

21.2.2 Cellular Mechanism of Vasodilation

There are two mechanisms involved in vasorelaxation: one via the nitric oxide (NO) synthase (NOS) enzyme and another via the cyclooxygenase (COX) enzyme in endothelial cells. Vasorelaxation induced via these pathways involves cyclic guanosine monophosphate (cGMP) as well as cyclic adenosine monophosphate (cAMP) to dilate the vascular smooth muscles. NO-induced endothelium-dependent vasorelaxation of the smooth muscle is mediated via decreasing intracellular calcium level, which is regulated by the endothelial NOS to convert the amino acid L-arginine to NO to eventually cause vasorelaxation as mentioned in Figure 21.2. eNOS synthesizes NO in endothelial cells is an endothelium-derived relaxing factor, which is produced at two sites, in endothelium as well as at the terminal end of cholinergic nerves. When required, NO can be synthesized at these sites and easily diffuse through cell membranes to cause vasorelaxation of smooth muscles. The endothelium-derived relaxing factor (EDRF) is an endogenous chemical substance produced by endothelial cells to respond against change in normal physiologic conditions by causing vasorelaxation. EDRF-induced vasorelaxation is mediated by activation of soluble *guanylate cyclase* to further increase the production of cyclic guanylate monophosphate in vascular smooth muscle. The EDRF is an endothelial NO or any substance that contains nitrogen oxide. This factor is synthesized from the L-arginine via an enzyme, which is dependent on calcium-calmodulin and NADPH. As mentioned in Figure 21.2, stimulation of endothelium via acetylcholine can lead to the production of NO, which can further activate signal-transducing guanylyl cyclase enzymes to enhance the production of cyclic guanosine monophosphate in the vascular smooth muscle to cause vascular dilation via reducing the level of intracellular Ca^{2+}. These pathways can be suppressed by L-arginine analogue.

In contrast, the COX-mediated pathway involves the prostacyclin (PGI2) synthesis from endogenous arachidonic acid (AA) to produce the high level of cAMP to further dilate the vascular smooth muscle. PGI2 and thromboxane (TXA2), produced by COX enzymes, work synergistically to regulate vascular tone. Out of two isoforms of COX, COX-1 is constantly expressed in endothelium, whereas COX-2 is expressed at the time of damage to endothelial cells or when they are exposed to inflammatory mediators such as cytokines. AA, which is a polyunsaturated fatty acid present in the phospholipids of the cell membrane, is an important inflammatory mediator, which is converted into various other inflammatory mediators by Lipoxygenases (LOX) (to produce leukotrienes) and Cyclooxygenase-2 (COX) (to produce prostaglandins and thromboxanes) enzymes. Cyclooxygenase-2 changes into AA to prostaglandin G2 also known as PGG2 (prostaglandins G), unstable prostaglandin endoperoxide and PGH2 (prostaglandin H2), which is further synthesized into PGI2 via *prostaglandin-I synthase*. After its formation, PGI2 binds to the prostaglandin I2 receptor (IP), present over both vascular smooth muscle and platelets cells. This binding allows the inhibition of platelet aggregation (in platelet cells) as well as activation of *adenylate cyclase* to stimulate the production of cAMP (in smooth muscle). Increase in production of cAMP stimulates cyclic AMP-dependent protein kinase, which facilitates dilation of the vascular smooth muscle. On the other hand, TxA2, which is produced by COX-1 via conversion of AA to PGH2, causes platelet aggregation and vasoconstriction. After its formation, TxA2 binds to a protein called

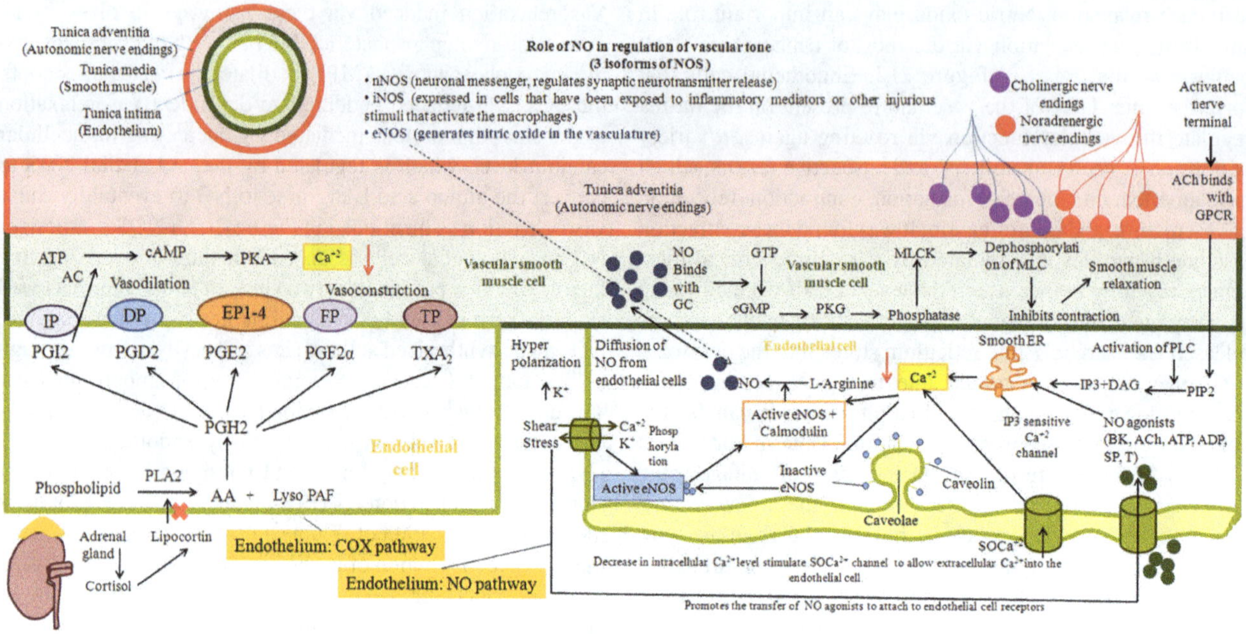

FIGURE 21.2 Nitric oxide-induced smooth muscle relaxation via IP3 pathway. NO: nitric oxide, MLCK: myosin light-chain kinase, ITP: inositol trisphosphate, DAG: diacylglycerol, GPCR: G protein-coupled receptors, ER: endoplasmic reticulum, cGMP: cyclic guanosine monophosphate, GTP: guanosine triphosphate, MLC: myosin light chain, PLC: phospholipase c, PIP2: phosphatidylinositol 4,5-bisphosphate, GC: guanylyl cyclase, Ach: acetylcholine, BK: bradykinin, ATP: adenosine triphosphate, ADP: adenosine diphosphate, SP: substance P, $SOCa^{2+}$: store-operated Ca^{2+} channel, ER: endoplasmic reticulum, PKG: cGMP-dependent protein kinase or protein kinase G, PGI2: prostacyclin, ATP: adenosine triphosphate, AC: adenylyl cyclase, AA: arachidonic acid, COX: cyclooxygenase, PGH2: prostaglandin H2, PGI2: prostaglandin I2 (prostacyclin), PGE2: prostaglandin E2, PGF2α: prostaglandin F2α, PGD2: prostaglandin D2, TxA2: thromboxane A2.

prostanoid thromboxane-prostanoid (TP) receptors, which are present over thrombocytes as well as smooth muscle cells to cause platelet aggregation and smooth muscle cell contraction. Calcium-mediated as well as calcium-independent contractions in the smooth muscles have been observed where calcium-mediated smooth muscle contractions facilitate the release of intracellular Ca^{2+} levels in the smooth muscle, resulting in constriction of vessels. The equilibrium in the level of TxA2 and PGI2 is required to retain stability as well as to maintain the vascular tone.

21.2.3 The Effect of EOs on the Vascular Tone to Regulate the Heart Rate and Arterial Pressure

Several reports, *in vitro* and *in vivo*, have suggested the role of EOs in the regulation of the vascular tone to further impact average blood pressure and HR via different mechanisms. Various studies (*in vivo* and/or *in vitro*) have been performed to understand the role of EOs in regulating HR. Based on these reports, the role of EO in the regulation of the vascular tone that affects the cardiovascular system is illustrated in Figure 21.3. It is suggested that increase in the intracellular potassium level causes depolarization of the smooth muscle cell membrane to further open VOCC, resulting in the inflow of extracellular Ca^{2+}. Increase in intracellular Ca^{2+} further causes vasoconstriction. Vasoconstriction can also result from the stimulation of the sympathetic nerve by epinephrine analogue such as phenylephrine; however, inhibition of the sympathetic nerve by antagonist or β-blocker like atenolol causes vasodilation. On the other hand, reserpine, an antihypertensive drug, prevents accumulation of catecholamines in adrenergic transmitter vesicles to reduce epinephrine, norepinephrine, and dopamine from peripheral sympathetic nerve terminals to further control the HR and induce myocardial contraction as well as systemic vascular resistance. Acetylcholine is the main neurotransmitter of the parasympathetic nervous system and can affect vasodilation by various pathways, such as activation of endothelial NO synthase and prostaglandin (PG) production. Atropine is a competitive antagonist of the actions of acetylcholine and other muscarinic agonists as it blocks the muscarine-mimicking effects of acetylcholine and other choline esters. Likewise, methylatropine is an anticholinergic drug that binds to cholinergic receptors to block the actions of acetylcholine. To facilitate vasodilation, calcium channel blockers such as verapamil inhibit voltage-operated Ca^{2+} channels have been used to reduce the intracellular level of calcium in smooth muscle cells. NSAIDs such as indomethacin and other analogs inhibit the synthesis of prostaglandins via suppressing the COX-2 effect to prevent vasodilation and cause vasoconstriction. Likewise, NG-nitro-L-arginine methyl ester (L-NAME) (a NOS inhibitor) inhibits NO synthesis to cause vasoconstriction. L-NAME is used as a negative control in experiments. Hyperpolarization is one of the key mechanisms to induce vasorelaxation in smooth muscles and can be mediated by the following mechanisms as illustrated in Figure 21.3:

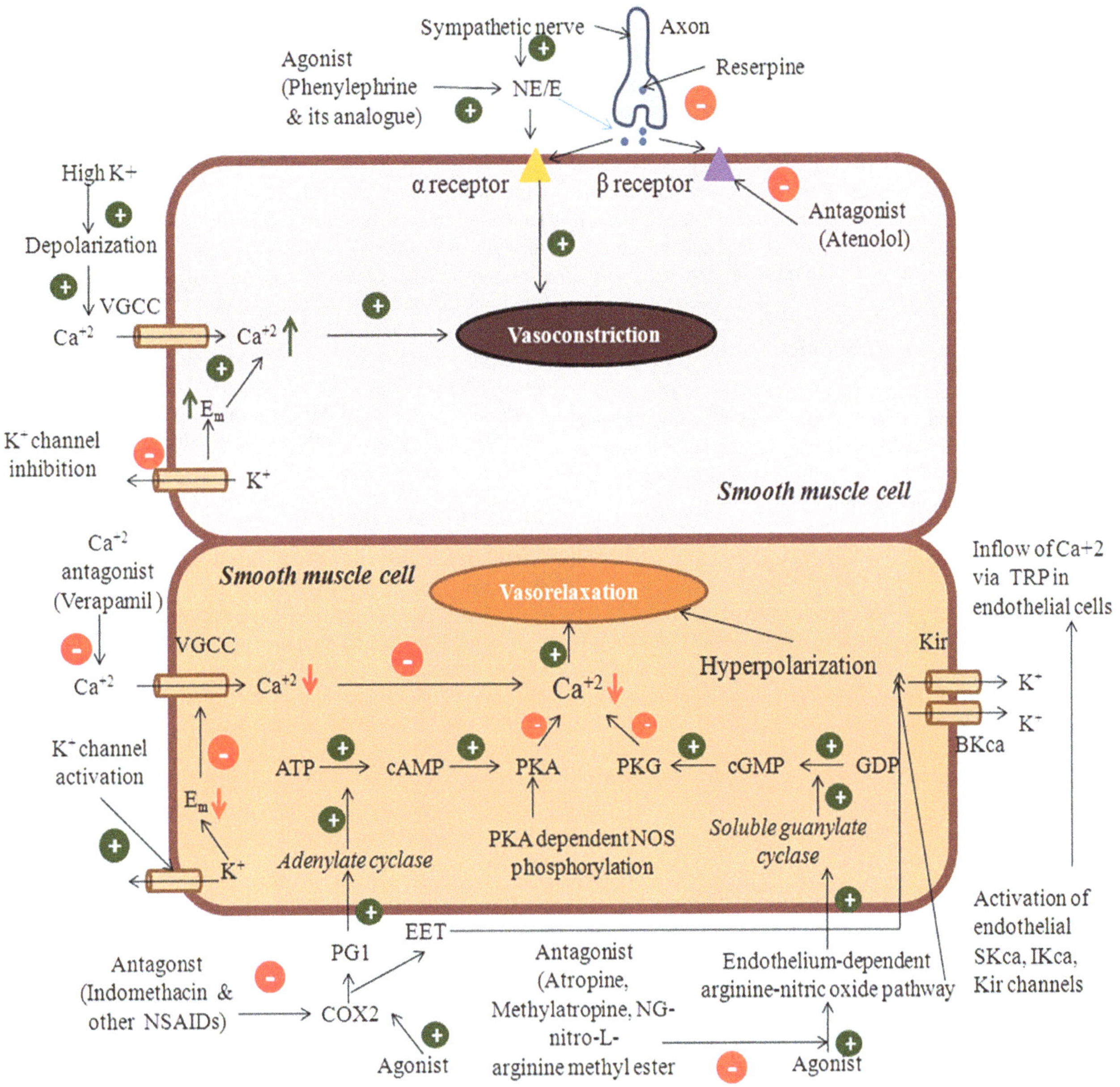

FIGURE 21.3 Molecular targets of EOs and their components to regulate smooth muscle contraction as well as relaxation to further regulate the HR and arterial pressure. PKA: protein kinase A, ATP: adenosine triphosphate, cGMP: cyclic guanosine monophosphate, GDP: guanosine diphosphate, PKG: protein kinase G, COX: cyclooxygenase, PG1: prostacyclin, NSAIDs: nonsteroidal anti-inflammatory drugs, NE: norepinephrine, VGCC: voltage-gated calcium channels, NOS: nitric oxide synthases, Em: vascular muscle cell membrane potential, EET: epoxyeicosatrienoic acids, SK: small-conductance calcium-activated potassium channels, IK: intermediate-conductance calcium-activated potassium channels, Kir: inward-rectifier potassium channels, BK: big potassium channels.

- Hyperpolarization of smooth muscle cells via the opening of potassium channels and/or Na^+/K^+-ATPase especially by diffusible factors including epoxyeicosatrienoic acids (via COX pathway), K^+ ions, and hydrogen peroxide.
- Endothelium-dependent hyperpolarization in endothelial cells with an increase in intracellular calcium, which can further activate small conductance (SK(Ca)) as well as intermediate conductance (IK(Ca)) Ca^{2+} activated K^+ channels.
- Via activation of inward-rectifier potassium channels (Kir) and big potassium (BK) channels of smooth muscles.

21.3 Vasodilator Effects of EOs

The cardiovascular effects of EOs over the heart rate as well as mean arterial pressure are listed in Table 21.1. Subsequent sections include descriptions of these EOs.

21.3.1 *Allium macrostemon*

The vasodilation effects of volatile oil from *Allium macrostemon* Bunge on isolated rat pulmonary arterials (PAs) were investigated in an earlier report to assess the underling mechanisms. The findings suggested that volatile oil showed vasorelaxation in rat PAs via an endothelium-dependent mechanism involving Ca^{2+} entry, PKA-dependent NOS phosphorylation, and NO signaling. The vasodilator activities of volatile oil could be due to its constituent dimethyl disulfide, which represents potential application in pulmonary hypertension [101].

21.3.2 *Chrysopogon zizanioides*

Recently, the vasorelaxation effect of root EO of *C. zizanioides* using rat-isolated thoracic aortic rings was investigated, and it was observed that the EO of *C. zizanioides* possesses vasorelaxant effect via the muscarinic pathway as well as acts as a calcium channel blocker [89].

21.3.3 *Croton argyrophylloides*

The EO of *Croton argyrophylloides* was found to stimulate the muscarinic receptor, liberate the endothelium-derived prostacyclin, and open KATP channels to induce vasorelaxation and further induce hypotension. It has been suggested that administration of *Croton argyrophylloides* EO into veins decreased blood pressure most likely via an active vascular relaxation rather than withdrawal of sympathetic tone whereas EO-induced tachycardia reported in conscious rats could be due to the reflex response via inhibition of vagal drive to the heart [102].

21.3.4 *Alpinia zerumbet*

The vasodilation property of *Alpinia zerumbet* EO as well as its component, 1,8-cineole, were investigated in an earlier report, and it was demonstrated that *A. zerumbet* EO can be used for the treatment of hypertension. It was suggested that the EO caused vasorelaxant effect, which might not be completely due to the actions of the main constituent, 1,8-cineole. It was also observed vasorelaxant effects were completely reliant on the functional integrity of the inner cellular lining of blood vessels and capillaries [12].

21.3.5 Asafoetida Oil

The vasorelaxant property of asafoetida EO over contraction reaction rings of rataorta and effect over NO, COX, and Ca^{+2}channels was studied. The findings demonstrated that asafoetida EO showed vasorelaxant activity on endothelium-intact as well as endothelium-denuded aortic rings with considerably more potency in endothelium-intact aortic rings. The vasorelaxant effects of asafoetida EO were decreased; however, simultaneous treatment of L-NG-Nitro arginine methyl ester or indomethacin and asafoetida EO did not cause full inhibition of vasodilatory effects. Moreover, treatment of asafoetida EO with a free-calcium medium also considerably decreased the $CaCl_2$-induced contractions. These findings suggest that asafoetida EO has vasodilatory effect via endothelium-dependent and endothelium-independent pathways. Additionally, asafoetida EO decreased the inflow of Ca^{+2}into the cell via plasma membrane Ca^{+2} [103].

21.3.6 *Aniba canelilla* Bark

The role of *Aniba canelilla* bark EO in causing cardiovascular complications using normotensive rodent model after IV injection was studied. It was found that IV injection caused dose-dependent hypotension (could be due to vasorelaxation) and bradycardia (could be due to parasympathetic drive to the heart) among pentobarbital-anesthetized as well as conscious rats. This vasodilation could be due to calcium inward current (endothelium-independent vasodilation) and due to endothelial L-arginine-NO cyclic-GMP pathway activation via peripheral muscarinic receptor (endothelium-dependent vasodilation) [15].

21.3.7 *Citrus aurantium*

Neroli, the *Citrus aurantium* EO, is well known for its possible therapeutic potential in various cardiovascular complications. Nevertheless, due to complex chemical profile as well as various therapeutic effects, its molecular mechanism has not been explored yet. A recent report suggested that *Citrus aurantium* EO caused vasorelaxation, which was partially facilitated via the nitric oxide-soluble guanylyl cyclase pathway, but the smooth muscle vasodilatory effects could be due to alteration of level of intracellular calcium via blockage of cation channel-operated extracellular calcium release and store-mediated calcium release (via ryanodine receptors signaling pathway) [104].

21.3.8 *Cymbopogon winterianus*

C. winterianus is a traditional plant that has been used for the management of various hypertensive disorders. In a previous study, the role of *Cymbopogon winterianus* EO in cardiovascular complications using rodent model was investigated. The findings demonstrated that the *Cymbopogon winterianus* EO-induced hypotension and vasorelaxation, mainly mediated via blocking of calcium channel. In addition, sinus bradycardia as well as arrhythmias due to treatment with *Cymbopogon winterianus* EO at high dose was due to cardiac muscarinic receptor stimulation.

It was observed that cardiovascular effects are not influenced by N omega-nitro-L-arginine methyl este or indomethacin, but these effects are partly decreased after administration of atropine [105].

In another study, the vasodilatory as well as hypotensive properties of dihydrogeraniol in rodent model were investigated. Dihydrogeraniol is a chemical component obtained from various medicinal plants such as Indian lemon grass, citronella grass, and Lippia, which have been considered for their antihypertensive effects. Treatment with dihydrogeraniol l caused hypotension in rats, which was been influenced by pretreatment with L-NAME hydrochloride or indomethacin, atropine, and hexamethonium. After treatment with hexamethonium and atropine, dihydrogeraniol induced response was reduced.

Also, dihydrogeraniol inhibited the contractions caused by phenylephrine caffeine at specific dose. Thus, findings from this report suggested that dihydrogeraniol acts directly on the vascular smooth muscle to reduce blood pressure and cause vasodilation [40].

21.3.9 *Croton nepetaefolius*

In an earlier report, it was suggested that *Croton nepetaefolius* EO (EOCN) reduced blood pressure in normotensive rats. This is due to its direct action on smooth muscle to reduce blood pressure and cause vasodilation. In another report, the role of the endothelium–NO pathway in the mediation of vasodilatory effects of the EOCN and two of its constituents, methyleugenol and α-terpineol, using rat-isolated thoracic aorta and mesenteric vascular bed preparations was explored. It was found that EOCN caused vasorelaxation of endothelium-intact aortic rings, which was precontracted with KCl, in a concentration-dependent manner. It was also discovered that either tissue pretreatment with L-N^G-nitro arginine methyl ester or removal of endothelium increased the IC50 value significantly. EOCN (10–200 µg/mL) also caused vasorelaxation effect in precontracted endothelium-intact aortic rings, which was reduced by the pretreatment with methylene blue. Thus, EOCN induced vasodilation response in both vascular bed as well as conducting artery. It was also demonstrated that these effects could be due to the presence of its major chemical component methyleugenol and α-terpineol. Moreover, vasorelaxant effects could also be partly dependent on the physiological state of a vascular endothelium [35].

One more study based on the hypotensive effect of the EOCN on rodents suggested that IV administration with EOCN reduced HR as well as MAP. Reducing rate of MAP mediated by EOCN was considerably high among hypertensive rodents. It was found that hexamethanium pretreatment, followed by the treatment of the EO, showed, hypotensive effects however unable to cause slow heart rate. Thus, it has been observed that effects induced by EO were independent of the hypothalamus to decrease blood pressure. 1,8-cineole, which is considered as a major constituent, has also been reported to cause hypotension with low HR (bradycardia) in a concentration-dependent manner. It was found that the mechanism causing hypotension and the one causing bradycardia by 1,8-cineole are different from each other. 1,8-cineole can cause hypotension via stimulating vascular relaxation; however, it is not mediated via deactivation of the sympathetic nerves. Moreover, several researchers have suggested that the duration required for reducing the maximum blood pressure has been found to be the same for both 1,8-cineole as well as acetylcholine; thus, it was believed that this response could be partially regulated by the L-arginine-nitric oxide pathway. One more study suggested that the hypotensive effect of methyleugenol is mediated via endothelial L-arginine-nitric oxide pathway.

21.3.10 *Ocimum gratissimum*

In an earlier report, the vasodilatory response of *Ocimum gratissimum* EO (OGEO) in aortas as well as mesenteric arteries excised from rodents was investigated. It was observed that the OGEO caused relaxation of the tonic contractions induced by phenylephrine in excised aortas in a dose-dependent manner (in both endothelium-intact and endothelium-denuded rings). However, this response was partly changed by L-NG-Nitro arginine methyl ester however indomethacin and tetraethylammonium unable to change response. This report demonstrated that OGEO has a concentration-dependent vasorelaxant effect response in aortas as well as mesenteric arteries excised from rodents. This response could be due to nitric oxide release in the rat mesenteric vasculature but aorta relaxation was partly dependent on nitric oxide release [106]. In another study, it was revealed that the same EO showed hypotensive responses in deoxycorticosterone acetate (DOCA)-salt hypertensive rats due to active vascular relaxation, which is partially dependent on the integrity of the vascular endothelium and seems to be mainly mediated via inhibition of plasmalemmal Ca^{2+} influx rather than Ca^{2+} induced Ca^{2+} release from the sarcoplasmic reticulum [78].

21.3.11 *Hyptis fruticose*

The report-related vasorelaxant effects of EO derived from bushmints (*Hyptis fruticose*) containing 1,8 cineole caryophyllene, and alpha-pinene as major components revealed that this EO caused vasorelaxation in rat mesenteric arterial rings pretreated with potassium chloride. Thus, it was proposed that bushmints EO may perhaps prevent Ca^{2+} release via acting against VOCCs. Based on this, it was speculated that the *Hyptis fruticose* EO might act as a calcium channel blocker due to its ability to inhibit the calcium chloride $_2$-mediated contractions.

21.3.12 *Lippia alba*

Lippia alba (Mill.) N.E. Brown (Verbenaceae) species popularly known as lemon balm was evaluated for its vasorelaxant effect on rat aorta. It was observed that the *L. alba* EO (EOLa) and its major constituent, citral, showed smooth muscle relaxant action in isolated aorta using several mechanisms of action, which was potentiated by the presence of the endothelium [69].

21.3.13 *Mentha × villosa*

In an earlier report, it was suggested that IV administration with the *Mentha × villosa* EO (MVEO) in rodents anesthetized with pentobarbitone reduced blood pressure due to the hypotensive activity of the MVEO, which could be due to the vasorelaxant effects directly on the vascular smooth muscle. In another study reported by the same researchers, it was observed that MVEO-induced hypotension is mediated via endothelial L-arginine/NO pathway. The findings from this study revealed that MVEO in a dose-dependent manner decreased blood pressure in conscious rats, and its action is due to active vascular relaxation. Vascular relaxation (aortic) was partially due to the NO release from vascular endothelial in the MVEO-treated rats, which supports the idea that MVEO-induced hypotension and bradycardia occur independently [70].

21.3.14 *Nigella sativa*

The EO obtained from *Nigella sativa* seeds exhibits smooth muscle relaxation, without involving endothelium and NO. Moreover, endothelium-independent vasorelaxant effects resulting from oil also block both voltage-sensitive and receptor-operated calcium channels, which may suggest its therapeutic importance and thus can be used as a potential antihypertensive agent [107].

21.3.15 *Nardostachyos radix*

Root as well as rhizome of Spikenard (*Nardostachys jatamansi*) has been extensively used for various ailments including neurological as well as cardiovascular complications. A recent report suggested that the vasodilation effects of Spikenard EO in isolated aorta ring are mediated via NO release as well as phosphorylation of endothelial nitric oxide synthase in human umbilical vein endothelial cells [73].

21.3.16 *Ocimum micranthum*

The cardiovascular effects of the (E)-methyl cinnamate from *Ocimum micranthum* in excised aortic rings of rodent were investigated in an earlier report. It was suggested that E-MC induced vasorelaxation in rat-isolated aorta in a concentration-dependent manner to relax endothelium-intact rat aortic rings (pretreated with phenylephrine). Thus, these findings suggested that E-MC showed vasorelaxation via endothelium-independent pathway, which is mediated by inhibition of plasmalemmal Ca^{2+} influx through voltage-dependent Ca^{2+} channels. Nevertheless, the participation of a myogenic mechanism in the effects of E-MC is also possible [80].

21.3.17 *Pogostemon elsholtzioides*

The vasodilatory as well as cardiovascular effects of the EO obtained from aromatic shrub, *Pogostemon elsholtzioides*, which is endemic to the eastern Himalaya region, was investigated in an earlier report. Findings obtained from this report suggested that the EO enriched with sesquiterpenes (such as benzophenone as well as curzerene), germacrone, and α-cadinol showed a considerable vasorelaxant effect in aortic rings precontracted with phenylephrine. The vasodilatory effect of the EO was reported with or without simultaneous treatment of L-NAME against aortic rings precontracted with phenylephrine. Moreover, the EO decreased HR, BP, and MAP. *P. elsholtzioides* EO showed considerable vasodilation against endothelium-intact rat aortic rings via releasing nitric oxide and decreasing BP [87].

21.3.18 *Protium heptaphyllum*

Almécega's resin (Protium heptaphyllum) EO has been studied for its vasorelaxation effect in the mesenteric artery of rat. Ortho-cymene para-cineole and limonene were found to be the active chemical components of this EO. It showed a vasorelaxant effect in intact rings precontracted with phenylephrine, and the EO also showed a dose-dependent vasorelaxation without participation of mediators synthesized by vascular endothelial cells [108].

21.3.19 *Pectis brevipedunculata*

The EO of *Pectis brevipedunculata* as well as its active component citral increased vasorelaxant effect on thoracic aortic rings via influencing the nitric oxide-cyclic GMP pathway and the calcium inflow via voltage-dependent L-type calcium channels (Cavl) [85].

21.3.20 *Pistacia integerrima*

Pistacia integerrima (Family: Anacardiaceae) galls are used in Indian ethno medicine for their antiasthmatic, sedative, and spasmolytic properties; nevertheless, there are no scientific reports supporting its spasmolytic activity. The vasorelaxant and spasmolytic activities of the EO isolated from the galls of *Pistacia integerrima* were evaluated in an earlier report.

Pistacia integerrima galls EO enhanced the relaxation of isoprenaline treated jejunum in rabbit. It was found that the EO induced effects was unaltered by its preincubation with hexamethonium, tetrodotoxin, indomethacin, and L-NAME. Moreover, it was also found that this EO inhibited calcium stimulated contraction of excised ileum of guinea pig in the Ca^{2+} free medium. The EO was reported for its potential in the reversal of a KCl-induced tonic contraction in the Ca^{2+} free medium. These findings suggested antispasmodic action of *Pistacia integerrima* oil mediated by calcium ion channels as well as β-adrenoceptors [109].

21.3.21 *Rosa damascene*

In previous reports, *Rosa damascene* showed various therapeutic effects such as anxiolytic and spasmolytic in the treatment of respiratory complications and improving cardiac strength. Vasorelaxant effects induced by *Rosa damascena* EOs on guinea pig tracheal chains have also been reported. In this report, EO of *Rosa damascena* showed a potent relaxant effect on guinea pig tracheal chains and this response was equivalent to theophylline [110].

21.4 The Role of EO Components in Vasodilation

Vasorelaxation caused by α-terpineol via NO-cGMP and COX pathways was investigated, and it was found that the vasorelaxation induced by α-terpineol was mediated by the NO-cGMP pathway whereas COX pathway metabolites were not involved in the vasorelaxant effect of α-terpineol. It was observed that the vasorelaxant effect of α-terpineol on superior mesenteric arteries mediated via NO-cGMP pathway reduced after the following:

- exclusion of the vascular endothelium
- treatment with L-NAME or NO scavenger
- treatment with L-NAME as well as L-arginine
- treatment with inhibitor of soluble *guanylate cyclase*

External supply of L-arginine has no effect on the induced vasorelaxant effect, which suggests that hypotension caused by α-terpineol could be due to the NO release from endothelium mediated by NO-cGMP pathway. One more study on various monoterpenes suggested their possible role in regulating rat MAP and HR [107]. It was found that monoterpenes (α & β pinene, citronellol, and linalool) showed hypotensive effect along with episode of tachycardia while sesquiterpene (α-bisabolol) showed hypotensive effect hypotension with bradycardia. It was also stated that the difference in the pharmacological activity could be due to the difference in structural configuration among different terpens as (–)-β-pinene has the exocyclic double bond whereas (+)-α-pinene contains endocyclic double bond. Owing to this, (–)-β-pinene possibly showed more therapeutic effect than (+)-α-pinene.

21.4.1 Thymoquinone

Thymoquinone is the major monoterpenoid derived from *Nigella sativa* L EO. The cardiovascular and antioxidant properties of this monoterpene were reported in various studies. It was found that treatment with thymoquinone decreased oxidative stress in systemic circulation of rats, which was estimated when rats underwent reperfusion injury or abdominal aorta ischemia [96]. Intraperitoneal treatment of rats with thymoquinone resulted in decrease in oxidative stress at systemic level and reduction in cardiac injuries. Free radical scavenging pathways of thymoquinone are regulated by reactive oxygen species, antioxidant enzymes, and pro-inflammatory mediators such as cytokine. It was found that thymoquinone-treated mice showed improved superoxide dismutase activity to break down potentially harmful oxygen molecules in cells and decreased proinflammatory cytokine, interleukin-6, level to further prevent cardiovascular complications caused by a pollutant. Isoproterenol-induced myocardial infarcted rats treated with thymoquinone showed a decrease plasma level of glutathione reductase, lactate dehydrogenase, and thiobarbituric acid reactive substance. However, superoxide dismutase activity was found to be decreased in the plasma. These findings showed cardioprotective effects of thymoquinone against the injury caused by isoproterenol.

Early vascular aging due to the changes taking place in the structure and function of vascular muscle or endothelial cells or extracellular matrix of blood vessels could lead to cardiovascular complications. Endothelial dysfunction, COX products (such as TXA2), NO, oxidative stress (increases NO breakdown), endothelium-derived hyperpolarizing factors, and extent of stimulation of parasympathetic/sympathetic usually determine vascular health. It was found that thymoquinone treatment in the mesenteric artery can reverse vascular aging by preventing aging-associated increase in oxidative stress in the artery as well as downregulation of the nitric oxide synthase in endothelium. It was also indicated that intake of thymoquinone restored the expression of eNOS, calcium-activated potassium channels, and the components of the angiotensin system in the mesenteric artery of middle-aged rats. Thus, thymoquinone-mediated restoration of NO- and EDHF-based vasorelaxation and normalization of oxidative stress via regulating function of endothelial cells suggests that thymoquinone can be potentially used for aging-related cardiovascular complications. Besides its potential in reducing oxidative stress, thymoquinone induced vasorelaxation in the aortas of rats via blocking voltage-operated Ca^{2+} channels. These previous findings suggest positive vascular as well as antioxidant properties of thymoquinone, which helps in providing protection against various cardiac complications.

21.4.2 Cinnamaldehyde

Cinnamaldehyde (3-phenylprop-2-enal) is not a terpene derivative but is an example of an aldehyde derived from cinnamon tree (*Cinnamomum cassia*) bark. As per a previous report, cinnamaldehyde prevented hypertension in animals resistant to insulin and those having inadequate level of via normalization of vascular contractility. Additionally, cinnamaldehyde treatment normalized response to KCl and phenylephrine; however, cinnamaldehyde could not normalize response against acetylcholine in the aortic rings of insulin-resistant animals. Cinnamaldehyde treatment restored normal Ca^{2+} influx but did not affect NO generation in insulin-resistant animals. In addition to its effect in preventing hypertension, cinnamaldehyde showed an insulinotropic effect in insulin-deficient or insulin-resistant animals via glucose uptake through glucose transporter (GLUT4) translocation in peripheral tissues. Another report suggested the cardiovascular protective effect of cinnamaldehyde via preservation of NO levels and upregulation of the transcription factor (Nuclear factor erythroid 2-related factor 2), which is responsible for the expression of endogenous antioxidant enzyme to enhance the antioxidant defense against reactive oxygen species (ROS). These results from the previous study suggested a protective effect of cinnamaldehyde to cause relaxation of vascular endothelium of hyperglycemic mice aortic rings. One more report showed that cinnamaldehyde caused vasorelaxation coronary arteries of porcine by reducing sensitivity as well as influx of calcium ion suggesting no involvement of endothelium for this response [26]. Additionally, cinnamaldehyde-containing micelles caused endothelium-dependent vasorelaxation by NO- and H_2O_2-dependent pathways. In 2014, Raffai demonstrated that cinnamaldehyde caused vasorelaxation via the following pathways in a concentration-dependent manner [26]:

- calcium-activated potassium-independent
- COX-independent
- endothelium-independent
- NO synthase-independent
- soluble guanylyl cyclase-independent
- TRPA1 channel-independent

From these findings, the authors concluded that cinnamaldehyde-loaded and poly(cinnamaldehyde) micelles induced vasodilation; however, its main mechanism of vasorelaxation differs from that of cinnamaldehyde. Likewise, another report demonstrated the vasorelaxant effect of cinnamaldehyde, possibly via affecting calcium transport or its release from intracellular stores. Cinnamaldehyde is also reported for its inhibitory action on the L-type Ca^{2+} channel to increase vasorelaxation in ventricular myocytes as well as vascular smooth muscle cells. The cardioprotective effect of cinnamaldehyde in isoproterenol-induced acute myocardial ischemic rats was investigated, and it was observed that pretreatment with cinnamaldehyde reduced ST-segment elevation and decreased creatine kinase, lactate dehydrogenase, tumor necrosis factor-α, and interleukin-6 and increased serum NO activity. Additionally, cinnamaldehyde upregulated the expression of superoxide dismutase as well as decreased the level of malondialdehyde in myocardium [28].

21.4.3 Cinnamic Acid

Cinnamic acid and its derivatives have been used for various pharmacological effects such as antimicrobial, antifungal, and antitumoral effects. A previous in vitro investigation revealed that cinnamic acid causes an endothelium-dependent vasodilation effect by the NO-cGMP-PKG-mediated mechanism in rat thoracic aorta [29]. Another report demonstrated anti-obesity as well as antihypertensive properties of cinnamic acid via suppressing the expression of lipid digestive as well as angiotensin-converting enzyme [111]. In vivo investigation revealed that cinnamic acid decreased ST-segment elevation and decreased *creatine kinase, lactate dehydrogenase*, tumor necrosis factor-α, and interleukin-6 and increased serum NO activity in ischemic rats (induced by isoproterenol) [28].

21.4.4 Cinnamyl Alcohol

Cinnamyl alcohol, a phytochemical diversely present in various herbal-based products and plants, possesses a broad range of pharmacological activities. In vitro studies performed by Kang et al. [30] demonstrated vasodilatory effects of cinnamyl alcohol using vascular endothelium, aortic rings preparation, as well as cultured smooth muscle cells. Findings suggested that aortic rings after cinnamyl alcohol treatment showed endothelium-dependent vasorelaxation. The vasodilatory effect was decreased by pretreatment with methylene blue, glibenclamide, and L-NAME, which demonstrates that the vasorelaxation effect could be mediated by guanylyl cyclase, nitric oxide, and potassium channel. Additionally, it has been suggested that cinnamyl alcohol treatment increased cGMP and increased the level of cGMP-dependent protein kinase 1 and influenced the Rho-kinase mediated signaling pathway. Thus, cinnamyl alcohol caused vasodilation by involving vascular endothelium, which could be due to stimulation of Nitric oxide – cyclic GMP signaling – protein kinase G mechanism in aorta of rat leading to opening of potassium ion channels as well as suppression of the rho-kinase mediated contraction.

21.4.5 α-Bisabolol

The cardioprotective effects of sesquiterpene, α-bisabolol, which is diversely present in various plants, are evidenced in various studies [20]. Vasorelaxant effects of (–) α-bisabolol on the aortic and mesenteric arteries were investigated in various reports. It was found that α-bisabolol induced vasorelaxant effects in various smooth muscle preparations (mainly in mesenteric vessels) as well as in precontracted aortic rings [20]. One more report authored by the same researchers showed that α-bisabolol induced vascular relaxation via involvement of calcium transport mediated by voltage-dependent channels. Likewise, one more report suggested the involvement of calcium-dependent vascular relaxation. In this report, α-bisabolol–induced vascular relaxation mediated via calcium influx was confirmed by removal of the calcium from the medium. Once calcium was totally removed, the α-bisabolol–induced vascular relaxation disappeared. Thus, this report clearly showed that α-bisabolol–induced vasorelaxation is caused by inhibition of calcium influx via voltage-dependent channels.

21.4.6 Carvacrol

Carvacrol (isomer of thymol) is a terpenoid phenol diversely present in EOs obtained from various medicinal plants. It was found that lead-induced hypercontraction in rat aortic rings was reduced by carvacrol [23]. Coincubation of aortic rings with carvacrol and did not induce alteration in the vasodilation patterns. Nevertheless, treatment of carvacrol with L-NAME reduced the vasodilation caused by carvacrol. These findings suggested that vasodilatory response could be due to the increase in NO synthesis and quenching of reactive oxygen species. In vitro studies on carvacrol-treated cells derived from parenchymal arterioles demonstrated that carvacrol augmented release calcium ions via stimulating the transient receptor potential vanilloid channel, to further stimulate intermediate and small-conductance calcium ion activated potassium ion (SK) channels. Activation of the SK channel induces hyperpolarization, which can further lead to vasorelaxation mediated by endothelium-dependent pathway [106]. Further investigations in nonanesthetized Wistar rats (*in vivo*) showed that carvacrol treatment caused hypotension and bradycardia via vasorelaxation mediated by inhibition of the Ca^{2+} influx through Cav and TRP channels. Ca^{2+} influx was reduced by affecting store-operated channels, voltage-gated ion channels, and transient receptor potentials channels [24]. A recent investigation suggested that carvacrol in rat aortic rings increased vasodilatation both in the presence and in the absence of endothelium. Thus, endothelial potassium channels were found to be possible targets of carvacrol because it was observed that voltage-operated potassium (Kv) channel blockers (4-aminopyridine and quinine) considerably decreased carvacrol vasorelaxant effects [112].

21.4.7 Borneol

A cyclic monoterpene alcohol, borneol, is diversely present in various medicinal plants especially *Cinnamomum camphora* (L.). It was found that treatment of aortic rings with borneol caused relaxation of precontracted phenylephrine or KCl–aortic rings via endothelium-independent pathway [21]. Also, borneol attenuated vasorelaxation in aortic rings after pretreatment with K^+ channel blockers. This vasorelaxant property could be, perhaps, due to inhibition of calcium release via regulating voltage-dependent calcium channels intracellular calcium store activation and activation of potassium channels. A Chinese traditional medicine pill called Suxiao Jiuxin-Wan (Suxiao Jiuxin Pill) containing borneol as a major chemical component has been widely used for the treatment of cardiovascular complications. It was observed that Suxiao Jiuxin induced vasorelaxation via both endothelium-dependent and independent pathways. *In vivo* studies on borneol showed neuroprotective effects against ischemic stroke [22] via downregulation of proinflammatory mediators (COX-2, IL-1β, iNOS, and TNF-α,). Moreover, it was found that borneol decreased the infarct area in a concentration-dependent manner. Borneol can activate the blood–brain barrier, which might be linked to the better expression of CD54 is a protein. Recently, it was also reported that (–)-borneol-dependent vasorelaxant effect could be due to the presence of vascular endothelium, with the direct involvement of NO and prostanoids. Additionally, (–)-borneol showed direct action on the vascular smooth muscle, and the mechanism of action is based on KATP channels [113].

21.4.8 Carvone

Carvone is the chemical compound derived from mentha, dill, caraway, and other plants. Carvone induced vasorelaxant effects in aortic rings and also showed protective effects in the artery when exposed to heavy metals [25]. A recent study demonstrated the vasorelaxant effect of (–)-carveol on human umbilical arteries, which is dependent on the opening of calcium and potassium channels. It was also reported that the vasorelaxant effect was decreased by tetraethylammonium. The antioxidant mechanism and its effect on calcium voltage-dependent channels as well as NO synthesis suggested its role in the vasorelaxation process. (+)- and (–)-carveol both are reported to have vasorelaxant effects in aortic rings and guinea pig tracheas without any considerable difference in therapeutic potential. It was also evidenced that both act directly on the smooth muscle, as vasorelaxant effects were not decreased in the aorotic rings without endothelium.

21.4.9 Eugenol

Eugenol, the main component of clove oil, belongs to the class of phenylpropanoids and presents a wide range of biological activities such as acting as a natural antioxidant. It was found that eugenol caused dilation of arteries present in rat cerebrum via suppression of voltage-gated calcium channels [114]. One more study suggested that eugenol produces smooth muscle relaxation resulting from the blockade of both voltage-sensitive and receptor-operated channels that are modulated by endothelial-generated NO [45,115]. Recent *in vivo* investigations showed antihypertensive action of eugenol via opening TRPV4 channels in mesenteric artery endothelial cells, resulting in vasorelaxation and decrease in systemic BP [116]. Eugenol pretreatment followed by the combined treatment of isoproterenol and eugenol leads to considerable reversal of cardiac hypertrophy, which was induced by isoproterenol and restored various changes caused by isoproterenol such as normalization of the heart weight, decreased apoptosis of myocytes with decreased accumulation of ROS, normalized glutathione contents, and normalized level of calcineurin and protein kinase C in ventricular tissue [117]. It was also observed that eugenol reduced vascular and neural complications in streptozotocin-induced diabetic rats [118]. The hypolipidemic effect of eugenol in rats fed with high-cholesterol and fat diet was found to be due to the considerable decrease in total cholesterol, low-density lipoproteins, and atherogenic index. Docking studies demonstrated that eugenol does not inhibit *HMG-CoA reductase* but rather induces its action by interaction with TRPV1 channels [119]. Eugenol is also reported to have an antioxidant and vasorelaxant effect, via blockage of calcium channels. It was observed that eugenol caused vasorelaxation of lead-treated aortic rings via increasing nitric oxide systemic absorption and reducing reactive oxygen species.

Eugenol caused hypotension and bradycardia in dose-dependent manner normotensive rats. The bradycardia is due to the involvement of parasympathetic nerve whereas the hypotensive effect is due to the vasorelaxant effect. It was also found that hypotension and bradycardia induced by eugenol in normotensive rats was not affected by pretreatment with L-NAME. Eugenol induced a reversible and concentration-dependent vasodilator effect in precontracted mesenteric bed preparations. The vasodilatory effect was not affected by atropine [120].

21.4.10 1-Nitro-2-Phenylethane

1-nitro-2-phenylethane is the NO_2 group containing phytochemical derived from *Aniba canelilla* EO. In vivo studies showed that 1-nitro-phenylethane induced bradycardic and hypotensive responses, and this response was fully gone after cervical bivagotomy. It was also suggested that the vasorelaxant effect might be due to the vagal reflex and a cholinergic mechanism. It was found that this nitro-based organic compound caused a vasovagal bradycardia and depressor reflex due to the activation of vagal afferent fibers in the respiratory tract rather than C fiber cardiac vagal efferent [121]. Another study showed that 1-nitro-2-phenylethane produces vasodilator effects by stimulating the soluble *guanylate cyclase*-cGMP pathway [122]. 1-nitro-phenylethane has been reported to have endothelium-independent vasorelaxant effects in mesenteric arteries from hypertensive rats [123].

21.4.11 Auraptene

Auraptene, a monoterpene coumarin derived from various Citrus plants, possesses cardioprotective activities. It was reported that auraptene significantly decreased mean systolic blood pressure in hypertensive rats, but not in normotensive rats [18]. Another study demonstrated that treatment of normotensive rats with single IV injections of auraptene showed a dose-dependent hypotensive effect. Additionally, it was found that nifedipine significantly decreased mean systolic blood pressure than auraptene [124].

21.4.12 Citral

Citral (3,7-dimethyl-2,6-octadienal) is the major chemical component of *Cymbopogon citratus* and also occurs in other plants and various citrus fruits. A recent review demonstrated the role of citral in reducing oxidative stress, inflammation and treatment of diabetes, dyslipidemia, endothelial dysfunction, and atherosclerosis [125]. Another study demonstrated antioxidant and cytoprotective effects of citral against oxidative damage induced by H_2O_2 in human endothelial cells [126].

It was observed that citral-induced vasodilatory effects aorta by influencing the nitric oxidel/cyclic GMP pathways. The authors reported that citral also affects calcium influx via voltage-dependent L-type Ca^{2+} channels. Findings from this report suggested that citral-inhibited contractions induced by high K^+ and phenylephrine and caused vasorelaxation by the endothelium-independent mechanism [85].

21.4.13 Citronellol

Citronellol is a monoterpene compound derived from the EO of Indian lemon grass, Citronella grass, and bushy matgrass that possesses cardioprotective effects. It was reported that citronellol induced hypotension in rats, which was not influenced after the treatment of rats with L-NAME hydrochloride, or indomethacin, hexamethonium, and atropine.

Citronellol strongly reduced the contractions induced by $CaCl_2$, phenylephrine, or caffeine. The results obtained from this study suggested that citronellol decreased BP via directly acting on the vascular smooth muscle leading to vasorelaxation [40]. Another study showed the cardioprotective effects of citronellal by reducing the MAP and inducing vasodilation of rat mesenteric arteries via involving endothelium in hypertensive rats.

21.4.14 Farnesene

Farnesene (sesquiterpene hydrocarbon) is the main chemical component of the German EO chamomile (*Matricaria chamomilla*). It was found that farnesene did not cause vasorelaxing even at higher concentration.

21.4.15 Limonene

Limonene is a cyclic monoterpene present in citrus, especially in citrus fruit peels, with a high level in its component of EOs [127]. D-limonene has been reported on for its various cardiovascular as well as antiarrhythmic effects in rodents. This study showed that D-limonene promotes hypotension with bradycardia in rodents as well as has antiarrhythmic effects [127]. Another report suggested that it has endothelium-independent vasorelaxant effects on the aortic rings as well as tracheas. Additionally, no significant differences were found in the pharmacological activity of both (+)-limonene and (–)-limonene enantiomers. Thus, this finding suggests that D-limonene might cause spasmolytic effects over trachea smooth muscle.

21.4.16 Linalool

Linalool is a naturally occurring monoterpene that is diversely present in various aromatic plant EOs. A recent investigation revealed that linalool showed a dose-dependent decrease in the incidence of arrhythmias in a rat model induced with myocardial infarction. It was suggested that the antiarrhythmic effect might be due to an increase in cardiac connexin expression as decrease in the Cx43 expression resulted in an increase in incidence of arrhythmias secondary to disordered cardiac electric conductivity [4]. An earlier report suggested that (–)-linalool may induce endothelium-dependent vasorelaxation in mouse thoracic aortae by activating soluble *guanylyl cyclase* and K^+ channels [128].

Another report revealed that linalool blocked the voltage-dependent calcium channel and elevated NO to induce vasorelaxation in arsenic and mercury-induced hypercontraction in rat aortas [25]. One more study suggested that linalool decreased BP without changing the HR in hypertensive rats. Linalool also induced vasorelaxation in a dose-dependent way in mesenteric artery of rats pretreated with phenylephrine, and response was not changed even after treatment with atropine. Furthermore, linalool decreased the vasocontractions caused by $CaCl_2$, phenylephrine, or caffeine. These findings suggest that the lowering effect on BP is possibly because linalool directly acts over the vascular smooth muscle resulting in vasorelaxation [129].

21.4.17 Linalyl Acetate

Linalyl acetate is the therapeutically active major ingredient of the EO derived from *Citrus bergamia, Lavandula angustifolia,* and *Salvia sclarea.* A previous report demonstrated that linalyl acetate induced vasorelaxation in the rabbit vascular smooth muscle via dephosphorylation of myosin light chain.

These effects were induced by partial stimulation of the NO/cGMP pathway, and partial myosin light chain dephosphorylation via stimulation of myosin light chain phosphatase [62]. An additional study suggested that treatment with linalyl acetate restored acetylcholine-induced vasorelaxation, blood pressure, HR, and AMP-activated protein kinase and serum nitrite levels. It was also found that treatment with linalyl acetate restores endothelial dysfunction and hemodynamic changes in diabetic rats exposed to chronic immobilization stress [130]. A recent study showed that treatment with linalyl acetate prevents olmesartan-induced intestinal hypermotility mediated by interference of the sympathetic inhibitory pathway in hypertensive rats [131,132]. It was also found that nicotine plus linalyl acetate or nifedipine treatment showed a constant relaxation effect on contraction of the mouse aorta. Additionally, treatment with linalyl acetate reduced nicotine-induced elevation in nitrite concentration. Thus, findings from this study suggested that linalyl acetate or nifedipine treatment recovered cell damage and restored or normalized cardiovascular changes induced by nicotine [133]. Likewise, treatment with LA prevented vascular damage and also reduced systolic blood pressure and decreased the level of serum malondialdehyde and serum lactate dehydrogenase in COPD-like and hypertensive rats [134].

21.4.18 Menthol

Menthol is a cyclic-monoterpene present in various *Mentha* species including and *M. piperita* as well as *M. arvensis* [73]. A recent report showed that menthol caused vasodilation in both normotensive and hypertensive subjects. It was observed that menthol-induced vasodilation in the normotensive group was not affected either by NOS or sensory nerve inhibition; nevertheless, menthol-induced vasorelaxation was attenuated with NOS and sensory nerve inhibition in the hypertensive group. It was also shown that the endothelium-derived hyperpolarizing factor inhibition attenuated menthol-induced vasodilation in both groups [135].

Menthol has been reported for its direct action act on the vascular endothelium as well as smooth muscle. Additionally, the latest reports showed that treatment with menthol indirectly affects the vascular tone via sensory fibers. As mechanisms of action of menthol involve various cellular targets and thus cross signaling between various pathways ultimately showed variation in response. The complex relationship between different pathways dependent on NO-dependent vasodilation and non-NO as well as nonprostaglandin-mediated endothelium-dependent vasodilation (due to endothelium-derived hyperpolarization factors) and sensory nerve responses produce variable response. Menthol-induced vasodilation involves activation of TRPM8 channels in the endothelial cell, which can result in an increase in cytosolic calcium. Increase in cytosolic calcium further increases cascades of reactions as mentioned below (⊗ = inhibition; ↑ = increase; ↓ = decrease; Ⓐ = activation; TRPM8 = transient receptor potential melastatin-8; cGMP = cyclic guanosine monophosphate; LCC = L-type calcium channels; NOS = nitric oxide synthase; EDHFs = endothelium-derived hyperpolarization factors) [136].

- Calmodulin-calcium binding → Ⓐ NOS → ↑ NO level in muscle cells → ↑ cGMP
- Activation of EDHFs → Ⓐ potassium channels on muscle cells → Ⓐ potassium channels on endothelial cells → hyperpolarization
- ⊗L-type Ca^{+2}channels in muscle cells → ↓ extracellular Ca^{+2}release
- Ⓐ membrane transient receptor potential cation channel subfamily M member 8 channels → ↑ extracellular Ca^{+2} release → ⊗ Rho/Rho-associated coiled-coil containing protein kinase signaling pathway
- ↑ Cytoplasmic Ca^{+2} activates mitochondrial uptake → ↓ ROS production → ⊗ L-type calcium channels
- ↑ cGMP → ↓ cytosolic calcium concentration → ⊗ RhoA/ROCK pathway → ↑ myosin phosphatase effect and relaxation of myocytes
- Ⓐ TRPM8 channels → ↑ cytosolic calcium level → ↑ calcitonin gene-associated peptide, ↑ neuropeptide (substance P), ↑ nitric oxide → ↑ vascular smooth muscle relaxation

21.4.19 N-Butylidenephthalide

n-Butylidenephthalide is a natural compound obtained from *Angelica sinensis* EO that has been studied for its various biological activities [74]. A recent study showed antiproliferating and apoptotic effects of n-butylidenephthalide over vascular smooth muscle cells. It was found that n-butylidenephthalide inhibited the platelet-derived growth factor-induced cytoskeleton reorganization of the vascular smooth muscle cells. n-butylidenephthalide was also found to inhibit thrombus formation and the expression of vimentin and collagen in vascular smooth muscle cells. An inhibitory effect of n-butylidenephthalide over the cytoskeleton reorganization of the vascular smooth muscle cells caused by platelet-derived growth factor, expression of vimentin and collagen, and migration ability induced by platelet-derived growth factor is also reported. Cell cycle studies showed that n-butylidenephthalide inhibited vascular smooth muscle cell proliferation caused by the platelet-derived growth factor and arrested the vascular smooth muscle cells in the G0/G1 phase. n-butylidenephthalide is also reported for its stimulatory effects on 5' adenosine monophosphate-activated protein kinase and suppressive effects over the mTOR phosphorylation [137].

Another report on this compound suggests that n-butylidenephthalide-induced vasorelaxation involves both endothelium-dependent and endothelium-independent components. It was found that n-butylidenephthalide acts via its suppressing effect over downstreaming of tol-type voltage-operated and prostanoid TP receptor-operated Ca^{2+} channels, which will become operational in a late contractile phase [138].

It was also found that this compound inhibits endothelial cell multiplication, vascular endothelial growth factor mediated wound healing, as well as development of tube on human umbilical vein endothelial cells via promoting programmed cell death and improving protection of the cell-division cycle (G0–G1 phase). Moreover, the authors also evidenced that the antiangiogenic effect of this compound could also be related to its inhibitory effect on angiogenesis and increase in the formation of blood vessels in zebra fish [74].

21.4.20 Rotundifolone

Rotundifolone, the most important component of *Mentha × villosa* EO, showed hypotensive effects, which may be due the lowering of HR and systemic vascular resistance, possibly because of nonselective muscarinic receptor stimulation. It was found that rotundifolone induced vasorelaxation in rat superior mesenteric arteries, which could be due to its stimulatory effects on calcium-activated potassium (BKCa) channel and inhibitory effects on Ca^{2+} release via L-type calcium channels, which can result in change in steady-state deactivation association for voltage-gated L-type Ca2+ channel toward more hyperpolarized membrane potentials. However, both mechanisms followed by rotundifolone to induce vasodilation are concentration dependent [76,77].

21.4.21 α-Terpineol

α-terpineol is a phytoconstituent obtained from the EOs of various aromatic plants. It has been reported that alpha-terpineol–induced hypotension and vasorelaxation are mediated by the endothelium, most likely via NO release and stimulation of the NO-cGMP pathway [139]. One more report demonstrated dose-dependent hypotensive effects (in vivo) of α-terpineol in hypertensive animals (induced by L-NAME). These effects were due to the vasorelaxant effects induced by α-terpineol in mesenteric rings, which were independent of the endothelium. It was observed that vasorelaxant effects could be associated with inhibitory effects of α-terpineol on voltage-dependent calcium channels.

21.5 Vasoconstrictor Effects of Various EOs

21.5.1 *Citrus bergamia*

Store-operated calcium ion entry was improved by the EO of *Citrus bergamia* Risso. *Citrus bergamia* RissoEO moves calcium ions from important intracellular stores via Ca^{2+}-stimulated and inositol 1,4,5-trisphosphate-facilitated Ca^{2+} release and affects increase in Ca^{2+} influx, possibly via the store-operated Ca^{2+} pathway. Thus, this EO is found to elevate intracellular Ca^{2+} in human vascular endothelial cells due to the release of Ca^{2+} from primary intracellular stores [32].

21.5.2 *Croton zehntneri*

Croton zehntneri EO is known for its cardiovascular effects in conscious rats. It was observed that administration of *Croton zehntneri* EO induced hypotensive effect followed by transient increase of blood pressure. These responses were due to the presence of estragole and anethole. Hypotensive effect induced by *Croton zehntneri* EO was mediated via the cholinergic mechanism or might be due to the simultaneous bradycardia. The pressor response of *Croton zehntneri* EO in the later phase might be due to the indirect vasoconstrictive action of *Croton zehntneri* EO most likely via inhibition of endothelial NO production [37].

21.5.3 Neryl Butyrate

Neryl butyrate is a component of EO isolated from aromatic plants. Neryl butyrate showed vasocontractile effects, and this effect was prevented by α-adrenergic antagonists, which represent the participation of α-adrenoceptors. *In vivo* investigation showed that neryl butyrate demonstrated hypotensive effect, indicating that additional systemic effect other than vasoconstriction might ensue [140].

21.6 EOs and Atherosclerosis

Various reports have suggested the role of EOs as well as their components in the treatment and prevention of atherosclerosis.

21.6.1 Onion and Garlic

Onion and garlic EOs are known to play a significant role as a dietary component for individuals susceptible to arteriosclerosis and thromboembolism. It was found that in comparison with clofibrate, onion as well as garlic EO showed more efficacies, whereas the low-density lipoprotein cholesterol-lowering effect of garlic EO in aorta of Indian albino rabbits was more effective than that of the onion EO [49–51]. It was also reported that the fibrinolytic activity of these EOs was due to the presence of organosulfur compounds in onion as well as garlic (diallyl disulfide, diallyl trisulfide, and allyl propyl disulfide). Moreover, the fibrinolytic activity of these EOs was found to be more significant than clofibrate, which suggests their possible inhibitory role in atherosclerosis progression [49–51]. A significant increase in fibrinolytic activity, considerable reduction in aortic atheroma, decrease in β/α lipoprotein ratio, and decrease in serum cholesterol and triglycerides were also reported in rabbits treated with EOs [49–51]. Previous reports showed that the protective effects of these EOs could be due to the following mechanisms [49–51]:

- Via regulating the rise in the systemic cholesterol as well as lipids
- Via inhibiting the decrease in the α-lipoprotein by maintaining the ratio between α and β human plasma lipoproteins
- Via increasing the fibrinolytic activity of the plasma

Moreover, the protective action of garlic EO on systemic lipid level as well as fibrinolytic activity in humans with the coronary artery complication was also investigated [49–51]. It was found that healthy as well as coronary artery patients when treated with garlic EO showed considerable decrease in serum cholesterol and triglycerides and increase in high-density lipoprotein levels. Treatment with the garlic EO was found to increase fibrinolysis among chronic infarction individuals.

21.6.2 *Satureja khuzestanica*

Satureja khuzestanica, an Iranian plant, is known for its antihyperlipidemic effects. Various reports based on the lipid-lowering effects of *Satureja khuzestanica* EO have been reported. An early report showed that treatment with EO derived from *Satureja khuzestanica* drastically reduced triglycerides levels, but did not affect blood total cholesterol levels significantly in Sprague–Dawley male rats. Likewise, another study showed that *Satureja khuzestanica* EO administration considerably reduced triglyceride levels in experimental animals. Studies based on the treatment of hyperlipidemic patients with type 2 diabetes mellitus with *Satureja khuzestanica* supplement showed a considerable decrease in cholesterol as well as low-density lipoprotein cholesterol and increased high-density lipoprotein cholesterol, whereas impact on the level of triglycerides was not seen. In contrast to this study, treatment of type 1 diabetic rats with *Satureja khuzestanica* EO considerably reduced cholesterol, low-density lipoprotein cholesterol, very-low-density lipoprotein, and triglycerides and increased high-density lipoprotein cholesterol.

21.6.3 Artemisia species

Several plants belonging to the Artemisia genus (Asteraceae) have been described for their cardioprotective effects. *Artemisia princeps* EO has been reported to have antiatherosclerotic effects. These authors observed that treatment with the wormwood EO increased the expression of LDL receptors (involved in metabolism of cholesterol), when HepG2 cells treated at lower concentration; however, concomitant treatment of HepG2 cells with EO at higher concentration and vitamin E decreased the expression of LDL receptor significantly. However, it was found that *HMG-CoA reductase* activity remained unaltered. Chung et al. [141] reported that the anti-atherogenic effects of EO with vitamin E could be due to the inhibition of LDL oxidation and upregulation of LDL receptor.

One more investigation showed that *Artemisia sieberi* EO treatment considerably decreased TC, TG, and LDL-C level and increased HDLC in alloxan-induced diabetic rats.

21.6.4 Asian Plantain (*Plantago asiatica*)

Polysaccharides derived from the *Semen plantaginis* (dried ripe seed of *Plantago asiatica*) have been evidenced for their cholesterol-lowering effects in blood. Phenolic compound-enriched *Asiatic plantain* administration can reduce postprandial oxidative stress, a form of nutritional oxidative stress in obese hyperlipidemic subjects. Treatment of human liver carcinoma cells with *Asian plantain* EO showed a change in the expression of the LDL receptor and HMG-CoA *reductase* with considerable reduction in low-density lipoprotein oxidation because of the presence of linalool. *Asian plantain* EO when administered orally reduced TC and TAG level in C57BL/6 mice. Furthermore, mRNA encoding functional LDL was found to be significantly high in the hepatocytes of EO-treated mice. Moreover, *Asian plantain* EO-treated mice showed considerably reduced protein as well as mRNA concentration of HMG-CoA *reductase* in contrast to the control group.

21.6.5 *Ocimum sanctum*

Eugenol- and methyleugenol-enriched *Ocimum sanctum* EO has been reported for its antilipidemic activities in various studies. It was found that treatment with *Ocimum sanctum* EO showed antilipidemic activities in rodents consuming a high-cholesterol diet. Findings from this study revealed that treatment with the EO considerably decreased cholesterol, low-density lipoprotein cholesterol, triglyceride, atherogenic index of plasma, lactate dehydrogenase, and creatine kinase. At the same time, it was found that TC and TG levels reduced by the EO did not appear in feces. Additionally, it was also found that EO treatment considerably reduced glutathione peroxidase, superoxide dismutase, and thiobarbituric acid reactive substances.

21.6.6 *Pinus koraiensis*

Pinus koraiensis (Korean pine) EO has been reported to have antihyperlipidemic effects in various studies. It was found that *Pinus koraiensis* EO increased the expression of mRNA that encodes for LDL receptors. Additionally, *Pinus koraiensis* EO decreased the level of various biomarkers involved in lipid metabolism:

- Fatty acid synthase that catalyzes fatty acid synthesis.
- Membrane-bound transcription factors such as sterol regulatory element-binding protein (SREBP)-1c, SREBP-2 that activate genes involved in cholesterol synthesis.
- 3-hydroxy-3-methyl-glutaryl-coenzyme A reductase, an enzyme of the metabolic pathway that regulates synthesizes of cholesterol.
- Glycerol-3-phosphate acyltransferase, an enzyme engaged in lipid metabolism.

It was also suggested that *Pinus koraiensis* EO decreased oxidative action of LDL and considerably suppressed acyl-CoA. *In vitro* findings over 3T3-L1 cells demonstrated that *Pinus koraiensis* EO inhibited increments in fat and triglycerides levels. This was mediated by decrease in the expression of adipogenic transcription factors, which are involved in regulating lipid homeostasis including peroxisome proliferator activated receptor and transcription factors including CCAAT enhancer binding protein α. In addition, it was also found that EO decreased transport proteins such as fatty acid-binding proteins to allow the transport of fatty acids between extracellular and intracellular membranes. This step was mediated by inhibiting the expression of PPARγ genes. Likewise, the EO also decreased the level of glycerol-3-phosphate dehydrogenase via inhibiting the upregulation of PPARγ genes. Treatment of high-fat diet-fed Sprague–Dawley rats with the *Pinus koraiensis* EO demonstrated considerable decrease in body weight gain, cholesterol, low-density lipoprotein cholesterol, triglyceride, and atherogenic index of plasma and increase in high-density lipoprotein in a concentration-dependent manner. Furthermore, it was shown that the EO considerably revoked the existing level of PPARγ in the hepatic tissue of abrogated-treated rats. Thus, considering all these findings, it has been suggested that *Pinus koraiensis* EO treatment exhibits hypolipidemic as well as antiobesity effects via suppression of the PPARγ-related pathway.

21.6.7 Fenugreek Seed

Terpenes-enriched fenugreek seed EO has been reported to have a crucial effect on the regulation of cholesterol metabolism via affecting the expression of important enzymes involved in lipid metabolism. It was also found that terpenoidal compounds present in fenugreek seed EO were found to be absorbed via gut membranes to affect cholesterol metabolism. A recent investigation showed the suppressive effects of a formulation containing fenugreek terpenes and omega-3 fatty acids on important enzymes involved in the metabolism of carbohydrate-n and hypertension in diabetic experimental animals. Findings from this study demonstrated that fenugreek terpenes with omega-3 fatty acids containing preparation treatment significantly suppressed an important enzyme associated with diabetes including α-amylase and maltase activity in pancreas and plasma. Furthermore, the findings from this study also indicated that this formulation protects the β-cells from damage and modulates the expression of the key enzyme involved in inducing hypertension such as angiotensin-converting enzyme in the plasma and kidney. Most importantly, this formulation considerably reduced the glucose, triglyceride, and total-cholesterol and LDL-cholesterol level in the plasma and liver of diabetic rats and elevated the HDL-cholesterol level to maintain the homeostasis of blood lipid, which suggests it has antihypertensive and hypolipidemic effects [142].

21.6.8 *Melissa officinalis*

Melissa officinalis EO mainly contains citral (neral as well as geranial), citronellal, and geraniol as the key components. An earlier report suggested an antihyperlipidemic effect of EO derived from *Melissa officinalis* in animals fed with high-cholesterol diet, and it was revealed that the EO considerably decreased the level of TC, LDL-C, VLDL-C, TG, and HDL-C. Another study indicated that the EO treatment considerably reduced the TG level in APOE2 mice and dose-dependent decrease in triglycerides as well as cholesterol level was found in liver hepatocellular carcinoma cells. Findings from transcriptome studies revealed that the *Melissa officinalis* EO treatment may possibly modify various lipid metabolism signaling pathways including cholesterol biosynthesis, bile acid, as well as fatty acid metabolism. It was also found that *Melissa officinalis* EO could downregulate translocation of membrane-bound transcription factors (sterol receptor element-binding protein-1c that activates genes involved in fatty acid synthesis).

21.6.9 *Nigella sativa*

Blood lipid-lowering effects of *Nigella sativa* EO were studied, and it was found that it improved the lipid profile without any adverse effects. Findings from this study showed that treatment of healthy volunteers with *Nigella sativa* EO significantly decreased fasting blood cholesterol, LDL, triglyceride, glucose, and HbA1C levels [143]. Another study showed that *Nigella sativa* seed oil, thymoquinone, and *Nigella sativa* seed extract decreased plasma levels of total cholesterol, low-density lipoprotein cholesterol, and triglycerides; nevertheless, the effect on high-density lipoprotein cholesterol was not considerable. It was also demonstrated that the lipid-modifying or antihyperlipidemic effects of *Nigella sativa* EO can be due to the suppression of intestinal cholesterol absorption, reduced hepatic cholesterol synthesis, and increase in the expression of LDL receptors [144]. The earlier study revealed that treatment of streptozotocin-induced diabetes mellitus rats with the *Nigella sativa* EO decreased the level of TC, TG, and LDL-C, which showed its hypocholesterolemic effects. It was also reported that treatment of Wistar rats with volatile oil derived from *Nigella sativa* normalized plasma triglycerides; decreased *HMG-CoA reductase* activity; blocked production of conjugated diene as well as malondialdehyde; and extended the lag times of low-density lipoprotein, small-dense LDL-C, and large-Buoyant LDL [76]. Likewise, treatment of hypercholesterolemic rabbits with *Nigella sativa* oil showed hypocholesterolemic and antiatherogenic cardioprotective properties by considerably reducing total cholesterol and low-density lipoprotein cholesterol levels, inhibiting plaque formation, and increasing high-density lipoprotein cholesterol levels [145].

21.6.10 *Citrus sp.*

Various reports demonstrated that citrus EO supplementation in diet improved the plasma lipid content and also elevated plasma antioxidant activity. A recent investigation showed that lime EO treatment increased the alanine aminotransferase, aspartate transaminase, low-density lipoprotein cholesterol, serum total cholesterol, and triglyceride levels in the hyperlipidemic rodents.

Additionally, it was also found that lime EO treatment improves health with regard to fatty liver atherogenic index and obesity [146]. It was also found that *Citrus aurantium* EO treatment significantly reduced the TC level in Swiss male mice.

21.6.11 Chios Mastic Gum (Derived from *Pistacia lentiscus*)

The hypocholesterolemic effects of *Pistacia lentiscus* have been evidenced in various reports. It was found that treatment of detergent-induced hyperlipidemia rats with EO derived from Chios mastic gum decreased the cholesterol as well as triglyceride levels in serum in a dose-dependent manner. Furthermore, it was also reported that the hypolipidemic effect possessed by the EO could be associated with camphene. Later, it was also found that treatment of hyperlipidemic rats with camphene decreased cholesterol, triglyceride, and low-density lipoprotein cholesterol. Additionally, treatment with camphene decreased cellular cholesterol in HepG2 cells with a significance rate equivalent to mevinolin.

21.6.12 Dill (*Anethum graveolens*)

A previous report demonstrated the hypolipidemic effects of *Anethum graveolens* powdered preparation as well as its EO on hypercholesterolemic male Wistar rats. It was found that *Anethum graveolens* EO treatment increased the high-density lipoprotein cholesterol level and considerably decreased cholesterol, triglycerides, and low-density lipoprotein cholesterol levels and hence can act as a potential cardioprotective agent.

21.6.13 Korean Mint (*Agastache rugosa*)

Nutrigenomics studies showed the lipoprotein-lowering effects of Korean mint EO in liver hepatocellular carcinoma cells and C57BL/6 mice. *Agastache rugose* EO treatment considerably reduced LDL oxidation in HepG2 cells. This action possessed by the EO can prevent reaction of LDL cholesterol with free radicals to form oxidized LDL, which can easily move into arterial walls and expand them with cholesterol. EO treatment of C57BL/6J mice also attenuated TC and TG levels considerably. Transcriptome studies showed that *Agastache rugose* EO treatment decreased membrane-bound transcription factors expression such as sterol regulatory element-binding factor (1, 2) and enzyme, *HMG-CoA reductase*, in HepG2 cells, which activate genes responsible for cholesterol synthesis. Additionally, it was also found that the EO increased the expression of gene that encodes for the low-density lipoprotein receptor in hepatocellular carcinoma cells and hepatic tissue of the rodent. Therefore, it has been demonstrated that the EO can prevent arteriosclerosis via the following:

- Inhibition of low-density lipoprotein oxidation
- Decrease in the expression of *HMG-CoA reductase* and sterol regulatory element-binding protein 2
- Increase the expression of low-density lipoprotein

21.7 Role of Biotechnology in Cardiovascular Complications

Gene transfer allows the overexpression of therapeutic genes either locally or systemically. Gene therapy can be used as a method to deliver vasoprotective molecules at the site of vascular injury. Due to the complexity of cardiovascular disorders, one of the major challenges could be identification of the gene to treat cardiovascular complications. For effective gene therapy, combination of therapeutic genes can be used rather than using a single gene to treat complications such as hypertension and atherosclerosis. Other effective approaches such as cell and gene therapies such as antisense and RNA interference can be used for the effective delivery of therapeutics [147–206].

21.7.1 Stem Cell Therapy

Stem cell therapy involves the transplantation of normal cardiac cells by using bone marrow precursor cells to restore its normal physiological state via repairing damaged cells and injured tissue and is considered a reliable method of treatment [147–206].

21.7.2 Nanotechnology

Nanomedicine in different forms can be used to promote cell-selective-targeted drug delivery to improve therapeutic potential of a drug by rigorously restricting its pharmacological activity to an injured site [147–206].

REFERENCES

1. Gaziano T, Reddy KS, Paccaud F, et al. Cardiovascular disease. In: Jamison DT, Breman JG, Measham AR, et al., editors. *Disease Control Priorities in Developing Countries*, 2nd edition. The International Bank for Reconstruction and Development/The World Bank, Washington, DC; 2006, Chapter 33. Available from: https://www.ncbi.nlm.nih.gov/books/NBK11767/, Co-published by Oxford University Press, New York.
2. Rastogi S, Pandey MM, Rawat AK. Traditional herbs: A remedy for cardiovascular disorders. *Phytomedicine.* 2016;23(11):1082–1089.
3. Nikolaevskiĭ VV, Kononova NS, Pertsovskiĭ AI, Shinkarchuk IF. Vliianie éfirnykh masel na techenie éksperimental'nogo ateroskleroza effect of essential oils on the course of experimental atherosclerosis. *Patol Fiziol Eksp Ter.* 1990;5:52–53. Russian.
4. Ke J, Zhu C, Zhang Y, Zhang W. Anti-arrhythmic effects of linalool via Cx43 expression in a rat model of myocardial infarction. *Front Pharmacol.* 2020;11:926.
5. Ziaee M, Khorrami A, Ebrahimi M, Nourafcan H, Amiraslanzadeh M, Rameshrad M, Garjani M, Garjani A. Cardioprotective effects of essential oil of *Lavandula angustifolia* on isoproterenol-induced acute myocardial infarction. *Rat Iran J Pharm Res.* 2015 Winter;14(1):279–289.
6. Sadeghzadeh J, Vakili A, Bandegi AR, Sameni HR, Zahedi Khorasani M, Darabian M. Lavandula reduces heart injury via attenuating tumor necrosis factor-alpha and oxidative stress in a rat model of infarct-like myocardial injury. *Cell J.* 2017;19(1):84–93.
7. Moon HK, Kang P, Lee HS, Min SS, Seol GH. Effects of 1,8-cineole on hypertension induced by chronic exposure to nicotine in rats. *J Pharm Pharmacol.* 2014;66(5):688–693.
8. Interaminense Lde F, de Siqueira RJ, Xavier FE, Duarte GP, Magalhães PJ, da Silva JK, Maia JG, Sousa PJ, Leal-Cardoso JH, Lahlou S. Cardiovascular effects of 1-nitro-2-phenylethane, the main constituent of the essential oil of *Aniba canelilla*, in spontaneously hypertensive rats. *Fundam Clin Pharmacol.* 2011;25(6):661–669.
9. Choisy S, Huchet-Cadiou C, Leoty C. Sarcoplasmic reticulum Ca(2+) release by 4-chloro-m-cresol (4-CmC) in intact and chemically skinned ferret cardiac ventricular fibers. *J Pharmacol Exp Ther.* 1999;290(2):578–586.
10. Suručić R, Kundaković T, Lakušić B, Drakul D, Milovanović SR, Kovačević N. Variations in chemical composition, vasorelaxant and angiotensin I-converting enzyme inhibitory activities of essential oil from aerial parts of seseli pallasii besser (apiaceae). *Chem Biodivers.* 2017;14(5):10.
11. da Cunha GH, de Moraes MO, Fechine FV, et al. Vasorelaxant and antihypertensive effects of methanolic fraction of the essential oil of *Alpinia zerumbet. Vasc Pharmacol.* 2013;58:337–345.
12. Pinto NV, Assreuy AM, Coelho-de-Souza AN, Ceccatto VM, Magalhães PJ, Lahlou S, Leal-Cardoso JH. Endothelium-dependent vasorelaxant effects of the essential oil from aerial parts of *Alpinia zerumbet* and its main constituent 1,8-cineole in rats. *Phytomedicine.* 2009;16(12):1151–1155.
13. da Cunha GH, de Moraes MO, Fechine FV, Frota Bezerra FA, Silveira ER, Canuto KM, de Moraes ME. Vasorelaxant and antihypertensive effects of methanolic fraction of the essential oil of *Alpinia zerumbet. Vascu Pharmacol.* 2013;58(5–6):337–345.
14. Lahlou S, Galindo CA, Leal-Cardoso JH, Fonteles MC, Duarte GP. Cardiovascular effects of the essential oil of *Alpinia zerumbet* leaves and its main constituent, Terpinen-4-ol, in rats: Role of the autonomic nervous system. *Planta Med.* 2002;68(12):1097–1102.
15. Lahlou S, Magalhães PJ, de Siqueira RJ, et al. Cardiovascular effects of the essential oil of *Aniba canelilla* bark in normotensive rats. *J Cardiovasc Pharmacol.* 2005;46(4):412–421.
16. Siqueira RJ, Rodrigues KMS, Silva MTB, et al. Linalool-rich rosewood oil induces vago-vagal bradycardic and depressor reflex in rats. *Phytother Res.* 2014;28:42–48.
17. Dib I, Fauconnier ML, Sindic M, Belmekki F, Assaidi A, Berrabah M, Mekhfi H, Aziz M, Legssyer A, Bnouham M, Ziyyat A. Chemical composition, vasorelaxant, antioxidant and antiplatelet effects of essential oil of *Artemisia campestris* L. from oriental morocco. *BMC Complement Altern Med.* 2017;17(1):82.
18. Razavi BM, Arasteh E, Imenshahidi M, Iranshahi M. Antihypertensive effect of auraptene, a monoterpene coumarin from the genus Citrus, upon chronic administration. *Iran J Basic Med Sci.* 2015;18(2):153–158.
19. You JH, Kang P, Min SS, Seol GH. Bergamot essential oil differentially modulates intracellular Ca^{2+} levels in vascular endothelial and smooth muscle cells: A new finding seen with fura-2. *J Cardiovasc Pharmacol.* 2013;61(4):324–328.
20. de Siqueira RJ, Freire WB, Vasconcelos-Silva AA, Fonseca-Magalhães PA, Lima FJ, Brito TS, Mourão LT, Ribeiro RA, Lahlou S, Magalhães PJ. In-vitro characterization of the pharmacological effects induced by (–)-α-bisabolol in rat smooth muscle preparations. *Can J Physiol Pharmacol.* 2012;90(1):23–35.
21. Silva-Filho JC, Oliveira NN, Arcanjo DD, Quintans-Júnior LJ, Cavalcanti SC, Santos MR, Oliveira Rde C, Oliveira AP. Investigation of mechanisms involved in (–)-borneol-induced vasorelaxant response on rat thoracic aorta. *Basic Clin Pharmacol Toxicol.* 2012;110(2):171–177.

22. Wu HY, Tang Y, Gao LY, Sun WX, Hua Y, Yang SB, Zhang ZP, Liao GY, Zhou QG, Luo CX, Zhu DY. The synergetic effect of edaravone and borneol in the rat model of ischemic stroke. *Eur J Pharmacol.* 2014;740:522–531.
23. Shabir H, Kundu S, Basir SF, Khan LA. Modulation of Pb(II) caused aortal constriction by eugenol and carvacrol. *Biol Trace Elem Res.* 2014;161(1):116–122.
24. Dantas BP, Alves QL, de Assis KS, Ribeiro TP, de Almeida MM, de Vasconcelos AP, de Araújo DA, de Andrade Braga V, de Medeiros IA, Alencar JL, Silva DF. Participation of the TRP channel in the cardiovascular effects induced by carvacrol in normotensive rat. *Vascul Pharmacol.* 2015;67–69:48–58.
25. Kundu S, Shabir H, Basir SF, Khan LA. Inhibition of As(III) and Hg(II) caused aortic hypercontraction by eugenol, linalool and carvone. *J Smooth Muscle Res.* 2014;50:93–102.
26. Raffai G, Kim B, Park S, Khang G, Lee D, Vanhoutte PM. Cinnamaldehyde and cinnamaldehyde-containing micelles induce relaxation of isolated porcine coronary arteries: Role of nitric oxide and calcium. *Int J Nanomed.* 2014;9:2557–2566.
27. Wang F, Pu C, Zhou P, Wang P, Liang D, Wang Q, Hu Y, Li B, Hao X. Cinnamaldehyde prevents endothelial dysfunction induced by high glucose by activating Nrf2. *Cell Physiol Biochem.* 2015;36(1):315–324.
28. Song F, Li H, Sun J, Wang S. Protective effects of cinnamic acid and cinnamic aldehyde on isoproterenol-induced acute myocardial ischemia in rats. *J Ethnopharmacol.* 2013;150(1):125–130.
29. Kang YH, Kang JS, Shin HM. Vasodilatory effects of cinnamic acid via the nitric oxide-cGMP-PKG pathway in rat thoracic aorta. *Phytother Res.* 2013;27(2):205–211.
30. Kang YH, Yang IJ, Morgan KG, Shin HM. Cinnamyl alcohol attenuates vasoconstriction by activation of K^+ channels via NO-cGMP-protein kinase G pathway and inhibition of Rho-kinase. *Exp Mol Med.* 2012;44(12):749–755.
31. Lu JX, Guo C, Ou WS, Jing Y, Niu HF, Song P, Li QZ, Liu Z, Xu J, Li P, Zhu ML, Yin YL. Citronellal prevents endothelial dysfunction and atherosclerosis in rats. *J Cell Biochem.* 2019;120(3):3790–3800.
32. Kang P, Suh SH, Min SS, Seol GH. The essential oil of *Citrus bergamia* Risso induces vasorelaxation of the mouse aorta by activating K(+) channels and inhibiting Ca(2+) influx. *J Pharm Pharmacol.* 2013;65(5):745–749.
33. Hasanzadeh F, Kashouk NM, Amini S, et al. The effect of cold application and lavender oil inhalation in cardiac surgery patients undergoing chest tube removal. *Excli J.* 2016;15:64–74.
34. Mehdizadeh R, Parizadeh MR, Khooei AR, Mehri S, Hosseinzadeh H. Cardioprotective effect of saffron extract and safranal in isoproterenol-induced myocardial infarction in wistar rats. *Iran J Basic Med Sci.* 2013;16(1):56–63.
35. Magalhães PJ, Lahlou S, Jucá DM, Coelho-de-Souza LN, da Frota PT, da Costa AM, Leal-Cardoso JH. Vasorelaxation induced by the essential oil of *Croton nepetaefolius* and its constituents in rat aorta are partially mediated by the endothelium. *Fundam Clin Pharmacol.* 2008;22(2):169–177.
36. Baccelli C, Martinsen A, Morel N, Quetin-Leclercq J. Vasorelaxant activity of essential oils from *Croton zambesicus* and some of their constituents. *Planta Med.* 2010;76(14):1506–1511.
37. de Siqueira RJ, Magalhães PJ, Leal-Cardoso JH, Duarte GP, Lahlou S. Cardiovascular effects of the essential oil of *Croton zehntneri* leaves and its main constituents, anethole and estragole, in normotensive conscious rats. *Life Sci.* 2006;78(20):2365–2372.
38. Singh V, Jain M, Misra A, et al. Curcuma oil ameliorates hyperlipidaemia and associated deleterious effects in golden *Syrian hamsters. Br J Nutr.* 2013;110:437–446.
39. Gayathri, K, Jayachandran, K, Vasanthi HR, Rajamanickam GV. Cardioprotective effect of lemon grass as evidenced by biochemical and histopathological changes in experimentally induced cardiotoxicity. *Hum Exp Toxicol.* 2011;30(8):1073–1082.
40. Bastos JF, Moreira IJ, Ribeiro TP, Medeiros IA, Antoniolli AR, De Sousa DP, Santos MR. Hypotensive and vasorelaxant effects of citronellol, a monoterpene alcohol, in rats. *Basic Clin Pharmacol Toxicol.* 2010;106(4):331–337.
41. Althurwi HN, Abdel-Kader MS, Alharthy KM, Salkini MA, Albaqami FF. Cymbopogon proximus essential oil protects rats against isoproterenol-induced cardiac hypertrophy and fibrosis. *Molecules.* 2020;25(8):1786.
42. Younis NS. D-Limonene mitigate myocardial injury in rats through MAPK/ERK/NF-κB pathway inhibition. *Korean J Physiol Pharmacol.* 2020;24(3):259–266.
43. Olivoto RR, Damiani CE, Kassouf Silva I, Lofrano-Alves MS, Oliveira MA, Fogaça RT. Effects of eugenol on resting tension of rat atria. *Braz J Med Biol Res.* 2014;47(4):328–333.
44. Lofrano-Alves MS, Oliveira EL, Damiani CE, Kassouf-Silva I, Fogaça RT. Eugenol-induced contractions of saponin-skinned fibers are inhibited by heparin or by a ryanodine receptor blocker. *Can J Physiol Pharmacol.* 2005;83(12):1093–1100.
45. Damiani CE, Moreira CM, Zhang HT, Creazzo TL, Vassallo DV. Effects of eugenol, an essential oil, on the mechanical and electrical activities of cardiac muscle. *J Cardiovasc Pharmacol* 2004;44:688–695.
46. Roberts RE, Allen S, Chang AP, Henderson H, Hobson GC, Karania B, Morgan KN, Pek AS, Raghvani K, Shee CY, Shikotra J, Street E, Abbas Z, Ellis K, Heer JK, Alexander SP. Distinct mechanisms of relaxation to bioactive components from chamomile species in porcine isolated blood vessels. *Toxicol Appl Pharmacol.* 2013;272(3):797–805.
47. Esmaeili H, Esmailidehaj M, Entezari Zarch S, Azizian H. Role of the potassium channels in vasorelaxant effect of asafoetida essential oil. *Avicenna J Phytomed.* 2020;10(4):407–416.
48. Tognolini M, Ballabeni V, Bertoni S, Bruni R, Impicciatore M, Barocelli E. Protective effect of *Foeniculum vulgare* essential oil and anethole in an experimental model of thrombosis. *Pharmacol Res.* 2007;56:254–260.
49. Bordia AK, Joshi HK, Sandya YK, Bhu N. Effect of essential oil of garlic on serum fibrinalytic activity in patients with coronary artery disease. *Atheroselerosis* 1977;28:379–386.
50. Bordia AK, Sodhya SK, Rathore AS, Bhu N. Essential oil of garlic on blood lipids and fibribolytic activity in patients with coronary artery disease. *J Assoc Phys India.* 1978;26:327–333.
51. Bordia AK, Sharma KD, Parmar VK, Varma SK. Protective effect of garlic oil on the changes produced by 3 weeks of fatty diet on serum cholesterol serum triglycerides, fibrimolyticacativity and platelet adhesiveness in man. *Indian Heart J.* 1982;34:86–88.

52. Yang C, Li L, Yang L, Lǚ H, Wang S, Sun G. Anti-obesity and hypolipidemic effects of garlic oil and onion oil in rats fed a high-fat diet. *Nutr Metab (London).* 2018;15:43.
53. Younis NS, Abduldaium MS, Mohamed ME. Protective effect of geraniol on oxidative, inflammatory and apoptotic alterations in isoproterenol-induced cardiotoxicity: Role of the Keapl/Nrf2/HO-1 and PI3K/Akt/mTOR pathways. *Antioxidants (Basel).* 2020;9(10):977.
54. Chen CJ, Kumar KJ, Chen YT, et al. Effect of hinoki and meniki essential oils on human autonomic nervous system activity and mood states. *Nat Prod Commun.* 2015;10(7):1305–1308.
55. Santos M, Carvalho A, Medeiros I, Alves P, Marchioro M, Antoniolli A. Cardiovascular effects of Hyptis fruticosa essential oil in rats. *Fitoterapia.* 2007;78:186–191.
56. Sadeghzadeh J, Vakili A, Bandegi AR, Sameni HR, Zahedi Khorasani M, Darabian M. Lavandula reduces heart injury via attenuating tumor necrosis factor-alpha and oxidative stress in a rat model of infarct-like myocardial injury. *Cell J.* 2017;19(1):84–93.
57. Nikolaevskiĭ VV, Kononova NS, Pertsovskiĭ AI, Shinkarchuk IF. Effect of essential oils on the course of experimental atherosclerosis. *Patol Fiziol Eksp Ter.* 1990;5:52–53.
58. Vakili A, Sharifat S, Akhavan MM, Bandegi AR. Effect of lavender oil (*Lavandula angustifolia*) on cerebral edema and its possible mechanisms in an experimental model of stroke. *Brain Res.* 2014;1548:56–62.
59. Shiina Y, Funabashi N, Lee K, Toyoda T, Sekine T, Honjo S, Hasegawa R, Kawata T, Wakatsuki Y, Hayashi S, Murakami S, Koike K, Daimon M, Komuro I. Relaxation effects of lavender aromatherapy improve coronary flow velocity reserve in healthy men evaluated by transthoracic Doppler echocardiography. *Int J Cardiol.* 2008;129(2):193–197.
60. Cho MY, Min ES, Hur MH, Lee MS. Effects of aromatherapy on the anxiety, vital signs, and sleep quality of percutaneous coronary intervention patients in intensive care units. *Evid Based Complement Alternat Med.* 2013;2013:381381.
61. Iokawa K, Kohzuki M, Sone T, Ebihara S. Effect of olfactory stimulation with essential oils on cardiovascular reactivity during the moving beans task in stroke patients with anxiety. *Complement Ther Med.* 2018;36:20–24.
62. Koto R, Imamura M, Watanabe C, Obayashi S, Shiraishi M, Sasaki Y, Azuma H. Linalyl acetate as a major ingredient of lavender essential oil relaxes the rabbit vascular smooth muscle through dephosphorylation of myosin light chain. *J Cardiovasc Pharmacol.* 2006;48(1):850–856.
63. Abdelhakim AM, Hussein AS, Doheim MF, Sayed AK. The effect of inhalation aromatherapy in patients undergoing cardiac surgery: A systematic review and meta-analysis of randomized controlled trials. *Complement Ther Med.* 2020;48:102256.
64. Rambod M, Rakhshan M, Tohidinik S, Nikoo MH. The effect of lemon inhalation aromatherapy on blood pressure, electrocardiogram changes, and anxiety in acute myocardial infarction patients: A clinical, multi-centered, assessor-blinded trial design. *Complement Ther Clin Pract.* 2020;39:101155.
65. de Siqueira RJ, Rodrigues KM, da Silva MT, Correia Junior CA, Duarte GP, Magalhães PJ, dos Santos AA, Maia JG, da Cunha PJ, Lahlou S. Linalool-rich rosewood oil induces vago-vagal bradycardic and depressor reflex in rats. *Phytother Res.* 2014;28(1):42–48.
66. Akrami A, Nikaein F, Babajafari S, Faghih S, Yarmohammadi H. Comparison of the effects of flaxseed oil and sunflower seed oil consumption on serum glucose, lipid profile, blood pressure, and lipid peroxidation in patients with metabolic syndrome. *J Clin Lipidol.* 2018;12:70–77.
67. Montero-Villegas S, Polo M, Galle M, et al. Inhibition of mevalonate pathway and synthesis of the storage lipids in human liver-derived and non-liver cell lines by *Lippia alba* essential oils. *Lipids.* 2017;52:37–49.
68. Maynard LG, Santos KC, Cunha PS, Barreto AS, Peixoto MG, Arrigoni-Blank F, Blank AF, Alves PB, Bonjardin LR, Santos MR. Chemical composition and vasorelaxant effect induced by the essential oil of *Lippia alba* (Mill.) N.E. Brown. (Verbenaceae) in rat mesenteric artery. *Indian J Pharmacol.* 2011;43(6):694–698.
69. da Silva RER, de Morais LP, Silva AA, Bastos CMS, Pereira-Gonçalves Á, Kerntopf MR, Menezes IRA, Leal-Cardoso JH, Barbosa R. Vasorelaxant effect of the *Lippia alba* essential oil and its major constituent, citral, on the contractility of isolated rat aorta. *Biomed Pharmacother.* 2018;108:792–798.
70. Lahlou S, Magalhães PJC, Carneiro-Leão RFL, Leal-Cardoso JH. Involvement of nitric oxide in the mediation of the hypotensive action of the essential oil of *Mentha×villosa* in normotensive conscious rats. *Planta Medica.* 2002;68:694–699.
71. Guedes DN, Silva DF, Barbosa-Filho JM, de Medeiros IA. Endothelium-dependent hypotensive and vasorelaxant effects of the essential oil from aerial parts of *Mentha×villosa* in rats. *Phytomedicine.* 2004;11(6):490–497.
72. Cheang WS, Lam MY, Wong WT, Tian XY, Lau CW, Zhu Z, Yao X, Huang Y. Menthol relaxes rat aortae, mesenteric and coronary arteries by inhibiting calcium influx. *Eur J Pharmacol.* 2013;702(1–3):79–84.
73. Maiwulanjiang M, Bi CW, Lee PS, et al. The volatile oil of nardostachyos radix et Rhizoma induces endothelial nitric oxide synthase activity in HUVEC cells. *PLoS One.* 2015;10:e0116761.
74. Yeh JC, Cindrova-Davies T, Belleri M, Morbidelli L, Miller N, Cho CW, Chan K, Wang YT, Luo GA, Ziche M, Presta M, Charnock-Jones DS, Fan TP. The natural compound n-butylidenephthalide derived from the volatile oil of Radix Angelica sinensis inhibits angiogenesis in vitro and in vivo. *Angiogenesis.* 2011;14(2):187–197.
75. Gilani AH, Shah AJ, Zubair A, Khalid S, Kiani J, Ahmed A, Rasheed M, Ahmad VU. Chemical composition and mechanisms underlying the spasmolytic and bronchodilatory properties of the essential oil of *Nepeta cataria* L. *J Ethnopharmacol.* 2009;121(3):405–411.
76. Ahmad S, Beg ZH. Elucidation of mechanisms of actions of thymoquinone-enriched methanolic and volatile oil extracts from *Nigella sativa* against cardiovascular risk parameters in experimental hyperlipidemia. *Lipids Health Dis.* 2013;12:86.
77. Lahlou S, Interaminense Lde F, Leal-Cardoso JH, Morais SM, Duarte GP. Cardiovascular effects of the essential oil of *Ocimum gratissimum* leaves in rats: Role of the autonomic nervous system. *Clin Exp Pharmacol Physiol.* 2004;31(4):219–225.
78. Interaminense LFL, Jucá DM, Magalhães PJC, Leal-Cardoso JH, Duarte GP, Lahlou S. Pharmacological evidence of calcium-channel blockade by essential oil of

Ocimum gratissimum and its main constituent, eugenol, in isolated aortic rings from DOCA-salt hypertensive rats. *Fundam Clin Pharmacol.* 2007;21:497–506.
79. Interaminense LFL, Leal-Cardoso JH, Magalhaes PJ, Duarte GP, Lahlou S. Enhanced hypotensive effects of the essential oil of *Ocimum gratissimum* leaves and its main constituent, eugenol, on DOCA-Salt hypertensive conscious rats. *Planta Med.* 2005;71:376–378.
80. Vasconcelos-Silva AA, Lima FJ, Brito TS, Lahlou S, Magalhães PJ. Vasorelaxation induced by methyl cinnamate, the major constituent of the essential oil of *Ocimum micranthum*, in rat isolated aorta. *Clin Exp Pharmacol Physiol.* 2014;41(10):755–762.
81. Ballabeni V, Tognolini M, Bertoni S, et al. Antiplatelet and antithrombotic activities of essential oil from wild *Ocotea quixos* (Lam.) Kosterm.(Lauraceae) calices from Amazonian Ecuador. *Pharmacol Res.* 2007;55:23–30.
82. De La Cruz J, Martin-Romero M, Carmona J, Villalobos M, De La Cuesta FS. Effect of evening primrose oil on platelet aggregation in rabbits fed an atherogenic diet. *Thrombosis Res.* 1997;87:141–149.
83. Moreno-Luna R, Muñoz-Hernandez R, Miranda ML, et al. Olive oil polyphenols decrease blood pressure and improve endothelial function in young women with mild hypertension. *Am J Hypertens.* 2012;25:1299–1304.
84. Cota DL, Rasal VP, Mishra S, Shengule S. Cardioprotective effect of oregano oil against doxorubicin-induced myocardial infarction in rats. *Phcog Mag.* 2018;14:363–368.
85. Pereira SL, Marques AM, Sudo RT, Kaplan MA, Zapata-Sudo G. Vasodilator activity of the essential oil from aerial parts of Pectis brevipedunculata and its main constituent citral in rat aorta. *Molecules.* 2013;18(3):3072–3085.
86. Kim JH, Lee HJ, Jeong SJ, Lee MH, Kim SH. Essential oil of *Pinus koraiensis* leaves exerts antihyperlipidemic effects via up-regulation of low-density lipoprotein receptor and inhibition of acyl-coenzyme A: Cholesterol acyltransferase. *Phytother Res.* 2012;26:1314–1319.
87. Shiva Kumar A, Jeyaprakash K, Chellappan DR, Murugan R. Vasorelaxant and cardiovascular properties of the essential oil of *Pogostemon elsholtzioides. J Ethnopharmacol.* 2017;199:86–90.
88. Rasheed HM, Khan T, Wahid F, Khan R, Shah AJ. Chemical composition and vascular and intestinal smooth muscle relaxant effects of the essential oil from *Psidium guajava* fruit. *Pharm Biol.* 2016;54(11):2679–2684.
89. Sivakumar L, Chellappan DR, Sriramavaratharajan V, Murugan R. Root essential oil of *Chrysopogon zizanioides* relaxes rat isolated thoracic aorta: An ex vivo approach. *Z Naturforsch C J Biosci.* 2020;76(3–4):161–168.
90. Rasheed HM, Khan T, Wahid F, Khan R, Shah AJ. Chemical composition and vasorelaxant and antispasmodic effects of essential oil from *Rosa indica* L. petals. *Evidence Based Complementary Altern Med.* 2015;2015:9.
91. Silva DF, Araújo IG, Albuquerque JG, Porto DL, Dias KL, Cavalcante KV, Veras RC, Nunes XP, Barbosa-Filho JM, Araújo DA, Cruz JS, Correia NA, De Medeiros IA. Rotundifolone-induced relaxation is mediated by BK(Ca) channel activation and Ca(v) channel inactivation. *Basic Clin Pharmacol Toxicol.* 2011;109(6):465–475.
92. Jeong J-W, Kim JW, Ku SK, et al. Essential oils purified from Schisandrae semen inhibits tumor necrosis factor-α-induced matrix metalloproteinase-9 activation and migration of human aortic smooth muscle cells. *BMC Complementary Alternat Med.* 2015;15:7.
93. Yan Y, Wuliji O, Zhao X, et al. Effect of essential oil of Syringa pinnatifolia Hemsl. var. Alashanensis on ischemia of myocardium, hypoxia and platelet aggregation. *J Ethnopharmacol.* 2010;131:248–255.
94. Al-Okbi SY, Mohamed DA, Hamed TE, Edris AE. Protective effect of clove oil and eugenol microemulsions on fatty liver and dyslipidemia as components of metabolic syndrome. *J Med Food.* 2014;17:764–771.
95. Peixoto-Neves D, Silva-Alves KS, Gomes MD, Lima FC, Lahlou S, Magalhães PJ, Ceccatto VM, Coelho-de-Souza AN, Leal-Cardoso JH. Vasorelaxant effects of the monoterpenic phenol isomers, carvacrol and thymol, on rat isolated aorta. *Fundam Clin Pharmacol.* 2010;24(3):341–350.
96. Aydin MS, Kocarslan A, Kocarslan S, Kucuk A, Eser İ, Sezen H, Buyukfirat E, Hazar A. Thymoquinone protects end organs from abdominal aorta ischemia/reperfusion injury in a rat model. *Rev Bras Cir Cardiovasc.* 2015;30(1):77–83.
97. Sargazi Zadeh G, Panahi N. Endothelium-independent vasorelaxant activity of *Trachyspermum ammi* essential oil on rat aorta. *Clin Exp Hypertens.* 2017;39(2):133–138.
98. Jung DJ, Cha JY, Kim SE, Ko IG, Jee YS. Effects of Ylang-Ylang aroma on blood pressure and heart rate in healthy men. *J Exerc Rehabil.* 2013;9(2):250–255.
99. Sabino CK, Ferreira-Filho ES, Mendes MB, et al. Cardiovascular effects induced by α-terpineol in hypertensive rats. *Flavour Fragr J.* 2013;28:333–339.
100. Younis NS, Mohamed ME. β-caryophyllene as a potential protective agent against myocardial injury: The role of toll-like receptors. *Molecules.* 2019;24(10):1929.
101. Han C, Qi J, Gao S, Li C, Ma Y, Wang J, Bai Y, Zheng X. Vasodilation effect of volatile oil from *Allium macrostemon* Bunge are mediated by PKA/NO pathway and its constituent dimethyl disulfide in isolated rat pulmonary arterials. *Fitoterapia.* 2017;120:52–57.
102. Alves-Santos TR, de Siqueira RJ, Duarte GP, Lahlou S. Cardiovascular effects of the essential oil of *Croton argyrophylloides* in normotensive rats: Role of the autonomic nervous system. *Evid Based Complement Alternat Med.* 2016;2016:4106502.
103. Esmaeili H, Sharifi M, Esmailidehaj M, Rezvani ME, Hafizibarjin Z. Vasodilatory effect of asafoetida essential oil on rat aorta rings: The role of nitric oxide, prostacyclin, and calcium channels. *Phytomedicine.* 2017;36:88–94.
104. Kang P, Ryu KH, Lee JM, Kim HK, Seol GH. Endothelium- and smooth muscle-dependent vasodilator effects of *Citrus aurantium* L. var. amara: Focus on Ca(2+) modulation. *Biomed Pharmacother.* 2016;82:467–471.
105. de Menezes IA, Moreira IJ, de Paula JW, Blank AF, Antoniolli AR, Quintans-Júnior LJ, Santos MR. Cardiovascular effects induced by *Cymbopogon winterianus* essential oil in rats: involvement of calcium channels and vagal pathway. *J Pharm Pharmacol.* 2010;62(2):215–221.
106. Pires AF, Madeira SV, Soares PM, Montenegro CM, Souza EP, Resende AC, Soares de Moura R, Assreuy AM, Criddle DN. The role of endothelium in the vasorelaxant effects

of the essential oil of *Ocimum gratissimum* in aorta and mesenteric vascular bed of rats. *Can J Physiol Pharmacol.* 2012;90(10):1380–1385.
107. Cherkaoui-Tangi K, Israili ZH, Lyoussi B. Vasorelaxant effect of essential oil isolated from *Nigella sativa* L. seeds in rat aorta: Proposed mechanism. *Pak J Pharm Sci.* 2016;29(1):1–8.
108. Mobin M, de Lima SG, Almeida LTG, Silva Filho JC, Rocha MS, Oliveira AP, Mendes MB, Carvalho FAA, Melhem MSC, Costa JGM. Gas chromatography-triple quadrupole mass spectrometry analysis and vasorelaxant effect of essential oil from *Protium heptaphyllum* (Aubl.) *March. Biomed Res Int.* 2017;2017:1928171.
109. Shirole RL, Shirole NL, Saraf MN. In vitro relaxant and spasmolytic effects of essential oil of *Pistacia integerrima* Stewart ex Brandis Galls. *J Ethnopharmacol.* 2015;168:61–65.
110. Boskabady MH, Kiani S, Rakhshandah H. Relaxant effects of Rosa damascena on guinea pig tracheal chains and its possible mechanism(s). *J Ethnopharmacol.* 2006;106(3):377–382.
111. Mnafgui K, Derbali A, Sayadi S, Gharsallah N, Elfeki A, Allouche N. Anti-obesity and cardioprotective effects of cinnamic acid in high fat diet- induced obese rats. *J Food Sci Technol.* 2015;52(7):4369–4377.
112. Testai L, Chericoni S, Martelli A, Flamini G, Breschi MC, Calderone V. Voltage-operated potassium (Kv) channels contribute to endothelium-dependent vasorelaxation of carvacrol on rat aorta. *J Pharm Pharmacol.* 2016;68(9):1177–1183.
113. Santos SE, Ribeiro FPRA, Menezes PMN, Duarte-Filho LAM, Quintans JSS, Quintans-Junior LJ, Silva FS, Ribeiro LAA. New insights on relaxant effects of (–)-borneol monoterpene in rat aortic rings. *Fundam Clin Pharmacol.* 2019;33(2):148–158.
114. Peixoto-Neves D, Leal-Cardoso JH, Jaggar JH. Eugenol dilates rat cerebral arteries by inhibiting smooth muscle cell voltage-dependent calcium channels. *J Cardiovasc Pharmacol.* 2014;64(5):401–406.
115. Damiani CE, Rossoni LV, Vassallo DV. Vasorelaxant effects of eugenol on rat thoracic aorta. *Vascul Pharmacol.* 2003;40(1):59–66.
116. Peixoto-Neves D, Wang Q, Leal-Cardoso JH, Rossoni LV, Jaggar JH. Eugenol dilates mesenteric arteries and reduces systemic BP by activating endothelial cell TRPV4 channels. *Br J Pharmacol.* 2015;172(14):3484–3494.
117. Choudhary R, Mishra KP, Subramanyam C. Prevention of isoproterenol-induced cardiac hypertrophy by eugenol, an antioxidant. *Indian J Clin Biochem.* 2006;21(2):107–113.
118. Nangle MR, Gibson TM, Cotter MA, Cameron NE. Effects of eugenol on nerve and vascular dysfunction in streptozotocin-diabetic rats. *Planta Med.* 2006;72(6):494–500.
119. Harb AA, Bustanji YK, Almasri IM, Abdalla SS. Eugenol reduces LDL cholesterol and hepatic steatosis in hypercholesterolemic rats by modulating TRPV1 receptor. *Sci Rep.* 2019;9(1):14003.
120. Lahlou S, Interaminense LF, Magalhães PJ, Leal-Cardoso JH, Duarte GP. Cardiovascular effects of eugenol, a phenolic compound present in many plant essential oils, in normotensive rats. *J Cardiovasc Pharmacol.* 2004;43(2):250–257.
121. de Siqueira RJ, Macedo FI, Interaminense Lde F, Duarte GP, Magalhães PJ, Brito TS, da Silva JK, Maia JG, Sousa PJ, Leal-Cardoso JH, Lahlou S. 1-Nitro-2-phenylethane, the main constituent of the essential oil of *Aniba canelilla*, elicits a vago-vagal bradycardiac and depressor reflex in normotensive rats. *Eur J Pharmacol.* 2010;638(1–3):90–98.
122. Brito TS, Lima FJ, Aragão KS, de Siqueira RJ, Sousa PJ, Maia JG, Filho JD, Lahlou S, Magalhães PJ. The vasorelaxant effects of 1-nitro-2-phenylethane involve stimulation of the soluble guanylate cyclase-cGMP pathway. *Biochem Pharmacol.* 2013;85(6):780–788.
123. Interaminense LF, dos Ramos-Alves FE, de Siqueira RJ, Xavier FE, Duarte GP, Magalhães PJ, Maia JG, Sousa PJ, Lahlou S. Vasorelaxant effects of 1-nitro-2-phenylethane, the main constituent of the essential oil of *Aniba canelilla*, in superior mesenteric arteries from spontaneously hypertensive rats. *Eur J Pharm Sci.* 2013;48(4–5):709–716.
124. Imenshahidi M, Eghbal M, Sahebkar A, Iranshahi M. Hypotensive activity of auraptene, a monoterpene coumarin from Citrus spp. *Pharm Biol.* 2013;51(5):545–549.
125. Mahmoud AM, Hernández Bautista RJ, Sandhu MA, Hussein OE. Beneficial effects of citrus flavonoids on cardiovascular and metabolic health. *Oxid Med Cell Longev.* 2019;2019:5484138.
126. Safaeian L, Sajjadi SE, Montazeri H, Ohadi F, Javanmard S. Citral protects human endothelial cells against hydrogen peroxide-induced oxidative stress. *Turk J Pharm Sci.* 2020;17(5):549–554.
127. Nascimento GAD, Souza DS, Lima BS, Vasconcelos CML, Araújo AAS, Durço AO, Quintans-Junior LJ, Almeida JRGDS, Oliveira AP, Santana-Filho VJ, Barreto AS, Santos MRVD. Bradycardic and antiarrhythmic effects of the D-limonene in rats. *Arq Bras Cardiol.* 2019;113(5):925–932.
128. Kang P, Seol GH. Linalool elicits vasorelaxation of mouse aortae through activation of guanylyl cyclase and K(+) channels. *J Pharm Pharmacol.* 2015;67(5):714–719.
129. Anjos PJ, Lima AO, Cunha PS, De Sousa DP, Onofre AS, Ribeiro TP, Medeiros IA, Antoniolli AR, Quintans-Júnior LJ, Santosa MR. Cardiovascular effects induced by linalool in normotensive and hypertensive rats. *Z Naturforsch C J Biosci.* 2013;68(5–6):181–190.
130. Shin YK, Hsieh YS, Kwon S, Lee HS, Seol GH. Linalyl acetate restores endothelial dysfunction and hemodynamic alterations in diabetic rats exposed to chronic immobilization stress. *J Appl Physiol.* 2018;124(5):1274–1283.
131. Kwon S, Hsieh YS, Shin YK, Kang P, Seol GH. Linalyl acetate prevents olmesartan-induced intestinal hypermotility mediated by interference of the sympathetic inhibitory pathway in hypertensive rat. *Biomed Pharmacother.* 2018;102:362–368.
132. Hsieh YS, Kwon S, Lee HS, Seol GH. Linalyl acetate prevents hypertension-related ischemic injury. *PLoS One.* 2018;13(5):e0198082.
133. Kim JR, Kang P, Lee HS, Kim KY, Seol GH. Cardiovascular effects of linalyl acetate in acute nicotine exposure. *Environ Health Prev Med.* 2017;22(1):42.
134. Hsieh YS, Shin YK, Han AY, Kwon S, Seol GH. Linalyl acetate prevents three related factors of vascular damage in COPD-like and hypertensive rats. *Life Sci.* 2019;232:116608.

135. Craighead DH, Alexander LM. Menthol-induced cutaneous vasodilation is preserved in essential hypertensive men and women. *Am J Hypertens.* 2017;30(12):1156–1162.
136. Silva H. Current knowledge on the vascular effects of menthol published correction appears. *Front Physiol.* 2020;11:298.
137. Yang HH, Xu YX, Chen JY, et al. N-butylidenephthalide inhibits the phenotypic switch of VSMCs through activation of AMPK and prevents stenosis in an arteriovenous fistula rat model. *Int J Mol Sci.* 2020;21:7403.
138. Chan SS, Choi AO, Jones RL, Lin G. Mechanisms underlying the vasorelaxing effects of butylidenephthalide, an active constituent of *Ligusticum chuanxiong*, in rat isolated aorta. *Eur J Pharmacol.* 2006;537(1–3):111–117.
139. Ribeiro TP, Porto DL, Menezes CP, Antunes AA, Silva DF, De Sousa DP, Nakao LS, Braga VA, Medeiros IA. Unravelling the cardiovascular effects induced by alpha-terpineol: A role for the nitric oxide-cGMP pathway. *Clin Exp Pharmacol Physiol.* 2010;37(8):811–816.
140. de Carvalho EF, Gadelha KKL, de Oliveira DMN, Lima-Silva K, Batista-Lima FJ, de Brito TS, Paula SM, da Silva MTB, Dos Santos AA, Magalhães PJC. Neryl butyrate induces contractile effects on isolated preparations of rat aorta. *Naunyn Schmiedebergs Arch Pharmacol.* 2020;393(1):43–55.
141. Chung MJ, Kang AY, Park SO, Park KW, Jun HJ, Lee SJ. The effect of essential oils of dietary wormwood (Artemisia princeps), with and without added vitamin E, on oxidative stress and some genes involved in cholesterol metabolism. *Food Chem Toxicol.* 2007;45(8):1400–1409. doi:10.1016/j.fct.2007.01.021.
142. Hamden K, Keskes H, Belhaj S, Mnafgui K, Feki A, Allouche N. Inhibitory potential of omega-3 fatty and fenugreek essential oil on key enzymes of carbohydrate-digestion and hypertension in diabetes rats. *Lipids Health Dis.* 2011;10:226.
143. Amini M, Fallah Huseini H, Mohtashami R, Sadeqhi Z, Ghamarchehre M. Hypolipidemic effects of *Nigella sativa* L. seeds oil in healthy volunteers: A randomized, double-blind, placebo-controlled clinical trial. *J Med Plants.* 2011;10(40):133–138.
144. Asgary S, Sahebkar A, Goli-Malekabadi N. Ameliorative effects of *Nigella sativa* on dyslipidemia. *J Endocrinol Invest.* 2015;38(10):1039–1046.
145. Al-Naqeep G, Al-Zubairi AS, Ismail M, Amom ZH, Esa NM. Antiatherogenic potential of *Nigella sativa* seeds and oil in diet-induced hypercholesterolemia in rabbits. *Evid Based Complement Alternat Med.* 2011;2011:213628.
146. Lin LY, Chuang CH, Chen HC, Yang KM. Lime (*Citrus aurantifolia* (Christm.) Swingle) essential oils: Volatile compounds, antioxidant capacity, and hypolipidemic effect. *Foods.* 2019;8(9):398.
147. Bhatia S. Bioinformatics. In: *Introduction to Pharmaceutical Biotechnology, Enzymes, Proteins and Bioinformatics.* IOP Publishing Ltd, Bristol, UK, 2018;2:1–16.
148. Bhatia S. Protein and enzyme engineering. In: *Introduction to Pharmaceutical Biotechnology, Enzymes, Proteins and Bioinformatics.* IOP Publishing Ltd, Bristol, UK, 2018;3:1–15.
149. Bhatia S. Introduction to genomics. In: *Introduction to Pharmaceutical Biotechnology, Enzymes, Proteins and Bioinformatics.* IOP Publishing Ltd, Bristol, UK, 2018;3:1–39.
150. Bhatia S. Characterization of cultured cells. In: *Introduction to Pharmaceutical Biotechnology: Animal Tissue Culture and Biopharmaceuticals.* IOP Publishing Ltd, Bristol, UK, 2019;3:1–47.
151. Bhatia S. Industrial enzymes and their applications. In: *Introduction to Pharmaceutical Biotechnology, Enzymes, Proteins and Bioinformatics.* IOP Publishing Ltd, Bristol, UK, 2018;3:1–21.
152. Bhatia S. Introduction to enzymes and their applications. In: *Introduction to Pharmaceutical Biotechnology, Enzymes, Proteins and Bioinformatics.* IOP Publishing Ltd, Bristol, UK, 2018;3:1–29.
153. Bhatia S. Biotransformation and enzymes. In: *Introduction to Pharmaceutical Biotechnology, Enzymes, Proteins and Bioinformatics.* IOP Publishing Ltd, Bristol, UK, 2018;3:1–13.
154. Bhatia S. Transgenic animals in biotechnology. In: *Introduction to Pharmaceutical Biotechnology, Volume 1: Basic Techniques and Concepts.* IOP Publishing Ltd, Bristol, UK, 2018;3:1–67.
155. Bhatia S. Applications of stem cells in disease and gene therapy. In: *Introduction to Pharmaceutical Biotechnology, Volume 1: Basic Techniques and Concepts.* IOP Publishing Ltd, Bristol, UK, 2018;3:1–40.
156. Bhatia S. Introduction to genetic engineering. In: *Introduction to Pharmaceutical Biotechnology, Volume 1: Basic Techniques and Concepts.* IOP Publishing Ltd, Bristol, UK, 2018;3:1–63.
157. Bhatia S. Modern DNA science and its applications. In: *Introduction to Pharmaceutical Biotechnology, Volume 1: Basic Techniques and Concepts.* IOP Publishing Ltd, Bristol, UK, 2018;3:1–70.
158. Bhatia S. Animal tissue culture facilities. In: *Introduction to Pharmaceutical Biotechnology: Animal Tissue Culture and Biopharmaceuticals.* IOP Publishing Ltd, Bristol, UK, 2019;3:1–32.
159. Bhatia S. Culture media for animal cells. In: *Introduction to Pharmaceutical Biotechnology: Animal Tissue Culture and Biopharmaceuticals.* IOP Publishing Ltd, Bristol, UK, 2019;3:1–33.
160. Bhatia S. Stem cell culture. In: *Introduction to Pharmaceutical Biotechnology: Animal Tissue Culture and Biopharmaceuticals.* IOP Publishing Ltd, Bristol, UK, 2019;3:1–24.
161. Bhatia S. Organ culture. In: *Introduction to Pharmaceutical Biotechnology: Introduction to Animal Tissue Culture Science.* IOP Publishing Ltd, Bristol, UK, 2019;3:1–28.
162. Kewal K. *Jain Applications of Biotechnology in Cardiovascular Therapeutics.* Humana Press, Bristol, UK, 2011.
163. Dishart KL, Work LM, Denby L, Baker AH. Gene therapy for cardiovascular disease. *J Biomed Biotechnol.* 2003;2003(2):138–148.
164. Sun R, Li X, Liu M, Zeng Y, Chen S, Zhang P. Advances in stem cell therapy for cardiovascular disease (review). *Int J Mol Med.* 2016;38(1):23–29.
165. Bhatia S. Application of plant biotechnology. In: *Modern Applications of Plant Biotechnology in Pharmaceutical Sciences.* Academic Press, Cambridge, MA; 2015:157–207.
166. Bhatia S. Somatic embryogenesis and organogenesis. In: *Modern Applications of Plant Biotechnology in Pharmaceutical Sciences.* Academic Press, Cambridge, MA; 2015:209–230.

167. Bhatia S. Classical and nonclassical techniques for secondary metabolite production in plant cell culture. In: *Modern Applications of Plant Biotechnology in Pharmaceutical Sciences*. Academic Press, Cambridge, MA; 2015 :231–291.
168. Bhatia S. Plant-based biotechnological products with their production host, modes of delivery systems, and stability testing. In: *Modern Applications of Plant Biotechnology in Pharmaceutical Sciences*. Academic Press, Cambridge, MA; 2015:293–331.
169. Bhatia S. Edible vaccines. In: *Modern Applications of Plant Biotechnology in Pharmaceutical Sciences*. Academic Press, Cambridge, MA; 2015:333–343.
170. Bhatia S. Microenvironmentation in micropropagation. In: *Modern Applications of Plant Biotechnology in Pharmaceutical Sciences*. Academic Press, Cambridge, MA; 2015:345–360.
171. Bhatia S. Micropropagation. In: *Modern Applications of Plant Biotechnology in Pharmaceutical Sciences*. Academic Press, Cambridge, MA; 2015:361–368.
172. Bhatia S. Laws in plant biotechnology. In: *Modern Applications of Plant Biotechnology in Pharmaceutical Sciences*. Academic Press, Cambridge, MA; 2015: 369–391.
173. Bhatia S. Technical glitches in micropropagation. In: *Modern Applications of Plant Biotechnology in Pharmaceutical Sciences*. Academic Press, Cambridge, MA; 2015:393–404.
174. Bhatia S. Plant tissue culture-based industries. In: *Modern Applications of Plant Biotechnology in Pharmaceutical Sciences*. Academic Press, Cambridge, MA; 2015: 405–417.
175. Bhatia S, Al-Harrasi A, Behl T, Anwer MK, Ahmed MM, Mittal V, Kaushik D, Chigurupati S, Kabir MT, Sharma PB, Chaugule B, Vargas-de-la-Cruz C. Anti-migraine activity of freeze dried-latex obtained from *Calotropis Gigantea* Linn. *Environ Sci Pollut Res Int*. 2021.
176. Al-Harrasi A, Bhatia S. Toxicity associated with essential oils. In: *Role of Essential Oils in the Management of Covid-19*. CRC Press, Boca Raton, FL; 2022:375–385.
177. Bhatia S. Development of broad spectrum mycosporine loaded sunscreen formulation from Ulva fasciata delile. *Biomedicine (Taipei)*. 2019;9(3):17.
178. Bhatia S. In vitro antioxidant and antinociceptive properties of *Porphyra vietnamensis*. *Biomedicine (Taipei)*. 2019;9(1):3.
179. Bhatia S, Sharma K, Nagpal K, Bera T. Investigation of the factors influencing the molecular weight of porphyran and its associated antifungal activity bioact. *Carb Diet Fiber*. 2015;5:153–168.
180. Bhatia S, Al-Harrasi A, Behl T, Anwer MK, Ahmed MM, Mittal V, Kaushik D, Chigurupati S, Kabir MT, Sharma PB, Chaugule B, Vargas-de-la-Cruz C. Unravelling the photoprotective effects of freshwater alga Nostoc commune Vaucher ex Bornet et Flahault against ultraviolet radiations. *Environ Sci Pollut Res Int*. 2021. doi:10.1007/s11356-021-16704-2.
181. Bhatia S, Sharma K, Sharma A, Nagpal K, Bera T. Anti-inflammatory, analgesic and antiulcer properties of Porphyra vietnamensis. *Avicenna J Phytomed*. 2015;5(1):69–77.
182. Bhatia S, Kumar V, Sharma K, Nagpal K, Bera T. Significance of algal polymer in designing amphotericin B nanoparticles. *Sci World J*. 2014;2014:564573.
183. Bhatia S, Rathee P, Sharma K, Chaugule BB, Kar N, Bera T. Immuno-modulation effect of sulphated polysaccharide (porphyran) from Porphyra vietnamensis. *Int J Biol Macromol*. 2013;57:50–56.
184. Bhatia S, Garg A, Sharma K, Kumar S, Sharma A, Purohit AP. Mycosporine and mycosporine-like amino acids: A paramount tool against ultra violet irradiation. *Pharmacogn Rev*. 2011;5(10):138–146.
185. Bhatia S, Sharma K, Namdeo AG, Chaugule BB, Kavale M, Nanda S. Broad-spectrum sun-protective action of Porphyra-334 derived from Porphyra vietnamensis. *Pharmacognosy Res*. 2010;2(1):45–49.
186. Bhatia S, Sharma K, Dahiya R, Bera T. *Modern Applications of Plant Biotechnology in Pharmaceutical Sciences*. Academic Press, Elsevier, Cambridge, MA; 2015:164–174.
187. Bhatia S. *Nanotechnology in Drug Delivery: Fundamentals, Design, and Applications*. CRC Press, Boca Raton, FL; 2016:121–127.
188. Bhatia S, Goli D. *Leishmaniasis: Biology, Control and New Approaches for Its Treatment*. CRC Press, Boca Raton, FL; 2016:164–173.
189. Bhatia S. *Natural Polymer Drug Delivery Systems: Nanoparticles, Plants, and Algae*. Springer Nature, Basingstoke, UK; 2016:117–127.
190. Bhatia S. *Natural Polymer Drug Delivery Systems: Nanotechnology and Its Drug Delivery Applications*. Springer International Publishing, Switzerland; 2016:1–32.
191. Bhatia S. *Natural Polymer Drug Delivery Systems: Nanoparticles Types, Classification, Characterization, Fabrication Methods and Drug Delivery Applications*. Springer International Publishing, Switzerland; 2016:33–93.
192. Bhatia S. *Natural Polymer Drug Delivery Systems: Natural Polymers vs Synthetic Polymer*. Springer International Publishing, Switzerland; 2016:95–118.
193. Bhatia S. *Natural Polymer Drug Delivery Systems: Plant Derived Polymers, Properties, and Modification & Applications*. Springer International Publishing, Switzerland; 2016:119–184.
194. Bhatia S. *Natural Polymer Drug Delivery Systems: Marine Polysaccharides Based Nano-Materials and Its Applications*. Springer International Publishing, Switzerland; 2016:185–225.
195. Bhatia S. *Systems for Drug Delivery: Mammalian Polysaccharides and Its Nanomaterials*. Springer International Publishing, Switzerland; 2016:1–27.
196. Bhatia S. *Systems for Drug Delivery: Microbial Polysaccharides as Advance Nanomaterials*. Springer International Publishing, Switzerland; 2016:29–54.
197. Bhatia S. *Systems for Drug Delivery: Chitosan Based Nanomaterials and Its Applications*. Springer International Publishing, Switzerland; 2016:55–117.
198. Bhatia S. *Systems for Drug Delivery: Advance Polymers and Its Applications*. Springer International Publishing, Switzerland; 2016:119–146.
199. Bhatia S. *Systems for Drug Delivery: Advanced Application of Natural Polysaccharides*. Springer International Publishing, Switzerland; 2016:147–170.

200. Bhatia S. *Systems for Drug Delivery: Modern Polysaccharides and Its Current Advancements*. Springer International Publishing, Switzerland; 2016:171–188.
201. Bhatia S. *Systems for Drug Delivery: Toxicity of Nanodrug Delivery Systems*. Springer International Publishing, Switzerland; 2016:189–197.
202. Bhatia S, Sharma K, Bera T. Structural characterization and pharmaceutical properties of porphyran. *Asian J Pharm*. 2015;9:93–101.
203. Bhatia S, Sharma A, Sharma K, Kavale M, Chaugule BB, Dhalwal K, Namdeo AG, Mahadik KR. Novel algal polysaccharides from marine source: Porphyran. *Pharmacogn Rev*. 2008;4:271–276.
204. Bhatia S. *Nanotechnology in Drug Delivery Fundamentals, Design, and Applications: Part 1: Protein and Peptide-Based Drug Delivery Systems*. Apple Academic Press, Palm Bay, FL; 2016:50–204.
205. Bhatia S. *Nanotechnology in Drug Delivery Fundamentals, Design, and Applications: Part 2: Peptide-Mediated Nanoparticle Drug Delivery System*. Apple Academic Press, Palm Bay, FL; 2016:205–280.
206. Bhatia S. *Nanotechnology in Drug Delivery Fundamentals, Design, and Applications: Part 3: CPP and CTP in Drug Delivery and Cell Targeting*. Apple Academic Press, Palm Bay, FL; 2016:309–312.

22

Pharmacokinetics of Essentials Oils

Ahmed Al-Harrasi
Natural and Medical Sciences Research Center, University of Nizwa

Saurabh Bhatia
Natural and Medical Sciences Research Center, University of Nizwa
University of Petroleum and Energy Studies

Mohammed Muqtader Ahmed and Md. Khalid Anwer
Prince Sattam Bin Abdul Aziz University

P.B. Sharma
Amity University Haryana

CONTENTS

22.1 Introduction

Essential oils (EOs) are complex mixtures of hydrophobic volatile components found in aromatic plants. So far, more than 3,000 compounds have been identified [1]. Owing to their volatile property and antimicrobial, spasmolytic, mucolytic, anti-inflammatory, and immune modulatory effects, EOs are suitable candidates to treat various respiratory complications such as obstruction and acute bronchitis. Various pharmacokinetic and pharmacodynamic properties of EOs have been established in vitro; however, data related with their pharmacodynamic as well as pharmacokinetic profile in targeted organ or tissue hasn't been established yet. Therefore, to correlate in vitro and in vivo findings it's important to study the pharmacodynamic as well as pharmacokinetic profiles of EOs. To determine the pharmacokinetic and pharmacodynamic effects of EOs as well as their components, oral administration to subjects is essential. Recently, to evaluate bioavailability as well as a ADME (absorption, distribution, metabolism, and excretion) of thymol, it was orally administered to 12 healthy volunteers. It was found that no thymol was detected in plasma or urine. Nevertheless, the metabolites of thymol sulfate and thymol glucuronide were present in urine [1]. There are a number of EO components with poor solubility such as linalool, which can lead to poor systemic availability, and thus resulting in reduced utilization. Thus, recently, to prevent the conversion of EOs into vapor phase and increase systemic availability, linalool-loaded lipid-based nanocarriers have been developed. It was found that these nanoformulations possessed sustained release effect and increased absorption of linalool [2]. A recent study also showed that EOs as well as their chemical components can cross the epidermis and increase the absorption of various medications present in topical formulation.

EOs and their components allow penetration into the lower skin layers via three mechanisms:

- By breaking down the lamellar lipid bilayer, also known as intercellular lipid structure or mortar, which holds together corneocytes in the stratum corneum
- By causing structural modification of intercellular protein

DOI: 10.1201/9781003175933-24

- By enhancing the lipophilic nature of the drug or whole preparation to facilitate its entry across biological membranes

22.2 Pharmacokinetics and Bioavailability of an EO

Various EOs and their components have been recommended over traditionally used synthetic permeation enhancers because of their safety profiles and ability to increase the penetration of hydrophilic as well as lipophilic medication from dermal preparation into the deep skin layers [3]. Furthermore, in some studies it was found that EOs can be used as penetration enhancer for a number of medications such as chuanxiong. Angelica and cinnamon EOs have been used as penetration enhancer for ibuprofen. It was found that these EOs considerably enhance the bioavailability of ibuprofen following transdermal administration.

Recently the effect of cinnamon EO as well as its key component, cinnamaldehyde, over percutaneous absorption of ibuprofen in vitro was studied and it was found that due to pull effect the absorption rate of cinnamaldehyde in cinnamon EO was found to be more than cinnamaldehyde alone [4]. A recent investigation also demonstrated that turpentine, Angelica, chuanxiong, Cyperus, cinnamon, and clove EOs showed considerably higher penetration effect and lower skin toxicity than azone. It was also found that EOs can improve the skin permeation of ibuprofen primarily by disturbing rather than extracting the stratum corneum lipids [5]. Furthermore, it has been reported that chuanxiong, Angelica, and cinnamon EOs as penetration enhancers could considerably increase the bioavailability of ibuprofen following transdermal administration [6]. Several validated procedures have been developed to simultaneously determine volatile components in the plasma of subject/s during in vivo studies after administration of the EOs. Maximum plasma concentration (C_{max}) and time to reach the maximum plasma concentration (T_{max}) for some EO components have been determined in some investigations to study pharmacokinetic parameters of various volatile components in rat plasma after oral administration of the EO. This lower limit of quantitation (lowest amount of an analyte in a sample that can be quantitatively determined with suitable precision and accuracy) is usually determined by using GC-MS.

Recently an accurate, selective as well as precise GC-MS procedure was developed for the simultaneous determination and pharmacokinetic investigation of volatile components (β-elemene,α-pinene, germacrone, curdione, curcumol, borneol, 1,8-cineole) after oral administration of *Rhizoma curcumae* EO. The developed method showed good recovery and stability outcomes [7].

Similarly, a validated, sensitive, and selective procedure using GC-MS method operated under selected ion monitoring mode for the simultaneous determination as well as pharmacokinetic investigation of cis-methyl isoeugenol, elemicin, α-asarone, and β-asarone in rat plasma after oral administration of the *Acorus tatarinowii* EO has been developed. It was found that analyte calibration curves were linear over a broad concentration range. The LOQ (limit of quantifications) was found to be cis-methyl isoeugenol (7.60 ng/mL), elemicin (3.10 ng/mL), α-asarone (6.50 ng/mL), and β-asarone (5.53 ng/mL) [8]. In another study the simultaneous determination of cinnamaldehyde, muscone, borneol, and isoborneol in rat plasma after oral administration of traditional Chinese medicine (Shexiang Baoxin pill) was done by an accurate, specific, and sensitive HS-SPDE GC-TMS (headspace, the solid-phase dynamic extraction method combined with gas chromatography-tandem mass spectrometry) procedure using naphthalene as an internal standard. It was found that this procedure can be used to study complex volatile samples [9]. Thus, the following parameters play an important role in determining pharmacokinetic parameters:

- Lowest limit of quantifications (LLOQ): a selective, accurate, and sensitive procedure by using HS-SPDE GC-TMS combined method
- Maximum plasma concentration (C_{max})
- Time to reach the maximum plasma concentration (T_{max})
- Analyte measurement by using calibration curves over a wide concentration range

Various formulations have been also developed recently to delay the release of EO components; such carvacrol-based formulations have been developed to prolong the release of carvacrol so as to attain a high level of carvacrol in the caeca of broiler chickens to prevent *Campylobacter jejuni* pathogenicity. It was found that the developed liquid preparation was as effective as carvacrol alone in vitro. *In vivo* results showed that solid preparation extended the release of carvacrol into the caeca and offered remarkable findings on *Campylobacter jejuni* population [10]. Other studies showed encapsulation methods of EOs to improve their stability and solubility as well as pharmacokinetic profiles. EOs such as turmeric and lemongrass have been encapsulated by using biopolymers (alginate and chitosan) to alter pharmacokinetic profile. The drug-release profiles showed slow and sustained release at neutral pH for 48 hours [11]. Pharmacokinetic studies on EO components offer information on absorption, distribution, metabolism, and excretion and on the enzymes, transporters, etc., involved in these processes. In the case of human studies, the profile of an EO/isolated component and its metabolites in blood and its half-lives and rates of elimination, for example, are studied. Several investigations based on pharmacokinetic parameters of menthol have been reported recently. Investigations based on rat model showed that peppermint oil is rapidly absorbed. Nevertheless, formulation like capsule delayed release, about 70% reaches the colon. Several EO-based formulations have been developed with an aim to control the release of EO components to extend or prolong their release for specific periods of time.

A study based on pharmacokinetic evaluation of peppermint EO (extended release preparations in comparison to nonextended release preparations) changed menthol pharmacokinetics parameters (related to urine) via extending the apparent lag phase as well as time to peak plasma levels. In this study, the developed preparation slowed down the release of the EO and did not change the total area under the curve as well as absorption half-life [12].

Another recent pharmacokinetic-based study of geraniol showed its high bioavailability in terms of the rate of absorption (peak of geraniol in systemic circulation at 30min) and amount of absorption (bioavailability of 92%) after its administration to rodents. It was also found that after oral administration geraniol can directly reach from systemic circulation the central nervous system. Also, without any hepatic toxicity, geraniol treatment increased activity of antioxidative enzymes in mice liver. Additionally, it was also found that geraniol somewhat altered cytochrome P450 enzyme effects [13].

Several studies showed the effect of EOs and their components over human cytochrome P450 enzymes (Cyt P3A4, Cyt P2D6, Cyt P1A2, and Cyt P2C9). Recently, the inhibitory effects of the EO of chamomile (*Matricaria recutita* L.) and its major components on human Cyt P450 enzymes were investigated.

A recent study also demonstrated that *Matricaria recutita* (chamomile) EO as well as its main components inhibit human CYP450 enzymes.

It was shown that chamomile EO comprising chemical components inhibits drug metabolizing enzymes and prevents their possible interactions with drugs whose route of removal from the body is primarily via CYP1A2 [14]. Similarly, inhibition of human Cyt P450 enzymes (mainly CYP1A2, CYP2A6, and CYP2E) by the natural hepatotoxin, safrole (methylenedioxy phenyl compound), present in sassafras and certain other EOs have been reported [15]. A recent *in vitro* study showed the inhibitory effect of farnesol, trans-nerolidol, and cis-nerolidol on the xenobiotic-metabolizing enzymes in human as well as rat liver. The findings obtained suggested that these phytochemicals can alter the Cy P3A, Cy P2B, and Cy P1A and facilitate metabolism of parallel administered medications as well as other xenobiotics [16]. Cedarwood EO contains key bioactive sesquiterpenes such as thujopsene, β-cedrene, and cedrol. Previous *in vivo* studies showed inhibitory effects on Cy P2B6 as well as Cy P3A4 by thujopsene, β-cedrene, and cedrol resulted in possible pharmacokinetic drug interactions [17]. Silexan is a preparation made from *Lavandula angustifolia*. A previous *in vivo* investigation showed that repeated treatment with silexan at 160 mg/day showed no inhibitory effects on the Cy P1A2, P3A4, P2D6, P2C19, and P2C9 enzymes [18]. A recent investigation showed that carvacrol binds to the active pocket of Cyt P450 and inhibits its expression and thus can be used as an adjuvant for the amelioration of alcohol-induced hepatotoxicity [19]. Another recent investigation showed an inhibitory effect of α-terpinyl acetate on human Cyt P450 2B6 enzymatic activity, an important hepatic enzyme for the metabolism of xenobiotics and clinical drugs [20]. A previous study showed that the rosemary EO comprising monoterpenes selectively modulates the activities of Cyt P450, mainly CYP2B in rat liver [21]. Moreover, a recent study showed that fennel, cumin, and clove EOs can reduce the expression of CYPs 2E1 and 3A4 but could not restore the expression of CYP 2C6 and 2C23 compared with cyclophosphamide-treated mice [22]. Another recent study showed that the *Nepeta cataria* EO was able to increase the mRNA expression of uridine diphosphate glucuronosyltransferases (UGTs) and sulfotransferases and inhibit CYP2E1 activities and thereby suppressed toxic intermediate formation [23]. A recent investigation showed that EOs obtained from basil and fennel seed considerably modified the expression of enzymes responsible for steroid biosynthesis and cholesterol transport, such as hydroxysteroid dehydrogenase 17 (β1,4,5), sulfotransferase 2A1, steroidogenic acute regulatory protein, Cy P11A1, and 3β- hydroxysteroid dehydrogenase 1/2, Also, basil as well as fennel EOs activate expression of placental-specific promoter I.1 and PIIderived mRNA (CY P19) in human placental (BeWo) and angiotensin-II-responsive steroid-producing adrenocortical cell lines (NCI-H295)R, and enhanced activity of Cy P19 enzyme [24]. Thus, a study based on determining the possible effects of EOs and their components over steroidogenic enzymes, human Cyt P450, and UGTs could help in understanding pharmacokinetics profile and bioavailability of an EO compound.

The EO and its components when used via aroma inhalation cause metabolic changes in people (31 females). The previous report based on metabolomics suggested that aroma inhalation for 10 consecutive days caused metabolic changes among the individuals, resulting in considerable increase of betaine, homocysteine, and arginine levels as well as reduced levels of organic acids, carbohydrates, and alcohols in urine. In particular, considerable change in products synthesized from gut microbial metabolism as well as tricarboxylic acid cycle has been reported [25]. Similarly, another report suggested metabolic changes when subjects were exposed to EOs.

Metabonomic examination of brain homogenate and urine samples after exposure to EO revealed transformation in metabolic profile such as augmented carbohydrates and lowered levels of fatty acids, amino acids, and neurotransmitters in the brain. Another study found increased levels of organic acids (lactate and pyruvate), carbohydrates (sucrose, maltose, fructose, and glucose), aspartate, and nucleosides in urine samples [26].

Further, metabolite profiling-based gas chromatography time-of-flight mass spectrometry studies help in revealing EO-induced metabolic changes in exposed subjects. Thus, based on the above findings in vitro studies of EOs alone are not sufficient to explore the pharmacokinetic profiles of EOs and their components. In vivo studies are required to investigate their pharmacokinetics and bioavailability in targeted organs. Therefore, a study based on ADME (absorption, distribution, metabolism, excretion) is essential to relate the in vitro findings to the in vivo results. This information could be helpful in understanding the safety profile of EOs. Thus, biotransformation, metabolite analysis, hepatic enzymes, bioavailability, pharmacokinetics, and pharmacodynamics studies of EOs along with advanced techniques used in assessment of these parameters are needed for assessing the toxicity and safety profiles of EOs.

22.3 Pharmacokinetic Parameters of EOs

22.3.1 Topical Absorption of EOs

EO constituents are small, lipophilic organic compounds that can infiltrate membranes such as the skin and reach systemic circulation, from where they can reach target organs [9,18]. Generally, pulmonary-mediated delivery of EOs offers the fastest route of admittance followed by dermal mode [19]. Topical administration of EOs can occasionally cause irritation to the dermis, particularly when they are used without any dilution. A number of EOs, including the bergamot EO, can also increase photosensitivity of skin and cause harmful changes such as skin inflammation or cancer. Thus, unnecessary topical application of preparations containing high amounts of EOs to injured skin or to large surface of the epidermis can lead to considerable absorption of EO in blood circulation and can raise risks of severe side effects [27,28]. Recent studies have focused on developing novel, safe, and effective skin penetration enhancers, especially from the natural origin for their several benefits over their synthetic counterparts such as less toxicity, sustainable mass production, and lower cost depending on the type of extraction used [29]. EOs have been considered as potential candidates to reversibly surmount the skin barrier to enhance penetration of drugs across skin layers.

A previous investigation showed skin penetration of terpenes such as α-pinene, terpinen-4-ol, linalool, citronellol, and linalyl acetate from EOs or from topical preparations (oil/gel/emulsion) constituting EOs (0.75% w/w). It was found that citronellol-enriched hydrogel showed promising results and crossed all skin barriers [30].

A recent study compared the transdermal penetration-enhancing effects of mentha haplocalyx EO with menthol. It was found that menthol acquire equivalent penetration-enhancing effects with the EO and had a similar effect on the morphology of the skin layers [31]. Another study showed the application of EO in enhancing delivery of chlorhexidine (an antiseptic known for poor absorption across the skin) across different skin layers including epidermis as well as dermis [32].

Similarly, 1,8-cineole (main component of the eucalyptus EO) has been reported to improve delivery of chlorhexidine. This combination was found to be effective in reducing several pathogenic microbes situated in the lower layers of the skin, which can possibly reduce the chances of infection [33].

Solid inclusion complexes with cyclodextrins can be used to overcome the volatility and solubility problems of EOs. A recent study showed that cyclodextrins alone can be effectively used in overcoming volatility and low aqueous solubility of thymol; however, they are ineffective in controlling marker release. Thus, nanostructured lipid carriers can be used as controlled drug release carriers to allow thymol penetration into the skin. As nanostructured lipid carriers alone were not efficient in preventing thymol volatility, especially at higher temperatures, this type of combined approach can be useful for the controlled release of thymol [34].

A recent study showed that in comparison with standard penetration enhancer (azone), the *Zanthoxyli pericarpium* EO, can be potentially used to promote diffusion via skin transdermal (of the two TCM (Traditional Chinese medicine) active constituents such as perarin and tetramethylpyrazine in a concentration-dependent manner) [35].

Furthermore, it was also found that EO derived from Chinese herbal medicine, namely *HonghuaJiao* (*Zanthoxylum bungeanum* Maxim), can actually improve the transdermal diffusion of medication and thus act as a biological skin penetration enhancer. In this study, the *Z. bungeanum* EO was used as a penetration enhancer for traditional Chinese medicine lipophilic active components such as osthole, tetramethylpyrazine, ferulic acid, puerarin, and geniposide. Also, *HonghuaJiao* EO demonstrated a lower level of toxicity in both human epidermal keratinocyte line and cellosaurus cell line (CCC-ESF-1) than the three terpene components used individually. The mechanisms of improvement in permeation demonstrated that these phytochemicals derived from EOs improved the skin penetration of medications primarily via influencing skin stratum corneum lipids [36]. A recent study showed that myrrh as well as frankincense EOs can enhance skin penetration by increasing drug distribution such as ferulic acid in the epidermis by altering the morphology of the epidermis [37]. Basil oil has also been reported as an effective skin permeation enhancer for enhanced drug delivery of labetalol via skin to systemic circulation [38]. Chuanxiong oil and Angelica EO have been recently reported for their considerable permeation enhancement for transdermal drug delivery of ibuprofen. Interestingly, it was found that the pain inhibitory effect of ibuprofen hydrogel was improved with chuanxiong oil when compared with ibuprofen alone [39]. Copaiba EO containing β-caryophyllene as a potent anti-inflammatory agent is mainly used for the treatment of inflammation; however, due to its unctuous character, skin penetration is always affected. A recent study showed that nanoemulsification of this EO converts it to a more acceptable hydrophilic formulation and also improves β-caryophyllene penetration via the skin due to the small droplet size and the high contact surface afforded by the nanoemulsions [40]. A previous study showed the toxicity profile and penetration effect of *Camellia oleifera* EO on percutaneous absorption of nitrendipine, baicalin, and nimesulide. It was found that the EO did not show any acute toxicity, irritation, or hypersensitive effects. In comparison with azone, more powerful enhancement effects of EOs were found at different concentrations of nitrendipine, baicalin, and nimesulide [41]. Another study showed that wintergreen EO can efficiently accelerate the diffusion of water-soluble and lipid-soluble medications (osthole and geniposide) via acting on the lipid layer present in stratum corneum, decrease condensed stratum corneum, and decrease function of skin layers [42].

22.3.2 EO Absorption via Oral Administration

Limited studies are available for the absorption of EO compounds after oral administration.

α-humulene from *Cordia verbenacea* EO was investigated for its absorption via topical route and its availability in plasma and tissue after administration in mice. The findings obtained demonstrated that α-humulene after 30 minutes showed peak in plasma, and the half-lives of alpha-humulene were very short (16.8 minutes after oral administration and 1.8 minutes after intravenous administration).

After 30 minutes of oral administration, the liver showed a high amount of α-humulene. It was found that via oral and topical routes, α-humulene showed rapid onset and comparatively greater absorption [43].

A validated procedure was developed for simultaneous determination of 2-methoxy cinnamic acid cinnamaldehyde and cinnamic acid in rodent systemic circulation after oral administration of *Cinnamomi ramulus* EO (CREO). The peak serum concentration and area under the curve of 2-methoxy cinnamic acid (0.01% CREO) were found to be greater than those of cinnamaldehyde (83.49% CREO), which suggested that 2-methoxy cinnamic acid might be the major bioactive component of CREO [44]. Oral administration of thymol (Bronchipret TP tablet = 1.08 mg thymol) to 12 healthy volunteers resulted in the detection of the metabolites such as thymol sulfate and thymol glucuronide in urine and thymol sulfate in plasma with peak plasma concentrations of 93.1 ± 24.5 ng/mL. Interestingly, after administration, thymol sulfate was found in the samples until 41 hours [1].

The pharmacokinetic investigations of Chinese medicine, *Pogostemonis herba* EO (PHEO), after oral administration was studied recently and it was found standard curve was linear in patchoulol (main chemical component of PHEO) and PHEO groups. The peak serum concentration and area under the curve of patchoulol were found to be higher at all doses of patchoulol than the PHEO doses. Additionally, the time taken to reach peak serum concentration was considerably high in the PHEO group [45].

A recent report revealed that a sesquiterpene, namely β-caryophyllene, is a naturally occurring cannabinoid found in various EOs preparations that selectively acts on the cannabinoid type 2 receptor. Due to this it has gained considerable attention in terms of its therapeutic potential. In contrast, various properties such as nonpolar nature, poor bioavailability, high sensitivity against acids, high volatility, and the fact that it is easily oxidized in the presence of air have restricted its applications. Therefore, various formulations have been developed to improve its bioavailability, solubility, controlled release, and stability [46].

A previous study indicated that d-limonene, a monoterpene that is widely distributed in several EOs, mainly citrus EOs, showed metabolic conversion into perillic acid, a major and biologically active metabolite of d-limonene, after a single dose administration of Mediterranean-style lemonade. It was found that plasma concentrations of perillic acid reached maximal levels at 1 h after the lemonade consumption with the terminal elimination half-life ranging from 0.82 to 1.84 hours. It was concluded that the major metabolite of d-limonene (i.e., perillic acid) is bioavailable after oral consumption of a citrus preparation rich in d-limonene content [47].

β-cyclodextrin, a cyclic oligosaccharide, has unique structural arrangements comprising hydrophobic space in its center with hydrophilic surface to form inclusion complex with various phytochemicals to improve their various properties such as stability, solubility, and bioavailability. Thus, β-cyclodextrin complex with EO has been used to improve volatility, instability, and poor water solubility and therefore improve its pharmacodynamic effects. Recently, β-cyclodextrin was used to improve the oral bioavailability of Xiang-Fu-Si-Wu decoction (containing EO as the major ingredient) drugs in rats. In vivo results from the same study demonstrated that Xiang-Fu-Si-Wu decoction EO/ β-cyclodextrin inclusion complex presented higher C_{max}, longer half-time, and more AUC [48]. In another study, to overcome volatility and poor water solubility of β-caryophyllene, β-caryophyllene/β-CD inclusion complex was developed. In vivo findings showed that β-caryophyllene/β-cyclodextrin complex considerably improved the oral bioavailability of β-caryophyllene in rats compared to β-caryophyllene alone [49]. An earlier investigation showed that the oral administration of 14C-citral and [1–14C]-trans-anethole to rodents resulted in its detection in feces or urine samples. Samples analysis by high-performance liquid chromatographic showed the presence of seven metabolites.

Administration of α-pinene, limonene, and 1,8-cineole, containing enteric-coated capsules uncrushed and crushed (as a substitute of a liquid preparation), to human volunteers showed the high absorption of 1,8-cineole, as found in the plasma of all subjects. Oral administration of uncrushed capsules to volunteers showed comparable area under the curve results of 1,8-cineole to those who administered with the crushed formulations. Further peak serum concentration values of crushed formulations was >25%, and time take to reach peak serum concentration was 0.75 hours compared to the 2.5 hours for uncrushed preparations.

22.3.3 EO Absorption via Pulmonary Route

EOs containing volatile compounds, mainly monoterpenes, are suitable for inhalation; thus, they can be used in the management of various respiratory complications. These volatile compounds can be absorbed via lungs where they can show their effects and reach systemic circulation for more benefits. α-Pinene, camphor, and menthol have been reported to follow the same absorption route. However, volatile compounds following this route are always criticized for their stability in vapor phase (such as chemical transformation in vapor phase) as well as mucosal drug deposition and metabolism. Furthermore, it was suggested that pulmonary absorption of volatile components is somehow dependent on the type of component and the breathing mechanics of the individuals [50]. Furthermore, it was found that after inhalation of the EO, distribution of the EO component could be different in different organs of the body as their ratio/proportion varies from one organ to another. It is important to identify the physiological parameters that allow the accumulation of respective chemical components and the properties of volatile components that make their accumulation different in different organs. Thus, it's essential to consider tissue-to-plasma ratios when studying the biological significance of inhalation after exposure to EO. An earlier study showed the tissue distribution of the inhaled *Alpinia zerumbet* EO in mice, and it was found that α-pinene (the major chemical component of the *Alpinia zerumbet* EO) showed similar rate of accumulation in both brain and liver. Nevertheless, the EO components showed high accumulation in the renal tissue [50].

Another study based on organ accumulation of the *Alpinia zerumbet* EO in mice after inhalation showed that distribution of EO components such as α-pinene, p-cymene, 1,8-cineole, and limonene varies considerably. It was found that the α-pinene level in the brain and liver was 2-fold higher after mixed-component inhalation than that after single-component inhalation. In contrast to mixed inhalation, the amount of α-pinene increased to around three times that of 1,8-cineole. It was assumed that absorption via inhalation significantly affects this phenomenon [51]. Another study showed the impact of inhalation in mice on behavioral changes as well as accumulation of α-pinene in both brain and hepatic tissue. It was found that the α-pinene accumulation reached peak level in the brain as well as in hepatic tissue on the third day of exposure to inhalation [52]. It was also found that inhalation of EO affects various systemic biochemical parameters such as the following:

- Affects postinhalation oxytocin levels during preinhalation and postinhalation [53].
- Inhalation of linalool and *Lavandula burnetii* influences plasma adrenocorticotropic hormone, adrenaline, noradrenaline, dopamine, and gonadotropin levels in experimental menopausal female rats [54]
- Pepper EO induces a 1.7-fold increase in plasma adrenaline concentration in comparison with the resting state ($p=0.06$), whereas fragrance inhalation of the rose EO caused a 30% decrease in adrenaline concentration ($p<0.01$) [55].
- Lavender EO affects the blood cortisol level among open-heart surgery patients [56].

22.3.4 Biotransformation of EOs

It is widely accepted that all organisms have their own intracellular machinery to metabolize organic compounds by involving them in a multistep biotransformation reaction system to eliminate them via the detoxification process. The detoxification process facilitates transformation of lipid-soluble substances into water-soluble metabolites, which can be easily excreted from the body. This metabolic process involves three different phases:

- Phase I: During Phase I of detoxification, xenobiotics are modified by detoxification enzymes (such as cyt. P450 enzymes) via biotransformation reactions such as oxidation (*dehydrogenases*), hydroxylation (*monoxygenases*), or hydrolysis (*carboxylesterase*). These all-biotransformation reactions are catalyzed by members of Cyt. P450 (I, II, III), and they are responsible for transformation of 75% of medications used in humans.
- Phase II: This phase involves the conjugation of Phase I metabolites with highly hydrophilic compounds such as glutathione, sugars, phosphates, or amino acids.
- Phase III: This phase involves transportation of conjugates synthesized in the second phase with the help of transporter proteins present in liver and intestine, which remove them from the cells. Phase III is mediated by protein transporters such as p-glycoproteins, multidrug resistance-associated proteins, and other ATP-binding cassette transporters usually present in liver, intestine, and renal tubular cells.

Metabolism of EO components via Phase I as well as Phase II biotransformation reactions is usually determined by their individual chemical structure. Thymol and carvacrol were metabolized by oxidation reaction, and their respective oxidized products were detected following oral delivery of the pure samples to rats. In experimental rodents as well as rabbits and human subjects metabolite study revealed the presence of Phase II metabolites such as glucuronides or sulfates. However, traces of unchanged components were identified in urine after 24 hours. Metabolite analysis in human subjects and experimental animals (especially rodents) showed the metabolism of trans-anethole. The presence of metabolites in the urine samples demonstrated that in human subjects this phenylpropene-based flavoring substance, namely trans-anethole, was totally metabolized by oxidative demethylation and experienced oxidative changes. End products detected in biological samples were removed as uncoupled and coupled metabolites (to glycine or glucuronic acid). In the urine sample, t-anethole in the unchanged form was not detected. However, the quantitative variation of metabolites excreted in humans in comparison with rodent urine has also been reported. Concentration-dependent difference in metabolites excreted in urine sample was reported for trans-anethole as well as14C-eugenol in rodents. It was also found that t-anethole forms metabolites from Phase I reaction in a concentration-dependent manner whereas 14C-eugenol metabolism demonstrated variation in conjugated metabolites in a dose-dependent manner. It was also found that the formation of Phase I metabolites from t-anethole was dose-dependent, whereas 14C-eugenol showed dose-dependent variations of conjugates.

Metabolite analysis of biological samples after treatment with peppermint as well as menthol EO was also studied in numerous human investigations. Menthol glucuronide formed via metabolic conversion of 35-50% of the menthol was removed and detected in the urine samples after oral administration of L-(–)-menthol or peppermint EO. Unchanged menthol and glucuronide were only detected by Bell et al [57]. However, in many reports, conjugated menthol metabolites along with traces of the sulfate conjugated metabolites were noticed. Because of the differences in absorption and dietary patterns from one individual to another, the amount of metabolites excreted in urine samples also differs. It was found that surgical opening of the abdominal wall (stoma) of the peppermint EO treatedpatient's decreased removal of menthol metabolite namely menthol glucuronide than after surgery administration individuals. This clearly suggests that absorption of menthol primarily occurred in the small intestine. This study failed to suggest that metabolism of other components of peppermint EO such as menthone or menthyl acetate occurs. Nevertheless, these compounds can be easily metabolized to menthol and eliminated as menthol glucuronide as well. Another study suggested the metabolite analysis of menthol after oral administration in rats. It was found that metabolite formation, particularly metabolites formed from oxidation reaction and their respective patterns, were comparable with thymol (conjugation at 3-OH). Additionally, menthol glucuronide can be considered as key urinary metabolite in rats as well as humans A study based on the metabolism of citral showed complete and stereoselective metabolic conversion in rodents. Besides the hepatic involvement, more organs also participated in the metabolic bioconversion of citral. When various modes of excretion after oral, intravenous, and topical administration were compared, it was found that citral showed a cutaneous first-pass effect [58].

At high concentration, a metabolic product of pulegone, namely menthofuran, as well as unmetabolized pulegone in peppermint EO showed possible toxicity. It was found that high doses of pulegone caused vacuolization of liver cells in rodents. As per the standards of the European pharmacopoeia peppermint EOs used for food applications should not contain pulegone and its metabolite, menthofuran more than 0.1%which is considered as tolerable daily intake. However, various herbal and food-based products still exceed this limit. It has been shown that menthol is metabolized in the hepatic cells by enzyme (i.e., Cyt.P2A6) glucuronidation as well as biotransformation reactions [58].

Tea tree EO has been widely used as an antimicrobial agent. Recently, a complete metabolomics survey was performed to find changes in the metabolite pattern in tea tree EO-treated Botrytis cinerea cells. Considerable differences were found among 91 metabolites out of which eight metabolites were unregulated and 83 were downregulated in the tea tree EO-treated cells. It was also found that tea tree EO suppresses primary metabolic pathways via inhibition of the TCA cycle and fatty acid metabolism. Also, it has been observed that tea tree EO treatment reduced the activities of important enzymes involved in the TCA cycle and unregulated the level of hydrogen peroxide [59]. A previous investigation based on metabolic profiling study showed metabolite formation in individuals subjected to EO inhalation (lavender, clary sage, sandalwood, and orange) for 10 continuous days. The findings obtained showed metabolic changes in the urine of females (n=31) with mild anxiety symptoms when exposed to aerial diffusion of EOs. Considerable changes in metabolites of individuals responsive to the EO were found, which was described by the upregulation of arginine, homocysteine, and betaine and reduced amounts of organic acids, alcohols, and carbohydrates in urine sample. In particular, considerable change in the patterns of metabolites formed via TCA pathway and gut microbial metabolism were also observed. Thus, metabolomics analysis or profiling after aromatherapy can be helpful in understanding unique metabolic signatures in human samples [25].

Metabolic changes were also evidenced after the exposure of rodents to aerial diffusion of EOs such as lavender, clary sage, sandalwood, and orange. Changes in the metabolites brain tissue and urinary samples were exposed to EOs. Metabolic alterations such as elevation in carbohydrates as well as reduced concentrations of neurochemicals, fatty acids, and amino acids in the brain were reported. Urine sample analysis showed higher levels of aspartate, nucleosides, carbohydrates, as well as organic acids [60]. Metabolism of curcumol, the major component of curcuma wenyujin EO, was investigated in rats by characterizing metabolites excreted into urine. Phase I metabolites of curcumol were isolated from the rodent urine samples after treatment with 40 mg/kg dose of curcumol [61].

EO components such as thymol as well as carvacrol showed quick absorption, were metabolized to form sulfate and glucuronic acid conjugates, and ultimately passed in the urine [62–64]. Apart from carvacrol and thymol, EO contains monoterpene compounds out of which p-cymene concentration was found to be high.

Generally, monoterpene compounds showed absorption via GIT. These compounds are oxidized to polar oxygenated metabolites by enzymes such as Cyt P450 enzymes, alcohol dehydrogenase, and aldehyde dehydrogenases. Hydroxylated metabolites and carboxylic acids formed from monoterpenes could be eliminated in the form of conjugates or oxidized further to produce metabolites. This may result in the production of further hydrophilic metabolites that can be eliminated in conjugated form via urine. Epoxide intermediates are initially formed after oxidation and are further subjected to hydrolysis to further produce diols or by conjugation with glutathione (WHO, 2005). Enzymes participating in these metabolic reactions allow chemical transformation of the parent or intermediate compounds into final metabolites that are excreted, eliminated, absorbed, or accumulated at one or more sites (tissues or biological solutions). Glucuronidation of the hydroxylated or oxygenated metabolites of *Origanum vulgare* EO is a key metabolic pathway that allows the removal of these components [65].

Additionally, five pathways (including glutamate-, alanine-, and aspartate biosynthesis- associated pathways, citric acid cycle, galactose-mediated Leloir pathway, fatty acid synthesis, biosynthesis of coenzyme A as well as pantothenate) were enriched by shared differential metabolites. The findings also revealed that EO can reduce inflammation by affecting glucose and amino acid biosynthesis pathways [66].

Geraniol metabolism in animals was initially evidenced in the 1980s [67]. In rodent model, geraniol was metabolized by hydroxylation at its allyl position to form different geraniol metabolites such as 3-hydroxycitronelic acid, 8-carboxygeraniol, geranoic acid, 3,7-dimethyl-octadiene-1,8-dioic acid, and 8-hydroxygeraniol. It is also known that Cyt. P1A1 as well as Cyt. P3A5 enzymes are responsible for metabolism of geraniol in the dermal layers as they are active in such environment [67]. However, on the other hand, geraniol inhibits Cyt P2B6 activity in a competitive manner, which is responsible for the metabolism of some important drugs in the liver [67].

22.3.5 Pharmacokinetic Parameters of EOs

The pharmacokinetic profile of EOs in some studies was determined in alpha and beta phases. The alpha phase is an early phase of quick drop of test compound in plasma level mainly due to drug distribution from the central compartment (systemic circulation) into the peripheral compartments (body tissues). The beta phase is usually characterized by gradual decrease in test compound in plasma after the alpha phase. Generally, the excretion profiles of the majority of EOs as well as their components are described as biphasic (i.e., removal of the EO components with simultaneous distribution of EO components in the tissues). This demonstrates that these constituents are distributed from systemic circulation to other tissues. Because of the high rate of elimination and short elimination half-lives, accumulation is unlikely. Pharmacokinetic studies in the context of EOs have been reported as EO–drug interaction between *Pimpinella anisum* EOs and acetaminophen and caffeine. This study was performed via oral administration of acetaminophen and caffeine after mice were treated with aniseed EO. Pharmacokinetic data showed aniseed EO treatment decreased peak plasma concentration of acetaminophen, reduced systemic availability of the drug, and decreased bioavailability of caffeine in comparison with control [68]. In traditional Chinese herbal medicine, osthole is usually used in combination with borneol to increase pharmacological effects.

A previous study showed that borneol (a component of various EOs such as Lavandula, Thymus vulgaris, and *Rosmarinus officinalis*) can increase gastrointestinal absorption and prevent the metabolism of osthole. Moreover, the promotional effect of (–)-borneol on the pharmacokinetic parameters of osthole was greater than that of (+)-borneol [69].

One of the best methods to evaluate the absorption, bioavailability, distribution, metabolism, and excretion of EO components is to determine their variations in blood-plasma levels over a period of time after administration into veins. In this context, in one study researchers measured levels of bronchosecretolytic ozothin in human blood-plasma after its administration into veins [70]. The plasma level was determined as total terpene concentration. Overall terpene level was determined in human blood-plasma. The findings obtained showed that terpene demonstrated short half-life (3–4 minutes) (α-phase), which represented rapid tissue distribution with β-half-life around 60–65 minutes because of metabolism and excretion.

An earlier study showed the pharmacokinetic profile after dermal application and inhalation of α-pinene. α-pinene showed short half-life (around 5 minutes); however, later on, half-life increased from 26 to 38 minutes. Even later, half-life of 695 minutes in the third γ-phase was found. One more study demonstrated an increase in α-pinene level in a small number of individuals 6–10 hours after dermal application; nevertheless, substantial changes because of the procedural challenges in determining low level stopped researchers from including these pieces of information in their pharmacokinetic calculation. Due to the high-level interaction with lipophilic membrane, α-pinene showed greater Vd (volume of distribution) suggesting a disposition in compartments. In spite of this, α-pinene showed a fast rate of elimination. Therefore, there would not be any chance of accumulation even after long-term application. A previous study revealed that inhalation of menthol and camphor demonstrated elimination data suited to a two-compartment model with half-life of 35.5 and 39.9 minutes, suggesting that after long-term application, there should be no accumulation. Inhalation of 1,8-cineole showed considerable variation of half-life among subjects (both genders), which could be due to subcutaneous fat (major factor in affecting elimination of 1,8-cineole). Recently, a more sensitive, simple, rapid, and specific HPLC procedure was established and corroborated for simultaneous quantitative estimation of cinnamaldehyde as well as cinnamic acid (its metabolite) in rat plasma. Findings from this study showed retention times of 6 and 7.1 minutes for cinnamic acid and cinnamaldehyde, respectively. The developed procedure was found to be linear around a blood-plasma level of 0.001–1 μg/ml) [71].

22.3.6 EO-Loaded Nanoparticles and Their Pharmacokinetic Studies

EOs are a group of multiple volatile component systems that have a variety of biological activities. Nevertheless, EOs have various disadvantages such as they are lipophilic in nature, have poor oral bioavailability, are vulnerable to various degradative pathways, and have high volatility. These disadvantages limit their wide applications. Encapsulation of EOs in polymeric nanoparticles could be an effective approach to protecting them from degradative pathways (such as oxidation and polymerization reaction in the presence of variation in light/temperature) to improve shelf-life and stability. Also, encapsulation offers controlled delivery and improved bioavailability and overall efficacy [71–99].

22.3.7 Elimination of EOs

Elimination of EO components has been determined for various samples such as urine, feces, or exhaled air. It was found that a majority of the EO components is eliminated by the renal system and the lung. Besides renal and pulmonary elimination, a minor proportion is eliminated by feces. Usually, unabsorbed as well as unmetabolized (i.e., unchanged polyphenolic compounds) are excreted through feces [100]. Linalool is excreted primarily in urine but is also excreted via feces and in expired air. For menthol and linalool elimination, it is evident that enterohepatic circulation delays their excretion. A number of investigations has shown the highest levels of EO components at 2 hours after administration, and after 5 hours, metabolites are successfully eliminated from systemic circulation. Blood plasma half-life of eugenol, thymol, and carvacrol varies between 1.84 and 2.05 hours, whereas t-cinnamaldehyde demonstrates quick elimination. Furthermore, one report showed simultaneous detection of two components from *Rhizoma curcumae* extract can alter the ADME profile [7]. Allaoua et al. found that metabolites of *Origanum vulgare* and *Thymus vulgaris* EOs were detected until 13 days in dairy cattle. It was found that early absorption can result in reduction of antimicrobial effects [10].

A majority of EO constituents are chemically transformed during metabolism and also removed via the renal system in hydrophilic form ensuing in limited Phase I metabolic reaction via coupling with sulfate or glucuronate exhaled via pulmonary system as carbon dioxide. As has been seen, after treatment with levorotatory menthol, 35% of the parent menthol was eliminated via renal system as its glucuronide metabolite [101]. Thymol, carvacrol, limonene, and eugenol also followed the same pathways after their treatment like menthol; glucuronide and sulfate metabolites were identified in urine and plasma samples [102]. Thus, short half-life as well as rapid metabolism of EO components demonstrates lower chances of accumulation in body tissues [1].

22.3.7.1 Pulmonary Elimination

Because of their volatile characteristics, EO components or their metabolic forms are expected to be eliminated by the pulmonary system by exhalation. Nevertheless, a mere 1.5 to 5% of monoterpene administration in veins eliminated in unchanged form via pulmonary system, and remaining 75%–95% of the EO was eliminated by pulmonary system via exhalation in 10 to 40 minutes. The overall proportion of exhaled terpenes was found to be reduced as the boiling point of individual components kept increasing. The maximum proportion of EO components was expected to be metabolized and breathed out as carbon dioxide or excreted via renal route as terpene conjugates. Citral and t-anethole showed elimination and urinary excretion of 50% of the dose after treatment and then was subjected to elimination via pulmonary route. As mentioned above, the fecal route of elimination adopted by EO components (usually nonmetabolized forms) is followed less by EO components as primary route of elimination. t-Anethole (about 60%) in metabolite form showed elimination via excretion through the renal system in humans. Only traces of t-anethole were metabolized and eliminated via the lung as $14CO_2$. Data obtained after complete excretion suggested that elimination was complete in 24 hours. It was found that increased dose had no effect on the excretion pathways of trans-anethole. On the other hand, excretion routes of trans-anethole among rodents as well as alpha-pinene among human subjects were found to be concentration dependent.

REFERENCES

1. Kohlert C, Schindler G, März RW, Abel G, Brinkhaus B, Derendorf H, Gräfe EU, Veit M. Systemic availability and pharmacokinetics of thymol in humans. *J Clin Pharmacol.* 2002;42(7):731–737.
2. Shi F, Zhao Y, Firempong CK, Xu X. Preparation, characterization and pharmacokinetic studies of linalool-loaded nanostructured lipid carriers. *Pharm Biol.* 2016;54(10):2320–2328.
3. Herman A, Herman AP. Essential oils and their constituents as skin penetration enhancer for transdermal drug delivery: A review. *J Pharm Pharmacol.* 2015;67(4):473–485.
4. Li Y, Yao JH, Shu YT, Dong J, Gu W, Xu F, Chen J. Comparative study of penetration-enhancing effect in vitro of cinnamon oil and cinnamaldehyde on ibuprofen. *Zhongguo Zhong Yao Za Zhi.* 2018;43(17):3493–3497.
5. Jiang Q, Wu Y, Zhang H, Liu P, Yao J, Yao P, Chen J, Duan J. Development of essential oils as skin permeation enhancers: Penetration enhancement effect and mechanism of action. *Pharm Biol.* 2017;55(1):1592–1600.
6. Jiang QD, Wu YM, Zhang H, Liu P, Chen J, Duan JA. Evaluation of pharmacokinetics and in vitro/in vivo correlation of ibuprofen with essential oils as penetration enhancer following transdermal administration. *Zhongguo Zhong Yao Za Zhi.* 2016;41(23):4362–4367.
7. Li W, Hong B, Li Z, Li Q, Bi K. GC-MS method for determination and pharmacokinetic study of seven volatile constituents in rat plasma after oral administration of the essential oil of *Rhizoma curcumae. J Pharm Biomed Anal.* 2018;149:577–585.
8. Wang Z, Wang Q, Yang B, Li J, Yang C, Meng Y, Kuang H. GC-MS method for determination and pharmacokinetic study of four phenylpropanoids in rat plasma after oral administration of the essential oil of *Acorus tatarinowii* Schott rhizomes. *J Ethnopharmacol.* 2014;155(2):1134–1140.
9. Chang W, Han L, Huang H, Wen B, Peng C, Lv C, Zhang W, Liu R. Simultaneous determination of four volatile compounds in rat plasma after oral administration of Shexiang Baoxin Pill (SBP) by HS-SPDE-GC-MS/MS and its application to pharmacokinetic studies. *J Chromatogr B Analyt Technol Biomed Life Sci.* 2014;963:47–53.
10. Allaoua M, Etienne P, Noirot V, Carayon JL, Téné N, Bonnafé E, Treilhou M. Pharmacokinetic and antimicrobial activity of a new carvacrol-based product against a human pathogen, *Campylobacter jejuni. J Appl Microbiol.* 2018;125(4):1162–1174.
11. Natrajan D, Srinivasan S, Sundar K, Ravindran A. Formulation of essential oil-loaded chitosan-alginate nanocapsules. *J Food Drug Anal.* 2015;23(3):560–568.
12. Chumpitazi BP, Kearns GL, Shulman RJ. Review article: the physiological effects and safety of peppermint oil and its efficacy in irritable bowel syndrome and other functional disorders. *Aliment Pharmacol Ther.* 2018;47(6):738–752.
13. Pavan B, Dalpiaz A, Marani L, Beggiato S, Ferraro L, Canistro D, Paolini M, Vivarelli F, Valerii MC, Comparone A, De Fazio L, Spisni E. Geraniol pharmacokinetics, bioavailability and its multiple effects on the liver antioxidant and xenobiotic-metabolizing enzymes. *Front Pharmacol.* 2018;9:18.
14. Ganzera M, Schneider P, Stuppner H. Inhibitory effects of the essential oil of chamomile (*Matricaria recutita* L.) and its major constituents on human cytochrome P450 enzymes. *Life Sci.* 2006;78(8):856–861.
15. Ueng YF, Hsieh CH, Don MJ. Inhibition of human cytochrome P450 enzymes by the natural hepatotoxin safrole. *Food Chem Toxicol.* 2005;43(5):707–712.
16. Špičáková A, Szotáková B, Dimunová D, et al. Nerolidol and farnesol inhibit some cytochrome P450 activities but did not affect other xenobiotic-metabolizing enzymes in rat and human hepatic subcellular fractions. *Molecules.* 2017;22(4):509.
17. Jeong HU, Kwon SS, Kong TY, Kim JH, Lee HS. Inhibitory effects of cedrol, β-cedrene, and thujopsene on cytochrome P450 enzyme activities in human liver microsomes. *J Toxicol Environ Health A.* 2014;77(22–24):1522–1532.
18. Doroshyenko O, Rokitta D, Zadoyan G, Klement S, Schläfke S, Dienel A, Gramatté T, Lück H, Fuhr U. Drug cocktail interaction study on the effect of the orally administered lavender oil preparation silexan on cytochrome P450 enzymes in healthy volunteers. *Drug Metab Dispos.* 2013;41(5):987–993.
19. Khan I, Bhardwaj M, Shukla S, Min SH, Choi DK, Bajpai VK, Huh YS, Kang SC. Carvacrol inhibits cytochrome P450 and protects against binge alcohol-induced liver toxicity. *Food Chem Toxicol.* 2019;131:110582.
20. Lee Y, Park HG, Kim V, Cho MA, Kim H, Ho TH, Cho KS, Lee IS, Kim D. Inhibitory effect of α-terpinyl acetate on cytochrome P450 2B6 enzymatic activity. *Chem Biol Interact.* 2018;289:90–97.
21. Debersac P, Heydel JM, Amiot MJ, Goudonnet H, Artur Y, Suschetet M, Siess MH. Induction of cytochrome P450 and/or detoxication enzymes by various extracts of rosemary: Description of specific patterns. *Food Chem Toxicol.* 2001;39(9):907–918.
22. Sheweita SA, El-Hosseiny LS, Nashashibi MA. Protective effects of essential oils as natural antioxidants against hepatotoxicity induced by cyclophosphamide in mice. *PLoS One.* 2016;11(11):e0165667.
23. Tan J, Li J, Ma J, Qiao F. Hepatoprotective effect of essential oils of *Nepeta cataria* L. on acetaminophen-induced liver dysfunction. *Biosci Rep.* 2019;39(8):BSR20190697.
24. Yancu D, Sanderson T. Essential oils disrupt steroidogenesis in a feto-placental co-culture model. *Reprod Toxicol.* 2019;90:33–43.
25. Zhang Y, Wu Y, Chen T, et al. Assessing the metabolic effects of aromatherapy in human volunteers. *Evid Based Complement Alternat Med.* 2013;2013:356381.

26. Wu Y, Zhang Y, Xie G, Zhao A, Pan X, Chen T, Hu Y, Liu Y, Cheng Y, Chi Y, Yao L, Jia W. The metabolic responses to aerial diffusion of essential oils. *PLoS One.* 2012;7(9):e44830.
27. Baser KHC, Buchbauer G. *Handbook of Essential Oils: Science, Technology, and Applications.* CRC Press, New York; 2010.
28. Moss M, Cook J, Wesnes K, Duckett P. Aromas of rosemary and lavender essential oils differentially affect cognition and mood in healthy adults. *Int J Neurosci.* 2003;113(1):15–38.
29. Fox LT, Gerber M, Plessis JD, Hamman JH. Transdermal drug delivery enhancement by compounds of natural origin. *Molecules.* 2011;16(12):10507–10540.
30. Cal K. Skin penetration of terpenes from essential oils and topical vehicles. *Planta Med.* 2006;72(4):311–316.
31. Lan Y, Wang JY, Tao Y, Ru QG, Wang YF, Yu JX, Liu Y, Wu Q. Comparison of essential oil from Mentha haplocalyx and menthol used as penetration enhancers. *Zhongguo Zhong Yao Za Zhi.* 2016;41(8):1516–1522.
32. Karpanen TJ, Conway BR, Worthington T, Hilton AC, Elliott TS, Lambert PA. Enhanced chlorhexidine skin penetration with eucalyptus oil. *BMC Infect Dis.* 2010;10:278.
33. Casey AL, Karpanen TJ, Conway BR, Worthington T, Nightingale P, Waters R, Elliott TSJ. Enhanced chlorhexidine skin penetration with 1,8-cineole. *BMC Infect Dis.* 2017;17(1):350.
34. Pires FQ, da Silva JKR, Sa-Barreto LL, Gratieri T, Gelfuso GM, Cunha-Filho M. Lipid nanoparticles as carriers of cyclodextrin inclusion complexes: A promising approach for cutaneous delivery of a volatile essential oil. *Colloids Surf B Biointerfaces.* 2019;182:110382.
35. Lan Y, Yang L, Shi DY, Wang YX, Wu XP, Xie X, Wu Q. In vivo transdermal penetration enhancing activity of essential oil from *Zanthoxyli pericarpium* by using microdialysis technique. *Zhongguo Zhong Yao Za Zhi.* 2017;42(14):2676–2682.
36. Lan Y, Li H, Chen YY, Zhang YW, Liu N, Zhang Q, Wu Q. Essential oil from *Zanthoxylum bungeanum* Maxim. and its main components used as transdermal penetration enhancers: a comparative study. *J Zhejiang Univ Sci B.* 2014;15(11):940–952.
37. Guan YM, Tao L, Zhu XF, Zang ZZ, Jin C, Chen LH. Effects of Frankincense and Myrrh essential oil on transdermal absorption of ferulic acid in Chuanxiong. *Zhongguo Zhong Yao Za Zhi.* 2017;42(17):3350–3355.
38. Jain R, Aqil M, Ahad A, Ali A, Khar RK. Basil oil is a promising skin penetration enhancer for transdermal delivery of labetolol hydrochloride. *Drug Dev Ind Pharm.* 2008;34(4):384–389.
39. Chen J, Jiang QD, Wu YM, Liu P, Yao JH, Lu Q, Zhang H, Duan JA. Potential of essential oils as penetration enhancers for transdermal administration of ibuprofen to treat dysmenorrhoea. *Molecules.* 2015;20(10):18219–18236.
40. Lucca LG, de Matos SP, Borille BT, de O Dias D, Teixeira HF, Veiga VF Jr, Limberger RP, Koester LS. Determination of β-caryophyllene skin permeation/retention from crude copaiba oil (*Copaifera multijuga* Hayne) and respective oil-based nanoemulsion using a novel HS-GC/MS method. *J Pharm Biomed Anal.* 2015;104:144–148.
41. Long ZH, Yang ZC, Yang XZ. Study on skin toxicology and penetration enhancement of skin absorption of volatile oil extracted from tender branchers of *Camellia oleifera. Zhongguo Zhong Yao Za Zhi.* 2007;32(17):1780–1783.
42. Gao XC, Tong Y. Effect of wintergreen oil on in vitro transdermal permeation of osthole and geniposide. *Zhongguo Zhong Yao Za Zhi.* 2017;42(7):1338–1343.
43. Chaves JS, Leal PC, Pianowisky L, Calixto JB. Pharmacokinetics and tissue distribution of the sesquiterpene alpha-humulene in mice. *Planta Med.* 2008;74(14):1678–1683.
44. Ji B, Zhao Y, Zhang Q, Wang P, Guan J, Rong R, Yu Z. Simultaneous determination of cinnamaldehyde, cinnamic acid, and 2-methoxy cinnamic acid in rat whole blood after oral administration of volatile oil of Cinnamoni Ramulus by UHPLC-MS/MS: An application for a pharmacokinetic study. *J Chromatogr B Analyt Technol Biomed Life Sci.* 2015;1001:107–113.
45. Zhang R, Yan P, Li Y, Xiong L, Gong X, Peng C. A pharmacokinetic study of patchouli alcohol after a single oral administration of patchouli alcohol or patchouli oil in rats. *Eur J Drug Metab Pharmacokinet.* 2016;41(4):441–448.
46. Santos PS, Oliveira TC, R Júnior LM, Figueiras A, Nunes LCC. β-caryophyllene delivery systems: Enhancing the oral pharmacokinetic and stability. *Curr Pharm Des.* 2018;24(29):3440–3453.
47. Chow HH, Salazar D, Hakim IA. Pharmacokinetics of perillic acid in humans after a single dose administration of a citrus preparation rich in d-limonene content. *Cancer Epidemiol Biomarkers Prev.* 2002;11(11):1472–1476.
48. Xi J, Qian D, Duan J, Liu P, Zhu Z, Guo J, Zhang Y, Pan Y. Preparation, Characterization and pharmacokinetic study of Xiangfu Siwu decoction essential oil/β-cyclodextrin inclusion complex. *Molecules.* 2015;20(6):10705–10720.
49. Liu H, Yang G, Tang Y, Cao D, Qi T, Qi Y, Fan G. Physicochemical characterization and pharmacokinetics evaluation of β-caryophyllene/β-cyclodextrin inclusion complex. *Int J Pharm.* 2013;450(1–2):304–310.
50. Satou T, Murakami S, Matsuura M, Hayashi S, Koike K. Anxiolytic effect and tissue distribution of inhaled *Alpinia zerumbet* essential oil in mice. *Nat Prod Commun.* 2010;5(1):143–146.
51. Satou T, Takahashi M, Kasuya H, Murakami S, Hayashi S, Sadamoto K, Koike K. Organ accumulation in mice after inhalation of single or mixed essential oil compounds. *Phytother Res.* 2013;27(2):306–311.
52. Satou T, Kasuya H, Maeda K, Koike K. Daily inhalation of α-pinene in mice: Effects on behavior and organ accumulation. *Phytother Res.* 2014;28(9):1284–1287.
53. Tadokoro Y, Horiuchi S, Takahata K. et al. Changes in salivary oxytocin after inhalation of clary sage essential oil scent in term-pregnant women: A feasibility pilot study. *BMC Res Notes* 2017;10:717.
54. Yamada K, Mimaki Y, Sashida Y. Effects of inhaling the vapor of *Lavandula burnatii* super-derived essential oil and linalool on plasma adrenocorticotropic hormone (ACTH), catecholamine and gonadotropin levels in experimental menopausal female rats. *Biol Pharm Bull.* 2005;28(2):378–379.

55. Haze S, Sakai K, Gozu Y. Effects of fragrance inhalation on sympathetic activity in normal adults. *Jpn J Pharmacol.* 2002;90(3):247–253.
56. Hosseini S, Heydari A, Vakili M, Moghadam S, Tazyky S. Effect of lavender essence inhalation on the level of anxiety and blood cortisol in candidates for open-heart surgery. *Iran J Nurs Midwifery Res.* 2016;21(4):397–401.
57. Bell G, Henry D, Richmond C. A specific G.L.C. assay for menthol in urine. *British Journal of Clinical Pharmacology.* 1981;12:281
58. Nair B. Final report on the safety assessment of *Mentha piperita* (peppermint) oil, *Mentha piperita* (peppermint) leaf extract, *Mentha piperita* (peppermint) leaf, and *Mentha piperita* (peppermint) leaf water. *Int J Toxicol.* 2001;20(Suppl 3):61–73.
59. Xu J, Shao X, Li Y, Wei Y, Xu F, Wang H. Metabolomic analysis and mode of action of metabolites of tea tree oil involved in the suppression of *Botrytis cinerea*. *Front Microbiol.* 2017;8:1017.
60. Wu Y, Zhang Y, Xie G, et al. The metabolic responses to aerial diffusion of essential oils. *PLoS One.* 2012;7(9):e44830.
61. Lou Y, Zhang H, He H, Peng K, Kang N, Wei X, Li X, Chen L, Yao X, Qiu F. Isolation and identification of phase 1 metabolites of curcumol in rats. *Drug Metab Dispos.* 2010;38(11):2014–2022.
62. WHO (World Health Organization). Evaluation of certain food additives and contaminants. Fifty-fifth report of the Joint FAO/WHO Expert Committee on Food Additives. WHO Technical Report Series, no. 901. Geneva, 6–15 June 2000. WHO, Geneva, Switzerland; 2001.
63. CIR (Cosmetic Ingredient Review). Final report on the safety assessment of sodium p-chloro-m-cresol, p-chloro-m-cresol, chlorothymol, mixed cresols, m-cresol, o-cresol, p-cresol, isopropyl cresols, thymol, o-cymen-5-ol, and carvacrol. *Int. J. Toxicol.* 2006;25: 29–127.
64. EFSA (European Food Safety Authority). Opinion of the scientific panel on food additives, flavourings, processing aids and materials in contact with food. Flavouring group evaluation 22: ring-substituted phenolic substances from chemical groups 21 and 25. *EFSA Journal.* 2006;393: 1–78.
65. EFSA Panel on Additives and Products or Substances used in Animal Feed (FEEDAP), Bampidis V, Azimonti G, Bastos ML, Christensen H, Kouba M, Kos Durjava M. Safety and efficacy of an essential oil from *Origanum vulgare* ssp. hirtum (Link) Ietsw. for all animal species. *Eur Food Safety Authority.* 2019;17(12):e05909.
66. Chen J, Tang C, Zhou Y, et al. Anti-inflammatory property of the essential oil from *Cinnamomum camphora* (Linn.) presl leaves and the evaluation of its underlying mechanism by using metabolomics analysis. *Molecules.* 2020;25(20):4796.
67. Mączka W, Wińska K, Grabarczyk M. One hundred faces of geraniol. *Molecules.* 2020;25(14):3303.
68. Samojlik I, Petković S, Stilinović N, Vukmirović S, Mijatović V, Božin B. Pharmacokinetic herb-drug interaction between essential oil of aniseed (*Pimpinella anisum* L. Apiaceae) and acetaminophen and caffeine: A potential risk for clinical practice. *Phytother Res.* 2016;30(2):253–259.
69. Luo DD, Chen XY, Zhang ZB, et al. Different effects of (+)-borneol and (–)-borneol on the pharmacokinetics of osthole in rats following oral administration. *Mol Med Rep* 2017;15:4239–4246.
70. Kleinschmidt J, Rommelt H, Zuber A. The pharmacokinetics of the bronchosecretolytic ozothin after intravenous injection. *Int J Clin Pharmacol Ther Toxicol.* 1985 Apr;23(4):200–203. PMID: 3997306.
71. Shetty V, Chellampillai B, Kaul-Ghanekar R. Development and validation of a bioanalytical HPLC method for simultaneous estimation of cinnamaldehyde and cinnamic acid in rat plasma: Application for pharmacokinetic studies. *New J Chem.* 2020;44:4346–4352.
72. Lammari N, Louaer O, Meniai AH, Elaissari A. Encapsulation of essential oils via nanoprecipitation process: Overview, progress, challenges and prospects. *Pharmaceutics.* 2020;12(5):431.
73. Bhatia S, Sharma A, Vargas De La Cruz CB, Chaugule B, Ahmed Al-Harrasi. Nutraceutical, antioxidant, antimicrobial properties of *Pyropia vietnamensis* (Tanaka et Pham-Hong Ho) J.E. Sutherl. et Monotilla. *Curr Bioact Compd.* 2020;16:1.
74. Bhatia S, Sardana S, Senwar KR, Dhillon A, Sharma A, Naved T. In vitro antioxidant and antinociceptive properties of *Porphyra vietnamensis*. *Biomedicine (Taipei).* 2019;9(1):3.
75. Bhatia S, Sharma K, Namdeo AG, Chaugule BB, Kavale M, Nanda S. Broad-spectrum sun-protective action of Porphyra-334 derived from *Porphyra vietnamensis*. *Pharmacognosy Res.* 2010;2(1):45–49.
76. Bhatia S, Sharma K, Sharma A, Nagpal K, Bera T. Anti-inflammatory, analgesic and antiulcer properties of *Porphyra vietnamensis*. *Avicenna J Phytomed.* 2015;5(1):69–77.
77. Bhatia S, Sardana S, Sharma A, Vargas De La Cruz CB, Chaugule B, Khodaie L. Development of broad spectrum mycosporine loaded sunscreen formulation from *Ulva fasciata* delile. *Biomedicine (Taipei).* 2019;9(3):17.
78. Bhatia S, Garg A, Sharma K, Kumar S, Sharma A, Purohit AP. Mycosporine and mycosporine-like amino acids: A paramount tool against ultra violet irradiation. *Pharmacogn Rev.* 2011;5(10):138–146.
79. Bhatia S, Namdeo AG, Nanda S. Factors effecting the gelling and emulsifying properties of a natural polymer. *SRP.* 2010;1(1):86–92.
80. Bhatia S, Sharma K, Bera T. Structural characterization and pharmaceutical properties of porphyran. *Asian J Pharm* 2015;9:93–101.
81. Bhatia S, Sharma A, Sharma K, Kavale M, Chaugule BB, Dhalwal K, Namdeo AG, Mahadik KR. Novel algal polysaccharides from marine source: Porphyran. *Pharmacogn Rev.* 2008;2:271–276.
82. Bhatia S, Sharma K, Nagpal K, Bera T. Investigation of the factors influencing the molecular weight of porphyran and its associated antifungal activity Bioact. *Carb Diet Fiber.* 2015;5:153–168.
83. Bhatia S, Kumar V, Sharma K, Nagpal K, Bera T. Significance of algal polymer in designing amphotericin B nanoparticles. *Sci World J.* 2014;2014:564573.

84. Bhatia S, Rathee P, Sharma K, Chaugule BB, Kar N, Bera T. Immuno-modulation effect of sulphated polysaccharide (porphyran) from *Porphyra vietnamensis. Int J Biol Macromol.* 2013;57:50–56.
85. Bhatia S. *Natural Polymer Drug Delivery Systems: Marine Polysaccharides Based Nano-Materials and Its Applications.* Springer International Publishing, Switzerland; 2016:185–225.
86. Bhatia S. *Natural Polymer Drug Delivery Systems: Plant Derived Polymers, Properties, and Modification & Applications.* Springer International Publishing, Switzerland; 2016:119–184.
87. Bhatia S. *Natural Polymer Drug Delivery Systems: Nanotechnology and Its Drug Delivery Applications.* Springer International Publishing, Switzerland; 2016:1–32.
88. Bhatia S. *Natural Polymer Drug Delivery Systems: Nanoparticles Types, Classification, Characterization, Fabrication Methods and Drug Delivery Applications.* Springer International Publishing, Switzerland; 2016:33–93.
89. Bhatia S. *Natural Polymer Drug Delivery Systems: Natural Polymers vs Synthetic Polymer.* Springer International Publishing, Switzerland; 2016:95–118.
90. Bhatia S. *Systems for Drug Delivery: Mammalian Polysaccharides and Its Nanomaterials.* Springer International Publishing, Switzerland; 2016:1–27.
91. Bhatia S. *Systems for Drug Delivery: Microbial Polysaccharides as Advance Nanomaterials.* Springer International Publishing, Switzerland; 2016:29–54.
92. Bhatia S. *Systems for Drug Delivery: Chitosan Based Nanomaterials and Its Applications.* Springer International Publishing, Switzerland; 2016:55–117.
93. Bhatia S. *Systems for Drug Delivery: Advance Polymers and Its Applications.* Springer International Publishing, Switzerland; 2016:119–146.
94. Bhatia S. *Systems for Drug Delivery: Advanced Application of Natural Polysaccharides.* Springer International Publishing, Switzerland; 2016:147–170.
95. Bhatia S. *Systems for Drug Delivery: Modern Polysaccharides and Its Current Advancements.* Springer International Publishing, Switzerland; 2016:171–188.
96. Bhatia S. *Systems for Drug Delivery: Toxicity of Nanodrug Delivery Systems.* Springer International Publishing, Switzerland; 2016:189–197.
97. Bhatia S. *Nanotechnology in Drug Delivery Fundamentals, Design, and Applications: Part 1: Protein and Peptide-Based Drug Delivery Systems.* Apple Academic Press, Palm Bay, FL; 2016:50–204.
98. Bhatia S. *Nanotechnology in Drug Delivery Fundamentals, Design, and Applications: Part 2: Peptide-Mediated Nanoparticle Drug Delivery System.* Apple Academic Press, Palm Bay, FL; 2016:205–280.
99. Bhatia S. *Nanotechnology in Drug Delivery Fundamentals, Design, and Applications: Part 3: CPP and CTP in Drug Delivery and Cell Targeting.* Apple Academic Press, Palm Bay, FL; 2016:309–312.
100. Bickers D, Calow P, Greim H, et al. A toxicologic and dermatologic assessment of linalool and related esters when used as fragrance ingredients. *Food Chem Toxicol.* 2003;41(7):919–942.
101. Bronaugh RL, Wester RC, Bucks D, Maibach HI, Sarason R. In vivo percutaneous absorption of fragrance ingredients in rhesus monkeys and humans. *Food Chem Toxicol.* 1990;28(5):369–373.
102. Guénette SA, Ross A, Marier JF, Beaudry F, Vachon P. Pharmacokinetics of eugenol and its effects on thermal hypersensitivity in rats. *Eur J Pharmacol.* 2007;562(1–2):60–67.

23

Hepatoprotective and Nephroprotective Effects of Essential Oils

Ahmed Al-Harrasi
Natural and Medical Sciences Research Center, University of Nizwa

Saurabh Bhatia
Natural and Medical Sciences Research Center, University of Nizwa
University of Petroleum and Energy Studies

Mohammed Muqtader Ahmed and Md. Khalid Anwer
Prince Sattam Bin Abdul Aziz University

CONTENTS

23.1 Introduction

Hepatic and renal injuries caused by different pathways involving various external or internal stimuli factors are considered as one of the most important reasons for morbidity as well as mortality. Present medications used for various hepatic and renal impairments cause serious side effects and toxicities. Alternatively, natural products, mainly essential oils (EOs), can be used to treat various hepatic and renal impairments. This chapter discusses the hepatoprotective and nephroprotective effects of EOs. The hepatoprotective and nephroprotective effects of various EOs are represented in Table 23.1.

23.2 Hepatoprotective and Nephroprotective Effects of EOs

Hepatoprotective and nephroprotective effects of EOs and their components via adopting following pathways:

- Effect of EOs on the expression of cytochromes P450: Cytochrome P450 (CYP): Cytochrome P450 (Cytochrome P450 2E1, 3A4, CYP 2C6, and 2C23) is a hemeprotein responsible for biotransformation of many medicines as well as endogenous substances. The hyperstimulation of CYPs in liver

DOI: 10.1201/9781003175933-25

TABLE 23.1
Hepatoprotective and Nephroprotective Effect of EOs

EOs	Biological Effects	Mechanism of Action (MOA)	References
Lemon *EO*	Averted hepatic and liver injury	Reduced oxidative stress, increase in antioxidant enzymes	[1]
Pinus halepensis L.	Protective effects on severe hepatic as well as renal injury	Reduced oxidative stress, increase in antioxidant enzymes	[2]
Origanum majorana	Ameliorate hepatic as well as renal functions and prevent genotoxic effects of lead	Decreased the amount of micronucleus, of aberrant cells number, and various types of chromosomal changes	[3]
Marjoram volatile oil	Protective effects on the brain, liver, and male fertility	Decrease in lipid peroxidative effects and increase glutathione level	[4]
Origanum vulgare L.	Cytotoxic activity (on hepatocarcinoma HepG2 and healthy human renal cells HEK293)	-	[5]
Cupressus sempervirens	Antiproliferative effects	Renal adenocarcinoma cell line	[6]
P. orientalis, P. asperula	Antiproliferative effects	Renal adenocarcinoma cell line	[6]
Artemisia sieberi	Protective effects on cardiac tissue, liver as well as kidney protective effects among diabetic rodents	Decrease glucose (in blood), cholesterol, triglyceride, glucagon, low-density lipoprotein C, uric acid, erythrocyte sedimentation rate, urea, and creatinine	[7]
Ginger and Turmeric Rhizomes	Nephroprotective activities	Modulation of renal associated biochemical markers as well as level of cytokines (IL-6, IL-10, and TNF-α)	[8]
Lavandula stoechas L	Hepatoprotective and nephroprotective effects	Abolish all malathion-induced weight increase, hepaticas well as renal weight gain	[9]
Trachyspermum ammi	Nephroprotective effects	Reduced creatinine and urea levels	[10]
Brassica oleracea L.	Hepatoprotective action	Antioxidant properties	[11]
Nepeta cataria L.	Hepatoprotective effect	Provide the protection to the hepatic tissue against hepatic damage caused by acetaminophen-	[12]
Coriandrum sativum L.	Antioxidant and hepatoprotective potential	Reduce the stable DPPH(*) and inhibit lipid peroxidation	[13]
Hyptis crenata	Hepatoprotective effect	EO restored levels of ALP, ALT, and bilirubin as well as suppressed cyto-skeleton alterations, suppressed rise in lipid peroxidation in hepatic cells	[14]
M. piperita	Hepatoprotective and nephroprotective effects	Decreased stress associated factors (ALT, AST, ALP, LDH, γGT, urea, and creatinine)	[15]
Satureja khuzestanica	Hepatoprotective effect	AST and ALT activities reduced, enzymes activities returned to normal, MDA was reduced, and GPx and GR activities increased	[16]
Foeniculum vulgare	Hepatoprotective effect	Reduced AST, ALT, ALP, and bilirubin levels	[17]
Rosemary (Rosmarinus officinalis L.)	Antioxidant and hepatoprotective activity	Diminish AST and ALT activities; considerably restored the of antioxidant enzymes activities	[18]
Nigella sativa oil	Nephroprotective effect	Reduced serum urea, potassium as well as creatinine levels and a considerable rise in sodium vitamin-D, as well as antioxidant enzymes	[19]
Thymus vulgaris	Hepatoprotective effects	Reduced the levels of the serum marker enzymes AST, ALT, and ALP and myeloperoxidase (MPO) activity and antioxidant activity	[20]
Artemisia Campestris EO+ vitamin E	Antioxidant potential and hepatoprotective effect	Decreased hepatic MDA, AST, ALP, and ALT levels with considerable increase in antioxidant enzyme activities	[21]

can result in various liver-associated complications. Biotransformation of medicines into toxic metabolites catalyzed by CYP can cause liver toxicity as found in the case of halothane as well as acetaminophen.

- Effects of EOs on modulation of the relationship between gut as well as its microbiota and liver (via altering gut flora arrangement, restoring increased intestinal permeability [which leads to leaking] to decrease the leak of toxins, modulating intestinal farnesoid X receptor mediated pathway or sirtuin 1 (SIRT1)-mediated pathway, or generating gut flora-based products).
- Effects of EOs on oxidative stress via activating nuclear factor erythroid 2-related factor 2: carbon tetrachloride (CCl_4), malathion, prallethrin, aspirin, sodium-valproic, deltamethrin, H_2O_2, cisplatin, cyclophosphamide, acetaminophen, etc.
- Effect of EOs on expression of genes: mRNA expression of uridine diphosphate glucuronosyltransferases and sulfotransferases, CYP 2E1, genes responsible for upregulation of antioxidant enzymes.
- Effects of EOs on histopathological damage in rats: Pathological lesions in the liver and kidney of rats, histomorphological damage, oxidative degradation of lipids and level of deoxyribonucleic acid (DNA)

damage, alterations in morphology of biological tissue, histomorphometric degeneration, histopathological changes such as hepatitis, binucleated hepatocytes induced liver toxicity, brain hemorrhage, and renal complications.

- Effects of EOs on hepatic inflammation mediated via anti-inflammatory pathway (via inhibiting toll-like receptors/myeloid differentiation primary response 88 or pyrin domain containing 3 inflammasome pathway), proinflammatory mediators such as cytokine IFN-γ, TNF have been reported.
- Effect of EOs over fat accumulation in the liver: Lipogenesis, lipophagy, β-oxidation, VLDL (very low-density lipoprotein) secretion, lipid metabolism modulation (via activating FXR (farnesoid X receptor), peroxisome proliferator-activated receptor α (PPARα), peroxisome proliferator-activated receptor gamma (PPARG), AMPK (5′-adenosine monophosphate-activated protein kinase), SIRT1 (homologue of Saccharomyces cerevisiae Sir2 protein), or antagonizing liver X receptors (LXR)).
- Effects of EOs on hepatocytes damage: Mitochondrial damage, ER damage, DNA damage, protein adducts, ROS accumulation.
- Effects of EOs on certain parameters: Hepatocyte apoptosis, macrophage infiltration, fibrosis (collagen production).
- Effects of EOs on hepatic and kidney lipid peroxidation (thiobarbituric acid reactive substances – TBARS): The level of thiobarbituric acid reactive substances and protein carbonyl in tissues.
- Effects of EOs on hemodialysis parameters: Study on hemodialysis patients who had pruritus, body gain or loss, and hemodynamic and metabolic disorders.
- Effects of EOs on biochemical markers: Antioxidant enzymes (superoxide dismutases – SOD [Cu/Zn-SOD, Mn-SOD, and Fe-SOD], catalase [CAT], glutathione reductase [GR], glutathione S-transferases [GST], and glutathione peroxidase [GPx]), level of albumin, lipoproteins (very low-density, low-density and high-density), total cholesterol and protein, blood urea, blood electrolyte or serum creatinine, bilirubin, liver enzymes (lactate dehydrogenase, creatinine aspartate transaminase, alkaline phosphatase, and alanine transaminase), LPO in kidney, glucose, malondialdehyde, hydrogen peroxide, sulfhydril group, dimethylnitrosamine N-demethylase I, hepatic aryl hydrocarbon hydroxylase, and 7-ethoxycoumarin-O-deethylase.

23.2.1 *Mentha piperita*

Bellassoued et al. [15] demonstrated that treatment with the *Mentha piperita* EO reduced renal as well as hepatic tissue from oxidative stress induced by CCl_4. It was found that pretreatment with the EO considerably decreased the oxidative stress parameters (creatinine, aspartate aminotransferase [AST], alanine aminotransferase [ALT], alkaline phosphatase [ALP], gamma glutamyl transferase [γGT], lactate dehydrogenase [LDH], and urea). Additionally, EO treatment considerably decreased oxidative degradation of lipids (prevent byproduct, thiobarbituric acid reactive substances formation) in kidney as well as liver and improved the antioxidant action of enzymes (catalase, superoxide dismutase, glutathione peroxidase), in contrast to CCl_4-treated rats. Also, EO pretreatment noticeably improved the renal as well as hepatic injuries caused by CCl_4.

23.2.2 *Citrus limon*

Hepatoprotective and nephroprotective effects of the *Citrus limon* EO were investigated in female Wistar albino rats pretreated with a high dose of aspirin to induce acute liver and kidney injuries. Findings from this study revealed that injurious effects caused by the high dose of aspirin were reduced after the administration of the EO. The authors reported that lipid peroxidation levels were reduced while activity of antioxidant enzymes such as superoxide dismutase, catalase, and glutathione peroxidase activities was improved. Thus, treatment with the citrus EO prevented the liver and kidney injuries caused by aspirin [1].

23.2.3 *Lavandula stoechas*

A previous study showed that the chemical composition of the *Lavandula stoechas* EO which allowed the identification of various compounds such as fenchone, α-pinene, camphor, camphene, and many others [22]. A previous report suggested that the *Lavandula stoechas* EO showed protective effects in liver and kidney from oxidative stress induced by malathion in rodent model. It was revealed that the *Lavandula stoechas* EO administration eradicated all malathion-induced hepatic and renal oxidative stress, body gain loss, altered dynamics of blood flow and metabolic malfunction, and liver- and kidney-associated increase in weight. EO administration also normalized levels of malondialdehyde, hydrogen peroxide, and sulfhydril group and improved activity of antioxidant enzymes [9].

23.2.4 *Origanum majorana*

An earlier report revealed that *Origanum majorana* EO treatment remarkably showed protective effects against oxidative stress, alteration in biochemical parameters, and histopathological changes in rodent model caused by prallethrin. It was indicated that concomitant treatment of the EO decreased kidney toxicity and excessive production of reactive oxygen species caused by prallethrin via reducing lipid peroxidation in renal tissue and serum level of uric acid creatinine and urea. Moreover, levels of glutathione, glutathione peroxidase, and superoxide dismutase were elevated in the rodents pretreated with prallethrin and EO [23].

23.2.5 Lavandula, Peppermint, and Melaleuca Oils

Massaging the hands of hemodialysis patients (three times/week) who had pruritus (scores >3) with a blend of Lavandula, peppermint, and melaleuca EOs significantly relieved pruritus. It was concluded that aromatherapy massage with these mixtures of oils (Lavandula, peppermint, and melaleuca EOs) can considerably alleviate pruritus among hemodialysis patients [24].

23.2.6 *Cinnamomum verum*

A recent study showed hepatoprotective and nephroprotective effects of the *C. verum* bark EO in vivo on CCl_4-induced hepatic and renal toxicity in rats. Also, in vitro antioxidant assay of the *C. verum* bark EO was investigated. It was indicated that treatment of rats with the *C. verum* bark EO significantly reduced CCl_4-induced increased levels of γ-glutamyl transferase, urea, triglycerides, total cholesterol, low-density lipoprotein, lactate dehydrogenase, creatinine aspartate transaminase, alkaline phosphatase, and alanine transaminase. Moreover, treatment with the EO enhanced the level of high-density lipoprotein in comparison with the untreated group. In vitro antioxidant activity showed that pretreatment with the EO decreased protein carbonyl and thiobarbituric acid reactive substance levels in tissues when compared with the untreated group. Furthermore, it was observed that EO administration inhibited the formation of pathological lesions in the liver and kidney of rats [25].

23.2.7 *Pinus halepensis*

Previous investigations showed that treatment of animals with *Pinus halepensis* L. (Pinaceae family) alleviated toxicity caused by aspirin in the tissue of the liver and kidney. A recent investigation showed that treatment of female Wistar albino rats with *P. halepensis* inhibited toxicity caused by aspirin in the liver and kidney. It was indicated that aspirin-induced histomorphological damage in the liver and kidney via elevating various biochemical parameters of the liver such as glucose, cholesterol, aspartate aminotransferase, alanine aminotransferase, and lactate dehydrogenase and via elevating the serum protein, urea, and creatinine level. EO treatment provided protection against toxicity caused by aspirin via normalizing all these parameters [2].

23.2.8 *Foeniculum vulgare*

Foeniculum vulgare (Apiaceae) oil has been recently reported for its hepatoprotective and nephroprotective effects against sodium valproate-induced toxicity in rodent model. It was found that treatment of male albino rats with fennel oil inhibited histomorphological changes caused by sodium valproate in the liver and kidney and normalized the level of biochemical markers such as alanine transaminase, alkaline phosphatase, aspartate transaminase urea, bilirubin, creatinine, and total proteins. It was suggested that these protective effects against toxicity induced by sodium valproate could be due to the presence of trans-anethole and antioxidant activity possessed by this organic compound [26].

23.2.9 *Salvia officinalis*

A recent investigation showed the protective effect of *Salvia officinalis* EO against hepatic and renal injury caused by CCl_4 in experimental rodent. The authors in this study revealed that the *Salvia officinalis* EO treatment at its higher concentrations reduced the level of the creatinine, hepatic enzymes, urea, and bilirubin accompanied by increase in the level of prothrombin total protein, globulin, and albumin. Furthermore, glutathione S-transferases elevation and reduction in oxidative degradation of lipids and DNA damage accompanied by restoration of the histoarchitectural distortions were also observed in *Salvia officinalis* EO–treated mice. These protective effects could be associated with antioxidant effects possessed by various phytochemicals present in the EO [27].

23.2.10 *Artemisia campestris*

A recent investigation showed that *A. campestris* EO reduced kidney as well neuron toxicity and oxidative stress induced by deltamethrin in male rodents. In this study, it was found that the *A. campestris* EO normalized the changed levels of serum uric acid, urea, creatinine, and acetylcholinesterase (AChE). In addition, it was also indicated that the *A. campestris* EO decreased oxidative stress and lipid peroxidation caused by deltamethrin. Moreover, it was revealed that EO treatment decreased deltamethrin-induced histopathology and histomorphometric degeneration. In this study, it was suggested that these protective effects of the EO could be related to its antioxidant properties [28].

23.2.11 *Syzygium aromaticum*

A recent investigation indicated the protective role of *Syzygium aromaticum* EO against the hepatic, renal, and neuro toxicity caused by hydrogen peroxide in Wistar rats. It was reported that *Syzygium aromaticum* EO treatment normalized the H_2O_2-caused imbalance in biochemical parameters. However, there were considerable changes seen on electrolyte composition of blood or creatinine level in serum. H_2O_2 triggered histopathological changes such as sinusoidal dilatation, inflammation, binucleate hepatocytes formation, brain hemorrhage, and renal congestion have been noticeably relieved by the *Syzygium aromaticum* EO. Thus, this study suggested the *Syzygium aromaticum* EO potential of decreasing oxidative stress caused by H_2O_2 could be associated with its protective effects [29].

23.2.12 *Pituranthos chloranthus*

In 2020, Lahmar et al. demonstrated the potential of *Pituranthos chloranthus* EO for reducing cisplatin-induced toxicity in BALB/c mice. It was revealed that *Pituranthos chloranthus* EO treatment noticeably alleviated cisplatin-induced toxicity, which was confirmed by reducing levels of serum biomarkers (creatinine, ALT, and AST) and reducing DNA damage in the liver and kidney tissue. Moreover, EO treatment was also found to restore the changes in the level of oxidative stress markers and proinflammatory cytokine, IFN-γ [30].

23.2.13 Rosemary EO

Hepatoprotective effects of the rosemary EO against liver injury caused by CCl_4 have been reported. It was found that treatment with rosemary EO showed hepatoprotective effects via reducing serum AST as well as ALT levels of rodents treated with CCl_4-. Also, it was observed that the EO inhibited CCl_4-induced elevation of lipid peroxides in the liver tissue. Additionally, EO treatment noticeably normalized the level of antioxidant enzymes (glutathione reductase, peroxidase, catalase, and glutathione peroxidase) in hepatic tissue. Hepatoprotection could be due to the presence of 1,8-cineole, camphor, and α-pinene via various pathways such as by reducing the tumor necrosis factor-α (TNF-α) level in serum. The authors concluded that the rosemary EO, in addition to its antioxidant effects, provides protection to hepatic tissue via activation of physiological defense mechanisms [18].

23.2.14 *Thymus vulgaris*

Grespan et al. [20] demonstrated the hepatoprotective effect of *Thymus vulgaris* EO in the experimental model of acetaminophen-induced injury. It was reported that treatment of experimental animals with the *Thymus vulgaris* EO decreased the levels of ALT, AST, ALP, and MPO in serum. Furthermore, findings from histopathological studies revealed that the *Thymus vulgaris* EO inhibited acetaminophen-induced necrosis. Results obtained from 2,2-diphenyl-1-picrylhydrazyl (DPPH) and lipid peroxidation assays showed that the EO possesses antioxidant activity by radical-scavenging effects and reduces lipid peroxidation significantly.

23.2.15 *Nepeta cataria*

A recent investigation based on the hepatoprotective effects of *Nepeta cataria* EO showed that this EO remarkably reduced acetaminophen-induced liver damage. Moreover, it was also found that the *Nepeta cataria* EO increased mRNA expression of uridine diphosphate glucuronosyltransferases (UGTs) and sulfotransferases, along with inhibition of CYP 2E1, and inhibited toxic intermediate formation. Also, upregulation of Phase II enzymes caused by the *Nepeta cataria* EO could be due to the activation of transcription factor such as nuclear factor erythroid-2-related factor 2 [12].

23.2.16 Fennel, Cumin and Clove

Sheweita et al. [31] demonstrated hepatoprotective effects of fennel, cumin, and clove via reducing hepatotoxicity induced by cyclophosphamide. In this study, it was found that concomitant fennel, cumin, and clove EO (FCC EO) treatment of male mice with cyclophosphamide partially attenuated the variations caused by cyclophosphamide in the activity of hepatic biochemical markers (AST, ALT, ALP), whereas treatment with the FCC EO alone could not alter liver function indices. Furthermore, it was also found that concomitant treatment of any of the EOs with cyclophosphamide reduced histopathological variations in hepatic tissue. Nevertheless, these changes were found to be not the same as those in the normal liver. In addition, EO treatment restored levels of antioxidant enzymes, altered by cyclophosphamide. Furthermore, it was observed that administration of the EO attenuated Cyt. (P2E1 & P3A4) expression but might not be able to affect the expression of Cyt. (P2C23 & P2C6) in comparison with cyclophosphamide-treated mice. Also, EO pretreatment normalized levels of dimethylnitrosamine N-demethylase I, hepatic aryl hydrocarbon hydroxylase, and 7-ethoxycoumarin-O-deethylase, which were altered by cyclophosphamide in mice [31].

23.2.17 *Nigella sativa*

Sultan et al. [32] showed the role of Nigella sativa fixed and essential oils in the modulation of hepatic enzymes and reduced the level of the nitric oxide to control the diabetes-associated complications. It was found that treatment of rodents with streptozotocin-induced diabetes mellitus with *Nigella sativa* fixed and essential oils increased the glutathione and tocopherol level as well as increased the expression of hepatic enzymes. The authors concluded that EO and FO derived from *N. sativa* could be effectively used in the treatment for hyperglycemia and its associated complications.

23.2.18 *Brassica oleracea*

A recent investigation showed the hepatoprotective effects of *Brassica oleracea* EO in CCl_4-induced liver damage in rats. The authors demonstrated that organic polysulfide (dimethyl trisulfide and dimethyl disulfide) enriched *Brassica oleracea* EO showed better hepatoprotective properties than diallyl disulfide. However, both preparations marginally affected the hepatic parenchyma, as detected by means of histopathology. Also, *Brassica oleracea* EO was found to be a potent TBARS inhibitor [11].

23.2.19 *Achillea biebersteinii*

In 2016, researchers demonstrated the effectiveness of α-terpinene and p-cymene enriched *A. biebersteinii* EO in the prevention of hepatotoxicity caused by CCl_4 in rats. The authors indicated that *Achillea biebersteinii* EO treatment noticeably restored biochemical profile (glutamic oxaloacetic transaminase (GOT), glutamic-pyruvic transaminase (GPT), gamma-glutamyl-transpeptidase (γ-GGT), alkaline phosphatase (ALP)), malondialdehyde (MDA), nonprotein sulfhydryl (NP-SH), and total protein (TP) and bilirubin levels in the liver to normal levels. Furthermore, the EO alleviated the histopathological changes caused by CCl_4 in the liver. Moreover, *A. biebersteinii* EO demonstrated insignificant antioxidant effects in β-carotene-linoleic acid as well as DPPH radical scavenging assays [33].

23.2.20 *Satureja khuzestanica*

Satureja khuzestanica EO has been reported for its hepatoprotective effects. In 2012, authors demonstrated inhibitory effects of *Satureja khuzestanica* EO over the activities of alanine aminotransferase and alkaline phosphatase in alloxan-induced Type 1 diabetic rats. Also, the *Satureja khuzestanica* EO decreased fasting blood glucose and exerted positive effects on lipid profile in diabetic rats [34–96].

23.3 Multi-Organ Protective Effects

EO-loaded nanomaterials can be prepared to target multiple organs to exert various biological cardioprotective, nephroprotective, hepatoprotective, and neuroprotective effects. These nanomaterials are designed to fabricate EO-loaded nanoparticles using various eco-friendly approaches. These oils can be used alone or in blend form or with main course medication to exert maximum therapeutic effects with minimum side effects. Natural polymers can be used to fabricate EO-loaded nanosystems, but interaction between polymers (as carrier) and core material must be assessed along with their physical and chemical properties [35–96].

REFERENCES

1. Bouzenna H, Dhibi S, Samout N, et al. The protective effect of *Citrus limon* essential oil on hepatotoxicity and nephrotoxicity induced by aspirin in rats. *Biomed Pharmacother.* 2016;83:1327–1334.
2. Bouzenna H, Samout N, Amani E, et al. Protective effects of *Pinus halepensis* L. essential oil on aspirin-induced acute liver and kidney damage in female Wistar albino rats. *J Oleo Sci.* 2016;65(8):701–712.
3. el-Ashmawy IM, el-Nahas AF, Salama OM. Protective effect of volatile oil, alcoholic and aqueous extracts of *Origanum majorana* on lead acetate toxicity in mice. *Basic Clin Pharmacol Toxicol.* 2005;97(4):238–243.
4. El-Ashmawy IM, Saleh A, Salama OM. Effects of marjoram volatile oil and grape seed extract on ethanol toxicity in male rats. *Basic Clin Pharmacol Toxicol.* 2007;101(5):320–327.
5. Elshafie HS, Armentano MF, Carmosino M, Bufo SA, De Feo V, Camele I. Cytotoxic activity of *Origanum vulgare* L. on hepatocellular carcinoma cell line HepG2 and evaluation of its biological activity. *Molecules.* 2017;22(9):1435.
6. Loizzo MR, Tundis R, Menichini F, Saab AM, Statti GA, Menichini F. Antiproliferative effects of essential oils and their major constituents in human renal adenocarcinoma and amelanotic melanoma cells. *Cell Prolif.* 2008;41(6):1002–1012.
7. Irshaid F, Mansi K, Bani-Khaled A, Aburjia T. Hepatoprotetive, cardioprotective and nephroprotective actions of essential oil extract of *Artemisia sieberi* in alloxan induced diabetic rats. *Iran J Pharm Res.* 2012;11(4):1227–1234.
8. Akinyemi AJ, Faboya OL, Paul AA, Olayide I, Faboya OA, Oluwasola TA. Nephroprotective effect of essential oils from ginger (*Zingiber officinale*) and turmeric (*Curcuma longa*) rhizomes against cadmium-induced nephrotoxicity in rats. *J Oleo Sci.* 2018;67(10):1339–1345.
9. Selmi S, Jallouli M, Gharbi N, Marzouki L. Hepatoprotective and renoprotective effects of lavender (*Lavandula stoechas* L.) essential oils against malathion-induced oxidative stress in young male mice. *J Med Food.* 2015;18(10):1103–1111.
10. Farzaei, MH, Zangeneh MM, Goodarzi N, Zangeneh A. Stereological assessment of nephroprotective effects of *Trachyspermum ammi* essential oil against carbon tetrachloride-induced nephrotoxicity in mice. *Int J Morphol.* 2018;36(2):750–757.
11. Morales-López J, Centeno-Álvarez M, Nieto-Camacho A, et al. Evaluation of antioxidant and hepatoprotective effects of white cabbage essential oil. *Pharm Biol.* 2017;55(1):233–241.
12. Tan J, Li J, Ma J, Qiao F. Hepatoprotective effect of essential oils of *Nepeta cataria* L. on acetaminophen-induced liver dysfunction. *Biosci Rep.* 2019;39(8):BSR20190697.
13. Samojlik I, Lakić N, Mimica-Dukić N, Daković-Svajcer K, Bozin B. Antioxidant and hepatoprotective potential of essential oils of coriander (*Coriandrum sativum* L.) and caraway (*Carum carvi* L.) (Apiaceae). *J Agric Food Chem.* 2010;58(15):8848–8853.
14. Lima GC, Vasconcelos YAG, de Santana Souza MT, et al. Hepatoprotective effect of essential oils from *Hyptis crenata* in sepsis-induced liver dysfunction. *J Med Food.* 2018;21(7):709–715.
15. Bellassoued K, Ben Hsouna A, Athmouni K, et al. Protective effects of *Mentha piperita* L. leaf essential oil against CCl_4 induced hepatic oxidative damage and renal failure in rats. *Lipids Health Dis.* 2018;17(1):9.
16. Assaei R, Zal F, Mostafavi-Pour Z, et al. Hepatoprotective effect of *Satureja khuzestanica* essential oil and vitamin e in experimental hyperthyroid rats: Evidence for role of antioxidant effect. *Iran J Med Sci.* 2014;39(5):459–466.
17. Ozbek H, Uğraş S, Dülger H, et al. Hepatoprotective effect of *Foeniculum vulgare* essential oil. *Fitoterapia.* 2003;74(3):317–319.
18. Rašković A, Milanović I, Pavlović N, Ćebović T, Vukmirović S, Mikov M. Antioxidant activity of rosemary (*Rosmarinus officinalis* L.) essential oil and its hepatoprotective potential. *BMC Complement Altern Med.* 2014;14:225.
19. Alsuhaibani AMA. Effect of *Nigella sativa* against cisplatin induced nephrotoxicity in rats. *Ital J Food Saf.* 2018;7(2):7242.
20. Grespan R, Aguiar RP, Giubilei FN, et al. Hepatoprotective effect of pretreatment with thymus vulgaris essential oil in experimental model of acetaminophen-induced injury. *Evid Based Complement Alternat Med.* 2014;2014:954136.
21. Saoudi M, Ncir M, Ben Ali M, et al. Chemical components, antioxidant potential and hepatoprotective effects of *Artemisia campestris* essential oil against deltamethrin-induced genotoxicity and oxidative damage in rats. *Gen Physiol Biophys.* 2017;36(3):331–342.
22. Sebai H, Selmi S, Rtibi K, Souli A, Gharbi N, Sakly M. Lavender (*Lavandula stoechas* L.) essential oils attenuate hyperglycemia and protect against oxidative stress in alloxan-induced diabetic rats. *Lipids Health Dis.* 2013;12:189.
23. Refaie AA, Ramadan A, Mossa AT. Oxidative damage and nephrotoxicity induced by prallethrin in rat and the protective effect of *Origanum majorana* essential oil. *Asian Pac J Trop Med.* 2014;7S1:S506–S513.
24. Shahgholian N, Dehghan M, Mortazavi M, Gholami F, Valiani M. Effect of aromatherapy on pruritus relief in hemodialysis patients. *Iran J Nurs Midwifery Res.* 2010;15(4):240–244.
25. Bellassoued K, Ghrab F, Hamed H, et al. Protective effect of essential oil of *Cinnamomum verum* bark on hepatic and renal toxicity induced by carbon tetrachloride in rats. *Appl Physiol Nutr Metab.* 2019;44(6):606–618.

26. Al-Amoudi WM. Protective effects of fennel oil extract against sodium valproate-induced hepatorenal damage in albino rats. *Saudi J Biol Sci.* 2017;24(4):915–924.
27. Fahmy MA, Diab KA, Abdel-Samie NS, Omara EA, Hassan ZM. Carbon tetrachloride induced hepato/renal toxicity in experimental mice: Antioxidant potential of Egyptian *Salvia officinalis* L essential oil. *Environ Sci Pollut Res Int.* 2018;25(28):27858–27876.
28. Saoudi M, Badraoui R, Bouhajja H, et al. Deltamethrin induced oxidative stress in kidney and brain of rats: Protective effect of *Artemisia campestris* essential oil. *Biomed Pharmacother.* 2017;94:955–963.
29. Bakour M, Soulo N, Hammas N, et al. The antioxidant content and protective effect of argan oil and *Syzygium aromaticum* essential oil in hydrogen peroxide-induced biochemical and histological changes. *Int J Mol Sci.* 2018;19(2):610.
30. Lahmar A, Dhaouefi Z, Khlifi R, Sioud F, Ghedira LC. *Pituranthos chloranthus* oil as an antioxidant-based adjuvant therapy against cisplatin-induced nephrotoxicity. *J Toxicol.* 2020;2020:7054534.
31. Sheweita SA, El-Hosseiny LS, Nashashibi MA. Protective effects of essential oils as natural antioxidants against hepatotoxicity induced by cyclophosphamide in mice. *PLoS One.* 2016;11(11):e0165667.
32. Sultan MT, Butt MS, Karim R, et al. Effect of *Nigella sativa* fixed and essential oils on antioxidant status, hepatic enzymes, and immunity in streptozotocin induced diabetes mellitus. *BMC Complement Altern Med.* 2014;14:193.
33. Al-Said MS, Mothana RA, Al-Yahya MM, et al. GC-MS analysis: In vivo hepatoprotective and antioxidant activities of the essential oil of *Achillea biebersteinii* Afan. Growing in Saudi Arabia. *Evid Based Complement Alternat Med.* 2016;2016:1867048.
34. Ahmadvand H, Tavafi M, Khalatbary AR. Hepatoprotective and hypolipidemic effects of *Satureja khuzestanica* essential oil in Alloxan-induced type 1 diabetic rats. *Iran J Pharm Res.* 2012;11(4):1219–1226.
35. Bhatia S, Sardana S, Sharma A, Vargas De La Cruz CB, Chaugule B, Khodaie L. Development of broad spectrum mycosporine loaded sunscreen formulation from Ulva fasciata delile. *Biomedicine (Taipei).* 2019;9(3):17.
36. Bhatia S, Sardana S, Senwar KR, Dhillon A, Sharma A, Naved T. In vitro antioxidant and antinociceptive properties of Porphyra vietnamensis. *Biomedicine (Taipei).* 2019;9(1):3.
37. Bhatia S, Sharma K, Nagpal K, Bera T. Investigation of the factors influencing the molecular weight of porphyran and its associated antifungal activity bioact. *Carb Diet Fiber* 2015;5:153–168.
38. Bhatia S, Sharma K, Sharma A, Nagpal K, Bera T. Anti-inflammatory, analgesic and antiulcer properties of Porphyra vietnamensis. *Avicenna J Phytomed.* 2015;5(1):69–77.
39. Bhatia S, Kumar V, Sharma K, Nagpal K, Bera T. Significance of algal polymer in designing amphotericin B nanoparticles. *Sci World J.* 2014;2014:564–573.
40. Bhatia S, Rathee P, Sharma K, Chaugule BB, Kar N, Bera T. Immuno-modulation effect of sulphated polysaccharide (porphyran) from Porphyra vietnamensis. *Int J Biol Macromol.* 2013;57:50–56.
41. Bhatia S, Garg A, Sharma K, Kumar S, Sharma A, Purohit AP. Mycosporine and mycosporine-like amino acids: A paramount tool against ultra violet irradiation. *Pharmacogn Rev.* 2011;5(10):138–146.
42. Bhatia S, Sharma K, Namdeo AG, Chaugule BB, Kavale M, Nanda S. Broad-spectrum sun-protective action of Porphyra-334 derived from Porphyra vietnamensis. *Pharmacognosy Res.* 2010;2(1):45–49.
43. Bhatia S, Sharma K, Dahiya R, Bera T. *Modern Applications of Plant Biotechnology in Pharmaceutical Sciences.* Academic Press, Elsevier, Cambridge, MA; 2015:164–174.
44. Bhatia S. *Nanotechnology in Drug Delivery: Fundamentals, Design, and Applications.* CRC Press, Boca Raton, FL; 2016:121–127.
45. Bhatia S, Goli D. *Leishmaniasis: Biology, Control and New Approaches for Its Treatment.* CRC Press, Boca Raton, FL; 2016:164–173.
46. Bhatia S. *Natural Polymer Drug Delivery Systems: Nanoparticles, Plants, and Algae.* Springer Nature, Basingstoke, UK; 2016:117–127.
47. Bhatia S. *Introduction to Pharmaceutical Biotechnology, Volume 2: Enzymes, Proteins and Bioinformatics.* IOP Publishing Ltd, Bristol, UK; 2018:1.
48. Bhatia S. *Introduction to Pharmaceutical Biotechnology, Volume 1: Basic Techniques and Concepts.* IOP Publishing Ltd, Bristol, UK; 2018:2.
49. Bhatia S. *Introduction to Pharmaceutical Biotechnology, Volume 3: Animal Tissue Culture Technology.* IOP Publishing Ltd, Bristol, UK; 2019:3.
50. Bhatia S. *Natural Polymer Drug Delivery Systems: Nanotechnology and Its Drug Delivery Applications.* Springer International Publishing, Switzerland; 2016:1–32.
51. Bhatia S. *Natural Polymer Drug Delivery Systems: Nanoparticles Types, Classification, Characterization, Fabrication Methods and Drug Delivery Applications.* Springer International Publishing, Switzerland; 2016:33–93.
52. Bhatia S. *Natural Polymer Drug Delivery Systems: Natural Polymers vs Synthetic Polymer.* Springer International Publishing, Switzerland; 2016:95–118.
53. Bhatia S. *Natural Polymer Drug Delivery Systems: Plant Derived Polymers, Properties, and Modification & Applications.* Springer International Publishing, Switzerland; 2016:119–184.
54. Bhatia S. *Natural Polymer Drug Delivery Systems: Marine Polysaccharides Based Nano-Materials and Its Applications.* Springer International Publishing, Switzerland; 2016:185–225.
55. Bhatia S. *Systems for Drug Delivery: Mammalian Polysaccharides and Its Nanomaterials.* Springer International Publishing, Switzerland; 2016:1–27.
56. Bhatia S. *Systems for Drug Delivery: Microbial Polysaccharides as Advance Nanomaterials.* Springer International Publishing, Switzerland; 2016:29–54.
57. Bhatia S. *Systems for Drug Delivery: Chitosan Based Nanomaterials and Its Applications.* Springer International Publishing, Switzerland; 2016:55–117.
58. Bhatia S. *Systems for Drug Delivery: Advance Polymers and Its Applications.* Springer International Publishing, Switzerland; 2016:119–146.

59. Bhatia S. *Systems for Drug Delivery: Advanced Application of Natural Polysaccharides.* Springer International Publishing, Switzerland; 2016:147–170.
60. Bhatia S. *Systems for Drug Delivery: Modern Polysaccharides and Its Current Advancements.* Springer International Publishing, Switzerland; 2016:171–188.
61. Bhatia S. *Systems for Drug Delivery: Toxicity of Nanodrug Delivery Systems.* Springer International Publishing, Switzerland; 2016:189–197.
62. Bhatia S, Sharma K, Bera T. Structural characterization and pharmaceutical properties of porphyran. *Asian J Pharm* 2015;9:93–101.
63. Bhatia S, Sharma A, Sharma K, Kavale M, Chaugule BB, Dhalwal K, Namdeo AG, Mahadik KR. Novel algal polysaccharides from marine source: Porphyran. *Pharmacogn Rev.* 2008;4:271–276.
64. Bhatia S. *Nanotechnology in Drug Delivery Fundamentals, Design, and Applications: Part 1: Protein and Peptide-Based Drug Delivery Systems.* Apple Academic Press, Palm Bay, FL; 2016:50–204.
65. Bhatia S. *Nanotechnology in Drug Delivery Fundamentals, Design, and Applications: Part 2: Peptide-Mediated Nanoparticle Drug Delivery System.* Apple Academic Press, Palm Bay, FL; 2016:205–280.
66. Bhatia S. *Nanotechnology in Drug Delivery Fundamentals, Design, and Applications: Part 3: CPP and CTP in Drug Delivery and Cell Targeting.* Apple Academic Press, Palm Bay, FL; 2016:309–312.
67. Bhatia S. *Systems for Drug Delivery: Safety, Animal, and Microbial Polysaccharides.* Springer Nature, Basingstoke, UK; 2016:122–127.
68. Bhatia S. Stem cell culture. In: *Introduction to Pharmaceutical Biotechnology, Volume 3: Animal Tissue Culture and Biopharmaceuticals.* IOP Publishing Ltd, Bristol, UK; 2019:1–24.
69. Bhatia S. Organ culture. In: *Introduction to Pharmaceutical Biotechnology, Volume 3: Introduction to Animal Tissue Culture Science.* IOP Publishing Ltd, Bristol, UK; 2019:1–28.
70. Bhatia S. Animal tissue culture facilities. In: *Introduction to Pharmaceutical Biotechnology, Volume 3: Animal Tissue Culture and Biopharmaceuticals.* IOP Publishing Ltd, Bristol, UK; 2019:1–32.
71. Bhatia S. Characterization of cultured cells. In: *Introduction to Pharmaceutical Biotechnology, Volume 3: Animal Tissue Culture and Biopharmaceuticals.* IOP Publishing Ltd, Bristol, UK; 2019:1–47.
72. Bhatia S. Introduction to genomics. In: *Introduction to Pharmaceutical Biotechnology, Volume 2: Enzymes, Proteins and Bioinformatics.* IOP Publishing Ltd, Bristol, UK; 2018:1–39.
73. Bhatia S. Bioinformatics. In: *Introduction to Pharmaceutical Biotechnology, Volume 2: Enzymes, Proteins and Bioinformatics.* IOP Publishing Ltd, Bristol, UK; 2018:1–16.
74. Bhatia S. Protein and enzyme engineering. In: *Introduction to Pharmaceutical Biotechnology, Volume 2: Enzymes, Proteins and Bioinformatics.* IOP Publishing Ltd, Bristol, UK; 2018:1–15.
75. Bhatia S. Industrial enzymes and their applications. In: *Introduction to Pharmaceutical Biotechnology, Volume 2: Enzymes, Proteins and Bioinformatics.* IOP Publishing Ltd, Bristol, UK; 2018:21.
76. Bhatia S. Introduction to enzymes and their applications. In: *Introduction to Pharmaceutical Biotechnology, Volume 2: Enzymes, Proteins and Bioinformatics.* IOP Publishing Ltd, Bristol, UK; 2018:1–29.
77. Bhatia S. Biotransformation and enzymes. In: *Introduction to Pharmaceutical Biotechnology, Volume 2: Enzymes, Proteins and Bioinformatics.* IOP Publishing Ltd, Bristol, UK; 2018:1–13.
78. Bhatia S. Modern DNA science and its applications. In: *Introduction to Pharmaceutical Biotechnology, Volume 1: Basic Techniques and Concepts.* IOP Publishing Ltd, Bristol, UK; 2018:1–70.
79. Bhatia S. Introduction to genetic engineering. In: *Introduction to Pharmaceutical Biotechnology, Volume 1: Basic Techniques and Concepts.* IOP Publishing Ltd, Bristol, UK; 2018:1–63.
80. Bhatia S. Applications of stem cells in disease and gene therapy. In: *Introduction to Pharmaceutical Biotechnology, Volume 1: Basic Techniques and Concepts.* IOP Publishing Ltd, Bristol, UK; 2018:1–40.
81. Bhatia S. Transgenic animals in biotechnology. In: *Introduction to Pharmaceutical Biotechnology, Volume 1: Basic Techniques and Concepts.* IOP Publishing Ltd, Bristol, UK; 2018:1–67.
82. Bhatia S. History and scope of plant biotechnology. In: *Modern Applications of Plant Biotechnology in Pharmaceutical Sciences.* Academic Press, Cambridge, MA; 2015:1–30.
83. Bhatia S. Plant tissue culture. In: *Modern Applications of Plant Biotechnology in Pharmaceutical Sciences.* Academic Press, Cambridge, MA; 2015:31–107.
84. Bhatia S. Laboratory organization. In: *Modern Applications of Plant Biotechnology in Pharmaceutical Sciences.* Academic Press, Cambridge, MA; 2015:109–120.
85. Bhatia S. Concepts and techniques of plant tissue culture science. In: *Modern Applications of Plant Biotechnology in Pharmaceutical Sciences.* Academic Press, Cambridge, MA; 2015:121–156.
86. Bhatia S. Application of plant biotechnology. In: *Modern Applications of Plant Biotechnology in Pharmaceutical Sciences.* Academic Press, Cambridge, MA; 2015:157–207.
87. Bhatia S. Somatic embryogenesis and organogenesis. In: *Modern Applications of Plant Biotechnology in Pharmaceutical Sciences.* Academic Press, Cambridge, MA; 2015:209–230.
88. Bhatia S. Classical and nonclassical techniques for secondary metabolite production in plant cell culture. In: *Modern Applications of Plant Biotechnology in Pharmaceutical Sciences.* Academic Press, Cambridge, MA; 2015:231–291.
89. Bhatia S. Plant-based biotechnological products with their production host, modes of delivery systems, and stability testing. In: *Modern Applications of Plant Biotechnology in Pharmaceutical Sciences.* Academic Press, Cambridge, MA; 2015:293–331.
90. Bhatia S. Edible vaccines. In: *Modern Applications of Plant Biotechnology in Pharmaceutical Sciences.* Academic Press, Cambridge, MA; 2015:333–343.
91. Bhatia S. Microenvironmentation in micropropagation. In: *Modern Applications of Plant Biotechnology in Pharmaceutical Sciences.* Academic Press, Cambridge, MA; 2015:345–360.

92. Bhatia S. Micropropagation. In: *Modern Applications of Plant Biotechnology in Pharmaceutical Sciences*. Academic Press, Cambridge, MA; 2015:361–368.
93. Bhatia S. Laws in plant biotechnology. In: *Modern Applications of Plant Biotechnology in Pharmaceutical Sciences*. Academic Press, Cambridge, MA; 2015:369–391.
94. Bhatia S. Technical glitches in micropropagation. In: *Modern Applications of Plant Biotechnology in Pharmaceutical Sciences*. Academic Press, Cambridge, MA; 2015:393–404.
95. Bhatia S. Plant tissue culture-based industries. In: *Modern Applications of Plant Biotechnology in Pharmaceutical Sciences*. Academic Press, Cambridge, MA; 2015:405–417.
96. Bhatia S, Al-Harrasi A, Behl T, Anwer MK, Ahmed MM, Mittal V, Kaushik D, Chigurupati S, Kabir MT, Sharma PB, Chaugule B, Vargas-de-la-Cruz C. Anti-migraine activity of freeze dried-latex obtained from *Calotropis Gigantea* Linn. *Environ Sci Pollut Res Int*. 2021.

24

Essential Oil Dispensing Methods

Ahmed Al-Harrasi
Natural and Medical Sciences Research Center, University of Nizwa

Saurabh Bhatia
Natural and Medical Sciences Research Center, University of Nizwa
University of Petroleum and Energy Studies

Md. Tanvir Kabir
BRAC University

Tapan Behl
Chitkara University

Deepak Kaushik
M.D. University

CONTENTS

24.1 Introduction

Dispersing natural antimicrobial components such as essential oils (EOs) in the gaseous phase by a process other than natural evaporation is challenging as the chemical components present are very sensitive to chemical transformation in the presence of different environmental conditions. Heating EOs is an inappropriate process, since, on the one hand, it can convert the liquid into gaseous dispersion, but on other hand, it can cause chemical transformation of chemical components, which can directly influence its biological properties [1]. In one study, it was found that a blend of 15 EOs when dispersed into gaseous phase by using heated fragrance lamp and volatile components confined to the headspace of the fragrance lamp had chemically transformed from solution containing monoterpene hydrocarbons (high volatility) to preparation having low-volatility monoterpene alcohols and sesquiterpenes [2]. EO-loaded candles could be a better alternative to directly heating EOs as such products can disperse EO effectively in a sustainable manner and ionize volatile compounds present in vapor phase. Ionization of volatile compounds has been reported to improve antibacterial activity. It was found that ionization of volatile compounds in vapor phase results in improved attachment of antimicrobial components to the bacterial cell membrane as well as enhanced penetration across the membrane leading to cell death [1]. EO enriched with a high level of β-pinene showed improvement

DOI: 10.1201/9781003175933-26

in antibacterial activity against *Escherichia coli* when the gaseous phase was ionized by candle flame [3]. Using water as a medium to improve EO dispersion is not recommended as phenolic components present in EOs have poor solubility leading to decreased antimicrobial effects. Another challenging part is water-loving components especially those containing hydroxyl groups in EOs show more solubility in water and remain in aqueous phase [4]. Various other dispersion procedures have been proposed such as use of aroma oil diffuser to disperse EO components. For instance, dispersion of linalool as well as carvacrol in gaseous phase resulted in decrease in bacterial number after 5 hours of dispersion [5]. A blend of geranium and lemongrass when dispersed via dynamic fragrance generator for 20 hours showed 80% decrease in airborne microbes but when dispersion was reduced to 30% an increase in microbial count in air was observed and ultimately microbial count in air went back to normal due to the termination of dispersion output [6]. This suggests that continuous dispersion plays an important role in killing airborne microorganisms. Another report showed the impact of evaporating blend of EOs (*Lavandula angustifolia, Eucalyptus globulus*, and *Melaleuca alternifolia*) on indoor environment in terms of the air quality and demonstrated time-dependent decrease in bacterial count (if dispersion was continuous microbial count decreased in air) [1].

24.2 Strategies Used in the Delivery of EOs

In spite of aspects related to the composition of EOs and stability parameters and their interactions, it is essential to study the delivery of EOs by using different inhalers, especially for better therapeutic outcomes. As per a previous report, for effective aromatherapy, it is essential to administer highly concentrated volatile mixtures of EOs via nasal route quickly within a limited time. The results obtained using this approach was promising as participants treated with EOs showed significant improvement in terms of certain health conditions such as arterial blood oxygenation, attentive concentration, blood pressure, chronic stress, cortisol, heart rate, pain, rhinitis, sleep disturbance, and affective states. By using EO-based inhalation, hyperthermia can be induced to reduce cerebral circulation, enhance cardiac output, and increase gaseous exchange in alveoli. A recent investigation showed the impact of inhalers on oxygen level in systemic circulation. In this study, direct delivery of aromatic compounds via nasal route surpassed the oxygenation impact of usual intense inhalation. This type of supraoptimal source of oxygen can increase metabolic performance of the cell, which can be further utilized in treating traumatic conditions.

24.3 Earlier Methods Used in the Delivery of EO via Inhalation

The design and material used for inhalers must be compatible with the EO and its components because the properties of EOs in vapor phase are different. It is important to develop a suitable device to produce dispersion under controlled conditions other than by natural evaporation. In earlier times, a few simple procedures for oil diffusion were used based on diffusion via evaporation. Natural EOs were absorbed into suitable material such as wood, fabric, or clay and allowed to vaporize in a defined space. This procedure is good for small areas, but in large areas, volatile components do not spread or emit much.

24.3.1 Room Diffusers

Recently, various EO-based dispensers have been used to diffuse vapors into environments using various mechanisms: nebulization (changes liquid preparation into a mist via nebulizer), heating, ultrasonication, vaporization, and humidification. Other approaches to disperse EOs have been used such as aroma oil diffusers to disperse the principle compounds of EOs such as carvacrol and linalool. It was found that using this type of dispersion causes a reduction in bacteria till 5 hours after spraying [5].

Likewise, an 8% decrease in microorganisms, especially bacteria, in air was found when a combination of EOs (*Pelargonium graveolens* and *Cymbopogon citratus*) was vaporized constantly for approximately 20 hours. Dispersion was distributed (100%) using a fragrance generator by using negative airflow to reduce fluid pressure. It was noted that when generation of EOs decreased up to 30%, bacterial counts of microorganisms increased; however, after exposure to EOs, bacterial counts gradually returned to normal [6], suggesting that continuous dispersion is essential for overall effectiveness. In 2007, a similar report showed the influence of EO (*Lavandula angustifolia, Eucalyptus globulus*, and *Melaleuca alternifolia*) vapors on indoor air quality. It was found that release of the volatile components in an environment happened in the first 20 minutes whereas the lowest count of airborne bacteria was found at 30 minutes. Afterward, the bacterial count was increased; this study suggested that continuous dispersion is important as discontinuation in exposure or production of EOs can lead to the reversal of the level of microorganisms. A previous investigation demonstrated that in an microbiological air sampler (made to accumulate the particulate matter) as well as an aroma oil diffuser for the evaporation of *Salvia officinalis* EO decreased the overall count of microorganisms as well as overall count of yeasts and molds in an indoor environment. *S. officinalis* EO demonstrated strong antibacterial effects in vapor phase against the investigated microbes and showed its potential as a natural disinfectant [7].

24.3.2 Heat Diffusers

Heat diffusers work in the same fashion as evaporative diffusers; nevertheless, in spite of using air, they are dependent on temperature to vaporize EOs in the surrounding environment. For evaporating EOs, heat diffusers cannot be considered as reliable source as heating can destroy the natural chemical composition of EOs, which can lead to loss of biological properties as well as the development of certain toxic compounds after postheating chemical transformation [1]. A previous investigation showed that when different EOs were vaporized by heated fragrance lamp and the chemical composition of vapor phase was examined, it was observed that these volatile components experienced chemical transformation (high volatility to low volatility) in the headspace of the heated fragrance lamp. [2]. EO diffusers based on heating phenomenon experience similar disadvantages as EO diffusers due to the evaporation phenomenon and the possible fractioning of EOs.

The most suitable heat diffusers are the ones that can effectively work at a temperature at which there will no or minimal chemical changes in volatile components. There are many types of heat diffusers such as candle diffusers and lamp ring diffusers.

24.3.3 EO Dispersion Using Candles

Another conventional approach to producing dispersion is by using candles. Candles can be used as a medium for EO dispersion [1]. It was found that this approach has a different effect on the composition of EOs as this approach is not restricted to only heat. It was proposed that using this method vapor molecules can be ionized, which allows greater attachment of components to the membrane of bacteria and hence increased absorptivity across the membranes resulting in efficient antibacterial effects. This was observed in the case of β-pinene. The antibacterial effect of β-pinene vapor was found to be improved against *E. coli* when the volatile components were exposed to ionizing source such as candle flame [3]. However, the use of candles is restricted as EOs have inflammable property which make an additional risk to increase their flammable property.

24.3.4 Water-Mediated Dispersion

Conventional approaches also include the use of water to produce dispersion; however, water is not an effective approach as phenolic compounds are nonpolar in nature, thus resulting in reduced antimicrobial activity. It is also known that the aqueous phase also decreases the volatility of components with more hydrophilic groups such as hydroxyl groups. These compounds show high solubility in water and stay in the aqueous layer [4]. In this method, EOs are mixed with water boiling in a room to allow the diffusion of EOs via steam. Boiled water at room temperature warms the EOs and allows their volatile components to vaporize quickly in the surrounding environment. This technique works very rapidly but needs continuous maintenance in replacing the evaporated water and oils.

24.3.5 Evaporative Diffusers

Evaporative diffusers work by evaporating EOs dripped onto a filter or other surface by using a small fan. Blowing air from the fan results in faster evaporation of EOs than normal dispersion of EOs at room temperature. Nevertheless, one of the major disadvantages of this procedure is that depending on volatility differences, low density fraction of EOs vaporize and diffuse more quickly in comparison with the heavier portions. This makes the process unstable. Moreover, fractioning could disturb the properties of EOs. The major advantage of this method is that without solely relying on the room air current, it allows quick distribution of the vapors across the space.

24.3.6 Ultrasonic Aroma Diffuser and Ionizer

Ultrasonic humidifiers work via high-frequency oscillation produced by using ultrasonic waves (Figure 24.1). The foremost function of an ultrasonic oscillator is to break the water droplets into ultrafine particles to create a fine mist of water, which is then further released into the room, generally via a small fan on the bottom of the unit. Ultrasonic diffusers function differently to produce mist or humidification of EOs. Ultrasonic diffusers have little disks that cause vibrations quickly in liquid medium that has been filled with EOs. The vibrations are sufficient to break up the EO and water into tiny droplets that can easily disperse in the air. Generally, for evaporation of EOs, heating is required; however, this method does not involve any heating procedure. Thus, due to the various limitations of evaporative humidifiers, an ultrasonic ionizer aromatherapy diffuser can be used for aroma evaporation (e.g., in one of the investigations, a natural bergamot EO was used to evaluate the effects of aromatherapy in improving work-related stress on elementary school teachers in Taiwan) [8].

24.3.7 Nebulizing EO Diffusers

Nebulizing diffusers supply continuous pressurized air through little ducts that have EOs. This gentle airflow builds a vacuum that draws the EOs from the ducts and delivers them in the form of air stream to disperse fine mist. However, this nebulization sometimes creates noise. Without diluting EOs or changing the EO composition, nebulization always disperses the complete EO into the air in the form of fine mist. Due to this, nebulization is always considered as the most effective

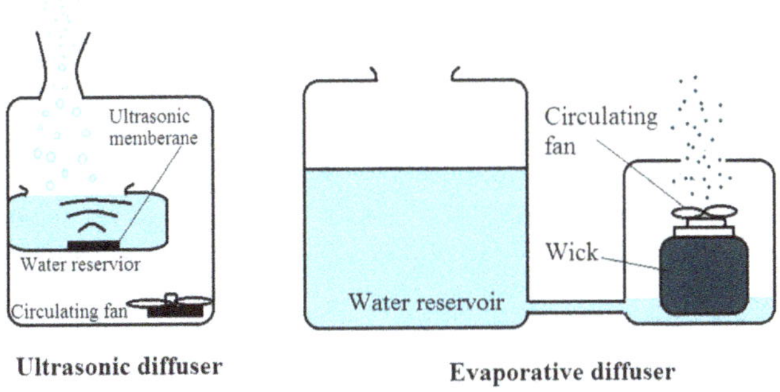

FIGURE 24.1 Ultrasonic diffuser and evaporative diffuser.

approach for EO diffusion. Because nebulization is also effective in dispersing EOs in an environment most nebulizers have the ability to control flow rate of air and timers to facilitate controlled delivery.

A recent investigation showed the effectiveness of EOs after nebulization in decreasing the load of microorganisms in nursing homes. Findings from this investigation showed decreases in microbial count (bacteria as well as fungi) after exposing rooms to nebulization using EOs alone or with sanitization treatment. It was concluded that the EO composition decreased both the microbial load in surroundings (in hospital) and pharmaceutical preparations [9].

24.3.8 Intranasal Decongestant EO Spray

Nasal spray preparations containing a mixture of EOs with or without main course medication can be used to treat various pulmonary or nonpulmonary conditions. EOs with anti-inflammatory, expectorant, spasmolytic as well as antiseptic and antimicrobial activities can be used for this purpose [10]. Recently, hypertonic EO-based intranasal spray on perennial allergic rhinitis symptoms was studied, and it was found that EO-based intranasal spray can be used in the management of perennial allergic rhinitis. Recent findings also suggest that the formulation of nasal spray for Radix Bupleuri EO can be potentially used in the treatment of fever [11,12]. A previous report also suggested that nasal spray containing five EOs (lemon-scented eucalyptus, eucalyptus, peppermint, green thyme, and rosemary) considerably decreased upper respiratory complications [13]. A previous study showed that community-based patients (including children, teenagers, and adults) treated with Rhinospray® Plus (a nasal spray containing tramazoline and EOs) had fewer viral infections of the nose and throat. It was also found that such treatment improved quality of life and that treatment was well tolerated [14]. However, it was also found that chronic inhalation of nasal sprays and decongestants containing compound menthol nasal drops (EOs of camphor, menthol, and liquid paraffin) could cause exogenous lipoid pneumonia. Thus, clinicians should be careful when recommending alternative EO approaches [15]. Recently, the effect of dispersion of *Citrus limon* and *Abies alba* EOs on airborne microorganisms including bacteria and fungi in hospitals was investigated. It was found that the antimicrobial effects of EOs in vapor phase can decrease contamination. A study was performed in two wards (1,227 beds) of an acute-care hospital in Austria. The findings showed decrease in microbial load (bacteria and fungi) initially for 2 hours by almost 40% and 30%–60%, respectively. It was found that these EO mixtures could efficiently decrease the load of microorganisms in indoor air [16]. Recently, lemongrass and geranium EOs were formulated to create BioScent, which was vaporized using an ST Pro machine and then tested for its efficacy to reduce surface and airborne levels of bacteria such as antibiotic sensitive/resistant bacteria, including vancomycin-resistant Enterococci, methicillin-resistant *Staphylococcus aureus, Clostridium difficile,* and *Acinetobacter baumanii* in air. It was found that antibacterial activities were altered depending on the type of assay used. Under controlled conditions (sealed box environment), methicillin-resistant *Staphylococcus aureus* count was decreased by 38% after 20 hours of exposure to BioScent vapor. Furthermore, the ST Pro machine responsible for the dispersion of BioScent decreased 89% of bacteria present in air in 15 hours when activated at a 100% continuous production [6]. Recently, inhalation of aerosol therapy containing EOs, saline, glucocorticoids, and antibiotics showed better subjective results in comparison with intranasal glucocorticoid therapy and saline irrigation in the treatment of chronic rhinosinusitis [16]. A recent investigation showed herbal spray (containing various EOs) considerably decreased the intensity of all evaluated factors (alopecia, skin-picking, secondary skin lesion, and itchy skin) among 20 adult horses. It was found that the developed EO-based spray showed promising results in horses suffering from pruritus without any side effects [17]. Pulmonary drug delivery has been known to be efficient at administering medication at local or systemic level to treat respiratory and nonrespiratory complications. Inhalation therapy via the lungs is considered as the most effective way to treat various lung complications [18]. This type of treatment decreases systemic side effects by using smaller doses of medicine [19]. Effective or reliable pulmonary drug delivery by using advance inhalers requires suitable interaction between the medication, the inhaler, and the patient [20]. In the last few decades, considerable scientific advancement has occurred in pulmonary drug delivery, a noninvasive approach, to target lungs as the medium for delivering medication in systemic circulation [21]. Pulmonary drug administration is a reliable mode of delivering medication in systemic circulation[22]. The pulmonary mode of administration is an effective route for systemic delivery as it allows the rapid absorption of medication by the substantial surface area offered by the alveoli, the rich vasculature (a network of capillaries) present over alveolar membrane, thin blood–air barrier, and the escaping first-pass effect [23]. The efficiency of an inhalation treatment is mainly reliant on the amount of medicine delivered at the target location [23]. Due to their volatile properties, EOs can be easily vaporized and effectively used via inhalation aerosol therapy.

In a previous investigation, tea tree and eucalyptus EOs were used as natural disinfectants in vapor phase against M13 bacteriophage and influenza A viruses and showed fruitful results [24].

Deposition of medication is primarily determined by the type of preparation, its composition as well as the device used to deliver the medication. The effectiveness of pulmonary administration is mainly dependent on phenomenon or mechanism used for delivering therapeutics as well as type of delivery devices such as dry powder inhalers (DPIs), pressurized metered-dose inhalers (pMDIs), and nebulizers. There are certain factors that should be considered when designing an effective inhaler such as:

- Good inspiratory flow rates
- Dispersion of volatile molecules
- Designing and materials used for the inhalers
- Good oropharyngeal deposition
- Good therapeutic outcome
- Preferably portable
- Easy to use

- Type of inhalator (jet, ultrasonic, mesh nebulizers, breath-enhanced and breath-actuated, nebulizers)
- Droplet size
- Viscosity of the EO solution
- Velocity of the volatile components produced from the nebulizer
- Impaction in the oropharynx
- Administration time
- The air stream as well as force possessed by aerosol components in the case of jet nebulizers
- Type of the material and design used for tubing and mask
- Overall volume of medication packed in the device

24.4 Strategies Used for Inhalation of EOs

EOs have been employed in the treatment of various ailments. Because of their volatile nature, EOs when inhaled can easily go to the upper as well as lower regions of the respiratory system. It is well known that inhalation of EOs can regulate brain health and functions associated with mood and neurodegeneration. Recent studies have shown that inhalation of EOs could have positive effects on different biological systems. However, on the other hand, EOs and their components can also cause toxicity by aggravating certain oxidative pathways, as was seen in the case of treatment of Wistar rats with geraniol as well as *Cymbopogon martinii* EOs. It was found that geraniol caused oxidative stress that may have triggered some degree of hepatic toxicity. Thus, considering safety and toxicity parameters, optimum delivery of EOs is required for positive therapeutic outcomes. As discussed above, various conventional and advanced approaches can be used to deliver EOs such as DPIs, pMDI, and nebulizers.

24.4.1 Particulate Entry to the Respiratory Tract

Advancements in pulmonary drug delivery systems via inhalation have been used to treat various complications associated with the lungs. Pulmonary formulations usually contain small molecules that can be administered effectively with very quick action. Via inhalation, these molecules have low metabolism and high bioavailability. Moreover, macromolecules such as proteins can also be delivered via this mode (e.g., first inhaled insulin product, Exubera, an inhaled form of rapid acting insulin developed by Pfizer) [25].

Before designing a suitable inhaler, it is important to understand lung architecture, lung conditions such as humidity, clearance mechanisms, and effects of aerosol deposition. On the other hand, it is also essential to know distribution of inhaled drugs in the lungs, parameters that can influence the distribution of inhaled drugs, and in what way these factors influence the therapeutic effects of the inhalation. Figure 24.2 demonstrates the major factors that must be considered when designing aerosol delivery devices.

Particle size is one of the most important factors that determine rate of deposition as well drug distribution in the respiratory tract. Particle size distribution (PSD) of fine solid particles or liquid droplets suspended in air is presented as mass median aerodynamic diameter of aerosols. Additionally, at the site of accumulation, geometric standard deviation of aerosols is also examined in the lungs.

Large particles (of size >6 μm) are likely to deposit in the upper airway (oropharynx and tracheal region), where flow of air is higher and unstable. This restricts the delivery of drugs to the lungs. The perfect particle size range for lung deposition is 2–6 μm diameter. Particles (2–6 μm) deposit mostly in the alveolar region and are more suitable as these particles can enhance accumulation at the targeted site and enhance the effectiveness of the medication.

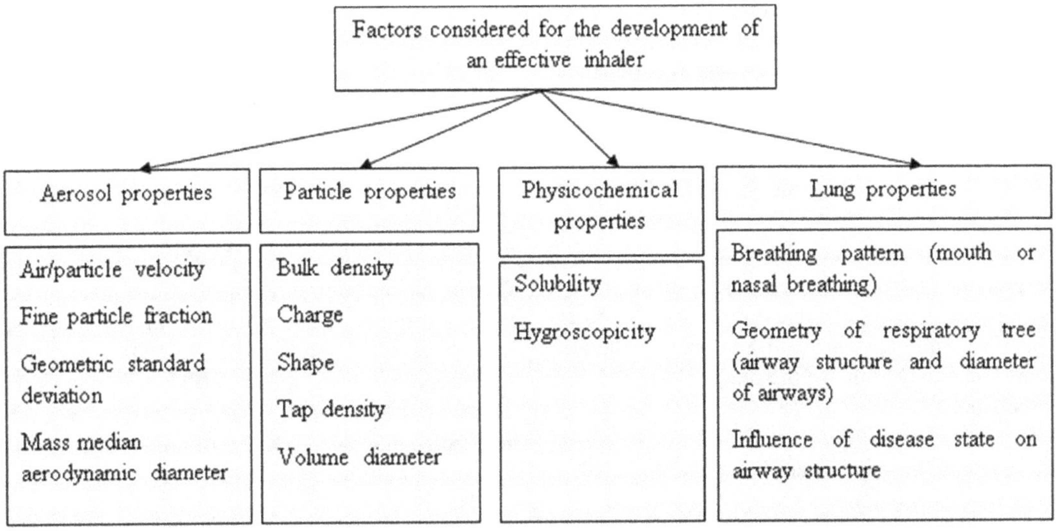

FIGURE 24.2 Factors considered for the development of an effective inhaler.

24.5 Modern Inhaler Devices and Their Challenges

One of the major challenges associated with modern inhalers is the accumulation of aerosol particles in the oropharynx and upper respiratory tract as well as the patient training required before its administration. pMDIs are small portable devices that deliver a measured amount of medication to the lungs. These inhalers produce aerosol quicker than can be inhaled. Thus, harmonization between rate of delivery of medication with its flow rate and inhalation of patient can be challenging in certain age groups such as children and the elderly.

24.5.1 Nebulizers for Liquid Material

Jet as well as ultrasonic nebulizers are different from each other in terms of pressures applied to produce the vapors from the liquid phase. Based on the type of model as well as the manufacturer, these nebulizers efficiently produce aerosols of size varying from 1 to 5 μm. These devices are a first choice when accurate harmonization between inhalation and actuation is required for the use of the pressurized regulated medication. Thus, these are suitable for children, aged, ventilated, coma, and ICU patients, and patients that are unable to use pressurized metered-dose inhalers or dry-powder inhaler. In comparison to other aerosol generators nebulizers efficiently deliver larger doses, but also require a large setup and are not portable and suitable doses need comparatively longer times for their administration. Jet nebulizers are based on the Venturi effect, which is based on creating constriction or cone in a pipe in order to reduce the pressure when it goes through the constriction site. Jet nebulization is based on movement of air (compressed gas) flow at high speed via a little duct (narrow passage or orifice) to reduce the pressure in order to convert the liquid into aerosols in the capillary tube. Air flow carrying the larger size droplets at high speed are allowed to pass through baffle to forms mist in form of smaller size droplets. These small droplets are renebulized and remain in the device until the size of the droplets is small enough to emit from the device. To prevent ill effects of high-velocity droplets in the oropharynx, baffles are installed in the nebulizer. Apart from their considerable advantages, jet nebulizer also have disadvantages such as considerable temperature drop in nebulized droplets due to vaporization, generation of noise, and the need for a compressor to move pressurized air stream from the tube for emission out of the nebulizer.

Ultrasonic nebulizers work in an opposite manner by increasing temperature of liquid using sound waves. They use vibration of piezoelectric crystals to create the sound waves that generate aerosol droplets with uniform size. However, since they require electricity and are not portable, are expensive, and can not nebulize viscous solutions or suspensions since they increase the temperature they are not frequently used.

- Ideally to release the appropriate dose from the nebulizer, the following parameters must be optimized:
- Pressure from the compressor in jet nebulizers as well as air stream must be optimized
- Design and material used in tube and mask must be validated and pretested
- Highly viscous solution resist nebulization because of this viscosity of the solution loaded must be optimized
- To avoid wasting drug solution, overall volume loaded in the nebulizer device must be optimized
- If these optimization procedures are not followed, there is a high chance of wasted drug solution in the form of dead volume, which can also cause inconsistency or dose variation. One of the major disadvantages of using nebulizers is that they have to be disassembled to be cleaned and then reassembled for each drug solution, which requires proper training. Liquid preparations are easier to administer via nebulizer than DPIs and pMDIs. Additionally, to improve therapeutic outcomes different EOs or medications can be blended and nebulized. Nevertheless, it is important to understand the viscosity of the solution and settings of the device to determine the size of the droplets.

A recent investigation showed the effect of inhalation via nebulization of rosemary, peppermint, and eucalyptus EOs on spirometry in 106 healthy participants. It was found that EOs did not show any effect on evaluated spirometric variables [26].

Recently, advanced nebulizer models have become available such as breath-enhanced (Pari LC® jet plus), breath-actuated (AeroEclipse®), and vibrating-mesh nebulizers (Pari eFlow® rapid, Omron U22, AKITA2® APIXNEB). These nebulizers have considerable advantages over conventional ones such as the following:

- Based on breathing pattern of individual emission of aerosol, which helps reduce loss of drug as well as enhances the inhaled mass
- Emission of medication in the environment must be prevented
- To avoid wasting drugs, nebulizes droplets at the time of the onset of inhalation
- Improves the output rate as well as reduces the delivery time
- Improves the amount of aerosol accumulated in the alveoli
- Decreases the dead volume of drug left in the nebulizer

24.5.2 Pressurized Metered-Dose Inhalers

Pressurized metered-dose inhalers are inhalers used to treat various respiratory complications. In one investigation, insulin nanoparticles were prepared by EOs (citral and cineole) as suspension stabilizers to form pMDI preparations. The findings demonstrated that the nanoparticles were suitable for peripheral accumulation in lungs and can be used to effectively administer therapeutics protein via inhalation for systemic effects [27].

Also, EOs including citral, menthol, eucalyptus oil, cinnamaldehyde, and cineole are being investigated as stabilizers for suspension metered-dose inhaler (MDI) formulations [28].

Remarkably, cineole with n-heptane [29] has been shown to improve suspension quality of a peptide nanoparticle, engineered by the mechanism developed by Tan et al [28–30]. A previous patented formulation for delivery via pMDIs was prepared that contained EO as the suspension stabilizer. In this invention, the EO was used as a nontoxic and miscible suspension stabilizer (because of its amphiphilic property, such as a ketone or aldehyde in nature) to deliver drug to the lungs [31].

24.5.3 Polymer-Mediated Encapsulation of EOs

Recently, EOs have gained a lot of attention due to their increased use in the pharmaceutical and cosmetic industries. However, EOs are often unstable in normal room conditions. This is mainly because of the presence of volatile and photo- and oxidation-sensitive compounds. Change in properties of these chemical compounds affects the stability and bioactivity of EOs. Nanoencapsulation of EOs by using synthetic or natural polymers is one of the most reliable approaches to improving their stability as well as shelf-life by protecting against external detrimental conditions [32–50]. Additionally, polymeric encapsulation of EOs improves water solubility and provides effective protection against external environmental variables such as degradation, oxidation, and temperature variation. Moreover, using this approach, EOs can be targeted and released in an in vivo environment at a specific site such as cell or tissue in a controlled manner. Out of all these approaches, polymeric nanoparticles, especially nanoprecipitation, have attracted great attention as they offer various advantages to EOs such as the following [32–50]:

- Shield against various detrimental factors
- Improve stability of whole formulation
- Control delivery of whole formulation
- Enhance bioavailability of whole formulation
- Improve efficacy of whole formulation
- Simple and reproducible technique

Various natural (derived from algal, mammalian, plant, marine, and other sources) and synthetic polymers can be used for this purpose [50–53]. An earlier report suggested improvement in antiherpetic activity when *Cymbopogon citratus* EO was encapsulated with poly (lactide-co-glycolide)-NP in comparison with non-capsulated oil [53]. Additionally, in a previous study, eugenol was encapsulated by poly-ε-caprolactone to improve its stability against light oxidation [54]. Another report suggested the use of natural polymers such as gelatin and Arabic gum to encapsulate *Jasminum officinale L.* EO to improve its heat resistance [55,56].

REFERENCES

1. Su HJ, Chao CJ, Chang HY, Wu PC. The effects of evaporating essential oils on indoor air quality. *Atmos Environ.* 2007;41:1230–1236.
2. Oberhofer B, Nikiforov A, Buchbauer G, Jirovetz L, Bicchi C. Investigation of the alteration of the composition of various essential oils used in aroma lamp applications. *Flavour Fragr J.* 1999;14:293–299.
3. Gaunt LF, Higgins SC, Hughes JF. Interaction of air ions and bactericidal vapours to control micro-organisms. *J Appl Microbiol.* 2005;99:1324–1329.
4. Sato K, Krist S, Buchbauer G. Antimicrobial effect of trans-cinnamaldehyde, (–)-perillaldehyde, (–)-citronellal, citral, eugenol and carvacrol on airborne microbes using an airwasher. *Biol Pharm Bull.* 2006;29:2292–2294.
5. Krist S, Sato K, Glasl S, Heoferl M, Saukel J. Antimicrobial effect of vapours of terpinol. (R)-(–)-linalool, carvacrol, (S)-(–)- perillaldehyde and 1,8-cineole on airborne microbes using a room diffuser. *Flavour Fragr.* 2008;23:353–356.
6. Doran AL, Morden WE, Dunn K, Edwards-Jones V. Vapour-phase activities of essential oils against antibiotic sensitive and resistant bacteria including MRSA. *Lett Appl Microbiol.* 2009;48(4):387–392.
7. Bouaziz M, Yangui T, Sayadi S, Dhouib A. Disinfectant properties of essential oils from *Salvia officinalis* L. cultivated in Tunisia. *Food Chem Toxicol.* 2009;47(11):2755–2760.
8. Liu SH, Lin TH, Chang KM. The physical effects of aromatherapy in alleviating work-related stress on elementary school teachers in Taiwan. *Evid Based Complement Alternat Med.* 2013;2013:853809.
9. Gelmini F, Belotti L, Vecchi S, Testa C, Beretta G. Air dispersed essential oils combined with standard sanitization procedures for environmental microbiota control in nosocomial hospitalization rooms. *Complement Ther Med.* 2016;25:113–119.
10. Remberg P, Björk L, Hedner T, Sterner O. Characteristics, clinical effect profile and tolerability of a nasal spray preparation of *Artemisia abrotanum* L. for allergic rhinitis. *Phytomedicine.* 2004;11(1):36–42.
11. Caimmi D, Neukirch C, Louis R, Malard O, Thabut G, Demoly P. Effect of the use of intranasal spray of essential oils in patients with perennial allergic rhinitis: A prospective study. *Int Arch Allergy Immunol.* 2020;182:1–8.
12. Xie Y, Lu W, Cao S, Jiang X, Yin M, Tang W. Preparation of bupleurum nasal spray and evaluation on its safety and efficacy. *Chem Pharm Bull (Tokyo).* 2006;54(1):48–53.
13. Ben-Arye E, Dudai N, Eini A, Torem M, Schiff E, Rakover Y. Treatment of upper respiratory tract infections in primary care: A randomized study using aromatic herbs. *Evid Based Complement Alternat Med.* 2011;2011:690346.
14. Katona G, Sultész M, Farkas Z. et al. Treatment of acute rhinitis with a nasal spray containing tramazoline and essential oils: A multicenter, uncontrolled, observational trial. *Clin Transl Allergy.* 2015;5:38.
15. Lu M, Yan W, Zhu X, Zhu H. Exogenous lipoid pneumonia induced by long-term usage of compound menthol nasal drops: A case report. *Beijing Da Xue Xue Bao Yi Xue Ban.* 2019;51(2):359–361.
16. Ghorat F, Shahrestani S, Tagabadi Z, Bazghandi M. The effect of inhalation of essential oils of polianthes tuberosa on test anxiety in students: A clinical trial. *Iran J Med Sci.* 2016;41(3 Suppl):S13.
17. Velepič M, Manestar D, Perković I, Škalamera D, Braut T. Inhalation aerosol therapy in the treatment of chronic rhinosinusitis: A prospective randomized study. *J Clin Pharmacol.* 2019;59(12):1648–1655.
18. Cox A, Wood K, Coleman G, Stewart AJ, Bertin FR, Owen H, Suen WW, Medina-Torres CE. Essential oil spray reduces clinical signs of insect bite hypersensitivity in horses. *Aust Vet J.* 2020;98(8):411–416.

19. Anderson PJ. History of aerosol therapy: Liquid nebulization to MDIs to DPIs. *Respir Care.* 2005;50(9):1139–1150.
20. Sanders M. Inhalation therapy: An historical review. *Prim Care Respir J.* 2007;16(2):71–81.
21. Labiris NR, Dolovich MB. Pulmonary drug delivery. Part I: Physiological factors affecting therapeutic effectiveness of aerosolized medications. *Br J Clin Pharmacol.* 2003;56(6):588–599.
22. Crompton G. A brief history of inhaled asthma therapy over the last fifty years. *Prim Care Respir J.* 2006;15(6):326–331.
23. Hess DR. Aerosol delivery devices in the treatment of asthma. *Respir Care.* 2008;53(6):699–723.
24. Chow AH, Tong HH, Chattopadhyay P, Shekunov BY. Particle engineering for pulmonary drug delivery. *Pharm Res.* 2007;24(3):411–437.
25. Usachev EV, Pyankov OV, Usacheva OV, Agranovski IE. Antiviral activity of tea tree and eucalyptus oil aerosol and vapour. *J Aerosol Sci.* 2013;59:22–30.
26. Patton JS, Byron PR. Inhaling medicines: Delivering drugs to the body through the lungs. *Nat Rev Drug Discov.* 2007;6(1):67–74.
27. Köteles F, Babulka P, Szemerszky R, Dömötör Z, Boros S. Inhaled peppermint, rosemary and eucalyptus essential oils do not change spirometry in healthy individuals. *Physiol Behav.* 2018;194:319–323.
28. Nyambura BK, Kellaway IW, Taylor KM. Insulin nanoparticles: Stability and aerosolization from pressurized metered dose inhalers. *Int J Pharm.* 2009;375(1–2):114–122.
29. Tan Y, Yang Z, Pan X, Chen M, Feng M, Wang L, Liu H, Shan Z, Wu C. Stability and aerosolization of pressurized metered dose inhalers containing thymopentin nanoparticles produced using a bottom-up process. *Int J Pharm.* 2012;427(2):385–392.
30. Kellaway IW, Taylor K, Nyambura BK, inventors; School of Pharmacy, University of London, assignee. Formulations for delivery via pressurised metered dose inhalers comprising an essential oil as suspension stabiliser. European patent EP 2,089,008. 20 July 2011.
31. Tan Y, Yang Z, Peng X, Xin F, Xu Y, Feng M, Zhao C, Hu H, Wu C. A novel bottom-up process to produce nanoparticles containing protein and peptide for suspension in hydrofluoroalkane propellants. *Int J Pharm.* 2011;413(1–2):167–173.
32. Kellaway IW, Taylor K, Nyambura BK. Formulations for delivery via pressurised metered dose inhalers comprising an essential oil as suspension stabiliser. WO2008053250A2.
33. Bhatia S, Kumar V, Sharma K, Nagpal K, Bera T. Significance of algal polymer in designing amphotericin B nanoparticles. *Sci World J.* 2014;2014:564573.
34. Bhatia S, Rathee P, Sharma K, Chaugule BB, Kar N, Bera T. Immuno-modulation effect of sulphated polysaccharide (porphyran) from Porphyra vietnamensis. *Int J Biol Macromol.* 2013;57:50–56.
35. Bhatia S. *Natural Polymer Drug Delivery Systems: Marine Polysaccharides Based Nano-Materials and Its Applications.* Springer International Publishing, Switzerland; 2016;185–225.
36. Bhatia S. *Natural Polymer Drug Delivery Systems: Plant Derived Polymers, Properties, and Modification & Applications.* Springer International Publishing, Switzerland; 2016;119–184.
37. Bhatia S. *Natural Polymer Drug Delivery Systems: Nanotechnology and Its Drug Delivery Applications.* Springer International Publishing, Switzerland; 2016;1–32.
38. Bhatia S. *Natural Polymer Drug Delivery Systems: Nanoparticles Types, Classification, Characterization, Fabrication Methods and Drug Delivery Applications.* Springer International Publishing, Switzerland; 2016;33–93.
39. Bhatia S. *Natural Polymer Drug Delivery Systems: Natural Polymers vs Synthetic Polymer.* Springer International Publishing, Switzerland; 2016;95–118.
40. Bhatia S. *Systems for Drug Delivery: Mammalian Polysaccharides and Its Nanomaterials.* Springer International Publishing, Switzerland; 2016;1–27.
41. Bhatia S. *Systems for Drug Delivery: Microbial Polysaccharides as Advance Nanomaterials.* Springer International Publishing, Switzerland; 2016;29–54.
42. Bhatia S. *Systems for Drug Delivery: Chitosan Based Nanomaterials and Its Applications.* Springer International Publishing, Switzerland; 2016;55–117.
43. Bhatia S. *Systems for Drug Delivery: Advance Polymers and Its Applications.* Springer International Publishing, Switzerland; 2016;119–146.
44. Bhatia S. *Systems for Drug Delivery: Advanced Application of Natural Polysaccharides.* Springer International Publishing, Switzerland; 2016;147–170.
45. Bhatia S. *Systems for Drug Delivery: Modern Polysaccharides and Its Current Advancements.* Springer International Publishing, Switzerland; 2016;171–188.
46. Bhatia S. *Systems for Drug Delivery: Toxicity of Nanodrug Delivery Systems.* Springer International Publishing, Switzerland; 2016;189–197.
47. Bhatia S. *Nanotechnology in Drug Delivery Fundamentals, Design, and Applications: Part 1: Protein and Peptide-Based Drug Delivery Systems.* Apple Academic Press, Palm Bay, FL; 2016;50–204.
48. Bhatia S. *Nanotechnology in Drug Delivery Fundamentals, Design, and Applications: Part 2: Peptide-Mediated Nanoparticle Drug Delivery System.* Apple Academic Press, Palm Bay, FL; 2016:205–280.
49. Bhatia S. *Nanotechnology in Drug Delivery Fundamentals, Design, and Applications: Part 3: CPP and CTP in Drug Delivery and Cell Targeting.* Apple Academic Press, Palm Bay, FL; 2016;309–312.
50. Turek C, Stintzing FC. Stability of essential oils: A review. *Compr Rev Food Sci Food Saf.* 2013;12:40–53.
51. Bilia, AR, Guccione C, Isacchi B, Righeschi C, Firenzuoli F, Bergonzi MC. Essential oils loaded in nanosystems: A developing strategy for a successful therapeutic approach. *Evid Based Complement Altern Med.* 2014;2014:1–14.
52. Pedro AS, Santo IE, Silva CV, Detoni C, Albuquerque E. The use of nanotechnology as an approach for essential oil-based formulations with antimicrobial activity. In: Méndez-Vila A, (editor). *Microbial Pathogens and Strategies for Combating Them: Science, Technology and Education.* Formatex Research Center, Badajoz, Spain; 2013;2:1364–1374.
53. Almeida, KB, Araujo JL, Cavalcanti JF, Romanos MTV, Mourão SC, Amaral ACF, Falcão, DQ. In vitro release and anti-herpetic activity of *Cymbopogon citratus* DC. volatile oil-loaded nanogel. *Rev Bras Farm.* 2018;28:498–502.

54. Choi M, Soottitantawat A, Nuchuchua O, Min S, Ruktanonchai U. Physical and light oxidative properties of eugenol encapsulated by molecular inclusion and emulsion-diffusion method. *Food Res Int*. 2009;42:148–156.
55. Lv Y, Yang F, Li X, Zhang X, Abbas S. Formation of heat-resistant nanocapsules of jasmine essential oil via gelatin/gum arabic based complex coacervation. *Food Hydrocoll*. 2014;35:305–314.
56. Miladi K, Sfar S, Fessi H, Elaissari A. Nanoprecipitation process: From particle preparation to in vivo applications. In: Vauthier C, Ponchel G (editors). *Polymer Nanoparticles for Nanomedicines*. Springer, Cham, Switzerland; 2016:17–53.

25

Toxicity Associated with Essential Oils

Ahmed Al-Harrasi
Natural and Medical Sciences Research Center, University of Nizwa

Saurabh Bhatia
Natural and Medical Sciences Research Center, University of Nizwa
University of Petroleum and Energy Studies

Tapan Behl
Chitkara University

Deepak Kaushik
M.D. University

Vineet Mittal
M.D. University

Ajay Sharma
Delhi Pharmaceutical Sciences and Research University

CONTENTS

DOI: 10.1201/9781003175933-27

25.1 Introduction

Essential oils (EOs) have gained increased attention due to their diverse applications in different sectors such as the pharmaceutical, cosmetic, and food industries. Due to the complex composition of EOs, they could be acutely toxic to humans and animals in small amounts. Regardless of the requirement, there are several reports of toxicity of EOs even at low dose, thus the toxicity as well as safety profiles of EOs in experimental models including animals and human subjects are required to ensure their safe use. The US FDA (United States Food and Drug Administration) designated a list of EOs as well as their components as GRAS (generally recognized as safe) along with their safe limits for food applications. The European Commission in 2012 officially sanctioned the utilization of EOs along with their permissible limits for their utilization in the food industry. Thus, considering their safety profiles, these EOs can be used in a small amount for medicinal use. In aromatherapy, EOs must be typically used with proper recommendations given by herbalist or aromatherapist or general physician. Use of several commonly used EOs could be rarely harmful or could be having very low systemic toxicity at 2% dilution (conditionally, they are not impure). Nevertheless, safety profiles and toxicity studies on different age groups, on different comorbid patients, and during pregnancy and childbirth have not been established. Topical complications such as hypersensitivity and allergic reactions, acute inflammation, itching, and sensitization are the major concerns. Combinations or blends (EO-EO, EO-EO-EO, EO-CC [chemical component of EO], EO-drug, EO-phytochemical, CC-drug, EO-drug-CC, EO-plant extract, EO-Vitamin) in different proportions make these multicomponent systems more complex, which can increase toxicity and impact safety [1].

25.2 Toxicity of EOs

Very few studies are available on the safety and toxicity of EOs. Because EOs are known for their antimicrobial effects mainly by causing injury to cell membrane, it is suspected that EOs are mainly lethal to prokaryotic cellular organisms and not for eukaryotic cells. The majority of EOs have not been tested for toxicity in animal models, cell lines, or animal cell–based assays. Most of the cited literature represents the antimicrobial potential of EOs. Due to the unknown toxicity and safety profiles of the majority of EOs, in comparison with antibiotics, EOs have limited use. Certainly, considerable investigations based on EO toxicity against eukaryotic cells, including fungi, larvae, and molluscs have been reported. Only a few reports are available on the effect of EOs in human cell lines in vitro. For assessing cytotoxic activity and effects of EOs in cell viability a tetrazole based 3-(4,5-dimethylthiazol-2-yl)-2,5-diphenyltetrazolium bromide method has been used against different cell lines. Thymol as well carvacrol have been found to be cytotoxic against human colorectal adenocarcinoma cell lines.

Another report showed that *Artemisia indica* EO showed dose-dependent suppression against human leukemia monocytic, adenocarcinoma alveolar basal epithelial cells, laryngeal cancer cells, and colorectal adenocarcinoma cell-based cell lines. An additional report showed that apple mint EO was found to be cytotoxic against human colon cancer, glioblastoma, and ovarian adenocarcinoma cell lines.

Reports also showed that oral administration of tea tree EO at high dose caused toxicity as well as irritation to the skin. It was also found that tea tree EO caused considerable skin allergy among susceptible individuals. This could be because of the various chemically transformed products that undergo oxidation from oil exposure to light and/or air [2]. The cytotoxic diterpene, 6,7-dehydroroyleanone, is the main component of *Plectranthus madagascariensis* EO [3]. In humans, several *in vivo* studies based on toxicity after the accidental ingestion of EOs (in large quantities) have been reported; however, accidental ingestion is not characteristic of toxic at likely curative doses. Posadzki et al. [4] studied the adverse effects of EOs used in aromatherapy. It was found that EO application usually via massage can cause allergic reactions or dermatitis, which are very common forms of adverse effects found with many EOs. Occurrence of other harmful effects such as kidney malfunction, lung stress, uncontrollable muscle contractions, unsteady movements, and prolonged unconsciousness was reported but less common. Evidence of mortality after topical and oral utilization of wintergreen EO in an 80-year-old male has been observed. However, a previous report did not reveal frequency or extent of common adverse effects related to EO application to assess safety in human subjects. It was realized that toxicity concerns related to some EOs cannot be generalized to a complete class of EOs as they depend on many factors, such as chemical composition of the EO, dose, route of administration, pharmacokinetic profile of EO, kind of interaction of EO in combination or blend form, health and age of an individual, and many other factors. Moreover, the toxicity profiles of EOs vary based on their different chemical components.

A monoterpenoidal ketone component, namely thujone, is extensively found in different plants such as *Artemisia artemisia, Salvia sclarea, Salvia officinalis, Tanacetum vulgare,* and *Thuja occidentalis L.* has been found to be toxic. Keton-based natural products are usually not toxic; nevertheless, thujone is the most toxic. Thus, safety assessment of EOs especially using standardized extracts or isolated components is essential.

There is little information available on the toxicity of EO vapors; however, toxicity profiles must be evaluated before their use as marketable antimicrobial agents. As EOs are multicomponent systems with various volatile components, each volatile component must be examined for its potential allergic effects. The European Flavor and Fragrance Association registered 24 allergens related to EOs; nevertheless, these allergic reactions are only observed after topical application and not inhalation. An investigation based on assessment of the volatile compounds of five EOs (rose, citrus limon, *Rosmarinus officinalis*, and *Melaleuca alternifolia*) in gaseous phase demonstrated that cancer causing agent, benzene, was found into that specific environment; however, the level was considerably less to cause any acute adverse reactions Hypersensitive individuals exposed to aromatic oil via pulmonary or ocular routes at 5 minutes (with overall exposure time of 30 minutes) showed increase in symptoms such as shortness of breath, coughing, and ocular irritation compared to placebo group. It was also found that volatile components present in EOs when vaporized in the form of aerosols encounter oxidizing agents resulting in the formation of pollutants (e.g., formaldehyde). These volatile components include ethers, hydrocarbons, terpenes, dextro-limonenes, and alcohols. EO components containing unsaturated hydrocarbons (alkenes as well as alkynes group), especially those with one or more double or triple bonds, are more vulnerable against reaction with oxidizing agents.

Therefore, this interaction between same or different EOs components always results in the formation of secondary pollutants along with the oxidation of components such as oxidation of limonene and linalool resulting into the formation of high molecular weight oxidation products such as aldehydes, ketones, and organic acids. On the other hand, the US EPA lists Citronella EO as an insect repellent because of its high effectiveness, low toxicity, and customer satisfaction [5]. Similarly, myrtle EO was not cytotoxic to human keratinocyte cell line, HaCaT; hepatocyte cell line, HepG2; and alveolar epithelial cell line, A549, at 0.64 mg/mL.

Phyllogonium viride EO containing germacrene B, beta-chamigrene, beta-caryophyllene, and beta-bazzanene also did not show cytotoxicity against colorectal tumor as well as breast cells at different doses [6].

Artemisia dracunculus EO containing methyl chavicol or tarragon (64.94%) did not cause any cytotoxicity (IC50 20 μL/mL) [7]. *Aloysia polystachya* EO containing dihydrocarvone, (R)-(−)-carvone, and R-(+)-limonene showed prominent toxicity against all cancerous cells (breast, colon, and prostate) [8].

Furthermore, Brazilian *Aniba rosaeodora* EO containing linalool did not cause any cytotoxicity among thioglycollate-elicited BALB/c mouse peritoneal macrophages and decreased levels of nitrite among unstimulated cells, suggesting a possible effect on nitic oxide synthesis [9].

Rhynchanthus beesianus EO containing 1,8-cineole (47.6%), borneol (15.0%), methyleugenol (11.2%), and bornyl formate (7.6%) at 128 μg/mL considerably reduced the level of interleukin-6, tumor necrosis factor-α, proinflammatory mediators, nitric oxide, and cytokines in lipopolysaccharide-stimulated RAW264.7 macrophages without any cytotoxic effect [10]. A previous study showed that treatment of human liver cancer cell line with estragole did not show any signs of cytotoxicity. In 2015, potential genotoxicity and mutagenicity caused by EOs and their constituents from aromatic plants and spices were investigated. It was found that except coriander, oregano, rosemary, carvacrol, and citral at high dose, the majority of EOs and their components did not show any mutagenic or genotoxic effects.

These and other investigations demonstrating cytotoxic and genotoxic effects of EOs and their related compounds are slowing the development of EOs as antimicrobial agents.

However, to develop the complete metabolic profiles of cytotoxic as well as genotoxic components from EOs in vivo investigations are required. In 2016, an in vivo (rodent) investigation showed that EOs and their components such as berberine, t-anethole, pulgeone, eugenol, and estragole are genotoxic, carcinogenic, or hepatotoxic. In contrast, various investigations have shown that EOs as well as their constituents are not harmful and are safe if used per the standard recommendations.

In 2011, a study demonstrated that 17 GRAS EO chemical compounds such as beta-caryophyllene, para-cymene, and camphene did not cause any toxicity to rodents. Furthermore, in 2017, a study revealed that treatment of rodents with *Oregano vulgare* EO at 200 mg/kg for 90 days did not produce any adverse effects. Similarly, it was found that treatment of rodents with *Piper glabratum* EO at high dose of 5,000 mg/kg did not cause adverse effects. *Foeniculum vulgare* EO at high dose of 0.5 mL/kg also did not considerably influence biochemical parameters such as tumor necrosis factor-alpha-a secretion, red blood cell count, white blood cell count, level of proteins, and also other parameters such as body weight and hepatic histopathological parameters in male rodents. Thus, it was concluded that EOs and their components could have protective or toxic effects, which are primarily dependent on the dose, chemical composition, and kind of interaction of EOs with each other or with main course medication.

25.3 Assessment of EO Toxicity

To meet the conditions of authorities such as the European Food Safety Authority, which assists in protecting against food-associated concerns such as food poisoning, toxicity etc., EOs and their components can be assessed by using the following parameters:

- *Allium cepa* assay: Common onion (*Allium cepa*) is used for the determination of different toxicity such as genotoxicity with the mitotic index.
- Comet assay: Occurrence of DNA damage as well as genotoxic effects can be determined by comet assay (standard and enzyme-modified). EOs can be examined for their potential to induce deoxyribonucleic acid (DNA) fragmentation in human cell lines by using this assay.
- Toxicity profiles of various EOs by *in vitro* (different normal or cancerous cell lines, cell cultures, harvested cells) assays and *in vivo* (*Caenorhabditis elegans* survival or toxicity assay, fertilized hen's egg chorioallantoic membrane assay) methods.
- Somatic mutation and the recombination test can be used to check the mutation frequency caused by EOs.
- Genotoxicity (by comet assay, DNA diffusion assays, etc.) can be performed by using different mammalian cell lines to test EOs.
- In vitro cytotoxicity (by trypan blue dye exclusion, MTT test, etc.) can be performed by using different mammalian cell lines to test EOs. Cell death assay, apoptosis, can be assessed by using Annexin/propidium iodide (PI) double staining.
- Sister chromatid exchange can be used to detect the genomic rearrangement or interchange of DNA between sister chromatids. This assay indicates interchange of DNA between replication products, which is an early sign of unstable chromosome after exposure to any genotoxic agents.

- Chromosome aberration examination can be used to evaluate the potential of a test compound (EO) to induce structural chromosomal abnormalities, including breaks and exchanges.
- Micronucleus assays are frequently used to assess chromosomal damage as a consequence of EO exposure.
- Oxidative stress [ROS (reactive oxygen species) generation] induced by the EO, modulation of catalase (CAT) and superoxide dismutase (SOD) activities by EO, malondialdehyde (MDA) levels by EO.
- Effect of EOs on changes in food and water intakes, body mass index, comparative organ weight, blood as well as serum biochemical parameters or histological (liver and kidneys) parameters in comparison with the control group can be evaluated. Histopathological changes including death of body tissue, swelling, and inflammation in the hepatic, renal, and spleen after EO administration can also be determined.
- In vivo zebrafish assay can be used to evaluate acute toxicity.

25.4 Protective and Toxic or Adverse Effects of EOs

Some important examples of EOs, their protective and toxic or adverse effects, are listed below.

25.4.1 *Achyrocline flaccida* EO

Achyrocline flaccida EO from southern Brazil containing α-pinene (41.10%) and caryophyllene (30.52%) as main components did not show any indications of DNA or chromosomal damage in single-cell gel electrophoresis and displayed significant antioxidant effects via preventing reactive oxygen species generation in the *Caenorhabditis elegans* assay [11].

25.4.2 *Aquilaria crassna*

Aquilaria crassna EO is known for its traditional uses to treat nausea, rheumatoid arthritis, complications associated with airways, and cough. Recently, acute toxicity investigations were performed in Swiss female mice by oral administration of EO (one time/day) at 2,000 mg/kg, and subchronic studies were performed at two different doses for 28 days. No considerable variations in body weight, food as well as water intake behavior, blood parameters, and biochemical findings, relative organ weights, macroscopic presentation of disease, or microscopic examination of tissue compared control group were found. These findings suggest that agarwood EO is safe and can be used therapeutically [12].

25.4.3 *Ayapana triplinervis* EO

Ayapana triplinervis contains thymohydroquinone dimethyl ether; both have been recently reported as reliable antiviral agents against mosquito-borne viral infection (ZIKV infection) responsible for causing neonatal microcephaly and neurological disorders in humans. To study acute toxicity of thymohydroquinone dimethyl ether in vivo, zebrafish assay was used. Time-of-drug-addition apparoacg for mechanism of action as well as target identification showed that thymohydroquinone dimethyl ether may possibly act by inhibiting virus entry. At the viral inhibitory dose, thymohydroquinone dimethyl ether administration in zebrafish did not cause stress and influence the existence of the fish, suggesting the nonexistence of severe toxicity for thymohydroquinone dimethyl ether [13].

25.4.4 *Achillea millefolium* EO

Achillea millefolium EO has been extensively used for various ailments. It is widely known for its antimicrobial effects against pathogenic microorganisms. A previous investigation showed genotoxicity after the administration of *Achillea millefolium* EO containing chamazulene, sabinene, terpin-4-ol, beta-caryophyllene, and eucalyptol as major components. Assessment of genotoxic effects induced by the EO was determined by study of diploid cells of *Aspergillus nidulans*. It was found that at 0.19–0.25 μL/mL the EO substantially induced mitotic recombination in diploid cells of *Aspergillus nidulans*. The genotoxicity of the EO could be due to the induction of mitotic nondisjunction or crossing over by the EO [14].

25.4.5 *Croton campestris* EO

Croton campestris EO contains germacrene-D, β-caryophyllene, and 1,8-cineol as key components. The administration of *Croton campestris* EO orally did not show any toxicity (LD_{50} >5,000 mg/kg). Additionally, due to chemical profile, the EO presented anti-inflammatory activity, which could be due to inhibitory effects on cytokines mediated by histamine and arachidonic acid-based pathways [15]. *Croton rhamnifolioides* EO containing spathulenol and 1,8-cineole as main components showed no significant toxicity after oral administration in mice and prevented gastric lesions in all mice models [16].

25.4.6 *Cymbopogon giganteus* EO

Based on findings obtained from oral acute toxicity (at 2,000 mg/kg body weight per day) and oral subacute toxicity studies (50 and 500 mg/kg), *Cymbopogon giganteus* EO was determined to have caused neither mortality nor toxicity (LD50>2,000 mg/kg) or significant changes in body and organ weight variation, blood parameters as well as biochemical findings, or histopathological findings compared to control group.

However, inhalation toxicity findings revealed that the EO caused death and acute lung inflammation after one treatment of EO (2%–5% v/v), whereas one treatment at 0.125%–0.5% v/v was found to be safe [17]. It was also found recently that *Cymbopogon khasianus* EO containing a high level of methyl eugenol has promising antimicrobial effects; nevertheless, the EO must be standardized for its methyl eugenol content and utilization must be within permissible limits. Recently, seed germination assay revealed the herbicidal effects of methyl eugenol-rich EO. Furthermore, genotoxicity of the EO has been shown by using Allium cepa test [18].

25.4.7 *Citrus aurantifolia* EO

Toxicity profile after treatment (P.O.) with C. aurantifolia EO containing nine components (i.e., anethole, anisole, citral, demitol, germacrene, linalool, bornane, pinene, safrole) was assessed via single-dose (acute toxicity) and multiple-dose administration. It was found that the EO did not show any acute toxic reaction but repeated dose systemic toxicity findings showed that the toxicity depended on dose and time. Histopathological findings indicated changes such as the death of body tissue, swelling due to fluid accumulation, and hepatic, renal, and spleen inflammation. Findings from in vivo studies demonstrated apart from its established profile that lime EO may possibly cause mild toxicity to blood cells, kidney, and liver [19].

25.4.8 *Curcuma caesia* EO

Recently, *Curcuma caesia* EO enriched with camphor, epicurzerenone, and eucalyptol was evaluated for genotoxic effects by using *Allium cepa* (onion) test. *Allium cepa* (onion) test demonstrated minimum genotoxic effects [20].

25.4.9 *Cinnamodendron dinisii* EO

Recently, *Cinnamodendron dinisii* EO was studied to evaluate toxic effects against cells, lytic effects on blood cells, and to determine its potential to cause fragmentation of DNA in human lymphocytes by using Comet assay. It was found that the EO demonstrated high toxic effects against kidney cells (Vero cells) as well as caused destruction of red blood cells and hemoglobin was also oxidized. *C. dinisii* EO also demonstrated genotoxicity resulting in dose-determined fragmentation of DNA in lymph cells. It was concluded that the *C. dinisii* EO has showed toxicity, proposing its application for clinical applications [21].

25.4.10 *Cinnamomum verum* Leaf EO

In vivo toxicity of this EO was determined using *Galleria mellonella* larvae, and it was found that it did not cause any toxicity at any concentration [22]. Another study based on acute and subacute toxicity demonstrated that *Cinnamomum osmophloeum* leaf EO at 1 ml/kg body weight and cinnamaldehyde at 4 mg/kg body weight did not show any considerable variations in hepatic as well as renal function and pathological parameters [23].

25.4.11 *Faeniculum vulgare* EO

Recently, th eprotective effects of fennel EO from *Faeniculum vulgare* against insecticide triflumuron pretreated human colon cancer cell line was evaluated. It was found that treatment of HCT116 cell with fennel EO increased cell viability, decreased reactive oxygen species production, and modulated catalase as well as and superoxide dismutase activities induced by triflumuron with decrease in MDA levels. Also, the fennel EO decreased DNA damage and there was considerable decrease in the membrane potential loss of mitochondria. Thus, it was concluded that *Faeniculum vulgare* EO could be a valuable shield against the lethal effects caused by insecticide in human colon cancer cells [24].

25.4.12 *Gautheria procumbens* EO

Gautheria procumbens EO containing linalool as well as methyl salicylate revealed no indications of nuclear abnormalities at various concentrations. Additionally, it was suggested that this EO can be considered as a potential option to develop preparations to deal with illnesses triggered by pathogenic microbes [25].

25.4.13 *Gallesia integrifolia* EO

Gallesia integrifolia has been proven to treat peptic ulcer. Gas chromatography–mass spectrometry (GC–MS) analysis showed that *Gallesia integrifolia* EO contains 27 components, mainly (–)-alpha-santalene. In vitro cytotoxicity and genotoxicity against CHO-K1 cells and in vivo oral acute toxicity studies revealed that *Gallesia integrifolia* EO is safe [26].

25.4.14 Lavender EO

Genotoxic effects of lavender EO as well as its main chemical compounds, linalyl acetate as well as linalool, have been recently assessed in vitro by the micronucleus test on peripheral human lymphocytes. It was found that this monoterpene ester namely linalyl acetate improved the incidence of micronuclei considerably while linalool did not show any genotoxic effects. The results demonstrated that the ability of lavender EO to cause mutation could be due to linalyl acetate [27]. Lavender and immortelle EOs are extensively used to treat health conditions. Recently, the cytogenic as well as genotoxic activities of immortelle as well as lavender EOs were evaluated by means of *Allium cepa* test and lymph cells. Findings from this study demonstrated that immortelle as well as lavender EO treatment increased the incidence of chromosome abnormalities compared to control group. Both EOs also enhanced the rate of programmed cell death and necrosis at varied concentrations. It was revealed that the studied EOs showed cytogenic as well as genotoxic activities in both human as well as plant cells [28].

25.4.15 *Litsea cubeba* EO

Litsea cubeba EO is obtained from of *Litsea cubeb* fruits. In a previous study, the toxicity (acute toxicity as well as genotoxicity tests) of *L. cubeba* EO was evaluated. Findings from this study showed that the lethal dose 50 (oral), the lethal dose 50 (skin), and the lethal concentration 50 (pulmonary) were around 4,000 mg/kg b. wt., 5,000 mg/kg, and ~12,500 parts per million, respectively. Thus, it was found that *L. cubeba* EO is somewhat lethal. Moreover, the genotoxicity findings showed that *Litsea cubeba* EO did not cause any genotoxicity when tested over *Salmonella typhimurium* [29].

25.4.16 *Mesosphaerum sidifolium* EO and Fenchone

Recently, *Mesosphaerum sidifolium* EO as well as its main component, fenchone (24.8%), were assessed for their toxic effects by using hemolysis assay and acute toxicity and micronucleus tests. *Mesosphaerum sidifolium* EO showed HC50

494.9 μg/mL whereas fenchone presented HC50 >3,000 μg/mL. *Mesosphaerum sidifolium* EO when administered in mice presented lethal dose 50 at about 500 mg/kg. It was found that this EO at 300 mg/kg caused rise in micronucleated erythrocytes, signifying mild genetic toxicity. Thus, it was concluded that this EO caused loss in weight but blood as well as biochemical findings and hepatic as well as renal histological findings showed no toxicity. However, fenchone treatment induced decrease of aspartate transaminase and alanine aminotransferase signifying liver injury [30].

25.4.17 *Origanum vulgare* EO

A recent study showed the antioxidant and antimicrobial effects of *Origanum spp.* EO, which makes it suitable for use as a food additive. To meet the specifications of the European Commission on Food Safety, recently, *Origanum vulgare* EO containing carvacrol (55.82%) and thymol (5.14%) was tested for genetic toxicity by Micronuclei testing as well as standard and enzyme-modified comet assay in rodents. Findings obtained from genotoxicity assays showed negative results in micronucleus test and comet assay (standard). Also, in enzyme-modified comet assay no evident destruction caused by oxidative stress was observed after treatment of rats with oregano EO. Thus, this oregano EO may be reliable and nontoxic and could be a valuable active agent in the food industry [31].

25.4.18 *Piper vicosanum* EO

Recently, the toxicological effects of *Piper vicosanum* EO via acute toxicity, genotoxicity, and mutagenicity tests were evaluated. It was found that *Piper vicosanum* EO did not show any acute toxicity (LD50 > 2,000 mg/kg). The results obtained from comet assay revealed that the Piper vicosanum EO did not show increase in the occurrence of DNA damage. Micronucleus analysis indicated that the EO-treated animals did not possess any cytotoxic or genotoxic changes in peripheral blood erythrocytes. These findings suggest that *Piper vicosanum* EO does not cause acute toxicity or genotoxicity [32].

25.4.19 Sandalwood EO

The cytotoxic and genotoxicity of sandalwood EO in human breast cancer (MCF-7) and human breast epithelial cell line (MCF-10A) cells were evaluated, and proteins linked to SEO genotoxicity were identified using a proteomics approach. The findings revealed that sandalwood EO caused genetic toxicity as well as induced DNA breaks (single and double) in human breast cancer cells [33].

25.4.20 *Satureja khuzistanica* EO

Satureja khuzistanica containing carvacrol (92.87%) and limonene (1.2%) has been used in folk medicine due to its antimicrobial and toxic effects to cancerous cells. This EO considerably decreased viability of cells (Vero, SW480, MCF7, and JET 3 cells) in a concentration-dependent way [34].

25.4.21 *Thymus vulgaris* EO

Algerian *Thymus vulgaris* EO (Lamiaceae) containing thymol (Mostaganem) as the major component showed acute toxicity in rodent at 4,500 mg/kg (via oral route), whereas Tlemcen EO at maximum dose of 5,000 mg/kg did not show any indications of acute toxicity [35].

25.4.22 *Xylopia langsdorffiana* EO

Xylopia langsdorffiana EO containing α-pinene (34.57%) and limonene (31.75%) was recently evaluated for its toxicity by using hemolysis, acute toxicity, and micronucleus assays. It was found that LD50 was about 351.09 mg/kg, with slight changes in liver (acute inflammation in liver) and caused no genetic toxicity [36].

25.4.23 Miscellaneous EOs

The cytotoxic/genotoxic effect of EOs such as rosemary, sage, thyme, yarrow, curry plant, mastic tree, and myrtle have been tested recently by human lymphocytes cytokinesis-block micronucleus test and cellular toxicity in ovarian cancer cell line (A2780). It was found that these EOs showed potent cellular toxicity and mild genetic toxicity against lymphocytes and presented marked cellular toxicity against ovarian cancer cells [37]. Similarly, cellular and genetic toxicity caused by EOs (*Cymbopogon martini*, Citronella, *Cymbopogon citratus*, and *Chrysopogon zizanioides*) and monoterpenoids (geraniol as well as citral) were evaluated in human peripheral lymphCells. Genotoxicity (by comet and DNA diffusion assays), cytotoxicity (trypan blue dye exclusion and MTT test), and apoptosis (by Annexin/PI double staining) studies were performed. It was found that four EOs as well as citral showed induced cytotoxic and genotoxic effects at greater dose. Additionally, EOs induced oxidative stress by ROS production. Except geraniol, apoptosis was induced by all tested samples. Thus, these EOs could be safe at low concentration [38]. A previous study revealed genotoxicity of the EOs obtained from *Anethum graveolens, Mentha piperita,* and *Pinus sylvestris.* Chromosome aberration examination revealed that the most active EO was from the seeds of *Anethum graveolens*, followed by EOs from *Anethum graveolens* herb, *Mentha piperita* herb, and *Pinus sylvestris.* Findings from sister chromatid exchange demonstrated that the effective EOs were from *Anethum graveolens* herb and seeds followed by EOs from *Pinus sylvestris* needles and *Mentha piperita* herb. It was observed that all EOs were cytotoxic for human lymphocytes. Additionally, somatic mutation and recombination test revealed a c-dependent increase in mutation frequency for pine and dill herb EOs. *Mentha piperita* EOs showed genetic changes in a concentration-independent way [39].

Recently, the toxicity profiles of various EOs (rosemary, citrus, and eucalyptus) were evaluated by using alternative *in vivo* (*Caenorhabditis elegans* and hen's egg test) and *in vitro* (cell cultures) methods to study the adverse effects on acute, developmental, and reproductive as well as irritant effects on mucous membrane. It was suggested that EOs can possess serious adverse effects at low dose [40]. Consequently, a thorough toxic effect evaluation is suggested for every EO. In this study, a slight increase in toxicity of rosemary EO was noticed with dose-dependent reduction of viability of the cells of each EO. The same findings were found from *C. elegans* test (LC50 value of 0.42% [v/v]); however, 10-fold greater lethal concentration 50 values were identified in wild nematodes [40]. Further development and reproduction of *C. elegans* were already considerably suppressed. Gene expression analysis showed considerable increase in the level of xenobiotic and oxidative stress pathways. Additionally, all EOs showed mucous membrane irritation potential for a short period [40]. Recently, the genotoxicity of the aforementioned EOs on human keratinocyte cells (HaCaT) was assessed using comet assay. It was found that none of the EOs caused considerable injury to DNA *in vitro* after 24 hours. Furthermore, human keratinocyte cell treatment with EOs augmented antioxidant effects. Overall, the findings suggested that these EOs have broad therapeutic effects [41].

25.4.24 EO-Loaded Nanosystem

Recently blending of EOs with main course medications and pure phytochemicals to improve therapeutic effects, reduce toxicity, improve the pharmacodynamic as well as pharmacokinetic effects, and improve the safety as well as stability profile of the whole preparation has been explored [42–62]. EO-based preparations are loaded in nanosystems using natural polymers. These EO-loaded nanosystems can efficiently deliver EOs at targeted sites with maximum therapeutic effects at lower concentrations and with minimal toxicity. EO-loaded nanosystems using natural polymers can also allow the sustained release of EOs at targeted sites [42–62].

REFERENCES

1. Lis-Balchin M. Possible health and safety problems in the use of novel plant essential oils and extracts in aromatherapy. *J R Soc Promot Health.* 1999;119(4):240–243.
2. Hammer KA, Carson CF, Riley TV, Nielsen JB. A review of the toxicity of *Melaleuca alternifolia* (tea tree) oil. *Food Chem Toxicol.* 2006;44(5):616–625.
3. Garcia C, Isca VMS, Pereira F, Monteiro CM, Ntungwe E, Sousa F, Dinic J, Holmstedt S, Roberto A, Díaz-Lanza A, Reis CP, Pesic M, Candeias NR, Ferreira RJ, Duarte N, Afonso CAM, Rijo P. Royleanone derivatives from *Plectranthus* spp. as a novel class of P-glycoprotein inhibitors. *Front Pharmacol.* 2020;11:557789.
4. Posadzki P, Alotaibi A, Ernst E. Adverse effects of aromatherapy: A systematic review of case reports and case series. *Int J Risk Saf Med.* 2012;24(3):147–161.
5. Sharma R, Rao R, Kumar S, Mahant S, Khatkar S. Therapeutic potential of citronella essential oil: A review. *Curr Drug Discov Technol.* 2019;16(4):330–339.
6. Klegin C, Klegin C, de Moura NF, de Sousa MHO, Frassini R, Roesch-Ely M, Bruno AN, Bitencourt TC, Flach A, Bordin J. Chemical composition and cytotoxic evaluation of the essential oil of *Phyllogonium viride* brid. (Phyllogoniaceae, Bryophyta). *Chem Biodivers.* 2021. doi: 10.1002/cbdv.202000794.
7. Mohammadi Pelarti S, Karimi Zarehshuran L, Babaeekhou L, Ghane M. Antibacterial, anti-biofilm and anti-quorum sensing activities of *Artemisia dracunculus* essential oil (EO): A study against *Salmonella enterica* serovar Typhimurium and *Staphylococcus aureus*. *Arch Microbiol.* 2021;203(4):1529–1537.
8. Moller AC, Parra C, Said B, Werner E, Flores S, Villena J, Russo A, Caro N, Montenegro I, Madrid A. Antioxidant and anti-proliferative activity of essential oil and main components from leaves of *Aloysia polystachya* harvested in central Chile. *Molecules.* 2020;26(1):131.
9. Teles AM, Silva-Silva JV, Fernandes JMP, Calabrese KDS, Abreu-Silva AL, Marinho SC, Mouchrek AN, Filho VEM, Almeida-Souza F. *Aniba rosaeodora* (Var. amazonica Ducke) essential oil: Chemical composition, antibacterial, antioxidant and antitrypanosomal activity. *Antibiotics (Basel).* 2020;10(1):E24.
10. Zhao X, Chen Q, Lu T, Wei F, Yang Y, Xie D, Wang H, Tian M. Chemical composition, antibacterial, anti-inflammatory, and enzyme inhibitory activities of essential oil from *Rhynchanthus beesianus* Rhizome. *Molecules.* 2020;26(1):167.
11. Machado VS, Verdi CM, Somacal S, Rossi GG, Machado ML, Klein B, Roos VC, Urquhart CG, Dalcol II, Sagrillo MR, Machado AK, Campos MM, Wagner R, Santos RCV. *Achyrocline flaccida* essential oil from Brazil: Phytochemical composition, genotoxicity, protective effects on Caenorhabditis elegans, and antimycobacterial activity. *Nat Prod Res.* 2020:1–5. https://pubmed.ncbi.nlm.nih.gov/32744075/
12. Dahham SS, Hassan LE, Ahamed MB, Majid AS, Majid AM, Zulkepli NN. In vivo toxicity and antitumor activity of essential oils extract from agarwood (*Aquilaria crassna*). *BMC Complement Altern Med.* 2016;16:236.
13. Haddad JG, Picard M, Bénard S, Desvignes C, Desprès P, Diotel N, El Kalamouni C. *Ayapana triplinervis* essential oil and its main component thymohydroquinone dimethyl ether inhibit zika virus at doses devoid of toxicity in Zebrafish. *Molecules.* 2019;24(19):3447.
14. de Sant'anna JR, Franco CC, Miyamoto CT, Cunico MM, Miguel OG, Côcco LC, Yamamoto CI, Junior CC, de Castro-Prado MA. Genotoxicity of *Achillea millefolium* essential oil in diploid cells of *Aspergillus nidulans*. *Phytother Res.* 2009;23(2):231–235.
15. Oliveira-Tintino CDM, Pessoa RT, Fernandes MNM, Alcântara IS, da Silva BAF, de Oliveira MRC, Martins AOBPB, da Silva MDS, Tintino SR, Rodrigues FFG, da Costa JGM, de Lima SG, Kerntopf MR, da Silva TG, de Menezes IRA. Anti-inflammatory and anti-edematogenic action of the *Croton campestris* A. St.-Hil (Euphorbiaceae) essential oil and the compound β-caryophyllene in in vivo models. *Phytomedicine.* 2018;41:82–95.
16. Vidal CS, Oliveira Brito Pereira Bezerra Martins A, de Alencar Silva A, de Oliveira MRC, Ribeiro-Filho J, de Albuquerque TR, Coutinho HDM, da Silva Almeida JRG, Quintans LJ Junior, de Menezes IRA. Gastroprotective effect and mechanism of action of *Croton rhamnifolioides* essential oil in mice. *Biomed Pharmacother.* 2017;89:47–55.

17. Toukourou H, Uwambayinema F, Yakoub Y, Mertens B, Laleye A, Lison D, Quetin-Leclercq J, Gbaguidi F. In vitro and in vivo toxicity studies on *Cymbopogon giganteus* Chiov. leaves essential oil from Benin. *J Toxicol.* 2020;2020:8261058.
18. Gogoi R, Loying R, Sarma N, Begum T, Pandey SK, Lal M. Comparative analysis of in-vitro biological activities of methyl eugenol rich *Cymbopogon khasianus* hack., leaf essential oil with pure methyl eugenol compound. *Curr Pharm Biotechnol.* 2020;21(10):927–938.
19. Adokoh CK, Asante DB, Acheampong DO, Kotsuchibashi Y, Armah FA, Sirikyi IH, Kimura K, Gmakame E, Abdul-Rauf S. Chemical profile and in vivo toxicity evaluation of unripe *Citrus aurantifolia* essential oil. *Toxicol Rep.* 2019;6:692–702.
20. Paw M, Gogoi R, Sarma N, Pandey SK, Borah A, Begum T, Lal M. Study of anti-oxidant, anti-inflammatory, genotoxicity, and antimicrobial activities and analysis of different constituents found in rhizome essential oil of *Curcuma caesia* Roxb., collected from North East India. *Curr Pharm Biotechnol.* 2020;21(5):403–413.
21. Andrade MA, Cardoso MDG, Preté PSC, Soares MJ, de Azeredo CMO, Trento MVC, Braga MA, Marcussi S. Toxicological aspects of the essential oil from *Cinnamodendron dinisii. Chem Biodivers.* 2018;15(5):e1800066.
22. Wijesinghe GK, Maia FC, de Oliveira TR, de Feiria SNB, Joia F, Barbosa JP, Boni GC, Sardi JCO, Rosalen PL, Höfling JF. Effect of *Cinnamomum verum* leaf essential oil on virulence factors of Candida species and determination of the in-vivo toxicity with Galleria mellonella model. *Mem Inst Oswaldo Cruz.* 2020;115:e200349.
23. Lin SS, Lu TM, Chao PC, Lai YY, Tsai HT, Chen CS, Lee YP, Chen SC, Chou MC, Yang CC. In vivo cytokine modulatory effects of cinnamaldehyde, the major constituent of leaf essential oil from *Cinnamomum osmophloeum* Kaneh. *Phytother Res.* 2011;25(10):1511–1518.
24. Timoumi R, Salem IB, Amara I, Annabi E, Abid-Essefi S. Protective effects of fennel essential oil against oxidative stress and genotoxicity induced by the insecticide triflumuron in human colon carcinoma cells. *Environ Sci Pollut Res Int.* 2020;27(8):7957–7966.
25. Verdi CM, Machado VS, Machado AK, Klein B, Bonez PC, de Andrade ENC, Rossi G, Campos MM, Wagner R, Sagrillo MR, Santos RCV. Phytochemical characterization, genotoxicity, cytotoxicity, and antimicrobial activity of *Gautheria procumbens* essential oil. *Nat Prod Res.* 2020:1–5. https://pubmed.ncbi.nlm.nih.gov/33356559/
26. Arunachalam K, Balogun SO, Pavan E, de Almeida GVB, de Oliveira RG, Wagner T, Cechinel Filho V, de Oliveira Martins DT. Chemical characterization, toxicology and mechanism of gastric antiulcer action of essential oil from *Gallesia integrifolia* (Spreng.) Harms in the in vitro and in vivo experimental models. *Biomed Pharmacother.* 2017;94:292–306.
27. Di Sotto A, Mazzanti G, Carbone F, Hrelia P, Maffei F. Genotoxicity of lavender oil, linalyl acetate, and linalool on human lymphocytes in vitro. *Environ Mol Mutagen.* 2011;52(1):69–71.
28. Mesic A, Mahmutović-Dizdarević I, Tahirović E, Durmišević I, Eminovic I, Jerković-Mujkić A, Bešta-Gajević R. Evaluation of toxicological and antimicrobial activity of lavender and immortelle essential oils. *Drug Chem Toxicol.* 2021;44(2):190–197.
29. Luo M, Jiang LK, Zou GL. Acute and genetic toxicity of essential oil extracted from *Litsea cubeba* (Lour.) *Pers J Food Prot.* 2005;68(3):581–588.
30. Rolim TL, Meireles DRP, Batista TM, de Sousa TKG, Mangueira VM, de Abrantes RA, Pita JCLR, Xavier AL, Costa VCO, Batista LM, da Silva MS, Sobral MV. Toxicity and antitumor potential of *Mesosphaerum sidifolium* (Lamiaceae) oil and fenchone, its major component. *BMC Complement Altern Med.* 2017;17(1):347. doi: 10.1186/s12906-017-1779-z. Erratum in: *BMC Complement Altern Med.* 2017;17 (1):364.
31. Llana-Ruiz-Cabello M, Puerto M, Maisanaba S, Guzmán-Guillén R, Pichardo S, Cameán AM. Use of micronucleus and comet assay to evaluate evaluate the genotoxicity of oregano essential oil (*Origanum vulgare* l. Virens) in rats orally exposed for 90 days. *J Toxicol Environ Health A.* 2018;81(12):525–533.
32. Hoff Brait DR, Mattos Vaz MS, da Silva Arrigo J, Borges de Carvalho LN, Souza de Araújo FH, Vani JM, da Silva Mota J, Cardoso CA, Oliveira RJ, Negrão FJ, Kassuya CA, Arena AC. Toxicological analysis and anti-inflammatory effects of essential oil from *Piper vicosanum* leaves. *Regul Toxicol Pharmacol.* 2015;73(3):699–705.
33. Ortiz C, Morales L, Sastre M, Haskins WE, Matta J. Cytotoxicity and genotoxicity assessment of sandalwood essential oil in human breast cell lines MCF-7 and MCF-10A. *Evid Based Complement Alternat Med.* 2016;2016:3696232.
34. Yousefzadi M, Riahi-Madvar A, Hadian J, Rezaee F, Rafiee R, Biniaz M. Toxicity of essential oil of *Satureja khuzistanica*: In vitro cytotoxicity and anti-microbial activity. *J Immunotoxicol.* 2014;11(1):50–55.
35. Abdelli W, Bahri F, Romane A, Höferl M, Wanner J, Schmidt E, Jirovetz L. Chemical composition and anti-inflammatory activity of algerian *Thymus vulgaris* essential oil. *Nat Prod Commun.* 2017;12(4):611–614.
36. Moura AP, Beltrão DM, Pita JC, Xavier AL, Brito MT, Sousa TK, Batista LM, Carvalho JE, Ruiz AL, Della Torre A, Duarte MC, Tavares JF, da Silva MS, Sobral MV. Essential oil from fruit of *Xylopia langsdorffiana*: Antitumour activity and toxicity. *Pharm Biol.* 2016;54(12):3093–3102.
37. Contini A, Di Bello D, Azzarà A, Giovanelli S, D'Urso G, Piaggi S, Pinto B, Pistelli L, Scarpato R, Testi S. Assessing the cytotoxic/genotoxic activity and estrogenic/antiestrogenic potential of essential oils from seven aromatic plants. *Food Chem Toxicol.* 2020;138:111205.
38. Sinha S, Jothiramajayam M, Ghosh M, Mukherjee A. Evaluation of toxicity of essential oils palmarosa, citronella, lemongrass and vetiver in human lymphocytes. *Food Chem Toxicol.* 2014;68:71–77.
39. Lazutka JR, Mierauskiene J, Slapsyte G, Dedonyte V. Genotoxicity of dill (*Anethum graveolens* L.), peppermint (*Menthaxpiperita* L.) and pine (*Pinus sylvestris* L.) essential oils in human lymphocytes and drosophila melanogaster. *Food Chem Toxicol.* 2001;39(5):485–492.
40. Lanzerstorfer P, Sandner G, Pitsch J, Mascher B, Aumiller T, Weghuber J. Acute, reproductive, and developmental toxicity of essential oils assessed with alternative in vitro and in vivo systems. *Arch Toxicol.* 2020;95:673–691.

41. Kozics K, Bučková M, Puškárová A, Kalászová V, Cabicarová T, Pangallo D. The effect of ten essential oils on several cutaneous drug-resistant microorganisms and their cyto/genotoxic and antioxidant properties. *Molecules.* 2019;24(24):4570.
42. Bhatia S, Namdeo AG, Nanda S. Factors effecting the gelling and emulsifying properties of a natural polymer. *SRP.* 2010;1(1):86–92.
43. Bhatia S, Sharma K, Bera T. Structural characterization and pharmaceutical properties of porphyran. *Asian J Pharm* 2015;993–101.
44. Bhatia S, Sharma A, Sharma K, Kavale M, Chaugule BB, Dhalwal K, Namdeo AG, Mahadik KR. Novel algal polysaccharides from marine source: Porphyran. *Pharmacogn Rev.* 2008;4:271–276.
45. Bhatia S, Sharma K, Nagpal K, Bera T. Investigation of the factors influencing the molecular weight of porphyran and its associated antifungal activity Bioact. *Carb Diet Fiber.* 2015;5:153–168.
46. Bhatia S, Kumar V, Sharma K, Nagpal K, Bera T. Significance of algal polymer in designing amphotericin B nanoparticles. *Sci World J.* 2014;2014:564573.
47. Bhatia S, Rathee P, Sharma K, Chaugule BB, Kar N, Bera T. Immuno-modulation effect of sulphated polysaccharide (Porphyran) from Porphyra vietnamensis. *Int J Biol Macromol.* 2013;57:50–56.
48. Bhatia S. *Natural Polymer Drug Delivery Systems: Marine Polysaccharides Based Nano-Materials and Its Applications.* Springer International Publishing, Switzerland; 2016:185–225.
49. Bhatia S. *Natural Polymer Drug Delivery Systems: Plant Derived Polymers, Properties, and Modification & Applications.* Springer International Publishing, Switzerland; 2016:119–184.
50. Bhatia S. *Natural Polymer Drug Delivery Systems: Nanotechnology and Its Drug Delivery Applications.* Springer International Publishing, Switzerland; 2016:1–32.
51. Bhatia S. *Natural Polymer Drug Delivery Systems: Nanoparticles Types, Classification, Characterization, Fabrication Methods and Drug Delivery Applications.* Springer International Publishing; Switzerland; 2016:33–93.
52. Bhatia S. *Natural Polymer Drug Delivery Systems: Natural Polymers vs Synthetic Polymer.* Springer International Publishing, Switzerland; 2016:95–118.
53. Bhatia S. *Systems for Drug Delivery: Mammalian Polysaccharides and Its Nanomaterials.* Springer International Publishing, Switzerland; 2016:1–27.
54. Bhatia S. *Systems for Drug Delivery: Microbial Polysaccharides as Advance Nanomaterials.* Springer International Publishing, Switzerland; 2016:29–54.
55. Bhatia S. *Systems for Drug Delivery: Chitosan Based Nanomaterials and Its Applications.* Springer International Publishing, Switzerland; 2016:55–117.
56. Bhatia S. *Systems for Drug Delivery: Advance Polymers and Its Applications.* Springer International Publishing, Switzerland; 2016:119–146.
57. Bhatia S. *Systems for Drug Delivery: Advanced Application of Natural Polysaccharides.* Springer International Publishing, Switzerland; 2016:147–170.
58. Bhatia S. *Systems for Drug Delivery: Modern Polysaccharides and Its Current Advancements.* Springer International Publishing, Switzerland; 2016:171–188.
59. Bhatia S. *Systems for Drug Delivery: Toxicity of Nanodrug Delivery Systems.* Springer International Publishing, Switzerland; 2016:189–197.
60. Bhatia S. *Nanotechnology in Drug Delivery Fundamentals, Design, and Applications: Part 1: Protein and Peptide-Based Drug Delivery Systems.* Apple Academic Press, Palm Bay, FL; 2016:50–204.
61. Bhatia S. *Nanotechnology in Drug Delivery Fundamentals, Design, and Applications: Part 2: Peptide-Mediated Nanoparticle Drug Delivery System.* Apple Academic Press, Palm Bay, FL; 2016:205–280.
62. Bhatia S. *Nanotechnology in Drug Delivery Fundamentals, Design, and Applications: Part 3: CPP and CTP in Drug Delivery and Cell Targeting.* Apple Academic Press, Palm Bay, FL; 2016:309–312.

www.ingramcontent.com/pod-product-compliance
Lightning Source LLC
Chambersburg PA
CBHW080653220326
41598CB00033B/5198